ANTIBODIES

Stimulation	Serology		Comp. Binding	Immunoglobin Class		Optimum Temperature	Clinical Significance		Comments
	Saline	AHG		IgM	IgG		HTR	HDN	
RBC	occ	yes	no	occ	yes	warm	yes	yes	Very rarely IgA anti-D may be produced; however, this is invariably with IgG.
RBC	occ	yes	no	occ	yes	warm	yes	yes	
RBC/NRBC	occ	yes	no	occ	yes	warm	yes	yes	Anti-E may often occur without obvious immune stimulation.
RBC	occ	yes	no	occ	yes	warm	yes	yes	
RBC	occ	yes	no	occ	yes	warm	yes	yes	Warm autoantibodies often appear to have anti-e-like specificity.
RBC	occ	yes	no	occ	yes	warm	yes	yes	
RBC	occ	yes	no	occ	yes	warm	yes	yes	
RBC/NRBC	occ	yes	no	occ	yes	warm	yes	yes	Anti-C^w may often occur without obvious immune stimulation.
RBC	occ	yes	no	occ	yes	warm	yes	yes	
RBC	occ	yes	no	occ	yes	warm	yes	yes	Antibodies to V and VS present problems only in the black population, where the antigen frequencies are in the order of 30 to 32.
RBC	occ	yes	no	occ	yes	warm	yes	yes	
RBC	occ	yes	some	occ	yes	warm	yes	yes	Some antibodies to Kell system have been reported to react poorly in low ionic media.
RBC	no	yes	no	rarely	yes	warm	yes	yes	
RBC	no	yes	no	no	yes	warm	yes	yes	Kell system antigens are destroyed by AET and by ZZAP.
RBC	rarely	yes	no	rarely	yes	warm	yes	yes	
RBC	rarely	yes	no	rarely	yes	warm	yes	yes	Anti-K1 has been reported to occur following bacterial infection.
RBC	no	yes	no	no	yes	warm	yes	yes	
RBC	no	yes	no	occ	yes	warm	yes	yes	The lack of Kx expression on RBCs and WBCs has been associated with the McLeod phenotype and CGD.
RBC	rare	yes	some	rare	yes	warm	yes	yes	Fy(a) and (b) antigens are destroyed by enzymes. Fy(a−b−) cells are resistant to invasion by *P. vivax* merozoites, a malaria-causing parasite.
RBC	rare	yes	some	rare	yes	warm	yes	yes	
RBC	no	yes	rarely	no	yes	warm	yes	yes	FY3 and 5 are not destroyed by enzymes.
RBC	no	yes	?	no	yes	warm			FY5 may be formed by interaction of Rh and Duffy gene products. FY6 is a monoclonal antibody which reacts with most human red cells except Fy(a−b−) and is responsible for susceptibility of cells to penetration by *P. vivax*.

(Continued on inside back cover)

Modern Blood Banking and Transfusion Practices

Fifth Edition

Modern Blood Banking and Transfusion Practices

Fifth Edition

DENISE M. HARMENING, PhD, MT(ASCP), CLS(NCA)

Professor

Department of Medical and Research Technology

University of Maryland, School of Medicine

Baltimore, Maryland

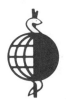

F.A. Davis Company • Philadelphia

F. A. Davis Company
1915 Arch Street
Philadelphia, PA 19103
www.fadavis.com

Printed in the United States of America

Last digit indicates print number: 10 9 8 7 6 5 4 3 2 1

Acquisitions Editor: Christa Fratantoro
Developmental Editor: Peg Waltner
Design Manager: Joan Wendt

As new scientific information becomes available through basic and clinical research, recommended treatments and drug therapies undergo changes. The author(s) and publisher have done everything possible to make this book accurate, up to date, and in accord with accepted standards at the time of publication. The author(s), editors, and publisher are not responsible for errors or omissions or for consequences from application of the book, and make no warranty, expressed or implied, in regard to the contents of the book. Any practice described in this book should be applied by the reader in accordance with professional standards of care used in regard to the unique circumstances that may apply in each situation. The reader is advised always to check product information (package inserts) for changes and new information regarding dose and contraindications before administering any drug. Caution is especially urged when using new or infrequently ordered drugs.

Library of Congress Cataloging-in-Publication Data

Modern blood banking and transfusion practices / [edited by] Denise M. Harmening.— 5th ed.
    p. ; cm.
 Includes bibliographical references and index.
 ISBN 0-8036-1248-6 (hardcover : alk. paper)
 1. Blood banks. 2. Blood—Transfusion. 3. Immunohematology.
 [DNLM: 1. Blood Banks—methods. 2. Blood Grouping and Crossmatching. 3. Blood Transfusion—methods. WH 460 M688 2005] I. Harmening, Denise.
RM172.M62 2005
615′.39—dc22

2004020021

Blood groups were discovered over a hundred years ago, but most of them have been recognized only in the last 50 years. Although transfusion therapy was used soon after the ABO blood groups were discovered, it was not until after World War II that blood transfusion science really started to become an important branch of medical science in its own right. Thus, compared with many sub-disciplines of medicine, blood transfusion science is an infant, growing fast, changing continually, and presenting a great potential for research and future development. To be able to grow, transfusion science needs to be nurtured with a steady flow of new knowledge generated from research. This knowledge then has to be applied at the bench. To understand and best take advantage of the continual flow of new information being generated by blood transfusion scientists and to apply it to everyday work in the blood bank, technologists and pathologists need to have a good understanding of basic immunology, genetics, biochemistry (particularly membrane chemistry), and the physiology and function of blood cells. To apply new concepts, they need technical expertise and enough flexibility to reject old dogma when necessary and to accept new ideas when they are supported by sufficient scientific data. High standards are always expected and strived for by technologists who are working in blood banks or transfusion services. I strongly believe that technologists should understand the principles behind the tests they are performing, rather than perform tasks as a machine does. Because of this, I do not think that "cookbook" technical manuals have much value in *teaching* technologists; they do have a place as reference books in the laboratory. During the years (too many to put in print) that I have been involved in teaching medical technologists, it has been very difficult to select one book that covers all that technologists in training need to know about blood transfusion science without confusing them. Dr. Denise Harmening has produced that single volume. She has been involved in teaching medical technologists for most of her career; after seeing how she has arranged this book, I would guess that her teaching philosophies are close to my own. She has gathered a group of experienced scientists and teachers who, along with herself, cover all the important areas of blood transfusion science. The chapters on the basic principles of cell preservation, genetics, immunology, and molecular biology provide a firm base for the learner to understand the practical and technical importance of the other chapters. The chapters on the blood groups and transfusion practice provide enough information for medical technologists without overwhelming them with esoteric and clinical details. Although this book is designed primarily for medical technologists, I believe it is admirably suited to pathology residents, hematology fellows, and others who want to review any aspect of modern blood transfusion science.

George Garratty, PhD, FIMLS, FRC Path
Scientific Director, American Red Cross Blood Services
Clinical Professor of Pathology and Laboratory Medicine
Los Angeles, California

This book is designed to provide the medical technologist, blood bank specialist, and resident with a concise and thorough guide to transfusion practices and immunohematology. This text, a perfect "crossmatch" of theory and practice, provides the reader with a working knowledge of modern routine blood banking. Forty contributors from across the country have shared their knowledge and expertise in 27 comprehensive chapters. Over 500 illustrations and tables facilitate the comprehension of difficult concepts not routinely illustrated in other texts. In addition, color plates provide a means for standardizing the reading of agglutination reactions and illustrating complex material. Several features of this textbook offer great appeal to students and educators. There are outlines and educational objectives at the beginning of each chapter; as well as each chapter ends with case histories and study guide questions. An extensive and convenient glossary is provided for easy access to definitions of blood bank terms. A blood group antibody characteristic chart is provided on the inside cover of the book to aid in retention of the vast amount of information and to serve as an easy access and guide to the characteristics of the blood group systems. Summary charts at the end of each chapter identify for students the most important information to know for clinical rotations. Original comprehensive step by step illustrations of ABO forward and reverse grouping, not found in any other book, help the student to quickly master this important testing, which represents the foundation of blood banking. The introduction to the historical aspects of blood transfusion and preservation is a prelude to the basic concepts of genetics, blood group immunology, molecular biology, and current overview of blood group systems. The next section of the book focuses on routine blood bank practices, including donor selection, component preparation, detection and identification of antibodies, compatibility testing, transfusion therapy, and apheresis. A chapter on transfusion safety and federal regulations clarifies the required quality assurance and inspection procedures. New to the fifth edition is Chapter 4, *Concepts in Molecular Biology,* which introduces the student to nucleic acid techniques and theory that govern molecular genetics in determining compatibility between donor and recipient, production of recombinant proteins such as growth factors utilized in certain apheresis procedures, and detection of transfusion-transmitted viruses in transfusion medicine. Certain clinical situations that are particularly relevant to blood banking are discussed in detail, including transfusion reactions, hemolytic disease of the newborn, autoimmune and drug-induced hemolytic anemia, transfusion-transmitted viruses, human leukocyte antigens, and paternity testing. Chapter 26, *Informational Systems in the Blood Bank,* helps prepare blood bankers for the responsibility of operating and maintaining a blood bank information system. Unique to this book is Chapter 27, *Medicolegal and Ethical Aspects of Providing Blood Collection and Transfusion Services.*

This book is a culmination of the tremendous efforts of a number of dedicated professionals who participated in this project by donating their time and expertise because they care about the blood bank profession. The book's intention is to foster improved patient care by providing the reader with a basic understanding of the function of blood, the involvement of blood group antigens and antibodies, the principles of transfusion therapy, and the adverse effects of blood transfusion. It has been designed to generate an unquenchable thirst for knowledge in all medical technologists, blood bankers, and practitioners, whose education, knowledge, and skills provide the public with excellent health care.

Denise M. Harmening, PhD, MT(ASCP), CLS(NCA)

Lucia M. Berte, MA, MT(ASCP)SBB, DLM, CQA(ASQ)CQMgr
Quality Systems Consultant
Elmhurst, Illinois

Maria P. Bettinotti, PhD, dip. ABHI
Molecular Immunology Laboratory
Department of Transfusion Medicine
National Institutes of Health
Bethesda, Maryland

Loni Calhoun, MT(ASCP)SBB
Senior Technical Specialist, Education and
Immunohematology
Division of Transfusion Medicine
ULCA Medical Center
Los Angeles, California

Cara L. Calvo, MS, MT(ASCP)SH, CLS(NCA)
Director and Assistant Clinical Professor
West Central Ohio Clinical Laboratory Science Program
Ohio Northern University, Department of Biological
Sciences
Ada, Ohio

Lorraine Caruccio, PhD, MT(ASCP)SBB
Laboratory of Molecular Immunology
Department of Transfusion Medicine
National Institutes of Health
Bethesda, Maryland

Judy Ellen Ciaraldi, BS, MT(ASCP)SBB, CQA(ASQ)
Consumer Safety Officer
Division of Blood Applications
Office of Blood Research and Review
Center for Biologics Evaluation and Research
U.S. Food and Drug Administration
Rockville, Maryland

Lloyd O. Cook, MD, MBA
Medical Director, Blood Bank and Transfusion Medicine
Assistant Professor, Department of Pathology
Medical College of Georgia
Augusta, Georgia

Deborah Firestone, MA, MT(ASCP)SBB
Chair, Clinical Laboratory Science
Stony Brook Health Sciences Center
School of Health Technology and Management
Division of Diagnostic and Therapeutic Sciences
State University of New York at Stony Brook
Stony Brook, New York

Ralph E.B. Green, B. App. Sci., FAIMLS, MACE
Associate Professor
Faculty Director of Teaching Quality
Department of Medical Laboratory Science
RMIT University
Melbourne, Australia

Denise M. Harmening, PhD, MT(ASCP), CLS(NCA)
Professor, Department of Medical and Research
Technology
University of Maryland, School of Medicine
Baltimore, Maryland

Chantal Ricaud Harrison, MD
Medical Director
Medical Center Blood Bank
Associate Professor
Department of Pathology
University of Texas—Health Center
San Antonio, Texas

Virginia C. Hughes, MS, MT(ASCP)SBB, CLS(NCA)I
Instructor, Division of Clinical Laboratory Sciences
Auburn University Montgomery
Montgomery, Alabama

Patsy C. Jarreau, MHS, CLS(NCA), MT(ASCP)
Associate Professor
Department of Clinical Laboratory Sciences
LSU Health Sciences Center
New Orleans, Louisiana

Melanie S. Kennedy, MD
Associate Professor, Department of Pathology
Ohio State University College of Medicine
Director of Transfusion Medicine
Ohio State University Medical Center
Columbus, Ohio

Dave Krugh, MT(ASCP)SBB, CLS, CLCP(NCA)
Compliance Officer, Transfusion Service
The Ohio State University Medical Center
Instructor, Department of Pathology
College of Medicine and Public Health
Columbus, Ohio

Patricia Joyce Larison, MA, MT(ASCP)SBB
Blood Bank Supervisor
Associate Professor, Department of Medical Technology
Medical College of Georgia
Augusta, Georgia

Regina M. Leger, MSQA, MT(ASCP)SBB, CQMgr(ASQ)
Research Associate II
American Red Cross Blood Services
Southern California Region
Los Angeles, California

Gary Moroff, PhD
Director, Blood Development
American Red Cross
Jerome H. Holland Laboratory for the Biomedical Sciences
Rockville, Maryland

Mary P. Nix, MS, MT(ASCP)SBB
Clinical Laboratory Sciences
Weber State University
Ogden, Utah

Deirdre DeSantis Parsons, MS, MT(ASCP)SBB, CLS(NCA)
Department of Medical and Research Technology
University of Maryland, School of Medicine
Baltimore, Maryland

Donna L. Phelan, BA, CHS(ABHI), MT(HEW)
Technical Supervisor, HLA Laboratory
Barnes-Jewish Hospital
St. Louis, Missouri

Lee Ann Prihoda, MA Ed., MT(ASCP)SBB
Manager, Education and SBB School
Gulf Coast Regional Blood Center
Houston, Texas

Francis R. Rodwig, Jr, MD, MPH
Chairman, Department of Pathology and Laboratory Medicine
Medical Director, Blood Bank
Ochsner Clinic Foundation
New Orleans, Louisiana

Kathleen Sazama, MD, JD, MS, MT(ASCP)
Vice President
Faculty Academic Affairs
UTMD Anderson Cancer Center
Houston, Texas

Burlin Sherrick, MT(ASCP)SBB
Blood Bank Supervisor and Adjunct Clinical Instructor
Lima Memorial Hospital
Lima, Ohio

Nancy B. Steffey, MT(ASCP)SBB
Assistant Director, Technical Services
Supervisor, Patient Services
American Red Cross Blood Services, Greater Alleghenies Region
Johnstown, Pennsylvania

Mitra Taghizadeh, MS, MT(ASCP)
Assistant Clinical Professor
Department of Medical and Research Technology
University of Maryland, School of Medicine
Baltimore, Maryland

Ann Tiehen, MT(ASCP)SBB
Educational Coordinator
Evanston Northwestern Healthcare
Evanston Hospital
Department of Pathology and Laboratory Medicine
Evanston, Illinois

Kathleen S. Trudell, MT(ASCP)SBB
Clinical Coordinator of Immunohematology
University of Nebraska Medical Center
School of Allied Health Professions
Division of Medical Technology
Omaha, Nebraska

Melissa Volny, MT(ASCP)SBB
Technical Specialist, Blood Bank Teaching Coordinator
Evanston Northwestern Healthcare
Evanston Hospital
Department of Pathology and Laboratory Medicine
Evanston, Illinois

Phyllis S. Walker, MS, MT(ASCP)SBB
Manager, Immunohematology Reference Laboratory
Blood Centers of the Pacific
San Francisco, California

Merilyn Wiler, MA Ed., MT(ASCP)SBB
Customer Regulatory Support Specialist
Gambro BCT
Lakewood, Colorado

Alan E. Williams, PhD
Director, Division of Blood Applications
Office of Blood Research and Review
Center for Biologics Evaluation and Research
U.S. Food and Drug Administration
Rockville, Maryland

Elizabeth F. Williams, MHS, CLS(NCA), MT(ASCP)SBB
Associate Professor
Department of Clinical Laboratory Sciences
LSU Health Sciences Center
New Orleans, Louisiana

Scott C. Wise, MSA, MT(ASCP)SBB
Supervisor, Blood Bank Apheresis and Donor Room
Medical College of Georgia
Augusta, Georgia

Patricia A. Wright, BA, MT(ASCP)SBB
Production Manager
American Red Cross
National Testing Laboratories
Dedham, Massachusetts

Haifens M. Wu, MD
Assistant Professor, Department of Pathology
Ohio State University College of Medicine
Director Coagulation Laboratory
Ohio State University Medical Center
Columbus, Ohio

Michele B. Zitzmann, MHS, CLS(NCA), MT(ASCP)
Associate Professor
Department of Clinical Laboratory Sciences
LSU Health Sciences Center
New Orleans, Louisiana

William B. Zundel, MS, MT(ASCP)SBB
Assistant Professor
Department of Clinical Laboratory Sciences
Weber State University
Ogden, Utah

CONTENTS

COLOR PLATES

1-6

A.

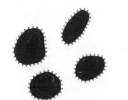

Human Sera

The Antihuman Globulin Test (AHG)

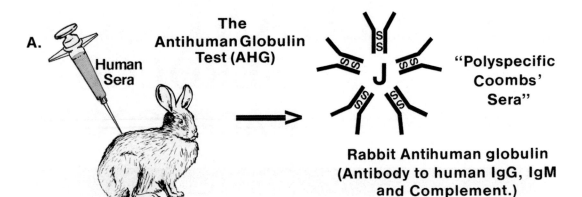

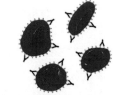

"Polyspecific Coombs' Sera"

Rabbit Antihuman globulin (Antibody to human IgG, IgM and Complement.)

B. Indirect AHG

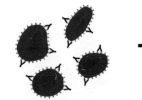

YY

Human Red Cells + human (Patient Serum) IgG Antibody ⟶ Red Cell (in Vitro) sensitization

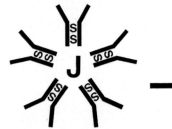

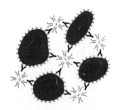

Sensitized Red Cells + (Coombs' Sera) AHG Reagent ⟶ Visual Red Cell Agglutination

C. Direct AHG

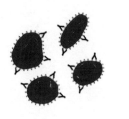

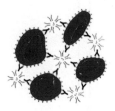

Washed (3x's) Patient Red Cells (sensitized in Vivo) + (Coombs' Sera) AHG Reagent ⟶ Visual Red Cell Agglutination.

Plate 1. The antihuman globulin (AHG) test (primary immunization). Note: The AHG reagents currently sold are the products of subsequent immunizations and contain primarily IgG rabbit antibody. Please note that monoclonal reagents are currently used in routine testing. These reagents may be a mixture of IgM and IgG, or IgG only.

RED CELL ANTIGEN-
SEROLOGIC
MACROSCOPIC

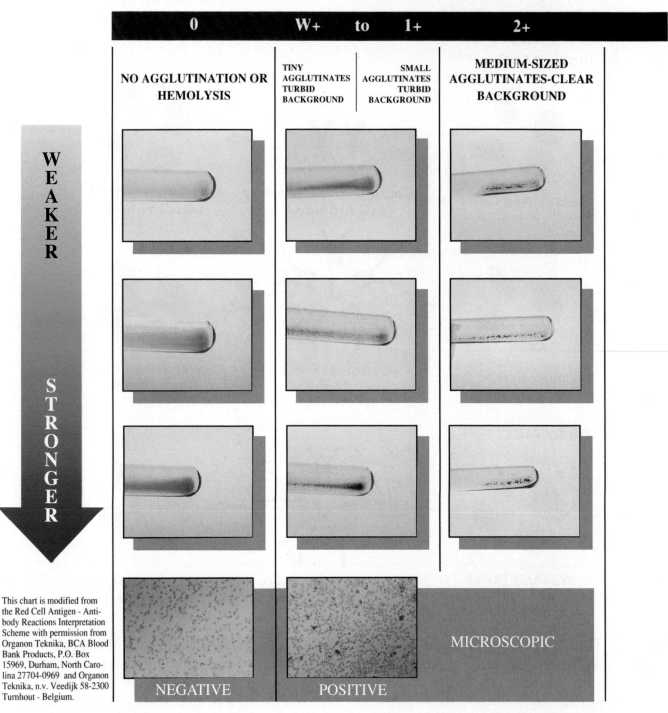

0	W+ to 1+	2+
NO AGGLUTINATION OR HEMOLYSIS	**TINY AGGLUTINATES TURBID BACKGROUND** / **SMALL AGGLUTINATES TURBID BACKGROUND**	**MEDIUM-SIZED AGGLUTINATES-CLEAR BACKGROUND**

WEAKER

STRONGER

This chart is modified from the Red Cell Antigen - Antibody Reactions Interpretation Scheme with permission from Organon Teknika, BCA Blood Bank Products, P.O. Box 15969, Durham, North Carolina 27704-0969 and Organon Teknika, n.v. Veedijk 58-2300 Turnhout - Belgium.

MICROSCOPIC

NEGATIVE

POSITIVE

Plate 2. Red cell antigen-antibody reactions: serologic grading and macroscopic evaluation.

ANTIBODY REACTIONS
GRADING
EVALUATION

3+	4+

SEVERAL LARGE AGGLUTINATES-CLEAR BACKGROUND

ONE SOLID AGGLUTINATE

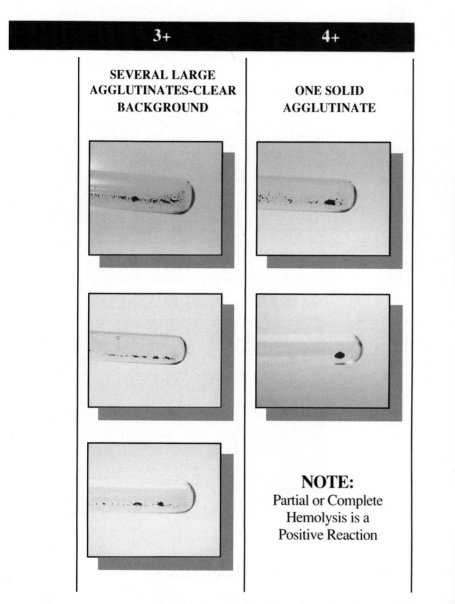

NOTE:
Partial or Complete Hemolysis is a Positive Reaction

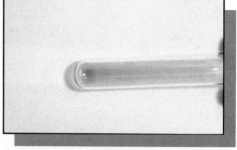

NEGATIVE: NO AGGREGATES

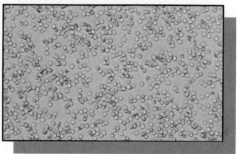

NEGATIVE: NO AGGREGATES (Microscopic)

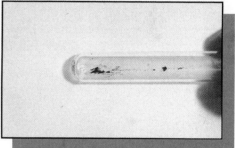

PSEUDOAGGLUTINATION OR STRONG ROULEAUX (2+)

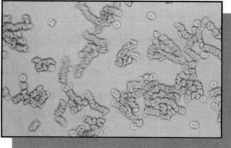

ROULEAUX:Microscopic (original magnification x10; enlarged 240%) NOTE: The "stack of coins" appearance of the agglutinates

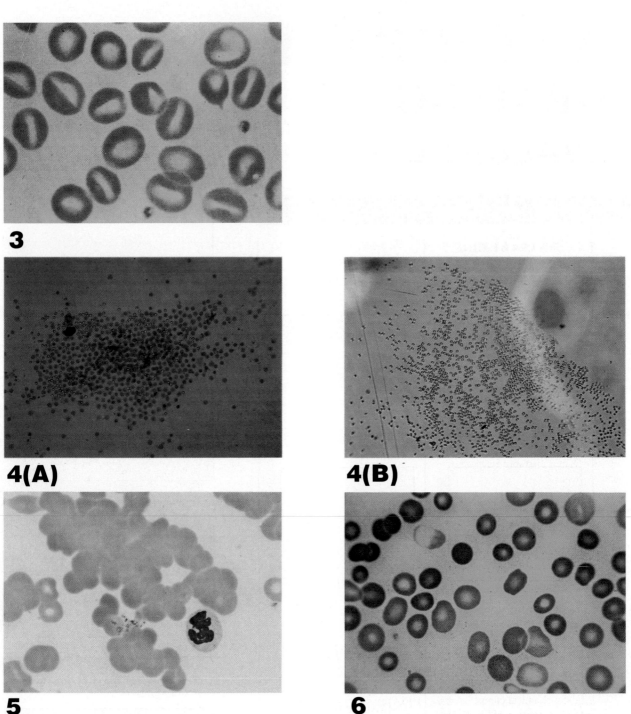

Plate 3. Stomatocytosis (original magnification × 100; enlarged 230%).

Plate 4. (A) Positive cytotoxic reaction. (B) Negative cytotoxic reaction.

Plate 5. Cold agglutinin disease (peripheral blood). (From Pittiglio, DH and Sacher, RS: *Clinical Hematology and Fundamentals of Hemostasis.* FA Davis, Philadelphia, 1987, with permission.)

Plate 6. Autoimmune hemolytic anemia (peripheral blood). (From Pittiglio, DH and Sacher, RS: *Clinical Hematology and Fundamentals of Hemostasis,* FA Davis Company, Philadelphia, 1987, with permission.)

one

Red Blood Cell and Platelet Preservation: Historical Perspectives, Review of Metabolism, and Current Trends

Denise M. Harmening, PhD, MT(ASCP), CLS(NCA), and Gary Moroff, PhD

OBJECTIVES

On completion of this chapter, the learner should be able to:

1. List the areas of red blood cell (RBC) metabolism that are crucial to normal RBC survival and functions.
2. Describe the chemical composition of the RBC membrane in terms of percentage of lipids, proteins, and carbohydrates.
3. List the two most important RBC membrane proteins, and describe their function and the characteristics of deformability and permeability.
4. List the various metabolic pathways involved in RBC metabolism, stating the specific function of each one.
5. List the globin chains found in HbA, HbA_2, HbF, and glycosylated hemoglobin and their respective concentrations (in percent) found in vivo.
6. Describe hemoglobin function in terms of the oxygen dissociation curve.
7. Define P_{50} and state normal in-vivo levels.
8. List the approved anticoagulant-preservative solutions and the maximum storage time for whole blood and RBCs in each preservative.
9. List three additive preservative solutions for RBCs and the maximum storage time with each solution.
10. List how the volume of anticoagulant-preservative solution and the volume of additive solution are modified when a 500-mL blood collection system is utilized, in contrast to when a 450-mL blood collection system is used.
11. List current/emerging concepts regarding freezing (including maximum storage time for frozen red cells and post-thaw storage) and rejuvenation of red cells.
12. List the advantages and disadvantages of RBC freezing.
13. List at least three areas of current research with RBCs.
14. List at least two hemoglobin-based oxygen carriers in advanced clinical testing as RBC substitutes.
15. Define perfluorochemicals and their potential use as a RBC substitute.
16. List the advantages and disadvantages of RBC substitutes.
17. Describe the metabolism and function of platelets.

18. List the maximum storage time and storage temperature range for platelet components prepared from whole blood and by apheresis. Discuss why platelets are no longer routinely stored at 1° to 6°C.

19. List the standards for the platelet content and the lowest acceptable pH (at the end of storage) for both types of platelet components (whole blood–derived and apheresis).

20. Discuss the trend in manufacturing two apheresis products from a unique apheresis collection.

21. List at least two methods for detecting bacterial contamination in platelet components.

22. List at least three areas of research with platelets.

23. List the principles, including constituents, in two methods that are being developed to reduce/inactivate residual pathogens in platelet components.

24. List at least one type of platelet substitute and the primary potential advantage of a hemostatically active platelet substitute.

Historical Aspects

People have always been fascinated by blood: ancient Egyptians bathed in it, aristocrats drank it, authors and playwrights used it as themes, and modern humanity transfuses it. The road to an efficient, safe, and uncomplicated transfusion technique has been rather difficult, but great progress has been made.

In 1492, blood was taken from three young men and given to the stricken Pope Innocent VII in the hope of curing him; unfortunately, all four died. Although the outcome of this event was unsatisfactory, it is the first time a blood transfusion was recorded in history. The path to the successful transfusions so familiar today is marred by many reported failures, but our physical, spiritual, and emotional fascination with blood is primordial. Why did success elude experimenters for so long?

Clotting was the principal obstacle to overcome. Attempts to find a nontoxic anticoagulant began in 1869, when Braxton Hicks recommended sodium phosphate. This was perhaps the first example of blood preservation research. Karl Landsteiner in 1901 discovered the ABO blood groups and explained the serious reactions that occur in humans as a result of incompatible transfusions. His work early in the 20th century won a Nobel Prize.

Next came appropriate devices designed for performing the transfusions. Edward E. Lindemann was the first to succeed. He carried out vein-to-vein transfusion of blood by using multiple syringes and a special cannula for puncturing the vein through the skin. However, this time-consuming, complicated procedure required many skilled assistants. It was not until Unger designed his syringe-valve apparatus that transfusions from donor to patient by an unassisted physician became practical.

An unprecedented accomplishment in blood transfusion was achieved in 1914, when Hustin reported the use of sodium citrate as an anticoagulant solution for transfusions. Later, in 1915, Lewisohn determined the minimum amount of citrate needed for anticoagulation and demonstrated its nontoxicity in small amounts. Transfusions became more practical and safer for the patient.

The development of preservative solutions to enhance the metabolism of the RBC followed. Glucose was tried as early as 1916, when Rous and Turner introduced a citrate-dextrose solution for the preservation of blood. However, the function of glucose in RBC metabolism was not understood until the 1930s. Therefore, the common practice of using glucose in the preservative solution was delayed.

World War II stimulated blood preservation research because the demand for blood and plasma increased. The pioneer work of Charles Drew during World War II on developing techniques in blood transfusion and blood preservation led to the establishment of a widespread system of blood banks. In February 1941, Dr. Drew was appointed director of the first American Red Cross Blood Bank at Presbyterian Hospital. The pilot program Dr. Drew established became the model for the national volunteer blood donor program of the American Red Cross.[1] In 1943, Loutit and Mollison of England introduced the formula for the preservative acid-citrate-dextrose (ACD). Efforts in several countries resulted in the landmark publication of the July 1947 issue of the *Journal of Clinical Investigation,* which devoted nearly a dozen papers to blood preservation. Hospitals responded immediately, and in 1947, blood banks were established in many major cities of the United States; subsequently, transfusion became commonplace. The daily occurrence of transfusions led to the discovery of numerous blood group systems. Antibody identification surged to the forefront as sophisticated techniques were developed. The interested student can review historic events during World War II in Kendrick's Blood Program in World War II, Historical Note.[2] In 1957, Gibson introduced an improved preservative solution, citrate-phosphate-dextrose (CPD), which was less acidic and eventually replaced ACD as the standard preservative used for blood storage.

Frequent transfusions and the massive use of blood soon resulted in new problems, such as circulatory overload. Component therapy has solved these problems. Before, a single unit of whole blood could serve only one patient. With component therapy, however, one unit may be used for multiple transfusions. Today, physicians can select the specific component for their patient's particular needs without risking the inherent hazards of whole blood transfusions. Physicians can transfuse only the required fraction in the concentrated form, without overloading the circulation. Appropriate blood component therapy now provides more effective treatment and more complete use of blood products. Extensive use of blood during this period, coupled with component separation, led to increased comprehension of erythrocyte metabolism and a new awareness of the problems associated with RBC storage.

The American Association of Blood Banks (AABB) estimates that 8 million volunteers donate blood each year.[3] Based on studies by the National Blood Data Resource Center (NBDRC), about 15 million units of whole blood and RBCs were donated in 2001 in the United States. The NBDRC reported that nearly 29 million units of blood components were transfused in 2001. With an aging population and advances in medical treatments requiring transfusions, the demand for blood/blood components can be expected to continue to increase.[3] These units are donated by fewer than 5 percent of healthy Americans who are eligible to donate each year, primarily through blood drives conducted at their place of work. Individuals can also donate at community blood centers (which collect approximately 88 percent of the nation's blood) or hospital-based donor centers (which collect approximately 12 percent of the nation's blood supply). Volunteer donors (who are not paid) provide nearly all of the blood used for transfusion in the United States. The amount of whole blood in a unit has been traditionally 450 mL +/−10 percent of blood (1 pint). More recently, 500 mL +/−10 percent of blood is also being collected. This has provided a small increase in the various components. Modified plastic collection systems are used when collecting 500 mL of blood, with the volume of anticoagulant-preservative solution being increased from 63 mL to 70 mL. The maximum amount of blood that can be donated or collected at one time is now guided by an AABB standard (22nd edition, 2003), which states that the volume of whole blood collected including an amount for samples shall be "10.5 mL/kg of donor weight." This means that for a 110-lb donor, a maximum volume of 525 mL can be collected.

The total blood volume of most adults is 10 to 12 pints, and donors can replenish the fluid lost from the donation of 1 pint in 24 hours. The donor red cells are replaced within 1 to 2 months after donation. A volunteer donor can donate whole blood every 8 weeks.

Units of the whole blood collected can be separated into three components: packed RBCs, platelets, and plasma. In recent years, less whole blood has been used to prepare platelets with the increased utilization of apheresis platelets. Hence, many units are converted only into RBCs and plasma. The plasma can be converted by cryoprecipitation to a clotting factor concentrate that is rich in antihemophilic factor (AHF, factor VIII) (refer to Chapter 11). A unit of whole blood/prepared RBCs may be stored for 21 to 42 days, depending on the anticoagulant-preservative solution to collect the whole blood unit and whether a preserving solution is added to the separated RBCs. Although most people assume that donated blood is free because most blood-collecting organizations are nonprofit, a fee is still charged for each unit to cover the costs associated with collecting, storing, testing, and transfusing blood.

The donation process consists of three steps or processes:

1. Educational reading materials,
2. The donor health history questionnaire, and
3. The abbreviated physical examination (**Box 1–1**).

The donation process, especially steps 1 and 2, has been

TABLE 1–1   Donor Screening Tests for Infectious Diseases

Test	Date Test Required
West Nile virus	2003
Human immunodeficiency virus (NAT)*,**	1999
Hepatitis C virus (NAT) **	1999
Human immunodeficiency virus antibodies (anti-HIV 1 and 2)	1992
Hepatitis C virus antibodies (anti-HCV)	1990
Human T-cell lymphotropic virus antibody (HTLV I and II)	1989
Hepatitis B core antibody (anti-HBc)	1986
Hepatitis B surface antigen (HBsAg)	1972
Syphilis	1945

*NAT-nucleic acid amplification testing
**Initially under IND starting in 1999

refined over time to allow carefully for the rejection of donors who may be at risk for transmission of transfusion-associated disease. For a more detailed description of donor screening and processing, refer to Chapter 11.

The nation's blood supply is safer than it has ever been because of the donation process and extensive laboratory screening (testing) of blood. Currently, nine screening tests for infectious disease are performed on each unit of donated blood (**Table 1–1**). A study by Dodd and colleagues[4] (2002) has estimated that the risk from repeat voluntary donors for the HCV and HIV viruses were 1 per 1,935,000 and 1 per 2,135,000 donations, respectively. It was noted that incidence rates are approximately two times greater for first-time donors. The use of nucleic acid amplification testing (NAT) under an Investigational New Drug Application (since 1999) and now as tests licensed by the Food and Drug Administration (FDA) (since 2002) is one reason for increased safety of the blood supply. Refer to Chapter 19 for a detailed discussion of transfusion-transmitted viruses.

RBC Biology and Preservation

Three areas of RBC biology are crucial for normal erythrocyte survival and function:

1. Normal chemical composition and structure of the RBC membrane
2. Hemoglobin structure and function
3. RBC metabolism

Defects in any or all of these areas will result in RBC survival of fewer than the normal 120 days in circulation.

RBC Membrane

The RBC membrane represents a semipermeable lipid bilayer supported by a protein meshlike cytoskeleton structure (**Fig. 1–1**).[5] Phospholipids, the main lipid components of the membrane, are arranged in a bilayer structure comprising the framework in which globular proteins traverse and move. Proteins that extend from the outer surface and span the entire membrane to the inner cytoplasmic side of the RBC are termed "integral" membrane proteins. Beneath the lipid bilayer, a second class of membrane proteins, called "periph-

---

BOX 1–1
The Donation Process

Step 1: Educational Materials
Educational material (such as the AABB pamphlet, "An Important Message to All Blood Donors") that contains information on the risks of infectious diseases transmitted by blood transfusion, including the symptoms and sign of AIDS, is given to each prospective donor to read.

Step 2: The Donor Health History Questionnaire
A uniform donor history questionnaire designed to ask questions that protect the health of both the donor and the recipient is given to every donor. The health history questionnaire is used to identify donors who have been exposed to other diseases (e.g.,variant Creutzfeldt-Jakob, West Nile fever, malaria, babesiosis, or Chagas disease).

Step 3: The Abbreviated Physical Examination
The abbreviated physical examination for donors includes blood pressure, pulse, and temperature readings, hemoglobin or hematocrit level, and the inspection of the arms for skin lesions.

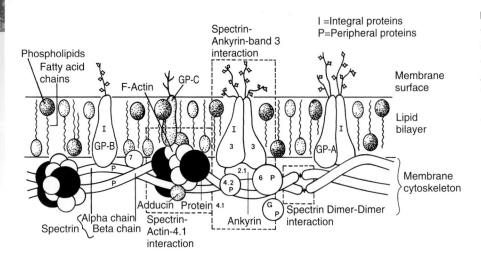

■ FIGURE 1–1   Schematic illustration of red blood cell membrane depicting the composition and arrangement of RBC membrane proteins. GP-A = glycophorin A; GP-B = glycophorin B; GP-C = glycophorin C; G = globin. Numbers refer to pattern of migration of SDS (sodium dodecyl sulfate) poly-acrylamide gel pattern stained with Coomassie brilliant blue. Relations of protein to each other and to lipids are purely hypothetical; however, the positions of the proteins relative to the inside or outside of the lipid bilayer are accurate. (Note: Proteins are not drawn to scale and many minor proteins are omitted.)

eral" proteins, is located and limited to the cytoplasmic surface of the membrane forming the RBC cytoskeleton (**Table 1–2**).[5] Both proteins and lipids are organized asymmetrically within the RBC membrane. Lipids are not equally distributed in the two layers of the membrane. The external layer is rich in glycolipids and choline phospholipids.[6] The internal cytoplasmic layer of the membrane is rich in amino phospholipids.[6] The biochemical composition of the RBC membrane is approximately 52 percent protein, 40 percent lipid, and 8 percent carbohydrate.[7]

As mentioned previously, the normal chemical composition and the structural arrangement and molecular interactions of the erythrocyte membrane are crucial to the normal length of RBC survival in circulation of 120 days. In addition, they maintain a critical role in two important RBC characteristics: deformability and permeability.

Deformability

To remain viable, normal RBCs must also remain flexible, deformable, and permeable. The loss of adenosine triphosphate (ATP) (energy) levels leads to a decrease in the phosphorylation of spectrin and, in turn, a loss of membrane deformability.[6] An accumulation or increase in deposition of membrane calcium also results, causing an increase in membrane rigidity and loss of pliability. These cells are at a marked disadvantage when they pass through the small (3 to 5 μm in diameter) sinusoidal orifices of the spleen, an organ that functions in extravascular sequestration and removal of aged, damaged, or less deformable RBCs or fragments of their

membrane. The loss of RBC membrane is exemplified by the formation of "spherocytes" (cells with a reduced surface-to-volume ratio) (**Fig. 1–2**) and "bite cells," in which the removal of a portion of membrane has left a permanent indentation in the remaining cell membrane (**Fig. 1–3**). The survival of these forms is also shortened.

Permeability

The permeability properties of the RBC membrane and the active RBC cation transport prevent colloid hemolysis and control the volume of the RBC. Any abnormality that increases permeability or alters cationic transport may lead to decrease in RBC survival.

The RBC membrane is freely permeable to water and anions. Chloride (Cl^-) and bicarbonate (HCO_3^-) can traverse the membrane in less than a second. It is speculated that this massive exchange of ions occurs through a large number of exchange channels located in the RBC membrane. The RBC membrane is relatively impermeable to cations such as sodium (Na^+) and potassium (K^+). RBC volume and water homeostasis are maintained by controlling the intracellular concentrations of sodium and potassium. The erythrocyte intracellular-to-extracellular ratios for Na^+ and K^+ are 1:12 and 25:1, respectively. The 300 cationic pumps, which active-

TABLE 1–2 RBC Membrane Integral and Peripheral Proteins	
Integral Proteins	**Peripheral Proteins**
Glycophorin A	Spectrin
Glycophorin B	Actin (band 5)
Glycophorin C	Ankyrin (band 2.1)
Anion-exchange-channel protein (band 3)	Band 4.1 and 4.2
	Band 6
	Adducin

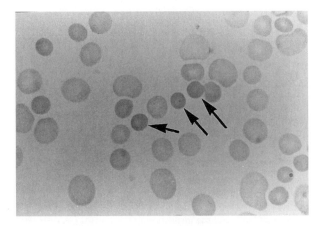

■ FIGURE 1–2   Spherocytes.

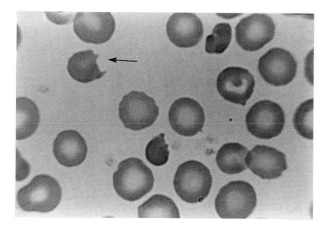

FIGURE 1–3 "Bite" cells.

ly transport Na⁺ out of the cell and K⁺ into the cell, require energy in the form of ATP. Calcium (Ca^{2+}) is also actively pumped from the interior of the RBC through energy-dependent calcium-ATPase pumps. Calmodulin, a cytoplasmic calcium-binding protein, is speculated to control these pumps and to prevent excessive intracellular Ca^{2+} buildup, which changes the shape and makes the RBC more rigid.

When RBCs are ATP-depleted, Ca^{2+} and Na⁺ are allowed to accumulate intracellularly, and K⁺ and water are lost, resulting in a dehydrated rigid cell subsequently sequestered by the spleen, resulting in a decrease in RBC survival.

Metabolic Pathways

The RBC's metabolic pathways that produce ATP are mainly anaerobic, because the function of the RBC is to deliver oxygen, not to consume it. Because the mature erythrocyte has no nucleus and there is no mitochondrial apparatus for oxidative metabolism, energy must be generated almost exclusively through the breakdown of glucose.

RBC metabolism may be divided among the anaerobic glycolytic pathway and three ancillary pathways that serve to maintain the structure and function of hemoglobin (**Fig. 1–4**). All of these processes are essential if the erythrocyte is to transport oxygen and to maintain critical physical characteristics for its survival.

Glycolysis generates about 90 percent of the ATP needed by the RBC. Approximately 10 percent is provided by the pentose phosphate pathway. The activity of this pathway increases following increased oxidation of glutathione or decreased activity of the glycolytic pathway.

When the pentose phosphate pathway is functionally deficient, the amount of reduced glutathione becomes insufficient to neutralize intracellular oxidants. The result is denaturation and precipitation of globin as aggregates (Heinz bodies) within the cell. The formation of Heinz bodies makes the RBC less deformable than a normal RBC and may cause the RBC to be caught in the spleen or capillaries, damaging the membrane. If membrane damage is sufficient, cell destruction occurs.

The methemoglobin reductase pathway is another important pathway of RBC metabolism. This pathway is necessary to

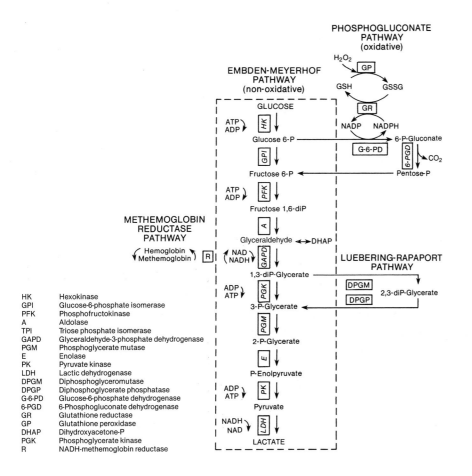

HK   Hexokinase
GPI   Glucose-6-phosphate isomerase
PFK   Phosphofructokinase
A   Aldolase
TPI   Triose phosphate isomerase
GAPD   Glyceraldehyde-3-phosphate dehydrogenase
PGM   Phosphoglycerate mutase
E   Enolase
PK   Pyruvate kinase
LDH   Lactic dehydrogenase
DPGM   Diphosphoglyceromutase
DPGP   Diphosphoglycerate phosphatase
G-6-PD   Glucose-6-phosphate dehydrogenase
6-PGD   6-Phosphogluconate dehydrogenase
GR   Glutathione reductase
GP   Glutathione peroxidase
DHAP   Dihydroxyacetone-P
PGK   Phosphoglycerate kinase
R   NADH-methemoglobin reductase

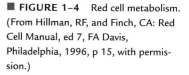

FIGURE 1–4 Red cell metabolism. (From Hillman, RF, and Finch, CA: Red Cell Manual, ed 7, FA Davis, Philadelphia, 1996, p 15, with permission.)

maintain the heme iron of hemoglobin in the ferrous (Fe^{2+}) functional state. In the absence of the enzyme methemoglobin reductase and the action of nicotinamide adenine dinucleotide (NAD), there is an accumulation of methemoglobin, which results from a conversion of ferrous iron to the ferric form (Fe^{3+}). Methemoglobin represents a nonfunctional form of hemoglobin and a loss of oxygen transport capabilities, inasmuch as metheme cannot bind with oxygen. To illustrate the efficiency of this system, normal healthy individuals have no more than 1 percent methemoglobin circulating in their RBCs. A defect in the methemoglobin reductase pathway is, therefore, significant to RBC posttransfusion survival and function.

Another pathway that is crucial to RBC function is the Luebering-Rapaport shunt. This pathway permits the accumulation of another important RBC organic phosphate, 2,3-diphosphoglycerate (2,3-DPG). The large amount of 2,3-DPG found within RBCs has a significant effect on the affinity of hemoglobin for oxygen.

Hemoglobin Structure and Function

Hemoglobin makes up approximately 95 percent of the dry weight of an RBC or approximately 33 percent of its weight by volume.[8] Because of its multichain structure, hemoglobin, which has a molecular weight of 68,000 daltons, is capable of considerable allosteric change as it loads and unloads oxygen. Normal hemoglobin consists of globin (a tetramer of two pairs of polypeptide chains) and four heme groups, each of which contains a protoporphyrin ring plus iron (Fe^{2+}).

Hemoglobin Synthesis

Normal hemoglobin production is dependent on three processes:

1. Adequate iron delivery and supply
2. Adequate synthesis of protoporphyrins (the precursor of heme)
3. Adequate globin synthesis

All adult normal hemoglobins are formed as tetramers consisting of two alpha (α) chains plus two (non-α) globin chains. Normal adult RBCs contain the following types of hemoglobin:

- 92 to 95 percent of the hemoglobin is HbA, which consists of two alpha, two beta ($\alpha_2\beta_2$) chains.
- 2 to 3 percent of the hemoglobin is HbA_2, which consists of two alpha, two delta ($\alpha_2\delta_2$) chains.
- 1 to 2 percent of the hemoglobin is fetal hemoglobin (HbF), which consists of two alpha, two gamma ($\alpha_2\gamma_2$) chains.

Each synthesized globin chain links with heme (ferroprotoporphyrin IX) to form hemoglobin, which normally consists of two α chains, two β chains, and four heme groups.

The rate of globin synthesis is directly related to the rate of porphyrin synthesis and vice versa: protoporphyrin synthesis is reduced when globin synthesis is impaired.

Hemoglobin Function

Hemoglobin's primary function is gas transport: oxygen delivery to the tissues and carbon dioxide (CO_2) excretion.

One of the most important controls of hemoglobin affinity for oxygen is the RBC organic phosphate 2,3-DPG. The unloading of oxygen by hemoglobin is accompanied by widening of a space between β chains and the binding of 2,3-DPG on a mole-for-mole basis, with the formation of anionic salt bridges between the chains. The resulting conformation of the deoxyhemoglobin molecule is known as the tense (T) form, which has a lower affinity for oxygen. When hemoglobin loads oxygen and becomes oxyhemoglobin, the established salt bridges are broken, and β chains are pulled together, expelling 2,3-DPG. This is the relaxed (R) form of the hemoglobin molecule, which has a higher affinity for oxygen.

These allosteric changes that occur as the hemoglobin loads and unloads oxygen are referred to as the respiratory movement. The dissociation and binding of oxygen by hemoglobin are not directly proportional to the partial pressure of oxygen (Po_2) in its environment but, instead, exhibit a sigmoid-curve relationship, known as the hemoglobin-oxygen dissociation curve (Fig. 1–5). The shape of this curve is very important physiologically because it permits a considerable amount of oxygen to be delivered to the tissues with a small drop in oxygen tension. For example, in the environment of the lungs, where the oxygen (Po_2) tension, measured in millimeters of mercury (mm Hg), is nearly 100 mm Hg, the hemoglobin molecule is almost 100 percent saturated with oxygen. As the RBCs travel to the tissues, where the Po_2 drops to an average 40 mm Hg (mean venous oxygen tension), the hemoglobin saturation drops to approximately 75 percent saturation, releasing approximately 25 percent of the oxygen to the tissues.

This is the normal situation of oxygen delivery at basal metabolic rate. The normal position of the oxygen dissociation curve depends on three different ligands normally found within the RBC: H^+ ions, CO_2, and organic phosphates. Of these three ligands, 2,3-DPG plays the most important physiologic role. The dependence of normal hemoglobin function on 2,3-DPG levels in the RBC has been well documented.[9–12] In situations such as hypoxia, a compensatory "shift to the right" of the hemoglobin-oxygen dissociation curve occurs to alleviate a tissue oxygen deficit (Fig. 1–6). This rightward

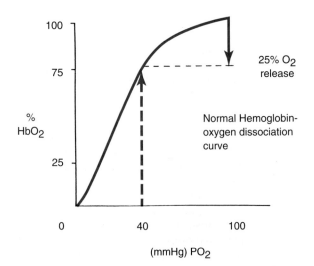

■ FIGURE 1–5 Hemoglobin-oxygen dissociation curve.

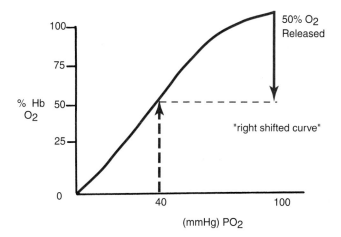

■ **FIGURE 1–6**   "Shift to the right" of the hemoglobin-oxygen dissociation curve.

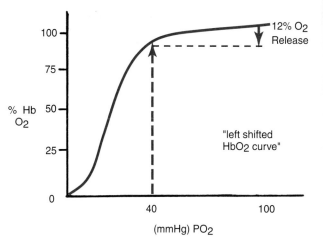

■ **FIGURE 1–7**   "Shift to the left" of the hemoglobin-oxygen dissociation curve.

shift of the curve, mediated by increased levels of 2,3-DPG, results in a decrease in hemoglobin's affinity for the oxygen molecule and an increase in oxygen delivery to the tissues. Note in **Figure 1–6** that the oxygen saturation of hemoglobin in the environment of the tissues (40 mm Hg Po_2) is now 50 percent; the other 50 percent of the oxygen is being released to the tissues. The RBCs thus have become more efficient in terms of oxygen delivery.

Therefore, a patient who is suffering from an anemia caused by loss of RBCs may be able to compensate by shifting the oxygen dissociation curve to the right, making the RBCs, although few in number, more efficient. Some patients may be able to tolerate anemia better than others because of this compensatory mechanism. A shift to the right may also occur in response to acidosis or a rise in body temperature. The shift to the right of the hemoglobin-oxygen dissociation curve is only one way in which patients may compensate for various types of hypoxia. Other ways include an increase in total cardiac output and an increase in the production of RBCs (erythropoiesis).

A "shift to the left" of the hemoglobin-oxygen dissociation curve results, conversely, in an increase in hemoglobin-oxygen affinity and a decrease in oxygen delivery to the tissues **(Fig. 1–7)**. With such a dissociation curve, RBCs are much less efficient because only 12 percent of the oxygen can be released to the tissues. Among the conditions that can shift the oxygen dissociation curve to the left are alkalosis; increased quantities of abnormal hemoglobins, such as methemoglobin and carboxyhemoglobin; increased quantities of hemoglobin F; and multiple transfusions of 2,3-DPG–depleted stored blood (attesting to the importance of 2,3-DPG in oxygen release).

Hemoglobin-oxygen affinity can also be expressed by P_{50} values, which designate the Po_2 at which hemoglobin is 50 percent saturated with oxygen under standard in-vitro conditions of temperature and pH. The P_{50} of normal blood is 26 to 30 mm Hg. An increase in P_{50} represents a decrease in hemoglobin-oxygen affinity, or a shift to the right of the oxygen dissociation curve. A decrease in P_{50} represents an increase in hemoglobin-oxygen affinity, or a shift to the left of the oxygen dissociation curve. In addition to the reasons listed for shifts in the curve, inherited abnormalities of the hemoglobin molecule can result in either situation; these

abnormalities are described by the P_{50} measurements. Abnormalities in hemoglobin structure or function can therefore have profound effects on the ability of the RBCs to provide oxygen to the tissues.

RBC Preservation

The goal of blood preservation is to provide viable and functional blood components for patients requiring blood transfusion. RBC viability is a measure of in-vivo RBC survival following transfusion. Because blood must be stored from the time of donation until the time of transfusion, the viability of RBCs must be maintained during the storage time as well. Seventy-five percent of cells that have been transfused should remain viable for 24 hours.[13] This criterion is used to evaluate new preservation solutions and storage containers. The measurements are made with RBCs that are taken from healthy subjects, stored and then labeled with radioisotopes, reinfused to the original donor, and measured 24 hours after transfusion.

To maintain optimum viability, blood is stored in the liquid state between 1° and 6°C for a specific number of days, as determined by preservative solution(s) used. The loss of RBC viability has been correlated with the "lesion of storage," which is associated with various biochemical changes. These changes include a decrease in pH, a decrease in glucose consumption, a buildup of lactic acid, a decrease in ATP levels, and a reversible loss of RBC function.[12] This loss of function is expressed as a shift to the left of the hemoglobin-oxygen dissociation curve or an increase in hemoglobin-oxygen affinity.

Because low 2,3-DPG levels profoundly influence the oxygen dissociation curve of hemoglobin,[14] DPG-depleted RBCs may have an impaired capacity to deliver oxygen to the tissues. As RBCs (in whole blood or RBC concentrates) are stored, 2,3-DPG levels decrease, with a shift to the left of the hemoglobin-oxygen dissociation curve, and therefore less oxygen is delivered to the tissues. It is well accepted, however, that 2,3-DPG is re-formed in stored RBCs, after in-vivo circulation resulting in restored oxygen delivery. The rate of restoration of 2,3-DPG is influenced by the acid-base status of the recipient, phosphorus metabolism, and the degree of anemia.

TABLE 1–3   Approved Anticoagulant Preservative Solutions

		Storage Time
Name	Abbreviation	Days
Acid-citrate-dextrose	ACD	21
Citrate-phosphate-dextrose	CPD	21
Citrate-phosphate-dextrose-adenine	CPDA-1	35
Citrate-phosphate–double dextrose	CP2D	21

Anticoagulant Preservative Solutions

ACD, CPD, and CP2D are approved anticoagulant preservative solutions for whole blood and RBC storage at 1° to 6°C for 21 days[15] (Table 1–3). Because of the lower pH in the ACD preservative, most of the 2,3-DPG is lost early in the first week of storage. Therefore, a substitute preservative, CPD, came into widespread use in the United States in the 1970s because it was superior for preserving this organic phosphate. This effect is the result of a higher pH (Table 1–4). Even in CPD, RBCs become low in 2,3-DPG by the second week.

Subsequent studies led to the addition of various chemicals, along with the currently approved anticoagulant-preservative CPD, in an attempt to stimulate glycolysis so that ATP levels were better maintained.[11] One of the chemicals, adenine, was approved for addition to CPD by the FDA in August 1978. The incorporation of adenine into the CPD solution(CPDA-1) increases ADP levels, thereby driving glycolysis toward the synthesis of ATP. CPDA-1 contains 0.25 mM of adenine plus 25 percent more glucose than CPD (see Table 1–4). Adenine-supplemented blood can be stored at 1° to 6°C for 35 days. The extra glucose was added because of the lengthened storage period. CP2D contains 100 percent more glucose than CPD, or 60 percent more glucose than CPDA-1. However, blood stored in all CPD preservatives also becomes depleted of 2,3-DPG by the second week of storage.

The reported pathophysiologic effects of the transfusion of RBCs with low 2,3-DPG levels and increased affinity for oxygen include an increase in cardiac output, a decrease in mixed venous Po_2 tension, or a combination of these. The physiologic importance of these effects is not easily demonstrated. This is a complex mechanism with numerous variables involved that are beyond the scope of this text.

Stored RBCs do regain the ability to synthesize 2,3-DPG after transfusion, but levels necessary for optimal hemoglobin oxygen delivery are not reached immediately. Approximately 24 hours are required to restore normal levels of 2,3-DPG after transfusion.[12] The 2,3-DPG concentrations after transfusion have been reported to reach normal levels as early as 6 hours posttransfusion.[13] Most of these studies have been performed on normal, healthy individuals. However, evidence suggests that, in the transfused subject whose capacity is limited by an underlying physiologic disturbance, even a brief period of altered oxygen hemoglobin affinity is of great significance.[14]

It is quite clear now that 2,3-DPG levels in transfused blood are important in certain clinical conditions. Several animal studies demonstrate significantly increased mortality associated with transfusing blood that is low in 2,3-DPG levels in subjects with persistent anemia, hypotension, hypoxia, and cardiac and hemorrhagic shock. Human studies demonstrate that myocardial function improves following transfusion of blood with high 2,3-DPG levels during cardiovascular surgery.[16]

Several investigators suggest that the patient in shock who is given 2,3-DPG–depleted erythrocytes in transfusion may have already strained the compensatory mechanisms to their limits.[16-18] Perhaps for this type of patient the poor oxygen delivery capacity of 2,3-DPG–depleted cells makes a significant difference in recovery and survival.

It is apparent that many factors may limit the viability of transfused RBCs. One of these factors is the plastic material used for the storage container. The plastic must be sufficiently permeable to CO_2 in order to maintain higher pH levels during storage. Glass storage containers are a matter of history in the United States. Currently, all blood is stored in polyvinyl chloride (PVC) plastic bags (Fig. 1–8). One issue associated with PVC bags relates to the plasticizer, di(ethylhexyl)-phthalate (DEHP), which is used in the manufacture of the bags. It has been found to leach into the blood from the plastic into the lipids of the plasma medium and RBC membranes during storage. However, its use or that of alternative plasticizers that leach are important because they have been

TABLE 1–4   Comparison of the Composition of Acid-Citrate-Dextrose (ACD) and Citrate-Phosphate-Dextrose (CPD) Anticoagulant Preservative Solutions

	ACD	CPD	CPDA-1	CP2D
Trisodium citrate (g)	22.0	26.30	26.35	26.35
Citric acid (g)	8.0	3.27	3.27	3.27
Dextrose (g)	24.5	25.50	31.90	51.10
Monobasic sodium phosphate (g)	–	2.22	2.22	2.22
Adenine (g)	–	–	0.27	–
Water (mL)	1000	1000	1000	1000
Volume/100 mL blood (mL)	15	14	14	14
Approximate volume of preservative solution/bag (mL)	67.5	63.0	63.0	63.0
Initial pH of solution*	5.0	5.6	5.6	5.6
pH of whole blood on initial day drawn into storage bag*	7.0	7.2	7.4	7.3
Storage time (days) 1°–6°C**	21	21	35	21

Note: Composition for 63 mL of anticoagulant-preservative solution which is mixed with 450 mL (±10%)of blood in each unit.

*Indicates measurement at room temperature. For 500 mL collections, 70 mL of anticoagulant-preservative solution is used.

**If additive preservative solutions are not utilized.

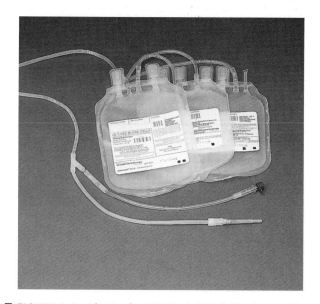

■ **FIGURE 1–8**   The Teruflex CPD/Optisol Triple blood bags with blood sampling arm. (Courtesy of Terumo Medical Corporation, Somerset, NJ.)

shown to stabilize the RBC membrane and therefore reduce the extent of hemolysis during storage. Research has been focused on the development of improved plastic blood bags as well as better preservative solutions. In addition to blood preservation issues, adverse effects and risks associated with blood transfusion have created concern and caution among clinicians when determining the need for blood and blood components (see Chapter 18).

Additive Solutions

Additive solutions are preserving solutions that are added to the RBCs after removal of the plasma with/without platelets. Additive solutions are now widely used. One of the reasons for their development related to the fact that removal of the plasma component during the preparation of RBC concentrates removed much of the nutrients needed to maintain RBCs during storage. This was dramatically observed when high hematocrit RBCs were prepared. The influence of removing substantial amounts of adenine and glucose present originally in, for example, the CPDA-1 anticoagulant-preservative solution led to a decrease in viability, particularly in the last 2 weeks of storage.[12] RBC concentrates prepared from whole blood units collected in primary anticoagulant-preservative solutions can be relatively void of plasma with high hematocrits, which causes the units to be more viscous and difficult to infuse, especially in emergency situations. Additive solutions (100 mL to the RBC concentrate prepared from a 450-mL blood collection) also overcome this problem. Additive solutions reduce hematocrits from around 70 to 85 percent to around 50 to 60 percent. The ability to pack RBCs to fairly high hematocrits before addition of additive solution also provides a means to harvest greater amounts of plasma with or without platelets.

The additive system concept was developed by Beutler[19] in the 1970s, and implementation of specific solutions was initiated in the early 1980s by Lovric[20] in Australia and Högman[21] in Sweden. The blood collection systems employed a primary

bag containing a standard anticoagulant-preservation solution and an accessory, or satellite, bag containing the additional nutrient solution that was added to the packed RBC component after the plasma was removed. The configuration of the additive solution approach remains essentially unchanged. In general, the additive solutions employed in the systems were composed of standard ingredients used intravenously: saline, dextrose, and adenine. The systems described by Högman and Lovric differ slightly in their approach. Högman's system uses the standard CPD anticoagulant in the primary bag with the additive solution containing saline, adenine, and glucose (SAG), which was modified further with the addition of mannitol (SAGM), which protected against storage-related hemolysis.[21] (SAGM is similar to Adsol AS-1; see **Table 1–6**.) Lovric doubled the dextrose concentration in the primary anticoagulant (CP2D) and used it in connection with an additive solution composed of saline, adenine, glucose, trisodium citrate, citric acid, and sodium phosphate.[20] It is thought the citrate and phosphate in this formulation may protect against hemolysis.

The formulations by Lovric and Högman provided the basis for the three additive solutions that are licensed in the United States:

1. AS-1 (Baxter Healthcare)
2. Nutricel (AS-3) (Pall Corporation, manufactured initially by the Cutter Biological and subsequently by Medsep Corporation)
3. Optisol (AS-5) (Terumo Corporation)

AS-1 solution contains SAGM to retard hemolysis. It is coupled with CPD as the primary bag anticoagulant-preservative. AS-3 contains SAG (as in AS-1) but at different concentrations and in addition to sodium phosphate, sodium citrate, and citric acid. It is coupled with CP2D as the primary bag anticoagulant-preservative. Optisol contains SAGM at different concentrations from AS-1 and uses CPD in the primary bag. All of these additive solutions are approved for 42 days of storage of RBCs. **Table 1–5** lists the currently approved additive solutions, and **Table 1–6** describes formulations for each one. The formulations listed in **Table 1–6** are for 100 mL of additive solution that is added to RBCs prepared from 450-mL blood collections. When the collection systems are for 500 mL of blood, the volume of the additive solution is 110 mL.

Initially, the AS-1 solution was used to store RBCs for up to 49 days. Conflicting data regarding in-vivo RBC survival from different studies with AS-1–stored RBCs resulted in the FDA convening a workshop on AS-1 and other additive solutions in 1985. The consensus of the FDA Advisory Panel resulted in changing the approval of AS-1 from 49 days to 42 days, which is the storage limit for all additive solutions in the

TABLE 1–5   Additive Solutions in Use in North America

Name	Storage Abbreviation	Time (Days)
Adsol (Baxter Healthcare)	AS-1	42
Nutricel (Pall Corporation)	AS-3	42
Optisol (Terumo Corporation)	AS-5	42

TABLE 1-6 Composition of Additive Solutions (mg/100mL)

	AS-1 (Adsol)	AS-3 (Nutricel)	AS-5 (Optisol)
Dextrose	2200	1100	900
Adenine	27	30	30
Monobasic sodium phosphate	0	276	0
Mannitol	750	0	525
Sodium chloride	900	410	877
Sodium citrate	0	588	0
Citric acid	0	42	0
Primary bag anticoagulant-preservative	CPD	CP2D	CPD

United States. Overall, data from clinical studies show that RBCs stored for 42 days in AS-1, AS-3, or AS-5 demonstrated a mean 24-hour postinfusion survival of greater than 75 percent, the minimum requirement for satisfactory RBC survival.

Table 1-7 shows the biochemical characteristics of RBCs stored in the three additive solutions after 42 days of storage.[22-24] Poststorage survival rates of greater than 80 percent were demonstrated in one study with less than 1 percent hemolysis. Additive system RBCs are used in the same way as traditional RBC transfusions. Blood stored in additive solutions is now routinely given to newborn infants and pediatric patients,[25] although some clinicians have continued to prefer CPDA-1 RBCs because of their concerns about one or more of the constituents in the additive solutions.

None of the additive solutions maintain 2,3-DPG throughout the storage time. As with RBCs stored only with primary anticoagulant-preservatives, 2,3-DPG is depleted by 2 weeks of storage.

Freezing and Rejuvenation

RBC Freezing

RBC freezing is primarily used for autologous units and the storage of rare blood types. Autologous transfusion allows individuals to donate blood for their own (autologous) use in meeting their needs for blood transfusion (see Chapter 16).

The procedure for freezing a unit of packed RBCs is not complicated. Basically, it involves the addition of a cryoprotective agent to RBCs that are less than 6 days old. Glycerol is used most commonly and is added to the RBCs slowly with

TABLE 1-7 Additive Red Cells: Biochemical Characteristics

	AS-1	AS-3	AS-5
Storage period (days)	42.00	42.00	42.00
pH (measured at 37°C)	6.6	6.5	6.5
24-hour survival*(%)	83.00	85.1	80.0
ATP (% initial)	68.00	67.0	68.5
2,3-DPG (% initial)	6.0	6.0	5.0
Hemolysis (%)	0.5	0.7	0.6

*Survival studies reported are from selected investigators and do not include an average of all reported survivals.

vigorous shaking, thereby enabling the glycerol to permeate the RBCs. The cells are then rapidly frozen and stored in a freezer. The usual storage temperature is below −65°C, although storage (and freezing) temperature depends on the concentration of glycerol used.[14] Two concentrations of glycerol have been used to freeze RBCs: a high-concentration glycerol (40 percent weight in volume [w/v]) and a low-concentration glycerol (20 percent w/v) in the final concentration of the cryopreservative.[23] Most blood banks that freeze RBCs use the high-concentration glycerol technique. **Table 1-8** lists the advantages of the high-concentration glycerol technique in comparison with the low-concentration glycerol technique. The reader is referred to Chapter 11 for a detailed description of the RBC freezing procedure.

Transfusion of frozen cells must be preceded by a deglycerolization process; otherwise the thawed cells would be accompanied by hypertonic glycerol when infused, and RBC lysis would result. Removal of glycerol is achieved by systematically replacing the cryoprotectant with decreasing concentrations of saline. The usual protocol involves washing with 12 percent saline, followed by 1.6 percent saline, with a final wash of 0.2 percent dextrose in normal saline.[23] A commercially available cell-washing system, such as one of those manufactured by several companies, has traditionally been used in the deglycerolizing process.

Excessive hemolysis is monitored by noting the hemoglobin concentration of the wash supernatant. Osmolality of the unit should also be monitored to ensure adequate deglycerolization. Traditionally, because a unit of blood is processed under open system conditions to add the glycerol (before freezing) or the saline solutions (for deglycerolization), the outdating period of thawed RBCs stored at 1° to 6°C has been 24 hours.

Generally, RBCs in CPD or CPDA-1 anticoagulant-preservatives or additive solutions are glycerolized and frozen within 6 days of whole blood collection. Red blood cells stored in additive solutions such as AS-1 and AS-3 have been frozen up to 42 days after liquid storage without rejuvenation.

The need for RBCs within 24 hours of thawing has limited the utilization of frozen RBCs. Recently, an instrument (ACP 215, Haemonetics) has been developed that allows the glycerolization and deglycerolization processes to be performed under closed system conditions.[26] This instrument utilizes a sterile connecting device for connections, in-line 0.22 micron filters to deliver solutions, and a disposable polycarbonate bowl with an external seal to deglycerolize the RBCs. Based on approval by the FDA, RBCs prepared from 450-mL collections and frozen within 6 days of blood collection with CPDA-1 can be stored after thawing at 1° to 6°C for up to 15 days when the processing is conducted with the ACP 215 instrument and the deglycerolized cells, prepared using salt solutions as in the traditional procedures, are suspended in the AS-3 additive solution as a final step, which is thought to provide stabilization to the thawed RBCs. These storage conditions are based on the parameters used in a study by Valeri and others that showed that RBC properties were satisfactorily maintained during a 15-day period.[26] Further studies will broaden the conditions that can be used to prepare RBCs for subsequent freezing with closed system processing.

Currently, the FDA licenses frozen RBCs for a period of 10 years from the date of freezing; that is, frozen RBCs may be stored up to 10 years before thawing and transfusion. Once thawed, these RBCs demonstrate function and viability near

TABLE 1–8   Advantages of High-Concentration Glycerol Technique Used by Most Blood Banks over Low-Concentration Glycerol Technique

Advantage	High Glycerol	Low Glycerol
1. Initial freezing temperature	−80°C	−196°C
2. Need to control freezing rate	No	Yes
3. Type of freezer	Mechanical	Liquid nitrogen
4. Maximum storage temperature	−65°C	−120°C
5. Shipping requirements	Dry ice	Liquid nitrogen
6. Effect of changes in storage temperature	Can be thawed and refrozen	Critical

those of fresh blood. Experience has shown that 10-year storage periods do not adversely affect viability and function.[15] Table 1–9 lists the advantages and disadvantages of RBC freezing.

Rejuvenation

Rejuvenation of RBCs is the process by which ATP and 2,3-DPG levels are restored or enhanced by metabolic alterations. The initial rejuvenation solution contained phosphate, inosine, glucose, pyruvate, and adenine (PIGPA).[27] Valeri and coworkers, the pioneers in developing rejuvenation studies with outdated RBCs, subsequently showed that glucose was not required and utilized a solution designated phosphate, inosine, pyruvate, and adenine (PIPA).[27] Currently, Rejuvesol (enCyte Systems, Inc.) is the only FDA-approved rejuvenation solution sold in the United States and contains the same biochemicals as the original PIPA solution.[28] Rejuvesol is currently approved for use with CPD, CPDA-1, and CPD/AS-1 RBCs.

Rejuvesol is being used primarily to salvage liquid-stored RBCs that have reached outdate, as rejuvenated RBCs can be frozen with glycerol as the cryoprotecting solution. Rare units and O-type units are primarily treated for subsequent cryopreservation. Autologous units that are not utilized during liquid storage are also rejuvenated and cryopreserved. It is also possible to transfuse rejuvenated RBCs within 24 hours of processing. In this case, although not widely used, the rejuvenated RBCs are washed to remove the excess rejuvenating solution and are held at 1° to 6°C until transfusion.

Rejuvenation is accomplished by incubating an RBC unit at 37°C for 1 hour (currently only RBCs prepared from 450-mL collection can be rejuvenated) with 50 mL of the rejuvenating solution. RBCs stored in the liquid state can be rejuvenated at outdate or up to 3 days after outdate and cryopreserved, depending on RBC preservative solutions used. The RBCs are washed during the post-freezing deglycerolization process to remove nonmetabolized rejuvenation solution

materials and deleterious amounts of extracellular potassium. Because the processing including the washing procedure is currently accomplished with open systems that are not specifically designed to prevent the entrance of bacteria, federal regulations require that rejuvenated/frozen RBCs are used within 24 hours of thawing.[15] The rejuvenation process is expensive and time-consuming; therefore, it is not used often but is invaluable for preserving selected autologous and rare units of blood for later use. It is possible that rejuvenated RBCs could be processed with the closed system ACP 215 instrument.

Current Trends in Blood/RBC Preservation Research

Research and development in RBC preparation and preservation is being pursued in four directions:

1. Development of modified/new additive solutions,
2. Development of procedures to reduce the level of pathogens that may be in RBC units,
3. Development of procedures to convert A-, B-, and AB-type RBCs to O-type RBCs, and
4. Development of RBC substitutes.

Improved Additive Solutions

Research is being conducted to develop improved additive solutions for RBC preservation. One reason is that longer storage periods could improve the logistics of providing RBCs for clinical use, including increased benefits associated with the use of autologous blood/RBCs. One approach by Hess and Greenwalt and coworkers,[29] involving customized solutions containing sodium bicarbonate, sodium phosphate, adenine, dextrose, mannitol, and sodium chloride and the use of a higher pH (alkaline range), is providing for better retention of ATP levels. Consequently, satisfactory 24-hour in-vivo survival (mean of 78 percent) was observed even after 12 weeks of storage, which is twice the current limit. Leukocyte-reduced RBCs were utilized for the storage studies.[29] It was shown that membrane loss could be prevented by maintaining higher concentrations of ATP. The authors noted that membrane loss reduces RBC deformability, which is correlated with reduced RBC survival. Högman and coworkers[30] have developed a hypotonic additive solution approach that does not include chloride ions in the additive solution. Their approach also uses a higher medium pH and has been shown to increase storage for at least 7 weeks. Their system also works, in part, through improved maintenance of ATP, and there is also better retention of 2,3-DPG. The anticoagulant-preservative solution used in the blood collection process for this system is either CPD or half-strength CPD. Half-strength

TABLE 1–9   Advantages and Disadvantages of RBC Freezing

Advantages	Disadvantages
Long-term storage (10 years)	A time-consuming process
Maintenance of RBC viability and function	Higher cost of equipment and materials
Low residual leukocytes and platelets	Storage requirements (−65°C)
Removal of significant amounts of plasma proteins	Higher cost of product

CPD is being evaluated because its use has been associated with higher pH levels.[30]

Procedures to Reduce/Inactivate Pathogens

Research is being conducted to develop procedures that would reduce the level of/inactivate residual viruses, bacteria, and parasites in RBC units. One objective is to develop robust procedures that would have the potential to inactivate unrecognized (unknown) pathogens that may be present, such as the viruses that have emerged in recent years. Two methods that utilize alkylating agents that react with the nucleic acids of pathogens (S-303, Cerus/Baxter; Inactine, Vitex) are being evaluated in clinical trials. Key to the utilzation of such chemicals will be the use of procedures that remove unreactive chemical and/or break-down products after the reaction period is complete. Removal is being accomplished by use of an absorbing material or by washing of the RBCs. There are three main areas of study that are being pursued to document that a pathogen-reduction procedure could be utilized. The extent of pathogen reduction/inactivation with a wide array of the actual pathogens that have been found in RBCs and models for specific pathogens, when necessary, is one key area being studied to show that routinely found pathogen titers can be satisfactorily reduced and inactivated. Retention of appropriate RBC viability and function with the conditions intended to be used to treat the RBCs must be shown. In addition, it is necessary to document that a treatment procedure has a satisfactory toxicologic profile based on wide-scope in-vitro and in-vivo animal model testing.

Formation of O-Type RBCs

The inadequate supply of O-type RBC units that is periodically encountered can hinder blood centers and hospital blood banks in providing RBCs for specific patients. Research over the last 20 years has been evaluating how the more available A and B type of RBCs can be converted to O-type RBCs. The use of enzymes that remove the carbohydrate moieties of the A and B antigens is the mechanism for forming O-type RBCs. The enzymes are removed by washing after completion of the reaction time. Specific enzymes are used to convert A- and B-type RBCs. A clinical study sponsored by the company that is developing the technology (ZymeQuest) has shown that O-type RBCs manufactured from B-type RBCs were effective when transfused to O- and A-type patients in need of RBCs.[31]

RBC Substitutes

Another area of blood research deals with the development of RBC substitutes (referred to in the past as blood substitutes). These formulations include hemoglobin-based oxygen carriers and the perfluorochemicals (PFCs).[32,33] The function of these products is to carry and transfer oxygen in the absence of intact RBCs. In recent years the term "oxygen therapeutics" has been used to more specifically describe the role for RBC substitutes, as they do not substitute for the entire RBC. Advantages and disadvantages of RBC substitutes are presented in (Tables 1–10 and 1–11).

Despite more than 30 years of research for acceptable RBC substitutes, an alternative to a unit of RBCs, even for specific clinical situations, is still not approved for human use. Originally developed to be used in trauma situations such as

TABLE 1-10   Advantages and Disadvantages of Stroma-Free Hemoglobin Solutions

Advantages	Disadvantages
Long shelf life	Short intravascular half-life
Very stable	Possible toxicity
No antigenicity (unless bovine)	Increased O_2 affinity
No requirement for blood-typing procedures	Increased oncotic effect

accidents, combat, and surgery, RBC substitutes have, until now, fallen short of meeting requirements for these applications. This is primarily due to the major complicating side effects, such as the vasoconstrictive effect, manifested as an increase in blood pressure upon infusion. Development of perfluorocarbon formulations has also been hindered by toxicity and manufacturing issues. Although RBC substitutes are still not in routine use today, specific products have been used for individual patients under compassionate use guidelines.

Hemoglobin-Based Oxygen Carriers

The hemoglobin-based oxygen carriers currently in advanced stages of development are the chemically modified hemoglobin formulations. These have replaced the unmodified formulations that were studied initially. There are also recombinant hemoglobin and encapsulated hemoglobin formulations being developed, although these products are in preclinical or early clinical testing, as are new types of modified hemoglobin.

There have been substantial improvements in the quality and purity of the hemoglobin formulations. The presence of stromal elements in earlier unmodified formulations caused a variety of toxicological reactions, based primarily on animal testing. In unmodified hemoglobin, the hemoglobin tetramers dissociated into dimers and monomers and lost their relationship with 2,3-DPG.[34] High oncotic effect is another problem that was associated with unmodified hemoglobins. As a result, significant toxicity characterized by renal dysfunction, systemic vasoconstriction, and gastrointestinal stress has been demonstrated.

Early formulations besides toxicity considerations exhibited a high oxygen affinity. The hemoglobin-oxygen dissociation curve showed a shift to the left, with P_{50} values ranging from 12 to 17 mm Hg.[34] Unmodified hemoglobins also exhibited low circulation times.

TABLE 1-11   Advantages and Disadvantages of Perfluorochemicals

Advantages	Disadvantages
Biologic inertness	Adverse clinical effects
Lack of immunogenicity	High O_2 affinity
Easily synthesized	Retention in tissues
	Requirement for O_2 administration when infused
	Deep-freeze storage temperatures

The products being prepared from RBCs are manufactured by procedures that exclude RBC stromal materials. Current formulations appear to have a half-life circulation time of approximately 24 hours. Cross-linking and/or polymerizing the hemoglobin chains has increased the circulation time by enlarging the molecule.[35] This inhibits hemoglobin breakup into smaller subunits, which are easily filtered by the kidney, and also decreases the kidney osmotic load. Depending on how the chemical modifications are made, oxygen affinity can also be altered. These chemical modifications are made using conventional chemical reactions. Recombinant techniques are also being used to manufacture hemoglobin formulations. The hemoglobin is made using modified human genes expressed in bacterial cells.

Chemically modified human and bovine hemoglobin being developed is summarized in **Table 1–12**. Clinical testing with the various products is being performed in different patient populations. It has been noted that a specific hemoglobin product may initially be approved for a specific clinical use. One product reviewed by the FDA in 2003 was a glutaraldehyde cross-linked bovine hemoglobin (Hemopure, Biopure Corporation).[36] From numerous clinical studies, it has been shown that the use of Hemopure reduces a need for RBC transfusions in surgery patients, especially cardiac patients. A glutaraldehyde cross-linked human hemoglobin product (Polyheme, Northfield Laboratories) is in Phase III clinical trial testing. This product contains an incorporated pyridoxal molecule that replaces 2,3-DPG to maintain satisfactory oxygen transport properties. Polyheme in relatively large amounts (up to 20 units) has been used successfully to treat trauma patients.[37] A third product, an o-raffinose polymerized human hemoglobin, is currently in Phase II/III clinical trial testing. This product has been studied in surgery patients, including coronary artery bypass graft patients. Other products are also in clinical testing. New concepts are being used to manufacture these products. The hemoglobin field received a setback in 1999 when one of the first products to reach Phase III clinical trials, a diaspirin cross-linked human hemoglobin (HemAssist, Baxter Healthcare), was removed from further development.[38] Use of this product for treatment of stroke and traumatic hemorrhage was associated with increased serious adverse effects and mortality compared with control protocols.

Another way to increase circulation time and to minimize osmotic effect is to encapsulate the hemoglobin in an artificial membrane.[39] This approach has not reached advanced clinical testing. Two manufacturing issues need to be considered when using an encapsulation approach; namely, preparing the hemoglobin molecule and preparing the membrane. Encapsulation may create an environment that would maintain the normal relationship between the hemoglobin tetramer and 2,3-DPG. In current products being developed, encapsulation is also being used to include RBC enzymes.

Perfluorochemicals

PFCs are hydrocarbon structures in which all the hydrogen atoms have been replaced with fluorine. They are chemically inert, are excellent gas solvents, and carry O_2 and CO_2 by dissolving them. Most PFCs can dissolve as much as 40 to 70 percent of oxygen per unit by volume, whereas whole blood can dissolve only about 20 percent.[40] The concentration of dissolved O_2 in the PFC solution is directly proportional to the concentration of O_2 in the environment. Because PFCs are immiscible with blood, these chemicals are injected as emulsions with albumin, fats, or other chemicals; otherwise, they may cause pulmonary embolism, asphyxia, and death.[40]

The ability of PFC to transport sufficient amounts of O_2 was first demonstrated when mice survived submersion in an oxygenated PFC. Shortly thereafter, Geyer exchanged the blood of rats with PFCs to a hematocrit of 1 percent without any sign of complication.[40] Reperfusion of the rats was also accomplished successfully. Numerous PFCs have been studied, each with different characteristics as far as emulsification capacity, ability to dissolve O_2, circulation half-life, and tissue half-life. Emulsifying agents also vary. The particle size of the emulsion should be small, 0.1 to 0.2 mm for biocompatibility.[40] Larger particle size emulsions are more rapidly removed from the circulation, increase the viscosity of the solution, and lessen the amount of O_2 dissolved. In addition, PFC emulsions of large size are unstable and may separate, thus causing embolization when transfused. Research has provided the means to develop a stable, small particle, 60 percent emulsion that appeared in studies to be well tolerated. This formulation (Oxygent, Alliance) has been used in a number of advanced clinical studies. In one Phase III clinical trial study with

---

TABLE 1–12   Hemoglobin-Based Oxygen Carriers (RBC Substitutes) Currently in Preclinical or Clinical Trials

Product Name	Chemistry/Source	Manufacturer
Hemopure	Glutaraldehyde-polymerized bovine Hb	Biopure
PolyHeme	Glutaraldehyde-polymerized human Hb with pyridoxal phosphate	Northfield Laboratories, Inc
Hemolink	O-Raffinose-polymerized human Hb	Hemosol, Inc
PHP	Pyridoxylated human Hb conjugated to polyoxyethylene	Curacyte, Inc (Apex BioSciences)
rHb2.0	Recombinant engineered	Baxter Healthcare Corporation
HemoTech	Covalent attachment of reduced glutathione, adenosine and adenosine-51-triphosphate molecules to bovine Hb	HemoBioTech, Inc
OxyVita	Sebacoyl cross-linked tetramers of human or bovine Hb	IPBL Pharmaceutics, Inc
Hemospan	Tetramers of human Hb conjugated with PEG	Sangart, Inc
HemoZyme	Polynitroxylated tetramers of human Hb	SynZyne Technologics, LLC
PolyHb-SOD-CAT	Tetramers of bovine Hb copolymerized with catalase and superoxide dismutase	McGill University

From Reid T, *Transfusion*, 2003, 43, p. 282.

patients undergoing noncardiac surgery, those receiving the perfluorocarbon emulsion needed less transfusions of allogeneic RBCs and autologously predonated RBCs.[33] The advantages and disadvantages of perfluorochemicals are summarized in **Table 1–11**.

Platelet Preservation

Introduction

Platelets are intimately involved in primary hemostasis, which is the interaction of platelets and the vascular endothelium in halting and preventing bleeding following vascular injury. Platelets are cellular fragments derived from the cytoplasm of megakaryocytes present in the bone marrow. They do not contain a nucleus, although the mitochondria contain DNA. Platelets are released and circulate approximately 9 to 12 days as small, disc-shaped cells with an average diameter of 2 to 4 μm. The normal platelet count ranges from 150,000 to 350,000 per μL. Approximately 30 percent of the platelets that have been released from the bone marrow into the circulation are sequestered in the microvasculature or in the spleen as functional reserves.

Platelets have specific roles in the hemostatic process that are critically dependent on an adequate number in the circulation as well as on normal platelet function. The role of platelets in hemostasis includes (1) initial arrest of bleeding by platelet plug formation and (2) stabilization of the hemostatic plug by contributing to the process of fibrin formation and maintenance of vascular integrity.

Platelet plug formation involves the adhesion of platelets to the subendothelium and subsequent aggregation with thrombin being a key effector of these phenomena. Platelets, like other cells, require energy in the form of ATP for cellular movement, active transport of molecules across the membrane, biosynthetic purposes, and maintenance of a hemostatic steady state.

Clinical Use of Platelets

Platelet components are effectively used to treat bleeding associated with thrombocytopenia, a marked decrease in platelet number. They are also transfused prophylactically to increase the circulating platelet count in hematology-oncology thrombocytopenic patients to prevent bleeding secondary to drug and radiation therapy. This is especially common in association with stem cell transplants after chemotherapy. It is interesting to note that a greater number of platelet units are used for prophylactic purposes compared with that used to treat bleeding, especially with hematology-oncology patients. Platelets are also utilized in some instances to treat other disorders in which platelets are qualitatively or quantitatively defective because of genetic reasons. In recent years coagulation factor VIIA has been used as an alternative to platelets when treating patients with congenital qualitative and quantitative disorders, such as Glanzmann thrombasthenia, who have bleeding episodes.[41]

In the 1950s/1960s, platelet transfusions were given as freshly drawn whole blood or platelet-rich plasma. Circulatory overload quickly developed as a major complication of this method of administering platelets. Since the 1970s, platelets are prepared from whole blood as concentrates in which the volume per unit is near 50 mL in constrast to the 250- to 300-mL volume of platelet-rich plasma units. Today platelets are prepared as concentrates from whole blood and increasingly by apheresis. Platelets still remain as the primary means of treating thrombocytopenia, even though therapeutic responsiveness varies according to patient conditions and undefined consequences of platelet storage conditions.

Whole blood–derived platelet concentrates (PC) are prepared from units of whole blood drawn into triple or quad collection bag systems. The anticoagulant-preservative solution used to collect units of whole blood also provide a preservative medium for the platelets. The citrate constituent helps to reduce unnecessary platelet activation. The harvesting of platelets from whole blood can be performed by two methods. In some parts of the world, including North America, the platelet-rich plasma (PRP) method is used. Units of PRP are separated by a slow centrifugation step, after which the PRP is centrifuged again with hard spin conditions to concentrate the platelets.[23] In Europe the buffy coat method is the predominant procedure in use. Units of whole blood are centrifuged with hard spin conditions to concentrate the platelets in the buffy coats. Subsequently, single or pooled buffy coats are centrifuged with slow spin conditions harvesting the platelets in the plasma supernatant.

It should be noted that the unit of blood must be kept at room temperature until the platelets have been prepared, which must be done within 8 hours after collection (within 24 hours in Europe before concentrating platelets in buffy coats), reflecting the need to store platelets at room temperature in view of the deteriorating effect of cold temperatures (see next section).

For PCs prepared in the United States by the PRP method, approximately 50 mL of plasma is retained with the platelets (volume usually between 45 and 65 mL) in order to maintain a pH of at least 6.2 during storage. The storage period is 5 days (expiration is midnight of day 5). Quality control testing guidelines requires that 90 percent of the sampled PCs contain a minimum of 5.5×10^{10} platelets and a pH of ≥ 6.2 at outdate.[23] Regulations require that at least four PCs be tested monthly for pH and platelet count at the time of expiration.[15] If the seal of any PC bag is broken, the platelets need to be transfused within 4 hours when stored at 20° to 24°C.

Whole blood–derived platelets, whether prepared by the PRP or the buffy coat method, are transfused as pools. Currently in most instances, 4 to 6 PCs are pooled in a container for transfusion. Previously, as many as 8 to 10 PCs were transfused as a dose. The lower number of PCs currently in use reflect, in part, the more efficient harvesting of platelets from whole blood.[42] Traditionally, in the United States pools are prepared at hospitals because they need to be transfused within 4 hours.[23] One reason for the limited storage period has been the concern for bacterial growth because storage is at room temperature (see section on bacterial growth issue). In Europe and others areas, PC pools, prepared with sterile docking, are being stored for up to 5 days.[43]

With plateletpheresis, platelets are harvested by drawing blood from a donor into an apheresis instrument (cell separator), which separates the blood into components using centrifugation; retaining the platelets; and returning the remainder of the blood to the donor. After repeated cycles the platelets are concentrated in storage containers. Apheresis components contain at least four to six times as many platelets as a unit of platelets obtained from whole blood. This translates into a product with 3.0 to 4.0×10^{11} platelets, which provides one transfusion dose. AABB Standards now require that 90 percent of the tested units have a minimum of 3.0×10^{11} platelets.[23] Similar to whole blood–derived platelets, a pH of at least 6.2 during storage (measured at time of issue or outdate) is required for apheresis components.

Frequently, the separation procedure is carried out in a way that allows collection (from appropriate donors) of sufficient platelets to prepare two unique separate products. The minimum number of collected platelets should be approximately 6.5×10^{11} if two apheresis components are to be prepared. The ability to prepare two apheresis components reflects, in part, the ability to harvest platelets more efficiently with the current generation of apheresis instruments. Each product needs to have at least 3.0×10^{11} platelets.[23]

The current generation of apheresis instruments also allows for the preparation of pre-storage leukocyte-reduced platelets (total leukocytes $<5.0 \times 10^6$) through specific processing without use of a leukocyte-reduction filter (Spectra, Trima, Gambro; Amicus, Baxter Healthcare) or by use of a leukocyte-reduction filter (MCS+, Haemonetics). Whole blood platelets can also be prepared to be pre-storage leukocyte-reduced. One system in routine use removes the leukocytes on expression of platelet-rich plasma from the separated RBCs through a leukocyte-reduction filter (PL filter, Pall). Under development are filters that remove leukocytes from RBCs, platelets, and plasma simultaneously during whole blood passage (see Chapter 11).

Current Conditions for Platelet Preservation (Platelet Storage)

Platelet concentrates prepared from whole blood and apheresis components are routinely stored at 20° to 24°C, with continuous agitation for up to 5 days on being prepared using a system classified as being closed, bags, and/or cell separator with apheresis collections. FDA standards define the expiration time as midnight of day 5. Although the principles for platelet preservation/storage have been developed primarily using whole blood–derived platelets, they also apply to apheresis platelets. Primarily flat-bed and circular agitators are in use. There are a number of containers in use for 5-day storage of whole blood–derived and apheresis platelets. In the United States, platelets are being stored in a 100 percent plasma medium. Although platelets can be stored at 1° to 6°C for 48 hours,[44] it does not appear that this is a routine practice.

History of Platelet Storage; Rationale for Current Conditions

The conditions utilized to store platelets have evolved since the 1960s as key parameters that influence the retention of platelet properties have been identified. Initially, platelets were stored in the cold at 1° to 6°C, based on the successful storage of RBCs, as whole blood or separated RBC components at this temperature range. A key study report in 1969 by Murphy and Gardner showed that cold storage at 1° to 6°C resulted in a marked reduction in platelet in-vivo viability, manifested as a reduction in in-vivo life span, after only 18 hours of storage.[45] This study also identified for the first time that 20° to 24°C (room temperature)should be the preferred range, based on viability results. The reduction in viability at 1° to 6°C was associated with conversion of the normal discoid shape to a form that is irreversibly spherical. This structural

change is considered to be the factor responsible for the deleterious effects of cold storage. When stored even for several hours at 4°C, platelets do not return to their disc shape upon rewarming. This loss of shape is probably a result of microtubule disassembly.

Based on many follow-up studies, platelets are still stored at room temperature. These studies provided an understanding of the factors that influenced the retention of platelet viability and the parameters that needed to be considered to optimize storage conditions.

One factor identified as necessary was the need to agitate platelet components during storage, although initially the rationale for agitation was not understood.[46, 47] Subsequently, agitation has been shown to facilitate oxygen transfer into the platelet bag and oxygen consumption by the platelets. The positive role for oxygen has been associated with the maintenance of platelet component pH.[48] Maintaining pH was determined to be a key parameter for retaining platelet viability in vivo when platelets were stored at 20° to 24°C. Although storage itself was associated with a small reduction in postinfusion platelet viability, an enhanced loss was observed when the pH was reduced from initial levels of near 7.0 to 6.5–6.8 with a marked loss when the pH was reduced to levels below 6.0.[47] A pH of 6.0 was initially the standard for maintaining satisfactory viability. The standard was subsequently changed to 6.2 with the availability of additional data. As pH is reduced from 6.8 to 6.2/6.0, the platelets progressively changed shape from discs to spheres. Much of this change was irreversible.

When whole blood–derived platelets were intially stored in the 1970s as concentrates, a major problem was a marked reduction in pH in many concentrates. This limited the storage period to 3 days. The reduction in pH, in the presence of agitation, was shown to be due to a decrease in plasma oxygen levels that was associated with the channeling of platelet metabolism from the aerobic respiratory pathway to the anaerobic glycolytic pathway. With glycolysis, glucose is converted to lactic acid, which depletes the plasma bicarbonate and hence the plasma constituent that allows for the maintenance of pH.[48] The reduction in pH was associated with platelet concentration/content. With total platelet content of approximately $5-8 \times 10^{10}$, pH levels were maintained at satisfactory levels during 3 days of storage. With content above approximately 8×10^{10}, pH levels were in most cases between 5.7–6.2 by 3 days of storage.[47] The containers being used for storage were identified as being responsible for the fall in pH because of their limiting gas transfer properties for oxygen and also for carbon dioxide. Carbon dioxide buildup from aerobic respiration and as the end product of plasma bicarbonate depletion also influenced the fall in pH. The gas transport properties of a container is known to reflect the container material, the gas permeability of the wall of the plastic container, the surface area of the container available for gas exchange, and the thickness of the container. Insufficient agitation may also have been a factor responsible for pH reduction because agitation facilitates gas transport into the containers.

Storage in Second Generation Containers

Gaining an understanding of the factors that led to the reduction in pH in first generation platelet containers resulted in the development of "second generation containers" starting around 1982. The second-generation containers, with increased gas transport properties (allowing increased oxygen transport and also carbon dioxide escape), are available and are being utilized for 5 days of storage of platelets without resulting in a substantial fall in pH (e.g., Baxter Healthcare, PL 732, PL 2410; Pall CLX; Terumo XT612). Such containers are in use for whole blood–derived PCs and apheresis components. Containers for platelet storage were originally constructed from polyvinyl chloride (PVC) plastic containing a phthalate plasticizer. The second generation containers are constructed in some cases with PVC and in other cases with polyolefin plastic. For most PVC containers, alternative plasticizers (trimellitate and citrate-based) have been used to increase gas transport. The nominal volumes of the containers are 300 to 400 mL and 1 to 1.5 L for whole blood–derived platelet concentrates and apheresis components, respectively. The size of the containers for apheresis components reflects the increased number of platelets that are being stored and, hence, the need for a larger surface area to provide adequate gas transport properties for maintaining pH levels near the initial level of 7.0 even after 5 days of storage. The higher oxygen tension reduces the glycolytic rate by accelerating oxidative metabolism (aerobic respiration), with better carbon dioxide efflux having a secondary influence. **Box 1–2** lists factors that should be considered when using 5-day platelet storage containers.

Storing Platelets Without Agitation for Limited Times

Although platelet components should be stored with continuous agitation, there are data that suggest that platelet properties, based on in-vitro studies, are retained when agitation is discontinued for at least 24 hours during a 5-day storage period.[49,50] This is probably related to the retention of satisfactory oxygen levels with the second generation containers when agitation is discontinued, as occurs by necessity when platelets are shipped over long distances by, for example, overnight courier.

Measurement of Viability and Functional Properties of Stored Platelets

Viability indicates the capacity of platelets to circulate after infusion without premature removal or destruction. Platelets have a lifespan of 8 to 10 days after release from megakaryocytes. Storage causes a reduction in this parameter, even when pH is maintained. Platelet viability of stored platelets is determined by measuring pretransfusion and posttransfusion platelet counts (1 hour and/or 24 hours) and expressing the difference based on the number of platelets transfused (corrected count increment) or by determining the disappearance rate of infused radiolabeled platelets to normal individuals whose donation provided the platelets. The observation of the swirling phenomenon caused by discoid platelets, when platelet suspensions, without sampling, are placed in front of a light source, has been used to obtain a qualitative evaluation of the retention of platelet viability properties in stored units.[51] The extent of shape change and the hypotonic shock response in in-vitro tests appear to provide some indication about the retention of platelet viability properties.[52]

Function is defined as the ability of viable platelets to respond to vascular damage in promoting hemostasis. Clinical assessment of hemostasis is being increasingly used. The template bleeding time test also has been used to assess the functional integrity of transfused platelets, but in recent years there have been questions about the specificity of this procedure.

The maintenance of pH during storage at 20° to 24°C has been associated with the retention of posttransfusion platelet viability and has been the key issue that has been addressed to improve conditions for storage at 20° to 24°C. There is also the issue of retaining platelet function during storage. Historically, room temperature storage has been thought to be associated with a reduction in platelet functional properties. However, the vast transfusion experience with room temperature platelets worldwide indicates that such platelets have satisfactory function. As has been suggested many times over the last 30 years, it is possible that room temperature–stored platelets undergo a rejuvenation of the processes that provide for satisfactory function upon in-vivo circulation.[53,54] The better functionality of cold-stored platelets, based on some studies, especially ones conducted in the 1970s, may have reflected an undesirable activation of platelet processes as a result of the temperature range of 1° to 6°C. Activation is a prerequisite for platelet function in hemostasis. During storage, it takes different forms. Even with storage at 20° to 24°C, there is some activation as judged by the release of granular proteins such as p-selectin (CD62) and platelet factor 4 and granular adenine nucleotides. There are some data that suggest that specific inhibitors of the activation processes may have a beneficial influence during storage.[55]

Platelet Storage and Bacterial Contamination

The major concern associated with storage of platelets at 20° to 24°C is the potential for bacterial growth, if the prepared platelets contain bacteria because of unremoved contamination at the phlebotomy site or the donor has an unrecognized bacterial infection.[56] Room temperature storage and the presence of oxygen provide a good environment for bacterial proliferation. Many studies have shown that approximately 1 to 3 of every 1000 prepared platelet units contain bacteria. Although the level of patient sepsis is much lower, particularly troublesome is the fact that some septic episodes have led to patient deaths.

Although there has been concern about bacterial proliferation for many years, until recently options to test for bacteria or inactivate bacteria, as part of a pathogen reduction procedure, have not been available. In the mid-1980s, the

BOX 1–2
Factors to be Considered when Using 5-Day Plastic Storage Bags

- Temperature control of 20°–24°C is critical during platelet preparation and storage.
- Careful handling of plastic bags during expression of platelet-poor plasma helps prevent the platelet button from being distributed and prevents removal of excess platelets with the platelet-poor plasma.
- Residual plasma volumes recommended for the storage of platelet concentrates from whole blood (45–65 mL).
- For apheresis platelets, the surface area of the storage bags needs to allow for the number of platelets that will be stored.

storage of platelets for 7 days was approved using containers developed for 5 days of storage. However, new evidence about the occurrence of transfusion-associated sepsis led to a reduction in the storage time a few years later (1986).

The major emphasis has been to develop systems that can be used to detect bacteria. Two systems that involve the culturing of platelet samples for approximately 24 to 30 hours have been documented to provide good sensitivity and specificity. As the level of bacteria at the time of platelet collection/preparation can be low, samples for determining the presence of bacteria are not obtained until approximately 24 hours of storage. One culturing system measures bacteria by detecting a change in carbon dioxide levels associated with bacterial growth (bioMerieux Corporation).[57] This system provides continuous monitoring of the platelet sample-containing culture bottles, one bottle being aerobic and one being anaerobic. The second system that provides results at one time point after the initiation of culturing documents the presence of bacteria by detecting a reduction in the oxygen level below a specific level in the culture air space (Pall Corporation).[58] These methods have been utilized in Europe and are starting to be employed in the United States. They can be used by blood centers that provide platelet components for transfusion purposes. There are also less sensitive methods that need to be used prior to transfusion. One method is gram staining. Another procedure involves the use of clinical chemistry dipsticks that measure pH and glucose levels, as substantial bacterial growth can be associated with low pH and glucose levels.[59]

The risk for bacterial contamination is also being reduced by collecting the first aliquot of collected blood for testing samples (sample first procedures). This should minimize the placement of contaminated skin plugs into the platelet products.

In view of the ability to test for bacterial contamination and sterile docking instruments, there is now interest in being able to store pools of platelets up to the outdate of the individual concentrates. The retention of platelet properties during storage of pools has been shown in a number of studies.

Current Trends in Platelet Preservation Research

Research and development in platelet preservation is being pursued in many directions, including the following:

1. New documentation that platelets can be stored for 7 days with the assumption that testing for bacteria would be an associated procedure
2. Development of additive solutions, also termed synthetic media
3. Development of procedures to reduce the level of pathogens that may be in platelet units
4. Development of platelet substitutes
5. New approaches for storage of platelets at 1° to 6°C
6. The development of processes to cryopreserve platelets

Storage for 7 Days at 20° to 24°C

With the use of procedures to detect bacteria, there is an interest in being able to store platelets for 7 days.[60] Although platelets were stored for 7 days at 20° to 24°C in the mid-

1980s for a few years, further data are needed to document the retention of platelet properties as new containers and new/modified methods for apheresis platelet collection are being used. One recent study showed that apheresis platelets stored for 7 days exhibited a reduction of 10 percent to 15 percent in in-vivo recovery and survival time relative to that observed with platelets stored for 5 days.[61]

Storage with Additive Solutions

Currently in Europe, additive (synthetic) solutions are being used to replace a large portion of the plasma in platelet suspensions prepared from whole blood by the buffy coat method. Residual plasma is about 20 percent to 35 percent.[62] One advantage is that this approach provides more plasma for fractionation. In addition, there are data indicating that optimal additive solutions may improve the quality of platelets during storage. Box 1–3 lists the main advantages of using a platelet additive solution for platelet storage. Research is being conducted to improve the additive solutions in use. Gulliksson recently suggested that platelets could be stored for at least 18 to 20 days at 20° to 24°C with an optimized additive medium based on considerations that indicate that storage could well inhibit platelet aging with the appropriate environments/medium.[63] Platelet additive solutions in use/being developed contain varying quantities of glucose, citrate, phosphate, potassium, magnesium, and acetate. Acetate is a primary constituent as it serves as a substrate for aerobic respiration (mitochondrial metabolism) while also providing a way to maintain pH levels as it reacts with hydrogen ions when it is first utilized.

Procedures to Reduce/Inactivate Pathogens

As for RBCs, procedures are being developed to treat platelet components to reduce/inactivate any residual pathogens (bacteria, viruses, parasites) that may be present. The procedures are using photochemical approaches that target nucleic acids. The targeting of nucleic acids is possible because platelets, like RBCs, do not contain functional nucleic acids. Two primary methods are used in testing. Both inactivate a wide array of pathogens while not causing significant toxicology based on in-vitro and animal testing. One method, currently approved for use in Europe and in Phase III testing in the United States, uses a psoralen termed amotosalen (also referred to as S-59) and ultraviolet light (UVA) (Cerus, Baxter).[64,65] For the pathogen reduction procedure, platelets are suspended in an additive solution that lowers the plasma to near 35 percent to facilitate the transmission of UVA. The UVA induces the psoralen to modify the nucleic acid of the pathogens so that replication is not possible. A special instrument for the treatment with UVA has been developed. After

---

BOX 1–3
Advantages of Using Platelet Additive Solutions

- Reduces plasma-associated transfusion side effects.
- Improves platelet storage conditions.
- Saves plasma for other purposes (e.g., transfusion or fractionation).
- Increases the efficiency of procedures for the decontamination of viruses and bacteria.

completion of the reaction period, residual, unreacted psoralen and psoralen breakdown products in the treatment medium are removed with an absorbing material. With pools of buffy coat–derived platelets, clinical hemostasis, hemorrhagic adverse events, and overall adverse events were comparable with those of patients receiving treated and control platelets.[64] Hemostatic effectiveness was also shown with S-59–treated apheresis platelets.[65] One negative feature is a reduction in the corrected count increments with treated platelets when compared with the use of untreated apheresis platelets. As a result, some thrombocytopenic recipients required more platelet transfusions.

A second method, involving riboflavin and light, is being used to treat apheresis platelets that are prepared with 20 percent plasma to facilitate light transmission (Navigant).[66]

Development of Platelet Substitutes

In view of the short shelf-life of liquid-stored platelet products, there has been a long-standing interest to develop platelet substitute products that maintain hemostatic function. It is understood that platelet substitutes may only have use in specific clinical situations because platelets have a complex biochemistry and physiology. Besides having a long shelf-life, platelet substitutes appear to have reduced potential to transmit pathogens as a result of the processing procedures. A number of different approaches have been utilized.[67] Apparently, one approach with the potential for providing clinically useful products is the use of lyophilization. Two products prepared from human platelets are apparently in preclinical testing. One preparation uses washed platelets treated with paraformaldehyde, with subsequent freezing in 5 percent albumin and lyophilization.[68] These platelets on rehydration have been reported to have hemostatic effectiveness in different animal models. A second method involves the freeze-drying of trehalose-loaded platelets.[69] Additional products that are apparently being developed include fibrinogen-coated albumin microcapsules/microspheres and modified RBCs with procoagulant properties as a result of fibrinogen binding. Fibrinogen is being used because in vivo this protein cross-links activated platelets to form platelet aggregates as part of the hemostatic process. Two other approaches include the development of platelet-derived microparticles that can stop bleeding and liposome-based hemostatic products.[67]

New Approaches for Storage of Platelets at 1° to 6°C

Although storage of platelets at 1° to 6°C was discontinued many years ago, there has been an interest to develop ways to overcome the storage lesion caused by 1° to 6°C.[70] The rationale for the continuing effort reflects concerns about storing and shipping platelets at 20° to 24°C, especially the chance for bacterial proliferation. Many approaches have been attempted without success, although early results showed some promise. The approaches primarily involve adding substances to inhibit cold-induced platelet activation, as this is thought to be the key storage lesion. Recently, two reports concluded that platelets stored at 1° to 6°C could conceivably have satisfactory in-vivo viability and function if the surface of the platelets were modified to prevent the enhanced clearance (unsatisfactory viability) from circulation.[71,72] Based on animal studies, it was suggested that cold-induced spherical

platelets can remain in the circulation if abnormal clearance is prevented. Spherical platelets, manifested as a result of cold storage, have been assumed to be a trigger for low viability. The specific approach involves the enzymatic galactosylation of cold-stored platelets to modify specifically one type of membrane protein. The addition of uridine diphosphate-galactose is the vehicle for the modificaiton.[72]

Frozen Platelets

There has been limited use of procedures that freeze platelets for clinical use (5 percent to 6 percent dimethyl sulfoxide and −80°C mechanical freezers). One clinical use has been the freezing of autologous platelets for subsequent utilization. Research on modified/easier-to-use procedures is being pursued, including an approach to reduce the DMSO concentration to 2 percent with the addition of a series of inhibitors of platelet activation.[73]

SUMMARY CHART:
Important Points to Remember (MT/MLT)

➤ Each unit of whole blood collected contains approximately 450 mL of blood and 63 mL of anticoagulant-preservative solution or approximately 500 mL of blood and 70 mL of anticoagulant-preservative solution.

➤ A donor can give blood every 8 weeks.

➤ Samples from donors of each unit of donated blood/apheresis are tested by nine screening tests for infectious diseases markers, as of 2003.

➤ Glycolysis generates approximately 90% of the ATP needed by RBCs, and 10% is provided by the pentose phosphate pathway.

➤ RBCs contain 92%–95% HbA, 2%–3% HbA_2, and 1%–2% HbF, and 75% posttransfusion survival of RBCs is necessary for a successful transfusion.

➤ ACD, CPD, and CP2D are approved preservative solutions for storage of RBCs at 1°–6°C for 21 days, and CPDA1 is approved for 35 days.

➤ Additive solutions (Adsol, Nutricel, Optisol) are approved in the United States for RBC storage for 42 days. Additive-solution RBCs have been shown to be appropriate for neonates and pediatric patients.

➤ RBCs have been traditionally glycerolized and frozen within 6 days of whole blood collection in CPD or CPD-A1 and can be stored for 10 years from the date of freezing. Now there is also freezing of 42-day additive-solution RBCs without rejuvenation. It has been necessary to transfuse thawed RBCs within 24 hours. With the recently developed ACP 215 closed system processing system for glycerolization and deglycerolization, the maximum post-thaw storage period at 1°–6°C is being/will be extended to 15 days.

➤ Rejuvesol is the only FDA-approved rejuvenation solution used in some blood centers to regenerate ATP and 2,3-DPG levels before RBC freezing. Rejuvenation is used primarily to salvage O-type and rare RBC units that are at outdate or with specific anticoagulant-preservative solution up to 3 days past outdate

➤ RBC substitutes being developed include hemoglobin-based oxygen carriers and PFCs.

➤ Hemoglobin-based oxygen carriers in advanced clinical testing are chemically modified hemoglobin solutions. One product is a polymerized bovine hemoglobin product, and other products are prepared from modified human hemoglobin.

➤ Research is being conducted to improve on the current additive solutions.

➤ Research is being conducted to develop procedures to reduce/inactivate any residual pathogens.

➤ PCs can be prepared from whole blood by centrifugation by the PRP method (United States) or by the buffy coat method. These platelet concentrates can be prepared to be pre-storage leukoreduced by filtration.

➤ A PC should contain a minimum of 5.5×10^{10} platelets (in 90% of the sampled units according to AABB Standards) in a volume routinely between 45 and 65 mL that is sufficient to maintain a pH of 6.2 or greater at the conclusion of the 5-day storage period.

➤ When PCs (usually 4–6) are pooled as a transfusible product/dose, the storage time changes to 4 hours. There is the thought that pools could be stored up to the time of outdating in conjunction with testing for bacterial contamination and the use of sterile docking to prepare the pools.

➤ Platelets are increasingly being prepared by apheresis using cell separators that can produce leukocyte-reduced products during the separation process or by subsequent filtration (depending on the cell separator).

➤ Apheresis components contain 4–6 times as many platelets as a PC prepared from whole blood. They should contain a minimum of 3.0×10^{11} platelets (in 90% of the sampled units).

➤ When appropriate and possible, apheresis procedures are harvesting from healthy donors enough platelets to prepare two unique products by division by weight (splitting), each with a minimum of 3.0×10^{11} platelets.

➤ Platelet components are stored for up to 5 days at 20°–24°C with continuous agitation. When necessary, as during shipping, platelets can be stored without continuous agitation for up to 24 hours (at 20°–24°C) during a 5-day storage period. Platelets are rarely stored at 1°–6°C.

➤ If a platelet bag is broken or opened, the platelets must be transfused within 4 hours when stored at 20°–24°C.

➤ Research is being conducted in many areas relating to the preparation and storage of platelets. These include documentation that platelets can be stored for up to 7 days at 20°–24°C with current technologies, development of procedures to reduce/inactivate any residual pathogens, development of additive (synthetic) solutions, and the development of platelet substitute products.

Review Questions

1. The loss of ATP leads to:
   a. An increase in phosphorylation of spectrin and a loss of membrane deformability
   b. An increase in phosphorylation of spectrin and an increase of membrane deformability
   c. A decrease in phosphorylation of spectrin and a loss of membrane deformability
   d. A decrease in phosphorylation of spectrin and an increase of membrane deformability

2. The majority of normal adult hemoglobin consists of:
   a. Two α chains and two β chains
   b. Two α chains and two δ chains
   c. Two α chains and two γ chains
   d. Four α chains

3. When RBCs are stored, there is a "shift to the left." This means:
   a. Hemoglobin oxygen affinity increases owing to an increase in 2,3-DPG
   b. Hemoglobin oxygen affinity increases owing to a decrease in 2,3-DPG
   c. Hemoglobin oxygen affinity decreases owing to a decrease in 2,3-DPG
   d. Hemoglobin oxygen affinity decreases owing to an increase in 2,3-DPG

4. Which of the following is (are) the role(s) of platelets?
   a. Maintain vascular integrity
   b. Initial arrest of bleeding
   c. Stabilizing the hemostatic plug
   d. All of the above

5. Which of the following anticoagulant-preservatives provide a storage time of 21 days at 1°–6°C for units of whole blood and prepared RBCs if an additive solution is not added?
   a. ACD
   b. CP2D
   c. CPD
   d. All of the above

6. What are the current storage time and storage temperature for platelet concentrates and apheresis platelet components?
   a. 5 days at 1°–6°C
   b. 5 days at 24°–27°C
   c. 5 days at 20°–24°C
   d. 7 days at 22°–24°C

7. What is the minimum number of platelets required in a PC prepared from whole blood by centrifugation (90% of sampled units)?
   a. 5.5×10^{11}
   b. 3.0×10^{10}
   c. 3.0×10^{11}
   d. 5.5×10^{10}

8. All but one of these factors will influence platelet metabolism and viability in a closed container system?
   a. Total platelet count
   b. Duration of storage
   c. Temperature of storage
   d. Fibrinogen concentration

9. What is the minimum number of platelets required in an apheresis component (90% of the sampled units)?
   a. 3×10^{11}
   b. 4×10^{11}
   c. 2×10^{11}
   d. 3.5×10^{11}

10. Whole blood and RBC units are stored at what temperature?
    a. 1°–6°C
    b. 20°–24°C
    c. 37°C
    d. 24°–27°C

11. Additive solutions are approved for blood storage for how many days?
    a. 21
    b. 42
    c. 35
    d. 7

12. Whole blood/RBCs can be stored in CPDA-1 at 1°–6°C for how many days?
    a. 21
    b. 42
    c. 35
    d. 7

13. What is the lowest allowable pH for a platelet component at outdate?
    a. 6.0
    b. 5.9
    c. 6.8
    d. 6.2

14. Frozen/thawed RBCs processed in an open system can be stored for how many days/hours?
    a. 3 days
    b. 6 hours
    c. 24 hours
    d. 15 days

15. What is the hemoglobin source for hemoglobin-based RBC substitutes in advanced clinical testing?
    a. Only bovine hemoglobin
    b. Only human hemoglobin
    c. Both bovine and human hemoglobins
    d. None of the above

REFERENCES

1. Parks, D: Charles Richard Drew, MD 1904–1950. J Natl Med Assoc 71:893–895, 1979.
2. Kendrick, DB: Blood Program in World War II, Historical Note. Washington Office of Surgeon General, Department of Army, Washington, DC, 1964, pp 1–23.
3. http://www.aabb.org, Facts about blood and blood banking, 2003.
4. Dodd, RY, Notari EP, and Stramer SL: Current prevalence and incidence of infectious disease markers and estimated window-period risk in the American Red Cross blood donor population. Transfusion 42:975–979, 2002.
5. Harmening, DM: Clinical Hematology and Fundamentals of Hemostasis, ed 3. FA Davis, Philadelphia, 1997, p 55.
6. Mohandas, N, and Chasis, JA: Red blood cell deformability, membrane material properties and shape: Regulation of transmission, skeletal and cytosolic proteins and lipids. Semin Hematol 30:171–192, 1993.
7. Mohandas, N, and Evans, E: Mechanical properties of the genetic defects. Ann Rev Biophys Biomol Struct 23:787–818, 1994.
8. Bunn, HF: Hemoglobin structure, function and assembly. In Embury, SH, Hebbel, RP, Mohandas, N, and Steinberg, MH (eds): Sickle Cell Disease: Basic Principles and Clinical Practice. Raven Press, New York, 1994.
9. Benesch, R, and Benesch, RE: The effect of organic phosphates from the human erythrocyte on the allosteric properties of hemoglobin. Biochem Biophys Res Commun 26:162, 1967.
10. Chanutin, A, and Curnish, RF: Effect of organic and inorganic phosphates on the oxygen equilibrium of human erythrocytes. Arch Biochem Biophys 121:96, 1967.
11. Beutler, E: Red cell metabolism and storage. In Anderson, KC, and Ness, PM (eds): Scientific Basis of Transfusion Medicine. WB Saunders, Philadelphia, 1994, pp 188–202.
12. Beutler, E: Preservation of liquid red cells. In Rossi, EC, et al (eds): Principles of Transfusion Medicine, ed 2. Williams & Wilkins, Baltimore, 1996, pp 51–60.
13. Petz, LD, and Swisher, SN: Clinical Practice of Transfusion Medicine, ed 3. Churchill Livingstone, New York, 1996.
14. Valeri, CR: Preservation of frozen red blood cells. In Simon, TL, Dzik WH, Snyder EL, Stowell CP, and Strauss RG (eds): Rossi's Principles of Transfusion Medicine, ed 3. Williams & Wilkins, Baltimore, 2002, pp 62–68.
15. Code of Federal Regulations, Section 21–Blood Products 600–680. US Government Printing Office, Washington, DC: 2002.
16. Sowade, O, et al: Evaluation of oxygen availability with oxygen status algorithm in patients undergoing open heart surgery treated with epoetin beta. J Lab Clin Med 129:97–105, 1997.
17. Gramm, J, et al: Effect of transfusion on oxygen transport in critically ill patients. Shock 5:190–193, 1996.
18. Yu, M: Invasive and noninvasive oxygen consumption and hemodynamic monitoring in elderly surgical patients. New Horiz 4:443–452, 1996.
19. Wood, L, and Beutler, E: Storage of erythrocytes in artificial media. Transfusion 11:122–133, 1971.
20. Lovric, VA: Modified packed red cells and the development of the circle pack. Vox Sang 51:1986.
21. Högman, CF: Additive system approach in blood transfusion birth of the SAG and Sagman systems. Vox Sang 51:1986.
22. Högman, CF: Recent advances in the preparation and storage of red cells. Vox Sang 67:243–246, 1994.
23. Technical Manual, ed 14. American Association of Blood Banks, Bethesda, MD, 2002, Chapter 8: Preparation, storage and distribution of components from whole blood donations.
24. Yasutake, M, and Takahashi, TA: Current advances of blood preservation—Development and clinical application of additive solutions for preservation of red blood cells and platelets. Nippon Rinsho 55:2429–2433, 1997.
25. Jain, R, and Jarosz, C: Safety and efficacy as AS-1 red blood cell use in neonates. Transfus Apheresis Sci 24:111–115, 2001.
26. Valeri, CR, et al: A multicenter study of in-vitro and in-vivo values in human RBCs frozen with 40-percent (wt/vol) glycerol and stored after deglycerolization for 15 days at 4°C in AS-3: assessment of RBC processing in the ACP 215. Transfusion 41:933–939, 2001.
27. Valeri, CR: Use of rejuvenation solutions in blood preservation. CRC Crit Rev Clin Lab Sci 17:299–374, 1982.
28. Szymanski, IO, et al: Effect of rejuvenation and frozen storage on 42-day-old AS-1 RBCs. Transfusion 41:550–555, 2001.
29. Hess, JR, et al: Twelve-week RBC storage. Transfusion 43:867–872, 2003.
30. Högman, CF, et al: Improved maintenance of 2,3-DPG and ATP in RBCs stored in a modified additive solution. Transfusion 42:824–829, 2002.
31. Kruskall, MS, et al: Transfusion to blood group A and O patients of group B RBCs that have been enzymatically converted to group O. Transfusion 40:1290–1298, 2000.
32. Reid, TJ: Hb-based oxygen carriers: Are we there yet? Transfusion 43:280–287, 2003.
33. Spahn, DR: Artificial oxygen carriers: Status 2002. Vox Sang 83:(Suppl 1):281–285, 2002.
34. Gould, SA, Lakshman, RS, and Moss, GS: Hemoglobin solutions as an acellular oxygen carrier. In Rossi, EC, et al (eds): Principles of Transfusion Medicine, ed 2. Williams & Wilkins, Baltimore, 1996, pp 51–60.
35. Vandegriff, KD, Malavalli, A, Wooldridge, J, Lohman, J, and Winslow, RM: MP4, a new nonvasoactive PEG-Hb conjugate. Transfusion 43:509–516, 2003.
36. Sprung, J, et al: The use of bovine hemoglobin glutamer-250 (Hemopure) in surgical patients: Results of a multicenter, randomized, single-blinded study. Anesth Analg 94:799–808, 2002.
37. Gould, SA, et al: The life-sustaining capacity of human polymerized hemoglobin as a blood substitute in massive blood loss when blood may be unavailable. J Am Coll Surg 195:445–452, 2002.
38. Winslow, RM: αα Crosslinked hemoglobins: Was failure predicted by preclinical testing? Vox 79:1–20, 2000.

39. Chang, TMS: Future generations of red blood cell substitutes. J Intern Med 253:527–537, 203.

40. Spence, RK: Perfluorocarbons. In Rossi, EC, et al (eds): Principles of Transfusion Medicine, ed 2. Williams & Wilkins, Baltimore, 1996, pp 189–196.

41. Poon, M-C: Recombinant Factor VIIa is effective for bleeding and surgery in patients with Glanzmann Thrombastenia. Blood 94:3951–3953, 1999.

42. Kelly, DL, et al: High-yield platelet concentrates attainable by continuous quality improvement reduce platelet transfusion cost and donor expense. Transfusion 37:482–486, 1997.

43. Van der Meer, PF, Pietersz, R, and Reesink, H: Leukoreduced platelet concentrates in additive solution: An evaluation of filters and storage containers. Vox Sang 81:102–107, 2001.

44. Code of Federal Regulations, Section 21, Subpart C–Platelets. US Government Printing Office, Washington, DC: 2002.

45. Murphy, S, and Gardner, FH: Platelet preservation: Effect of storage temperature on maintenance of platelet viability—deleterious effect of refrigerated storage. N Engl J Med 280:1094–1098, 1969.

46. Slichter, SJ, and Harker, LA: Preparation and storage of platelet concentrates II: Storage variables influencing platelet viability and function. Br J Haematol 34:403–412, 1976.

47. Murphy, S: Platelet storage for transfusion. Semin Hematol 22:165–177, 1985.

48. Murphy, S, and Gardner, FH: Platelet storage at 22°C: Role of gas transport across plastic containers in maintenance of viability. Blood 46:209–218, 1975.

49. Moroff, G, and George, VM: The maintenance of platelet properties upon limited discontinuation of agitation during storage. Transfusion 30:427–430, 1990.

50. Hunter, S, Nixon, J, and Murphy, S: The effect of interruption of agitation on platelet quality during storage for transfusion. Transfusion 41:809–814, 2001.

51. Bertolini, F, and Murphy, S: A multicenter inspection of the swirling phenomenon in platelet concentrates prepared in routine practice. Transfusion 36:128–132, 1996.

52. Holme, S, Moroff, G, and Murphy, S: A multi-laboratory evaluation of in vitro platelet assays: The tests for extent of shape change and response to hypotonic shock. Transfusion 38:31–40, 1998.

53. Filip, DJ, and Aster, RH: Relative hemostatic effectiveness of human platelets stored at 4°C and 22°C. J Lab Clin Med 91:618–624, 1978.

54. Owens M, et al: Post-transfusion recovery of function of 5-day stored platelet concentrates. Br J Haematol 80:539–544, 1992.

55. Holme, S, et al: Improved maintenance of platelet in vivo viability during storage when using a synthetic medium with inhibitors. J Lab Clin Med 119:144–150, 1992.

56. Brecher, ME, and Hay, SN: The role of bacterial testing of cellular blood products in light of new pathogen inactivation technologies. Blood Therapics Med 3:49–55, 2003.

57. Macauley, A, et al: Operational feasibility of routine bacterial monitoring of platelets. Transfusion Med 13:189–195, 2003.

58. Ortolano, GA, et al: Detection of bacteria in WBC-reduced PLT concentrates using percent oxygen as a marker for bacteria growth. Transfusion 43:1276–1284, 2003.

59. Wagner, SJ, and Robinette, D: Evaluation of swirling, pH and glucose tests for the detection of bacterial contamination in platelet concentrates. Transfusion 36:989–993, 1996.

60. Cardigan, R, and Williamson, LM: The quality of platelets after storage for 7 days. Transfusion Med 13:173–187, 2003.

61. Dumont, LJ, et al: Seven-day storage of single-donor platelets: Recovery and survival in an autologous transfusion study. Transfusion 42:847–854, 2002.

62. De Wildt-Eggen, J, and Gulliksson, H: In vivo and in vitro comparison of platelets stored in either synthetic media or plasma. Vox Sang 84:256–264, 2003.

63. Gulliksson, H: Defining the optimal storage conditions for the long-term storage of platelets. Transfusion Med Rev17:209–215, 2003.

64. Van Rhenen, D, et al: Transfusion of pooled buffy coat platelet components prepared with photochemical pathogen inactivation treatment: The euroSPRITE trial. Blood 101:2426–2433, 2003.

65. McCullough, J, et al: Pathogen inactivated platelets using Helinx™ technology are hemostatically effective in thrombocytopenic patients: The SPRINT trial. Blood 98:450a (abstract), 2001.

66. Corbin, F: Pathogen inactivation of blood components: Current status and introduction of an approach using riboflavin as a photosensitizer. Int J Hematol 76 (Suppl 2):253–257, 2002.

67. Blajchman, MA: Substitutes and alternatives to platelet transfusions in thrombocytopenic patients. J ThrombHaemostasis 1:1637–1641, 2003.

68. Fischer TH, et al: Intracellular function in rehydrated lyophilized platelets. Brit J Haematol 111:167–174, 2000.

69. Crowe, JH, et al: Stabilization of membranes in human platelets freeze-dried with trehalose. Chem Phys Lipids 122:41–52, 2003.

70. Vostal, JG, and Mondoro, TH: Liquid cold storage of platelets: A revitalized possible alternative for limiting bacterial contamination of platelet products. Transfus Med Rev 11:286–295, 1997.

71. Hoffmeister KM, et al: The clearance mechanism of chilled blood platelets. Cell 112:87–97, 2003.

72. Hoffmeister, KM, et al: Glycosylation restores survival of chilled blood platelets. Science 301:1531–1534, 2003.

73. Currie, LM, et al: Enhanced circulatory parameters of human platelets cryopreserved with second-messenger effectors: An in vivo study of 16 volunteer donors. Br J Haematol 105:826–831, 1999.

two

Basic Genetics for Blood Bankers

Lorraine Caruccio, PhD, MT(ASCP)SBB

OBJECTIVES

On completion of this chapter, the learner should be able to:

1. Understand Mendel's laws of independent segregation and random assortment and how he developed them.
2. Correlate the ideas of dominant and recessive traits with examples of the inheritance of blood group antigens.
3. Understand the Hardy-Weinberg principle and how it applies to genetic traits.
4. Be able to solve Hardy-Weinberg problems for any blood group antigen, given the necessary information.
5. Determine the inheritance pattern of a given trait by examination of the pedigree analysis.
6. Describe the processes of mitosis and meiosis and the differences between them.
7. Distinguish between X-linked and autosomal traits and how each is inherited.
8. Describe in detail the processes of replication, transcription, and translation and know the basic mechanism of each.
9. Be familiar with the various types of genetic mutations and how they can change the function of living cells and organisms.
10. Understand the cell's different mechanisms to correct mutations.
11. Discuss some of the ways genetics can be used in the modern transfusion laboratory and have the necessary background information to understand modern genetic testing techniques.

Introduction

One of the most important areas of modern biology is the science of genetics. Genetics is highly important in many areas of our lives today. It plays a critical role in testing for inherited diseases as well as in the search for new genetic markers, in determining legal outcomes via forensic pathology and genotyping for paternity cases, in nutrition with the development of modern genetic techniques of disease- and drought-resistant crops, in national safety with the latest vaccines and critical screening methods for weapons of bioterrorism, and most recently, developing advanced treatment options with

the advent of gene therapy. The modern blood bank is no exception in respect to the importance of genetics. All the different areas of transfusion medicine rely on an understanding of blood group genetics as well as on accurate and sensitive methods of pathogen testing to keep the blood supply safe. Historically, the major focus and role of genetics in blood banking has been more so in population genetics and inheritance patterns, but now cellular and molecular genetics are equally important. The student of transfusion medicine must know not only how to interpret a familial inheritance pattern but also modern methods that require a high level of training and skill, such as in restriction mapping, sequencing, and polymerase chain reactions (PCR). The scientific importance attributed to genetics can be noted in the number of Nobel laureates that have built their careers on research with a strong genetics emphasis. The science of genetics has opened up new frontiers in biology.

In this chapter, a general overview of genetics at three different levels (*population*, concerning large numbers of individuals; *cellular*, which pertains to the cellular organization of genetic material; and *molecular*, based on the biochemistry of the structures that comprise genes, or "traits," and the structures that support them) are explained in some detail. This is very adequate as a basis for understanding the chapter on modern genetics techniques as well as a study of the inheritance of blood groups; however, students highly interested in the topic are invited to pursue further study using any one of the excellent texts listed in the bibliography or one of the many high-level journals that are available at most major university libraries. Those students desiring a career in or who wish to make a significant contribution to blood banking research should make it a priority to understand at great depth the science of modern genetics and cellular biology.

Classic Genetics

The science of genetics is one of the most important areas of modern biology. The understanding of the inheritance of blood group antigens and the testing for disease markers at the molecular level, both of which are vitally important in transfusion medicine, are based on the science of genetics. Modern genetics is concerned not only with the biochemical nature of nucleic acids including deoxyribonucleic acid (DNA), ribonucleic acid (RNA) and the various proteins that are part of the chromosomal architecture but also with population genetics and epidemiology. The understanding of inheritance patterns in which genetic traits are followed and analyzed as well as the biochemical reactions that result in gene mutations that can give rise to disease states are all-important in the study of genetics. This chapter will review a few of the major developments in the history of genetics and will discuss both population and biochemical genetics. It will also give a brief overview of modern molecular techniques. More detailed discussions can be found in advanced texts, and the reader is encouraged to search out the original literature and become familiar with it. A separate chapter will explain the modern testing methods of molecular biology including recombinant DNA technology, Southern and Northern blotting, restriction fragment length polymorphism analysis, PCR techniques, and cloning and sequencing in greater detail.

All areas of transfusion medicine, including HLA typing, cell processing, parentage studies, viral testing, and blood services, would not be completely successful without a clear understanding of the principles of genetics and the laws of inheritance. The antigens present on all blood cells are expressed as a phenotype, but it is the genotype of the organism that controls what antigens may be expressed on the cell. For example, when it is impossible to have a clear picture of the red cell antigens present on the red cells of a donor or recipient, or if an antibody screening test gives ambiguous results, genotyping the donor or recipient leukocytes can let technologists know what antigens may be present on the cells and what antibodies can be made against them. Thus, genetics can have an important role in blood banking.

Population Genetics

Mendel's Laws of Inheritance

The science of genetics had its modern development in the work of Gregor Mendel. Mendel was an Austrian monk and mathematician who used sweet pea plants growing in a monastery garden to study physical traits in organisms and how they are inherited. He determined the physical traits to be due to factors he called "elementen" within the cell. In modern genetics we know the physical basis of these so-called "elementen" are genes within the nucleus of the cell. Mendel was fortunate enough to have chosen a good model organism for his studies and had help cultivating his plants. He studied the inheritance of several readily observable pea plant characteristics, notably flower color, seed color, and seed shape and based his first law of inheritance, the law of independent segregation, on these results. The first generation in the study, called the parental, pure, or P1 generation, consisted of all red or all white flowers that bred true for many generations. The plants were either homozygous for red flowers (RR, a dominant trait; dominant traits are usually written with an uppercase letter) or homozygous for white flowers (rr, a recessive trait; recessive traits are usually written with a lowercase letter). When these plants were crossbred, the second generation, called first-filial, or F1, had flowers that were all red. When plants from the F1 generation were crossbred to each other, the second-filial, or F2 generation, of plants had flowers that were red and white in the ratio of 3:1 **(Fig. 2–1)**. All the plants from the F1 generation are heterozygous (or hybrid) for flower color (Rr). The F2 generation has a ratio of 3 red flowered plants to 1 white flowered plant. This is because the plants that have the R gene, either RR homozygous or Rr heterozygous, will have red flowers because the red

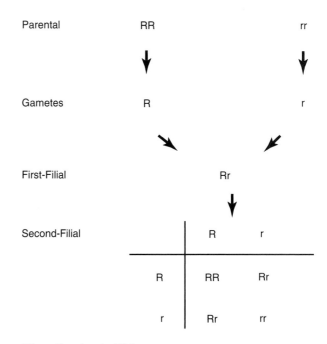

Where R=red and r=White

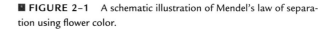

■ **FIGURE 2–1**   A schematic illustration of Mendel's law of separation using flower color.

gene is dominant. Only when the red gene is absent and the white gene occurs in duplicate, as in the rr homozygous white flowered plant, will the recessive white gene expression be visible as a phenotype. This illustrates Mendel's first law, the law of independent segregation, which determines that individual traits are inherited separately from each other. Specifically, Mendel's first law shows that alleles of genes have no permanent effect on one another when present in the same plant but segregate unchanged by passing into different gametes.

An intermediate situation can also occur when alleles exhibit partial dominance. This is observed when the phenotype of a heterozygous organism is a mixture of both homozygous phenotypes seen in the P1 generation. An example of this is plants with red and white flowers that have offspring with pink flowers or flowers with red and white sections. It is important to remember that although the phenotype does not show dominance or recessive traits, the F1 generation has the heterozygous genotype of Rr.

Unlike the flower color of many types of plants, most blood group genes are inherited in a codominant manner. In codominance both alleles are expressed, and their gene products are seen at the phenotypic level. In this case, one gene is not dominant over its allele, and the protein products of both genes are seen at the phenotypic level. An example of this is seen in (Fig. 2–2) with the MNSs blood group system where a heterozygous MN individual would type as both M- and N-antigen-positive.

Mendel's second law is called the law of independent assortment and states "genes for different traits are inherited separately from each other." Specifically, if a homozygote that is dominant for two different characteristics is crossed with a homozygote that is recessive for both characteristics, the F1 generation consists of plants whose phenotype is the same as that of the dominant parent. However, when the F1 generation is crossed in the F2 generation, two general classes of offspring are found. One is the parental type; the other is a new phenotype called a reciprocal type and represents plants with the dominant feature of one plant and the recessive feature of

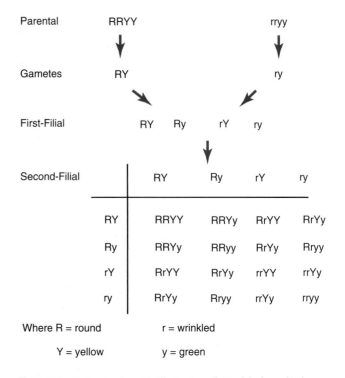

Where R = round   r = wrinkled

Y = yellow   y = green

■ **FIGURE 2–3**   A schematic illustration of Mendel's law of independent assortment using seed types.

another plant. Recombinant types occur in both possible combinations. Mendel formulated this law by doing studies with different types of seeds produced by peas and noted that they can be colored green or yellow and textured smooth or wrinkled in any combination. An illustration of independent assortment of Mendel's second law is given in **Figure 2–3** using his system of pea plant seed types as the example.

Mendel's laws apply to all sexually reproducing diploid organisms whether they are microorganisms, insects, plants, animals or people. However, there are exceptions to the Mendelian laws of inheritance. If the genes for separate traits are closely linked on a chromosome, they can be inherited together as a single unit. The expected ratios of progeny in F1 matings may not be seen if the various traits being studied are linked. There can also be differences in the gene ratios of progeny of F1 matings if recombination has occurred during the process of meiosis. An example of this in blood banking is the MNSs system, in which the MN alleles and the Ss alleles are physically close on the same chromosome and are therefore linked together. Recombination happens when DNA strands are broken and there is exchange of chromosomal material followed by activation of DNA repair mechanisms. The exchange of chromosomal material results in new hybrid genotypes that may or may not be visible at the phenotypic level.

Mendel's laws of inheritance give us an appreciation of how diverse an organism can be through the variations in its genetic material. The more complex the genetic material of an organism, including the number of chromosomes and the number of genes on the chromosomes, the greater the potential uniqueness of any one organism from another organism of the same species. Also, the more complex the genetic material, the more complex and varied its responses to conditions

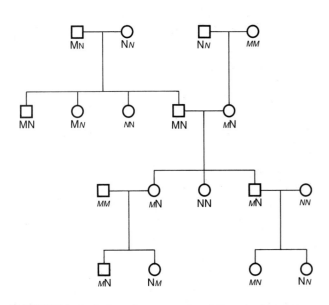

■ **FIGURE 2–2**   Independent segregation of the codominant genes of M and N.

in the environment. Therefore, as long as control is maintained during cell division and differentiation, organisms with greater genetic diversity and number can have an advantage over other organisms in a given setting.

Hardy-Weinberg Principle

G.H. Hardy, a mathematician, and W. Weinberg, a physician, developed a mathematical formula that allowed the study of Mendelian inheritance in great detail. The Hardy-Weinberg formula, $p+q = 1$, in which p equals the gene frequency of the dominant allele and q is the frequency of the recessive allele, can also be stated $p^2+2pq+q^2 = 1$ and specifically addresses questions about recessive traits and how they can be persistent in populations (Fig. 2–4). Like many mathematical formulations, however, certain ideal situations and various conditions must be met in order to use the equations appropriately. These criteria can be generally stated:

1. The population studied must be large, and mating among all individuals must be random.
2. Mutations must not occur in parents or offspring.
3. There must be no migration, differential fertility, or mortality of the genotypes being studied (Box 2–1).

In any normal human population, it is almost impossible to meet these demanding criteria. Although large populations exist, collecting sample data from a significantly large enough segment of a population that correctly represents the members of the population is not always feasible. Also, mating is not always random, and there is mixing of populations on a global scale that leads to "gene flow" on a constant basis. Recently, sequencing of the human genome has revealed that gene mutations occur much more commonly than originally thought possible. Some of these mutations affect the phenotype of an individual, such as loss of enzyme function, and some do not. Despite these drawbacks, Hardy-Weinberg is still one of the best tools for studying inheritance patterns in human populations and is a cornerstone of population genetics. Most of the various genes controlling the inheritance of blood group antigens can be studied using the Hardy-Weinberg equations. A relevant example that shows how to use the Hardy-Weinberg formula is the frequency of the Rh antigen, D in a given population.

In this simple example, there are two alleles, D and d, and to determine the frequency of each allele, we count the number of individuals that have the corresponding phenotype, remembering that both Dd and DD will appear as Rh-positive,

BOX 2–1
Criteria for Use of the Hardy-Weinberg Formula

- Population studied must be large.
- Mating among all individuals must be random.
- Mutations must not occur in parents or offspring.
- There must be no migration, differential fertility, or mortality of genotypes studied.

and divide this number by the total number of alleles. This value is represented by p in the Hardy-Weinberg equation. Again, counting the alleles lets us determine the value of q. When p and q are added, they must equal 1. The ratio of homozygotes and heterozygotes is determined using the other form of the Hardy-Weinberg equation $p^2+2pq+q^2 = 1$. If in our example, we tested 1000 random blood donors for the Rh antigen and found that DD and Dd (Rh-positive) occurred in 84 percent of the population and dd (Rh-negative) occurred in 16 percent, the gene frequency calculations would be performed as follows:

$$p = \text{gene frequency of D}$$

$$q = \text{gene frequency of d}$$

$$p^2 = DD, 2pq = Dd, \text{ which combined are } 0.84$$

$$q^2 = dd, \text{ which is } 0.16$$

$$q = \text{square root of } 0.16, \text{ which is } 0.4$$

$$p+q = 1$$

$$p = 1-q$$

$$p = 1-0.4$$

$$p = 0.6$$

The above example is for a two-allele system only. A three-allele system would require use of the expanded binomial equation $p+q+r = 1$ or $p^2+2pq+2pr+q^2+2qr+r^2 = 1$. More complex examples using this formula can be found in more advanced genetics textbooks.

Inheritance Patterns

The interpretation of pedigree analysis requires the understanding of various standard conventions in the representation of data figures. Males are always represented by squares and females by circles. A line joining a male and female indicates a mating between the two, and offspring are indicated by a vertical line. A double line between a male and female indicates a consanguineous mating. A stillbirth or abortion is indicated by a small black circle. Deceased family members have a line crossed through them. The propositus in the pedigree is indicated by an arrow pointing to it and indicates the most interesting or important member of the pedigree. Something unusual about the propositus is often the reason the pedigree analysis is undertaken. Figure 2–5 has

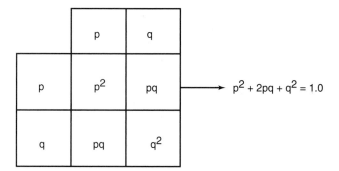

■ FIGURE 2–4   Common inheritance patterns.

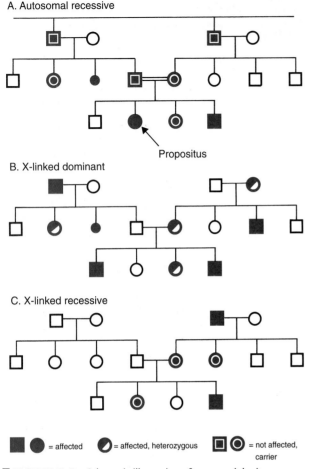

A. Autosomal recessive

B. X-linked dominant

C. X-linked recessive

■ ● = affected   ◐ = affected, heterozygous   ▣ ◉ = not affected, carrier

■ **FIGURE 2–5**   Schematic illustration of common inheritance patterns.

examples of different types of inheritance patterns seen in pedigree analysis. Almost all pedigrees will follow one of these patterns or, rarely, a combination of them.

The first example is a pedigree demonstrating autosomal-recessive inheritance. "Autosomal" refers to traits that are not carried on the sex chromosomes. A recessive trait is carried by either parent or both parents but is not generally seen at the phenotypic level unless both parents carry the trait. In some cases a recessive trait can be genetically expressed in a heterozygous individual but is often not seen at the phenotypic level. When two heterozygous individuals mate, they can produce a child who inherits a recessive gene from each parent, and therefore the child is homozygous for that trait. An example from blood banking is when both parents are Rh-type Dd and have a child that is dd and therefore Rh-negative.

In the second example there is a case of a dominant X-linked trait. If the father carries the trait on his X chromosome, he has no sons with the trait, but all his daughters will have the trait. This is due to the fact that a father always passes his Y chromosome to his sons and his X chromosome to his daughters. Women can be either homozygous or heterozygous for an X-linked trait, and therefore when mothers have an X-linked trait, their daughters inherit the trait in a manner identical to autosomal inheritance. The sons have a 50-percent chance of inheriting the trait or not. Because the trait is dominant, the sons who inherit it will express the trait. The

Xg^a blood group system is one of the few blood group systems that follow an X-linked inheritance pattern.

The third example illustrated is of X-linked recessive inheritance. In this case the father always expresses the trait but never passes it on to his sons. The father always passes the trait to all his daughters, who are then carriers of the trait. The female carriers will pass the trait on to half of their sons, who will be carriers. In the homozygous state, X'Y, the males will express the trait, whereas only the rare homozygous females, X'X', will express the trait. In this situation, with an X-linked recessive trait, a disease-carrying gene can be passed from generation to generation with many individuals not affected. A classic example of this is the inheritance of hemophilia A, which affected many of the royal houses of Europe.

In addition, there is autosomal-dominant, in which all the members of a family that carry the allele show the physical characteristic. Generally, each individual with the trait has at least one parent with the trait. Unlike X-linked traits, autosomal traits usually do not show a difference in the distribution between males and females, and this can be a helpful clue in their evaluation. Also, in autosomal and X-linked traits, if an individual does not have the trait, that individual is a carrier and can pass it on to offspring. This is why recessive traits seem to skip generations, which is another helpful clue in determining inheritance patterns. A third clue is that dominant traits are usually present in every generation. Finally, unusually rare traits that occur in every generation and in much greater frequency than the general population are often the result of matings between related individuals (**Box 2–2**).

Cellular Genetics

Organisms can be divided into two major categories: prokaryotic, without a defined nucleus, and eukaryotic, with a defined nucleus. Human beings and all other mammals are included in the eukaryotic group, as are birds, reptiles, amphibians, fish, and some fungus species. The nucleus of a cell contains most of the genetic material important for replication and is a highly organized complex structure. The nuclear material is organized into chromatin consisting of nucleic acids and structural proteins and is defined by staining patterns. Heterochromatin stains as dark bands, and achromatin stains as light bands and consists of highly condensed regions of chromosomes that are usually not transcriptionally active. Euchromatin is the swollen form of chromatin in cells, which is considered to be much more active in the synthesis of RNA for transcription. Most cellular nuclei contain these different types of chromatin. The chromatin material itself, which chiefly comprises long polymers of DNA and various basic

---

BOX 2–2
Examples of Inheritance Patterns in Transfusion Medicine

- Autosomal-dominant   *In (Lu)* suppressor gene
- Autosomal-recessive   *dd* genotype
- X-linked dominant   Xg^a blood group system
- X-linked recessive   Hemophilia A

proteins called histones, is compressed and coiled to form chromosomes during cell division. Each organism has a specific number of chromosomes, some as few as 4, some as many as 50. In humans, there are 46 chromosomes. The 46 chromosomes are arranged into pairs, with one of each being inherited from each parent. Humans have 22 autosomes and 1 set of sex chromosomes, XX in the female and XY in the male, and this comprises the 2N state of the cell, which is normal for all human cells except the gametes (sex cells). N refers to the number of pairs of chromosomes in a cell.

Mitosis

During cell division, the chromosomes are reproduced in such a way that all daughter cells are genetically identical to the parent cell. Without maintaining the same number and type of chromosomes, the daughter cells would not be viable. The process by which cells divide to create identical daughter cells is called mitosis. The chromosomes are duplicated, and one of each pair is passed on to the daughter cells. During the process of mitosis, quantitatively and qualitatively identical DNA is delivered to daughter cells formed by cell division. The complex process of mitosis is usually divided into a series of stages characterized by the appearance and movement of the chromosomes. The stages are interphase, prophase, metaphase, anaphase, and telophase. The different phases of mitosis include interphase at the beginning, in which DNA is in the form of chromatin and is dispersed throughout the nucleus. This is the stage of the DNA when cells are not actively dividing. New DNA is synthesized by a process called replication in the next stage called prophase, in which the chromatin condenses to form chromosomes. In prophase, the nuclear envelope starts to break down. In the next stage, metaphase, the chromosomes are lined up along the middle of the nucleus and paired with the corresponding chromosome. It is this stage that is used to make chromosome preparations for chromosome analysis in cytogenetics. In anaphase, which comes next, the cellular spindle apparatus is formed and the chromosomes are pulled to opposite ends of the cell. The cell begins to be pinched in the middle, and cell division starts to take place. In the last stage, telophase, the cell is pulled apart, division is complete, and the chromosomes and cytoplasm are completely separated into two new daughter cells. The process of mitosis is illustrated in **Fig. 2–6** and outlined in **Box 2–3**.

Meiosis

A different process is used to produce the gametes. The process is called meiosis and results in four unique, rather than two identical, daughter cells. If cells with 2N chromosomes were paired, the resulting daughter cells would have 4N chromosomes, which would not be viable. Therefore, gametes carry a haploid number of chromosomes, 1N, so that when they combine the resulting cell has a 2N configuration. Meiosis only occurs in the germinal tissues and is important for reproduction. Without the complicated process of meiosis, there would be no change from generation to generation, and evolution would not occur or happen too slowly for organisms to adapt to environmental changes. Meiosis has first stages nearly identical to those in mitosis, in which chromatin is condensed, homologous chromosomes are paired in

---

BOX 2–3
Stages of Mitosis (A) and Meiosis (B)

(A) Mitosis

Interphase (2N)	Resting stage between cell divisions; during this period cells are synthesizing RNA and proteins, and chromatin is uncondensed.
Prophase (4N)	First stage of mitotic cell division. Chromosomes become visible and condense. Each chromosome has two chromatids from duplication of DNA and chromatids are linked via the centromere.
Metaphase (4N)	Chromosomes move toward the equator of the cell and are held in place by microtubules attached at the mitotic spindle apparatus.
Anaphase (4N)	The two sister chromatids separate. Each one migrates to opposite poles of the cell and the diameter of cell decreases at equator.
Telophase (2N)	Chromosomes are at the poles of the cell and the cell membrane divides between the two nuclei. The cell divides and each cell contains a pair of chromosomes identical to the parent cell.

(B) Meiosis

Interphase (2N)	Resting stage between cell divisions; during this period cells are synthesizing RNA and proteins, and chromatin is uncondensed.
Prophase I (4N)	First stage of meiotic division. Chromosomes condense. Homologous chromosomes pair to become bivalent. Chromosome crossing over occurs at this stage.
Metaphase I (4N)	Bivalent chromosomes align at cell equator. Bivalent chromosomes contain all four of the cell's copies of each chromosome.
Anaphase I (4N)	Homologous pairs move to opposite poles of the cell. The two sister chromatids separate.
Telophase I (2N)	The cell separates to become two daughter cells. The new cells are now 2N.
Metaphase II (2N)	Homologues line up at the equator.
Anaphase II (N)	Homologues move to opposite poles of the cell equator.
Telophase II (N)	Each cell separates into two new cells. There are now four (N) cells with a unique genetic constitution.

---

prophase, and chromosomes are aligned along the center of the cell; however, there is no centromere division, and at anaphase and telophase the cell divides and enters once again into interphase, in which there is no replication of DNA. This is followed by the second prophase, in which chromosomes are condensed, and then the second metaphase, with the centromeres dividing. Finally, in the second anaphase and telophase stages, the two cells divide, giving rise to four 1N

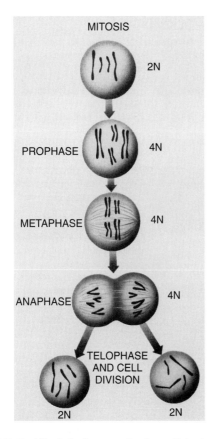

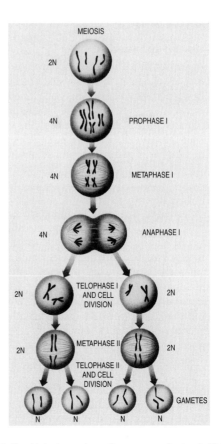

■ **FIGURE 2-6** Mitosis leads to two daughter cells having the same number of chromosomes as the parent cell. (From Watson, JD, Tooze, J, and Kurtz, DT: Recombinant DNA: A Short Course. © 1983 by James D. Watson, John Tooze, and David T. Kurtz. Reprinted by permission of WH Freeman and Company, New York, p 7.)

■ **FIGURE 2-7** Meiosis produces four gametes having half the number of chromosomes present in the parent cell. (From Watson, JD, Tooze, J, and Kurtz, DT: Recombinant DNA: A Short Course. © 1983 by James D. Watson, John Tooze, and David T. Kurtz. Reprinted by permission of WH Freeman and Company, New York, p 7.)

daughter cells. In addition, during meiosis, crossing over and recombination can happen between maternal- and paternal-derived chromosomes. This allows for the creation of new DNA sequences that are different from the parent strains. Combined with random segregation, it is possible to have very large numbers of new DNA sequences, and in humans with 23 pairs of chromosomes the total possible number is several million. Meiosis is illustrated in **Figure 2-7** and outlined in **Box 2-3**.

Cell Division

Cell division is also a complicated process and one that is important to understand. It also occurs with various specific stages. In eukaryotic cells such as human cells, the cell cycle is divided into four distinct stages and is represented by a clock or circular scheme indicating that it can repeat itself or can be stopped at any one point in the cycle. The first step or stage is the resting stage or G_0 and is the state of cells not actively dividing. The pre-replication stage is next and is called G_1. The step at which DNA is synthesized is the next stage, called the S stage. It is followed by the G_2 stage or post-replication stage. Finally, there is the M phase, in which mitosis occurs. Chromosomes are in the interphase stage of mitosis in the span from G_0 to the end of the G_2 phase. Cells that are completely mature and no longer need to divide to

increase their numbers, such as nerve cells, can remain in the G_0 stage for a very long time. It is a hallmark of cancer cells, such as the transformed cells seen in the various leukemias and solid tumors, that they can go through the stages of cell division much faster than nontransformed, normal cells and therefore outgrow them. In this way, they take up the bulk of nutrients needed by the nontransformed cells and crowd them out of existence as well as overgrow the adult organism in which they occur (Box 2-4).

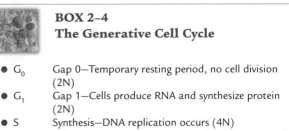

BOX 2-4
The Generative Cell Cycle

- G_0 Gap 0—Temporary resting period, no cell division (2N)
- G_1 Gap 1—Cells produce RNA and synthesize protein (2N)
- S   Synthesis—DNA replication occurs (4N)
- G_2 Gap 2—During the gap between DNA synthesis and mitosis, the cell continues to synthesize RNA and produce new proteins (4N)
- M   Mitosis—Cell division occurs (2N)

Molecular Genetics

Deoxyribonucleic Acid (DNA)

The study of genetics at the molecular level requires an understanding of the biochemistry of the molecules involved. This includes knowledge of the physical conformation of chromosomes as well as the biological and chemical nature of the polymers the different nucleic acids and of nuclear proteins. DNA is a masterpiece of architectural evolution and the "backbone" of heredity. Chromatin is actually a type of polymer structure. Chromosomes are composed of long linear strands of deoxyribonucleic acid (DNA) tightly coiled around highly basic proteins called histones (Fig. 2–8), and each single chromosome is a single extremely long strand of duplex DNA. Remember that DNA is a nucleic *acid*, and therefore most of the proteins that interact with it have an overall *basic* pH. This helps to stabilize the overall complex structure. The complex of DNA and histone protein is referred to as a nucleosome. The DNA and protein complex is bound together so tightly and efficiently that extremely long stretches of DNA several inches in length can be packaged inside of the nucleus a cell on a microscopic level. The DNA and histones are held together by various proteins that keep the DNA in a very specific helical conformation. This conformation also protects the DNA from degradation when it is not being replicated or transcribed.

All DNA in human cells is in the form of a two-stranded duplex, with one strand in one direction and its complementary strand in the opposite direction (the strands are said to be "antiparallel"). DNA is composed of four nitrogenous bases, a sugar molecule called deoxyribose and a phosphate group. The sugar and phosphate moieties comprise the backbone of the DNA molecule while the nitrogenous bases face in to each other and are stabilized by hydrogen bonding and Van der Waals forces. The backbone of a DNA molecule is joined by phosphodiester linkages. Unlike in proteins with an α–helical structure, there is little bonding force between bases on the same strand, which allows DNA to be strong but flexible. The four different bases are adenine (A), cytosine (C), guanine (G), and thymine (T). Adenine and guanine are purines, consisting of double-ring structures, and cytosine and thymine are pyrimidines, single-ring structures (Fig. 2–9). The hydrogen bonding in DNA is specific, in which A only bonds to T with two hydrogen bonds, thus forming the weaker pairing, and

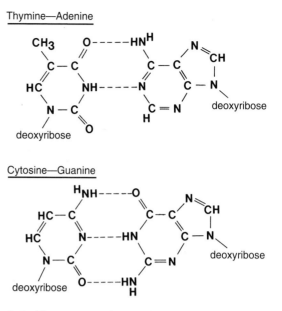

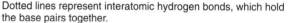

Dotted lines represent interatomic hydrogen bonds, which hold the base pairs together.

■ FIGURE 2–9   The pyrimidine and purine bases found in the DNA molecule.

C only bonds with G with three hydrogen bonds, forming the stronger pairing. This is the classic Watson-Crick base pairing that occurs in the B-form, right-handed helical structure of DNA; it was first postulated by James Watson and Francis Crick at Cambridge University in the early 1950s (Fig. 2–10).[1] Since then, it has been discovered that DNA can also occur in modified forms such as Z-DNA, which is a type of left-handed helix with a different three-dimensional

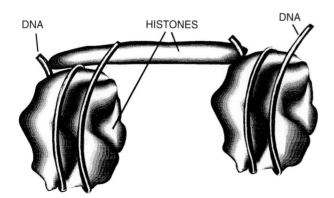

■ FIGURE 2–8   Nucleosomes consist of stretches of DNA wound around histone proteins.

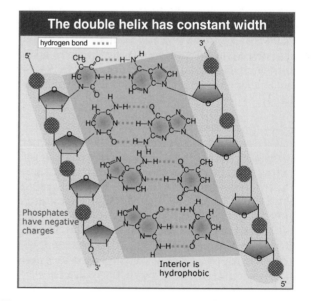

■ FIGURE 2–10   Base pairing in DNA and DNA structure. (From Lewin B: Genes VIII. Copyright 2004 Benjamin Lewin. Published by Prentice Hall/Pearson Education, NY. Reprinted with permission of the author, p 6.)

conformation but that contains the same four nitrogenous bases.[2] In addition, there are some unusual forms of nitrogenous bases that can be incorporated into DNA templates.

The phosphates in the DNA backbone attach to the sugar at the third and fifth carbon atoms. Remember, all atoms in a molecular structure are numbered. The linkage of the purine or pyrimidine nitrogenous base to the sugar is at carbon one. Therefore, the two DNA strands are antiparallel; that is, one strand is 5′ to 3′ in one direction (pronounced 5 prime to 3 prime), and the complementary strand is 5′ to 3′ in the other direction. During transcription, only one strand is copied, which is the complementary strand that gives the correct 5′ to 3′ sequence of messenger RNA (mRNA) that corresponds to the template, or coding strand, of the DNA molecule.

As there are only 4 different bases used to make up DNA templates and there are 20 different amino acids that are used to construct proteins, it is evident that any single nucleotide cannot code for any specific amino acid. What has been discovered is that triplets of nucleotides, called a codon, such as ATG, code for one specific amino acid. However, there is a redundancy to the genetic code in that some amino acids have more than one triplet, which codes for their addition to the peptide chain formed during translation. Generally, the more common the amino acid is in proteins, the greater the number of codons it has. There are four special codons, including the only one specific codon for the initiation of transcription and translation and three different codons that are used to stop the addition of amino acids in the process of peptide synthesis called translation. The genetic code is illustrated in (Fig. 2–11).

Replication

Replication is the complex process by which DNA is copied before mitosis can occur. DNA is copied in such a way that each daughter cell will have the same amount of DNA and the same sequence. Nearly all DNA replication is done in a bidirectional manner and is semiconservative in nature.[3] Specifically, as enzymes involved in the replication process open the double-stranded DNA helix, one strand of DNA is copied in a 5′ to 3′ manner, while the other strand is opened partially in sections and is copied 5′ to 3′ in sections as the double-stranded template continuously opens. In addition, each newly synthesized DNA will be paired with one of the parent strands. The replication process is pictured in **Figure 2–12**.

In order for DNA to be faithfully replicated, with exact copying of the template and its sequence into a new double-stranded helix, many enzymes and proteins must participate in the process. DNA replication occurs in specific steps, and certain enzymes and other molecules are required at each step. First, DNA must be uncoiled from its super-coiled (or double-twisted) nature, and the two strands must be separated and kept apart; this is done by enzymes called DNA gyrase (undoes the super coils) and DNA helicase (separates the two strands of duplex DNA). These enzymes, using energy derived from ATP hydrolysis, accomplish the feat of opening the DNA molecules. In the next step, DNA polymerase III can synthesize a new strand in the 5′ to 3′ direction on the leading strand. Proteins called single-stranded binding proteins interact with the opened strands of DNA to prevent hydrogen bonding when it is not needed during replication. DNA polymerase III also proofreads the addition of new bases to the

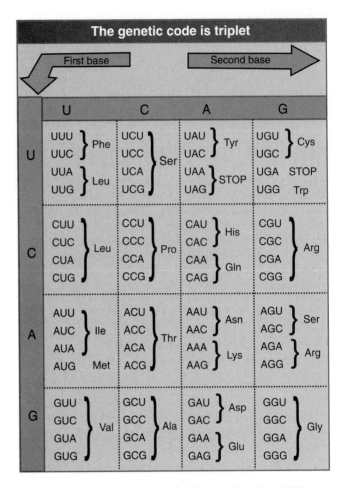

■ FIGURE 2–11 The genetic code. (From Lewin B: Genes VIII. Copyright 2004 Benjamin Lewin. Published by Prentice Hall/Pearson Education, NY. Reprinted with permission of the author, p 168.)

growing DNA strands and can remove an incorrectly incorporated base, such as G paired to T. In order for replication to take place on any piece of DNA, there must first be a short oligonucleotide (composed of RNA) piece that binds to the beginning of the region to be replicated. This "primes" the replication process; therefore, these short oligonucleotide sequences are called primers. All DNA is replicated in a

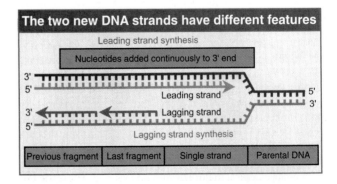

■ FIGURE 2–12 DNA replication. (From Lewin B: Genes, VIII, Copyright 2004 Benjamin Lewin. Published by Prentice Hall/Pearson Education, NY. Reprinted with permission of the author, p 392.)

5′ to 3′manner. Replication of the other parent strand, called the lagging strand, is more complicated because of this restriction. As the helix is opened up, RNA primer sequences are added to the area of the opening fork, and the RNA primers are extended in a 5′ to 3′ manner until the polymerase reaches the previously synthesized end. Rather than being replicated in a continuous manner, these replication forks open up all along the lagging strand and are extended in this way. These small regions of newly replicated DNA are known as Okazaki fragments. The fragments must be joined together to make a complete and continuous strand. This is accomplished by two enzymes called DNA polymerase I and DNA ligase. The RNA primers are synthesized and added to the DNA strands by an enzyme called primase that anneals to the parent strands. After replication of the leading and lagging strands is complete, DNA ligase joins the phosphodiester bonds of the DNA backbone to complete the intact molecule. Isomerase enzymes recoil the DNA; once this is completed and the DNA is proofread, the cell can continue with mitosis and cell division.

Repair

DNA must be copied exactly or the information it contains will be altered, possibly resulting in a decrease in vitality of the organism. However, mistakes in the complex process of replication do occasionally occur, and a number of efficient mechanisms have evolved to correct these mistakes. The mechanisms can detect the mistakes and correct the actual DNA sequence. One of the most important mechanisms for correcting DNA replication errors is the proofreading ability of DNA polymerases. The proofreading occurs in both the 5′ to 3′ and 3′ to 5′ directions and allows the polymerase to backtrack on a recently copied DNA strand and remove an incorrect nucleotide and insert the correct one in its place. In addition to the proofreading ability of DNA polymerase enzymes, there is a second type of editing called mismatch repair in which an incorrect nucleotide is removed and the correct one is inserted in its place.

In addition to errors in the primary sequence of DNA molecules, there are other possible alterations that can have an effect on the way the sequence information is processed. Many common chemicals and environmental factors can alter DNA by modifying it chemically or physically. These include alkylating agents, which react with guanine and result in depurination. Some cancer treatments are often based on this principle. Ionizing radiation and strong oxidants such as peroxides can cause single-strand breaks. Ultraviolet radiation can alter thymine bases, resulting in thymine dimers. Certain drugs such as the antibiotic mitomycin C can form covalent linkages between bases on opposite strands; therefore, during replication there will not be separation of the strands at that site, and the resulting daughter strands will have mutations. Nearly all defects in DNA replication can be corrected by the various mechanisms used by the cell to maintain DNA integrity. However, if too many mistakes occur, the repair systems can be overwhelmed, and mistakes will not be corrected. The cell in which these mutations occur may or may not be viable.

There are several major DNA repair systems. These include photo reactivation (PR), excision repair (also referred to as cut and patch repair), recombinational repair, mismatch repair, and SOS repair **(Box 2–5)**. DNA repair systems can recognize

BOX 2–5
DNA Repair Systems

- Photo reactivation
- Excision repair
- Recombinatorial repair
- Mismatch repair
- SOS repair

mismatched base pairs, missing nucleotides, and altered nucleotides in DNA sequences. For example, when thymine dimers are formed after exposure to ultraviolet (UV) light, the PR enzyme becomes active and enzymatically cleaves the thymine dimers. In addition to the PR system of DNA repair, thymine dimers can be removed by the rather complex process of excison repair, in which the disrupted section of the DNA is removed. A cut is made on one side of the thymine dimer that bulges out from the rest of the duplex DNA. DNA polymerase I synthesizes a short replacement strand for the damaged DNA section. The old strand is removed by DNA polymerase I as it moves along the DNA. Finally, the old DNA strand is removed, and the newly formed DNA segment is ligated into place. Recombinational repair uses the correct strand of DNA to fill in the strand where the error was deleted. Polymerase I and DNA ligase then fill in the other strand. Mismatch repair is activated when base pairing is incorrect and a bulge occurs in the duplex DNA. Mismatch repair enzymes are able to remove the incorrect nucleotides and insert the correct ones. Methyl groups on adenines are used by the mismatch enzyme systems to determine which nucleotide is correct and which is a mistake. SOS repair is induced when DNA and cell damage occurs. Damage can be caused by UV radiation, chemical mutagens, and excessive heat, as well as by such treatments as exposure to cross-linking agents. There are certain sections of highly conserved DNA that are activated when DNA is damaged and the genes that are part of the SOS response system must work in a coordinated manner to repair the damaged DNA through recombination events that remove the damaged sections and replace them with the correct sequences. Some repair systems have been studied more closely in prokaryotes than eukaryotes. All of these systems are available to maintain the integrity of the DNA.

Mutations

Although many effective DNA proofreading and repair systems help to keep newly synthesized DNA from having mutations, none of the systems are foolproof and occasional mutations occur. Once a mutation is introduced into a DNA coding strand, the information in that strand is now altered. It may be altered at the protein level if the mutation encodes for a different amino acid or a change in reading frame. In general, a mutation is any change in the structure or sequence of DNA, whether it is physical or biochemical. An organism, whether it is as simple as a single-celled protozoan or as complex as a human being, is referred to as a mutant if its DNA sequence is different from that of the parent organism. The original form of the DNA sequence and the organism in which it occurs is called the wild type. The various chemicals and conditions that can cause mutations are referred to as mutagens. Many mutagens are also carcinogens in that the cells in which they occur have an advantage in growth patterns that allows them to dominate the cells around them.

There are different types of mutations, and they may have very different consequences for the organisms in which they occur. Also, remember that mutations can be spontaneous; if they occur in the germinal tissue, they are passed on from one generation to the next. The simplest type of mutation is the point mutation in which only one nucleotide in the DNA sequence is changed. Point mutations include substitutions, insertions, and deletions. Certain substitutions, although they change the DNA sequence and the triplet codon(s), may not change the amino acid sequence in the corresponding protein because of redundancy in the genetic code. Recall that some of the amino acids have more than one codon that represents them and, therefore, that if the new codon is for the same amino acid, the mutation will be silent, and the protein sequence will be the same. An example of this is the amino acid threonine, which has ACA, ACC, ACG, and ACU as possible codons. Therefore, a substitution of C, G, or U for A at the third position of the codon would still have a peptide with threonine at that position. A type of "silent mutation" also occurs when a mutation happens that causes a change in the peptide sequence, but that part of the peptide does not seem critical for its function; therefore, no mutation is seen at the phenotypic level, such as enzyme function. A transition is a type of mutation in which one purine-pyrimidine substituted for another purine-pyrimidine. When a purine is substituted for a pyrimidine or a pyrimidine for a purine, it is called a transversion (Fig. 2–13).[4]

Another type of mutation that can have a deleterious effect on the peptide sequence is called a missense point mutation. A missense mutation results in a change in a codon, and this change results in a change of amino acid in the corresponding peptide. These changes cannot be accommodated by the peptide while still maintaining its function. Typical examples of missense mutations are the alterations in the hemoglobin molecule at a single base pair, resulting in different types of inherited anemias.[5] A very specific type of serious mutation is called a nonsense mutation; this results when a point change in one of the nucleotides of a DNA sequence causes one of the three possible stop codons to be formed. The three stop codons are called amber, opal, and ochre and cause the termination of the reading of the DNA sequence so that the resulting peptide is truncated at its 3' end.

A more severe type of mutation happens when there is an insertion or deletion of one or more (but never three) nucleotides in the DNA sequence. The result of this type of mutation is a change in the triplet codon sequence and therefore an alteration in the frameshift reading so that a large change in the amino acid sequence occurs. In transfusion medicine, it has been shown that there is a single base pair deletion in the gene encoding for the transferase protein of the A blood group.[6] The frameshift mutation results in a nonfunctional transferase protein that is seen phenotypically as the O blood group.

Unusual genetic changes can also happen that result in gross mutations in the DNA sequence. Duplications, recombinations, and large deletions have a lower frequency rate than the mutations in the replication of DNA noted above. Duplications can occur quite frequently and give rise to pseudogenes and other "junk" DNA that does not code for proteins. A large part of DNA consists of such junk DNA without apparent ill effects and may even be necessary to some extent for the structural integrity of DNA and chromosomes. Also, there are sequences "left over" from earlier evolution that are still present in human DNA, such as *Alu* sequences. There may also be evolutionary pressures forcing duplications to occur. In blood banking, there are two good examples of duplications. The first involves the *glycophorin A* and *B* genes, the second involves the *Rh* genes *D* and *CcEe*. The Chido and Rodgers blood group antigens, carried on the complement components of the *C4A* and *C4B* genes, arose from duplications and mutations of the *C4* genes.

Mutations involving recombination or crossing over take place during the process of meiosis in the formation of gametes. It is very important to generate sex cells that are different from the parental cells. Recombination involves breaking both double-stranded DNA homologues, exchanging both strands of DNA, and then resolving the new DNA duplexes by reconnecting phosphodiester bonds. Crossing over can be single, double, or triple events (Fig. 2–14). An example of such an event resulting in a hybrid formation is seen in the MNSs blood group system. Single and double crossover events have formed the genes for the Stones, Dantu, and Mi V blood groups. One of the most important events in the immune system is the recombination of the *D, V,* and *J* genes that occurs to give rise to the vast array of immunoglobulin genes that are necessary to form the antibodies of the humoral system.

Deletion of large segments of DNA sequences covering hundreds and possibly even thousands of nucleotides is also possible. It is a type of mutation that is not capable of being corrected by any of the DNA repair systems due to the size and complexity of the mutation. Such mutations can result in complete loss of a peptide, a severely truncated peptide, or the formation of a nonfunctional peptide. An example of this type of mutation in transfusion medicine is the Rodgers negative phenotype, which results from a 30 kD deletion of both the complete *CD4* (Rodgers) and *21-hydroxylase* genes.[7]

Ribonucleic Acid (RNA)

Ribonucleic acid (RNA) is similar to DNA but has certain key differences. One of the differences is that unlike DNA, which is usually a double-stranded helix, RNA occurs most often as

Transition

	S antigen	s̄ antigen
amino acid	methionine	threonine
mRNA code	AUG	ACG
DNA code	TAC	TGC

Transversion

	N antigen	He antigen
amino acid	leucine	tryptophan
mRNA code	UUG	UGG
DNA code	AAC	ACC

■ **FIGURE 2–13** Examples of DNA mutations (transversions and transitions) in blood groups.

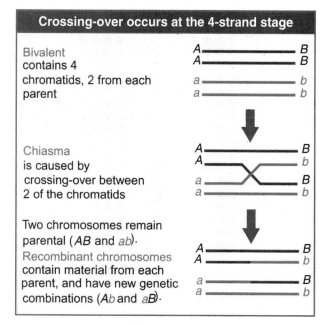

Crossing-over occurs at the 4-strand stage

Bivalent
contains 4
chromatids, 2 from each
parent

Chiasma
is caused by
crossing-over between
2 of the chromatids

Two chromosomes remain
parental (*AB* and *ab*).
Recombinant chromosomes
contain material from each
parent, and have new genetic
combinations (*Ab* and *aB*).

■ **FIGURE 2–14**   Crossing over of DNA strands and chiasma formation to create new sequences. (From Lewin B: Genes VIII. Copyright 2004 Benjamin Lewin. Published by Prentice Hall/Pearson Education, NY. Reprinted with permission of the author, p 20.)

a single-stranded structure, although internal hydrogen bonding occurs frequently, probably to stabilize the RNA molecules. Both DNA and RNA are made up of nucleotides, but in place of thymine in DNA there is uracil in RNA. Uracil is very similar to thymine except that it lacks a methyl group. Another major difference is the substitution of the sugar ribose for deoxyribose in the backbone structure. The sugar in DNA, deoxyribose, lacks a hydroxyl group (-OH) at the 2′ carbon position (thus, de-oxy-ribose nucleic acid, or DNA). Ribose in RNA has the hydroxyl group at this carbon position, whereas DNA has hydrogen. In eukaryotes, RNA is always used to transmit genetic information from the nucleus, where it is stored as DNA, to the cytoplasm, where it is translated into peptides and proteins. DNA is copied into RNA by a process called transcription, then modified and transported out of the nucleus to the ribosomes, where it is translated into protein, which is then modified if necessary for its proper function. Therefore, RNA is the "go between" of DNA, which stores genetic information, and protein, which is the final product of the expression of that genetic information. In prokaryotes, there are specific differences in how DNA is processed to make RNA, but because we are interested in human genetics we will not go into detail on these differences. It is worth mentioning that certain viruses can store genetic information as RNA, whereas others use DNA, either single- or double-stranded, and some viruses use both during the different parts of their infectious cycles.

In eukaryotes there are three major types of RNA; each has a specific function as well as its corresponding polymerase. The first class of RNA molecule is ribosomal RNA (rRNA), which makes up a large part of the ribosomal structure on the endoplasmic reticulum in the cytoplasm. It is here that RNA is translated into peptide. RNA polymerase I transcribes rRNA. It is the most abundant and consistent form of

RNA in the cell. The second class of RNA is messeger RNA (mRNA); it is the form that is transcribed from DNA that encodes specific genes, such as those determining the various blood groups. RNA polymerase II transcribes mRNA. The third major class of RNA is transfer RNA (tRNA); it is involved in bringing amino acids to the mRNA bound on the ribosome. Other small RNA molecules have other various functions within the cell but are beyond the general scope of this text.

Transcription

Transcription is the cellular process by which DNA is copied to RNA. Although mRNA accounts for only about 5 percent of the total RNA inside a eukaryotic cell, it has the extremely important role of being a "transportable" and disposable form of the genetic code. Messenger RNA allows for highly efficient processing of the genetic code into proteins that play nearly all the functional roles within a cell. Transcription begins when the enzyme RNA polymerase II binds to a region upstream (to the left of the 5′ start site) of a gene. Certain DNA short sequences, called consensus sequences, are located at specific sections upstream of the gene to be transcribed; these are used to position RNA polymerase properly so transcripton of a gene is started correctly. This region is referred to as the promoter and is important in how and when a gene is expressed. It is not part of the mRNA itself and is never transcribed, but it controls transcription. Promoters can be positively or negatively regulated by various transcription factors and other transcription-specific protein effectors. Also, regions of DNA sequence called enhancers can affect transcription rates without being close to the coding regions of the genes they influence. RNA is synthesized in a 5′ to 3′ direction; transcription starts at the 3′ end of the coding (or template) strand of the DNA duplex after it is opened to two single strands and proceeds to the 5′ end. In this way, a 5′ to 3′ coding strand is generated with U in place of T. The RNA transcript is complementary to the template strand and is equivalent to the coding strand of the DNA molecule. Transcription is illustrated in **Figure 2–15**.

After RNA is transcribed, it is further processed before it is transported to the ribosome and translated into protein. One major modification to eukaryotic mRNA is the 5′ 7-methyl guanosyl cap that is added to protect the mRNA from

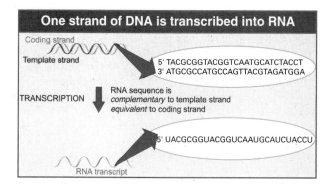

One strand of DNA is transcribed into RNA

Coding strand
Template strand

5′ TACGCGGTACGGTCAATGCATCTACCT
3′ ATGCGCCATGCCAGTTACGTAGATGGA

TRANSCRIPTION

RNA sequence is
complementary to template strand
equivalent to coding strand

5′ UACGCGGUACGGUCAAUGCAUCUACCU

RNA transcript

■ **FIGURE 2–15**   Transcription of RNA from DNA. (From Lewin B: Genes VIII. Copyright 2004 Benjamin Lewin. Published by Prentice Hall/Pearson Education, NY. Reprinted with permission of the author, p 241.)

degradation by nucleases. The 3' end of mRNA is modified by the addition of a string of adenines that form a polyadenylation signal (poly-A tail), which can vary in length from about 20 to 200 nucleotides and is believed to increase mRNA stability. In addition to these steps, eukaryotic mRNA has intervening sequences called introns that do not code for protein or peptide and must be removed before translation can begin. The process by which introns are removed from mRNA is called RNA splicing. Specific sequences at the beginning and end of each intron signal the necessary enzymes to remove the introns from the mRNA and degrade them. The remaining sequences, which contain only exons that code for peptides and proteins, are then joined together by a process called ligation to form a mature mRNA molecule. The mature mRNA is then transported out of the nucleus and to the ribosomes, where translation takes place **(Fig. 2–16)**.

Translation

Translation is the process by which RNA transcripts are turned into proteins and peptides, the structural and functional molecules of the cell. Like DNA and RNA, proteins have a direction, reading their sequences left to right from the amino terminal to the carboxy terminal. Peptides and proteins (polypeptides) are composed of amino acids (aa) joined to make a linear chain. Peptides consist of one strand of aa, and polypeptides consist of more than one strand. Many peptide strands have only primary and secondary structure. Proteins can also have more complicated tertiary and quaternary structure. The making of the peptide chain(s) in the correct sequence is complicated and requires many molecules to carry it out. Translation takes place on the rough endoplasmic reticulum (ER) in the cytoplasm. Also called the rough ER, it is the site of the ribosomes (rRNA), which are the subcellular structural organelles that process mRNA into peptides and proteins. In eukaryotic organisms, translation is "monocistronic" in that only one ribosome reads the mRNA transcript at any time. Translation is a complicated process and involves three major steps: initiation, elongation, and termination. The first event of the initiation sequence is the attachment of a free methionine to a transfer RNA molecule called tRNA^{met}, which requires the presence of a high-energy molecule called guanine triphosphate (GTP) and a special protein called initiation factor IF2. When GTP, IF2, and factors IF1 and IF3 are present at the ribosome, tRNA^{met} is able to bind the small 40S subunit of the ribosome to form an initiation complex. The larger subunit of the ribosome, the 60S, also binds to the complex and hydrolyzes the GTP, and then the IFs are released. Translation is illustrated in **Figures 2–17 and 2–18.**

There are two sites present on the 60S ribosome unit, the A site and the P site. During translation, the charged tRNA^{met} must occupy the P site, and the A site next to the P site must have a charged tRNA with its correct matching amino acid in position. Peptide bond formation occurs by transferring the polypeptide attached to the tRNA in the P site to the aminoacyl-tRNA in the A site. All tRNA molecules have a similar secondary structure with intramolecular hydrogen bonding; are long, single-stranded RNAs; and are often described as having a cloverleaf-shaped conformation no matter which aa they are carrying to the translation machinery. There are two major functional areas of the tRNA molecule. The first is the part

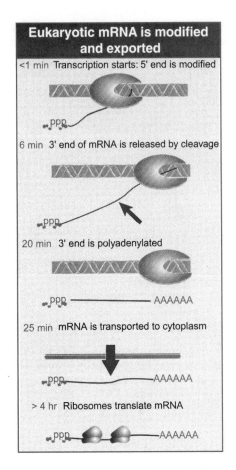

■ **FIGURE 2–16** Translation of RNA into protein. (Lewin B: Genes VIII. Copyright 2004 Benjamin Lewin. Published by Prentice Hall/Pearson Education, NY. Reprinted with permission of the author, p 122.)

called the anticodon; it consists of three nucleotides that hydrogen-bond to the corresponding correct site on the mRNA. It is this hydrogen bonding that makes sure the correct aa is joined in the peptide chain by allowing only the correct tRNA molecule with the right anticodon to bond to the correct mRNA codon. The second part of the tRNA molecule is at the 3' hydroxyl end and binds an amino acid. Only one aa

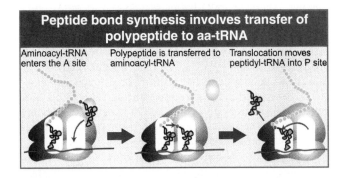

■ **FIGURE 2–17** Peptide bond synthesis in translation. (Lewin B: Genes VIII. Copyright 2004 Benjamin Lewin. Published by Prentice Hall/Pearson Education, NY. Reprinted with permission of the author, p 137.)

Protein synthesis has 3 stages

Initiation 40s subunit on mRNA binding site is joined by 60s subunit, and aminoacyl tRNA binds next

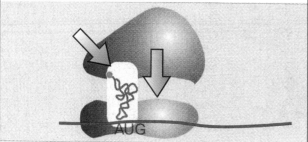

Elongation Ribosome moves along mRNA and length of protein chain extends by transfer from peptidyl-tRNA to aminoacyl-tRNA

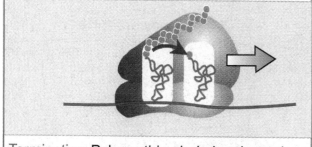

Termination Polypeptide chain is released from tRNA, and ribosome dissociates from mRNA

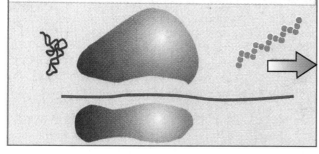

■ **FIGURE 2–18** Stages of protein synthesis in translation. (Lewin B: Genes VIII. Copyright 2004 Benjamin Lewin. Published by Prentice Hall/Pearson Education, NY. Reprinted with permission of the author, p 137.

can bind to one tRNA molecule; specificity is determined by the 3′ hydroxyl end. According to the recognition region, an aminoacyl synthase enzyme adds the specific aa to the correct tRNA molecule. Only when the tRNA is charged with an amino acid can it transport it to the ribosome for translation. During the elongation step of translation, the incoming tRNA binds to the A site in presence of the elongation factor called E2F. Again, GTP is hydrolyzed as the energy source to move the tRNA in the A position to the P position. As the tRNA in the A site is moved to the P site, the tRNA in the P site is released back to the cytoplasm to pick up another aa. The ribosomes move down the codons on the mRNA one at a time, adding correct aa to the growing peptide chain. As the ribosome moves down the mRNA, it eventually comes to one of

the three stop codons UAA, UGA, or UAG, and translation of that mRNA is finished. Termination factors help the ribosome units to separate, and the peptide chain is further processed. Post-translational processing can consist of glycosylation, the addition of sugar groups, or the removal of leader peptide sequences that are used to traffic proteins to the cell membrane; processing can also consist of complicated folding schemes that ensure the protein is in its correct tertiary form. A large family of proteins called the heat shock proteins helps new proteins to be folded correctly by binding to hydrophobic (water-avoiding) sections of the nascent protein chain. Hydrogen bonding, van der Waals forces, and hydrophilic (water-attracting) regions of proteins also help to give the new protein its correct three dimensional conformation. After translation is complete, the mRNA is often rapidly degraded by enzymes, a process that helps to control gene expression, or it may attach to another ribosome and the entire translation process starts all over again. See **Figure 2–19**.

Modern Genetics Techniques

Over the last three decades, the knowledge of genetics has advanced at a seemingly exponential level. Understanding the biochemical and biophysical nature of DNA, RNA, and peptides and proteins has allowed techniques to be developed to study these important molecules in great detail and to define the ways in which they interact in a living entity, whether it be a cell, groups of cells, or complex multicellular organisms. Most of the techniques used in molecular biology (the science of studying and manipulating genetic material) are based on the biochemical properties of genes and chromosomes. Chapter 4 of this text goes into greater detail about molecular biology techniques; however, they are presented here for a quick preview to that chapter.

tRNA is an adaptor

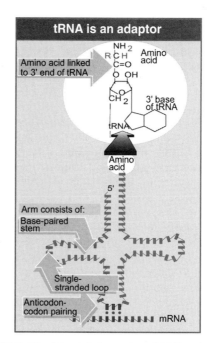

■ **FIGURE 2–19** Schematic illustration of tRNA molecule and base pairing. (Lewin B: Genes VIII. Copyright 2004 Benjamin Lewin. Published by Prentice Hall/Pearson Education, NY. Reprinted with permission of the author, p 115.)

DNA Typing

Basic Techniques

The following steps are common to most techniques of molecular biology:

First, any material that is to be studied must first be isolated intact with a minimum of structural damage. This is often done with chemicals that interact with one part of the cellular material and not another.

Second, there must be a way to visualize and locate the molecular species to be studied. This is often done with probes (signal) that will bind specifically to the species, such as DNA, by hybridization of hydrogen bonds of the DNA.

Third, a method to separate out different species, such as different sequences of DNA, must be available. This often involves running nucleic acids through gels, binding them to columns, hybridizing them to membranes, or binding them to other molecules.

Fourth, a method to quantify the isolated and studied species has to be used to get differences exact as possible in the process studied. Changes in optical density when exposed to UV irradiation, radioisotope levels, fluorescence emission, and other methods are readily used.

DNA Isolation

Most of the nucleic acids are isolated by alkaline denaturation and precipitated with alcohol. They can also be further purified from other unwanted cellular components, such as the cytoplasmic membrane, by use of specific columns that will bind nucleic acids based on charge-charge interactions. Column chromatography has been in use for many years, and different materials are used to prepare columns, depending on the nature of the materials to be separated. In less recent times, DNA was isolated after treatment of cells with harsh agents, such as phenol and chloroform, and then high-speed centrifugation on cesium chloride gradients. RNA requires greater care than DNA as it is a single-stranded molecule and much more labile. Chemicals that will inactivate ever-present RNases (anywhere that fingertips go, so go RNases) must be used to obtain RNA that is not degraded or "chewed." As mRNA is only a small part of the total RNA isolated, it can be purified by nature of its poly-A tail, using a column that contains poly-T attached to resin bead molecules. Methods such as complementary DNA (cDNA) synthesis, in which RNA is converted into a DNA copy in vitro, allows greater study of RNA sequences by making a more stable version of it. RNA isolation also requires greater disruption of the cellular material, usually with chaotropic agents such as guanidine thiocyanate, lithium salts, and mechanical means to disrupt cell membranes, such as douncing or shearing with a needle and syringe. Once DNA has been isolated, it can be stored in low salt buffers at $-20°C$ and RNA at $-80°C$ for many months to years. Storage in water is not recommended because the nucleic acids are polymers and hydrolysis reactions will degrade them.

Sequence Determination

There are many different types of analysis of DNA. One of the most important is determining its sequence, either by direct sequencing (which chemically cleaves DNA based on the nucleotides present at the reaction site) or by termination with dideoxy-nucleotides using DNA polymerase. Also important are restriction enzyme digestion (type II endonucleases, also referred to as restriction enzymes, isolated from bacteria that break open the DNA backbone depending on a specific sequence) and Southern blotting (in which DNA is digested and then bound to a membrane followed by hybridization with a sequence-specific probe, usually a short DNA piece).[8] Because genes have unique sequences, it is important to get every nucleotide correct. Mutations will be identified with these techniques because, for example, a restriction enzyme will not cut a sequence of DNA if there is a mutation but will cut the DNA without the mutation. The two sequences can then be compared and analyzed.

Electrophoresis

Comparison of DNA and RNA is often done by a process called gel electrophoresis. In this process, agarose or acrylamide is used to cast a porous gel, the DNA is put into openings in the gel, and the gel is put into a tank with a suitable tris-based buffer. The gel has a consistency of jello or gelatin. Next, an electric current is applied to electrodes on the tank; based on differences in size and conformation, the negatively charged DNA or RNA species will move through the gel at different rates toward the positive pole. The DNA pieces in the gel (termed "bands") can be visualized by using ethidium bromide, propidium iodide, or fluorescent dyes that bind to or intercalate inside of the DNA base pairs.

Cloning and PCR

Cloning is a way to make an exact copy of a desired DNA sequence and to obtain large amounts of it in pure form. Cloning relies on isolating DNA segments of interest and making copies of them when they are introduced into another larger DNA vehicle, such as a bacterial plasmid that can be replicated without restriction on number, and grown to high density.[9] New techniques allow the study of DNA with sequence-specific proteins such as transcription factors that control gene expression; these techniques also include isolating chromatin and looking at its conformation and analysis tools for studying the newly found enzymatic nature of small RNA molecules. PCR is very important and is used to amplify isolated pieces of DNA, or RNA after it is converted into cDNA. The amplified pieces are referred to as *amplicons*. The PCR uses DNA polymerase and heating and cooling steps to amplify a target DNA sequence with primers that bind to the sequence.[10] The DNA is heated to separate the strands, and then cooled to allow primers to bind to target sequences. An extension step follows at a temperature optimal for special enzymes that add nucleotides to the annealed primers. The "cycle" of heating (*denaturation*), cooling (*annealing*), and extending (*extension*) is repeated many times, and the amount of DNA made can be increased exponentially. Many types of PCR are now in use for various applications in molecular biology.

Advanced Techniques

The techniques developed in more recent years as well as older techniques still valuable in the study of nucleic acids and the cellular processes they are involved in keep improving and expanding. While it is necessary to have the exact sequence of DNA that is of interest (for example, if it is associated with an inherited disease), it is equally important to understand how that DNA is expressed inside of a living cell. As technology is developed, it will be interesting to see what new methods become available and occur in common use. Methods to silence genes, to look at single live cells, and to analyze the different signaling pathways in the cell that genes control and that control genes are all being actively developed. Of particular interest are the development of *nanotechnology*, high throughput DNA "chip" technology, and computational biology in which enormously complex models of expression and regulation (such as proteosomes) are being assembled and analyzed.

Finally, without the most modern methods, computer aids, and great skills of the people currently in the field of genetics, the human genome projects of the National Institutes of Health and the Celera Corporation would not have been possible. The future of genetics is very bright indeed, and we are fortunate to be able to witness a revolution in biology taking place. Let us hope our enthusiasm and technical skills are matched by good ethics and a sincere desire for the betterment of all people.

Summary Overview

This chapter covers the basic concepts of genetics necessary to understand its role in modern blood banking. Knowledge of modern methods of analysis is also required to appreciate how problems in genetics are solved and explained. The more medical technologists become familiar with these techniques, the faster they can be applied in general use in blood bank laboratories and the faster they can be used to address questions and solve problems in transfusion medicine. A solid understanding of classic genetics, including Mendel's Laws and Hardy-Weinberg formulas, cellular concepts that control chromosomes and cellular division such as mitosis and meiosis, as well as the biochemistry of the molecular structures of the nucleic acids and the proteins that are complexed with them is required to fully understand modern genetics. How these theories, concepts, and principles apply to transfusion medicine should be understood as clearly as possible as genetics is a very dynamic science that has its greatest potential in direct applications. Most of the antigens in the various blood group systems (i.e., ABO, Rh, Kell, Kidd, etc.) generally follow straightforward inheritance patterns, usually of a codominant nature. For more detailed explanations, refer to the corresponding chapters for the specific blood group systems. However, to aid the reader's overall comprehension, certain key basic concepts are reviewed here.

Terminology

Just as it takes "two to tango," it takes two gametes to make a fertilized egg with the correct (2N) number of chromosomes (46 in the human animal) in the nucleus of a cell. Therefore, each parent contributes only half (1N) of the inherited genetic information, or genes, to each child. Whether children are conceived naturally or with the assistance of modern technology such as in-vitro fertilization, each child must have the correct number of genes and chromosomes (2N), without major mutations affecting necessary biochemical systems, in order to be healthy and complete. The genetic material has a complex pattern of organization that has been evolving for

millions of years to a magnificent level of coordination and control. At the smallest level, genes are composed of discrete units of DNA (deoxyribonucleic acid) arranged in a linear fashion, similar to a strand of pearls, with structural proteins wrapped around the DNA at specific intervals to pack it into tightly wound bundles. The DNA is organized at a higher level into chromosomes, with each chromosome being one incredibly long strand of duplex (double-stranded) DNA. A gene is a section, often a very large section, of DNA along the chromosome. The specific sequence of nucleotides, as well as the location on the chromosome, determines a gene. In addition, each gene has specific and general sequences that occur upstream (before the start site) and downstream (after the termination signals) that contribute to how a gene functions. The specific location of a gene on a chromosome is called a *locus* (plural = *loci*), and at each locus there may be only one (rare) or several different forms of the gene, which are called *alleles*. A simple and relevant example is the ABO blood group system, discovered by Landsteiner, the gene that codes for the A, B, or O blood type located on the terminal portion of the long arm of chromosome 9; the alleles for inheritance at this locus are A, B, or O, depending on the enzyme inherited. (See the chapter on the ABO blood group for a more complete explanation of the inheritance of ABO.)

It is important to keep in mind the distinction between *phenotype* and *genotype*. Genotype is the sequence of DNA that is inherited. The phenotype is anything that is produced by the genotype, including an enzyme to control a blood group antigen, thickness of the skin, the curvature of the spine, the length of the muscles, the level of insulin produced, and such obvious traits as eye, skin and hair color. Keep in mind that more than one gene can have an effect on a particular trait (part of a phenotype), such as the height of an individual; all relevant genes can be considered as part of the genotype for that trait.

Depending on the alleles inherited, an organism (or a child for that matter) can be either *homozygous* or *heterozygous* for a specific trait. The presence of two identical alleles (the same allele from both parents (e.g., A from the mother and A from the father) results in a *homozygous (AA)* genotype, and the phenotype is group A blood. On the other hand, the inheritance of different alleles from each parent gives a *heterozygous* genotype, which could be AB, A_1A_2, or AO, depending on the alleles of each parent (e.g., A from the mother and B from the father in the first example, AB). In the second example, the A_1 allele results in more enzyme than A_2 and therefore more "A" antigen on the red cell, so without careful serology or genotyping methods to detect the presence of A_2, the blood group would appear to be A_1.

Another important concept is that of the "silent" gene, or *amorph*. An amorph is a gene that does not produce any obvious, easily detectable traits and is only seen at the phenotypic level when the individual is homozygous for the trait. A good example of this is found with the Rh blood group antigen D ("big D") and its amorph d ("little d"). In the case of Rh type, when an individual inherits the gene for D, whether homozygous (DD) or heterozygous for D (Dd), D antigens appear on the surface of the RBCs, and this individual is said to be Rh-positive. However, if this person is homozygous for the amorph d, no detectable D antigens will be observed at the phenotypic level, and this individual is said to be Rh-negative. In this case, both phenotype and genotype would give the same conclusion: lack of the Rh gene and antigen, respectively. Other blood groups, such as the Ii, Kell, Lutheran, Duffy, and Kidd systems, also encompass the principle of an amorphic allele. Refer to the respective chapters on these blood groups for more detailed information.

Blood Group Nomenclature

The common nomenclature used for blood group systems is not the same as the more standardized nomenclature used for Mendelian genetics. Several points should be made clear so that blood bank technologists are not confused when reading literature that is not solely focused on transfusion medicine. Specifically, Mendel's laws indicate that *dominant* genes are denoted with capitalized letters, and *recessive* genes are denoted with lowercase letters. This is not always true in the blood group nomenclature. Notably, in some blood group systems the antigens that have detectable traits can be represented by both upper- and lowercase letters. This is most likely due to the codominant nature of many blood group traits where the products of both alleles are seen. Good examples are the Rh family Cc and Ee antigens. In this case, if C ("big C") and c ("little c") are inherited, the genotype is heterozygous, and the phenotype is also heterozygous, and the distinction is made that C and c are two different alleles that are expressed equally due to their codominant nature. Therefore, neither one is completely dominant or recessive. The same condition is true for E ("big E") and e ("little e") inheritance and expression. In the MNSs system, a different nomenclature is used, with a single letter for the blood group and a plus (+) or minus (−) sign to indicate the presence or absence of the detectable, respective antigen. For example, M+N+S−s+ would be an individual that is positive for the M, N, and s antigens and negative for S antigen.

There are some blood group systems, such as Kidd, Lutheran, Lewis, and Duffy, that may use two letters to denote the system and a plus or minus sign. An example is given with the Duffy system, where a superscript or, more correctly, an a or b letter indicates the allele, and a plus or minus symbol represents the allele's presence or absence, e.g., Fy(a+b−), where this individual is positive for the Duffy a antigen and negative for the Duffy b antigen. To make matters even worse, in a few allelic pairs, a lower-incidence antigen, such as Wr^a, is designated with a superscript a. In some others, such as Co^a, the superscript a denotes an antigen that is of higher incidence in the general population. Unfortunately, it seems necessary to commit these examples and such others to memory or to a handy written log so as to keep them straight. Despite this possible drawback, remember the correct terminology: a genotype always refers to a blood group gene, and a phenotype always refers to a blood group antigen.

Finally, the ISBT (International Society of Blood Transfusion) Working Party on Terminology for Red Cell Surface Antigens has provided a more standardized, numerical system of nomenclature, and although not yet used rigorously, it helps to solve this problem by giving blood group antigens specific numbers. Although not the same as Mendelian methods of nomenclature, it at least keeps the system of naming the myriad blood bank antigens consistent for all users in all languages. It is a somewhat painful idea to give up the old familiar names and colloquialisms in terminology but one that is in the right direction for modern blood banking practices. There are correct and incorrect ways to designate blood group antigens and the antibodies that are used to identify them, as well as all the common and colloquial ways that have been in use for a long time. The blood bank student should refer to the most current edition of the AABB (American Association of Blood Banks) Technical Manual for more information on correct use of current nomenclature as well as the specific chapters in this text dealing with the different blood groups in greater detail.

SUMMARY CHART:
Important Points to Remember (MLT/MT/SBB)

➤ Genetics is defined as the study of inheritance or the transmission of characteristics from parents to offspring. It is based on the biochemical structure of chromatin, which includes nucleic acids and the structural proteins that constitute the genetic material as well as various enzymes that assist in genetic processes such as replication.

➤ All living organisms have specific numbers of chromosomes. Humans have 22 pairs of autosomes and one set of sex chromosomes, females (XX) and males (XY), giving a total of 46 chromosomes in diploid cells.

➤ Mendel's law of independent assortment states that factors for different characteristics are inherited independent of each other if they reside on different chromosomes.

➤ Human chromosomes are composed of the genetic material chromatin, a complex of the nucleic acid polymer DNA wrapped around highly basic proteins called histones. The helical structure of DNA allows a lot of information to be packaged in a very small amount of space.

➤ Replication of DNA is semiconservative and is accomplished via the enzyme DNA polymerase, which produces a complementary duplicate strand of nucleic acid. Therefore, each strand of DNA can act as a template to be copied to make the opposite strand. DNA has a direction and is always read and written in the 5' (left) to 3' (right) direction.

➤ Mutation refers to any structural alteration of DNA in an organism (mutant) that is caused by a physical or chemical agent (mutagen). Mutations can be beneficial or deleterious. Some mutations are lethal and therefore cannot be passed on to another generation. Some mutations are silent and have no consequence on the organism in which they occur and therefore have no selective pressure against them in the population.

➤ Transcription is an enzymatic process whereby genetic information in a DNA strand is copied into an mRNA complementary strand. Eukaryotic mRNA is altered after it is made by various processing steps, such as the removal of introns and addition of a poly-A tail to the 3' end. These processing steps take place in the nucleus of the cell before the mRNA is exported to the cytoplasmic ribosomes for translation.

➤ Translation is the complex process by which mRNA, which contains a mobile version of the DNA template encoding the genes for an organism, is turned into proteins, which are the functional units of an organism and the cells that it consists of. Translation occurs on the ribosomes, and additional steps may be necessary to get a specific protein into its final correct form, such as with the insulin molecule that requires disulfide linkages. Proteins are made of strings of amino acids and are always read in an amino terminal (left) to carboxyl terminal(right) direction.

➤ Various methods have been developed to manipulate DNA; these make up the part of genetics known as genetic engineering. Southern blotting, sequencing, and cloning analyze DNA, whereas Northern blotting and RNase protection assays analyze RNA. Western blotting and immunoprecipitation as well as mass spectometry and 2-D gel analysis are used to study proteins. Blotting and various biochemical assays are used to analyze carbohydrates and lipids.

➤ Restriction endonucleases are enzymes found in various strains of bacteria and used in molecular techniques to cut DNA at specific sites. Restriction digests have a particular and unique pattern characteristic of the DNA that was used as a template. This is a very useful technique because mutations in DNA often destroy or create new restriction patterns.

➤ A DNA probe is a piece of DNA having a sequence for the specific gene of study that can be labeled in various ways, such as with a radioactive substance or by fluorescent compounds, and visualized by autoradiography or a type of fluorescent imaging system.

➤ The polymerase chain reaction (PCR) is an in-vitro method for enzymatic synthesis and amplification of specific DNA sequences using a pair of primers, usually short nucleotide sequences, that hybridize to opposite DNA strands and flank the region of interest. Various modifications have made the PCR reaction more efficient and specific and allow more complex analysis.

➤ A cloning vector is an extra-chromosomal genetic element that can carry a recombinant DNA molecule (bacteriophages, plasmids, or cosmids) into a host cell (bacteria, yeast, plant, or mammal). It can replicate on its own and may be very concentrated in a single cell. Most vectors contain markers for selection such as antibiotic resistance or fluorescent proteins.

➤ Sources of DNA for analysis by molecular techniques may include any prokaryotic, nonnucleated cells, such as bacteria, or eukaryotic, nucleated cells, such as leukocytes, and may come from living or dead tissue, such as cell samples, cell cultures, or forensic material. Good sources of RNA include any active or dividing cell source, such as reticulocytes or fetal liver. Care must be taken to avoid RNA degradation by naturally occurring RNases. Nonactive cells often have low levels of mRNA, and greater care must be used to harvest sufficient good quality mRNA. Once the mRNA is isolated it can be transcribed into cDNA (complementary DNA) for further study by use of well-known reverse transcription techniques.

➤ Many new techniques are now in use and are being developed for understanding the complete nature of the genetic material and how it functions in complex ways to control the nature of a living organism. This area of biology is growing very fast and will help to elucidate all the interactions, pathways, signals, and structures that make up the living cell and allow it to function in such a complex and sophisticated manner.

Review Questions

1. Which of the following best describes mitosis:
   a. Genetic material is quadruplicated, equally divided between four daughter cells
   b. Genetic material is duplicated, equally divided between two daughter cells
   c. Genetic material is triplicated, equally divided between three daughter cells
   d. Genetic material is halved, doubled, then equally divided between two daughter cells

2. When a recessive trait is expressed, it means that:
   a. One gene carrying the trait was present
   b. Two genes carrying the trait were present
   c. No gene carrying the trait was present
   d. The trait is present but difficult to observe

3. In a pedigree, the "index case" is another name for:
   a. Stillbirth
   b. Consanguineous mating
   c. Propositus
   d. Monozygotic twins

4. What four nitrogenous bases make up DNA:
   a. Adenine, leucine, guanine, thymine
   b. Alanine, cytosine, guanine, purine
   c. Isoleucine, lysine, uracil, leucine
   d. Adenine, cytosine, guanine, thymine

5. Proteins and peptides are composed of:
   a. Golgi bodies grouped together
   b. Paired nitrogenous bases
   c. Nuclear basic particles
   d. Linear arrangements of amino acids

6. Which phenotype could not result from the mating of a Jk(a+b+) female and a Jk(a+b+) male:
   a. Jk(a+b−)
   b. Jk(a+b+)
   c. Jk(a−b+)
   d. Jk(a−b−)

7. Exon refers to:
   a. The part of a gene that contains non-sense mutations
   b. The coding region of a gene
   c. The noncoding region of a gene
   d. The enzymes used to cut DNA into fragments

8. PCR technology can be used to:
   a. Amplify small amounts of DNA
   b. Isolate intact nuclear RNA
   c. Digest genomic DNA into small fragments
   d. Repair broken pieces of DNA

9. Transcription can be defined as:
   a. Introduction of DNA into cultured cells
   b. Reading of mRNA by the ribosome
   c. Synthesis of RNA using DNA as a template
   d. Removal of external sequences to form a mature RNA molecule

10. When a man possesses a phenotypic trait that he passes to all his daughters and none of his sons, the trait is said to be:
    a. X-linked dominant
    b. X-linked recessive
    c. Autosomal dominant
    d. Autosomal recessive

11. When a woman possesses a phenotypic trait that she passes to all of her sons and none her daughters, the trait is said to be:
    a. X-linked dominant
    b. X-linked recessive
    c. Autosomal dominant
    d. Autosomal recessive

12. DNA is replicated:
    a. Semiconservatively from DNA
    b. In a random manner from RNA
    c. By copying protein sequences from RNA
    d. By first copying RNA from protein

13. RNA is processed:
    a. After RNA is copied from DNA template
    b. After protein folding and unfolding on the ribosome
    c. Before DNA is copied from DNA template
    d. After RNA is copied from protein on ribosomes

14. Translation of proteins from RNA takes place:
    a. On the ribosomes in the cytoplasm of the cell
    b. On the nuclear membrane
    c. Usually while attached to nuclear pores
    d. Inside the nucleolus of the cell

15. Meiosis is necessary to:
    a. Keep the N number of the cell changing within populations
    b. Prepare RNA for transcription
    c. Generate new DNA sequences in daughter cells
    d. Stabilize proteins being translated on the ribosome

REFERENCES

1. Watson, JD, and Crick, FHC: Molecular structure of nucleic acids: A structure for deoxyribose nucleic acid. Nature 171:737, 1953.
2. Garret, RH, and Grisham, CM: Structure of nucleic acids. In Roskoski, JR: Biochemistry. WB Saunders, Philadelphia, 1995, pp 222–224.
3. Knippers, R, and Ruff, J: The initiation of eukaryotic DNA replication. In DNA Replication and the Cell Cycle. Springer-Verlag, New York, 1992, pp 2–10.
4. Vogel, F, and Motulsky, AG: Gene mutation: Analysis at the molecular level. In Human Genetics Problems and Approaches, ed 3. Springer, New York, 1997, pp 413–414.
5. Caskey, CT, et al: Triplet repeat mutations in human disease. Science 256:784–789, 1992.
6. Yamamoto, F, et al: Molecular genetic basis of the histo-blood group ABO system. Nature 345:229, 1990.
7. de Van Kim, C, et al: Molecular cloning and primary structure of the human blood group RhD polypeptide. Proc Natl Acad Sci USA 89:10929, 1992.
8. Southern, EM: Detection of specific sequences among DNA fragments separated by gel electrophoresis. J Mol Biol 98:503, 1975.
9. Monaco, AP: Isolation of genes from cloned DNA. Curr Opin Genet Dev 4:360–365, 1994.
10. Vosberg, HP: The polymerase chain reaction: An improved method for analysis of nucleic acids. Hum Genet 83:1–15, 1989.

BIBLIOGRAPHY

Alberts, B, et al: Molecular Biology of the Cell. Garland Publishing, New York, 1983.
Allen, RW, and AuBuchon, JP: Molecular Genetics in Diagnosis and Research. American Association of Blood Banks, Bethesda, MD, 1995.
American Association of Blood Banks: Blood Group Genetics: Technical Manual, ed 13. Bethesda, MD, 1999.
American Association of Blood Banks: Molecular Biology in Transfusion Medicine: Tech Manual. Bethesda, MD, 1996.
Calladine, CR, and Drew, HR: Understanding DNA, the Molecule and How it Works, ed 2. Academic Press, San Diego, 1997.
Clark, DP, and Russell, LD: Molecular Biology Made Simple and Fun, ed 2. Cache River Press, St. Louis, 2000.
Freifelder, D: Molecular Biology: A Comprehensive Introduction to Prokaryotes and Eukaryotes. Jones & Bartlett, Boston, 1983.
Giblett, ER: Genetic Markers in Human Blood. Blackwell Scientific, Oxford, 1969.
Glick, BR, and Pasternak, JJ: Molecular Biotechnology: Principles and Applications of Recombinant DNA, ed 2. ASM Press, Washington, DC, 1998.
Harmening, DM: Modern Blood Banking and Transfusion Practices, ed 4. FA Davis, Philadelphia, 1994.
Hillyer, CD, Silberstein, LE, Ness, PM, Anderson, KC, and Roush, KS: Blood Banking and Transfusion Medicine, Basic Principles and Practice. Churchill Livingstone, Philadelphia, 2003.
Lehninger, AL: Principles of Biochemistry. Worth Publishers, New York, 1982.
Lewin, B: Genes III. John Wiley and Sons, New York, 1987.
Lewin, B: Genes VIII. Prentice Hall, New York, 2003.
Maxson, LR, and Daugherty, CH: Genetics: A Human Perspective. Wm. C. Brown, Dubuque, IA, 1985.
Nicholl, DST: An Introduction to Genetic Engineering. Cambridge University Press, Cambridge, MA, 1994.
Pines, M: The New Human Genetics: How Gene Splicing Helps Researchers Fight Inherited Disease. National Center of General Medical Sciences, Bethesda, MD, 1984.
Quinley, ED: Immunohematology: Principles and Practice. JB Lippincott, Philadelphia, 1993.
Race, RR, and Sanger, R: Blood Groups in Man, ed 5. Blackwell Scientific, Oxford, 1975.
Rothwell, NV: Understanding Genetics: A Molecular Approach. Wiley-Lissler, New York, 1993.
Stansfield, WD: Schaum's Outline Series: Theory and Problems of Genetics. McGraw-Hill, New York, 1991.
Trent, RJ: Molecular Medicine: An Introductory Text, ed 2. Churchill Livingstone, Edinburgh, 1999.
Vogel, F, and Motulsky, AG: Human Genetics: Problems and Approaches. Springer, New York, 1997.
Watson, JD, Tooze, J, and Kurtz, DT: Recombinant DNA: A Short Course. WH Freeman and Co., New York, 1983.
Winnacker, EL: From Genes to Clones: Introduction to Gene Technology. VCH, Weinheim, Germany, 1987.
Zubay, G: Biochemistry, ed 2. Macmillan, New York, 1988.

three

Fundamentals of Immunology for Blood Bankers

Lorraine Caruccio, PhD, MT(ASCP)SBB

OBJECTIVES

On completion of this chapter, the learner should be able to:

1. Describe the different components of the immune system (IS) and outline their functions.
2. Know the characteristics of the major cells of the IS and their functions.
3. List the major effector molecules and the roles they play in the immune response; for example, cytokines.
4. Understand the basic steps of hematopoiesis in the IS.
5. Briefly explain the function of the major histocompatibility complex (MHC) class I and II molecules.
6. Describe the physical characteristics of immunoglobulins in relation to structure and know the different subtypes.

7. Explain the activation sequences of the three major complement pathways and describe how they come to a common starting point.
8. List the methods used in the blood bank to detect antibodies and complement bound to red blood cells (RBCs).
9. Characterize the immune response, including antigen-antibody reactions, lymphocyte functions, and host factors that can activate and suppress the IS.
10. Discuss traditional and nontraditional laboratory techniques.
11. Know the various factors affecting agglutination reactions.
12. Be familiar with some of the more common diseases that can affect blood bank testing.

Introduction

The *immune system* (IS) is one of the most interesting, complex, and important systems in the human body. The immune system is also very old in an evolutionary sense. *Immunity* refers to the process by which a host organism protects itself from attacks by both external and internal agents. Immunity is necessary to protect the host from obvious invaders such as parasites and also against external noxious elements and sun exposure. Protection from *nonself* and abnormal *self* is controlled at different levels. The number of different types of nonself organisms includes uni- and multicellular organisms such as viroids, viruses, bacteria, mycoplasma, fungi, and parasites. Protection from these organisms historically has been the area of greatest concern in immunology research. Tumor cells, cells that are too old or misshapen to function, and cells destined for termination by apoptosis (genetically programmed cell death) within the host must be recognized and eliminated. The process of removing damaged host cells is a more recent area of immunity research. The IS must first recognize a myriad of unwanted cells, either nonself or self, and then respond correctly to remove them without destroying or damaging the host organism beyond repair. The immune system is really part of a greater system that also includes the hematopoietic, nervous, digestive, and respiratory systems. In a way, it can be said that the immune system is an integral part of every other system in the body, and without it the other systems would not be able to function. This is in part due to the complexity of the challenges it faces as well as the complexity of the organism of which it is a part.

The Role of the Immune System

The work of the IS can be divided into two separate but compatible roles. One part is the defense against foreign, external organisms and objects, and the second is to keep abnormal, damaged cells from causing havoc. The IS must first recognize abnormal cells; this can be done if they are coated with antibody, complement, or other proteins, have unusual physical conformations such as damaged red blood cells (RBCs) or have certain immune markers present on their surfaces. After the IS recognizes abnormal cells and invading agents, it must become active to remove them efficiently. There are various specialized cells and highly organized molecular cascades to accomplish this. The final result is removal of the offending agent and a return to immune equilibrium. Because the number of different agents that the IS must deal with is so large, the IS has evolved into one of the most complex systems. There are many types of cells and highly coordinated processes, as well as specialized molecules, for its use. All of the systems are interrelated and coordinated, resulting in exceptional control and versatility. Traditionally in transfusion medicine, the major focus of understanding the IS has been in the areas of antigen and antibody reactions, including indirect and direct antibody screening and crossmatching. Immunology in transfusion medicine today is often focused on hematopoietic precursor cell collection and purification, in addition to highly complex, demanding protocols for new testing methods and newer technologies to look at antigen and antibody interactions as well as reagent production. The technologist must be familiar with all of these and maintain expertise with older methods still in use. The test complexity and levels of material to be mastered directly reflects the complexity of the IS itself. It is one of the most interesting and complicated areas of modern biology and the one that historically has been most important for transfusion medicine.

This chapter can only begin to give an overall introduction to the many different areas of immunology. It will include in the first sections the biology and biochemistry of the IS, with the cells and molecules involved in its function and how they interact; the later sections will look at the testing methods used and how our IS knowledge was and is used to develop those methods. A brief discussion of immune-mediated diseases important to blood banking is included at the end. Students interested in this chapter and desiring further study can refer to any of the classic texts and publications on the IS as well as the excellent current journals with articles by the leading immunologists in the field. There are also many well-developed Web sites devoted to the subject of immunology. A good starting point for further reading is any of the noteworthy reference texts listed at the end of this chapter.

Overview of the Immune System

All organisms at all levels of life are challenged constantly by various factors from their environment and must protect against them. The host organism is a rich source of nutrients and protection for an organism that is able to avoid the host's IS. One of the most fundamental concepts in immunology is the idea of self versus nonself: how the IS distinguishes between the two and what is actually being described when we refer to these two terms. The two terms have now been broadened in meaning. In current terms, self refers to anything within the organism that derives from the host genome and the rearrangement of host genes. It includes cells, fluids, molecules, and more complex structures of a host organism. Anything put into the host body, even a close genetic match, can be regarded as nonself and can therefore be rejected by an immune response. The nonself description refers to anything outside the host physically, whether a living organism (parasites, fungus) or nonliving toxin (poison ivy fluid, insect venom). The IS also responds against damaged (senescent RBCs) or diseased cells (tumors) in the host body. In this context, because a growing fetus has a different genetic make-up than that of the mother's IS, the fetus is considered nonself and must be protected from immune responses by the placenta. When foreign objects or damaged host cells are detected by the IS, an immune response occurs. Immune responses occur at different levels and consist of the *innate* (or natural, primary) and the *acquired* (or adaptive, secondary) responses. The overall mechanisms and components of

TABLE 3–1   Comparison of the Major Mechanisms of the Immune System

Innate or Natural Immunity	Acquired or Adaptive Immunity
• Primary lines of defense	• Supplements protection provided by innate immunity
• Early evolutionary development	• Later evolutionary development—seen only in vertebrates

• Nonspecific
  • Natural—present at birth
  • Immediately available
  • May be physical, biochemical, mechanical, or a combination of defense mechanisms
	• Specific
	  • Specialized
	  • Acquired by contact with a specific foreign substance
	  • Initial contact with foreign substance triggers synthesis of specialized antibody proteins resulting in reactivity to that particular foreign substance

• Mechanism does not alter on repeated exposure to any specific antigen	• Memory
	  • Response improves with each successive encounter with the same pathogen
	  • Remembers the infectious agent and can prevent it from causing disease later
	  • Immunity to withstand and resist subsequent exposure to the same foreign substance is acquired

each are outlined in (Tables 3–1 and 3–2). The innate immune response consists of physical barriers, biochemical effectors, and immune cells. The first step of innate defense is external, including skin and enzymes present on the skin's surface. The second line of innate defense is internal and can recognize common invaders with a *nonspecific* response, such as phagocytosis that does not have to be primed. The last line of defense is the acquired immune response that needs time and reorganization to mount an effective and *specific* reaction and that protects against a repeat attack by the same organism using immune memory. The IS's specificity also prevents the host from becoming attacked and damaged during an immune response. The localized nature of an immune reaction also prevents systemic damage throughout the host organism. The wide variety of potential organisms and substances that can invade the host requires a vast array of means to recognize and remove them. The acquired

immune response must be capable of generating a near-infinite level of specific responses to all the different complex organisms and substances that the host can encounter over its lifetime. Finally, the different types of effector responses of the IS allow it to have diverse responses to self and nonself invaders.

Cellular and Humoral Immunity

The two major components of the vertebrate IS are cellular and humoral immunity. The cellular part of the system is mediated by various cells of the IS, such as macrophages, T cells, and dendritic cells. Lymphokines are other effector molecules that play critical roles in the cellular system by activating and deactivating different cells as well as allowing cells to communicate throughout the host body. Lymphokines are powerful molecules that include cytokines and chemokines.

TABLE 3–2   Cellular and Humoral Components of the Immune System

Innate or Natural Immunity		Acquired or Adaptive Immunity
First Line of Defense	**Second Line of Defense**	**Third Line of Defense**

Internal Components
Physical
• Intact skin
• Mucous membranes
• Cilia
• Cough reflex
Biochemical
• Secretions
  • Sweat
  • Tears
  • Saliva
  • Mucus
• Very low pH of vagina and stomach
	Internal Components
	• Cellular
	  • Phagocytic cells
	    • Macrophages
	    • Monocytes
	    • PMNs: Large granular leukocytes
	    • NK cells
	• Humoral (fluid)/biochemical
	  • Complement-alternate pathway
	  • Cytokines
	    • Interferons
	    • Interleukins
	• Acute inflammatory reaction
		Internal Components
		• Cellular
		  • Lymphocytes
		    • T cells
		      • T_H
		      • T_C
		    • T memory cells
		    • B cells
		    • B memory cells
		    • Plasma cells
		  • APCs
		    • Macrophages
		    • Monocytes
		    • Dendritic cells
		    • B cells
		  • Humoral
		    • Antibodies
		    • Complement-classic pathway
		    • Cytokines

APCs = antigen-presenting cells

The humoral part of the system consists of the fluid parts of the IS, such as antibodies and complement components found in plasma, saliva, and other secretions. One of the most important and key parts of humoral immunity is the antibody, a large, complex protein structure with specific effector functions. Antibodies are also called immunoglobulins, *immuno* because of their function and *globulin* because they are a type of globular soluble protein. They are found in the gamma globulin portion of plasma, or serum when it is separated by fractionation or electrophoresis. The function of the antibody is to bind to foreign molecules (usually proteins) called antigens. Most antigens are found on the surface of foreign cells or damaged internal cells. A key feature of antigen-antibody reactions is their specificity. Only one antibody reacts with one antigen, or one part (an *epitope*) of a complex antigen. An immune reaction against an antigen stimulates the production of antibodies that will match the epitope (or *antigenic determinant*) present on the antigen. The binding reaction of antigen and antibody has often been called a *lock and key* mechanism, referring to its specificity and conformity. Antigen-antibody complex formation inactivates the antigen and elicits a number of complicated effector mechanisms that will ultimately result in the destruction of the antigen and the cell to which it is bound. The laboratory study of antigen-antibody reactions is called *serology* and has been the basis of blood banking technology for many years. Antibody screening methods and crossmatching techniques rely on the detection of antigen-antibody complexes; the direct antiglobulin (*Coombs*) test relies on the detection of antibodies (and complement) bound to the surface of RBCs. **Tables 3–1** and **3–2** list the immune mechanisms and components.

Innate Immunity and Acquired Immunity

One of the ways to characterize the immune system is by its cellular and humoral components; another is by the two major ways the IS works to prevent infection and damaged cells from destroying the host. The innate part of the system is less complicated and more primitive. It does not function in a specific way, but rather it recognizes certain complex repeating patterns present on common invading organisms, such as the lipopolysaccharide coat of gram-negative bacteria. The innate part can function immediately to stop host organisms from being infected. The more advanced acquired immune response developed after vertebrates had evolved; it relies on the formation of specific antigen-antibody complexes and specific cellular responses to keep the host organism infection-resistant. Acquired immunity allows for a specific response, and IS memory allows resistance to a pathogen that was previously encountered. *Innate immunity* is the immediate line of immune defense. There are two important features of innate immunity. First, the innate immune system is nonspecific. The same response is used against invading organisms no matter what the source is as long as the innate IS can recognize them as nonself. Innate immunity is named because it is innate, or present, at birth and does not have to be learned or acquired. Second, it does not need modifications to function and is not altered with repeated exposure to the same antigen. As they developed early in evolution, certain parts of the innate immunity are seen in invertebrates as well as in vertebrates, but because innate immunity functions so

well as a first line of defense, it was maintained in the IS of vertebrates.

Physical and biochemical barriers as well as various cells make up the innate IS. Physical barriers include intact skin, mucous membranes, cilia lining the mucous membranes, and cough reflexes. Biochemicals of the innate system include bactericidal enzymes such as lysozyme and RNases, fatty acids, sweat, digestive enzymes in saliva, stomach acid, and vaginal low pH. Important innate immune cells include certain phagocytic leukocytes and natural killer (NK) cells, a type of large, granular lymphocyte. Phagocytic cells of different types are found in most tissues of the human organism such as the brain, liver, intestines, lungs, and kidneys. Phagocytes include circulating monocytes in the blood and peripheral, mobile macrophages (activated monocytes) that can move between vessel walls. Phagocytes recognize complex molecular structures on the surface of invading cells or in the secretions and fluids of the host body and are able to remove the invading organisms by engulfing and digesting them with vesicle enzymes. Two major cells that can use phagocytosis to remove pathogens are the polymorphonuclear cells, which include neutrophils, basophils, and eosinophils, and the mononuclear cells, which include the monocytes in plasma and the macrophages in tissues. Various molecules of the IS collaborate with the innate IS's cells. *Opsonins* are complex factors including antibodies and complement components in plasma that coat pathogens and facilitate phagocytosis. When phagocytes ingest foreign cells and destroy them, they can become activated to release soluble polypeptide substances called cytokines that have various effects (such as activation and proliferation) on other cells of the immune and vascular systems. There is a large number of different cytokines, some having unique functions and others having overlapping functions. Some work together, and some oppose the functions of other cytokines. Many are secreted, and some are membrane receptors. Overall, cytokines help to regulate the immune response in terms of specificity, intensity, and duration.

NK cells can recognize host cells that have been infected with virus or bacteria or abnormal host cells, such as tumor cells, because of the macromolecules on the cell's surface. NK cells are a type of large, granular T lymphocyte and probably evolved to protect the host from tumor cells and infected cells before the acquired immune response can be activated. NK cells can secrete very potent cytokines such as interferons that are specially designed to destroy virally infected cells. Virally infected cells, when lysed by the infection, release many more active virions and viral particles that can infect many more host cells. Interferon helps stop this rapid progression of disease. However, interferons only work on current infections and do not prevent a future infection from happening. Interleukins are another type of cytokine that can act by signaling other leukocytes to become active and to divide to increase their numbers. One of the most important interleukins is interleukin-2 (IL-2), which is needed by T lymphocytes to function properly in vivo and is also required to grow T lymphocytes in in-vitro conditions. Most cytokines are required at certain levels to be optimal as too few do not help to maintain a strong immune response, and too many of some cytokines can actually be detrimental to the survival and functioning of immune cells and toxic to the host organism.

Another important component of the innate immune system is the *complement system*. Complement has three major roles in immunity, including the final lysis of abnormal and pathogenic cells via the binding of antibody, opsonization of phagocytosis, and mediation of inflammation. The proteins of the complement system are enzymes that are normally found in the plasma in a *proenzyme* inactive state. Three ways the complement proteins can be activated are the classic, alternative, and lectin pathways, all with essentially the final result of cell lysis and inflammation. The classic pathway uses antigen-antibody binding and therefore is a specific activator of complement. The alternative pathway activates complement by means of recognition of polysaccharides and liposaccharides found on the surfaces of bacteria and tumor cells and therefore uses nonspecific methods of activation. The lectin pathway is activated by mannose binding proteins bound to macrophages. The inflammatory response, or inflammation, is also a critical component of the innate IS and is familiar to most people when they have a minor wound as redness and warmth at the wound site. Inflammation is initiated by any type of tissue damage, whether to the skin or to an internal organ. Burns, infection, fractures, necrosis, and superficial wounds all elicit an inflammatory response, which is characterized by an increase in blood flow to the wounded area, increased blood vessel permeability at the site to allow for greater flow of cells, a mobilization of phagocytic cells into the site, and a possible activation of heat-shock proteins and other agents that maintain the healing process at the site of tissue damage. The wound is repaired, new tissue grows in place of the damaged tissue, and inflammation is stopped. Uncontrolled inflammation can result in damage to healthy tissue as well as diseased tissue. The regulation of inflammation is tightly controlled and requires signals to turn it on and off to be effective.

The innate system also has acute phase response factors. These factors are proteins that are increased in plasma (and serum) during the early stages of an infection. They include C-reactive protein, fibrinogen, and serum amyloid protein. They are made in the liver in response to certain highly inflammatory cytokines.

Acquired immunity is the other major arm of the host's IS and is the most highly evolved. It is also the most specific and allows the IS to have memory of pathogens it has encountered previously and therefore acquire immunity with repeat exposure to an antigen. The acquired system is present only in vertebrates. The term acquired refers to the fact that the immunity is acquired via specific contact with a pathogen or aberrant cell. The adaptive term refers to the nature of this part of the IS's ability to adapt to and destroy new complex pathogens, although it must first react to them through complex recognition processes. Acquired immunity is specific in recognition of the new pathogen, and it also has specific responses depending on the type of pathogen it encounters. The acquired IS uses antibodies as specific immune effectors. Antigen specificity and uniqueness determine the particular antibody that will bind to it. The antigen-antibody complex is a three-dimensional interaction that does not allow near-misses to bind. For example, antibodies against one blood group antigen do not react against another blood group antigen. An antigen that an antibody is made against is sometimes referred to as its *antithetical* antigen. Due to the fact that acquired immunity has memory, medical histories of patients that require transfusions are absolutely critical. Antibodies do not always remain in plasma at levels seen with serologic test-ing, and if antigen-positive RBC units are transfused in a sensitized patient, the second antibody response against the transfused cell antigens can be more vigorous and may even result in intravascular RBC hemolysis, a very dangerous condition.

Cells and Organs of the Immune System

The immunization process requires many different types of cells and tissues, including phagocytic granulocytes of the innate system; the neutrophils, eosinophils, and basophils; as well as monocytes and macrophages. Lymphocytes, a type of mononuclear cell, are important in acquired immunity. They are divided into two major types, the *T lymphocyte* (T cell) and the *B lymphocyte* (B cell). The T lymphocyte matures in the thymus gland and is responsible for making cytokines and destroying virally infected host cells. B lymphocytes mature in the bone marrow, and when they are stimulated by antigen they evolve into *plasma cells* that secrete antibody. *NK cells* are a type of lymphocyte that plays a role in immune protection against viruses. *Dendritic cells* are present throughout many systems of the body and are responsible for antigen processing and are sometimes referred to as *antigen presenting cells*. Macrophages can also process antigen. T and B cells communicate with each other and are both necessary for antibody production. B cells undergo gene rearrangement in order to have the correct antibody made that can react with the correct antigen. T cells also have receptors that undergo gene rearrangement in order to react with antigens correctly. There are different types of T cells; they are distinguished by the membrane markers they possess. These markers are referred to as *clusters of differentiation* (CD) markers and are detected by immunotyping. The receptors on the cell membranes of T and B lymphocytes allow them to recognize foreign substances. Lymphocytes recognize only one specific antigen, which is determined by the genetic programming of that lymphocyte. Because there are so many different antigens that pathogens can carry, the IS has adapted to be able to recognize *millions* of different antigens, with a specific antibody that will match *only one* particular antigen. Therefore, if a foreign antigen is present, only a small percentage of the host's antibodies and T-cell receptors will recognize it. The way the IS gets around this is by activating host cells that recognize the antigen and multiplying them to great numbers. The cells that result from this multiplication are called clones and result from one single progenitor cell that divides many times. A clone is a genetic copy so all clones attack the same antigenic target as the progenitor cell. In cases where an antigen is recognized by more than one antibody, a process of clonal selection happens, in which the different cells that recognize the different epitopes of the antigen are expanded. The cells that have weak interactions with the antigen are often removed or made inactive. In transfusion medicine, this plays a role in selecting the best antibody reagents for testing as not all epitopes of a complex antigen, such as a blood group, will be equally reactive.

The maturation of B and T cells occurs after antigen is encountered. Both B and T cells mature into what are called *effector* cells, which are the functional units of the IS. The final *effect* that B and T cells bring about is the elimination of pathogens and foreign cells. Immune memory is also acquired when lymphocytes mature into memory cells after antigenic stimulation; this allows the IS to recognize antigens from previous encounters. Once an infection is cleared, some of the cells that can recognize the antigen remain in circulation. The lymphocytes are permanently set to respond to the same antigen again by the process of memory. The second time this antigen is encountered, memory allows for a more effective and rapid immune response. Memory cells can persist for the lifetime of the host. It is one of the reasons that some immunizations with vaccines do not have to be repeated except on a cautionary basis to keep the immunization active.

B Cells

Antibodies can be secreted or membrane-bound. Antibodies are secreted by mature B cells called *plasma cells* and bind to antigens in a specific manner. The antigens are usually in soluble form in the plasma. The receptor on the B cell that recognizes antigen is a membrane-bound antibody. When the receptor antibody on the B cell reacts with a specific antigen and recognizes it, the B cell is activated to divide, and the cells produced from this rapid division mature into plasma cells and memory B cells. Memory B cells can remain in the host for many years, thus providing life-long immunity. Memory B cells have antibody on their surfaces that is of the same conformation as that of the progenitor B cell from which they were derived. Plasma cells are antibody factories that make large amounts of antibody in a soluble form that remains in circulation in the plasma, body secretions, and lymphatics. Each plasma cell makes only one specific type of soluble antibody, and that antibody has the same specificity as that of the B cell from which it was derived. Antibodies can neutralize toxic substances and antigens that are encountered by binding to them and therefore preventing them from interacting with the host. When the antigenic site is nonreactive by the binding of antibody, it cannot interact with host cells to infect them or damage them. Also, binding of antigen by antibody brings about opsonization, which aids in direct killing of pathogens by cell lysis. When complement is activated by an antigen-antibody complex, the pathogen can be destroyed. Pathogens can be destroyed intra- or extravascularly. Antibodies are one of the most important components of the IS and blood bank testing procedures.

T Cells

Just as B cells are the key elements of the humoral part of the acquired IS, T cells are the most important arm of the cellular part of acquired immunity. One of the major and important differences of cellular immunity is that T cells recognize antigens that are internalized within a host cell. The antigens are then processed and presented on the host cell surface in small peptide fragments. T cell–mediated immunity is involved in the response against fungal and viral infections, intracellular parasites, tissue grafts, and tumors. T-cell receptors do not recognize foreign antigen on their own as B cells do; they require help in the form of cell membrane proteins known as major histocompatibility complex (MHC) molecules. Therefore, there is a certain level of restriction placed on the acquired cellular branch of the IS as determined by the inherited MHC molecules on host cells. The MHC genes determine the human leukocyte antigens (HLA) present on leukocytes and other cells; they have been known for many years to cause rejection of tissue grafts. There are two major classes of MHC genes and antigens, MHC class I and MHC class II. MHC class I antigens are found on most nucleated cells in the body, and MHC class II antigens are found on most antigen-presenting cells. In humans, MHC class I genes code for the HLA-A, HLA-B, and HLA-C antigens, whereas MHC class II genes code for HLA-DR, HLA-DQ, and HLA-DC antigens. Both MHC class I and MHC class II are important in the recognition of foreign substances and the immune reactions against them as well as antigen presentation processes.

There are two major functions of T cells. The first major function is to produce immune mediating substances such as cytokines, which influence many immune functions throughout the body. The second major function is to kill cells that contain foreign antigen. When T cells are activated by meeting antigen, they start to secrete cytokines and change their cellular interactions (**Table 3–3** has a list of important cytokines). T cells are also grouped into two major categories with two major functions called T helper (TH) cells and T cytotoxic (TC) cells. TH cells are also distinguished by the membrane marker CD4; TC cells are distinguished by the marker CD8. TH cells are further grouped into TH1 and TH2 and respond to different cytokines. TH cells have the ability to recognize antigen, along with MHC class II molecules, and provide help to B cells to evolve into plasma cells and make antibodies. TH cells therefore determine which antigens become IS targets as well as determine which immune mechanisms will be used against the target antigens. TH cells aid in the proliferation of immune cells after they encounter antigen and help determine which responses will happen. TH cells, in addition to helping B cells and macrophages, can also help TC cells by causing them to proliferate and differentiate and therefore become effector cells. Immune effector cells are capable of destroying pathogens, and TC cells are capable of cytotoxicity, or cell killing. Unlike TH cells that interact with MHC class II, TC cells interact with MHC class I molecules. TC cells in general do not secrete lymphokines as much as TH cells do; they are the cells that receive help from the TH cells and are then able to destroy tumor cells, virally infected cells, and tissue grafts. Like all other aspects of the acquired IS, TH cell activation must be carefully regulated to avoid attacks against the host cells. This is accomplished in part by having TH activation only in the context of the appropriate MHC class II antigen presentation as well as requiring two signals for complete activation.

Antigen-Presenting Cells (APCs)

There are several types of leukocytes that function as antigen-presenting cells (APCs), including macrophages and granulocytes such as neutrophils, as well as some B cells. In addition to leukocytes, there are specialized immune cells capable of antigen presentation. These include the different types of dendritic cells present in the skin (Langerhans cells), nervous tissue (glial cells), lymph nodes, spleen, intestines, liver (Kupffer cells), bone (osteoclasts), and thymus. These APCs first phagocytize the foreign antigen, process it internally, and then with the help of MHC molecules present short peptide sequences of the antigen on their cell membranes. TH cells can then recognize the antigen in the context of MHC presentation and respond to it by the appropriate immune reaction.

TABLE 3–3 Cytokines

Cytokine	Source	Stimulatory Function
Interleukins		
IL-1	Mφ, fibroblasts	Proliferation-activated B cells and T cells Induction PGE$_2$ and cytokines by Mφ Induction neutrophil and T-cell adhesion molecules on endothelial cells Induction IL-6, IFN-β1, and GM-CSF Induction fever, acute phase proteins, bone resorption by osteoclasts
IL-2	T	Growth-activated T cells and B cells; activation NK cells
IL-3	T, MC	Growth and differentiation hematopoietic precursors Mast cell growth
IL-4	CD4, T, MC, BM stroma	Proliferation-activated B cells, T cells, mast cells, and hematopoietic precursor Induction MHC class II and Fc∈R on B cells, p75 IL-2R on T cells Isotype switch to IgG1 and IgE Mφ APC and cytotoxic function, Mφ fusion (migration inhibition)
IL-5	CD4, T, MC	Proliferation-activated B cells; production IgM and IgA Proliferation eosinophils; expression p55 IL-2R
IL-6	CD4, T, Mφ, MC, fibro-blasts	Growth and differentiation B-cell and T-cell effectors and hemopoietic precursors Induction acute phase proteins
IL-7	BM stromal cells	Proliferation pre-B cells, CD4 cells, CD8 cells, and activated mature T cells
IL-8	Monocytes	Chemotaxis and activation neutrophils Chemotaxis T cells Inhibits IFN-γ secretion
IL-9	T	Growth and proliferation T cells
IL-10	CD4, T, B, Mφ	Inhibits mononuclear cell inflammation
IL-11	BM stromal cells	Induction acute phase proteins
IL-12	T	Activates NK cells
IL-13	T	Inhibits mononuclear phagocyte inflammation
Colony Stimulating Factors		
GM-CSF	T, Mφ, fibroblasts, MC, endothelium	Growth of granulocyte and Mφ colonies Activated Mφ, neutrophils, eosinophils
G-CSF	Fibroblasts, endothelium	Growth of mature granulocytes
M-CSF	Fibroblasts, endotheli-um, epithelium	Growth of macrophage colonies
Steel factor	BM stromal cells	Stem cell division (c-kit ligand)
Tumor Necrosis Factors		
TNF-α	Mφ, T	Tumor cytotoxicity; cachexia
TNF-β	T	Induction acute phase proteins Antiviral and antiparasitic activity Activation phagocytic cells Induction IFN-γ, TNF-α, IL-1, GM-CSF, and IL-6
Interferons		
IFN-α	Leukocytes	Antiviral; expression MHC I
IFN-β	Fibroblasts	
IFN-γ	T	Antiviral; Mφ activation Expression MHC class I and II on Mφ and other cells Differentiation of cytotoxic T cells Synthesis IgG2a by activated B cells Antagonism several IL-4 actions
Other		
TGF-β	T, B	Inhibition IL-2R upregulation and IL-2 dependent T-cell and B-cell proliferation Inhibition (by TGF-β1) of IL-3 and CSF induced hematopoiesis Isotype switch to IgA Wound repair (fibroblast chemotaxin) and angiogenesis Neoplastic transformation of certain normal cells
LIF	T	Proliferation of embryonic stem cells without affecting differentiation Chemoattraction and activation of eosinophils

Roitt, I: Essential Immunology, ed 8. Blackwell Scientific Publications, London, 1994, with permission.

APC = antigen-presenting cells; BM = bone marrow; CSIF = cytokine synthesis inhibitory factor, Fc∈R = immunoglobulin Fc receptor for IgE; G-CSF = granulocyte colony stimulating factor; GM-CSF = granulocyte monocyte/macrophage colony stimulating factor; IFN = interferon; IL = interleukin; LIF = leukocyte inhibitory factor; MC = mast cell; M-CSF = monocyte colony stimulating factor; MHC = major histocompatibility complex; Mφ = macrophage; NK = natural killer cells; PGE$_2$ = prostaglandin E$_2$; T = T lymphocyte; TGF = transforming growth factor; TNF = tumor necrosis factor.

TABLE 3–4   Lymphoid Organs Associated with the Acquired Immune System

Primary Lymphoid Organs	Secondary Lymphoid Organs
• Thymus • Bone marrow	• Lymph nodes • Spleen • Mucosa-associated tissues
Site of maturation for T and B cells Lymphocytes differentiate from stem cells, then migrate to secondary lymphoid organs	Site of cell function for mature T and B cells Cells interact with each other, accessory cells, and antigens

Immune System Organs

The organs of the IS are divided into two sections called the primary and the secondary. The primary lymphoid organs are the thymus and bone marrow, where immune cells differentiate and mature, and the secondary lymphoid organs include the lymph nodes and spleen, in which immune cells interact with each other and process antigens (Table 3–4).

Immune Maturation

Because of the complexity and diversity of immune responses, a specific immediate immune response is not always possible. It usually takes days to months for all the aspects of an efficient immune response to happen from the moment that antigen is first encountered. The lag phase until an appropriate immune response occurs is called the *latency* or *window period*. It is during this time that antibody cannot be detected with serologic testing. During the latency period, however, T and B cells are very active in processing antigen and initiating the primary response to the antigen. The first antibodies made against the new antigen are different from the antibodies of the secondary response. The primary antibodies are of the immunoglobulin M (IgM) subclass, whereas the antibodies of the secondary response are of the immunoglobulin G (IgG) subclass and have a different structure (**Fig. 3–1**). After the antigen is cleared, memory cells are stored in immune organs of the host. When the same antigen is encountered again, the memory cells are activated and produce a stronger and more rapid response. IgG antibodies are formed during the secondary response and are made in great quantities, and although IgM is made during the primary response, there is a period when it overlaps with the production of IgG antibodies at the beginning of the secondary response. IgG secondary antibodies have a higher avidity for antigen and can be produced by much lower concentrations of antigen. Secondary antibodies can usually be measured within 1 to 2 days. For example, a primary antibody may require more than 100-fold excess of antigen to initiate the first response. Many of the antigens that stimulate the primary response have multiple repeating epitopes such as polysaccharides and are therefore good immune stimulators at lower concentrations.

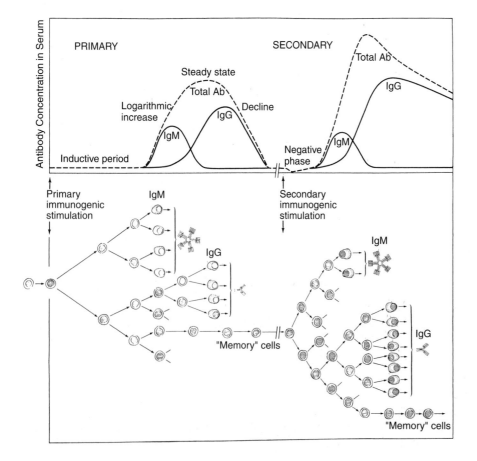

■ **FIGURE 3–1** Schematic representation of primary and secondary antibody responses. Note the enhanced antibody production and expanded antibody-producing cell population during the secondary antibody response. (From Herscowitz, HB: Immunophysiology. In Bellanti, JA [ed]: Immunology III. WB Saunders, Philadelphia, 1985, p 117, with permission.)

Cell Lineages and Markers

Nearly all cells of the host's body, especially the various leukocytes, have specific cell markers or *receptors* with which they interact with other cells and receive signals from cellular messenger systems. Macrophages, NK cells, T and B cells, and APCs can interact directly with cell-to-cell communication or indirectly by specific, soluble mediators through a complex system. These cell surface molecules are classified by complex in-vitro testing using monoclonal antibodies. They specify cellular definitions and functions including maturation levels and lineage specificity and are designated as CD markers. These markers on cells can change during the lifetime of the cell or in response to infection or activation. Currently, there are nearly 200 different CD markers known; the first were identified on immune cells. CD markers are critical to identify hematopoietic cell maturation stages and lineages.

All immune cells originate from pluripotent hematopoietic progenitors (also called hematopoietic stem cells, or CD34-positive cells) through one of two pathways of lineage, the *myeloid* and the *lymphoid*. Various growth factors are responsible for differentiating and maturing stem cells into the many different cells of the IS. Growth factors also allow progenitor stem cells to reproduce themselves as well as to develop into more differentiated types of cells. The cells of the myeloid lineage consist of phagocytic cells such as the monocytes and macrophages, often referred to as the mononuclear phagocytic system (MPS), and the granulocytes or polymorphonuclear cells (PMNs), the neutrophils, eosinophils, and the basophils, in addition to the APCs such as the dendritic cells in the skin and liver. Erythrocytes as well as platelets originate from this system. The lymphoid lineage consists of the various subpopulations of lymphoid cells, the T cells, B cells, and NK cells.

The myeloid-monocyte precursors originate in the bone marrow and then differentiate into circulating blood monocytes. When monocytes encounter antigen, they can differentiate into tissue macrophages. One of the main functions of the MPS cells is processing of antigen, which is required to remove pathogen by the acquired IS. Phagocytic cells can directly kill many pathogens such as bacteria and fungi as part of the innate IS. As mentioned above, MPS cells present antigen to lymphocytes after processing it and interact with other immune cells via cell membrane receptors. The Fc part of the antibody receptor and the complement receptor CR1 are used by phagocytes during opsonization.[1] When these cells are functioning as APCs, they express the MHC class II molecules on their membranes and lack the Fc receptor. Granulocytes originate in the bone marrow. They are the predominant leukocyte in the circulation of the mature adult (60 to 70 percent). Granulocytes all have granules in their cytoplasm and are of three types, distinguished by the hematologic staining of their granules. The neutrophils stain a faint purple or neutral color (neutral granules), the eosinophils a reddish orange color (acidic granules), and the basophils a bluish black color (basic granules). The main role of these cells is phagocytosis; they function primarily in acute inflammatory responses and have enzymes and other molecules that allow them to destroy engulfed pathogens. All three types of granulocytes possess receptors for the Fc portion of IgG (CD16) and complement receptors C5a, CR1(CD35), and CR3(CD11b). Additionally, eosinophils possess low-affinity Fc receptors for IgE and therefore play a critical role in allergic reactions and inflammation in parasitic infections. Basophils and mast cells (a type of tissue basophil) possess high-affinity Fc immunoglobulin E (IgE) receptors, are powerful effectors of inflammation and allergic reactions, and can cause the release of localized histamine.

Lymphocytic cells are generated in the thymus or bone marrow and travel through the circulatory system to the lymph nodes and spleen, where they mature and differentiate. In a mature adult, the lymphocytes account for about 20 to 30 percent of the circulating leukocytes. In primary organs, these cells acquire receptors that enable them to interact with antigens and also to differentiate between self and nonself antigens, a very critical part of lymphocyte maturation and the acquired IS in general. In the secondary organs, immune cells are provided with a highly interactive environment in which immune responses are exchanged and made specific. Remember, there are two primary classifications of lymphocytes, T and B cells, and these similar-looking cells can be distinguished by the presence of specific cell markers by means of using sophisticated immunologic methods of testing, such as flow cytometry (discussed later in this chapter). Specific to the T cell is the T cell antigen receptor (TCR), which is in proximity to and usually identified with the CD3 complex on the T-cell membrane. The TCR is a heterodimer of two polypeptides, the α and β. It associates in cell-to-cell contacts and interacts with both antigenic determinants and MHC proteins. In addition to CD3 on T cells, there is the separate CD2 marker, also referred to as the T11 or the leukocyte function antigen-3 (LFA-3), and it seems to be involved in cell adhesion. It has the unique ability to bind with sheep erythrocytes in-vitro. One of the most important discoveries about T cells is the distinction that TH cells have the CD4 marker and recognize antigen together with the MHC class II molecules, and TC cells possess CD8 markers and interact with MHC class I molecules. The ratios of T cells with CD4 versus CD8-positive cells can be a marker for particular diseases. One of the defining features of AIDS is a reversal of the typical CD4 to CD8 ratio, which helped to explain some of the pathology of AIDS.

There are also compounds referred to as superantigens, which can stimulate multiple T cells, causing them to release large amounts of cytokines. Certain bacteria toxins are superantigens and can lead to lethal reactions in the host if the immune system is overstimulated.

B cells are defined by the presence of immunoglobulin on their surface; however, they also possess MHC class II antigens (antigen presentation), the complement receptors CD35 and CD21, Fc receptors for IgG, and CD19, CD20, and CD22 markers, which are the CD markers used to identify B cells. Membrane-bound immunoglobulin may act as an antigen receptor for binding simple structural antigens or antigens with multiple repeating determinants (referred to as T cell–independent antigens, meaning they do not require the intervention of T cell help). When T cell–dependent antigens (structurally complex and unique substances, such as virus particles) are encountered, B cells require the intervention of T cells to assist in the production of antibody. When B cells become activated, they mature and develop into plasma cells, which produce and secrete large quantities of soluble Ig into tissue or plasma.

The third major class of lymphocytes, the NK cells, are sometimes referred to as *third population cells* because they originate in the bone marrow from a developmental line distinct from those of T and B lymphocytes. They are also referred to as large granular lymphocytes. Unlike B cells, NK cells do not have surface Ig or secrete Ig, nor do they have antigen receptors like the TCR of T cells. NK cells have the CD56 and CD16 markers and do not require the presence of an MHC marker to respond to an antigen. They are thymus-independent and are able to lyse virally infected cells and tumor cells directly in a process known as *antibody-dependent cell-mediated cytotoxicity* (ADCC) by anchoring immunoglobulin to the cell surface membrane through an Fc receptor.

Cytokines and Immunoregulatory Molecules

Cytokines are soluble protein or peptide molecules that function as powerful mediators of the immune response. There are two main cytokine types, *lymphokines*, which are produced by lymphocytes, and *monokines*, which are produced by monocytes and macrophages. Cytokines function in a complex manner by regulating growth, mobility, and differentiation of leukocytes. One cytokine may act by itself or together with other cytokines. Other cytokines oppose the actions of one or more cytokines and function to quantitatively increase or decrease a particular immune reaction. Some cytokines are synergistic and need each other to have their full effect. The effects of cytokines can be in the immediate area of their release or at a point quite distant from it as they can travel through the plasma to affect distant cells and tissues. There is often significant overlap in how cytokines function.

The major classes of cytokines include the interleukin (IL), interferon (IFN), tumor necrosis factor (TNF), and colony-stimulating factor (CSF); each class has several members (see **Table 3–3**). Cytokines act by binding to specific target cell receptors. When cytokines bind to their receptors on cells, the number of receptors is often increased as the cell is stimulated. Internal cellular signaling pathways become activated. The cell is no longer in a resting state and can have a new function. The initial signal for this transformation may be the binding of antigen. For example, interleukin-2 (IL-2), a cytokine necessary for lymphocyte function, requires an initial signal to be the antigen presented by an APC to a T cell; the production and response of IL-2 receptor, therefore, is maximized by an antigen activated T cell. After cytokine binding, both the receptor and the cytokine become internalized, which induces the target cell to grow and *differentiate*. Differentiated cells have specialized functions such as secreting antibodies or producing enzymes. Immune cells and other host cells respond to cytokines and can react with chemoattraction, as well as antiviral, antiproliferation, and immunomodulation. Cytokines fine-tune the IS and also function as critical cell activators. In addition to the cytokines, other mediator substances of the IS, including chemokines, immunoglobulins, complement proteins, kinins, clotting factors, acute phase proteins, stress-associated proteins, and the fibrinolytic system, are cellular products that can have powerful cellular effects. Cytokines typically communicate between cells through the plasma. Chemokines are attractant molecules that interact between cells, immunoglobulins, and complement proteins and are important in destroying pathogens, kinins, and clotting factors. Acute phase proteins and fibrinolytic proteins play a role in inflammation, a process that recruits appropriate cells to an immune site and modifies the vascular system. In addition to inflammation and cell-to-cell communication, some cytokines are immunosuppressive. One of the important chemokine receptors in blood banking is the Duffy antigen group present on RBCs; the lack of these antigens can prevent certain types of malaria parasites from infecting the host. Another important chemokine receptor is CCR5, which plays a role in resistance to HIV-1 infection.

Basic Immune System Genetics

Individuals have a unique immune response based on their genetic inheritance. In experimental animals, such as guinea pigs, there are familial patterns of susceptibility and resistance. In blood banking this is important because not all transfusion recipients make antibodies to alloantigens on transfused RBCs. *Responders* are people who have a tendency based on their inheritance to make antibodies. The terms *high responders* and *low responders* describe individual responses to antigen challenges. Both T and B cells have antigen receptor molecules on their membranes, and these molecules consist of two polypeptide chains. These proteins are synthesized by two genes located on two different chromosomes. The T and B cell antigen receptor protein genes are both found on chromosome 14 but at separate loci. The second locus for B cells may be on chromosome 2 or chromosome 22, and the second T-cell locus is found on chromosome 7.[2] The enormous level of diversity of the immune response cannot be explained by only one gene coding for every immunoglobulin or T-cell receptor; research on IS genetics has revealed that antibody and T-cell receptor genes can move and rearrange themselves to very high levels of diversity and are genetically mobile. The *germ line DNA* is found at the same locus as in an unmodified gene of an inherited chromosome and is identical to all genetic information of all other body cells. During early development and differentiation, lymphocyte germ line DNA can move to another position on the chromosome. The germ line DNA also possesses immense repetition. The mechanism of rearrangement during differentiation is necessary to bring together sets of genes that result in complete new protein arrangements. This random rearrangement and assortment are what generate much of the diversity in antibody and T-cell receptor specificity. Once DNA rearrangement has occurred, the antigenic specificity of that particular cell is fixed, and the unnecessary and unused genetic material is eliminated.[3] When antigenic stimulation occurs, one B cell forms an antibody with a single specificity. During the lifetime of the cell, the cell can switch to make a different isotype (class) of antibody that has the same antigen specificity. Isotype switching requires further DNA rearrangement in mature B cells. Class switching is dependent on antigenic stimulation as well as the presence of cytokines released by T cells and reflects the further adaptation of the immune response. Isotype switching is seen in blood banking when antibodies react at different temperatures and phases.

The genetic recombination events that are required to produce mature B and T cells that secrete antibodies and have TCRs, respectively, with defined specificity are under control of the RAG-1 and RAG-2 genes. These are the recombination-activating genes 1 and 2 and are necessary for maturation of B and T cells as well as production of specific effector molecules.

The *major histocompatibility complex* (MHC) is the region of the genome that encodes the *human leukocyte antigen* (HLA) proteins and is extremely important in immunology. The MHC is critical in immune recognition and regulation of antigen presentation in cell-to-cell interactions, transplantation, paternity testing, and specific HLA patterns. It also seems to correlate with susceptibility for certain diseases. HLA molecules are categorized into two classes: MHC class I and MHC class II. Class I molecules are found on all nucleated cells except trophoblasts and sperm and play a key role in cytotoxic T-cell function. MHC class I molecules consist of a peptide binding region, a transmembrane portion, and an intracellular signaling region. β_2-Microglobulin, a thymic-derived peptide, is noncovalently linked to the MHC class I molecule. It helps to stimulate T cells. When antigen is recognized by a CD8 T cell, it must be recognized within the context of a class I molecule (**Figs. 3–2** and **3–3**); after recognition, the cytotoxic cell destroys the target cell bearing the antigen. Class II molecules are found on antigen-presenting cells such as B lymphocytes, activated T cells, and the various dendritic cells. They consist of a peptide binding region, a transmembrane portion, and an intracellular section for signaling. Class II molecules on APCs are essential for presenting processed antigen to CD4 T cells and are necessary for T-cell functions and B-cell help (**Figs. 3–4** and **3–5**). In addition, there are class III molecules that encode complement components such as C2, C4, and factor B. The genes for MHC classes I–III molecules are located on the short arm of chromosome 6 and are highly *polymorphic* in nature with multiple alleles.

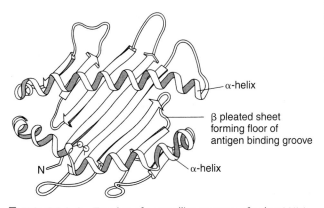

■ **FIGURE 3–3**   Top view of a crystalline structure of a class I HLA molecule. The molecule is shown as the T-cell receptor would see it. The antigen-binding site formed by the α helices (ribbonlike structures) and β pleated strands (broad arrows) is shown. N indicates the amino terminus. (From Swartz, BD: The human major histocompatibility human leukocyte antigen (HLA) complex. In Stites, DP, and Terr, AL: Basic and Clinical Immunology, ed. 7. Appleton & Lange, Norwalk, CT, 1991, p 48, with permission.)

Immune Suppression

Immune suppression can be due to a number of factors. Certain cytokines, including interleukins and some growth factors, can cause a decrease in immune responsiveness. Suppression of some IS components is critical at certain times so that the IS does not become overactivated and attack host cells. T and B cells that recognize host cells and might

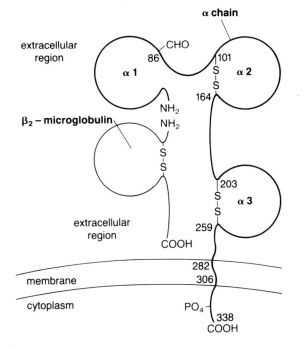

■ **FIGURE 3–2**   Class I HLA molecule. Molecule consists of an MW 44,000 polymorphic transmembrane glycoprotein, termed the α *chain,* which bears the antigenic determinant, in noncovalent association with an MW 12,000 nonpolymorphic protein termed β_2 *microglobulin.* The α chain has three extracellular domains termed α_1, α_2, and α_3. NH_2 = amino terminus; COOH = carboxy terminus; CHO = carbohydrate side chain; -SS- = disulfide bond; PO_4 = phosphate radical. (From Swartz, BD: The human major histocompatibility human leukocyte antigen (HLA) complex. In Stites, DP, and Terr, AL: Basic and Clinical Immunology, ed 7. Appleton & Lange, Norwalk, CT, 1991, p 47, with permission.)

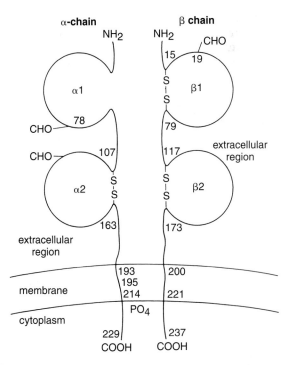

■ **FIGURE 3–4**   Class II (HLA–DR) molecule. The molecule consists of an MW 34,000 glycoprotein (the α chain) in a noncovalent association with an MW 29,000 glycoprotein (the β chain). (From Swartz, BD: The human major histocompatibility human leukocyte antigen (HLA) complex. In Stites, DP and Terr, AL: Basic and Clinical Immunology, ed 7. Appleton & Lange, Norwalk, CT, 1991, p 49, with permission.)

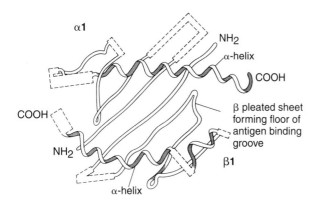

■ FIGURE 3-5   Top view of a crystalline structure of a class II HLA molecule. The molecule is shown as the T-cell receptor would see it. The antigen-binding site formed by the α chain, α₁ domain, and β chain β₁ domain consists of the β pleated sheet platform (thin strands) supporting two α helices (ribbonlike structures) and is very similar to that of the class I molecule (see Fig. 3-3). (From Swartz, BD: The human major histocompatibility human leukocyte antigen (HLA) complex. In Stites, DP, and Terr, AL: Basic and Clinical Immunology, ed. 7. Appleton & Lange, Norwalk, CT, 1991, p 50, with permission.)

destroy them must be removed before they can develop into mature lymphocytes. After much debate, specific suppressor cells have recently been isolated and seem to have unique CD profiles. They probably play a role in modulating lymphocyte function. Immune suppression can also occur when there is too little immunoglobulin made or too many T and B cells are lost through severe infection, extreme immune stimulation, or IS organ failure. Various drugs such as corticosteroids and AZT have immune-suppressive functions, and some are used to treat autoimmune diseases and graft recipients. Certain infectious diseases such as AIDS can also cause host immunosuppression. In addition, it has been observed that transfusion of blood products, especially if not leukoreduced, can cause a temporary immunomodulation. The reasons behind this are not clear. Immunosuppresion can occur due to inherited diseases such as the genetic lesions that cause severe combined immunodeficiency disease. Other forms of immunosuppression are acquired such as with drugs (steroids) or disease conditions (AIDS). Immunosuppression can also be due to severe

malnutrition. Immunosuppression is important in blood banking because immunosuppressed and immunocompromised patients must receive irradiated blood products so that the donor lymphocytes do not engraft and attack the recipient's IS and destroy it.

Characteristics of Immunoglobulins

Immunoglobulin (Ig), also called antibody, is a complex protein produced by plasma cells, with specificity to antigens (or immunogens), that stimulates their production. An Ig is a specific host self protein produced in response to a specific foreign nonself protein or other complex molecule not found in or tolerated by the host. Immunoglobulins make up a high percentage of the total proteins in disseminated body fluids, about 20 percent in a normal individual. Antibodies bind antigen, fix complement, facilitate phagocytosis, and neutralize toxic substances in the circulation. Thus, antibodies have multiple functions, some more highly specialized and specific than others. Immunoglobulins are classified according to the molecular structure of their heavy chains. The five classifications are IgA (α [alpha] heavy chain), IgD (δ [delta] heavy chain), IgE (ε [epsilon] heavy chain), IgG (γ [gamma] heavy chain), and IgM (μ [mu] heavy chain). Table 3-5 illustrates some of the various differences in the classes of immunoglobulins, such as molecular weight, percentage in serum, *valency* (number of antigen-binding sites), carbohydrate content, half-life in the blood, and whether they exist as monomers or multimers. IgG is the most concentrated in serum, approximately 80 percent of the total serum Ig; next is IgA, at about 13 percent (although it is the major Ig found in body secretions); 6 percent is IgM; 1 percent is IgD; and IgE is the least common and is present at less than 1 percent.[4]

Immunoglobulin (IG) Structure

All classes and subclasses of immunoglobulins have a common biochemical structural configuration with structural similarities and are probably derived from a common evolutionary molecular structure with well-defined function (Fig. 3-6). The basic Ig structural unit is composed of four polypeptide chains: two identical light chains (molecular weights of approximately 22,500 daltons) and two identical

TABLE 3-5 Characteristics of Serum Immunoglobulins					
Characteristic	**IgA**	**IgD**	**IgE**	**IgG**	**IgM**
Heavy chain type	Alpha	Delta	Epsilon	Gamma	Mu
Sedimentation coefficient(s)	7–15*	7	8	6.7	19
Molecular weight (kD)	160–500	180	196	150	900
Biologic half-life (d)	5.8	2.8	2.3	21	5.1
Carbohydrate content (%)	7.5–9.0	10–13	11–12	2.2–3.5	7–14
Placental transfer	No	No	No	Yes	No
Complement fixation (classic pathway)	–	–	–	+	+++
Agglutination in saline	+	–	–	±	++++
Heavy chain allotypes	A$_m$	None	None	G$_m$	None
Proportion of total immunoglobulin (%)	13	1	0.002	80	6

*May occur in monomeric or polymeric structural forms.
kD = kilodaltons; d = days; – = absent; ± = weak reactivity; + = slight reactivity; +++ = strong reactivity; ++++ = very strong reactivity.

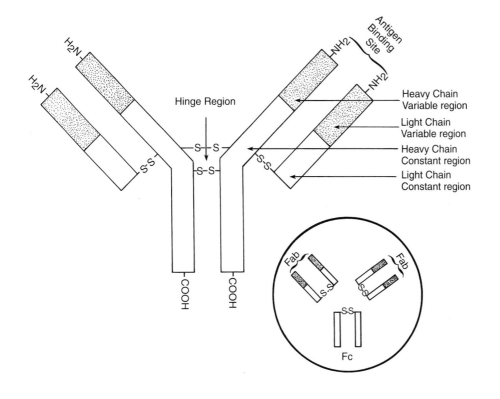

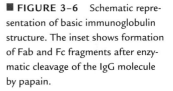

■ **FIGURE 3–6**   Schematic representation of basic immunoglobulin structure. The inset shows formation of Fab and Fc fragments after enzymatic cleavage of the IgG molecule by papain.

heavy chains (molecular weights from approximately 50,000 to 75,000 daltons). Covalent disulfide bonding holds both the light and heavy chains together, and the covalent disulfide linkages in Ig molecules provide greater structural strength than do hydrogen bonding and van der Waals forces. However, they limit the flexibility of the Ig molecule **(Fig. 3–7)**. The heavy chains are also interconnected by disulfide linkages in the hinge region of the molecule. Although there are five types of heavy chains, there are only two types of light chains, κ (kappa) and λ (lambda); both types are found in all classes of immunoglobulins regardless of heavy chain classification.

Ig molecules are proteins and therefore have two terminal regions, the *amino* (-NH$_2$) terminal, when written from the left, and the *carboxyl* (-COOH) terminal, when written from the right of the sequence. The carboxyl region of all heavy chains has a relatively constant amino acid sequence; this region is named the *constant* region. It has a constant structure because it binds to relatively constant regions on receptors. Like the heavy chain, the light chain also has a constant region. Due to certain common Ig structures, enzyme treatment yields specific cleavage products of defined molecular weight and structure. The enzyme papain splits the antibody molecule at the hinge region to give three fragments, the crystalizable fragment, the *Fc* fragment, and two that are called antigen-binding fragments, *FAB*. The Fc fragment encompasses that portion of the Ig molecule from the carboxyl region to the hinge region and is responsible for complement fixation as well as monocyte binding by Fc receptors on cells and placental transfer (IgG only). In contrast to the carboxyl terminal regions, the amino terminal regions of both light and heavy chains of immunoglobulins are known as the *variable* regions because they are structured according to the great variation in antibody specificity. Structurally and functionally the Fab fragments encompass the portions of the

Ig from the hinge region to the amino terminal and are the regions responsible for binding antigen **(Fig. 3–6)**.

The *domains* of immunoglobulins are the regions of the light and heavy chains that are folded into compact globular loop structures **(Fig. 3–7)**. The domains are held together by intrachain covalent disulfide bonds; the V region of the domain specifies the variable region, and the C is the constant region. The domains are also specified according to light and heavy chains. Looking at one half of an Ig molecule, one domain (V$_L$) is the variable region, and one domain (C$_L$) is in the constant region of each light chain, and one variable domain (V$_H$) is also on each heavy chain. The number of domains is determined by the isotype. There are three constant domains, C$_H$1 to C$_H$3, on the heavy chains of IgA, IgD, and IgG, and four constant domains, C$_H$1 to C$_H$4, on the heavy chains of IgE and IgM. The antigen-binding, or *idiotypic*, regions (which distinguish one V domain from all other V domains) are located within the three-dimensional structures formed by the V$_L$ and V$_H$ domains together. Certain heavy chain domains are associated with particular biologic properties of immunoglobulins, especially those of IgG and IgM, and include complement fixation. They are identified with the C$_H$2 domain and the C$_H$3 domains, which serve as attachment sites for the Fc receptor of monocytes and macrophages.

Immunoglobulins Significant for Blood Banking

All immunoglobulins can be significant for transfusion medicine; however, IgG, IgM, and IgA have the most significance for the blood bank. Most *clinically significant* antibodies react at body temperature (37°C), are IgG isotype, and are capable of destroying transfused antigen-positive RBCs and causing anemia and transfusion reactions of various severities. IgM antibodies are most commonly encountered as *naturally*

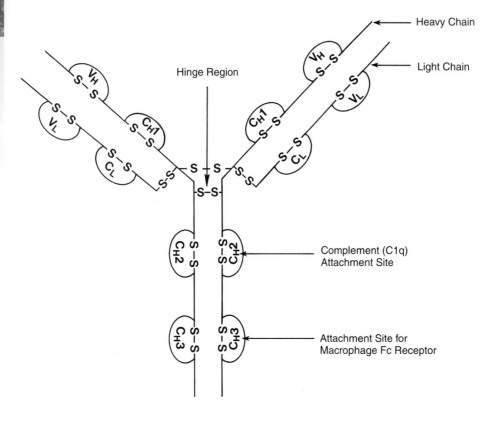

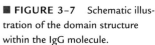

■ **FIGURE 3–7** Schematic illustration of the domain structure within the IgG molecule.

occurring antibodies in the ABO system and are believed to be produced in response to commonly occurring antigens like intestinal flora and pollen grains. They are to be *expected* in plasma and are therefore important in reverse group (or back type) testing. Other blood groups such as Lewis, Ii, P, and MNS may also produce IgM antibodies, which usually react best at ambient temperature (22°–24°C). The primary testing problem encountered with IgM antibodies is that they can interfere with the detection of clinically significant IgG antibodies by masking their reactivity. Unlike IgG, IgM exists in both monomeric and polymeric forms (as pentamers) containing a J (joining) chain. The pentameric form can be dissociated through cleavage of covalent bonds interconnecting the monomeric subunits and the J chain by chemical treatment with sulfhydryl reducing reagents such as β-2-mercaptoethanol (2-ME) or dithiothreitol (DTT) **(Fig. 3–8)**. These reagents can distinguish a mixture of IgM and IgG antibodies because only IgM is removed by the use of such compounds; therefore, the removal allows unexpected IgG to be detected. IgG antibodies are significant in transfusion medicine because they are the class of immunoglobulins that are made in response to transfusion with nonself and therefore are incompatible RBCs and other blood products. IgG antibodies are important in hemolytic disease of the newborn (HDN) because antibodies can be formed in response against alloantigens on fetal RBCs that enter the mother's circulation, usually during delivery. HDN can be fatal. It is one area of medicine where immunohematology has provided prevention and treatment. Antibody screening, Rh typing, and passive anti-D antibody have prevented HDN from developing in D-negative mothers who give birth to D-positive babies. IgG has the greatest number of subclasses: IgG$_1$, IgG$_2$, IgG$_3$, and IgG$_4$, and all four are easily separated by electrophoresis. The small differences in the chemical structure within the con-

stant regions of the gamma heavy chains designate the various subclasses, and the number of disulfide bonds between the two heavy chains in the hinge region of the molecule constitutes one of the main differences between subclasses. Functional differences between the subclasses include the ability to fix complement and cross the placenta **(Table 3–6)**. IgG blood group antibodies of a single specificity are not necessarily one specific subclass; all four subclasses may be present, or one may predominate. For example, the antibodies to the Rh system antigens are mostly of the IgG$_1$ and IgG$_3$ subclasses, whereas anti-K (Kell), and anti-Fy (Duffy) antibodies are usually of the IgG$_1$ subclass. Anti-Jk (Kidd) antibodies are mainly IgG$_3$ and may account for the unusual nature of these different antibodies with regard to testing and clinical significance. The purpose for the existence of biologic differences in subclass expression is as yet unknown. Especially important in blood banking, severe HDN has been most often associated with IgG$_1$ antibodies.[5]

Like IgM, IgA exists in two main forms, a monomer and polymer form, as dimers or trimers composed of two or three identical monomers, respectively, joined by a J chain. IgA is located in different parts of the IS depending on subclass. Serum IgA is found in both monomeric and polymeric forms; however, secretory IgA is usually found in the mucosal tissues of the body. Its polymer form acquires a glycoprotein secretory component as it passes through epithelial cell walls of mucosal tissues and appears in nearly all body fluids, including saliva, tears, bronchial secretions, prostatic fluid, vaginal secretions, and the mucous secretions of the small intestine. IgA is important in immunohematology because about 30 percent of anti-A and anti-B antibodies are of the IgA class (the remaining percentages are IgM and IgG) **(Fig. 3–9)**.[6] Also, anti-IgA antibodies can cause severe problems if transfused in plasma products to patients who are deficient in IgA,

TABLE 3–6 Biologic Properties of IgG Subclasses

Characteristic	IgG$_1$	IgG$_2$	IgG$_3$	IgG$_4$
Proportion of total serum IgG (%)	65–70	23–28	4–7	3–4
Complement fixation (classic pathway)	++	+	+++	−
Binding to macrophage Fc receptors	+++	++	+++	±
Ability to cross placenta	+	±	+	+
Dominant antibody activities:				
Anti-Rh	++	−	+	±
Anti-factor VII	−	−	−	+
Anti-dextran	−	+	−	−
Anti-Kell	+	−	−	−
Anti-Duffy	+	−	−	−
Anti-platelet	−	−	+	−
Biologic half-life (days)	21	21	7–8	21

− = absent; ± = weak (or unusual) reactivity; + = slight (or usual) reactivity; ++ = moderate (or more common) reactivity; +++ = strong reactivity.

as potentially fatal anaphylaxis can result. Another reason for the importance of IgA is that IgA can increase the effect of IgG-induced RBC hemolysis.[7]

IgE is normally found only in monomeric form in trace concentrations in serum, about 0.004 percent of total immunoglobulins, and is important in allergic reactions. The Fc portion of the IgE molecule attaches to basophils and mast cells and facilitates histamine release when an allergen binds to the Fab portion of the molecule and cross-links with a second molecule on the cell surface. Histamine is critical for bringing about an allergic reaction. Although hemolytic transfusion reactions are not caused by IgE, urticaria may occur because of the presence of IgE antibodies. Because IgE causes transfusion reactions by release of histamines, patients who have several allergic reactions to blood products can be pretreated with antihistamines to counteract the response when receiving blood products.[8] IgD, present as less than 1 percent of serum immunoglobulins, appears to have functions that deal primarily with maturation of B cells into plasma cells. IgD is usually found bound to the membrane of immature B cells. Therefore, IgD may be necessary for regulatory roles during B-cell differentiation and antibody production but is probably the least significant for blood banking.[9]

ISOTYPES OF ABO ANTIBODIES

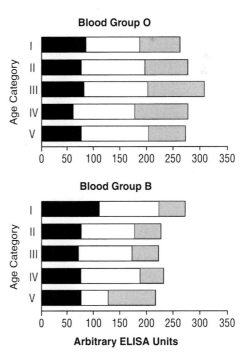

FIGURE 3–9 Distribution of anti-A IgM, IgG, and IgA antibodies by age categories, IgM (black), IgG (white), IgA (gray), expressed as arbitrary ELISA units. Age categories: I = 20–30 years; II = 31–40 years; III = 41–50 years; IV = 51–60 years; V = 61–67 years. (Adapted with permission from Transfusion, published by American Association of Blood Banks. Rieben, R, et al: Antibodies to histo-blood group substances A and B: Agglutination titers, Ig class, and IgG subclasses in healthy persons of different age categories. Transfusion 31:613, 1991.)

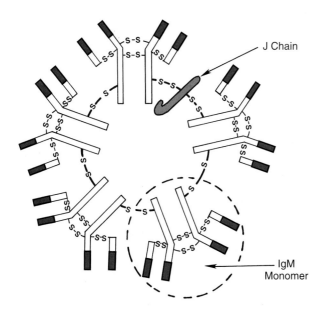

FIGURE 3–8 Schematic representation of the pentameric configuration of the IgM immunoglobulin.

Ig Variations

There are three main types of antibody-inherited variation: isotype, allotype, and idiotype. Isotype (or class variation) refers to variants present in all members of a species, including the different heavy and light chains and the different subclasses. All humans have the same Ig classes and subclasses. Allotypic variation is present primarily in the constant region; not all variants occur in all members of a species. Idiotypic variation, which determines the antigen-binding specificity (or *complementary determining regions*, [CDRs]) of antibodies and T-cell receptors, is found only in the variable (and *hypervariable*) regions and is specific for each antibody molecule.

Allotypic determinants have been defined at specific locations on the C_L domains of kappa light chains (K_m markers), on the constant domains of IgA_2 (A_{2m} markers), and on the constant domains of IgG (G_m markers). Three K_m, two A_m, and 28 G_m markers have been described. G_m markers are important and have been typed in paternity cases and population genetics. In addition, the inheritance of certain G_m phenotypes may influence the ability to produce an antibody response of a given Ig subclass. Certain disease associations, especially autoimmune diseases such as rheumatoid arthritis, have been shown with some G_m phenotypes. The genes that define allotype expression, therefore, may play an analogous role to that of other immune response genes found within the HLA system.

The allotypes of a growing fetus may cause the maternal IS to become immunized to paternal allotypic determinants on fetal immunoglobulins.[10] Just as alloimmunization can occur during pregnancy, it can occur from transfusions, especially in patients who have received multiple transfusions of blood, plasma, or gamma globulin. Specifically, antibodies against A_{2m} allotypes have been implicated in some transfusion reactions in patients who may have an IgA deficiency. Idiotypes can be seen as nonself because they are often present at concentrations too low to induce self tolerance. Idiotypes are determined by the antigens that react with them and exist in a type of equilibrium with anti-idiotypic antibodies. The presence of antigen disrupts this equilibrium and may be important in controlling an immune response.

Overall there is variation unique to a species (isotype), unique to an individual (allotype), and unique to a molecule (idiotype) (the antibody or T-cell receptor) of an individual.

Ig Fc Receptors

Macrophages and monocytes have receptors for the attachment of IgG and can bind the C_H3 domain of the Fc portion. Only the IgG_1 and IgG_3 subclasses are capable of attachment to phagocytic receptors. This is one way that incompatible RBCs coated with IgG antibody are removed by phagocytosis. The other phagocytic cells with Fc receptors include neutrophils, NK cells, and mature B cells.[10,11]

Complement System

The complement system, or *complement*, is a complex group of over 20 circulating and cell membrane proteins that have a multitude of functions within the immune response. Primary roles include direct lysis of cells, bacteria, and enveloped viruses as well as assisting with opsonization to facilitate phagocytosis. Another role is production of peptide fragment split products, which are capable of mediating inflammatory and immune responses such as increased vascular permeability, smooth muscle contraction, chemotaxis, migration, and adherence. The complement components circulate in inactive form as *proenzymes,* with the exception of factor D of the alternate pathway. The complement proteins are activated in a *cascade* of events through three main pathways: the classical pathway, the alternative pathway, and the lectin pathway. The three pathways converge at the activation of the component C3. The classical pathway is activated by the binding of an antigen with an IgM, IgG_1, or IgG_3 antibody. The alternative pathway is activated by high molecular weight molecules with repeating units such as polysaccharides and lipopolysaccharides found on the surfaces of target cells such as bacteria, fungi, parasites, and tumor cells. The lectin pathway is activated by attachment of plasma mannose-binding lectin (MBL) to microbes. MBL in turn activates proteins of the classical pathway.

Complement components are sequentially numbered C1 through C9, but this refers to their discovery date, not to their activation sequence. The four unique serum proteins of the alternative pathway are designated by letters: factor B, factor D, factor P (properdin), and IF (initiating factor). Some activation pathways require Ca^{2+} and Mg^{2+} cations as cofactors for certain components and in certain nomenclature complement components or complexes that are active enzymatically are designated by a short bar placed over the appropriate number or letter. The cleavage products of complement proteins are distinguished from parent molecules by suffixes such as C3a and C3b. The complement system is able to modulate its own reactions by inhibitory proteins such as C1 inhibitor (C1INH), factor H, factor I, C4-binding protein (C4BP), anaphylatoxin inactivator, anaphylatoxin inhibitor, membrane attack complex (MAC) inhibitor, and C3 nephritic factor (NF). This regulation of complement is important so that complement proteins do not destroy healthy host cells and inflammation is controlled.

Classical Complement Pathway

The activation of the classic complement pathway is initiated when antibody binds to antigen. This allows the binding of the complement protein C1 to the Fc fragment of an IgM, IgG_1, or IgG_3 subclass antibody. Complement activation by IgG antibody depends on concentration of cell surface antigen and antigen clustering, in addition to antibody avidity and concentration. IgM is large and has Fc monomers close to each other on one immunoglobulin molecule; therefore, only one IgM molecule is necessary to activate complement. The C1 component is actually a complex composed of three C1 subunits, C1q, C1r, and C1s, which are stabilized by calcium ions. Without calcium present, there is no stabilization of the C1q, r, s complex, and complement is not activated. In the C1 complex bound to antigen antibody, C1q is responsible for catalyzing the C1r to generate activated C1s. Activated C1s is a serine-type protease. The C1q, r, s complex (actually as a $C1q[r, s]_2$ unit) acts on C2 and C4 to form C4b2a. C4b2a uses component C3 as a natural substrate. By-products that result from the activation of the classical sequence include C3a; C4b, which binds to the cell surface; C4a, which stays in the medium and has modest anaphylatoxin activity; and C3b, which attaches to the microbial surface. Note that complement fragments that have the *b* type are usually bound to membranes whereas the *a* fragments often have anaphylatoxic activity. Human RBCs have CR1 receptors for C4d and C3b, and some of the cleavage products will attach to the RBC membrane. Eventually these fragments are further degraded to C4d and C3d through the action of C4BP, factor H (which binds C3b), and factor I (which degrades both C4b and C3b). Some of C3b binds to the C4b2a complex, and the resulting C4b2a3b complex functions as a C5 convertase. The C5 convertase then acts on C5 to produce C5a (a strong stimulator of anaphylatoxis) and C5b, which binds to the cell membrane and recruits C6, C7, C8, and C9 to the cell membrane. C5b with C6, C7, C8, and C9 bound for the membrane attack complex, which causes cell lysis **(Figs. 3–10 and 3–11)**.

Alternative Complement Pathway

The alternative pathway is older in evolution and allows complement to be activated without acquired immunity. The alternative pathway is activated by surface contacts with complex molecules and artificial surfaces such as dialysis membranes, dextran polymers, and tumor cells. There are four important proteins in this pathway, factor D, factor B, properdin, and C3. In this pathway, complement component factor D is analogous to C1s in the classical pathway; factor B is analogous to C2; and the cleavage product C3b is analogous to C4. Also, factor C3bBbP is analogous to C4b2a, and C3b$_2$BbP is analogous to C4b2a3b in the classical pathway. Activation of the alternative pathway requires that a C3b molecule be bound to the surface of a target cell. Small amounts

of C3b are generated continuously owing to the spontaneous hydrolytic cleavage of the C3 molecule. When C3b encounters normal cells, it is rapidly eliminated through the combined interactions of factors H and I. The accumulation of C3b on microbial cell surfaces is associated with attachment of C3b to factor B. The complex of C3b and factor B is then acted on by factor D. As a result of this action, factor B is cleaved, yielding a cleavage product known as Bb. The C3bBb complex is stabilized by the presence of properdin (P), yielding C3bBbP. This complex acts as an esterase that cleaves C3 into additional C3a and C3b. C3b, therefore, acts as a positive feedback mechanism for driving the alternative pathway. The C3b$_2$BbP complex acts as a C5 convertase and initiates the later steps of complement activation (see **Fig. 3–10**).

Lectin Complement Pathway

The third pathway of activation, the lectin pathway, is activated by the attachment of MBL to microbes. The subsequent reactions are the same as those of the classical pathway. Remember that all three methods of activation lead to a final common pathway for complement activation and membrane attack complex (MAC) formation.

Membrane Attack Complex

The final step of complement activation is the formation of the MAC, which is composed of the terminal components of the complement sequence. There are two different ways in which the MAC is initiated. In either classical or alternative

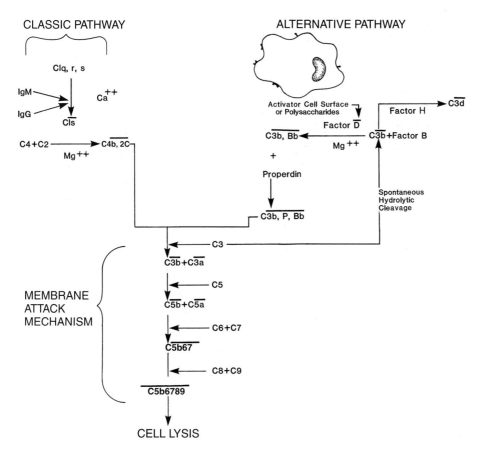

■ **FIGURE 3–10**   Schematic diagram illustrating the sequential activation of the complement system via the classic and alternative pathways.

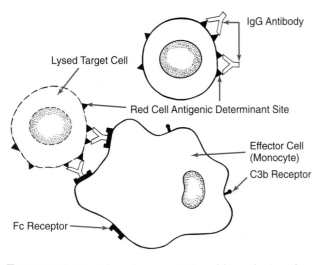
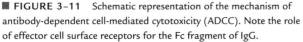

■ FIGURE 3–11   Schematic representation of the mechanism of antibody-dependent cell-mediated cytotoxicity (ADCC). Note the role of effector cell surface receptors for the Fc fragment of IgG.

to complement-mediated intravascular hemolysis. However, extravascular hemolysis usually occurs as a result of antibody coating of RBCs, and the split products of complement activation can stimulate the reticuloendothelial system and cause anaphylatoxic effects. Antibody-coated RBCs, either self or nonself, are removed by cells of the mononuclear phagocyte system, as well as the cells lining the hepatic and splenic sinusoids. These phagocytic cells are able to clear antibody-coated RBCs because they have cell surface receptors for complement CR1 (C3b) and Ig Fc receptors (see **Fig. 3–11**). IgM-coated RBCs are not eliminated through Fc receptor–mediated phagocytosis, but if erythrocytes are coated with IgG and complement, they will be cleared rapidly from circulation by monocytes and macrophages. If RBCs are coated with only C3b, they may not be cleared but only sequestered temporarily. Interesting to blood bankers is the fact that the CR1 (C3b/C4b, CD35) receptor on RBCs, which is important in the attachment of immune complexes to erythrocytes, is also the blood group antigen Knops/McCoy, which generates high-titer low-avidity antibodies in immunized transfusion recipients.[12,13]

Characteristics of Antigens

The immune response is initiated by the presentation of an *antigen* (can initiate formation of and react with an antibody) or *immunogen* (can initiate an immune response) to the IS and the IS determining that the antigen is nonself. The term antigen is more commonly used in blood banking because the primary testing concern is the detection of antibodies to blood group antigens. The immune reaction to any immunogen, including antigens, is determined by the host response as well as by several biochemical and physical characteristics of the immunogen. Properties such as size, complexity, conformation, charge, accessibility, solubility, digestibility, and biochemical composition influence the amount and type of immune response **(Box 3–1)**. Molecules that are too small cannot stimulate antibody production. Immunogens having a molecular weight (MW) less than 10,000 daltons (D), for example, are called *haptens* and usually do not elicit an immune response on their own. A hapten coupled with a carrier protein having a MW greater than 10,000 D, however, can produce a reaction. Usually, the more chemically complex molecules produce more rigorous immune responses. Antibodies and cellular responses are very specific for an antigen's physical, globular conformation as opposed to its linear sequence. Overall charge is important as antibody response is also formed to the net charge of a molecule, whether it has positive, negative, or neutral antigenic determinants.

Binding of Complement by RBC Antibodies

Disruption in the activation of either complement pathway can result in damage to the host's own cells. Concern to transfusion medicine specialists is the formation of antibodies with complement capacity that can bring about the destruction of RBCs. Recall that in order to initiate activation, C1 molecules bind with two adjacent Ig Fc regions. A pentameric IgM molecule provides two Fc regions side by side, thereby binding complement. A monomeric IgG molecule, on the other hand, binds C1q less efficiently, and two IgG molecules are needed in close proximity to bind complement. For example, as many as 800 IgG anti-A molecules may need to attach to one adult A RBC to bind a single C1 molecule, and so there is little complement activation by IgG anti-A immunoglobulins.[4] Also, IgG antibodies against the Rh antigens usually do not bind complement due to the low level of Rh antigens on RBC surfaces. An example of an efficient IgG hemolysin is found in patients with the disease paroxysmal cold hemoglobinuria in which antibodies are directed against P blood group determinants. Also, antibodies to the Lewis blood group system are generally IgM, and they can activate complement but rarely cause hemolytic transfusion reactions due to their low optimal reactivity temperature. Therefore, in blood banking, with the exception of the ABO system, only a few antibodies activate the complement sequence that leads

pathways the formation of C5 convertase is necessary. In the activation of the classical pathway, the MAC is initiated by the enzymatic activity of component C4b2a3b on C5. In the alternative pathway it is C3b$_2$Bb that has the ability to cleave C5. The next step in either pathway is the same. Component C5 is split into the fragments C5a (a potent anaphylatoxin) and C5b; C5b fragment attaches to cell membranes and can continue the complement cascade by initiating the membrane attachment of C6, C7, and C8. After the attachment of C9 to the C5b678 complex, a small transmembrane channel or pore is formed in the lipid bilayer of the cell membrane, and this allows for osmotic lysis and subsequent death of the cell.

BOX 3–1
Characteristics of Antigens: Properties that Influence Immune Response

- Size
- Complexity
- Conformation
- Charge
- Accessibility
- Solubility
- Digestibility
- Chemical composition

Obviously, if an antigen cannot be seen by the IS, no immune reaction will take place, and so the accessibility of epitopes influences the immune response. Also, antigenic substances that are less soluble are less likely to elicit an immune response. The biochemical composition of the stimulus plays a role in immune stimulation. Remember that RBC antigens are very diverse in structure and composition and may be proteins (such as the Rh, M, and N blood group substances) or glycolipids (such as the ABH, Lewis, Ii, and P blood group substances). Human leukocyte antigens (HLAs) are glycoproteins. Because of these differences in structure, conformation, and molecular nature, not all blood group substances are equally immunogenic in-vivo **(Table 3–7)**. Fifty to 70 percent of D-negative recipients of D-positive blood would be expected to form anti-D antibodies; however, only about 5 percent of K-negative individuals are likely to develop anti-K after being transfused with K-positive blood. The varying immunogenicity of different blood group antigens has practical significance because RBCs from donors need to be routinely typed only for A, B and D antigens, and other blood group antigens are generally unlikely to elicit an immune response in a transfusion recipient.

Characteristics of Blood Group Antibodies

There are many different and important characteristics of blood group antibodies such as whether they are polyclonal or monoclonal, naturally occurring or immune, and allo- or autoantibodies.

Polyclonal and Monoclonal Antibodies

In laboratory testing, there are two types of antibody (reagent antibodies are called *antisera*) that are available for use; they are manufactured differently and have different properties. Recall that an antigen usually consists of numerous epitopes. It is the epitopes and not the entire antigen that a B cell recognizes as nonself and is stimulated to produce antibody against. Therefore, these different epitopes on a single antigen

induce the proliferation of a variety of B-cell clones, resulting in a heterogeneous population of serum antibodies. These antibodies are referred to as *polyclonal* or *serum* antibodies and are produced in response to a single antigen with more than one epitope. In vivo, the polyclonal nature of antibodies improves the immune response with respect to quality and quantity. Antibodies against more than one epitope are needed to give immunity against an entire antigen, such as a pathogenic virus or tumor cell. However, this diversity is not optimal in the laboratory, and in-vitro reagents produced by animals or humans can give confusing test results. Consistency and reliability are needed in laboratory testing; due to the individual variability in immune responses, polyclonal sera can vary in antibody concentration from person to person and animal to animal. Sera from the same animal can also vary somewhat, depending on the animal's overall health and age and strength of its immune response. Individual sera also differ in the serologic properties of the antibody molecules they contain, the epitopes they recognize, and the presence of additional nonspecific or cross-reacting antibodies. One way to avoid this problem is to use monoclonal antibodies produced by isolating individual B cells from a polyclonal population and propagating them in cell culture with *hybridoma* technology. The supernatant from the cell culture contains antibody from a single type of B cell, clonally expanded, and therefore with the same variable region and having a single epitope specificity. This results in a *monoclonal* antibody suspension. Monoclonal antibodies are preferred in testing because they are highly specific, well characterized, and uniformly reactive. Most reagents used today are monoclonal in nature.

Naturally Occurring and Immune Antibodies

There are two types of antibodies that concern blood banking: one is *naturally* occurring and the other is *immune*. Both are produced in reaction to encountered antigens. RBC antibodies are considered naturally occurring when they are found in the serum of individuals who have never been previously exposed to RBC antigens by transfusion, injection, or pregnancy. These antibodies are probably produced in response to substances in the environment that are highly similar to RBC antigens such as pollen grains and parts of bacteria membranes. The common occurrence of naturally occurring antibodies suggests that their antigens are widely found in nature and have a repetitive complex pattern. Most naturally occurring antibodies are IgM cold agglutinins, which react best at room temperature or lower, activate complement, and when active at 37°C may be hemolytic. In blood banking, the common naturally occurring antibodies react with antigens of the ABH, Hh, Ii, Lewis, MN, and P blood group systems. Some naturally occurring antibodies found in normal serum are manufactured without a known environmental stimulus.[14] In contrast to natural antibodies, RBC antibodies are considered immune when found in the serum of individuals who have been transfused or pregnant. These antigens are not generally found in nature, and their molecular makeup is unique to human RBCs. Most immune RBC antibodies are IgG antibodies that react best at 37°C and require the use of antihuman globulin sera (Coombs sera) for detection. The most common immune antibodies encountered in testing include those that react with the Rh, Kell, Duffy, Kidd, and Ss blood group systems.[15]

Blood Group Antigen	Blood Group System	Immunogenicity (%)*
D (Rh$_0$)	Rh	50.00
K	Kell	5.00
c (hr')	Rh	2.05
E (rh'')	Rh	1.69
k	Kell	1.50
e (hr'')	Rh	0.56
Fy^a	Duffy	0.23
C (rh')	Rh	0.11
Jk^a	Kidd	0.07
S	MNSs	0.04
Jk^b	Kidd	0.03
s	MNSs	0.03

TABLE 3–7   Relative Immunogenicity of Different Blood Group Antigens

Adapted from Williams, WJ, et al (eds): Hematology. McGraw-Hill, New York, 1983, p 1491.

*Percentage of transfusion recipients lacking the blood group antigen (in the first column) who are likely to be sensitized to a single transfusion of red cells containing that antigen.

Unexpected Antibodies

Naturally occurring anti-A and anti-B antibodies are routinely detected in human serum; however, which antibodies are present depends on the blood type of the individual. Blood group A has anti-B; blood group B has anti-A; blood group O has both as well as anti-A,B; and blood group AB has neither. These naturally occurring antibodies, or *isoagglutinins*, are significant and useful tools in the confirmation of blood typing. They are easily detected by use of A and B reagent RBCs with a direct agglutination technique. In normal, healthy individuals, anti-A and anti-B are generally the only RBC antibodies expected to be found in a serum sample. People with an IS that does not function normally may not have the expected naturally occurring antibodies (Chapter 6, The ABO Blood Group System, has more detail on these antibodies). All other antibodies directed against RBC antigens are considered unexpected and must be detected and identified before blood can be safely transfused, even if antibodies react at room temperature or only with Coombs sera. Also, autoreactive antibodies must be investigated. The reactivity of unexpected antibodies is highly varied and unpredictable as they may be either isotype IgM or IgG; rarely, both may be present in the same sample. These antibodies may be able to hemolyze, agglutinate, or sensitize RBCs. Some antibodies require special reagents to enhance their reactivity and detection. Due to the enormous polymorphism of the human population, a diversity of RBC antigens exists, requiring a variety of standardized immunologic techniques and reagents for their detection and identification.

The in-vitro analysis of unexpected antibodies involves the use of antibody screening procedures to optimize antigen-antibody reactions. The majority of these procedures includes reacting unknown serum from a donor or patient sample with known reagent cells at various amounts of time, temperature, and media. All routine blood bank testing requires the use of samples for both expected and unexpected antibodies. (Refer to Chapter 12, Detection and Identification of Antibodies, for a more detailed discussion.)

Alloantibodies and Autoantibodies

Antibodies can be either allo- or autoreactive. *Alloantibodies* are produced after exposure to genetically different, or non-self, antigens of the same species, such as a different RBC antigen after transfusion. Transfused components may elicit the formation of alloantibodies against antigens (red cell, white cell and platelets) not present in the recipient. *Autoantibodies* are produced in response to self antigens. They can cause reactions in the recipient if they have a specificity that is common to the transfused blood. Some autoantibodies do not have a detectable specificity and are referred to as *pan-* or *polyagglutinins*. Autoantbodies can react at different temperatures, and cold or warm autoantibodies may both be present. Patients with autoantibodies frequently have autoimmune diseases and may require considerable numbers of blood products and special techniques to find the most compatible units possible. A potentially serious problem for blood bankers is transfused patients who have made alloreactive antibodies that are no longer detectable in the patient's plasma or serum. If these individuals are transfused with the immunizing antigen again, they will make a much stronger immune response against those RBC antigens, which can cause severe and possibly fatal transfusion reactions. These recipients will then have a positive autocontrol or *direct antiglobulin test* (DAT). This is why the previous history of any patient is a critical part of the testing. Autoantibodies can be removed from RBCs by special elution techniques and then tested against reagent RBCs. Remember that in order to transfuse blood safely, the identity of alloantibodies must always be determined!

Characteristics of Antigen-Antibody Reactions

There are many complex properties of antigen and antibody reactions that influence serologic and other testing methods involving antibodies. The final result of antibody production after an immune stimulation depends on many factors, including intermolecular binding forces and factors such as antibody properties. Note that although antigens are present in *circulating* blood, the immune response only reacts with them and clears them from the *peripheral* tissues. The antigen-binding site of the antibody molecule is uniquely designed to recognize a corresponding antigen; this antibody amino acid sequence cannot be changed without altering its specificity. The extent of the reciprocal relationship, also called the *fit* between the antigen and its binding site on the antibody, is often referred to as a *lock and key* mechanism.

Intermolecular Binding Forces

Intermolecular binding forces such as hydrogen bonding, electrostatic forces, van der Waals forces, and hydrophobic bonds, are all involved in antigen-antibody binding reactions. Stronger covalent bonds are not involved in this reaction, although they are important for the intramolecular conformation of the antibody molecule. Hydrogen bonds result from weak dipole forces between hydrogen atoms bonded to oxygen or nitrogen atoms in which there is incomplete transfer of the electronic energy to the more electronegative atom (oxygen or nitrogen). When two atoms with dipoles come close to each other, there is a weak attraction between them. Although hydrogen bonds are singularly weak, many of them together can be very strong. They are found in many complex molecules throughout the human body. Electrostatic forces result from weak charges on atoms in molecules that have either a positive or negative overall charge (like charges repel, unlike charges attract). This is seen in the formation of salt bridges. Van der Waals forces appear to be a type of weak interaction between atoms in larger molecules. *Hydrophobic* (water-avoiding) bonds result from the overlap of hydrophobic amino acids in proteins. The hydrophobic amino acids bury themselves together to avoid water and salts in solution. The repulsion of these amino acids to prevent contact with water and aqueous solutions can be very strong collectively. Many proteins have bonds of these types. In addition, there are *hydrophilic* (water-loving) bonds that allow for the overlap of amino acids that are attracted to water. Hydrophobic and hydrophilic bonds repel each other, and these repulsive forces play a role in the formation of the antigen-antibody bond also. All of these bonds play roles in the total conformation and strength of antigen-antibody reactions and IS molecules.

Antibody Properties

There are many important terms that refer to the properties of antibody reactions. The first term is antibody *affinity;* it is often defined as the strength of a single antigen-antibody bond produced by the summation of attractive and repulsive forces. The second term is *avidity,* which is used to express the binding strength of a multivalent antigen with antisera produced in an immunized individual. Avidity, therefore, is a measure of the *functional affinity* of an antiserum for the whole antigen and is sometimes referred to as a combination of affinities. Avidity can be important in blood banking because high-titer low-avidity antibodies exhibit low antigen-binding capacity but still show reactivity at high serum dilutions.[16] The *specificity* of an antiserum (or antibody) is one of its most important characteristics and is related to its relative avidity for antigen. Antibody specificity can be further classified as a specific reaction, cross-reaction, or no reaction. A specific reaction implies reaction between similar epitopes. A cross reaction results when certain epitopes of one antigen are shared by another antigen and the same antibody can react with both antigens. No reaction occurs when there are no shared epitopes **(Fig. 3–12).** In addition, there is the *valency* of an antibody, which is the number of antigen-binding sites on an antibody molecule or the number of antibody binding sites on an antigen. Antigens are usually multivalent, but antibodies are usually bivalent. IgM and IgA antibodies can have higher valences due to the multimeric nature of some of their structures.

Because the biochemistry controlling the forces of antibody binding are well understood, the influence of these forces can be manipulated by using various reagents and methods to enhance the reactivity of certain RBC antigens with antibodies. When more than one antibody is present in a blood bank sample, it is often necessary to use special techniques to identify all the antibodies. These techniques and reagents were developed with an understanding of antibody reactivity.

Host Factors

In addition to antigen characteristics and antibody properties, host factors play a key role in an individual's immune response. These factors are important in the host's overall immune response as well as various specific immune reactions. Each individual's immune system is unique to that individual and will help determine how that individual is able to resist disease. There are many factors that can influence

the host's IS. These include nutritional status, hormones, genetic inheritance, age, race, sex, physical activity level, environmental exposure, and the occurrence of disease or injury. One of the most critical is nutritional status as severe malnutrition can lead to a considerable reduction in TH cells and therefore antibody responses of lower affinity. Hormone receptors are found on various immunologic cells; hormone-signaling mechanisms can both enhance and suppress immune responses. Genetic influences are due to the inheritance of the genes of the MHC. Immune response genes help control T- and B-cell reactions to individual antigens. MHC genes control the way an individual processes antigen; as pathogens are processed by the IS, the MHC genes an individual has will play a strong role in how that individual responds to a pathogen. In addition to individual factors, aging has an influence on immune response. It is believed that immune function decreases as age increases; this may be one reason why so many diseases such as cancer and autoimmune conditions are seen at a later time in life. A decrease in antibody levels in older individuals may result in false-negative reactions, especially in reverse ABO blood typing. In some instances an individual's race may be a factor in susceptibility to certain diseases. A dramatic example of this is seen in malaria infection. The majority of African American individuals who do not inherit the Duffy blood system antigens, Fy^a or Fy^b, are resistant to malarial invasion with *Plasmodium knowlesi* and *Plasmodium vivax.* The absence of these antigens may make these individuals ideal donors for those who have developed Duffy system antibodies. Strenuous exercise, traumatic injury, and the presence of certain diseases are other factors that may have an immunomodulatory effect on the immune response. This may be observed as negative or weak serum test results, notably with reverse ABO groupings as in other immunomodulatory conditions or nonspecific reactions **(Box 3–2).** This illustrates once again the importance of the historical record of the patient or donor.

Tolerance

Tolerance is defined as the lack of an immune response or an active immunosuppressive response. It has been observed post-transfusion for many years, but its mechanism is still unclear. Tolerance can be either naturally occurring or experimentally induced. Exposure to an antigen during fetal life usually produces tolerance to that antigen. An example of this type of tolerance is found in the chimera, an individual who receives an in utero cross-transfusion of ABO-incompatible blood from a dizygotic (nonidentical) twin.[17] The chimera does not produce antibodies against the A and B antigen of

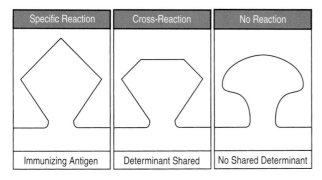

Specific Reaction	Cross-Reaction	No Reaction
Immunizing Antigen	Determinant Shared	No Shared Determinant

■ **FIGURE 3–12** Types of antigen-antibody reactions: specific reaction, cross-reaction, and no reaction.

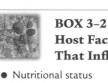

BOX 3–2
Host Factors: Properties of the Host That Influence Immune Response

- Nutritional status
- Hormones
- Genetics
- Age
- Race
- Exercise level
- Disease
- Injury

the twin, and ABO group of such an individual may appear as a testing discrepancy.

The induction of tolerance is used to prevent D-negative mothers from developing anti-D antibodies after delivery of Rh-positive infants. When a D-negative woman gives birth to a D-positive infant, she is exposed to D-positive RBCs, most of which occurs during the delivery of the baby. Approximately 50 to 70 percent of Rh-negative mothers develop anti-D antibodies on first exposure to D-positive cells. These antibodies can result in HDN upon later pregnancies with a D-positive fetus. Use of passive immunization to prevent the formation of these antibodies can prevent HDN. This is accomplished by administering IgG Rh-immune globulin (RHIG) within 48 to 72 hours after the birth of the infant. About 25 to 30 percent of D-negative individuals are nonresponders and do not produce anti-D antibodies, even when subjected to repeated exposure to D-positive cells. Because it is not known who will respond, it is recommended that all D-negative mothers who deliver D-positive newborns receive RHIG to prevent immunization.

Detection of RBC Antigen-Antibody Reactions

Various factors influence detection of RBC antigen-antibody reactions. These include having a correct sample (a sample that is stored under the right conditions) and the proper reagents performing the correct test and understanding how the test should be done.

Blood Samples Required for Testing

One of the most important steps in obtaining the correct and valid results of an analytical or diagnostic test is to have the correct sample. Different tests in the blood bank may require different samples. Some tests require the use of serum to ensure that adequate amounts of viable complement are available for fixation by blood group antibodies. Serum is obtained when no anticoagulant is used in the sample collection tube. The sample clots and is centrifuged to separate the clotted cells and the liquid serum fraction. An anticoagulated sample would not be conducive to complement activation studies because anticoagulants bind divalent Ca^{2+} and Mg^{2+} ions and inhibit complement activity. The commonly used anticoagulant ethylenediaminetetraacetic acid (EDTA) at a ratio of 2 mg to 1 mL of serum will totally inhibit complement activation by binding calcium and, to a lesser extent, magnesium. Another anticoagulant, sodium heparin, inhibits the cleavage of C4. These problems can be avoided by using serum instead of plasma for blood bank procedures that require fresh complement. Currently, however, plasma is used routinely in place of serum; years of testing with both samples have shown that, for most tests, plasma is comparable to serum. Plasma samples are preferred for DAT and elution studies because they lack fibrin strands, which can cause false-positives. Serum should be removed as soon as possible from a clotted blood sample; if testing cannot begin immediately, then serum should be removed and stored at 4°C for no longer than 48 hours. After this time, serum should be frozen at −50°C or lower to retain complement activity. If required, complement can be deactivated in serum samples by heating serum at 56°C for 30 minutes which destroys C1 and C2 and damages C4. Also, factor B of the alternate pathway is inactivated by heating at 50°C for 20 minutes. Serum also has an inhibitor present that blocks the action of activated C1 by binding to and removing C1s and C1r from the activated complex of C1qrs. The complement system may become activated during storage of preserved RBC products. In citrate-phosphate-dextrose-adenine (CPDA-1)–preserved RBCs, for example, activation of the alternate pathway can be caused by contact of plasma C3 with plastic surfaces of blood bags, and this may cause hemolysis that will become visible as the RBCs settle upon storage.[18]

Traditional Laboratory Methods

The various complex immunologic responses that are important to blood banking have been studied by a number of immunologic methods. These in-vitro testing methods were developed with a solid understanding of the in-vivo biochemistry and biophysics of the IS. Many of the methods used today are modifications of previous blood bank techniques or more generalized immunologic testing methods that have been adapted to the needs of immunohematology laboratories. The routine methods used today have to be highly efficient to meet clinical laboratory requirements. Many different types of tests are available, and it is important to be familiar with the different purposes of each. In-vitro testing for the detection of antigens or antibodies may be accomplished by commonly used techniques including hemagglutination (a special type of agglutination), precipitation, agglutination inhibition, and hemolysis. Other techniques such as radioimmunoassay (RIA), enzyme-linked immunosorbent assay (ELISA) or enzyme immunoassay (EIA), and immunofluorescence (IF), which quantifies antigen or antibody with the use of a radioisotope, enzyme, or fluorescent label, respectively, may be used in automated or semiautomated blood banking instrumentation.[19] These techniques are very important in testing for viral pathogens in donor units as well as patient samples. Recently, blood bank automated methods for the typing of whole blood units and patient samples have become more popular and may become routine in the near future.

In most transfusion laboratory testing, hemagglutination reactions are the major technique used. Hemagglutination methods for the analysis of blood group antigen-antibody responses and typing for ABO, Rh, and other blood group antigens is accomplished by *red cell agglutination* reactions. Agglutination is a straightforward process and can be shown to develop in two stages. In the first stage, called *sensitization*, antigen binding to the antibody occurs. Epitopes on the surfaces of RBC membranes combine with the antigen-combining sites (Fab region) on the variable regions of the immunoglobulin heavy and light chains (see **Figs. 3–6** and **3–7**). Antigen and antibody are held together by various noncovalent bonds, and no visible agglutination is seen at this stage. In the second stage, a *lattice*-type structure composed of multiple antigen-antibody bridges between RBC antigens and antibodies is formed. A network of these bridges forms, and visible agglutination is present during this stage. The development of an insoluble antigen-antibody complex, resulting from the mixing of equivalent amounts of soluble antigen and antibody, is known as a *precipitation reaction.*

Agglutination inhibition is a method in which a positive reaction is the opposite of what is normally observed in agglutination. Agglutination is inhibited when an antigen-antibody reaction has previously occurred in a test system and prevents agglutination. The antigen and antibody cannot bind because another substrate has been added to the reaction mixture and blocks the formation of the antigen-antibody agglutinates. Inhibition reactions in the blood bank are used in *secretory studies* to determine whether soluble ABO substances are present in body fluids and secretions. The secreted substrate can combine with the antibody and block RBC antigen-antibody reactions. People who have blood group antibodies in their body fluids are called *secretors*. See Chapter 6, The ABO Blood Group System, for more information on this phenomenon.

Hemolysis represents a strong positive result and indicates that an antigen-antibody reaction has occurred in which complement has been fixed and RBC lysis occurs. The Lewis blood group antibodies anti-Le[a] and anti-Le[b] may be regarded as clinically significant if hemolysis occurs in their in-vitro testing reactions.

RIA, ELISA (or EIA), and IF techniques are immunologic methods based on quantization of antigen or antibody by the use of a radioisotope, enzyme, or fluorescent label, respectively. Either the antigen or the antibody can be labeled in these tests. These techniques measure the interaction of the binding of antigen with antibody and are extremely sensitive. Most of these techniques employ reagents that use either antigen or antibody, which is bound in a solid or liquid phase in a variety of reaction systems ranging from plastic tubes or plates to microscopic particles or beads. These methods use a separation system and washing steps to isolate bound and free fractions and a detection system to measure the amount of antigen-antibody interaction. The values of unknown samples are then calculated from the values of standards of known concentration.

Factors That Influence Agglutination Reactions

Various factors can influence reactivity of antigen-antibody reactions, but as the majority of blood bank reactions are (RBC) agglutinations, the main emphasis in this discussion will be on these factors. Typical of most biochemical reaction systems, agglutination reactions are influenced by the concentration of the reactants (antigen and antibody) as well as by factors such as pH, temperature, and ionic strength. The surface charge, antibody isotype, RBC antigen dosage, and the use of various enhancement media, antihuman globulin reagents, and enzymes are all important in antigen-antibody reactions. The most important factors are discussed in the following sections.

Centrifugation

Centrifugation is an effective way to enhance agglutination reactions because it decreases reaction time by increasing the gravitational forces on the reactants as well as bringing reactants closer together. High-speed centrifugation is one of the most efficient methods used in blood banking. Under the right centrifugation conditions, sensitized RBCs overcome their natural repulsive effect (zeta potential) for each other and agglutinate more efficiently (discussed in the section on Enhancement Media). Having RBCs in closer physical proximity allows for an increase in antigen-antibody lattice formation, which results in enhanced agglutination.

Antigen-Antibody Ratio

Antigen and antibody have optimal concentrations; in ideal reactive conditions, an equivalent amount of antigen and antibody binds. Any deviation from this decreases the efficiency of the reaction and a loss of the *zone of equivalence* between antigen and antibody ratio that is necessary for agglutination reactions to occur. An excess of unbound immunoglobulin leads to a *prozone* effect, and a surplus of antigen (antigen-binding sites) leads to a *postzone* effect **(Fig. 3–13)**. In either situation, the lattice formation and subsequent agglutination may not occur, which can give false-negative results. If this is suspected, simple steps can be taken to correct it. If the problem is excessive antibody, the plasma or serum may be diluted with appropriate buffer, and each serial dilution of serum tested against RBCs. The problem of excessive antigen can be solved by increasing the serum-to-cell ratio, which tends to increase the number of antibodies available to bind with each RBC. Antigen-antibody test systems, therefore, can be manipulated to overcome the effects of excessive antigen or antibody.

Another reason antigen amount may be altered is due to weak expression of antigen on RBCs (*dosage effect*). Weak expression occurs as a result of the inheritance of genotypes that give rise to heterozygous expression of RBC antigens and resultant weaker phenotypes. For example, M-positive RBCs from an individual having the genotype *MM* (homozygous) have more M antigen sites than M-positive cells from an individual having the *MN* (heterozygous) genotype. In the Kidd system, Jk[a] homozygous inheritance has greater RBC antigen expression than Jk[a] heterozygous. The same is true for Jk[b] homo- and heterozygous expression. In the Rh system, the C, c, E, and e antigens also show dosage effects.

Effect of pH

The ideal pH of a test system for antigen-antibody reactions is a range between 6.5 and 7.5, which is similar to the pH of normal plasma or serum. Exceptions include some anti-M and some Pr(Sp$_1$) group antibodies that show stronger reactivity below pH 6.5.[20]

Temperature

Different isotypes of antibodies may exhibit optimal reactivity at different temperatures. IgM antibodies usually react optimally at ambient temperatures or below 22°C, whereas IgG antibodies usually require 37°C. Because clinically significant antibodies may be in both these temperature ranges, it is important to do testing with a range of temperatures **(Fig. 3–14)**.

Ig Type

Examples of IgM antibodies that have importance in blood banking include those against the ABH, Ii, MN, Lewis (Le[a], Le[b]), Lutheran (Lu[a]), and P blood group antigens. Important IgG antibodies are those directed against Ss, Kell (Kk, Js[a], Js[b], Kp[a], Kp[b]), Rh (DCEce), Lutheran (Lu[b]), Duffy (Fy[a], Fy[b]), and Kidd (Jk[a], Jk[b]) antigens (see **Fig. 3–14**). IgM antibodies are generally capable of agglutinating RBCs suspended in 0.85 to 0.90 percent saline medium. The IgM antibody is 160 Å larger than an IgG molecule and approximately 750 times as effi-

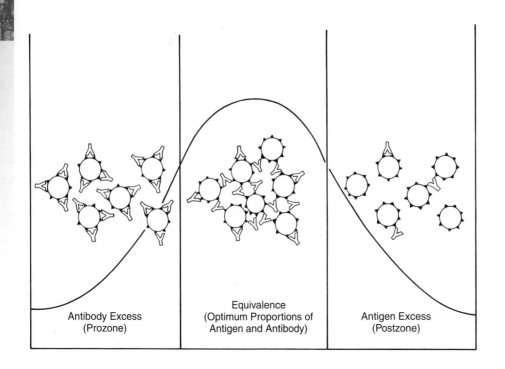

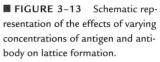

■ **FIGURE 3–13**   Schematic representation of the effects of varying concentrations of antigen and antibody on lattice formation.

cient as IgG in agglutination reactions; this allows it to easily bridge the distance between two RBCs.[20] Another factor that contributes to the difference in reactivity between the IgM and IgG molecules is the number of antigen-combining sites on each type of immunoglobulin. The IgM molecule has the potential to bind 10 separate antigen sites; however, an IgG molecule has only 2 binding sites per molecule, which implies that an IgG molecule would have to bind 2 RBCs with only 1 binding site on each cell.[20] IgM molecules rarely bind 10 sites owing to the size and spacing of antigens in relation to the

size and configuration of the IgM molecule (see **Fig. 3–8**). Typically, when the IgM molecule attaches to two RBCs, probably two or three antigen-combining sites attach to each RBC. Agglutination reactions involve more than one immunoglobulin molecule, and these conditions are multiplied many times in order to represent its relevance in the agglutination reaction (**Fig. 3–15**). Because of the basic differences in the nature of reactivity between IgM and IgG antibodies, different serologic systems must be used to detect optimally both classes of clinically significant antibodies. An overview of the serologic methods traditionally used for antibody detection in the blood bank laboratory is outlined in **Table 3–8**.

Enhancement Media

Agglutination reactions for IgM antibodies and their corresponding RBC antigens are easily accomplished in saline medium as these antibodies usually do not need enhancement or modifications to react strongly with antigens. Detection of IgM antibodies, however, may not have the same clinical significance as the detection of most IgG antibodies because IgG antibodies react best at 37°C and are generally responsible for hemolytic transfusion reactions and HDN. To discover the presence of IgG antibodies, there are many enhancement techniques available (**Table 3–9**).

One of the key ways to enhance the detection of IgG antibodies is to increase their reactivity. Many of the commercially available enhancement media accomplish this by reducing the *zeta potential* of RBC membranes. The net negative charge surrounding RBCs (and most other human cells) in a cationic media is part of the force that repels RBCs from each other and is due to sialic acid molecules on the surface of RBCs. Most acids have a negative charge, and the large concentration of these molecules on RBCs creates a "zone" of negative charge around the RBC. This zone is protective and keeps RBCs from adhering to each other in the peripheral

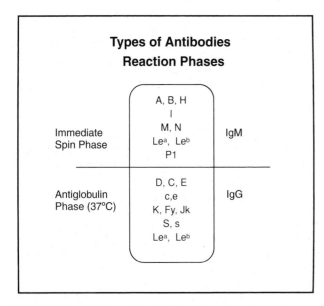

**Types of Antibodies
Reaction Phases**

| Immediate Spin Phase | A, B, H
I
M, N
Leᵃ, Leᵇ
P1 | IgM |
| Antiglobulin Phase (37°C) | D, C, E
c,e
K, Fy, Jk
S, s
Leᵃ, Leᵇ | IgG |

■ **FIGURE 3–14**   Types of antibodies and reaction phases. (From Kutt, SM, Larison, PJ, and Kessler, LA: Solving Antibody Problems, Special Techniques, Ortho Diagnostic Systems, Raritan, NJ, 1992, p 10, with permission.)

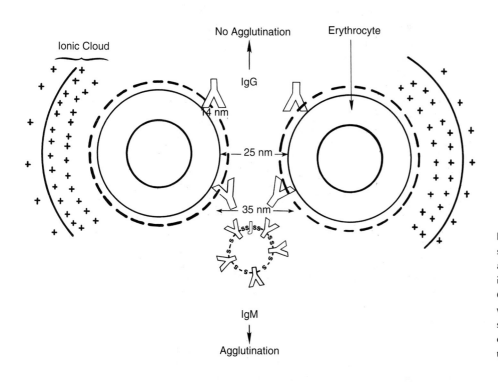

■ **FIGURE 3–15** Schematic representation of the ionic cloud concept and its relevance to hemagglutination induced by IgM and IgG antibodies. Compare the size of the IgG antibody with that of the IgM molecule. The size of the IgG molecule is not large enough to span the distance between two adjacent RBCs.

TABLE 3–8 Serologic Systems Used in Traditional Laboratory Methods for Red Cell Antibody Detection				
Reaction Phase	**Ig Class Commonly Detected**	**Purpose and Mechanism of Reaction**	**Tests That Use Serologic System**	**Type of Antibodies Commonly Detected**
Immediate spin	IgM	IgM antibodies react best at cold temperatures. IgM is an agglutinating antibody that has the ability to easily bridge the distance between red cells.	ABO reverse testing Cross-match Antibody screening/identification Autocontrol	Expected ABO alloantibodies Unexpected cold-reacting alloantibodies or autoantibodies
37°C incubation	IgG	IgG antibodies react best at warm temperatures. No visible agglutination commonly seen. IgG is sensitizing antibody with fewer antigen binding sites than IgM and cannot undergo the second stage of agglutination, lattice formation. Complement may be bound during reactivity, which may or may not result in visible hemolysis.	Antibody screening/ identification Cross-match (if needed) Autocontrol	
Antiglobulin test	IgG	Antihuman globulin (AHG) has specificity for the Fc portion of the heavy chain of the human IgG molecule and/or complement components. AHG acts as a bridge cross-linking red cells sensitized with IgG antibody or complement.	Antibody screening/identification Cross-match (if needed) Autocontrol Direct antiglobulin test (DAT)	Unexpected warm-reacting alloantibodies or autoantibodies

TABLE 3–9   Potentiators

Reagent	Action	Procedure	Type of Antibody ID
Saline		4–22°C (IgM) immediate spin (IS) up to 60 min; 37°C (IgG) for 45–60 min	Primarily IgM; IgG if incubated at 37°C
AHG	Cross-links sensitized cells, resulting in visible agglutination	1. DAT: AHG added directly to washed RBCs 2. IAT: serum + screen cells; incubation at 37°C for time determined by additive used; cell washing before addition of AHG	1. Polyspecific; anti-IgG + anticomplement 2. IgG monospecific: anti-IgG only
22% Albumin*	Causes agglutination by adjusting zeta potential between RBCs	Incubation at 37°C for 15–60 min; cell washing prior to indirect antiglobulin test (IAT)	IgG
LISS*	Low ionic strength environment causes RBCs to take up antibody more rapidly	Incubation at 37°C for 5–15 min; cell washing before IAT	IgG
PEG*	Increases test sensitivity; Aggregates RBCs causing closer proximity of RBCs to one another assisting in antibody cross-linking	Incubation at 37°C for 10–30 min; cell washing before IAT NOTE: The test mixture cannot be centrifuged and examined reliably for direct agglutination after 37°C incubation.	IgG
Enzymes	Reduces RBC surface charge; Destroys or depresses some RBC antigens; enhances other RBC antigens	1. One-step: enzymes added directly to serum/RBC mixture 2. Two-step: RBC pretreated with enzymes before addition of serum	Destroys Fy^a, Fy^b, MNS; enhances reactivity to Rh, Kidd, P_1, Lewis, and I antibodies

*All additives should be added after the IS phase immediately before 37°C incubation

LISS = low Ionic strength solutions; PEG = polyethylene glycol

blood. A potential is created because of the ionic cloud of cations (positively charged ions) that are attracted to the zone of negative charges on the RBC membrane (see **Fig. 3–15**).[20] The potential around the RBC is called the zeta potential and is an expression of the difference in electrostatic charges at the RBC surface and the surrounding cations. IgM and IgG antibodies have differences in how they react to the same zeta potential. Reducing the zeta potential allows the more positively charged antibodies to get closer to the negatively charged RBCs and therefore increases RBC agglutination by IgG molecules.

Protein Media

Colloidal substances, or *colloids*, are a type of clear solution that contains particles permanently suspended in solution. Colloidal particles are usually large moieties like proteins as compared with the more familiar *crystalloids*, which usually have small, highly soluble molecules, such as glucose, that are easily dialyzed. The colloidal solutes can be charged or neutral and go into solution because of their microscopic size. There are several colloidal solutions currently in use in blood bank testing, and they are all used to enhance agglutination reactions. Colloids include albumin, polyethylene glycol (PEG), polybrene, polyvinylpyrrolidone (PVP), and protamine. These substances work by increasing the *dielectric constant* (a measure of electrical conductivity), which then reduces the zeta potential of the RBC.

Low Ionic Strength Solution (LISS) Media

Low ionic strength solutions (LISS), or low salt media, generally contain 0.2 percent sodium chloride. They decrease the ionic strength of a reaction medium, which reduces the zeta potential and therefore allows antibodies to react more efficiently with RBC membrane antigens. LISS media are often used because they result in an increased rate of antibody uptake during sensitization and a decreased reaction incubation time (from 30 to 60 minutes to 5 to 15 minutes as compared with protein potentiators such as albumin).[20, 21] However, they can result in false-positive reactions and may cause wasted time if reactions have to be repeated with albumin.

Polyethylene Glycol (PEG) and Polybrene

PEG and polybrene are macromolecule additives used with LISS to bring sensitized RBCs closer to each other to facilitate antibody cross-linking and agglutination reactions. They are often used in place of albumin and have some advantages and possible drawbacks. Polybrene can detect ABO incompatibility as well as clinically significant IgG alloantibodies, whereas PEG produces very specific reactions with reduction in false-positive or nonspecific reactions. PEG is considered to be more effective than albumin, LISS, or polybrene for detection of weak antibodies. These reagents have been used in automated and manual testing systems.

Proteolytic Enzymes

Enzymes are protein molecules that function by altering reaction conditions and bring about changes in other molecules without being changed themselves. Only a small part of a large enzyme molecule reacts with a small part of another molecule, called its substrate. They are specific for the molecules they target and can modify proteins, nucleic acids, carbohydrates, or lipids. Proteolytic enzymes target protein molecules. Certain enzymes have been found to modify various blood group antigens and are useful in testing, especially in cases in which there are multiple antibodies present in a sample. Enzymes used in the detection and identification of blood group antibodies include ficin (isolated from fig plants), papain (from papaya), trypsin (from pig stomach), and bromelin (from pineapple). There is no clear consensus of how reagent enzymes work; it is thought that treating RBCs with enzymes results in the release of sialic acid from the membrane, with a subsequent decrease in the negative charges and zeta potential of the RBCs. It has also been suggested that enzyme treatment removes hydrophilic (water attracting) glycoproteins from the membrane of RBCs, causing the membrane to become more hydrophobic (water avoiding), which would allow RBCs to come closer together. Also, because of the removal of glycoproteins from the membrane, antibody molecules may no longer be subject to physical obstruction and steric hindrance from reacting with RBC antigens. The use of enzymes provides enhanced antibody reactivity to Rh, Kidd, P_1, Lewis, and I antigens and destroys or decreases reactivity to Fy^a, Fy^b, M, N, and S antigens.[21]

Antihuman Globulin (AHG) Reagents

When RBCs become coated with antibody or complement or both but do not agglutinate in regular testing, special reagents are needed to produce agglutination. The direct antihuman globulin (AHG) test is designed to determine if RBCs are coated with antibody or complement or both. *Polyspecific* AHG can determine if RBCs have been sensitized with IgG antibody or complement (components C3b or C3d) or both. *Monospecific* AHG reagents react only with RBCs sensitized with IgG or complement.[21] Some AHG reagents are manufactured by injecting animals, usually goats or rabbits, with human globulin, which in turn makes *antihuman* antibodies against the foreign human protein. For the manufacture of polyspecific AHG, both the gamma (IgG) and beta (C3b and C3d) globulin fractions of plasma are processed. For monospecific AHG, animals are injected only with IgG and produce antibodies directed against the gamma heavy chain. Blood bank reagents can be either *polyclonal* or *monoclonal* in source and are discussed in greater detail in this chapter. In the indirect antiglobulin test, the same AHG reagents are used to detect antibodies or complement that have attached to RBC membranes but with a prior incubation step with serum (or plasma). If the antibodies present in serum cannot cause RBC agglutination but only sensitize the RBCs, then the AHG reagents will allow for agglutination to occur by cross-linking the antibodies on the RBCs. The use of AHG reagents allows blood bank testing to be more sensitive. AHG is one of the most important reagents, and the development of AHG is one of the milestones in blood bank testing (see Tables 3–8 and 3–9 and Chapter 5, The Antiglobulin Test, for a more detailed discussion).

Chemical Reduction of IgG and IgM Molecules

There are special reagents available that can be used to help identify the different antibodies present in a mixture of alloantibodies or alloantibodies occurring with autoantibodies. The reagents generally act on covalent sulfhydryl bonds and facilitate antibody identification by removal of either IgG or IgM antibodies. Dithiothreitol (DTT) and β-2-mercaptoethanol (2-ME) are thiol reducing agents that break the disulfide bonds of the J (joining) chain of the IgM molecule but leave the IgG molecule intact.[22] Another reagent, ZZAP, which consists of a thiol reagent plus a proteolytic enzyme, causes the dissociation of IgG molecules from the surface of sensitized RBCs and alters the surface antigens of the RBC.[23] Chemical reduction of the disulfide bond of the IgG molecule is also used to produce chemically modified reagents that react with RBCs in saline. Sulfhydryl compounds reduce the strong but less flexible covalent disulfide bonds in the hinge region of the IgG molecule, allowing the Fab portions more flexibility in facilitating agglutination reactions.[24]

Monoclonal Versus Polyclonal Reagents

Traditional polyclonal antisera reagents have been produced by immunizing donors with small amounts of RBCs positive for an antigen that they lack and then collecting the serum, which should contain antibodies against that antigen. AHG reagents were originally made by injecting animals (usually rabbits) with human globulin components and then collecting the antihuman antibodies. One antigen can have a number of different epitopes, and polyclonal reagents are directed against multiple epitopes found on the original antigen used to stimulate antibody production and can have multiple reactivities. Monoclonal reagents are directed against specific epitopes and therefore are a potential solution. They are made by *hybridoma* technology with spleen lymphocytes from immunized mice, which are fused with rapidly proliferating myeloma cells. The spleen lymphocytes have single epitope specificity; the myeloma cells (a type of immortalized, cultured cell) make vast amounts of antibody. These very efficient hybrid cells, after extensive screening and testing, are selected and cultured to produce lines of immortal cell clones that make a lot of one type of antibody that reacts with one specific epitope. Monoclonal reagents do not use human donors and therefore do not use a human source for reagent purposes. They have several important advantages over polyclonal reagents. Because monoclonal reagents are produced from immortal clones maintained in-vitro, no batch variation exists, and nearly unlimited high titers of antibodies can be produced. Also, the immortal clones can be kept growing in in-vitro culture for years without loss of production and are therefore cost-efficient. Monoclonal antibodies react very specifically and often have higher affinities. For these reasons, monoclonal reagents are not subject to cross-reactivity and interference from nonspecific reactions and can react strongly with the small quantities of antigen in some antigen subgroups. AHG phase testing may not be needed. Unfortunately, there are some disadvantages of monoclonal antisera use, which include *overspecificity*, the fact that complement may not be fixed in the antigen-antibody reaction, both of which can cause false-negative results, and problems with *oversen-*

sitivity, which can cause false-positive results. Some of the disadvantages of monoclonal reagents may be overcome by using blends of different monoclonal reagents or by using polyclonal reagents and monoclonal reagents together.[25] Monoclonal antisera have generally replaced most of the polyclonal antisera and have been used for HLA typing, AHG testing, and phenotyping RBC and lymphocyte antigens.

New and Nontraditional Laboratory Methods

In more recent years, some of the sophisticated testing methods used in immunology research laboratories have become more commonplace in transfusion laboratories. Many of the techniques do not use traditional hemagglutination as the final reaction point. Although many of these methods are more complex to perform, they are highly sensitive and specific. In the not-too-distant future, they may become standardized for routine blood bank use, although most of these methods are now employed primarily in reference laboratories.

Flow Cytometry

Some of the most important techniques to study immunologic reactions and systems are fluorescence-assisted cell sorting (FACS) and flow cytometry. Flow cytometry makes use of antibodies that are tagged with a fluorescent dye. Fluorescence occurs when the compound absorbs light energy of one wavelength and emits light of a different wavelength. Cells that are coated with fluorescent-labeled antibody emit a brightly fluorescent color of a specific wavelength. Fluorescent dyes such as fluorochromes are used as markers in immunologic reactions and a fluorochrome-labeled antibody and can be visualized by an instrument that detects emitted light. There are many different fluorochromes available that have different colors, and they can be coupled to nearly any antibody. Care must be taken not to use colors that have similar spectral overlaps. Flow cytometry can be used to obtain quantitative and qualitative data on cell populations and to sort different cell populations.

There are direct and indirect procedures for labeling with fluorochromes. In a direct procedure, the specific antibody, called the primary antibody, is directly conjugated (or chemically bound) with a fluorescent dye and reacts with a specific antigen. Indirect procedures need a secondary antibody that is conjugated to a fluorochrome; this reacts with an unlabeled specific primary antibody that has reacted with antigen. Indirect methods often require more complex analysis because these reactions have higher amounts of nonspecificity. The secondary antibody is usually made against the species of the primary antibody, such as goat anti-mouse antibody labeled with a fluorochrome.

The principle of flow cytometry is based on the scattering of light as cells are bathed in a fluid stream through which a laser beam enters. The cells move into a chamber one at a time and absorb light from the laser. The light absorbed is different from light emitted. If labeled antibody is bound to the cell, then the light emitted is different from light emitted by cells without antibody. The distinction must be made by the cytometer (a sophisticated cell counter) between different wavelengths of light. The light signal is amplified and analyzed. There are a number of components to the flow cytometry system: these include one or more lasers for cell illumination, photodetectors for signal detection, a possible cell sorting device, and a computer to manage the data.[26] Fluorescence is used in place of hemagglutination as the endpoint of the reaction. Immunofluorescent antibodies and flow cytometry have been used to quantify fetomaternal hemorrhage, identify transfused cells and follow their survival in recipients, measure low levels of cell-bound IgG, and distinguish homozygous from heterozygous expression of blood group antigens.[27]

Solid-Phase Adherence Test

Solid-phase adherence techniques can be used to identify both antigens and antibodies. These tests use antigen-antibody reactions and adherence to a solid phase support system as opposed to hemagglutination in solution to determine if a reaction is positive or negative. Various plastic materials, such as polystyrene, polypropylene, and polyvinyl, are used to make microplates with wells that may be coated with either antibody or monolayers of cellular material for more efficient reactions.[28] Coating reagents include glutaraldehyde, lysine (a positively charged amino acid), and serum-specific antibodies.[29] There are both direct and indirect solid phase testing procedures. The *direct test* consists of reagent antibody of known specificity fixed to the microplate wells with the addition of RBCs with unknown antigen. If an antigen-antibody reaction occurs, the RBCs cover the entire well, and the reaction is considered positive. If no antigen-antibody reaction occurs, no adherence occurs, and the RBCs are free to fall to the bottom of the well and form a button. The direct test may be used for RBC typing for specific antigens. The *indirect test* uses RBCs of known antigenic composition bound to pretreated microplate wells. The unknown test serum is added, incubated, and washed free of unbound serum proteins. IgG-coated indicator cells are then added. A positive reaction is demonstrated if the IgG-coated cells cover the well in a uniform pattern, and a negative reaction is noted when indicator cells settle to the bottom in a button. Remember that with solid phase adherence tests, the button on the well bottom is a negative reaction, unlike with hemagglutination tests where a button is positive and indicates antibody cross-linking.

Gel Test

The gel test uses a type of gel matrix instead of saline to separate positive and negative reactions. A dextran acrylamide gel that can separate particles (or cells) based on size is contained in a plastic microtube. The microtube takes the place of a glass test tube and has an upper reaction chamber and a gel column with a tapered bottom.[30] Whatever is being tested is added to the upper chamber, including cells, plasma (or serum), or both. The reaction is incubated if necessary and then centrifuged. During centrifugation, the inert gel particles act as a filter or sieve to trap RBC agglutinates of different sizes at different levels within the microtube gel column. Larger agglutinates remain at the top, smaller agglutinates filter out toward the lower part of the column, and unagglutinated cells are centrifuged to the bottom of the microtube. Different gel materials are available and can be neutral, specific, or for antiglobulin testing.[30] The gel technique may be used for cell antigen detection and identification, serum antibody detection and identification, and crossmatching and is applicable to automated blood bank methods.[31]

RBC Affinity Column Test

The affinity column test is similar to the gel test in that it uses a plastic microtube filled with a gel-like substance. Affinity column test cards have an immunoreactive gel with a mixture of the high affinity Fc receptor binding reagents, protein G and protein A (isolated from bacteria), covalently bonded to agarose beads (a type of carbohydrate in a matrix) suspended in a viscous solution. Protein G binds to all four subclasses of human IgG, and protein A binds to the subclasses IgG_1, IgG_2, and IgG_4. Protein G and protein A reactions are comparable to reactions seen with AHG and are used in place of AHG in this test system. As in other gel column technology, the serum and cells are mixed and incubated in an area above the gel column. The higher specific gravity of the gel prevents the test sample from entering the reaction gel column. The microtubes are centrifuged; as the test mixture passes through the viscous buffer solution, the RBCs coated with IgG antibodies adhere to the immunoreactive protein/gel beads. Positive reactions produce a band of RBCs at the top of the immunoreactive gel column or a band of RBCs at the top of the gel column and a button of RBCs at the bottom. The thickness of this band of RBCs at the top of the gel column is indicative of the strength of the antigen-antibody reactions. Negative reactions result in all the RBCs passing through the column and forming a button at the bottom. The binding of IgG with protein G and protein A gels has been used in immunologic testing for a long time and has been used in the blood bank for the detection of IgG antibodies.[32]

Diseases Important in Blood Bank Serologic Testing

A number of diseases that are immune-mediated are important in blood bank testing and merit a brief mention here. Some of these will be discussed in greater detail in later chapters in this text.

Immunodeficiency

Immunodeficiency diseases can result from various defects in the IS at many different levels of immune function and may be congenital or acquired. They can result from defects in either innate or adaptive immunity or both; the cause is often not known. Some of the more well-known immunodeficiencies are listed in **Box 3–3**.[33] Immunodeficiencies can influence blood bank test results and transfusion decisions, such as when there is a false-negative reverse grouping for ABO due to low immunoglobulin levels.

Hypersensitivity

Hypersensitivity (or allergy) is an inflammatory response to a foreign antigen and can be cell- or antibody-mediated or both. There are four different types of hypersensitive reactions, and the symptoms and treatment required for each are different. All four types can be caused by blood product transfusions and may be the first sign of a transfusion reaction.

Type I reaction, also called *anaphylaxis* or *immediate* hypersensitivity, involves histamine release by mast cells or

---

BOX 3–3
Classification of Immunodeficiency Disorders

Antibody (B cell) Immunodeficiency, Disorders
X-linked hypogammaglobulinemia (congenital hypogamma-globulinemia)
Transient hypogammaglobulinemia of infancy
Common, variable, unclassifiable immunodeficiency (acquired by hypogammaglobulinemia)
Immunodeficiency with hyper-IgM
Selective IgA deficiency
Selective IgM deficiency
Selective deficiency of IgG subclasses
Secondary B cell immunodeficiency associated with drugs, protein-losing states
X-linked lymphoproliferative disease

Cellular (T cell) Immunodeficiency Disorders
Congenital thymic aplasia (DiGeorge syndrome)
Chronic mucocutaneous candidiasis (with or without endocrinopathy)
T cell deficiency associated with purine nucleoside phosphorylase deficiency
T cell deficiency associated with absent membrane glycoprotein
T cell deficiency associated with absent class I or II MHC antigens or both (base lymphocyte syndrome)

Combined Antibody-mediated (B cell) and Cell-mediated (T cell) Immunodeficiency Disorders
Severe combined immunodeficiency disease (autosomal recessive, X-linked, sporadic)
Cellular immunodeficiency with abnormal immunoglobulin synthesis (Nezelof syndrome)
Immunodeficiency with ataxia-telangiectasia
Immunodeficiency with eczema and thrombocytopenia (Wiskott-Aldrich syndrome)
Immunodeficiency with thymoma
Immunodeficiency with short-limbed dwarfism
Immunodeficiency with adenosine deaminase deficiency
Immunodeficiency with nucleoside phosphorylase deficiency
Biotin-dependent multiple carboxylase deficiency
Graft-versus-host disease
Acquired immunodeficiency syndrome (AIDS)

Phagocytic Dysfunction
Chronic granulomatous disease
Glucose-6-phosphate dehydrogenase deficiency
Myeloperoxidase deficiency
Chédiak-Higashi syndrome
Job's syndrome
Tuftsin deficiency
Lazy leukocyte syndrome
Elevated IgE, defective chemotaxis, and recurrent infections

Ammann,[33] p 319, with permission.

---

basophils with surface IgE antibody. It can occur in IgA-deficient individuals who receive plasma products containing IgA. *Urticarial* reactions (skin rashes) may also result from transfusion of certain food allergens or drugs in plasma products. A type II reaction can involve IgG or IgM antibody with complement, phagocytes, and proteolytic enzymes. HDN or transfusion reactions caused by blood group antibodies as well as autoimmune hemolytic reactions are all type II reactions. Like type II reactions, type III reactions involve phagocytes and IgG and IgM and complement. Type III reactions result in tissue damage from the formation of immune complexes of antigen-antibody aggregates, complement, and phagocytes and are therefore very serious. Penicillin and other drug-induced antibodies can lead to hemolytic reactions through type III hypersensitivity. The type IV reaction involves only T-cell–mediated responses and their cytokines and can be fatal if untreated. The most important type IV reaction is *graft-versus-host,* of which there is also more than one type. Immunocompromised patients must receive irradiated blood products so that T lymphocytes do not engraft and attack the host tissues. Type IV reactions are a problem for bone marrow transplant and stem cell transfusion recipients.

Monoclonal and Polyclonal Gammopathies

Plasma cell neoplasms result in proliferation of abnormal immunoglobulin (or *gamma globulin*) from either a single B cell clone (monoclonal gammopathies) or multiple clones (in polyclonal gammopathies) and may be a specific isotype or only light or heavy chain molecules. Increased serum viscosity is a result of these diseases and can interfere with testing. The increased concentrations of serum proteins can cause nonspecific aggregation (as opposed to agglutination) of erythrocytes called *rouleaux,* which is seen as a stacking of RBCs, like a stacking of coins. It often occurs in multiple myeloma patients. If rouleaux is suspected, the saline replacement technique may be needed to distinguish true cell agglutination from nonspecific aggregation.

Autoimmune Disease

Autoantibodies are produced against the host's own cells and tissues. It is unknown why this loss of tolerance to self antigens occurs, but there are many possible explanations such as aberrant antigen presentation, failure to obtain clonal deletion, anti-idiotypic network breakdown, and cross reactivity between self and nonself antigens. Autoimmune hemolytic anemias are an important problem in testing and transfusion. They may produce antibodies that cause RBC destruction and anemia and result in antibody- or complement-sensitized RBCs. The direct antiglobulin test should be done to detect sensitized RBCs and determine if the cells are coated with antibody or complement. Special procedures such as elution or chemical treatment to remove antibody from cells may be required to prepare RBCs for antigen typing. Serum autoantibodies may interfere with alloantibody detection and compatibility testing. Special reagents and procedures to denature immunoglobulins may be required to remove autoantibodies from serum so they do not interfere with the testing for clinically significant antibodies.

Hemolytic Disease of the Newborn

HDN can result when the maternal IS produces an antibody directed at an antigen present on fetal cells but absent from maternal cells. The mother is exposed to fetal RBCs as a result of fetomaternal transfer of cells during pregnancy or childbirth. Maternal memory cells can cause a stronger response during a second pregnancy if the fetus is positive for the sensitizing antigens. IgG_1, IgG_3, and IgG_4 are capable of crossing the placenta and attaching to fetal RBCs whereas IgG_2 and IgM are not. Severe HDN is most often associated with IgG_1 antibodies and may require exchange transfusion. Antigens of

the ABO, Rh, and other blood groups systems such as Kell have been shown to cause HDN.

Summary

The immune response consists of a complicated and tightly controlled system of many factors including tissues, organs, cells, and biologic mediators that coordinate to defend a host organism against intrusion by a foreign substance or abnormal cells of self origin. The IS functions under the genetic control of the MHC-HLA system to recognize and react to immune stimuli. Immunoglobulins, or antibodies, have special significance for transfusion medicine because antigens present on transfused cells may cause deleterious reactions in the recipient and complicate therapy. The majority of blood bank testing is focused on the prevention, detection, and identification of blood group antibodies as well as the typing of RBC antigens. In addition to antibodies, the complement system is important because of its interaction with the antibody response and the in-vivo and in-vitro effects of complement activation and possible RBC destruction. Antigen characteristics as well as host factors have an impact on the immune response; knowledge of them enables testing problems to be resolved. Understanding the IS and its responses is essential to understanding the factors that can affect agglutination reactions between RBCs and antibodies, especially in testing conditions and media selection. There are routine as well as more sophisticated methods now available for transfusion medicine testing. High throughput testing aided by computer systems may one day be the norm for all immunohematology assays. Finally, it is important to be aware of certain disease conditions that can affect blood bank testing and transfusion and how to handle them.

SUMMARY CHART:
Important Points to Remember (MLT/MT/SBB)

➤ The immune system is very old and complex:
  ➤ It interacts with other host systems and maintains the host equilibrium

➤ The two major roles for the IS are:
  ➤ Protection from pathogens and foreign substances
  ➤ Removal of abnormal and damaged host cells

➤ The two major branches of the IS are:
  ➤ Innate, or natural; the nonspecific primitive IS
  ➤ Acquired, or adaptive; the specific, evolved IS

➤ The two major arms of the acquired IS are:
  ➤ Humoral, mediated by B cells and antibody production
  ➤ Cellular, mediated by T cells and lymphokines

➤ The basic mechanisms used by the IS are:
  ➤ Recognition of self and nonself organisms, cells, and tissues
  ➤ Removal of unwanted organisms, cells, and tissues (self/nonself)
  ➤ Repair of damaged host tissues

- The acquired IS demonstrates:
  - Diversity and uniqueness:
  - Individual B and T cells have vast arrays of unique membrane molecules
  - These molecules can have configurations to match nearly any antigen in the environment
  - Each individual lymphocyte has one unique receptor per cell that recognizes one epitope
  - Recognition:
  - Lymphocytes can differentiate self molecules from nonself molecules
  - Specificity:
  - Antibodies and T cell receptors recognize and react only with the antigen that matches and fits their specific configuration
  - Memory:
  - Selected T and B cells can remain dormant and later respond more rigorously upon second exposure of a previously recognized antigen
  - Tolerance:
  - Immune responses against the host are either removed or downregulated
- There are three types of lymphocytes: T cells, B cells, and NK cells
  - T cells (or lymphocytes) have the TCR, which is usually associated with the CD3 complex. T cells require APCs to respond to antigens. There are two well-characterized subpopulations of T cells distinguished by CD markers, T helper (T_H, CD4-positive) and T cytotoxic (Tc, CD8-positive) lymphocytes. In laboratory testing, T cells can be distinguished from B cells by their ability to bind sheep erythrocytes (called the CD2 marker) as well as specific markers
  - T_H lymphocytes:
    — have CD4 markers on their cell membranes
    — provide B cell help to stimulate the immune response
    — release lymphokines when stimulated
    — recognize antigens in association with MHC class II molecules
  - Tc lymphocytes:
    — have the CD8 marker on their membranes
    — can eliminate specific target cells without the help of antibody (cytotoxicity)
    — recognize antigens in association with MHC class I molecules
- B lymphocytes (or cells) make up about 5 to 15 percent of circulating lymphocytes and are characterized by their membrane-bound antibodies (or immunoglobulins). Membrane-bound antibodies are manufactured by B cells and inserted into their cell membranes where they act as antigen receptors
  - Stimulated B cells differentiate into plasma cells to secrete humoral immunoglobulin
  - B cells receive T cell help for antibody production and for immunologic memory
  - A single B cell clone manufactures Ig of a single specificity for a specific antigen for its entire cell lifetime
- NK cells:
  - Also called large granular lymphocytes; play a role in host resistance to tumors and viral infections

- The primary, or original, immune response occurs after the first exposure to an antigen. The secondary, or anamnestic, immune response happens after a second exposure with the same specific antigen
  - Complement consists of a large group of different enzymatic proteins (convertases/esterases) that circulate in an inactive proenzyme form. Once the cascade is started, they activate each other in a sequence to form products that are involved in optimizing phagocytosis and cell lysis. Complement can be activated through three pathways:
  - The *classical* pathway is initiated by antigen-antibody complexes and requires C1q for activation to proceed
  - The *alternative* pathway is activated by certain macromolecules on the cell walls of bacteria, fungi, parasites, and tumor cells and requires C3b, serum factors B, D, properdin, and initiating factor
  - The *lectin* pathway is activated by binding of MBL to microbes
- All three pathways meet at a common point in the cascade and result in formation of the membrane attack complex to remove unwanted cells.
  - There are three different types of complement receptors on cells, CR1 on RBCs and platelets, CR2 on B cells, and CR3 on myeloid cells
  - There are five classes (or isotypes) of immunoglobulins, all of which have a basic four-chain protein structure, consisting of two identical light and two identical heavy chains. Disulfide (covalent) bonds link each light chain to a heavy chain and the two heavy chains to each other
  - Antibody molecules are isotypic (based on heavy chain subtype), allotypic (based on one heavy chain mutation), or idiotypic (based on hypervariable and variable regions of light and heavy chains) and are reflected in the Ig sequences
  - The N-terminal domains of both heavy and light chains are the variable regions that make up the antigen-binding site of the antibody and vary according to the antibody specificity (the CDR or complementary determining regions) and contain the Fab portion of the Ig molecule. The rest is the C-terminal domains of heavy chains that contain the constant (C) and Fc regions that bind the antibody to cell membrane receptors
- An immune reaction is determined by host response as well as various characteristics of foreign substances. Many factors such as size, complexity, conformation, charge, accessibility, and biochemical composition influence the amount and type of immune response. Blood group antigens may be proteins, glycolipids, or glycoproteins. Not all blood group substances are equally immunogenic in vivo. Generally, molecules of a certain size and complexity as well as significant doses are necessary for a good immune response
- Blood group antibodies may be characterized by such factors as epitope and variable region diversity (monoclonal or polyclonal), mode of sensitization (naturally occurring or immune), expected or unexpected presence in routine serum samples, isotype class (IgM or IgG or, rarely, IgA), activity (warm or cold reactive or both,

agglutinating or sensitizing), clinical significance, alloantibody or autoantibody specificity, serum titer, and chemical reactivity (influence of enzymes, sensitivity to pH, DTT or 2-ME reagents

► RBC antigen-antibody reactions are most commonly detected by hemagglutination procedures. Hemagglutination occurs after sensitization and lattice formation. The final step is precipitation of RBC antigen-antibody complexes. A number of traditional and nontraditional methods may be used to detect and identify serum antibodies and RBC antigenic composition. Hemagglutination reactions are excellent for a clinical laboratory setting as they are fast, simple, and inexpensive and have an obvious endpoint. They also make use of the fact that RBC antigens are clinically important.

Review Questions

1. Characteristics of the acquired IS include:
   a. Immediate defense mechanism
   b. Lack of an inflammatory response
   c. Production of antibody and lymphokines
   d. Primary and secondary responses being the same

2. Substances that participate in the regulation of the immune response are called:
   a. Haptens
   b. Haptoglobin
   c. Cytokines
   d. Lysozymes

3. Which cell is identified primarily by the presence of immunoglobulin on its surface?
   a. Neutrophil
   b. NK cell
   c. B cell
   d. Monocyte

4. Which cell functions primarily in antigen processing and presentation?
   a. Tc cell
   b. Macrophage
   c. Plasma cell
   d. NK cell

5. Which of the following is a signal for the expression of IL-2 receptors on a T_H cell?
   a. Antigen internalized by a B cell in a T-independent process
   b. Presentation of antigen by a monocyte to a T_H cell
   c. Binding of immunoglobulin on the surface of a macrophage
   d. Cross-linking of antigen on surface of a mast cell

6. Which classes of HLA marker(s) are important in immune recognition of antigen in cell-to-cell interactions?
   a. Class II
   b. Class I
   c. Class III
   d. Class I and Class II

7. Which immunoglobulin class would be most important in the study of immune-mediated transfusion reactions due to the presence of alloantibodies?
   a. IgA
   b. IgM
   c. IgE
   d. IgG

8. Which immunoglobulins can activate the classic pathway of the complement system?
   a. IgA and IgM
   b. IgG (all subgroups) and IgA
   c. IgG1, IgG3, and IgM
   d. IgE and IgD

9. Which complement factor is common to both classic and alternative pathways and will result in formation of the MAC?
   a. Factor B
   b. Factor C3
   c. Factor C1
   d. Factor C4

10. Which of the following patient samples for blood bank testing is *most likely* to contain active complement?
    a. EDTA-anticoagulated sample
    b. Heparin-anticoagulated sample
    c. Serum sample drawn 2 days ago
    d. Serum sample drawn 2 hours ago

11. Which one of the following statements is true concerning the formation of antibodies to blood group antigens?
    a. All blood group antigens are equally immunogenic
    b. Only ABO and Rh blood group antigens are immunogenic
    c. Antibodies may form against any foreign blood group antigen
    d. Antibodies formed against Kidd antigens are always IgM

12. Antibody idiotype is determined by the:
    a. Constant region of heavy chain
    b. Constant region of light chain
    c. Constant regions of heavy and light chains
    d. Variable regions of heavy and light chains

13. Which antibody is produced rapidly and in highest amounts during secondary response?
    a. IgG
    b. IgM
    c. IgA
    d. Both IgM and IgG are produced rapidly and in equal amounts

14. Which of the following is *most likely* to account for the failure of a visible RBC antigen-antibody reaction?
    a. Homozygous expression of antigen on an RBC
    b. pH of 7.2

c. Incubation at 37°C for suspected IgG antibody

d. Excess antibody or antigen levels

15. What is the main advantage of LISS media over other types of enhancement media?
    a. Increases speed of antibody sensitization
    b. Increases saturation of antigens on RBCs
    c. May be used for either manual or automated systems
    d. Selectively enhances or suppresses certain blood group antigen-antibody reactions

16. What is the action of AHG reagent?
    a. Reduces the zeta potential of the RBC, allowing closer approach of RBCs
    b. Cross-links RBCs that have become sensitized with antibody or complement
    c. Renders the RBC membrane more hydrophobic, allowing RBCs to come closer together
    d. Enzymatically releases sialic acid from the RBC membrane

17. Monoclonal antibodies:
    a. Have specificity for a single epitope
    b. May be manufactured using hybridoma technology
    c. Develop from a single B-cell clone
    d. All of the above

18. A cellular product is irradiated to prevent the transfusion of viable lymphocytes to an immunocompromised patient. What type of reaction is prevented by this action?
    a. Type I, anaphylaxis
    b. Type II, transfusion reaction
    c. Type III, immune complex formation
    d. Type IV, graft-versus-host reaction

19. From a blood bank testing perspective, what is the main problem with a patient who has autoantibodies?
    a. Large amounts of excess protein may coat RBCs
    b. Autoantibodies are formed rapidly and to many blood group determinants
    c. Autoantibodies may interfere with the detection of clinically significant alloantibodies
    d. Rouleaux of RBCs make antigen typing difficult

20. Which IgG subclass is most important in causing HDN?
    a. IgG_1
    b. IgG_2
    C. IgG_3
    d. IgG_4

21. Secreted IgA exists as a:
    a. Monomer only
    b. Dimer only
    c. Trimer only
    d. Both monomeric and polymeric forms

22. IgM antibody has 10 antigen-binding sites but its valency is:
    a. Pentameric

b. Twofold pentameric

c. Trimeric

d. Hexameric

23. IgD antibody is found on the cell membranes of:
    a. All lymphocytes in circulation
    b. B cells
    c. T cells
    d. Mast cells

24. Some of the characteristics of hybridomas include:
    a. They can be grown in culture for many passages
    b. They produce an antibody with a single specificity
    c. They are produced from fusions of plasma cells and myeloma cells
    d. All of the above

25. Unactivated complement proteins in circulation are in the form of:
    a. Proenzymes
    b. Carbohydrates complexed to lipids
    c. Denatured enzymes
    d. Nucleic acid polymers

26. Which of the following is a list of the five heavy chain constant region amino acid sequences of immunoglobulins:
    a. alpha, gamma, delta, epsilon, mu
    b. alpha-1, alpha-2, alpha-3, epsilon, mu
    c. alpha, beta, gamma, delta, epsilon
    d. alpha, beta, omega, delta, mu

27. Circulating C1 macromolecule complement protein complex consists of which three proteins?
    a. C1q, C1r, C1s
    b. C1q, C2q, C3q
    c. C1q-a, C1r-a, C1s-a
    d. C1q, C5r, C9s and properdin

28. Which complement proteins are good at initiating inflammation?
    a. C1q, C1r, C1s
    b. C3a and C5a
    c. C4a
    d. C3b and C5b

29. The ionic strength of a reaction medium is dependent on:
    a. The number of RBCs in the reaction
    b. The amount of antibody in the reaction
    c. The number of IgM antibodies
    d. The level of ions in the reaction medium

30. PEG increases the strength of agglutination reactions by:
    a. Increasing the ionic strength of the reaction
    b. Increasing water removal from the surface of the RBC
    c. Increasing the concentration of antigen on the RBC surface
    d. Precipitating excess ions from the reaction

REFERENCES

1. Waytes, AT, et al: Preligation of CR1 enhances IgG-dependent phagocytosis by cultured human monocytes. J Immunol 146:2694, 1991.
2. Vengelen-Tyler, V: AABB Technical Manual, ed 12. American Association of Blood Banks, Arlington, VA, 1996, p 189.
3. Benjamini, E, Sunshine, G, and Leskowitz, S: Immunology: A Short Course, ed 3. Wiley-Liss, New York, 1996, pp 93–106.
4. Goodman, JW: Immunoglobulin structure and function. In Stites, DP, and Terr, AL: Basic and Clinical Immunology, ed 7. Appleton & Lange, Norwalk, CT, 1991, pp 109–118.
5. Nance, SJ, Arndt, PA, and Garratty, G: Correlation of IgG subclass with the severity of hemolytic disease of the newborn. Transfusion 30:381, 1990.
6. Rieben, R, et al: Antibodies to histo-blood group substances A and B: Agglutination titers, Ig class, and IgG subclasses in healthy persons of different age categories. Transfusion 31:607, 1991.
7. Sokol, RJ, et al: Red cell autoantibodies, multiple immunoglobulin classes, and autoimmune hemolysis. Transfusion 30:714, 1990.
8. Vengelen-Tyler, V: AABB Technical Manual, ed 12. American Association of Blood Banks, Arlington, VA, 1996, pp 548–549.
9. Kerr, WG, Hendershot, LM, and Burrows, PD: Regulation of IgM and IgD expression in human B-lineage cells. J Immunol 146:3314, 1991.
10. Goodman, JW: Immunoglobulin structure and function. In Stites, DP, and Terr, AL: Basic and Clinical Immunology, ed 7. Appleton & Lange, Norwalk, CT, 1991, p 115.
11. Mollison, PL: Red cell antigens and antibodies and their interactions. In Blood Transfusion in Clinical Medicine, ed 9. Blackwell Scientific, London, 1993, pp 132–134.
12. Moulds, JM, et al: The C3b/C4b receptor is recognized by the Knops, McCoy, Swain-Langley, and York blood group antisera. J Exp Med 173:1159, 1991.
13. Rao, N, et al: Identification of human erythrocyte blood group antigens on the C3b/C4b receptor. J Immunol 146:3502, 1991.
14. Mollison, PL: ABO, Lewis, ii, and P groups. In Blood Transfusion in Clinical Medicine, ed 9. Blackwell Scientific, Oxford, 1993, pp 100–102.
15. Mollison, PL: ABO, Lewis, ii, and P groups. In Blood Transfusion in Clinical Medicine, ed 9. Blackwell Scientific, Oxford, 1993, pp 110–113.
16. Turgeon, ML: Fundamentals of Immunohematology. Williams & Wilkins, Philadelphia, 1995, pp 135, 137, 156.
17. Vengelen-Tyler, V: AABB Technical Manual, ed 12. American Association of Blood Banks, Arlington, VA, 1996, p 539–540.
18. Schleuning, M, et al: Complement activation during storage of blood under normal blood bank conditions: Effects of proteinase inhibitors and leukocyte depletion. Blood 79:3071, 1992.
19. Vengelen-Tyler, V: AABB Technical Manual, ed 12. American Association of Blood Banks, Arlington, VA, 1996, pp 224–225.
20. Issitt, PD, and Anstee, DJ: Applied Blood Group Serology, ed 3. Montgomery Scientific, Durham, NC, 1998, pp 34–35.
21. Kurt, SM, et al: Rh Blood Group System Antigens, Antibodies, Nomenclature, and Testing. Ortho Diagnostic Systems, Raritan, NJ, 1990, pp 13–14.
22. Mollison, PL: ABO, Lewis, ii, and P groups. In Blood Transfusion in Clinical Medicine, ed 9. Blackwell Scientific, London, 1993, pp 99–100.
23. Vengelen-Tyler, VV: AABB Technical Manual, ed 12, American Association of Blood Banks, Arlington, VA, 1996, pp 666–667.
24. Issitt, PD, and Anstee, DJ: Applied Blood Group Serology, ed 3. Montgomery Scientific, Durham, NC, 1998, p 68.
25. Vengelen-Tyler, V: AABB Technical Manual, ed 12. American Association of Blood Banks, Arlington, VA, 1996, pp 204–205.
26. Stevens, CD: Clinical Immunology and Serology. FA Davis Company, Philadelphia, 1996, p 37.
27. Vengelen-Tyler, V: AABB Technical Manual, ed 12. American Association of Blood Banks, Arlington, VA, 1996, p 224.
28. Turgeon, ML: Fundamentals of Immunohematology. Williams & Wilkins, Baltimore, 1995, p 397.
29. Vengelen-Tyler, V: AABB Technical Manual, ed 12. American Association of Blood Banks, Arlington, VA, 1996, p 225.
30. Turgeon, ML: Fundamentals of Immunohematology. Williams & Wilkins, Baltimore, 1995, p 396.
31. Vengelen-Tyler, V: AABB Technical Manual, ed 12. American Association of Blood Banks, Arlington, VA, 1996, p 227.
32. Frame, T: Personal communication, August, 1997.
33. Ammann, AJ: Mechanisms of immunodeficiency. In Stites, DP, and Terr, AL: Basic and Clinical Immunology, ed 7. Appleton & Lange, Norwalk, CT, 1991, p 319.

BIBLIOGRAPHY

Abbas, AK, and Lichtman, AH: Basic Immunology: Functions and Disorders of the Immune System. WB Saunders, Philadelphia, 2001.

Abbas, AK, and Lichtman, AH: Cellular and Molecular Immunology, ed 5. Elsevier Science (USA), Philadelphia, 2003.

Alberts, B, et al: Molecular Biology of the Cell, ed 4. Garland Science, New York, 2002.

Benjamini, E, Sunshine, G, and Leskowitz, S: Immunology: A Short Course, ed 3. Wiley-Liss, New York, 1996.

Brecher, ME: AABB Technical Manual, ed 14. American Association of Blood Banks, Bethesda, MD, 2002.

Bryant, NJ: Laboratory Immunology and Serology, ed 3. WB Saunders, Philadelphia, 1992.

Cochet, O, Teillaud, J-L, and Sautes, C: Immunological Techniques Made Easy. John Wiley & Sons, Chichester, England, 1998.

Cruse, JM, and Lewis, RE: Illustrated Dictionary of Immunology. CRC Press, Boca Raton, 1995.

Elliott, MJ, et al: Inhibition of human monocyte adhesion by interleukin 4. Blood 77:2739, 1991.

Harmening, DM: Modern Blood Banking and Transfusion Practices, ed 4. FA Davis Company, Philadelphia, 1999.

Hybridomas and Monoclonal Antibodies. Bioeducational Publications, Rochester, NY, 1982.

Issitt, PD, and Anstee, DJ: Applied Blood Group Serology, ed 3. Montgomery Scientific, Durham, NC, 1998.

Kerr, WG, Hendershot, LM, and Burrows, PD: Regulation of IgM and IgD expression in human B-lineage cells. J Immunol 146:3314, 1991.

Kuby, J: Immunology. WH Freeman & Co, New York, 1992.

Kutt, SM, et al: Rh Blood Group System Antigens, Antibodies, Nomenclature and Testing. Ortho Diagnostic Systems, Raritan, NJ, 1990.

Lau, P, et al: Group A variants defined with a monoclonal anti-A reagent. Transfusion 30:142, 1990.

Mollison, PL: Blood Transfusion in Clinical Medicine, ed 9. Blackwell Scientific, London, 1993.

Moulds, JM, et al: The C3b/C4b receptor is recognized by the Knops, McCoy, Swain-Langley, and York blood group antisera. J Exp Med 173:1159, 1991.

Nance, SJ, Arndt, PA, and Garratty, G: Correlation of IgG subclass with the severity of hemolytic disease of the newborn. Transfusion 30:381, 1990.

Paul, W: Fundamental Immunology, ed 4. Lippincott-Raven, Philadelphia, 1999.

Rao, N, et al: Identification of human erythrocyte blood group antigens on the C3b/C4b receptor. J Immunol 146:3502, 1991.

Rieben, R, et al: Antibodies to histo-blood group substances A and B: Agglutination titers, Ig class, and IgG subclasses in healthy persons of different age categories. Transfusion 31:607, 1991.

Roitt, I: Essential Immunology, ed 8. Blackwell Scientific, Oxford, 1994.

Roitt, I, Brostoff, J, and Male, D: Immunology, ed 4. Mosby, London, 1996.

Rose, NR, Hamilton, RG, and Detrick, B: Manual of Clinical Laboratory Immunology, ed 6. ASM Press, Washington DC. 2002.

Schleuning, M, et al: Complement activation during storage of blood under normal blood bank conditions: Effects of proteinase inhibitors and leukocyte depletion. Blood 79:3071, 1992.

Sokol, RJ, et al: Red cell autoantibodies, multiple immunoglobulin classes, and autoimmune hemolysis. Transfusion 30:714, 1990.

Stevens, CD: Clinical Immunology and Serology. FA Davis Company, Philadelphia, 1996.

Stites, DP, and Terr, AL: Basic and Clinical Immunology, ed 7. Appleton & Lange, Norwalk, CT, 1991.

Turgeon, ML: Fundamentals of Immunohematology. Williams & Wilkins, Baltimore, 1995.

Waytes, AT, et al: Preligation of CR1 enhances IgG-dependent phagocytosis by cultured human monocytes. J Immunol 146:2694, 1991.

four

Concepts in Molecular Biology

Maria P. Bettinotti, PhD, dip. ABHI

Introduction

Molecular biology is the science that studies the complex molecular interactions that take place in the living cell. For the molecular biologist, *life is chemistry*. Life's master molecule, deoxyribonucleic acid (DNA), encodes the information that directs all of the living chemical machinery.

According to the "central dogma" of molecular biology, first formulated by Francis Crick, the basic information of life flows from DNA through ribonucleic acid (RNA) to proteins. By means of the genetic code, a sequence of nucleotides is translated into a sequence of amino acids, better known as a protein. The key to the chemistry of life is the conformational variety of protein molecules, that is to say, the many complex shapes that protein molecules contort themselves into.

A protein may be shaped into a building block or a structural component of a cell. For example, spectrin is a main structural protein of the red blood cell (RBC) skeleton. The RBC skeleton provides the mechanical strength and deformability necessary for the RBC to move through capillaries with a diameter half the size of the RBC. Spectrin is important to RBC function, a fact made clear by diseases such as hereditary spherocytosis (HS), which may be caused by defects in the spectrin gene. Patients with HS have fragile, spherical RBCs, which the spleen traps and destroys.

A protein may have pockets that temporarily bind or "host" particular substrate molecules, enabling the substrate molecules to chemically react with each other. The protein that acts as a catalyst is called an "enzyme." A good example is the ABO blood group system. The *H* gene codes for fucosyl transferase, an enzyme that adds L-fucose to a series of precursor structures. Once L-fucose has been added, the *A* and *B* gene-specified enzymes can add sugars to the chains that now carry the *H* residue. The A allele encodes a galactosaminyl transferase. The B allele encodes a galactosyl transferase. The O allele is silent. Thus, the immunodominant carbohydrates of the H, A, and B antigens are L-fucose, N-acetylgalactosamine, and D-galactose, respectively. In other words, these genes determine a carbohydrate structure through the action of their encoded proteins acting as enzymes.

A protein may be shaped to bind to DNA itself at specific nucleotide sequences in the chromatin to influence or "regulate" a gene's transcription. This is a protein acting as a transcription factor.

Through all these mechanisms, the genotype of a cell is translated into its phenotype.

Transfusion medicine is tied to three branches of molecular biology: (1) to molecular genetics because donor-recipient compatibility depends on the genetic transmission of polymorphic tissue markers, such as blood groups and human leukocyte antigens (HLA); (2) to biotechnology because of the production of recombinant proteins relevant to blood banking, such as growth factors, erythropoietin, and clotting factors; and (3) to molecular diagnostics used to detect transfusion transmitted viruses. Therefore, blood bankers must learn the basic principles of molecular biology.

Chapter 2 describes in detail the biochemistry of gene replication, transcription, and translation. In this chapter, some of the experiments that led to the discovery and the understanding of the mechanisms underlying these phenomena are reviewed. These experiments are direct antecessors of modern benchtop molecular techniques relevant to transfusion medicine. This brief introduction to molecular biology provides the basis for understanding the applications of this discipline elsewhere in this book.

DNA Is the Genetic Material

Living organisms can replicate and pass hereditary traits (genes) to successive generations; this is their most distinctive characteristic.

In 1928, the British microbiologist Fred Griffith presented a model system that was key to demonstrating that DNA is the genetic material (**Fig. 4–1**). He used two naturally occurring strains of pneumococcus bacterium that differed in their infectivity of mice. The virulent smooth (S) strain, which has a smooth polysaccharide capsule, kills mice through pneumonia. The nonvirulent rough (R) strain lacks the outer capsule and is nonlethal to mice. Neither living R strain nor heat-killed S strain causes illness. However, the co-injection of both is lethal, and virulent S strain bacteria can be recovered from mice infected with this mixture. A "transforming principle" from the heat-killed S strain is able to change the living R strain from innocuous to virulent (S).

Oswald T. Avery and his group at Rockefeller Institute

were able to reproduce this transformation in vitro. They observed microscopically the formation of polysaccharide coats in R pneumococci when cultured bacteria were treated with extracts purified from the heat-killed S strain. The rough pneumococci (R) were transformed into smooth (S). In 1944, they reported that they had purified the transforming principle. By molecular composition and weight, it was mainly DNA. Moreover, treatment with RNA or protein hydrolytic enzymes did not degrade it, but treatment with DNAse caused loss of activity. Avery correctly interpreted that the inducing substance was a gene composed of nucleic acid and that the capsular antigen was a gene product (we now know that several genes are necessary to produce the capsule).

However, Avery's discovery was not accepted immediately. The reasoning was that DNA, a monotonous molecule formed by only four nucleotides, could not be the genetic material. By contrast, proteins, formed by 20 different amino acids with many conformations and important structural and functional activities, were better candidates. Perhaps a few proteins that contaminated the isolated DNA were responsible for Avery's transformation experiment.

Confirmation that DNA was the genetic material came from the "phage group." By the end of World War II, Max Delbrück of Vanderbilt University, Salvador Luria of Indiana University, and Alfred Hershey of Carnegie's Department of Genetics at Cold Spring Harbor coincided in their interest to research bacteriophages, viruses that infect bacteria. Bacteriophages are very small viruses that consist only of a DNA core enclosed in a protein capsule. It was known that, during bacterial infection, the phage particles reproduce inside the cell and lyse the bacteria to release a new generation of viruses. These three remarkable scientists considered this an ideal model for studying the mechanism of heredity because of the simplicity of the organisms. In 1945, Delbrück started a course at Cold Spring Harbor Laboratory to introduce other researchers to their new field of study. The "phage course" was for more than 25 years a training ground for the first generations of molecular biologists.

In 1952, Alfred Hershey and Martha Chase reported an experiment that convinced the scientific community that DNA was indeed the genetic material (**Fig. 4–2**). They infected in parallel two bacterial cultures with phages in which either the protein capsule was labeled with radioactive sulfur (^{35}S) or the DNA core was labeled with radioactive phosphorus (^{32}P). After dislodging the phage particles from the bacteria with a blender, they pelleted the bacteria by centrifugation. The phage particles were left in the supernatant. ^{35}S (protein) was found only in the supernatant of the ^{35}S-labeled culture. ^{32}P (DNA) was found only in the bacterial pellet of the ^{32}P-labeled culture. From this pellet, a new generation of phages arose. The investigators concluded that the phage protein removed from the cells by stirring was the empty phage coat, whose mission was to transport the DNA from cell to cell. The DNA was the material of life, containing the phage genetic information necessary for the viral reproduction inside the bacteria.

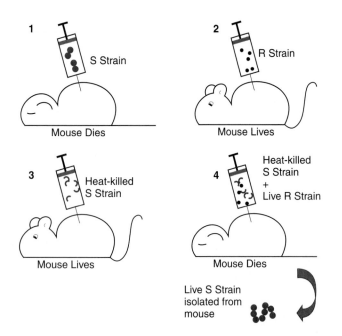

■ FIGURE 4–1 Griffith's Transformation Experiment. Bacterial cells can be transformed from nonpathogenic to virulent by an inert component of the virulent strain (1) Mice injected with pneumococcus strain S die. The strain is virulent. (2) Mice injected with pneumococcus strain R live. The strain is nonvirulent. (3) Mice injected with heat-killed S strain live. (4) Mice injected with a mixture of R live strain and heat-killed S strain die, and live S strain can be isolated from them.

DNA Structure

By 1950, the chemical composition of nucleic acids was known. Nucleic acids were known to be long molecules composed of three distinct chemical subunits: a five-carbon sugar,

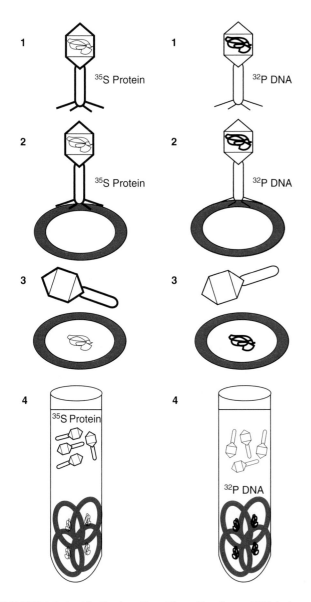

■ **FIGURE 4–2**   The Hershey-Chase Phage Experiment. DNA is the molecule that carries genetic information (1) Bacteriophages were labeled with ^{35}S or with [32]P. [35]S was incorporated into proteins and ^{32}P into DNA. (2) Two *Escherichia coli* (*E. coli*) cultures were infected in parallel with the two different phages. (3) Phages were dislodged from bacteria by treatment with a blender. (4) After centrifugation, [35]S (proteins) was detected only in the supernatant of the first culture and [32]P (DNA) only in the pellet of the second culture. The phages remained in the supernatant and the bacteria in the pellet. From the bacterial pellet, a new generation of viruses could be raised.

acidic phosphate, and four types of nitrogen-rich bases. Two forms of nucleic acids were differentiated by their sugar composition: RNA contained ribose and DNA 2-deoxyribose. Both possessed adenine, guanine, and cytosine. RNA contained uracil, and DNA contained thymine.

In 1950, Erwin Chargaff of Columbia University reported a consistent one-to-one ratio of adenine to thymine and guanine to cytosine in DNA samples from different organisms.

In 1951, Maurice Wilkins and Rosalind Franklin produced x-ray diffraction photographs of DNA, which suggested a hel-

ical molecule with repeats of 34 angstroms (Å) and a width of 20 Å.[1,2]

In 1953, James Watson, trained in the phage group, and Francis Crick, a physicist trained in x-ray crystallography, published a paper in the journal *Nature* in which they assembled the puzzle pieces of DNA structure.[3] They proposed that the DNA molecule was an α helix (see Chapter 2). DNA was a helical ladder, the rails of which were built from alternating units of deoxyribose and phosphate. Each rung of the ladder was composed of a pair of nucleotides (a base pair) held together by hydrogen bonds. The double helix consisted of two strands of nucleotides that ran in opposite directions (antiparallel). Consistent with the 34-Å repeat from x-ray diffraction, 10 base pairs were stacked on top of each other at each turn of a helix. In agreement with Chargaff's observation, adenine always paired with thymine, and guanine always paired with cytosine. Thus the nucleotide alphabet of one half of the DNA helix determined the alphabet of the other half.

DNA Function

Genes must be replicated and passed down to each new cell and each new generation. Genes must also provide the information for protein synthesis. How do DNA molecules function as genes? The search for the answer to this question fueled the advance of molecular biology and introduced the era of biotechnology.

DNA Replication

The Watson-Crick structure revealed how DNA could replicate. The DNA molecule is made of two antiparallel complementary strands. Cytosine always pairs with guanine, and thymine always pairs with adenine. The information in one DNA strand predicts the information in the other strand. During replication, the hydrogen bonds break, the strands separate, and each one functions as template for the synthesis of another complementary half molecule. Two identical DNA molecules are generated, each containing an original strand and a new complementary strand, each to be passed to a daughter cell. Because each daughter double helix contains an "old" strand and a newly synthesized strand, this model of replication is called semiconservative.

The first experiment supporting the semiconservative mode of replication was reported in 1958 by Matthew Meselson and Frank Stahl of the California Institute of Technology (**Fig. 4–3**). *Escherichia coli* cultures were grown for several generations in a medium containing the heavy isotope ^{15}N as the sole source of nitrogen. The bacteria were then switched to medium containing the light isotope [14]N. DNA was extracted from each sample and centrifuged in a solution of cesium chloride, forming a density gradient. DNA molecules of different densities settled to form discrete bands at the point at which their densities equaled the density of the cesium chloride gradient. The DNA of bacteria grown in the "heavy" nitrogen culture medium, in which both strands contained ^{15}N, gave one heavy band. The first generation of bacteria after the switch to "light" nitrogen culture medium gave one intermediate band. All the molecules of DNA were now formed by one "old heavy" strand, with ^{15}N, and one "new light" strand, with [14]N. In the second generation of bacteria, two kinds of DNA molecules were synthesized. One "old

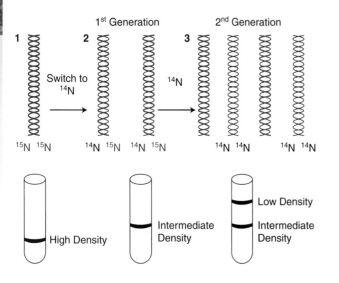

1ˢᵗ Generation   2ⁿᵈ Generation

Switch to ^{14}N

^{14}N

^{15}N ^{15}N ^{14}N ^{15}N ^{14}N ^{15}N ^{14}N ^{14}N ^{14}N ^{14}N

High Density

Intermediate Density

Low Density

Intermediate Density

■ **FIGURE 4–3** Meselson-Stahl demonstration of DNA replication in a semiconservative way. Genomic DNA was extracted from *E. coli* (1) grown in culture medium containing "heavy" ^{15}N, (2) one generation after switching the bacteria to medium with "light" ^{14}N, or (3) two generations after the change of medium. The bottom row shows the different DNA fractions after centrifugation in a cesium chloride gradient. The first tube contains only one high-density band. The second tube contains only one band of intermediate density corresponding to DNA formed by one "old heavy" and one newly synthesized "light" strand. The third tube contains two bands. The intermediate band corresponds to DNA formed by an "old heavy" strand and a "new light" strand. The low-density band corresponds to molecules of DNA containing an "old light" strand and a "new light" strand.

heavy" DNA strand was paired with one "new light" strand, or one "old light" strand was paired with one "new light" strand, rendering two bands in the gradient centrifugation: one intermediate and one light. Thus, in the successive generations DNA was copied over and over following the semiconservative model.

The mechanism of DNA replication was further studied using cellular components to reconstruct in vitro the biochemical reactions that occur within the cell. In this way, the whole process was dissected. In *E. coli* DNA polymerase III is able to form a new strand using deoxyribonucleoside triphosphates (dNTPs) as substrates, double-stranded DNA as template, and magnesium as cofactor. This enzyme can add nucleotides only onto the hydroxyl group (OH) at the 3′ end of an existing nucleic acid fragment. Both strands are synthesized at the same time. The "leading strand" grows continuously in the 5′ to 3′ direction. In the "lagging strand," the enzyme primase, an RNA polymerase, catalyzes the synthesis of a small piece of RNA called a *primer* that provides the 3′OH to which DNA polymerase III can add nucleotides **(Fig. 4–4)**. Finally, enzymes with RNAse activity remove the RNA fragment, DNA polymerase I fills in the gap with DNA, and DNA ligase links the fragments into a continuous DNA strand. Several other components are necessary for DNA synthesis. For example, the enzyme helicase unwinds the helix, allowing the polymerase to gain access to the DNA, and strand binding proteins (SSB) bind to single-stranded DNA, maintaining the double helix in open configuration. This brief overview of DNA replication provides the basis for understanding the techniques of DNA sequencing and polymerase chain reaction (PCR), described later in this chapter.

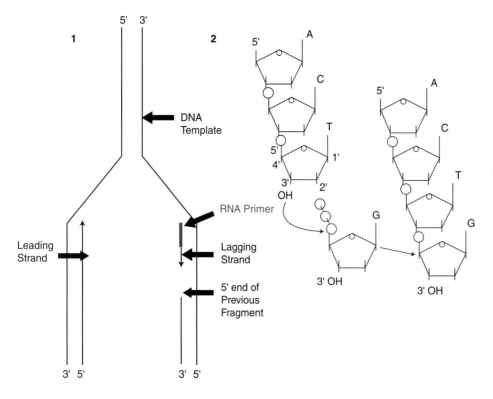

■ **FIGURE 4–4** DNA replication. (1) In the cell, both strands of DNA are replicated simultaneously. Synthesis of the "leading strand" is continuous. Synthesis of the lagging strand is discontinuous. RNA primers function as anchors to which DNA polymerase adds nucleotides complementary to the sequence of the template strand. (2) DNA polymerase adds the nucleoside 5′ monophosphate moiety of a nucleoside-5′-triphosphate to the 3′-OH end of the RNA primer or to the growing DNA chain.

Expression of Genetic Information

Genes act by determining the sequence of amino acids and therefore the structure of proteins. Knowledge of the structure of DNA revealed that the genetic information must be specified by the order of the four bases (A, C, G, and T). Proteins are polymers of 20 amino acids, the sequence of which determines their structure and function. Could the sequence of nucleotides determine the sequence of amino acids?

The discovery of the molecular basis of sickle cell anemia provided the first experimental evidence that the nucleotide sequence of a DNA molecule indeed determined the amino acid sequence of a protein. Sickle cell anemia is a genetic-recessive disease. Patients with this disease have two copies of the mutated gene. Individuals with only one mutated copy of the gene show only mild or no clinical manifestation at all and are called carriers. In 1949, Linus Pauling and Vernon Ingram showed that the hemoglobin of individuals with and without sickle cell anemia had different electrophoretic mobility. This indicated that hemoglobin from the patients had a different charge and therefore a structure different from normal hemoglobin. Carriers of the disease had both types of hemoglobin. In 1957 Ingram identified that substituting valine for glutamic acid in the sixth amino acid of the β-globin chain was the cause of the defective hemoglobin.[4] Thus, a direct link was established between a gene mutation and the structure of a protein.

How is the genetic information transmitted from a sequence of nucleotides into a sequence of amino acids? Work done mainly in the laboratory of Paul Zamecnik showed that proteins were synthesized in the cytoplasm in eukaryotic cells. He worked with cell-free extracts obtained by lysis of rat liver cells followed by centrifugation, which separated the soluble cytoplasmic fraction from the nuclei and from nonsoluble materials such as membranes and mitochondria. His studies established that the microsomal fraction, which we now call ribosomes, was the major cellular component required for protein synthesis.

Because DNA was in the nucleus, separated from the cytoplasm by the nuclear membrane, an intermediary molecule had to be responsible for conveying the genetic information from the nucleus to the cytoplasm. RNA was a good candidate for this role. Its structure suggested that RNA could be produced from a DNA template and that RNA was located mainly in the cytoplasm, where protein synthesis occurred.

Experimental evidence supporting the role of RNA as the intermediary molecule came from the prokaryotic world. When bacteriophage T4 infects *E. coli,* the synthesis of bacterial RNA stops, and the only new RNA synthesized is transcribed from T4 DNA. Using radioactive labeling, Sidney Brenner, François Jacob, and Matthew Meselson showed that the newly synthesized T4 RNA associated with bacterial ribosomes but, unlike ribosomal RNA, it was very unstable.[5] These RNA molecules, which served as templates for protein synthesis, were given the name messenger RNAs (mRNAs).

How could the sequence of four different nucleotides direct the sequence of 20 different amino acids? If the unit of information, called a codon, was one nucleotide, it could encode only four amino acids. If the codon was 2 nucleotides long, it could code for $4^2 = 16$ amino acids. A 3-nucleotide codon could code for $4^3 = 64$ amino acids, more than enough to account for the 20 different amino acids present in proteins. But how could a triplet of nucleotides direct the incorporation of an amino acid into a protein? Direct complementary pairing between nucleotides and amino acids was not possible because both molecules are chemically unrelated.

The experimental answer to these questions came again from studying cell-free extracts. In these experiments, a third type of RNA molecule, which we now call transfer RNA (tRNA), was isolated. These were short molecules, 70 to 80 nucleotides long, and some displayed the remarkable characteristic of having amino acids covalently attached to their 3' end. The enzymes responsible for attaching a specific amino acid to a specific tRNA were also isolated from cell-free extracts and were given the name aminoacyl tRNA synthetases. Sequencing of several tRNAs showed that they all had a common three-dimensional structure, but a unique three-nucleotide-long sequence was always present in a loop region. This sequence, which we now call anticodon, provided the specificity for each tRNA, carrying its specific amino acid to align with the corresponding codon in the mRNA.

The next question was which triplet of nucleotides of the mRNA corresponded to which amino acid; in other words, it was time to decipher the genetic code. By 1966, Marshall Nirenberg and Gobind Khorana cracked the code. Nirenberg used cell-free extracts containing ribosomes, amino acids, tRNAs, and aminoacyl tRNA synthetases and added synthetic mRNA polymer containing only uracil. He was able to produce in vitro a polymer protein containing only phenylalanine. In this way, he showed that UUU was the codon for phenylalanine.[6] During the next few years, all possible mRNA combinations were tried, and the 61 different triplets were assigned to their corresponding amino acids; 3 triplets were found to code for a stop signal **(Table 4–1)**. The genetic code is called "degenerate" because one amino acid may be encoded by more than one nucleotide triplet.

The Central Dogma of Molecular Biology, Expanded

Deciphering the genetic code confirmed the central dogma of molecular biology first formulated by Francis Crick. The genetic material is DNA. DNA is self-replicating and is transcribed into mRNA, which in turn serves as a template for the synthesis of proteins. Although Crick's central dogma remains true, the knowledge acquired in the following years has refined and enlarged it, a process that continues now and into the future.

First, a different method of information flow in biological systems was discovered. By the early 1950s, scientists knew that many viruses contain RNA. Was RNA the genetic material of the so-called "RNA viruses"? The first experiment that proved this hypothesis used the tobacco mosaic virus. RNA isolated from this virus could infect new host cells and generate new viruses. Subsequently, a novel enzyme, which directed RNA synthesis using an RNA molecule as a template, was isolated from RNA bacteriophages infecting *E. coli.* In the following years, scientists found that most RNA viruses, including plant and animal viruses, used an RNA-based mode of replication.

However, this mechanism did not explain the mode of replication of a particular group of animal RNA viruses: the tumor viruses. These viruses can cause cancer in infected ani-

TABLE 4–1 Amino Acid Codons and STOP Codons

Amino Acid	Codon	Amino Acid	Codon
Arginine	CGA	Valine	GUA
	CGC		GUC
	CGG		GUU
	CGU		GUG
	AGA	Lysine	AAA
	AGG		AAG
Leucine	CUA	Asparagine	AAC
	CUC		AAU
	CUG		
	CUU	Glutamine	CAA
	UUA		CAG
	UUG	Histidine	CAC
Serine	UCA		CAU
	UCC	Glutamic Acid	GAA
	UCG		GAG
	UCU	Aspartic Acid	GAC
	AGC		GAU
	AGU	Tyrosine	UAC
Threonine	ACA		UAU
	ACC		
	ACG	Cysteine	UGC
	ACU		UGU
Proline	CCA	Phenylalanine	UUC
	CCC		UUU
	CCG	Isoleucine	AUA
	CCU		AUC
Alanine	GCA		AUU
	GCC	Methionine	AUG
	GCG	Tryptophan	UGG
	GCU	**STOP**	UAA
Glycine	GGA		UAG
	GGC		UGA
	GGG		
	GGU		

mals. In the early 1960s, Howard Temin discovered that replication of these viruses required DNA synthesis in the host cells. He formulated the hypothesis that RNA tumor viruses replicated via the synthesis of a DNA intermediate or "provirus." In 1970 Temin and David Baltimore showed independently that these viruses contain an enzyme that catalyzes the synthesis of DNA using RNA as a template.[7,8] The presence of viral DNA in replicating host cells was also demonstrated. The synthesis of DNA from RNA, now called reverse transcription, was thus definitely established as a mode of biologic information transfer.

Reverse transcription is an important tool in molecular biology techniques. Reverse transcriptases can be used to generate DNA copies of any RNA molecule. As we will see later in this chapter, using reverse transcriptase, mRNAs can be transcribed to its complementary DNA (cDNA) and studied by recombinant DNA techniques.

Scientists have added further qualifications to the central dogma:

1. Genes are not "fixed." There are many transposable genetic elements in the eukaryotic genome. Another mechanism of physical rearrangement is DNA recombination. An example is the genetic rearrangements that generate the coding regions of the immunoglobulin binding site (Chapter 3).
2. DNA sequences and protein amino acid sequences are not entirely collinear. In many organisms, including humans, coding sequences (exons) are interrupted by noncoding sequences (introns). This introduces the possibility of alternative splicing to create different proteins from the same gene. Also, different reading frames can generate different mRNAs and therefore different proteins. Viruses frequently use this last mechanism.
3. Scientists have discovered further roles for RNA. Some RNA molecules display catalytic activity; by "RNA interference," small RNA molecules help to regulate gene expression.

Recombinant DNA

The classic experiments in molecular biology, which we have described, used simple and rapidly replicating organisms (bacteria and viruses) as study models. The genomes of eukaryotes are, however, much more complicated, and scientists had to explore new ways to isolate and study individual genes of these organisms. The big breakthrough came with the development of recombinant DNA technology. DNA from one organism, humans for example, can be "cut and pasted" into a carrier DNA molecule or vector. The new DNA molecule, which is a "recombinant" of the original DNA with the vector DNA, can be introduced into another, usually simpler, host organism. Because the genetic code is almost universal, the host organism treats the gene as its own. This technique is called molecular cloning.

Cloning is the reproduction of daughter cells from one single cell by fission or mitotic division, giving rise to a population of genetically identical clones. In DNA cloning, the DNA fragment of interest carried by the vector is introduced into a host cell. Successive divisions of the host cell create a population of clones containing the DNA fragment of interest. The gene or genes of interest can be studied using the techniques available for the host organism. These techniques have allowed detailed molecular studies of the structure and function of eukaryotic genes and genomes.

The Coding Sequence of a Gene

In humans and most other eukaryotes, the coding part of a gene consists of exons, which in the genomic DNA alternate with noncoding introns. The mRNA contains only the exons, the coding sequence of nucleotides that directs the process of translation into the amino acid sequence of the corresponding protein. Both the genomic DNA and the coding sequence of a gene can be cloned. First, the mRNA is transcribed in vitro to its cDNA, using the enzyme reverse transcriptase. Because all eukaryotic mRNAs end in a poly-A tail, a short synthetic poly-T nucleotide can be used as a universal primer. The final product is a hybrid double strand of mRNA and cDNA. The mRNA is degraded, and a DNA strand complementary to the cDNA is synthesized using DNA polymerase. The cDNA, which has the information for the coding gene sequence, can be subjected to the same techniques as genomic DNA.

DNA Cloning

The next several paragraphs describe the essential tools for molecular cloning: restriction endonucleases, gel electrophoresis, vectors, and host cells. An example of gene cloning follows.

Restriction Endonucleases

The first breakthrough in the production of recombinant DNA came with the discovery and isolation of restriction endonucleases, enzymes that cleave DNA at specific sequences and allow scientists to "cut and paste" DNA in a controlled and predetermined fashion.

Restriction endonucleases are isolated from bacteria. From the early 1950s it was observed that certain strains of *E. coli* were resistant to infection by various bacteriophages. This form of primitive bacterial immunity was called "restriction" because the host was able to restrict the growth and replication of the virus. The resistant bacteria had enzymes that selectively recognized and destroyed foreign DNA molecules by cutting it into pieces (endonuclease activity). At the same time, these enzymes modified (by methylation) the host's chromosomal DNA, protecting it from self-destruction. Numerous restriction endonucleases have been isolated from different bacteria. These enzymes have been classified as type I, II, and III according to their mechanism of action. Only the type II enzymes are relevant for our description of molecular cloning.

In 1970, Hamilton Smith and Kent Wilson at Johns Hopkins University isolated the first type II restriction endonuclease. Type II restriction enzymes are extremely useful for the molecular biologist because they cut DNA at a precise position within its recognition sequence and have no modifying activity.[9] More than 200 restriction endonucleases covering more than 100 different recognition sites are available commercially. The name given to each enzyme reflects its origin. For example, Smith and Wilson's endonuclease was called *HindII* because it was obtained from *Haemophilus influenzae* strain R_d. The number II indicates that it was the second endonuclease to be identified in these bacteria.

Restriction endonucleases usually recognize sequences 4 to 8 nucleotides in length. The recognition sequences are "palindromic;" that is, they read the same in the 5' to 3' direction on both strands of the double helix. Some enzymes cut both strands in the middle of the target sequence, generating, "blunt ends." Some enzymes cut both strands off the center, generating staggered ends. For example *EcoRI* recognizes the sequence:

5'GAATTC3'
3'CTTAAG5'

EcoRI cuts after the first G in both strands, generating fragments with the following ends:

5'G   AATTC3'
3'CTTAA   G5'

The single-strand-overhanging ends are complementary to any end cut by the same enzyme. These "sticky" or cohesive ends are extremely useful for "cutting and pasting" DNA from different origins and therefore creating recombinant DNA. Examples of other restriction endonucleases and corresponding recognition sequences are listed in **Table 4–2.**

Gel Electrophoresis

Another technique fundamental for DNA cloning is gel electrophoresis **(Fig. 4–5)** because it allows the isolation and purification of DNA fragments of a defined length.

The word electrophoresis means "to carry with electricity."

TABLE 4–2   Examples of Type II Restriction Endonucleases

Enzyme	Recognition Sequence
*Alu*I	AG↓CT
*Aos*I	TGC↓GCA
*Apy*I	CC↓(A,T)GG
*Asu*I	G↓GNCC
*Asu*II	TT↓CGAA
*Avr*II	C↓CTAGG
*Bal*I	TGG↓CCA
*Bam*HI	G↓GATCC
*Bcl*I	T↓GATCA
*Bgl*II	A↓GATCT
*Bst*EII	G↓GTNACC
*Bst*NI	CC↓(A,T)GG
*Bst*XI	CCANNNNN↓NTGG
*Cla*I	AT↓CGAT
*Dde*I	C↓TNAG
*Eco*RI	G↓AATTC
*Eco*RII	↓CC(A,T)GG
*Fnu*4HI	GC↓NGC
*Fnu*DII	CG↓CG
*Hae*I	(A,T)GG↓CC(T,A)
*Hae*II	PuGCGC↓Py
*Hae*III	GG↓CC
*Hha*I	GCG↓C
*Hinc*II	GTPy↓PuAC
*Hind*II	GTPy↓PuAC
*Hind*III	A↓AGCTT
*Hinf*I	G↓ANTC
*Hpa*I	GTT↓AAC
*Hpa*II	C↓CGG
*Mbo*I	↓GATC
*Mst*I	TGC↓GCA
*Not*I	GC↓GGCCGC
*Pst*I	CTGCA↓G
*Rsa*I	GT↓AC
*Sac*I	GAGCT↓C
*Sac*II	CCGC↓GG

Agarose gel electrophoresis is a simple and rapid method of separating DNA fragments according to their size. The DNA sample is introduced into a well in a gel immersed in buffer and is exposed to electric current. The DNA molecules run at different speeds according to their size. After staining with a fluorescent dye, bands of DNA of specific length can be seen under ultraviolet (UV) light and isolated from the gel.

In solution, at a neutral pH, DNA is negatively charged because of its phosphate backbone. When placed in an electric field, DNA molecules are attracted toward the positive pole (anode) and repelled from the negative pole (cathode).

To make a gel, molten agarose is poured into a mold where a plastic comb is suspended. As it cools, the agarose hardens to form a gel slab with preformed wells. The gel is placed in a tank full of buffer and with electrodes at opposing ends. The samples containing the DNA fragments are pipetted into the wells after mixing them with a loading solution of high density, such as sucrose or glycerol. The dense solution helps the DNA sink when loaded into the wells.

When voltage is applied, the DNA fragments migrate toward the anode. The porous gel matrix acts as a sieve through which larger molecules move with more difficulty than smaller ones. The distance run by a DNA fragment is inversely proportional to its molecular weight and therefore to its length or number of nucleotides.

DNA bands can be detected in the gel after staining with a

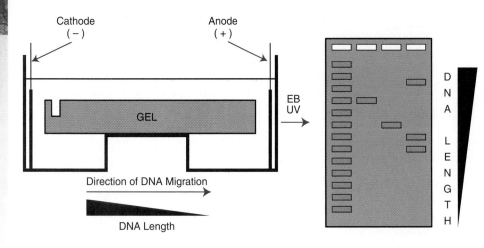

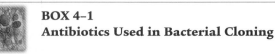

■ **FIGURE 4–5** Agarose gel electrophoresis. Negatively charged DNA molecules migrate toward the positive pole. The agarose gel acts as a molecular sieve: the shorter the DNA molecule, the longer the distance of migration. DNA bands are detected by exposure to ultraviolet light (UV) after staining with the fluorescent dye ethidium bromide (EB).

fluorescent dye, such as ethidium bromide (EB). The gel is soaked in a diluted EB solution or, alternatively, the electrophoresis is run with a gel and buffer containing EB. EB is a planar molecule, which intercalates between the stacked nucleotides of the DNA helix. When the gel is exposed to ultraviolet light of 300 nm, the stained DNA fragments are seen as fluorescent orange bands and can be documented by photography. Each band of DNA is formed by millions of DNA molecules of equal length.

Gel electrophoresis is used in molecular cloning to isolate and purify the vector and insert that which will be used to form a recombinant DNA vector.

Vectors

A vector is a DNA molecule used to carry a foreign DNA fragment into a host organism. Vectors can be used to produce large quantities of a target DNA fragment or to get a foreign gene expressed in a host cell. We will describe in detail plasmid vectors and mention other usual vectors.

Plasmids

Plasmids are the simplest kind of vectors. Plasmids are bacterial circular genetic elements that replicate independently from the chromosome. Naturally occurring plasmids contribute significantly to bacterial genetic diversity by encoding functions such as resistance to certain antibiotics, which provides the bacterium with a competitive advantage over antibiotic-sensitive strains. The plasmid vectors used in molecular cloning are "designer plasmids," modified to make perfect recombinant DNA carriers. A vast selection of plasmids are commercially available that are useful for different purposes, such as DNA sequencing, protein expression in bacteria, and protein expression in mammalian cells.

Plasmids contain an origin of replication from which their DNA replicates. Plasmid vectors can be under "stringent" control of replication, in which case they replicate only once per cell division. By contrast, the so-called "relaxed" plasmids replicate autonomously and can grow as hundreds of copies per cell. Relaxed plasmids are used to amplify large amounts of cloned DNA.

Plasmid vectors contain genes that encode for antibiotic resistance. When bacteria grow in a culture medium with the given antibiotic, only host cells containing the plasmid will survive. Thus, a pure population of bacteria can be obtained. Examples of antibiotics used for bacterial cloning are listed in **Box 4–1**.

Cloning a DNA fragment requires inserting it into the plasmid vector. Plasmids are designed to contain one or more cloning sites, also called polylinkers, a series of recognition sequences for different restriction endonucleases. Most commonly, these are recognition sites for enzymes that cut both strands off the center, which generates cohesive ends. The circular DNA is cut (or linearized) with a chosen restriction enzyme. The DNA fragment to be inserted is cut with the same enzyme. The sticky ends of the linearized plasmid can form hydrogen bonds with the complementary nucleotides in the overhang of the DNA fragment to be inserted. Both fragments are run in a preparative agarose gel. The bands corresponding to the expected size of the linearized plasmid and insert are cut, and the purified DNA fragments are isolated. Both fragments are "pasted" together with DNA ligase, which forms phosphodiester bonds between adjacent nucleotides **(Fig. 4–6)**.

Typical plasmid vectors consist of DNA 2 to 4 kb long and can accommodate inserts up to 15 kb long. Several other vectors are available for cloning fragments of DNA of different sizes.

Other Vectors

λ Vectors contain the part of the bacteriophage's genome necessary for lytic replication in *E. coli* and one or more restriction endonuclease sites for insertion of the DNA fragment of interest. They can accommodate foreign DNA 5 to 14 kb long. The recombinant DNA is "packaged" into viral particles (see the Hershey-Chase experiment, **Fig. 4–2**) and used to infect *E. coli.*

BOX 4–1
Antibiotics Used in Bacterial Cloning

- Ampicillin
- Carbenicillin
- Chloramphenicol
- Hydromycin B
- Kanamycin
- Tetracycline

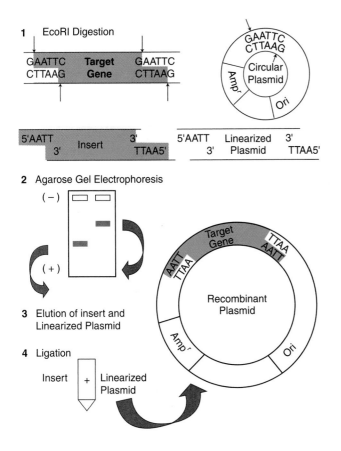

■ FIGURE 4–6   Gene cloning: Part I. (1) The target DNA and the vector plasmid are digested with *EcoRI*. (2) The insert and linearized plasmid are submitted to agarose gel electrophoresis.(3) The bands containing the insert and linearized plasmid are cut from the gel and the DNA fragments eluted. (4) Insert and linearized plasmid are ligated together and a recombinant plasmid containing the target gene is obtained.

Cosmids are vectors that can accept DNA 28 to 45 kb long. They are useful for producing large-insert genomic libraries. Cosmids have a small region of bacteriophage λ necessary for packaging viral DNA into λ particles. The linear genomic DNA fragment is inserted into the vector and packaged into bacteriophage particles. After infecting the *E. coli* cells, the vector circularizes into a large plasmid containing the DNA fragment of interest.

Bacterial artificial chromosomes (BACs) are circular DNA molecules that contain a unit of replication, or "replicon," capable of carrying fragments as large as a quarter of the *E. coli* chromosome. BACs are capable of maintaining DNA inserts of up to 350 kb. A typical BAC library contains inserts of 120 kb.

The Host Cell

The recombinant DNA molecule, which was produced in vitro, must now be introduced into a living cell. The typical host organism is *E. coli*. As we have previously seen, the uptake and expression of foreign DNA by a cell, first described by Griffith and Avery, is called transformation. However, natural transformation is a rare event. The efficiency of the bacterial transformation can be increased by chemical or electrical (electroporation) methods that modify the cellular membrane. The bacteria treated by these methods are called "competent."

Because *E. coli* is a normal inhabitant of the human colon, it grows best in vitro at 37°C in a culture medium containing nutrients similar to those available in the human digestive tract. For example, the Luria-Bertani (LB) medium contains carbohydrates, amino acids, nucleotide phosphates, salts, and vitamins derived from yeast extracts and milk protein.

To isolate individual colonies, cells are spread on the surface of LB agar plates containing an antibiotic used as a selectable marker. A suspension of the cells is diluted enough so that each single cell will give rise to an individual colony. Plates are incubated at 37°C. After 12 to 24 hours (at the maximum rate, cells divide every 22 minutes), visible colonies of identical daughter cells appear. Individual colonies are picked and further propagated in liquid LB culture medium with antibiotic. The incubation proceeds with continuous shaking to maintain the cells in suspension and to promote aeration.

Plasmid Isolation

Plasmids can be easily separated from the host's chromosomal DNA because of their small size and circular structure. A rapid method for making a small preparation of purified plasmid from 1 to 5 mL of culture is called a miniprep. The overnight culture is centrifuged, and the pellet containing the bacteria is treated with a solution containing sodium dodecyl sulfate (SDS) and sodium hydroxide. SDS is an ionic detergent that lyses the cell membrane, releasing the cell contents. Sodium hydroxide denatures DNA into single strands. Treating the solution with potassium acetate and acetic acid causes an insoluble precipitate of detergent, phospholipids, and proteins and neutralizes the sodium hydroxide. At neutral pH, the long strands of chromosomal DNA renature only partially and become trapped in the precipitate. The plasmid DNA renatures completely and remains in solution. After centrifugation, the pellet is discarded. Ethanol or isopropanol is added to the supernatant to precipitate the plasmid DNA out of the solution. After centrifugation, the DNA pellet is washed with 70 percent ethanol and dissolved in water or buffer. RNase is used to destroy the RNA that coprecipitates with the plasmid.

A miniprep provides enough material for some downstream applications such as sequencing or subcloning into a different plasmid vector. However, it can be easily scaled up to a "maxiprep" when more plasmid DNA is needed.

DNA Cloning: An Example

To summarize the process of DNA cloning, we will describe a hypothetical example in which a gene of interest, or "target gene," is obtained from genomic DNA for sequencing purposes. In **Figure 4–6** the target gene, flanked by two *EcoRI* restriction sites, is cut from genomic DNA and inserted into a plasmid vector. The plasmid contains an origin of replication (Ori) so it can be copied by the bacteria's DNA replication machinery. It also contains a gene that provides resistance to the antibiotic ampicillin (Amp^r); therefore, the bacteria that have the plasmid will be able to grow in culture medium with the antibiotic, whereas the bacteria that did not get the plasmid will die. In **Figure 4–7**, competent *E. coli* are transformed with the plasmid and plated at a very low dilution in a Petri dish in solid LB medium with ampicillin. Only the bac-

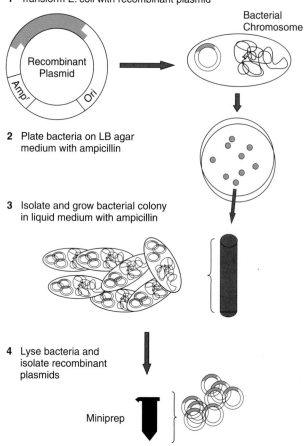

1 Transform E. coli with recombinant plasmid

Bacterial Chromosome

Recombinant Plasmid

Amp^r Ori

2 Plate bacteria on LB agar medium with ampicillin

3 Isolate and grow bacterial colony in liquid medium with ampicillin

4 Lyse bacteria and isolate recombinant plasmids

Miniprep

■ **FIGURE 4–7**   Gene cloning: Part II. (1) The recombinant plasmid is used to transform competent *E. coli*. (2) E. coli bacteria are plated onto solid agar LB medium containing ampicillin. Only bacteria containing the plasmid survive. Isolated colonies, each from a single cell, grow after overnight incubation at 37°C. (3) A colony is picked and cultured overnight in 1 to 5 mL of liquid LB medium containing ampicillin. (4) The recombinant plasmid is isolated from the bacterial culture ("miniprep").

teria containing the plasmid are able to grow and form colonies, visible after overnight incubation at 37°C. A colony is isolated and grown in liquid LB medium with ampicillin. The plasmid replicates independently from the bacterial chromosome, and several plasmids are formed inside each bacterium. From this cell suspension, the recombinant plasmid is isolated. The resulting miniprep contains abundant copies of the gene of interest (target gene) that can be used as a template for obtaining the sequence of the target gene.

Expression of Cloned Genes: Recombinant Proteins in Clinical Use

Large amounts of proteins ("recombinant proteins") can be obtained for biochemical studies or for therapeutic use by molecular cloning. The cost and effort necessary to isolate these proteins from their original source makes their use impractical. Also, the risk of viral contamination is a fundamental consideration in any therapeutic product that is purified from mammalian cells, in particular from human tissues. For these reasons, the use of recombinant proteins is

a major improvement in the treatment of several diseases. The cloned gene is inserted into an expression vector, usually a plasmid, which directs the production of large amounts of the protein in either bacteria or eukaryotic cells. A great variety of expression vectors are available for recombinant protein expression in *E. coli*, yeast, insect cells, and mammalian cells.

The list of recombinant proteins used as therapeutic agents increases constantly. Interferon-α used to treat hairy cell leukemia and hepatitis C and B, recombinant hepatitis B vaccine, recombinant antihemophiliac factor, and recombinant coagulation factor IX are some examples of recombinant proteins useful for transfusion medicine. Granulocyte colony-stimulating factor (GCSF) is used to increase the production of hematopoietic stem cells (HSC) for HSC transplantation (HSCT). Epoetin alfa is used to treat anemia caused by chronic renal failure (**Box 4–2**).

Gene Therapy

Gene therapy is the introduction of new genetic material into the cells of an organism for therapeutic purposes. In the United States, only somatic gene therapy is allowed in humans: that is, the treated cells are somatic and not germ line cells.

The obvious clinical use of gene therapy is the treatment of inherited diseases. In the first clinical trial of that kind, the gene coding for adenosine deaminase was introduced into lymphocytes of children suffering from severe combined immunodeficiency disease. However, several current clinical trials are focused on oncology. These treatments seek to enhance the host antitumor responses by overexpression of cytokines or by genetic alteration of the tumor cell.

One approach for introducing DNA into mammalian cells is by physical or chemical methods. Electroporation and liposome-mediated gene transfer are widely used in the laboratory, but they are not feasible for clinical gene therapy. The second approach is the use of viral vectors, such as retroviruses, adenoviruses, herpesviruses, and lentiviruses. Most human clinical trials to date have used retroviral vectors. However, the use of these vectors carries serious risks that must be weighed against the severity of the underlying illness. The exogenous gene may cause disease if overexpressed or expressed in a certain cell type. Contaminants may be introduced during vector manufacture. Also of concern is the potential for recombination of gene therapy vectors with human endogenous retroviral sequences. The search for bet-

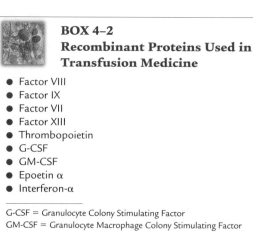

BOX 4–2
Recombinant Proteins Used in Transfusion Medicine

- Factor VIII
- Factor IX
- Factor VII
- Factor XIII
- Thrombopoietin
- G-CSF
- GM-CSF
- Epoetin α
- Interferon-α

G-CSF = Granulocyte Colony Stimulating Factor
GM-CSF = Granulocyte Macrophage Colony Stimulating Factor

ter vectors is under way in animal models and holds promise for a safer and more effective gene therapy.

The Polymerase Chain Reaction (PCR)

An alternative to cloning for isolating large amounts of a single DNA fragment or gene is the polymerase chain reaction (PCR), which was developed by Kary Mullis at Cetus Corporation in 1985.[10] As opposed to cloning, performed in a living cell, PCR is carried out completely in vitro. Provided that some sequence of the DNA molecule is known, PCR can be used to amplify a defined segment of DNA several millions times.

In PCR, DNA is replicated in the test tube, replacing the steps that normally occur within a cell by adding synthetic or recombinant reagents and by changes in the reaction temperature. The role of the enzyme primase, which generates the primers to which DNA polymerase attaches the successive nucleotides, is replaced by synthetic oligonucleotides. The primers are usually 15 to 20 nucleotides long and span the target region to be amplified. In other words, the primers are designed to anneal to complementary DNA sequences at the 5' end of each strand of the DNA fragment. The product obtained will have the sequence of the template bracketed by the primers.

The two primers are mixed with a DNA sample containing the target sequence, Taq DNA polymerase, the four deoxyribonucleoside triphosphates (dNTPs), and magnesium, which acts as a cofactor. Taq polymerase is the DNA polymerase of *Thermus aquaticus*, a bacterium that grows in hot springs and therefore resists high temperatures. The first step of the reaction is *denaturation*. Applying high temperatures plays the role of the helicases and gyrases that unwind the DNA so that the DNA polymerase complex can reach the template. At 94°C, the double strand is denatured into single strands. In the second step, annealing of the primers to the target sequences flanking the fragment of interest is achieved by cooling to a temperature of 50° to 60°C. The third step, primer extension by DNA polymerase, is done at 72°C. This is the optimal temperature for the Taq polymerase, which incorporates nucleotides to the 3' OH end of the primers using the target DNA as template. The cycles of DNA synthesis, which consist of denaturation, annealing, and extension, are repeated simply by repeating the cycle of temperatures. The reaction is carried out in a programmable heating and cooling machine called a thermocycler.

Figure 4–8 shows a schematic PCR reaction. In each cycle, an original template strand is copied to generate a complementary strand, which begins at the 5' end of the primer and ends wherever the Taq polymerase ceases to function. After the second cycle, DNA is synthesized, using the newly copied strands as templates. In this case, synthesis stops when it reaches the end of the molecule defined by the primer. By the end of the third cycle, a new blunt-ended double-stranded product is formed, with its 5' and 3' ends precisely coinciding with the primers. These blunt-ended fragments accumulate exponentially during subsequent rounds of amplification. Thus, the majority of fragments in the later PCR cycles have

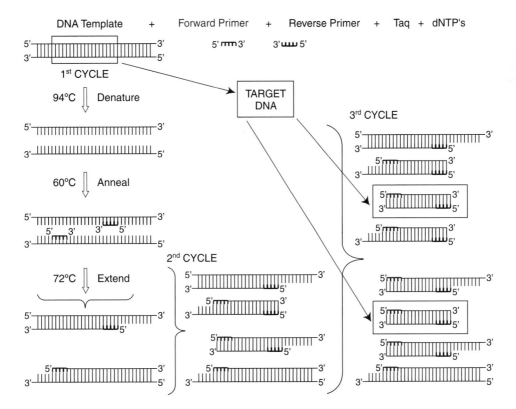

■ **FIGURE 4–8**   Polymerase chain reaction (PCR). Each cycle of PCR consists of denaturation of the double-stranded DNA by heating at 94°C, annealing of the forward and reverse primers to the template by cooling to 60°C, and extension at 72°C of the growing complementary strand catalyzed by the enzyme Taq polymerase. The target DNA sequence, bracketed by the forward and reverse primers, is indicated by a black box in the template DNA. In the third cycle, blunt-ended double-stranded products (also indicated by a black box) are formed with its 5' and 3' ends coinciding with the primers. These target DNA fragments continue to grow exponentially with each cycle.

both ends defined. For example, a single DNA molecule amplified through 30 cycles of replication would theoretically yield 2^{29} (approximately 1 billion) progeny molecules. In reality, the exponential phase of product accumulation during PCR is not indefinite; therefore, the theoretical number of product molecules is not reached. After a certain number of cycles, the accumulation of product reaches a plateau, the level of which depends on the initial number of target sequences, the quantity of reagents, and the efficiency of extension.

DNA Sequencing

Individual fragments of DNA can be obtained in sufficient amount for determining their nucleotide sequence either by molecular cloning or by PCR. Current methods of DNA sequencing are rapid and efficient. As the coding sequence of a gene can be unequivocally translated into the amino acid sequence of its encoded protein, the easiest way of determining a protein sequence is the sequencing of a cloned gene.

Modern sequencing is based on the chain termination method developed in 1977 by Fred Sanger at the Medical Research Council's Laboratory of Molecular Biology in Cambridge, England.[11] The Sanger method is based on two facts of DNA synthesis. First, when a short primer is hybridized to a single-stranded template in the presence of the four dNTPs, DNA polymerase is able to synthesize a new strand of DNA complementary to the template. Second, if 2′, 3′-dideoxyribonucleoside triphosphates (ddNTPs) are included in the reaction, elongation will stop when a ddNTP is incorporated because the ddNTP lacks the 3′ hydroxyl group necessary to form the phosphodiester linkage with the following nucleotide.

We will describe the automated fluorescent cycle sequencing method (**Fig. 4–9**), which is currently used by most laboratories. The reaction, which is carried out in a thermocycler, contains a DNA template, a primer, Taq DNA polymerase, the four dNTPs, and four ddNTPs, each labeled with a different fluorescent dye. The primer is a synthetic oligonucleotide, complementary to the beginning of the fragment to be sequenced. For example, if the gene is cloned in a plasmid vector, the primer will correspond to a region of the plasmid close to the cloning site. The reaction is heated to 94°C, which causes DNA denaturation to single strand, followed by cooling to 65°C to allow annealing and extension. Several cycles are repeated. Working from the primer, the polymerase randomly adds dNTPs or ddNTPs that are complementary to the DNA template. The ratio of dNTPs to ddNTPs is adjusted so that a ddNTP is incorporated into the elongating DNA chain approximately once in every 100 nucleotides. Each time a ddNTP is incorporated, synthesis stops, and a DNA fragment of a discrete size and labeled fluorescently according to its last nucleotide is produced. At the end of 25 cycles of the reaction, millions of copies of the template DNA sequence are terminated at each nucleotide. These fragments are separated by size by polyacrylamide gel electrophoresis in the presence of urea as denaturing agent, creating a "ladder" of DNA fragments, each longer than the previous one by one nucleotide. The fluorescent labels are detected as the terminated fragments pass a laser aimed at the bottom of the gel. When the fluorescent terminators are struck by the laser beam, each emits a colored light of a characteristic wavelength, which is collected by the detector and

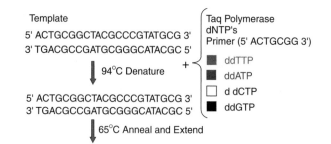
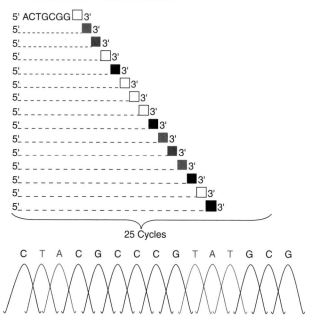

FIGURE 4–9 DNA sequencing: automated fluorescent cycle method. The double-stranded DNA template is denatured by heating at 94°C. Cooling to 65°C allows the annealing of the oligonucleotide primer. In the presence of the four dNTPs and the four fluorescently labeled ddNTPs, Taq polymerase incorporates nucleotides into the growing chain, following the template sequence in a 5′ to 3′ direction. Once in approximately 100 nucleotides, a ddNTP will be incorporated and synthesis will stop. A fragment of DNA is generated that contains a fluorescent tag in its last nucleotide. After polyacrylamide gel electrophoresis, a ladder of DNA fragments with tags of different colors according to its 3′ labeled end nucleotide can be "read" as an electrophoregram.

interpreted by the computer software as A (green), T (red), C (blue), or G (yellow). The final output is an electrophoregram showing colored peaks corresponding to each nucleotide position. Modern sequencers use multiple capillary electrophoresis instead of a gel slab, allowing nearly complete automation of the electrophoresis and data collection process.

Detection of Nucleic Acids and Proteins

Up to now, techniques to isolate and characterize individual genes have been described. To study the role of genes within cells, however, the expression of individual genes and their encoded proteins must be analyzed. In the following paragraphs, methods for detecting specific nucleic acids and proteins will be described.

Nucleic Acid Hybridization

Base pairing between complementary strands of DNA or RNA allows the specific detection of nucleic acid sequences. Double-stranded nucleic acids denature at high temperature (90° to 100°C) and renature when cooled to form double-stranded molecules as dictated by complementary base pairing. This process is called nucleic acid hybridization. Nucleic acid hybrids can be formed between two strands of DNA, two strands of RNA, or one strand of RNA and one of DNA. DNA or RNA sequences complementary to any purified DNA fragment can be detected by nucleic acid hybridization. The DNA fragment, which for example can be a cloned gene or a PCR product, is labeled using radioactive, fluorescent, or chemiluminescent tags. The labeled DNA is used as a probe for hybridization with any DNA or RNA complementary sequence. The resulting hybrid double strand will be labeled and can easily be detected by autoradiography or digital imaging.

Southern Blotting

In this technique developed by E. M. Southern, the DNA to be analyzed is digested with one or more restriction endonucleases and the fragments separated by agarose gel electrophoresis.[12] The gel is then placed over a nitrocellulose or nylon membrane and overlaid with transfer buffer. The DNA fragments are transferred or "blotted" when vacuum is applied by the flow of transfer buffer. The membrane-bound fragments have the same relative positions as the fragments separated by size on the gel. The filter is then hybridized with a labeled probe, and the fragments containing the sequence of interest are detected as labeled bands **(Fig. 4–10)**.

Northern Blotting

This technique is a variation of the Southern blotting and is used for detection of RNA instead of DNA. Total cellular RNAs are extracted and fractioned by size through gel electrophoresis. The RNAs are then blotted onto a filter and detected by hybridization with a labeled probe. This technique is used for studying gene expression.

DNA Microarrays

DNA microarrays, also called gene chips, allow tens of thousands of genes to be analyzed simultaneously.[13] A gene chip consists of a glass slide or a membrane filter onto which oligonucleotides or fragments of cDNA are printed by a robot in small spots at high density. Because a chip can contain more than 10,000 unique DNA sequences, scientists can produce DNA microarrays containing sequences representing all the genes in a cellular genome. A common application of this technique is the study of differential gene expression; for example, the comparison of the genes expressed by a normal cell as opposed to those of a tumor cell. RNA is extracted from both types of cells, and cDNA is reverse transcribed from the mRNA. The two sets of cDNAs are labeled with different fluorescent dyes (typically red and green), and a mixture of the cDNAs is hybridized to the gene chip that contains many of the genes already known in the human genome. The array is analyzed using a laser scanner. The ratio of red to green fluorescence at each specific spot on the array indicates the relative extent of transcription of the given gene in the tumor cells compared with the normal cells.

Fluorescent in situ Hybridization (FISH)

In this technique, scientists use fluorescent probes to detect homologous DNA or RNA sequences in chromosomes or

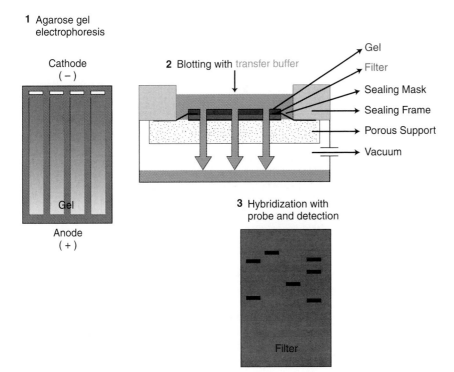

1 Agarose gel electrophoresis

Cathode (−)

Gel

Anode (+)

2 Blotting with transfer buffer

Gel
Filter
Sealing Mask
Sealing Frame
Porous Support
Vacuum

3 Hybridization with probe and detection

Filter

■ **FIGURE 4–10** Southern blotting. (1) The DNA restriction digest is submitted to agarose gel electrophoresis.(2) The DNA fragments are transferred from the gel to a filter membrane by flow of buffer with negative pressure under vacuum. (3) The filter is hybridized with a labeled probe and the labeled DNA bands detected by digital imaging.

intact cells. In this case, the hybridization of the probe to specific cells or subcellular structures is determined by direct microscopic examination.

PCR-Based Techniques

Amplification of DNA by PCR allows the detection of even single copies of DNA molecules. By contrast, Southern blotting has a limit of detection of around 100,000 copies. The specificity of the PCR amplification depends on the primers that hybridize to complementary sequences of the template molecule spanning the target DNA fragment. With carefully chosen primers, PCR can be used to selectively amplify DNA molecules from complex mixtures, such as genomic DNA from cell extracts.

Reverse Transcription-PCR (RT-PCR)

By adding a step of cDNA synthesis by reverse transcription (RT) prior to the PCR amplification, single copies of RNA can be detected. By RT-PCR, RNA molecules can be specifically amplified from total RNA obtained from cell extracts or tissue sections.

Real-Time PCR

In real-time PCR (also called RT-PCR), the product formed in each cycle of amplification is detected by fluorescence at the same time that it is produced. Combined with reverse transcription, this method allows the quantification of specific mRNA in complex mixtures and is extremely useful in the study of gene expression.

The high sensitivity of PCR-based DNA and RNA detection techniques makes them valuable for early detection of transfusion-transmitted viruses, such as HIV and hepatitis B and C. Nucleic acid testing (NAT) is rapidly becoming a standard method in blood banks. It allows the detection of pathogens before the appearance of a testable immune response, such as screening of antibodies. Reducing the "window" period (during which donors can be infected but do not yet test positive) helps to enhance the safety of blood products.

Antibodies as Probes for Proteins

Gene expression at the protein level can be studied by using labeled antibodies as probes. In particular, monoclonal antibodies[14] are widely used in the technique called immunoblotting. By analogy to Southern blotting, immunoblotting is also known as Western blotting. Proteins in cell extracts are separated by polyacrylamide gel electrophoresis in the presence of the ionic detergent SDS. In SDS-PAGE electrophoresis, each protein binds many detergent molecules, which causes its denaturation and provides a negative charge. Proteins will migrate to the anode; the rate of migration depends on their size. The proteins are then transferred from the gel into a filter membrane. The protein of interest is detected by incubation with a specific labeled antibody.

Recombinant DNA Libraries

A way of isolating single genes is by the production of recombinant DNA libraries. Instead of trying to fish one gene out of a mass of genomic DNA or cDNA, each gene is physically separated and introduced into a vector. The target gene is selected by screening each of the individual pieces with a specific probe. Recombinant DNA libraries are collections of clones that contain all genomic or mRNA sequences of a particular cell type. Clones containing a specific gene are identified by hybridization with a labeled probe, such as a cDNA or genomic clone or a PCR product.

As seen in the section on vectors, different vectors are useful for isolating DNA fragments of different sizes. For example, the Human Genome Project used BAC vectors to produce recombinant human genomic libraries. Genomic DNA was isolated from cells and partially digested with restriction enzymes, obtaining large fragments of around 100 to 200 kb. Inserts of these cloned BACs were subcloned as smaller fragments into phage or plasmid vectors, which were used for sequencing.

Complementary DNA libraries can be used to determine gene-coding sequences from which the amino acid sequence of the encoded protein can be deduced.

Oligonucleotides can be synthesized on the basis of partial amino acid sequence of the protein of interest and used to screen a recombinant cDNA library. The clones that contain the gene encoding the target protein are isolated and sequenced. The complete protein sequence can thus be obtained by translating the mRNA codons into amino acids. This approach was used in 1990 by Fumi-Chiro Yamamoto and his colleagues to isolate the gene that codes for the group A transferase.[15]

Another approach for isolating a gene on the basis of the protein that it encodes is by using antibodies specific against the target protein to screen expression libraries. In this case, the cDNA library is generated in an expression vector that drives protein synthesis in E. coli.

Techniques for Studying Gene Polymorphism

By recombinant DNA techniques, experimental analysis proceeds either from DNA into protein or from protein into DNA. An important consequence for transfusion medicine has been the introduction of techniques for typing molecular polymorphism not only at the protein level but also at the genetic level. These techniques are usually grouped under the name of DNA typing.

Restriction Fragment Length Polymorphism

Genomic DNA is usually obtained from peripheral blood mononuclear cells (PBMC) after lysis of the cellular membranes with a hypotonic solution containing detergents and proteinase K. The proteins and cell debris are separated by "salting out" while the DNA remains in solution. Genomic DNA is obtained by precipitation with absolute ethanol or isopropanol. The pellet of DNA is separated after centrifugation and is dissolved in water or buffer.

Genomic DNA is digested with a restriction enzyme and submitted to Southern blotting using a probe specific for the gene under study. DNA from different individuals may render a different pattern of bands. These restriction fragment length polymorphisms (RFLPs) result from a change in the nucleotide sequence of DNA, which is recognized by the restriction enzyme. A restriction site may disappear or be

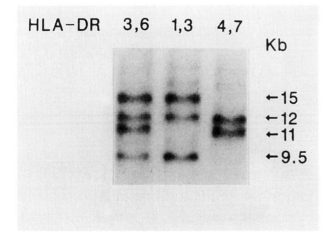

■ **FIGURE 4–11** RFLP. Southern blot analysis of genomic DNA to determine HLA-DR genotype.

created by a mutation, and this results in a change in the size of the DNA fragments.

For example, RFLP can be used to detect the glycosyl transferase gene in a person who is type AO or BO. The nucleotide deletion of the O allele results in the loss of a *BstEII* site (GGTGACC) and creation of a new *KpnI* site (GGTACC). RFLP can also be used to determine if an individual carries the mutation for sickle cell anemia. The gene that codes for Hb$_s$ has one nucleotide difference with the normal β-globin coding allele. The sixth codon of the defective gene is GTG (Val). The sixth codon of the normal gene is GAG (Glu). The restriction site for *MstII* (CCTGAGG) is lost in the mutated gene (CCTGTGG).

RFLP is widely used in HLA typing for transplantation (**Fig. 4–11**), in paternity testing, and in forensic science.

PCR and Allele-Specific Probes

PCR can be used to amplify polymorphic genes from genomic DNA. The PCR products are blotted in a nylon filter and hybridized with specific probes that allow the distinction of the different known alleles. This method, usually called dot blotting or sequence-specific oligonucleotide probe (SSOP) is commonly used for HLA typing (**Fig. 4–12**).

A variation of this method is sequence-specific PCR (SSP), in which the alleles are distinguished by PCR amplification with primer pairs specific for one allele or a group of alleles. Genomic DNA is submitted to PCR amplification with a battery of primer pairs. The products of the different PCR reactions are run in an agarose gel and stained with EB. The presence of fluorescent bands of a defined size in the gel indicates the presence of the allele for which the primer pair is specific (**Fig. 4–13**).

DNA Sequencing

Alleles of polymorphic genes can also be specifically amplified by PCR and sequenced after cloning into plasmid vectors. Alternatively, direct sequencing of PCR products can be done without previous cloning, if the product obtained is pure enough. This procedure is currently used in HLA typing for allogeneic HSCT.

DNA Profiling or "Fingerprinting"

"Minisatellites" and "microsatellites" are regions of DNA interspersed in the human genome formed by variable tandem repeats of short nucleotide sequences. The variability depends on the number of repeat units contained within each "satellite." Minisatellites or variable tandem repeats are composed of repeated units ranging in size from 9 to 80 bp. Microsatellites or short tandem repeats contain repeat units of 2 to 5 nucleotides.

The polymorphism of these loci in the human population is so high that there is a very low probability that two individuals will have the same number of repeats. When several loci are analyzed, the probability of finding two individuals in the human population with the same polymorphic pattern is extremely low. The independence of inheritance of the different loci tested is ensured by choosing loci on different chromosomes. The pattern of polymorphism (the differences in number of repeats or length) can be determined by RFLP or PCR analysis. In 1997, the Federal Bureau of Investigation

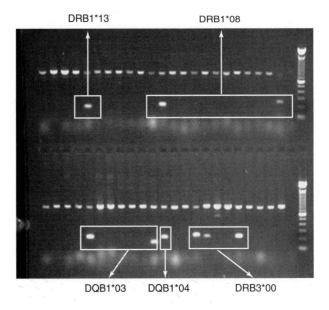

■ **FIGURE 4–13** SSP. Genomic DNA was PCR amplified with primer-pairs specific for different HLA class II alleles or group of alleles. Courtesy of HLA laboratory, Department of Transfusion Medicine, NIH

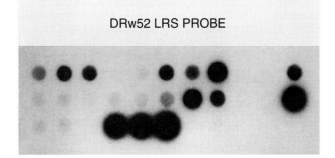

■ **FIGURE 4–12** SSOP. Dot-blot of PCR products hybridized to an allelic-specific HLA probe.

recommended a 13-panel of STRs, plus an XY marker, for criminal investigations. With this number of independently inherited polymorphisms, the probability of even the most common combinations is less than 1 in 10 billion. Thus, modern DNA testing can uniquely identify each person; hence the name "DNA fingerprinting." DNA profiling is used in forensic applications, paternity testing, and in following chimerism after HSCT.

Systems Biology

Some of the most exciting recent advances in molecular biology have been the result of analyzing the complete nucleotide sequence of both the human genome and the genome of several model organisms including *E. coli*, *Saccharomyces cerevisiae* (yeast), Drosophila (the fruit fly), Caenorhabiditis elegans (the worm), and Mus musculus (the mouse).

A draft sequence of the human genome was published in 2001 by two independent teams of researchers[16,17]. The public effort was led by the International Human Genome Project and used BAC libraries, as we briefly described in the section on recombinant libraries. The other group, led by Craig Venter of Celera Genomics, used a "shotgun" approach in which small fragments of genomic DNA were cloned and sequenced. Overlaps between the fragment sequences were used to assemble the whole genome. This draft encompassed about 90% of the euchromatin portion of the human genome. Continuing work by researchers around the world has rendered a high-quality human genome sequence in 2003, 50 years after the *Nature* paper in which Watson and Crick described the structure of DNA. This wealth of information, which is constantly updated, can be accessed through the National Center for Biotechnology Information (NCBI) Web site (www.ncbi.nlm.nih.gov).

In its first 50 years, molecular biology has been primarily an analytical science, concerned mainly with reducing biologic problems to the level of individual genes. This approach has been extraordinarily successful in finding the key genes involved in cellular replication and development as well as identifying the genes involved in genetic disorders such as sickle cell anemia and hereditary spherocytosis. The challenge for the next few decades is to understand the synchronized activity of numerous genes during key biologic events, such as development and memory, and to understand the multiple genes presumably involved in complex diseases such as cancer and diabetes. A further complication is the fact that several different proteins can be produced from a single gene by alternative RNA splicing and that additional forms are created by post-translational modifications.

To solve these complex questions, biologists are turning to more synthetic approaches that allow them to examine the coordinated expression of multiple genes. Experiments performed using DNA and protein chips are starting to show how hundreds or thousands of genes are expressed coordinately in response to different developmental and environmental stimuli. Analysis of these data is one of the applications of bioinformatics, a discipline that uses computer algorithms to manage and analyze large-scale experiments. The functions of genes implicated in a specific pathway can be further explored by "reverse genetics." Genes can be "knocked out" or inserted as wild-type or mutated into the germ line of a mouse or other animal model[18,19]. The resulting knockout or transgenic animal can be analyzed for metabolic or behavioral changes, which can give clues to the mechanism of function of the gene under study. A novel way of studying specific gene function is RNA interference, by which small synthetic RNA molecules can be used to silence a specific target gene.[20] The new biology that is emerging, systems biology,[21] requires integration of knowledge from experiments done in vitro, in vivo, and in silico (in a computer).

SUMMARY CHART:
Important Points to Remember (MT/SBB)

➤ The central dogma of molecular biology: DNA→ RNA → protein.

➤ Proteins have structural, enzymatic, and gene regulatory function. Through these mechanisms the genotype of a cell is translated into its phenotype.

➤ DNA is the genetic material.

➤ DNA is a double helix, consisting of two antiparallel strands of stacked nucleotides paired through hydrogen bonds. Adenine (A) always pairs with thymine (T), and cytosine (C) always pairs with guanine (G).

➤ The structure of DNA determines its function. The sequence of nucleotides of one strand determines the sequence of its complementary strand, the basis for the semiconservative way of replication.

➤ A gene is transcribed into precursor RNA, and the spliced mRNA is translated into the amino acid sequence of the coded protein. The sequence of mRNA unequivocally determines the sequence of the protein.

➤ Recombinant DNA is the DNA of one organism "cut and pasted" into a carrier vector. The foreign gene introduced in a host organism is functional because the genetic code is universal.

➤ By DNA cloning, recombinant genes of complex animals, such as humans, are introduced into simple organisms, such as bacteria, and other model organisms, such as mice, allowing structural and functional studies.

➤ Restriction endonucleases, bacterial enzymes that recognize and cut specific DNA sequences, are fundamental tools for DNA cloning.

➤ Gel electrophoresis separates nucleic acids by size.

➤ The most common host cell is the bacterium *E. coli*.

➤ Plasmids, the most commonly used vectors, are independently replicating circular DNA molecules modified to provide the host cell with resistance to antibiotics (selectable marker) and one or more restriction enzyme sites for inserting the recombinant gene.

➤ By reverse transcription, mRNA is transcribed into complementary DNA (cDNA).

➤ Automated fluorescent DNA sequencing based on the Sanger method is a standard laboratory procedure.

➤ DNA sequencing of a cloned cDNA corresponding to a given gene is the easiest way to determine the amino acid sequence of a protein.

➤ Genomic and cDNA libraries are collections of clones containing the genetic material of a cell.

➤ Base pairing between complementary strands of DNA or RNA (hybridization with a labeled probe) is used to detect specific nucleic acid sequences in complex mixtures.

➤ Southern blotting, Northern blotting, and dot blotting are hybridization-based techniques for nucleic acid sequence specific recognition.

➤ The polymerase chain reaction (PCR) is an in-vitro method for DNA amplification.

➤ Molecular polymorphism is studied at the genetic level by DNA typing. Methods for DNA typing relevant for transfusion medicine are restriction fragment length polymorphism, allele-specific oligonucleotide probe hybridization, allele-specific PCR amplification, DNA sequencing, and DNA profiling (DNA fingerprinting).

➤ PCR is used for the early detection of transfusion-transmitted pathogens.

➤ Other therapeutic uses of molecular biology are gene therapy and the clinical use of recombinant proteins, such as interferons, coagulation factors, and growth factors.

REVIEW QUESTIONS

1. The central dogma of molecular biology states that:
   a. DNA is the genetic material
   b. RNA is the genetic material
   c. DNA is translated to mRNA
   d. Proteins are transcribed from mRNA

2. Recombinant-DNA technology is possible because:
   a. Restriction endonucleases cut RNA
   b. Restriction endonucleases cut proteins
   c. The genetic code is universal
   d. Bacteria are difficult to culture

3. Agarose gel electrophoresis is a technique used for:
   a. DNA synthesis
   b. RNA synthesis
   c. Separation of DNA molecules by size
   d. Oligonucleotide synthesis

4. Restriction fragment length polymorphism (RFLP) is based on the use of the enzymes:
   a. Reverse transcriptases
   b. Bacterial endonucleases
   c. DNA polymerases
   d. RNA polymerases

5. The polymerase chain reaction (PCR):
   a. Is carried out *in vivo*
   b. Is used for peptide synthesis
   c. Requires RNA polymerase
   d. Is used for the amplification of DNA

6. Plasmids are:
   a. Vectors used for molecular cloning
   b. Antibiotics
   c. Enzymes
   d. Part of chromosomes

7. Some model organisms:
   a. Simplify the study of human disease
   b. Are used to produce recombinant proteins
   c. Are prokaryotes and some are eukaryotes
   d. All of the above

8. DNA sequencing:
   a. Is more difficult than peptide sequencing
   b. Requires the use of RNA polymerase
   d. Is an enzymatic *in vitro* reaction

9. RFLP and SSP are techniques used for:
   a. Protein isolation
   b. RNA isolation
   c. DNA typing
   d. Protein typing

10. Recombinant DNA techniques:
    a. Are not used in a clinical setting
    b. Are useful research tools
    c. Are not used in blood banking
    d. Are useful only for research

REFERENCES

1. Franklin, RE, and Gosling, RG: Molecular configuration in sodium thymonucleate. Nature 171: 740 – 741, 1953.
2. Wilkins, MHF, Stokes, AR, and Wilson, HR: Molecular structure of deoxypentose nucleic acids. Nature 171: 738 – 740, 1953.
3. Watson, JD, and Crick, FHC: Molecular structure of nucleic acids: A structure for deoxyribose nucleic acid. Nature 171: 737 – 738, 1953.
4. Ingram, VM: Gene mutations in human hemoglobin: The chemical difference between normal and sickle cell hemoglobin. Nature 180: 326 – 328, 1957.
5. Brenner, S, Jacob, F, and Meselson, M: An unstable intermediate carrying information from genes to ribosomes for protein synthesis. Nature 190: 576 – 581, 1961.
6. Nirenberg, M, and Leder, P: RNA codewords and protein synthesis. Science 145: 1399 – 1407, 1964.
7. Temin, HM, and Mizutani, S: RNA-dependent DNA polymerase in virions of Rous sarcoma virus. Nature 226: 1211 – 1213, 1970.
8. Baltimore, D: RNA-dependent DNA polymerase in virions of RNA tumour viruses. Nature 226: 1209 – 1211, 1970.
9. Nathans, D, and Smith, HO, Restriction endonucleases in the analysis and restructuring of DNA molecules. Ann Rev Biochem 44: 273 – 293, 1975.
10. Saiki, RK, Gelfand, DH, Stoffel, S, Scharf R, Higuchi, R, Horn, GT, Mullis, KB, and Ehrlich, HA: Primer-directed enzymatic amplification of DNA with a thermostable DNA polymerase. Science 239: 487 – 491, 1988.
11. Sanger, F, Nicklen, S, and Coulson, AR: DNA sequencing with chain-terminating inhibitors. Proc Natl Acad Sci USA 74: 5463 – 5467, 1977.
12. Southern, EM: Detection of specific sequences among DNA fragments separated by gel electrophoresis. J Mol Biol 98: 503 – 517, 1975.
13. Brown, PO, and Botstein, D: Exploring the new world of the genome with DNA microarrays. Nature Genetics 21: 33 – 37, 1999.
14. Kohler, G, and Milstein, C: Continuous cultures of fused cells secreting antibody of predefined specificity. Nature 256: 495 – 497, 1975.
15. Yamamoto, F, et al: Cloning and characterization of DNA complementary to human Histo-blood group A transferase mRNA. J Biol Chem 265: 1146 – 51, 1990.
16. International Human Genome Sequencing Consortium: Initial sequencing and analysis of the human genome. Nature 409: 860 – 921, 2001.
17. Venter, J C et al: The sequence of the human genome. Science 291: 1304 – 1351, 2001.
18. Capecchi, MR: Altering the genome by homologous recombination. Science 244: 1288 – 1292, 1989.
19. Bronson, SK, and Smithies, O: Altering mice by homologous recombination using embryonic stem cells. J Biol Chem 269: 27155 – 27158, 1995.
20. Sharp, PA: RNA interference-2001. Genes Dev 15: 485 – 490, 2001.
21. Kitano, H, (ed.): Foundations of Systems Biology. The MIT Press, Cambridge, Massachusetts, 2001.

BIBLIOGRAPHY

Alberts, B et al: Molecular biology of the cell. 4th edition. Garland Publishing, New York, 2002.

American Association of Blood Banks Technical Manual. 14th edition. AABB, Bethesda, MD, 2002.

Anderson, KC, and Ness, PM: Scientific basis of transfusion medicine. Second edition. W. B. Saunders Company, Philadelphia, 2000.

Birren B et al.: Analyzing DNA: a laboratory manual. Cold Spring Harbor Laboratory Press, Cold Spring Harbor, NY, 1997.

Cooper, GM, and Hausman, RE: The cell: a molecular approach. 3rd edition. ASM Press, Washington, D.C., 2004.

Harmening, DM: Modern blood banking and transfusion practices. 4th edition. F.A. Davis Company, Philadelphia, 1999.

Issitt, PD, and Anstee, DJ: Applied blood group serology. 4th edition. Montgomery Scientific Publications, Durham, NC, 1998.

Lewin, B: Genes VII. Oxford University Press, Oxford, UK, 2000.

Micklos DA, and Freyer, GA: DNA Science. A first course. 2nd edition. Cold Spring Harbor Laboratory Press, Cold Spring Harbor, NY, 2003.

Sambrook, J, and Russell, DW: Molecular cloning: A laboratory manual. Third edition. Cold Spring Harbor Laboratory Press, Cold Spring Harbor, New York, 2001.

The human genome: *Nature* 409: 745–964, 2001.

The human genome: *Science*, 291: 1145–1434, 2001.

five

The Antiglobulin Test

**Ralph E.B. Green, B. App. Sci., FAIMLS, MACE, and
Virginia C. Hughes, MS, MT(ASCP)SBB, CLS(NCA)I**

OBJECTIVES

On completion of this chapter, the learner should be able to:

1. State the principle of the antiglobulin test.
2. Differentiate monoclonal from polyclonal and monospecific from polyspecific antihuman globulin (AHG) reagents.
3. Describe the preparation of monoclonal and polyclonal AHG reagents.
4. Explain the antibody requirements for AHG reagents.
5. Discuss the use of polyspecific versus monospecific AHG in the indirect antiglobulin test (IAT).
6. Discuss the advantages and disadvantages of anticomplement activity in polyspecific AHG.

7. Compare and contrast the IAT and the direct antiglobulin test (DAT).
8. Include an explanation of (1) principle, (2) applications, and (3) red blood cell sensitization.
9. List the reasons for the procedural steps in the DAT and IAT.
10. Interpret the results of a DAT panel.
11. List the factors that affect the antiglobulin test.
12. List the sources of error associated with the performance of the antiglobulin test.
13. Discuss new techniques for antiglobulin testing.

Introduction

The antiglobulin test (also called Coombs' test) is based on the principle that antihuman globulins (AHGs) obtained from immunized nonhuman species bind to human globulins such as IgG or complement, either free in serum or attached to antigens on red blood cells (RBCs).

There are two major types of blood group antibodies, IgM and IgG. Because of their large pentamer structure, IgM antibodies bind to corresponding antigen and directly agglutinate RBCs suspended in saline. IgG antibodies are termed *nonagglutinating* because their monomer structure is too small to agglutinate sensitized RBCs directly. The addition of AHG containing anti-IgG to RBCs sensitized with IgG antibodies allows for hemagglutination of these sensitized cells. Some blood group antibodies have the ability to bind complement to the RBC membrane. Antiglobulin tests detect IgG and/or complement-sensitized RBCs.

History of the Antiglobulin Test

Before the discovery of the antiglobulin test, only IgM antibodies had been detected. The introduction of the antiglobulin test permitted the detection of nonagglutinating IgG antibodies and led to the discovery and characterization of many new blood group systems.

In 1945, Coombs and associates[1] described the use of the antiglobulin test for the detection of weak and nonagglutinating Rh antibodies in serum. In 1946, Coombs and coworkers[2] described the use of AHG to detect in-vivo sensitization of the RBCs of babies suffering from hemolytic disease of the newborn (HDN). Although the test was initially of great value in the investigation of Rh HDN, its versatility for the detection of other IgG blood group antibodies soon became evident. The first of the Kell blood group system antibodies[3] and the associated antigen were reported only weeks after Coombs had described the test.

Although Coombs and associates[1] were instrumental in introducing the antiglobulin test to blood group serology, the principle of the test had in fact been described by Moreschi[4] in 1908. Moreschi's studies involved the use of rabbit antigoat serum to agglutinate rabbit RBCs that were sensitized with low nonagglutinating doses of goat anti-rabbit RBC serum.

Coombs' procedure involved the injection of human serum into rabbits to produce antihuman serum. After absorption to remove heterospecific antibodies and dilution to avoid prozone, the AHG serum still retained sufficient antibody activity to permit cross-linking of adjacent RBCs sensitized with IgG antibodies. The cross-linking of sensitized RBCs by AHG produced hemagglutination, indicating that the RBCs had been sensitized by an antibody that had reacted with an antigen present on the cell surface.

The antiglobulin test can be used to detect RBCs sensitized with IgG alloantibodies, IgG autoantibodies, and complement components. Sensitization can occur either in vivo or in vitro. The use of AHG to detect in-vitro sensitization of RBCs is a two-stage technique referred to as the indirect antiglobulin test (IAT). In-vivo sensitization is detected by a one-stage procedure, the direct antiglobulin test (DAT). The IAT and DAT still remain the most common procedures performed in blood group serology.

AHG Reagents

Several AHG reagents have been defined by the Food and Drug Administration (FDA) Center for Biologics Evaluation and Research (CBER). These are listed in **Table 5–1** and are

TABLE 5–1 Antihuman Globulin Reagents	
Reagent	**Definition**
Polyspecific	
1. Rabbit polyclonal	Contains anti-IgG and anti-C3d (may contain other anticomplement and other anti-immunoglobulin antibodies).
2. Rabbit/murine monoclonal blend	Contains a blend of rabbit polyclonal antihuman IgG and murine monoclonal anti-C3b and -C3d.
3. Murine monoclonal	Contains murine monoclonal anti-IgG, anti-C3b, and anti-C3d.
Monospecific Anti-IgG	
1. Rabbit polyclonal	Contains anti-IgG with no anti-complement activity (not necessarily gamma-chain specific).
2. IgG heavy-chain specific	Contains only antibodies reactive against human gamma chains.
3. Monoclonal IgG	Contains murine monoclonal anti-IgG
Anticomplement	
Rabbit polyclonal 1. Anti-C3d and anti-C3b 2. Anti-C3d, anti-C4b, anti-C4d	Contains only antibodies reactive against the designated complement component(s), with no anti-immunoglobulin activity.
Murine Monoclonal 1. Anti-C3d 2. Anti-C3b, anti-C3d	Contains only antibodies reactive against the designated complement component, with no anti-immunoglobulin activity.

Modified from Tyler, V (ed): Technical Manual, ed 12. American Association of Blood Banks, Bethesda, MD, 1996.

discussed in the following paragraphs. Antihuman globulin reagents may be polyspecific or monospecific.

Polyspecific AHG

Polyspecific AHG contains antibody to human IgG and to the C3d component of human complement. Other anticomplement antibodies, such as anti-C3b, anti-C4b, and anti-C4d, may also be present. Commercially prepared polyspecific AHG contains little, if any, activity against IgA and IgM heavy chains. However, the polyspecific mixture may contain antibody activity to kappa and lambda light chains common to all immunoglobulin classes, thus reacting with IgA or IgM molecules.[5]

Monospecific AHG

Monospecific AHG reagents contain only one antibody specificity: either anti-IgG or antibody to specific complement components such as C3b or C3d. Licensed monospecific AHG reagents in common use are anti-IgG and anti-C3b-C3d.[5]

Anti-IgG

Reagents labeled anti-IgG contain no anticomplement activity. Anti-IgG reagents contain antibodies specific for the Fc fragment of the gamma heavy chain of the IgG molecule. If not labeled "gamma heavy chain–specific," anti-IgG may contain anti–light chain specificity and therefore react with cells sensitized with IgM and IgA as well as with IgG.[5]

Anti-Complement

Anti-complement reagents, such as anti-C3b-C3d reagents, are reactive against the designated complement components only and contain no activity against human immunoglobulins.[5]

Preparation of AHG

The classic method of AHG production involves injecting human serum or purified globulin into laboratory animals, such as rabbits. The human globulin behaves as foreign antigen, the rabbit's immune response is triggered, and an antibody to human globulin is produced. For example, human IgG injected into a rabbit results in anti-IgG production; human complement components injected into a rabbit result in anticomplement. This type of response produces a polyclonal antiglobulin serum. Polyclonal antibodies are a mixture of antibodies from different plasma cell clones. The resulting polyclonal antibodies recognize different antigenic determinants (epitopes), or the same portion of the antigen but with different affinities. Hybridoma technology can be used to produce monoclonal antiglobulin serum. Monoclonal antibodies are derived from one clone of plasma cells and recognize a single epitope.

Preparation of Polyspecific AHG

Polyclonal AHG Production

Polyclonal AHG is usually prepared in rabbits, although when large volumes of antibody are required, sheep or goats may be used. In contrast with the early production methods, in which a crude globulin fraction of serum was used as the immunogen, modern production commences with the purification of the immunogen from a large pool of normal sera.

Conventional polyspecific antiglobulin reagents are produced by immunizing one colony of rabbits with human immunoglobulin (IgG) antigen and another colony with human C3 antigen. Because of the heterogeneity of IgG molecules, the use of serum from many donors to prepare the pooled IgG antigen to immunize the rabbits and the pooling of anti-IgG from many immunized rabbits are essential in producing reagents for routine use that are capable of detecting the many different IgG antibodies. This is an advantage of using anti-IgG of polyclonal origin for antiglobulin serum.[6]

Both colonies of animals are hyperimmunized to produce high-titer, high-avidity IgG antibodies. Blood specimens are drawn from the immunized animals, and if the antibody potency and specificity meet predetermined specifications, the animals are bled for a production batch of reagent. Separate blends of the anti-IgG and anticomplement antibodies are made, and each pool is then absorbed with A_1, B, and O cells to remove heterospecific antibodies. The total antibody content of each pool is determined, and the potency of the pools is analyzed to calculate the optimum antibody dilution for use. Block titrations for anti-IgG pools are performed by reacting dilutions of each antibody against cells sensitized with different amounts of IgG. This is a critical step in the manufacturing process because excess antibody, especially with anti-IgG, may lead to prozoning and, hence, false-negative test results.

Because it is not possible to coat cells with measured amounts of complement, the potency of anti-C3 pools is measured using at least two examples each of a C3b- and C3d-coated cell. Both anti-C3b (C3c) and anti-C3d are present in the polyclonal anti-C3 pool. The level of anti-C3d is particularly critical in keeping false-positive tests to a minimum yet detecting clinically significant amounts of RBC-bound C3d. Additionally, if the dilution of the anti-C3 pool is determined on the basis of the amount of anti-C3d present, the level of anti-C3b (C3c) varies. The inability to determine the potency of anti-C3b and anti-C3d individually is one of the difficulties with polyclonal reagents that can be avoided with monoclonal products.[6] Once the required performance characteristics of the trial blend are obtained, a production blend of the separate anti-IgG and anticomplement pools is made.

Monoclonal AHG Production

The monoclonal antibody technique devised by Kohler and Milstein[7] has been used to produce AHG and has proved particularly useful in producing high-titer antibodies with well-defined specificities to IgG and to the fragments of C3.[8–10]

Monoclonal antibody production begins with the immunization of laboratory animals, usually mice, with purified human globulin. After a suitable immune response, mouse spleen cells containing antibody-secreting lymphocytes are fused with myeloma cells. The resulting "hybridomas" are screened for antibodies with the required specificity and affinity. The antibody-secreting clones may then be propagated in tissue culture or by inoculation into mice, in which case the antibody is collected as ascites. Because the clonal line produces a single antibody, there is no need for absorption to remove heterospecific antibodies. All antibody molecules produced by a clone of hybridoma cells are identical in terms of antibody structure and antigen specificity. This has advantages and disadvantages in AHG production. Once an antibody-secreting clone of cells has been established, antibody with the same specificity and reaction characteristics will be available indefinitely. This allows the production of a consistently pure and uncontaminated AHG reagent. The disadvantage is that all antibodies produced by a clone of cells recognize a single epitope present on an antigen. For antigens composed of multiple epitopes such as IgG, several different monoclonal antibodies reacting with different epitopes may need to be blended, or a monoclonal antibody specificity for an epitope on all variants of a particular antigen may need to be selected to ensure that all different expressions of the antigen are detected. Monoclonal antibodies to human complement components anti-C3b and anti-C3d may be blended with polyclonal anti-IgG from rabbits to achieve potent reagents that give fewer false-positive reactions as a result of anticomplement; Gamma Biologicals manufactures AHG reagents from an entirely monoclonal source. The anti-IgG component is produced by exposing mice to RBCs coated with IgG. The resulting monoclonal anti-IgG reacts with the C_H3 region of the gamma chain of IgG subclasses 1, 2, and 3. The antibody does not react with human antibodies of subclass IgG_4, but these are not considered to be clinically significant. Blending the monoclonal anti-IgG with a monoclonal anti-C3b and monoclonal anti-C3d results in a polyspecific AHG reagent. The preparation of polyclonal and monoclonal AHG is dia-

grammed in **Figure 5–1**. Before the AHG is available for purchase, manufacturers must subject their reagents to an evaluation procedure, and the results must be submitted to the United States Food and Drug Administration for approval. Whether produced by the polyclonal or monoclonal technique, the final polyspecific product is one that contains both anti-IgG and anticomplement activity at the correct potency for immediate use. The reagent also contains buffers, stabilizers, and bacteriostatic agents and may be dyed green for identification.

Preparation of Monospecific AHG

Monospecific AHG is prepared by a production process similar to that described for polyspecific AHG; however, it contains only one antibody specificity. Monospecific anti-IgG is usually of polyclonal origin; however, monoclonal anti-IgG has been prepared effectively by hybridoma technology. Monospecific anticomplement reagents are often a blend of monoclonal anti-C3b and monoclonal anti-C3d.

Antibodies Required in AHG

Anti-IgG

AHG must contain antibody activity to nonagglutinating blood group antibodies. The majority of these antibodies are a mixture of IgG_1 and IgG_3 subclass. Rarely, nonagglutinating

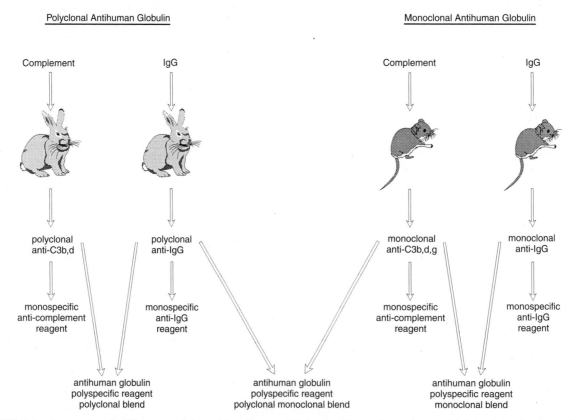

■ **FIGURE 5–1**   Preparation of AHG reagents. Polyspecific antihuman globulin may be manufactured by combining polyclonal anti-IgG with either polyclonal or monoclonal anticomplement components. A monoclonal blend may be manufactured by blending monoclonal anti-C3b, monoclonal anti-C3d, and monoclonal anti-IgG. Monospecific antihuman globulin reagents can be manufactured by conventional or hybridoma technology.

IgM antibodies may be found; however, they have always been shown to fix complement and may be detected by anticomplement.[11] IgA antibodies with Rh specificity have been reported; however, IgG antibody activity has always been present as well. The only RBC alloantibodies that have been reported as being solely IgA have been examples of anti-Pr,[12] and those antibodies were agglutinating. IgA autoantibodies have been reported, although very rarely.[13] Therefore, anti-IgG activity must be present in the AHG reagent. Anti-IgM and anti-IgA activity may be present, but neither is essential. The presence of anti–light-chain activity allows detection of all immunoglobulin classes.

Anti-Complement

Some antibodies "fix" complement components to the RBC membrane after complexing of the antibody with its corresponding antigen. These antibodies are listed in **Table 5–2**. These membrane-bound complement components can be detected by the anticomplement activity in AHG.

Early AHG reagents were prepared using a crude globulin fraction as the immunogen. In 1947, Coombs and Mourant demonstrated that the antibody activity that detected Rh antibodies was associated with the anti–gamma globulin fraction in the reagent. The first indication that there might be another antibody activity present that had an influence on the final reaction was presented by Dacie in 1951.[14] He observed that different reaction patterns were obtained when dilutions of AHG were used to test cells sensitized with "warm" as compared with "cold" antibodies. In 1957, Dacie and coworkers[15] published data showing that the reactivity of AHG to cells sensitized with "warm" antibodies resulted from anti–gamma globulin activity, whereas anti–nongamma globulin activity was responsible for the activity of cells sensitized by "cold" antibodies. The nongamma globulin component was shown to be beta globulin and had specificity for complement. Later studies[16,17] revealed that the complement activity was a result of C3 and C4.

During the 1960s many reports were published indicating the need for anticomplement activity in AHG to allow the detection of antibodies by the IAT.[18–21] Many of the specificities mentioned in these reports were ones that are now generally considered to be of little clinical significance (e.g., anti-Le[a], anti-P[1], and anti-H). However, one specificity that

TABLE 5–2 Antibodies Capable of Binding Complement		
Most	**Some**	**Rare**
ABO	S	S
Le[a]	Xg[a]	P[1]
Le[b]	LKE	Lu[a]
Jk[a]	Lan	Lu[b]
Jk[b]		Kell
Sc1		Fy[a]
Co3		Fy[b]
Ge2		Co[b]
Ge3		
Ii		
P		
P[k]		
Vel		

Note: These antibodies are discussed in detail in Chapters 6 through 9.

was consistently mentioned and that is considered clinically significant was anti-Jk[a]. Evidence was also presented showing that the presence of anticomplement activity would enhance the reactions of clinically significant antibodies (e.g., anti-Fy[a] and anti-K).[18]

Use of Polyspecific Versus Monospecific AHG in the IAT

As previously stated, polyspecific AHG contains both anti-IgG activity and anti-C3 activity. There is considerable debate among immunotransfusionists over the use of monospecific anti-IgG versus polyspecific AHG for routine antibody detection and pretransfusion testing. Because most clinically significant antibodies detected during antibody screening are IgG, the most important function of polyspecific AHG is the detection of IgG antibodies.

There have been numerous reports of clinically significant RBC alloantibodies that were not detectable with monospecific anti-IgG but were detected with the anticomplement component of AHG.[22] Unfortunately, polyspecific AHG has also been associated with unwanted positive reactions that are not caused by clinically significant antibodies. To investigate these variables, Petz and coworkers[23] examined 39,436 sera comparing monospecific anti-IgG with polyspecific AHG. They also compared the albumin technique with low ionic strength solutions (LISS)-suspended RBCs. Four Jk[a] antibodies were detected with polyspecific but not with monospecific anti-IgG using albumin or LISS-suspended RBCs. An additional anti-Jk[a] was detected only with polyspecific AHG when using LISS but not with albumin. Also, five antibodies of anti-Kell, anti-Jk[a], and Fy[a] specificities were detected when using LISS, but not albumin, with both polyspecific AHG and anti-IgG. Their results concluded that some clinically significant antibodies are detected with the anticomplement component of AHG but not with anti-IgG. This is especially true for anti-Jk[a], a complement-binding IgG antibody often associated with delayed hemolytic transfusion reactions.

Petz and others[22] also determined the number of false-positive reactions obtained when using polyspecific AHG versus anti-IgG with LISS and albumin. False-positive reactions were defined as those caused by antibodies with no definable specificity or by antibodies considered to be clinically insignificant because of optimum reactivity at cold temperatures (anti-I, anti-H, anti-P[1], anti-M). Of the unwanted positive reactions, 93 percent were shown to be caused by C3 on the cells. The authors emphasize that, if the first step in evaluating a weakly positive AHG reaction is to repeat using the prewarmed technique, about 60 percent of the false-positive weak reactions become negative.

In a 3-year study, Howard and associates[24] found eight patients whose antibodies were detected primarily or solely by AHG containing anticomplement activity. Seven of these antibodies had anti-Jk[a] or anti-Jk[b] specificity. Some of them could be detected using homozygous Jk[a] or Jk[b] cells and an AHG containing only anti-IgG activity. Two of the anti-Jk[a] antibodies were associated with delayed hemolytic transfusion reactions. The complement-only Kidd antibodies represented 23 percent of all Kidd antibodies detected during the study. The authors concluded that they would continue to use polyspecific AHG reagent for routine compatibility testing.

In summary, one must balance the advantage of detecting

clinically significant complement-only antibodies with the disadvantages resulting from using antiglobulin serum containing anti-complement activity.[22] A decision on the use of the AHG reagent for indirect tests is the prerogative of the individual blood bank. Many blood banks have adopted the use of monospecific anti-IgG for routine pretransfusion testing, citing cost containment measures necessitated by the high number of repeats versus the rarity of complement-only detected antibodies such as anti-Jk[a]. Milam[25] states rare clinical transfusion intolerance when using monospecific anti-IgG over polyspecific AHG reagents to screen for unexpected antibodies and to test for blood group compatibility offers reliability without interference from common and clinically insignificant IgM-complement fixing antibodies.

AHG Reagents and the DAT

The DAT detects in vivo sensitization of RBCs with IgG and/or complement components. During complement activation, C3 and C4 are split into two components. C3b and C4b bind to the RBC membrane, whereas C3a and C4a pass into the fluid phase. Further degradation of membrane-bound C3b and C4b occurs by removal of C3c and C4c to leave C3d and C4d firmly attached to the RBC membrane.[26–28] Anti-C3c was considered by the ISBT/ICSH Joint Working Party[29] to be the most important anticomplement component, because of its limited capacity to cause nonspecific reactions. However, when RBCs are incubated with serum for longer than 15 minutes, the number of C3c determinants falls rapidly because C3c is split off the C3bi molecule. This finding further supports the use of anti-C3d in international reference reagents by the Joint Working Party. The final degradation step has been shown to occur in vivo[30] and, in fact, is a common occurrence in both warm and cold autoimmune hemolytic anemias. Engelfriet and others[31] have also shown that degradation of C3b to C3d can occur in vitro, providing that the incubation period is greater than 1 hour. In 1976, Garratty and Petz[32] confirmed the need for anti-C3d activity in AHG for use in the DAT. They also confirmed Engelfriet's observation that, given sufficient time, cell-bound C3b could be degraded to C3d in vitro.

The detection of C3d on the RBC membrane is important in the investigation of both warm and cold autoimmune hemolytic anemia (AIHA). Many cases of warm AIHA are associated with both IgG and C3d coating the RBCs. In cold AIHA, C3d may be the only globulin detectable on the RBC. Characterization of AIHA requires the detection of the specific globulin sensitizing the RBCs in vivo, usually IgG or C3d or both. In the investigation of AIHA, a DAT is performed initially with polyspecific AHG. If globulins are detected on the RBC membrane, follow-up testing with monospecific AHG (anti-IgG, anti-C3d) is performed to identify the coating proteins. Although the RBCs of most patients with AIHA are coated with IgG, the cells of some patients will exhibit both IgG and complement coating or complement alone. The presence of complement alone may support the diagnosis of AIHA, rendering the finding significant.[25]

Principles of the Antiglobulin Test

The antiglobulin test is based on the following simple principles:[33]

1. Antibody molecules and complement components are globulins.
2. Injecting an animal with human globulin stimulates the animal to produce antibody to the foreign protein (i.e., AHG). Serologic tests employ a variety of AHG reagents reactive with various human globulins, including anti-IgG, antibody to the C3d component of human complement, and polyspecific reagents that contain both anti-IgG and anti-C3d activity.
3. AHG reacts with human globulin molecules, either bound to RBCs or free in serum.
4. Washed RBCs coated with human globulin are agglutinated by AHG.

The complete procedures for the direct and indirect antihuman globulin tests can be found in the procedural appendix at the end of this chapter. **Color Plate 1** summarizes the methodology of both tests. **Figure 5–2** illustrates in-vitro sensitization detected in the IAT and in-vivo sensitization detected by the DAT.

DAT

Principle and Application of the DAT

The DAT detects in-vivo sensitization of RBCs with IgG and/or complement components. Clinical conditions that can result in in-vivo coating of RBCs with antibody and/or complement are:

1. Hemolytic disease of the newborn (HDN)
2. Hemolytic transfusion reaction (HTR)
3. Autoimmune and drug-induced AIHA.

Table 5–3 lists the clinical application and in-vivo sensitization detected for each situation.

The DAT is not a required test in routine pretransfusion protocols. In a study by the College of American Pathologists in 1998,[34] 54 percent of 4299 laboratories surveyed reported

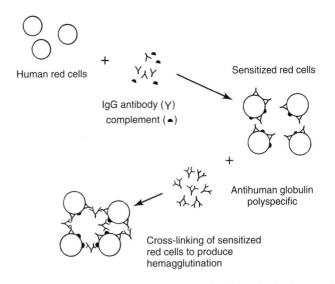

Human red cells

IgG antibody (Y)
complement (•)

Sensitized red cells

Antihuman globulin polyspecific

Cross-linking of sensitized red cells to produce hemagglutination

■ **FIGURE 5–2**   AHG test. The IAT is used to determine in-vitro sensitization of RBCs, whereas the DAT is used to detect in-vivo sensitization. Polyspecific AHG contains anti-IgG and anti-complement activity.

TABLE 5–3   Direct Antiglobulin Test

Principle: Detects In-Vivo RBC Sensitization	
Application	**In-Vivo Sensitization**
HDN	Maternal antibody coating fetal RBCs
HTR	Recipient antibody coating donor RBCs
AIHA	Autoantibody coating individual's RBCs

using the DAT in pretransfusion testing, the primary rationale being early detection of alloimmunization. Eder[35] tested the clinical utility of the DAT at a large tertiary care hospital in Philadelphia. A retrospective study was performed from 1999 to 2002. DATs with anti-IgG were performed on 15,662 pretransfusion patient samples; 15 percent were positive. Subsequent eluate testing revealed nonreactivity in 76 percent; 9 percent panreactive; and 12 percent passively acquired ABO or D antibodies. Only one case demonstrated an RBC antibody in the eluate that was not detected in the serum, concluding that even in a tertiary care setting the routine DAT is inefficient yielding a positive predictive value of 0.16 percent. Judd and coworkers revealed similar findings on 65,049 blood samples in a 29-month period, where only 5.5 percent of samples resulted in a positive DAT.[36]

DAT Panel

Initial DATs include testing one drop of a 3 to 5 percent suspension of washed RBCs with polyspecific (anti-IgG, anti-C3d) reagent. Positive results are monitored by a DAT panel using monospecific anti-IgG and anti-C3d to determine the specific type of protein sensitizing the cell. Some institutions choose to run polyspecific and monospecific reagents at one time as well as a saline control. The saline control serves to detect spontaneous agglutination of cells or reactions occurring without the addition of AHG reagents. In warm AIHA, including drug-induced hemolytic anemia, the RBCs may be coated with IgG or C3d, or both. Patterns of reactivity and the type of protein sensitization in AIHA are summarized in Table 5–4. In a transfusion reaction workup, the DAT may demonstrate IgG or C3d, or both, depending on the nature and specificity of the recipient's antibody. In the investigation of HDN, testing for complement proteins is not necessary inasmuch as the

TABLE 5–4   DAT Panel: Patterns of Reactivity in Autoimmune Hemolytic Anemia*

Anti-IgG	Anti-C3d	Type of AIHA
+	+	WAIHA (67%)
+	−	WAIHA (20%)
−	+	CHD; PCH, WAIHA (13%)

Modified from Walker, RH (ed): Technical Manual, ed 10. American Association of Blood Banks, Arlington, VA, 1990.
*The DAT with monospecific antiglobulin reagents is helpful in classifying AIHAs. Other procedures and studies are necessary to diagnose and characterize which form of autoimmune disease is present.
WAIHA = warm autoimmune hemolytic anemia; CHD = cold hemagglutinin disease; PCH = paroxysmal cold hemoglobinuria

protein sensitizing the newborn RBCs is presumed to be maternal IgG. Problems can arise in accurate D typing in the case of a newborn with a positive DAT. If the DAT is positive due to IgG and the immediate spin for D typing is negative, a test for weak D cannot be performed. The same is true for a patient with AIHA due to a warm IgG antibody coating the patient cells. The antibody must be removed from the RBCs for accurate phenotyping. Other techniques can be used to remove antibody from the patients RBCs. These include chloroquine diphosphate, EDTA-glycine, and a method using murine monoclonal antibodies.

Evaluation of a Positive DAT

Clinical consideration should dictate the extent to which a positive DAT is evaluated. Interpreting the significance of a positive DAT requires knowledge of the patient's diagnosis, drug therapy, and recent transfusion history. A positive DAT may occur without clinical manifestations of immune-mediated hemolysis. Table 5–5 describes the in-vivo phenomena that may be associated with a positive DAT.

The American Association of Blood Banks *Technical Manual*[33] states that "results of serological tests are not diagnostic; their significance can only be assessed in relationship to the patient's clinical condition." Answering the following questions before investigating a positive DAT for patients other than neonates will help determine what further testing is appropriate:

1. Is there evidence of in-vivo hemolysis?
2. Has the patient been transfused recently?
3. Does the patient's serum contain unexpected antibodies?
4. Is the patient receiving any drugs?
5. Has the patient received blood products or components containing ABO-incompatible plasma?
6. Is the patient receiving antilymphocyte globulin or antithymocyte globulin?
7. Is the patient receiving IVIG or IV RhIG?

IAT (Indirect Antiglobulin Test)

Principle and Application of the IAT

The IAT is performed to determine in-vitro sensitization of RBCs and is used in the following situations:

1. Detection of incomplete (nonagglutinating) antibodies to potential donor RBCs (compatibility testing) or to screening cells (antibody screen) in serum
2. Determination of RBC phenotype using known antisera (e.g., Kell typing, weak D testing)
3. Titration of incomplete antibodies

Table 5–6 lists the IATs and the in-vitro sensitization detected for each application.

For in-vitro antigen-antibody reactions, the IAT tasks are listed and explained in Table 5–7.

The DAT does not require the incubation phase because of the antigen-antibody complexes formed in vivo.

Factors Affecting the Antiglobulin Test

The DAT can detect a level of 100 to 500 IgG molecules per RBC and 400 to 1100 molecules of C3d per RBC.[31]

TABLE 5–5   In-Vivo Phenomena Associated with a Positive DAT

Transfusion	1. Recipient alloantibody and donor antigen	Alloantibodies in the recipient of a recent transfusion that react with antigen on donor RBC.
	2. Donor antibody and recipient antigen	Antibodies present in donor plasma that react with antigen on a transfusion recipient's RBCs.
Drug induced	1. Drug adsorption	Penicillin adsorbed to RBCs in vivo. Antipenicillin reacts with the penicillin bound to the RBCs. Penicillin-coated RBCs become coated with IgG.
	2. Immune complex adsorption mechanism	Drug and specific antibody form complexes that attach nonspecifically to RBCs and initiate complement activation on the RBC surface.
	3. Membrane modification	RBCs coated with cephalothin (Keflin) adsorb albumin, IgA, IgG, IgM, and α and β (i.e., complement) globulins. The DAT is reactive with anti-IgG and anti-C3d.
	4. Autoimmunity	Following α-methyldopa therapy, autoantibodies are formed, which react with intrinsic RBC antigens. DAT is reactive with anti-IgG.
	Type (DAT Reactivity)	
Autoimmune hemolytic anemia	1. WAIHA (IgG and/or C3)	Autoantibody reacts with patient's RBCs in vivo.
	2. CHD (C3)	Cold-reactive IgM autoagglutinin binds to RBCs in peripheral circulation (32°C). IgM binds complement as RBCs return to warmer parts of circulation; IgM dissociates, leaving RBCs coated only with complement.
	3. PCH (IgG)	The IgG autoantibody reacts with RBCs in colder parts of body, causes complement to be bound irreversibly to RBCs, and then elutes at warmer temperature.
Hemolytic disease of newborn	1. Maternal alloantibody crosses placenta (IgG)	Maternal (IgG) alloantibody, specific for fetal antigen, coats fetal RBCs. DAT is reactive with anti-IgG.
Miscellaneous	1. Administration of equine preparations of antilymphocyte globulin and antithymocyte globulin	Heterophile antibodies that are present in ALG or ATG coat recipient's RBCs.
	2. Administration of high-dose IV gamma globulin	Non–antibody-mediated binding of immunoglobulin to RBCs in patients with hypergammaglobulinemia

Modified from Walker, RH (ed): Technical Manual, ed 10. American Association of Blood Banks, Arlington, VA, 1990.
AIHA = autoimmune hemolytic anemia; CHD = cold hemagglutinin disease; PCH = paroxysmal cold hemoglobinuria.

For the IAT there must be between 100 and 200 IgG or C3 molecules on the cell to obtain a positive reaction. The number of IgG molecules that sensitize an RBC and the rate at which sensitization occurs can be influenced by several factors, outlined as follows:

Ratio of serum to cells. Increasing the ratio of serum to cells increases the sensitivity of the test system. Generally, a minimum ratio of 40:1 should be aimed for, and this can be achieved by using 2 drops of serum and 1 drop of a 5 percent volume of solute per volume of solution (v/v) suspension of cells.[35] When using cells suspended in saline, it is often advantageous to increase the ratio of serum to cells in an effort to detect weak antibodies (e.g., 4 drops of serum with

1 drop of a 3 percent [v/v] cell suspension will give a ratio of 133:1).

Reaction medium. *Albumin:* The macromolecules of albumin allow antibody-coated cells to come into closer contact with each other so that aggregation occurs. In 1965, Stroup and MacIlroy[37] reported on the increased sensitivity of the IAT if albumin was incorporated into the reaction medium. Their reaction mixture, consisting of 2 drops of serum, 2 drops of 22 percent (w/v) bovine albumin, and 1 drop of 3 to 5 percent (v/v) cells, was shown to provide the same sensitivity at 30 minutes of incubation as a 60-minute saline test. The use of albumin does not seem to provide any advantage over LISS techniques and adds to the cost of the test.[37] Petz and cowork-

TABLE 5–6   Indirect Antiglobulin Test

Principle: Detects In-Vitro Sensitization		
Application	**Tests**	**In-Vitro Sensitization**
Antibody detection	Compatibility testing	Recipient antibody reacting with donor cells
	Antibody screening	Antibody reacting with screening cells
Antibody identification	Antibody panel	Antibody reacting with panel cells
Antibody titration	Rh antibody titer	Antibody and selected Rh cells
RBC phenotype	RBC antigen detection (ex: weak D, K, Fy)	Specific antisera + RBCs to detect antigen

TABLE 5–7   Tasks and Purposes of the Indirect Antigloblin Test

Task	Purpose
Incubate RBCs with antisera	Allows time for antibody molecule Attachment to RBC antigen
Perform a minimum of three saline washes	Removes free globulin molecules
Add antiglobulin reagent	Forms RBC agglutinates (RBC Ag + Ab + anti-IgG)
Centrifuge	Accelerates agglutination by bringing cells closer together
Examine for agglutination	Interprets test as positive or negative
Grade agglutination reactions	Determines the strength of reaction
Add antibody-coated RBCs to negative reactions	Checks for neutralization of antisera by free globulin molecules (Coombs' control cells are D-positive RBCs coated with anti-D)

ers[23] also showed that an albumin technique may miss a number of clinically significant antibodies.

LISS: These enhance antibody uptake and allow incubation times to be decreased. Some LISS also contain macromolecular substances. The LISS technique introduced by Low and Messeter[38] has critical requirements with respect to the serum-to-cell ratio. Moore and Mollison[39] showed that optimum reaction conditions were obtained using 2 drops of serum and 2 drops of a 3 percent (v/v) suspension of cells in LISS. Increasing the serum-to-cell ratio increased the ionic strength of the reaction mixture, leading to a decrease in sensitivity, thus counteracting the shortened incubation time of the test. A LISS medium may be achieved by either suspending RBCs in LISS or using a LISS additive reagent.

Polyethylene glycol (PEG): PEG is a water-soluble linear polymer and is used as an additive to increase antibody uptake. Its action is to remove water, thereby effectively concentrating antibody. Anti-IgG is the AHG reagent of choice with PEG testing to avoid false-positive reactions.[5] Because PEG may cause aggregation of RBCs, reading for agglutination following 37°C incubation in the IAT is omitted. Several investigators[40] compared the performance of PEG as an enhancement media with that of LISS. Findings indicated that PEG increases the detection of clinically significant antibodies while decreasing detection of clinically insignificant antibodies. Barrett and associates[41] reported that as PEG has been used for pretransfusion antibody screening, 6353 RBC components have been transfused without any reported acute or delayed HTRs.

Temperature. The rate of reaction for the majority of IgG antibodies is optimal at 37°C; therefore, this is the usual incubation temperature for the IAT. This is also the optimum temperature for complement activation.

Incubation time. For cells suspended in saline, incubation times may vary between 30 and 120 minutes. The majority of clinically significant antibodies can be detected after 30 minutes of incubation, and extended incubation times are usually not necessary. If a LISS technique is being used,[38,39] incubation times may be shortened to 10 to 15 minutes. With these shortened times, it is essential that tubes be incubated at a temperature of 37°C. Extended incubation (i.e., up to 40 minutes) in the LISS technique has been shown to cause antibody to elute from the RBCs, causing a decrease in the sensitivity of the test.[42] However, this could not be confirmed by Voak and coworkers.[43]

Washing of RBCs. When both the DAT and IAT are performed, RBCs must be saline-washed a minimum of three times before the addition of AHG reagent. Washing the RBCs removes free unbound serum globulins. Inadequate washing may result in a false-negative reaction because of neutralization of the AHG reagent by residual unbound serum globulins.

Washing should be performed in as short a time as possible to minimize the elution of low-affinity antibodies. The cell pellet should be completely resuspended before adding the next saline wash. All saline should be discarded completely after the final wash because residual saline dilutes the AHG reagent and therefore decreases the sensitivity of the test.

Centrifugation at each wash should be sufficient to provide a firm cell pellet and therefore minimize the possible loss of cells with each discard of saline.

Saline for washing. Ideally, the saline used for washing should be fresh or, alternatively, buffered to a pH of 7.2 to 7.4. Saline stored for long periods in plastic containers has been shown to decrease in pH, which may increase the rate of antibody elution during the washing process.[44] Changes in pH may have important implications when monoclonal AHG is used, inasmuch as monoclonal antibodies have been shown to have narrow pH ranges for optimum reactivity. Significant levels of bacterial contamination in saline have been reported[45]; this situation can contribute to false-positive results.

Addition of AHG. AHG should be added to the cells immediately after washing to minimize the chance of antibody eluting from the cell and subsequently neutralizing the AHG reagent. The volume of AHG added should be as indicated by the manufacturers. However, Voak and associates[46] have shown that adding two volumes of AHG may overcome washing problems when low levels of serum contamination remain. These authors indicated that the neutralization of AHG is a problem only with free IgG left in serum following inadequate saline washings and not with residual serum complement components. The complement fragments free in serum are not the same as the complement fragments bound to RBCs, and therefore residual serum does not contain C3b and C3d to neutralize the anti-C3b and anti-C3d in AHG reagent.

Centrifugation for reading. Centrifugation of the cell pellet for reading of hemagglutination along with the method used for resuspending the cells is a crucial step in the technique. The CBER-recommended method for the evaluation of AHG uses 1000 relative centrifugal forces (RCFs) for 20 seconds, although the technique described in this chapter suggests 500 RCFs for 15 to 20 seconds. The use of higher RCFs yields more sensitive results; however, depending on how the pellet is resuspended, it may give weak false-positive results because of inadequate resuspension or alternatively may give a negative result if resuspension is too vigorous. The optimum centrifugation conditions should be determined for each centrifuge.

Sources of Error

Some of the more common sources of error associated with the performance of the AHG test have been outlined in the previous section. **Box 5–1** lists reasons for false-negative and false-positive AHG reactions. An anticoagulant such as EDTA should be used to collect blood samples for the DAT in order to avoid the in-vitro complement attachment associated with refrigerated clotted specimens.

All negative antiglobulin test reactions must be checked by the addition of IgG-sensitized cells. Adding IgG-coated RBCs to negative test reactions should demonstrate hemagglutination of these RBCs with the anti-IgG in the AHG reagent. If no hemagglutination follows the addition of IgG-coated RBCs, the test result is invalid and the test must be repeated. The most common technical errors that result in failure to demonstrate hemagglutination after the addition of IgG-coated RBCs are inadequate washing, nonreactive AHG reagent, and failure to add AHG reagent. While most blood banks do not check monospecific anti-C3d reactivity with the addition of C3d-coated RBCs to negative reactions, these cells are available and may be produced in-house.[47]

BOX 5–1
Sources of Error in the Antihuman Globulin Technique

False-Positive Results

- Improper specimen (refrigerated, clotted) may cause in-vitro complement attachment
- Autoagglutinable cells
- Bacterial contamination of cells or saline used in washing
- Cells with a positive direct AHG test used for the IAT
- Saline contaminated by heavy metals or colloidal silica
- Dirty glassware
- Overcentrifugation and overreading
- Polyagglutinable cells
- Preservative-dependent antibody in LISS reagents (IAT)
- Contaminating antibodies in the AHG reagent
- Centrifugation of test with polyethylene glycol prior to washing

False-Negative Results

- Inadequate or improper washing of cells
- AHG reagent nonreactive because of deterioration or neutralization
- AHG reagent not added
- Serum not added in the indirect test
- Serum nonreactive because of deterioration of complement
- Inadequate incubation conditions in the IAT
- Cell suspension either too weak or too heavy
- Undercentrifuged or overcentrifuged
- Poor reading technique
- Low pH of saline

Rosenfield, RE, et al: Solid phase serology for the study of human erythrocytic antigen-antibody reactions. Proc Fifteenth Congr Int Soc Blood Trans, Paris, 1976, p 27.

Modified and Automated Antiglobulin Test Techniques

Modifications to the antiglobulin test technique (LISS, PEG, and albumin) have been mentioned; however, some other modifications may be used in special circumstances.

Low Ionic Polybrene Technique

In 1980, Lalezari and Jiang[48] reported on the adaptation of the automated low ionic polybrene (LIP) technique for use as a manual procedure. The technique relies on low ionic conditions to rapidly sensitize cells with antibody. Polybrene, a potent rouleaux-forming reagent, is added to allow the sensitized cells to approach each other to permit cross-linking by the attached antibody. A high ionic strength solution is then added to reverse the rouleaux; however, if agglutination is present, it will remain. The test can be carried through to an AHG technique if required. If this is performed, a monospecific anti-IgG reagent must be used because the low ionic conditions cause considerable amounts of C4 and C3 to coat the cells and would give false-positive reactions if a polyspecific reagent were used.

The antiglobulin test has also been performed using microplates. Crawford and colleagues[49] used microplates for a number of different grouping procedures, including the IAT. Microplate technology is used increasingly in blood group serology, and many techniques are being adapted for it. Redman and associates[50] have adapted the LIP technique for use in microplates. Although their report does not include the use of an AHG phase, this additional step could easily be included.

Enzyme-Linked Antiglobulin Test

In the enzyme-linked antiglobulin test (ELAT), an RBC suspension is added to a microtiter well and washed with saline. AHG, which has been labeled with an enzyme, is added. The enzyme-labeled AHG will bind to IgG-sensitized RBCs. Excess antibody is removed, and enzyme substrate is added. The amount of color produced is measured spectrophotometrically and is proportional to the amount of antibody present. The optical density is usually measured at 405 nm. The number of IgG molecules per RBC can also be determined from this procedure.

Solid Phase

Solid-phase technology may be used for the performance of antiglobulin tests. Several different techniques have been reported using either test tubes[51] or microplates.[52,53] With the availability of microplate readers, this modification lends itself to the introduction of semiautomation. Direct and indirect tests can be performed using solid-phase methodology. In the former, antibody is attached to a microplate well, and RBCs are added. If antibody is specific for antigen on RBCs, the bottom of the well will be covered with suspension; if no such specificity occurs, RBCs will settle to the bottom of the well. In the latter, known RBCs are bound to a well that has been treated with glutaraldehyde or poly L-lysine. Test serum is added to RBC-coated wells, and if antibody in serum is specific for antigen on fixed RBCs, a positive reaction occurs as described above.

Immucor Incorporated manufactures a solid-phase system for the detection and identification of alloantibodies. Group O reagent RBC membranes are bound to the surfaces of polystyrene microtitration strip wells. IgG antibodies from patient or donor sera are bound to the membrane antigens. After incubation, unbound immunoglobulins are rinsed from the wells; then a suspension of anti-IgG–coated indicator RBCs is added to the wells. Centrifugation brings the indicator RBCs in contact with antibodies bound to the reagent RBC membranes. If the test result is negative, a pellet of indicator RBCs forms in the bottom of the wells. A positive test causes adherence of the indicator RBCs, forming anti–IgG-IgG complexes and a second immobilized RBC layer.

The Gel Test

The gel test is a process to detect RBC antigen-antibody reactions by means of using a chamber filled with polyacrylamide gel. The gel acts as a trap; free unagglutinated RBCs form pellets in the bottom of the tube, whereas agglutinated RBCs are trapped in the tube for hours. Therefore, negative reactions appear as pellets in the bottom of the microtube, and positive reactions are fixed in the gel.

There are three different types of gel tests: neutral, specific, and antiglobulin. A neutral gel does not contain any specific reagent and acts only by its property of trapping agglutinates. The main applications of neutral gel tests are antibody screening and identification with enzyme-treated or untreated RBCs and reverse ABO typing. Specific gel tests use a specific reagent incorporated into the gel and are useful for antigen determination. The low ionic antiglobulin test (GLIAT) is a valuable application of the gel test and may be used for the IAT or the DAT. AHG reagent is incorporated into the gel. For example, in an IAT gel, 50 μL of a 0.8 percent RBC suspension is pipetted onto a gel containing AHG, serum is added, and the tube is centrifuged after a period of incubation. At the beginning of centrifugation, the RBCs tend to pass through the gel, but the medium in which they are suspended remains above. This results in separation between the RBCs and the medium without a washing phase. RBCs come in contact with AHG in the upper part of the gel, and the positive and negative reactions are separated. The detection of unexpected antibodies by GLIAT compares favorably with conventional AHG methods and provides a safe, reliable, and easy-to-read AHG test.[54]

For the DAT, 50 μL of a 0.8 percent RBC suspension in LISS solution (ID-Diluent 2) is added to the top of each microtube of the LISS/Coombs ID cards. The cards are centrifuged at 910 rpm for 10 minutes.[55] In the case of a positive reaction, monospecific reagents (anti-IgG, anti-C3d) can be used in the gel test.

Traditional Tube Technique Versus the Gel Test in the DAT

There have been numerous studies comparing the tube and gel test when performing DATs. The main difference in the two techniques is that the former requires washing, and the latter omits a washing stage, resulting in discrepant results between the two methods. Chuansumrit et al[56] compared the conventional tube technique with the gel test in evaluating ABO HDN. Sixty infants with hyperbilirubinemia were tested: 22 cases were ABO-incompatible (A or B infants born to group O mothers), and 38 were ABO-compatible with the mother. Whereas the positive rates of the DAT in the incompatible group were comparable, 54.5 percent (tube) and 50 percent gel test; the second group showed a positive DAT rate of 2.6 percent (tube) and 10.5 percent (gel). The infants were shown to have hyperbilirubinemia, and the antibody coating the cells was found to be IgG only, using monospecific reagents. The authors concluded the DAT via the gel test is beneficial in detecting ABO HDN.

Lai et al[57] described a case of AIHA with a negative DAT using the traditional tube test and a positive result using the gel test. The study found a warm low affinity antibody in the patient's serum, by means of the gel test, that was lost in the tube technique through washing when performing the DAT. The authors concluded that because the gel test does not include washing steps, the elution of low-affinity autoantibody may be avoided but the eluate may yield a negative result. Additionally, the gel test, because of its no-wash nature, might be warranted in the case of a suspected AIHA. Mitek et al[58] compared the gel test to the tube and ELAT techniques. They found the gel test to be more sensitive in the case of hypergammagloblinemic patients, yielding positive results due to IgG in the gel test and negative results in the tube and ELAT. Blood banks should be aware of the differences in the DAT when using the very popular gel test over and tube technique. Additional comparative studies will add to the current body of knowledge.

The changes in blood bank technology, along with the changes in emphasis on the importance of crossmatching versus antibody screening, will probably further modify the role of the antiglobulin test over the coming years. At present, however, it still remains the most important test in the blood bank for the detection of clinically significant antibodies to RBCs and for the detection of immune hemolysis.

CASE STUDIES

Case One

A 32-year old white female gave birth to a 5 lb 3 oz healthy male. The mother was an RhIg candidate in that she typed as O, D-negative. A cord blood was sent down to the blood bank for ABO, Rh, and DAT. The baby forward-typed as A negative, weak D-positive. The DAT was also positive with polyspecific AHG and monospecific anti-IgG. The technologist realized the test for weak D could not be reported in the presence of a positive DAT and reported the type as A unknown.

Questions

1. What further testing is indicated?
2. Why is a weak test for the D antigen not performed in the presence of a positive DAT?

Case Two

A 54-year old white male is admitted for an exploratory laparotomy. A type and antibody screen is ordered prior to his scheduled surgery. ABO and Rh typing reveal the patient is O-positive, and the blood bank technologist performed an antibody screen using the patient serum and a 3-screening cell kit. Reactions were all negative at 37° and AHG. One drop of Coombs' check cells was added to each tube, and the results were nonreactive.

Questions

1. What is the correct course of action in this case?
2. Give reasons why the addition of Coombs' check cells resulted in nonreactivity.
3. What do Coombs' control cells consist of?

SUMMARY CHART:

Important Points to Remember (MT/MLT)

➤ The antiglobulin test is used to detect RBCs sensitized by IgG alloantibodies, IgG autoantibodies, and/or complement components.

➤ AHG reagents containing anti-IgG are needed for the detection of IgG antibodies because the IgG monomeric structure is too small to directly agglutinate sensitized RBCs.

➤ Polyspecific AHG sera contain antibodies to human IgG and the C3d component of human complement.

➤ Monospecific AHG sera contain only one antibody specificity: either anti-IgG or antibody to anti–C3b-C3d.

➤ Classic AHG sera (polyclonal) are prepared by injecting human globulins into rabbits, and an immune stimulus triggers production of antibody to human serum.

➤ Hybridoma technology is used to produce monoclonal antiglobulin serum.

➤ The DAT detects in-vivo sensitization of RBCs with IgG and/or complement components. Clinical conditions that can result in a positive DAT include HDN, HTR, and AIHA.

➤ The IAT detects in-vitro sensitization of RBCs and can be applied to compatibility testing, antibody screen, antibody identification, RBC phenotyping, and titration studies.

➤ A positive DAT is followed by a DAT panel using monospecific anti-IgG and anti-C3d to determine the specific type of protein sensitizing the RBC.

➤ EDTA should be used to collect blood samples for the DAT to avoid in-vitro complement attachment associated with refrigerated clotted specimens.

REVIEW QUESTIONS

1. A principle of the antiglobulin test is:
   a. IgG and C3d are required for RBC sensitization
   b. Human globulin is eluted from RBCs during saline washings
   c. Injection of human globulin into an animal engenders passive immunity
   d. AHG reacts with human globulin molecules bound to RBCs or free in serum

2. Polyspecific AHG reagent contains:
   a. Anti-IgG
   b. Anti-IgG and anti-IgM
   c. Anti-IgG and anti-C3d
   d. Anti-C3d

3. Monoclonal anti-C3d is:
   a. Derived from one clone of plasma cells
   b. Derived from multiple clones of plasma cells
   c. Derived from immunization of rabbits
   d. Reactive with C3b and C3d

4. Which of the following is a clinically significant antibody whose detection may be dependent on anticomplement activity in polyspecific AHG?
   a. Anti-Jk^a
   b. Anti-Le^a
   c. Anti-P$_1$
   d. Anti-H

5. After the addition of IgG-coated RBCs to a negative AHG reaction during an antibody screen, a negative result is observed. Which of the following is a correct interpretation?
   a. The antibody screen is negative
   b. The antibody screen needs to be repeated
   c. The saline washings were adequate
   d. Reactive AHG reagent was added

6. RBCs must be washed in saline at least three times before the addition of AHG reagent to:
   a. Wash away any hemolyzed cells
   b. Remove traces of free serum globulins
   c. Neutralize any excess AHG reagent
   d. Increase the antibody binding to antigen

7. An in-vitro phenomenon associated with a positive IAT is:
   a. Maternal antibody coating fetal RBCs
   b. Patient antibody coating patient RBCs
   c. Recipient antibody coating transfused donor RBCs
   d. Identification of alloantibody specificity using panel of reagent RBCs

8. False-positive DAT results are most often associated with:
   a. Use of refrigerated, clotted blood sample in which complement components coat RBCs in vitro
   b. A recipient of a recent transfusion manifesting an immune response to recently transfused RBCs
   c. Presence of heterophile antibodies from administration of globulin
   d. A positive autocontrol caused by polyagglutination

9. Polyethylene glycol enhances antigen-antibody reactions by:
   a. Decreasing zeta potential
   b. Concentrating antibody by removal of water
   c. Increasing antibody affinity for antigen
   d. Increasing antibody specificity for antigen

10. Solid-phase antibody screening is based on:
    a. Adherence
    b. Agglutination
    c. Hemolysis
    d. Precipitation

11. A positive DAT may be found in which of the following situations?

   a. A weak D-positive patient

   b. A patient with anti-K

   c. HDN

   d. An incompatible crossmatch

12. What do Coombs' control cells consist of?

   a. Type A-positive cells coated with anti-D

   b. Type A-negative cells coated with anti-D

   c. Type O-positive cells coated with anti-D

   d. Type O-negative cells coated with anti-D

REFERENCES

1. Coombs, RRA, et al: A new test for the detection of weak and "incomplete" Rh agglutinins. Br J Exp Pathol 26:255, 1945.
2. Coombs, RRA, et al: In vivo isosensisation of red cells in babies with haemolytic disease. Lancet i:264, 1946.
3. Race, RR, and Sanger, R: Blood Groups in Man, ed 6. Blackwell Scientific, Oxford, 1975, p 283.
4. Moreschi, C: Neue Tatsachen über die Blutkorperchen Agglutinationen. Zentralbl Bakteriol 46:49, 1908.
5. Brecher, ME (ed): Technical Manual, ed 14. American Association of Blood Banks, Bethesda, MD, 2002.
6. Issitt, C: Monoclonal Antiglobulin Reagents. Dade International Online, 1997. http://www.dadeinternational.com/hemo/papers/ monoanti.htm.
7. Kohler, G, and Milstein, C: Continuous cultures of fused cells secreting antibody of predefined specificity. Nature 256:495, 1975.
8. Lachman, PJ, et al: Use of monoclonal antibodies to characterize the fragments of C3 that are found on erythrocytes. Vox Sang 45:367, 1983.
9. Holt, PDJ, et al: NBTS/BRIC 8: A monoclonal anti-C3d antibody. Transfusion 25:267, 1985.
10. Voak, D, et al: Monoclonal antibodies—C3 serology. Biotest Bull 1:339, 1983.
11. Mollison, PL: Blood Transfusion in Clinical Medicine, ed 7. Blackwell Scientific, Oxford, 1983, p 502.
12. Garratty, G, et al: An IgA high titre cold agglutinin with an unusual blood group specificity within the Pr complex. Vox Sang 25:32, 1973.
13. Petz, LD, and Garratty, G: Acquired immune hemolytic anemias. Churchill Livingstone, New York, 1980, p 193.
14. Dacie, JF: Differences in the behaviour of sensitized red cells to agglutination by antiglobulin sera. Lancet ii:954, 1951.
15. Dacie, JV, et al: "Incomplete" cold antibodies: Role of complement in sensitization to antiglobulin serum by potentially haemolytic antibodies. Br J Haematol 3:77, 1957.
16. Harboe, M, et al: Identification of the component of complement participating in the antiglobulin reaction. Immunology 6:412, 1963.
17. Jenkins, GC, et al: Role of C4 in the antiglobulin reaction. Nature 186:482, 1960.
18. Polley, MJ, and Mollison, PL: The role of complement in the detection of blood group antibodies: Special reference to the antiglobulin test. Transfusion 1:9, 1961.
19. Polley, MJ, et al: The role of 19S gamma-globulin blood group antibodies in the antiglobulin reaction. Br J Haematol 8:149, 1962.
20. Stratton, F, et al: The preparation and uses of antiglobulin reagents with special reference to complement fixing blood group antibodies. Transfusion 2:135, 1962.
21. Stratton, F, et al: Value of gel fixation on Sephadex G-200 in the analysis of blood group antibodies. J Clin Pathol 21:708, 1968.
22. Petz, LD, et al: Clinical Practice of Transfusion Medicine, ed 3. Churchill Livingstone, New York, 1996, p 207.
23. Petz, LD, et al: Compatibility testing. Transfusion 21:633, 1981.
24. Howard, JE, et al: Clinical significance of the anti-complement component of antiglobulin antisera. Transfusion 22:269, 1982.
25. Milam JD: Laboratory Medicine Parameter: Utilizing monospecific antihuman globulin to test blood group compatibility. Am J Clin Pathol 104:122, 1995.
26. Lachman, PJ, and Muller-Eberhard, HJ: The demonstration in human serum of "conglutinogen-activating-factor" and its effect on the third component of complement. J Immunol 100:691, 1968.
27. Muller-Eberhard, HJ: Chemistry and reaction mechanisms of complement. Adv Immunol 8:1, 1968.
28. Cooper, NR: Isolation and analysis of mechanisms of action of an inactivator of C4b in normal human serum. J Exp Med 141:890, 1975.
29. Case, J, et al: International reference reagents: Antihuman globulin, an ISBT/ICSH Joint Working Party Report. Vox Sang 77:121, 1999.
30. Brown, DL, et al: The in vivo behaviour of complement-coated red cells: Studies in C6-deficient, Ce-depleted and normal rabbits. Clin Exp Immunol 7:401, 1970.
31. Engelfriet, CP, et al: Autoimmune haemolytic anemias: 111 preparation and examination of specific antisera against complement components and products, and their use in serological studies. Clin Exp Immunol 6:721, 1970.
32. Garratty, G, and Petz, LD: The significance of red cell bound complement components in development of standards and quality assurance for the anti-complement components of antiglobulin sera. Transfusion 16:297, 1976.
33. Brecher, ME (ed): Technical Manual, ed 14. American Association of Blood Banks, Bethesda, MD, 2002.
34. College of American Pathologists: Transfusion medicine survey set J: A final critique, 1998, 1-5.
35. Eder, AF: Evaluation of routine pretransfusion direct antiglobulin test in a pediatric setting. Lab Med 24:680, 2003.
36. Judd, WJ, et al: The evaluation of a positive direct antiglobulin test in pretransfusion testing revisited. Transfusion 26:220, 1986.
37. Stroup, M, and Macilroy, M: Evaluation of the Albumin antiglobulin technique in antibody detection. Transfusion 5:184, 1965.
38. Low, B, and Messeter, L: Antiglobulin test in low-ionic strength salt solution for rapid antibody screening and cross-matching. Vox Sang 26:53, 1974.
39. Moore, HC, and Mollison, PL: Use of a low-ionic strength medium in manual tests for antibody detection. Transfusion 16:291, 1976.
40. Shirley, R, et al: Polyethylene glycol versus low-ionic strength solution in pretransfusion testing: A blinded comparison study. Transfusion 34:5, 1994.
41. Barrett, V, et al: Analysis of the routine use of polyethylene glycol (PEG) as an enhancement medium. Immunohematology 11:1, 1995.
42. Jorgensen, J, et al: The influence of ionic strength, albumin and incubation time on the sensitivity of indirect Coombs' test. Vox Sang 36:186, 1980.
43. Voak, D, et al: Low-ionic strength media for rapid antibody detection: Optimum conditions and quality control. Med Lab Sci 37:107, 1980.
44. Bruce, M, et al: A serious source of error in antiglobulin testing. Transfusion 26:177, 1986.
45. Green, C, et al: Quality assurance of physiological saline used for blood grouping. Med Lab Sci 43:364, 1968.
46. Voak, D, et al: Antihuman globulin reagent specification: The European and ISBT/ICSH view. Biotest Bull 3:7, 1986.
47. Mallory, D, et al: Immunohematology methods and procedures. The American National Red Cross, 1993, pp 40–41.
48. Lalezari, P, and Jiang, RF: The manual polybrene test: A simple and rapid procedure for detection of red cell antibodies. Transfusion 20:206, 1980.
49. Crawford, MN, et al: Microplate system for routine use in blood bank laboratories. Transfusion 10:258, 1970.
50. Redman, M, et al: Typing of red cells on microplates by low-ionic polybrene technique. Med Lab Sci 43:393, 1986.
51. Rosenfield, RE, et al: Solid phase serology for the study of human erythrocytic antigen-antibody reactions. Proc 15th Congr Int Soc Blood Trans, Paris, 1976, p 27.
52. Moore, HH: Automated reading of red cell antibody identification tests by a solid phase antiglobulin technique. Transfusion 24:218, 1984.
53. Plapp, FV, et al: A solid phase antibody screen. Am J Clin Pathol 82:719, 1984.
54. Lapierre, Y, et al: The gel test: A new way to detect red cell antigen-antibody reactions. Transfusion 30:2, 1990.
55. Tissot, JD, et al: The direct antiglobulin test: Still a place for the tube technique? Vox Sang 77:223, 1999.
56. Chuansumrit, A, et al: The benefit of the direct antiglobulin test using gel technique in ABO hemolytic disease of the newborn. Southeast Asian J Trop Med Pub Health 28:428, 1997.
57. Lai, M, et al: Clinically significant autoimmune hemolytic anemia with a negative direct antiglobulin test by routine tube test and positive by column agglutination method. Immunohematology 18:109, 2002.
58. Mitek, JF, et al: The value of the gel test and ELAT in autoimmune haemolytic anaemia. Clin Lab Haem 17:311, 1995.

BIBLIOGRAPHY

Beck, ML, and Marsh, WL: Letter to the editor: Complement and the antiglobulin test. Transfusion 17:529, 1977.
Black, D, and Kay, J: Influence of tube type on the antiglobulin test. Med Lab Sci 43:169, 1986.
Freedman, J, et al: Further observations on the preparation of antiglobulin reagents reacting with C3d and C4d on red cells. Vox Sang 33:21, 1977.
Freedman, J, and Mollison, PL: Preparation of red cells coated with C4 and C3 subcomponents and production of anti-C4d and anti-C3d. Vox Sang 31:241, 1976.
Federal Register 42:41920, 1977.
Federal Register 50:5579, 1985.
Garratty, G, and Petz, LD: An evaluation of commercial antiglobulin sera with particular reference to their anticomplement properties. Transfusion 11:79, 1971.
Giles, C, and Engelfriet, CP: Working party on the standardization of antiglobulin reagents of the expert panel of serology. Vox Sang 38:178, 1980.
Graham, HA, et al: A new approach to prepare cells for the Coombs test. Transfusion 22:408, 1982.
Issitt, PD, et al: Evaluation of commercial antiglobulin sera over a two-year

period. Part 1: Anti-beta 1A, anti-alpha 2D, and anti-beta 1E levels. Transfusion 14:93, 1974.

Judd, WJ, et al: Paraben-associated autoanti-Jk^a antibodies: Three examples detected using commercially prepared low-ionic strength saline containing parabens. Transfusion 22:31, 1982.

Petz, LD: Complement in immunohaematology and in neurologic disorders.

International Symposium on the Nature and Significance of Complement Activation. Ortho Research Institute of Medical Science, Raritan, NJ, 1976, p 87.

Plapp, FV, et al: Solid phase red cell adherence tests in blood banking. In Smit Bigings, C Th, Das, PC, and Greenwalt, TJ: Future Development in Blood Banking. Martinus Nijhoff, Boston, 1986, p 177.

PROCEDURAL APPENDIX

Manual Antiglobulin Test Techniques

I. DAT

A. Procedure

1. Label two 10 or 12 × 75 mm glass test tubes. Test and control, respectively, and add 1 drop of a 3% v/v suspension of test cells to each.
2. Wash the cells a minimum of three times with saline, and *ensure that all saline is completely decanted after the last wash.*
3. To the tube labeled "test," add 1 to 2 drops of AHG as recommended by the manufacturer and mix.
4. To the control tube add 1 to 2 drops of 3% w/v bovine albumin in saline and mix.
5. Centrifuge both tubes at 500 RCF for 15 to 20 seconds.
6. Following centrifugation, completely resuspend the cell pellet by gently tipping and rolling the tube. Read and score agglutination macroscopically with the aid of a background light source and low-power magnification.
7. Incubate the tubes for another 5 minutes at room temperature and repeat steps 5 and 6. Most manufacturers recommend this additional step because it has been shown that some negative or even weak reactions may increase in strength. These reactions have been attributed to the presence of C3d and, to a lesser extent, IgA on the cell surface. Conversely, the reaction with some cells may weaken after the extra incubation; this has been attributed to either detachment of IgG antibody or prozoning when excess anti-IgG has been added.

B. Controls

To all negative tubes add 1 drop of control cells weakly sensitized with IgG, mix the cells, and repeat Steps 5 and 6. A mixed-field weakly positive reaction should now be obtained, indicating that the AHG had been added to the tube and that it was still reactive. All negative results could therefore be considered valid. If a negative result was obtained after addition of the control cells, it would indicate that the AHG had not been added or that, if added, it was nonreactive. This could occur if:

1. The reagent had deteriorated in storage.
2. The reagent had been contaminated by serum and the antibody activity neutralized.

3. The cells had been insufficiently washed and residual serum or plasma had neutralized the AHG reagent when added to the tube.

Control cells weakly sensitized with complement should be used with monospecific anti-C3d reagent to validate negative results.

The control tube containing cells and 3% w/v bovine albumin should give a negative result. If the result is positive, it indicates that the cells are autoagglutinable and that the test cannot be properly interpreted.

For reasons previously outlined, the cells used for DATs should be collected into either EDTA or citrates containing anticoagulant to minimize the possibility of the in-vitro attachment of complement components.

II. IAT

A. Procedure

1. Into a labeled glass 10 or 12 × 75 mm test tube, place 2 to 4 drops of test serum and 1 drop of a washed 3% v/v suspension of RBCs.
2. Mix the cell suspension, and incubate for 30 minutes in a 37°C water bath.
3. Centrifuge the tube at 500 RCF for 15 to 20 seconds.
4. After centrifugation, completely resuspend the cell pellet by gently tapping and rolling the tube. Read and score agglutination macroscopically with the aid of a background light source and low-power magnification.
5. Wash the cells at least three times with saline, and *ensure that all saline is completely decanted following the final wash.*
6. Add 1 to 3 drops of AHG as recommended by the manufacturer and mix.
7. Repeat Steps 3 and 4.

B. Controls

To all negative tubes, add 1 drop of control cells weakly sensitized with IgG, mix the cells, and repeat Steps 3 and 4. Negative results can be considered valid if a weakly positive mixed-field reaction is obtained after addition of the control cells. If this reaction is not obtained, the test should be repeated.

When phenotyping RBCs using an AHG-reactive typing serum, it is important to follow the antisera manufacturer's recommendations for the use of the reagent.

SiX

The ABO Blood Group System

**Denise M. Harmening, PhD, MT(ASCP), CLS(NCA), and
Deborah Firestone, MA, MT(ASCP)SBB**

OBJECTIVES

On completion of this chapter, the learner should be able to:

1. Describe the reciprocal relationship between ABO antigens and antibodies for blood types O, A, B, and AB.
2. Identify the frequencies of the four major blood types in the white, black, Mexican, and Asian populations.
3. Explain the effect of age on the production of ABO isoagglutinins.
4. Describe the immunoglobulin classes of ABO antibodies in group O, A, and B individuals.
5. Predict the ABO phenotypes and genotypes of offspring from various ABO matings.
6. Explain the formation of H, A, and B antigens on the red blood cells (RBCs) from precursor substance to immunodominant sugars.
7. Describe the formation of H, A, and B soluble substances.
8. Explain the principle of the hemagglutination inhibition assay for the determination of secretor status.
9. Describe the qualitative and quantitative differences between the A_1 and A_2 phenotypes.
10. Describe the reactivity of *Ulex europaeus* with the various ABO groups.
11. Describe the characteristics of the weak subgroups of A (A_3, A_x, A_{end}, A_m, A_y, A_{el}).
12. Describe the characteristics of the Bombay phenotypes.
13. Explain the effects of disease on the expression of ABH antigens and antibodies.
14. Interpret the results from an ABO typing and resolve any discrepancies if present.

Historical Perspective

Karl Landsteiner truly opened the doors of blood banking with his discovery of the first human blood group system, ABO. This marked the beginning of the concept of individual uniqueness defined by the RBC antigens present on the RBC membrane. The ABO system is the most important of all blood groups in transfusion practice. It is the only blood group system in which individuals predictably have antibodies in their serum to antigens that are absent from their RBCs. This occurs without any exposure to RBCs by transfusion or pregnancy. Due to the presence of these antibodies, transfusion of an incompatible ABO type can result in the almost immediate lysis of donor RBCs. This produces a very severe, if not fatal, transfusion reaction in the patient. Even today, transfusion of the wrong ABO group remains the leading cause of death reported to the Food and Drug Administration (FDA).[1,2] Testing to detect ABO incompatibility between a donor and potential transfusion recipient is the foundation on which all other pretransfusion testing is based. ABO forward and reverse grouping tests are required to be performed on all donors and patients.[3] ABO grouping is the most frequently performed test in the blood bank. There is always a reciprocal relationship between the forward and reverse type; thus, one serves as a check on the other.

In 1901 Landsteiner drew blood from himself and five associates, separated the cells and serum, and then mixed each cell sample with each serum.[4] He was inadvertently the first individual to perform the forward and reverse grouping. Forward grouping (front type) is defined as using known sources of commercial antisera (anti-A, anti-B) to detect antigens on an individual's RBCs. **Figure 6–1** (see color insert following page 112) outlines the steps of performing the forward grouping for ABO, and **Table 6–1** lists the results of the forward grouping procedure. Reverse grouping (back type) is defined as detection of ABO antibodies in the patient's serum by using known reagent RBCs; namely, A1 and B cells. **Figure 6–2** (see color insert following page 112) outlines the steps of performing the reverse ABO grouping, and **Table 6–2** summarizes the results of the procedures. **Table 6–3** lists the characteristics of the routine reagents used for ABO testing in the blood bank laboratory.

It has been postulated that bacteria are chemically similar to A and B antigens. Bacteria are widespread in the environment, providing a source of constant exposure of individuals to A-like and B-like antigens. This exposure serves as a source of stimulation of anti-A and anti-B. All other defined blood group systems do not regularly have in their serum "naturally occurring" antibodies to antigens they lack on their RBCs. Antibody production in most other blood group systems requires the introduction of foreign RBCs by transfusion or pregnancy, although some individuals can occasionally have antibodies present that are not related to the introduction of foreign RBCs. (These antibodies are usually of the IgM type and are not consistently present in everyone's serum). Performance of serum grouping is, therefore, unique to the ABO blood group system. The regular occurrence of anti-A and/or anti-B in persons lacking the corresponding antigen(s) serves as a confirmation of results in RBC grouping. **Table 6–4** summarizes the forward and reverse grouping for the common ABO blood groups.

The frequency of these blood groups in the white population is as follows: group O, 45 percent; group A, 40 percent; group B, 11 percent; and group AB, 4 percent **(Table 6–5)**.[5] Therefore, O and A are the most common blood group types, and blood group AB is the rarest. However, frequencies of ABO groups differ in a few selected populations and ethnic groups **(Table 6–6)**.[5] For example, group B is found twice as frequently in Blacks and Asians as in Whites, and subgroup A$_2$ is rarely found in Asians.[6]

ABO Antibodies

Individuals normally produce antibodies directed against the A and/or B antigen(s) absent from their RBCs. These antibodies have been described as naturally occurring because they are produced without any exposure to RBCs. The ABO antibodies are predominantly IgM, activate complement, and react at room temperature or colder.[6] ABO antibodies produce strong direct agglutination reactions during ABO testing. The production of ABO antibodies is initiated at birth, but titers are generally too low for detection until the individual is 3 to 6 months of age.[6] Therefore, most antibodies found in cord blood serum are of maternal origin. Results of serum ABO testing before 3 to 6 months of age cannot be considered valid because some or all of the antibodies present may be IgG maternal antibodies that have crossed the placenta. As a result, it is logical to perform only forward grouping on cord blood from newborn infants. Antibody production peaks when an individual is between 5 and 10 years of age and declines later in life.[6] Elderly people usually have lower levels of anti-A and anti-B; antibodies may be undetectable in the reverse grouping. ABO antibodies can cause rapid intravascular

TABLE 6–1 ABO Forward Grouping: Principle—Detection of Antigens on Patient's RBCs with Known Commercial Antisera

Patient RBCs with Anti-A	Patient RBCs with Anti-B	Interpretation of Blood Group
0	0	O
4+	0	A
0	4+	B
3+	3+	AB

+ = visual agglutination
0 = negative
Note: Reaction gradings vary from patient to patient.

TABLE 6–2 ABO Reverse Grouping: Principle—Detection of ABO Antibodies (Isoagglutinins) in Serum of Patient with Known Commercial RBCs

Patient Serum with Reagent A$_1$ Cells	Patient Serum with Reagent B Cells	Interpretation of Blood Group
4+	4+	O
0	3+	A
3+	0	B
0	0	AB

+ = visual agglutination
0 = negative
Note: Reaction gradings vary from patient to patient.

TABLE 6-3   Characteristics of Routine Reagents Used for ABO Testing

	Anti-A Reagent	Anti-B Reagent
Forward Grouping	• Monoclonol antibody* • Highly specific • IgM • Clear blue colored reagent • Expected 3+ to 4+ reaction • Usually use 1–2 drops	• Monoclonal antibody* • Highly specific • IgM • Clear yellow colored reagent (contains an Acroflavin dye) • Expected 3+ to 4+ reaction • Usually use 1–2 drops

Reagent A₁ and B Cells

Reverse Grouping	• Human source • 4%–5% red cell suspension • Expected 2+ to 4+ reaction usually use one drop

*General rule: Always drop clear solutions first, RBCs second, to make sure you have added both a source of antibody and antigen.

hemolysis if the wrong ABO group is transfused and can result in death of the patient.

Although anti-A (from a group B individual) and anti-B (from a group A individual) contains predominantly IgM antibody, there may be small quantities of IgG present.[6] Serum from group O individuals contains not only anti-A and anti-B but also anti-A,B, which reacts with A and B cells. Anti-A,B antibody activity, originally thought to be just a mixture of anti-A and anti-B, cannot be separated into a pure specificity when adsorbed with either A or B cells. For example, if group O serum is adsorbed with A or B cells, the antibody eluted will react with both A and B cells.[7,8] Anti-A,B therefore possesses serologic activity not found in mixtures of anti-A plus anti-B. The predominant immunoglobulin class of antibodies in group O serum is IgG.[6] Knowledge of the amount of IgG anti-A, anti-B, or anti-A,B in a woman's serum sometimes allows prediction or diagnosis of hemolytic disease of the newborn caused by ABO incompatibility (see Chapter 20).

Testing RBCs with reagent anti-A,B is not required as a routine part of RBC testing. It is believed by some, however, that anti-A,B is more effective at detecting weakly expressed A and B antigens than reagent anti-A or anti-B. Reagent anti-A,B can be prepared using blended monoclonal anti-A and anti-B, polyclonal human anti-A,B or a blend of monoclonal anti-A, anti-B and anti-A,B.[8] Consult the manufacturer's package insert in order to determine if a reagent anti-A,B reacts with a specific weak A phenotype.

Both immunoglobulin classes of ABO antibodies react preferentially at room temperature (20°–24°C) or below and efficiently activate complement at 37°C.

Inheritance of the ABO Blood Groups

The theory for the inheritance of the ABO blood groups was first described by Bernstein in 1924. He demonstrated that an individual inherits one *ABO* gene from each parent and that these two genes determine which ABO antigens are present on the RBC membrane. The inheritance of *ABO* genes, therefore, follows simple mendelian genetics. ABO, like most other blood group systems, is codominant in expression.[9] (For a review of genetics, see Chapter 2.) One position, or locus, on each chromosome 9 is occupied by an *A, B,* or *O* gene.[10] The *O* gene is considered an amorph as no detectable antigen is produced in response to the inheritance of this gene. The designations A and B refer to phenotypes, whereas *AA, BO,* and *OO* denote genotypes. In the case of an O individual, both

TABLE 6-4   Summary of Forward and Reverse Groupings

Blood Group	Forward Group Patient's Cells with Reagents			Reverse Group Patient's Serum with Reagents		
	Anti-A	Anti-B	Antigen(s) on RBCs	A₁ cells	B cells	Antibody(ies) in serum
O	0	0	No A or B antigen on cell	4+	4+	A and B antibodies in serum
A	4+	0	A antigen on cell	0	2+	B antibodies in serum
B	0	4+	B antigen on cell	3+	0	A antibodies in serum
AB	3+	3+	A and B antigens on cell	0	0	No A or B antibodies in serum

Note: Reaction gradings vary from patient to patient.
0 = negative (no agglutination)
+ = visual agglutination

TABLE 6-5 Frequency of ABO Blood Groups		
	Race	
Blood Group	Whites	Blacks
O	45%	49%
A	40%	27%
B	11%	19%
AB	4%	4%

TABLE 6-6 Additional ABO Genotypes, Phenotypes, and Frequencies			
		U.S. Frequencies	
Genotype	Phenotype	Whites	Blacks
A_1A_1 A_1A_2 A_1O	A_1	33%	19%
A_2A_2 A_2O	A_2	7%	5%
A_1B	A_1B	2%	2%
A_2B	A_2B	1%	2%

phenotype and genotype are the same, because that individual would have to be homozygous for the *O* gene. An individual who has the phenotype A (or B) can have the genotype *AA* or *AO* (or *BB* or *BO*). The phenotype and genotype are the same in an AB individual because of the inheritance of both the *A* and *B* gene. **Table 6–7** lists possible ABO phenotypes and genotypes from various matings.

Formation of A, B, and H RBC Antigens

The formation of ABH antigens results from the interaction of genes at three separate loci (ABO, Hh, and Se). These genes do not actually code for the production of antigens but rather produce specific glycosyltransferases that add sugars to a basic precursor substance **(Table 6–8)**. A, B, and H antigens are formed from the same basic precursor material (called a paragloboside) to which sugars are attached in response to specific enzyme tranferases elicited by an inherited gene.[11–13]

The precursor substance on erythrocytes is referred to as type 2. This means that the terminal galactose on the precursor substance is attached to the *N*-acetylglucosamine in a beta $1 \rightarrow 4$ linkage **(Fig. 6–3)**. A type 1 precursor substance refers to a beta $1 \rightarrow 3$ linkage between galactose and *N*-acetylglucosamine and will be discussed later. ABH antigens on the RBC are constructed on oligosaccharide chains of type 2 precursor substance.[14]

The ABH antigens develop as early as the 37th day of fetal life but do not increase much in strength during the gestational period. The RBCs of the newborn have been estimated to carry anywhere from 25 to 50 percent of the number of antigenic sites found on the adult RBC. As a result, reactions of newborn RBCs with ABO reagent antisera are frequently weaker than reactions with adult cells. The expression of A and B antigens on the RBCs is fully developed by 2 to 4 years of age and remains constant for life.[8] As well as age, the phenotypic expression of ABH antigens may vary with race, genetic interaction, and disease states.[15]

Interaction of *Hh* and *ABO* Genes

Individuals who are blood group O inherit at least one *H* gene (genotype *HH* or *Hh*) and two O genes. The *H* gene elicits the production of an enzyme, α-2-L-fucosyltransferase, which transfers the sugar L-fucose to an oligosaccharide chain on the terminal galactose of type 2 chains.[13] The sugars that occupy the terminal positions of this precursor chain and confer blood group specificity are called the immunodominant sugars. Therefore, L-fucose is the sugar responsible for H specificity (blood group O) **(Fig. 6–4)**. The *O* gene at the ABO

TABLE 6-7 ABO Groups of the Offspring from the Various Possible ABO Matings		
Mating Phenotypes	Mating Genotypes	Offspring Possible Phenotypes (and Genotypes)
A × A	*AA × AA*	A (AA)
	AA × AO	A (AA or AO)
	AO × AO	A (AA or AO) or O(OO)
B × B	*BB × BB*	B (BB)
	BB × BO	B (BB or BO)
	BO × BO	B (BB or BO) or O (OO)
AB × AB	*AB × AB*	AB (AB) or A (AA) or B (BB)
O × O	*OO × OO*	O (OO)
A × B	*AA × BB*	AB (AB)
	AO × BB	AB (AB) or B (BO)
	AA × BO	AB (AB) or A (AO)
	AO × BO	AB (AB) or A (AO) or B (BO) or O (OO)
A × O	*AA × OO*	A (AO)
	AO × OO	A (AO) or O (OO)
A × AB	*AA × AB*	AB (AB) or A (AA)
	AO × AB	AB (AB) or A (AA or AO) or B (BO)
B × O	*BB × OO*	B (BO)
	BO × OO	B (BO) or O (OO)
B × AB	*BB × AB*	AB (AB) or B (BB)
	BO × AB	AB (AB) or B (BB or BO) or A (AO)
AB × O	*AB × OO*	A (AO) or B (BO)

TABLE 6–8   Glycosyltransferases and Immunodominant Sugars Responsible for H, A, and B Antigen Specificities

Gene	Glycosyltransferase	Immunodominant Sugar	Antigen
H	α-2-L-fucosyltransferase	L-fucose	H
A	α-3-N-acetylgalactosaminyltransferase	N-acetyl-D-galactosamine	A
B	α-3-D-galactosyltransferase	D-galactose	B

locus, which is sometimes referred to as an amorph, does not elicit the production of a catalytically active polypeptide, and therefore the H substance remains unmodified.[13] As a result, the O blood group has the highest concentration of H antigen. The H substance (L-fucose) must be formed for the other sugars to be attached in response to an inherited A and/or B gene.

The *H* gene is present in more than 99.99 percent of the random population. The allele of H, "h," is quite rare, and the genotype, *hh*, is extremely rare. The term "Bombay" has been used to refer to the phenotype that lacks normal expression of the ABH antigens because of the inheritance of the *hh* genotype. The *hh* genotype does not elicit the production of α-2-L-fucosyltransferase; as a result, L-fucose is not added to the type 2 chain, and H substance is not expressed on the RBC. Even though Bombay (*hh*) individuals may inherit *ABO* genes, normal expression, as reflected in the formation of A, B, or H antigens, does not occur. (A discussion of the Bombay phenotype occurs later in this chapter.)

In the formation of blood group A, the *A* gene (*AA* or *AO*) codes for the production of α-3-N-acetylgalactosaminyltransferase, which transfers an N-acetyl-D-galactosamine (GalNAc)

sugar to the H substance. This sugar is responsible for A specificity (blood group A) **(Fig. 6–5)**. The A-specific immunodominant sugar is linked to a type 2 precursor substance that now contains H substance through the action of the *H* gene.

The *A* gene tends to elicit higher concentrations of transferase than the *B* gene. This leads to the conversion of practically all of the H antigen on the RBC to A antigen sites. As many as 810,000 to 1,170,000 antigen sites exist on an A₁ adult RBC in response to inherited genes.

Individuals who are blood group B inherit a *B* gene (*BB* or *BO*) that codes for the production of α-3-D-galactosyltransferase, which then attaches D-galactose (Gal) sugar to the H substance previously placed on the type 2 precursor substance through the action of the *H* gene.[14] This sugar is responsible for B specificity (blood group B) **(Fig 6–6)**. Anywhere from 610,000 to 830,000 B antigen sites exist on a B adult RBC in response to the conversion of the H antigen by the α-3-D-galactosyltransferase produced by the B gene.[6]

When both *A* and *B* genes are inherited, the B enzyme (α-3-D-galactosyltransferase) seems to compete more efficiently

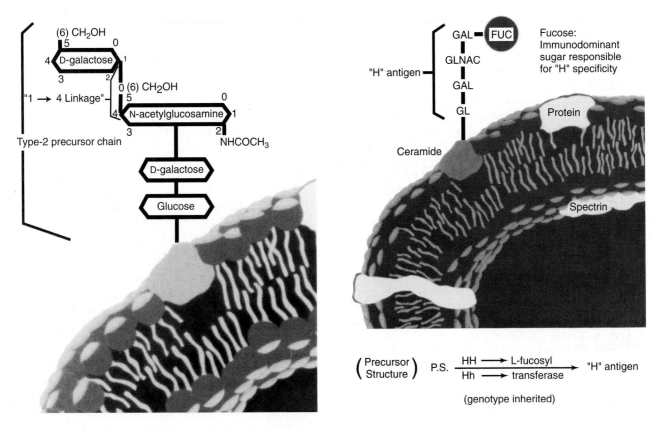

■ FIGURE 6–3   Type-2 precursor chain.

■ FIGURE 6–4   Formation of the H antigen.

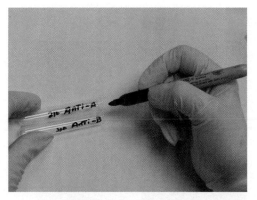

Step 1: Label test tubes.

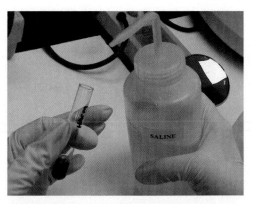

Step 2: Make a 2-5% patient red cell suspension.

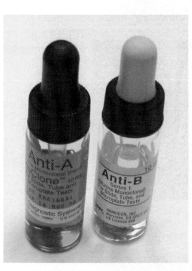

Step 3: Add reagent antisera*
(approximately 2 drops).

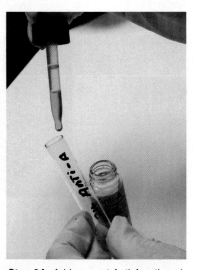

Step 3A: Add reagent Anti-A antisera*
(approximately 2 drops).

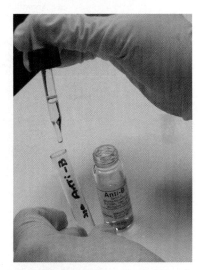

Step 3B: Add Anti-B reagent antisera*
(approximately 2 drops).

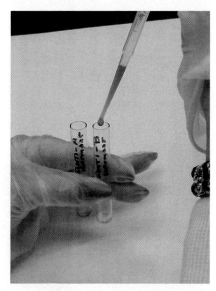

Step 4: Add one drop of 2-5%
suspension of patient red cells to
each tube.

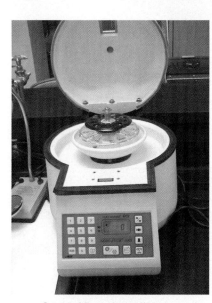

Step 5: Mix and centrifuge
(approximately 20 seconds).

* Consult manufacturer's package insert for specifics.

■ **FIGURE 6–1** Procedure for forward grouping. Principle: Detection of antigens on the patient's RBCs with known commercial antisera. *(Continued on the following page)*

Step 6: Read and record agglutination reactions.

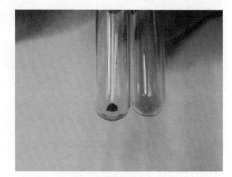

Group B
4+ Agglutination with Anti-B
0 Agglutination with Anti-A

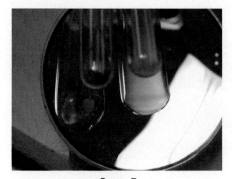

Group B
4+ Agglutination with Anti-B
0 Agglutination with Anti-A

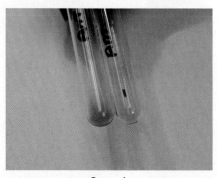

Group A
4+ Agglutination with Anti-A
0 Agglutination with Anti-B

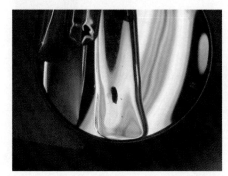

Group A
4+ Agglutination with Anti-A
0 Agglutination with Anti-B

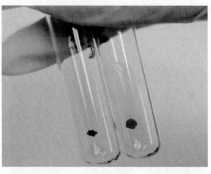

Group AB
4+ Agglutination with Anti-A and Anti-B

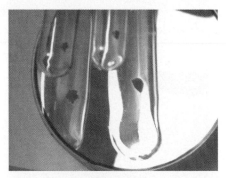

Group AB
4+ Agglutination with Anti-A and Anti-B

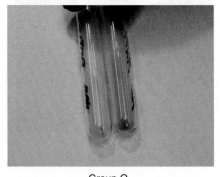

Group O
No Agglutination with Anti-A or Anti-B

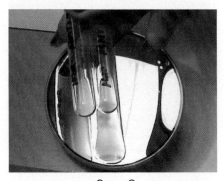

Group O
No Agglutination with Anti-A and Anti-B

■ **FIGURE 6–1** *(continued)* Procedure for forward grouping. Principle: Detection of antigens on the patient's RBCs with known commercial antisera.

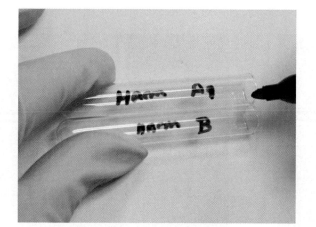

Step 1: Label Test Tubes

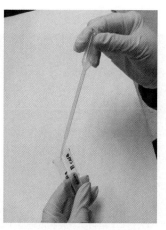

Step 2: Add two drops of patient serum to each tube

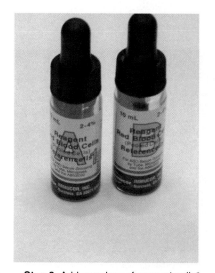

Step 3: Add one drop of reagent cells* to each test tube

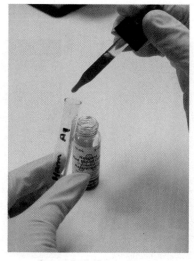

Step 3A: Add one drop of Reagent A₁ cells

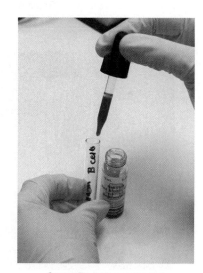

Step 3B: Add one drop of Reagent B cells

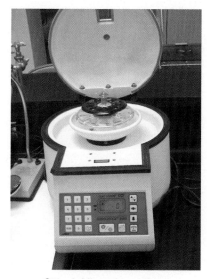

Step 4: Mix and centrifuge (approximately 20 seconds)

* Consult manufacturer's package insert for specifics.

■ **FIGURE 6–2** Procedure for reverse grouping. Principle: Detection of antibodies in the patient's serum with known commercial antisera. *(Continued on the following page)*

Step 5: Resuspend cells button; interpret and record results.

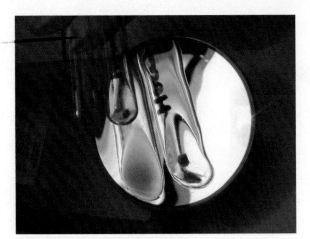

Group A
4+ Agglutination with B Cells
0 Agglutination with A_1 Cells

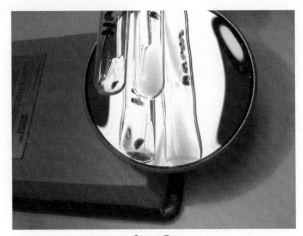

Group B
4+ Agglutination with A_1 Cells
0 Agglutination with B Cells

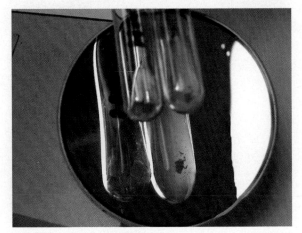

Group O
4+ Agglutination with A_1 Cells
3+ Agglutination with B Cells

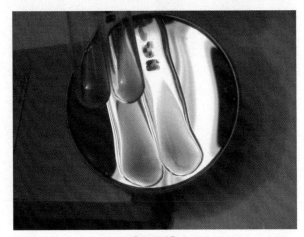

Group AB
0 Agglutination with A_1 Cells
No Agglutination with A_1 and B Cells

■ **FIGURE 6–2 *(continued)*** Procedure for reverse grouping. Principle: Detection of antibodies in the patient's serum with known commercial antisera.

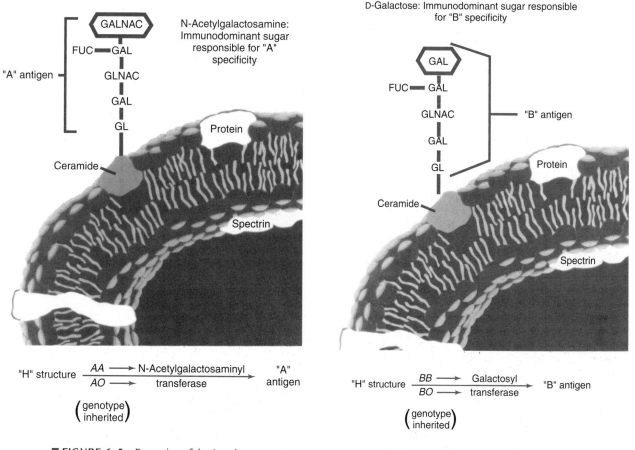

■ FIGURE 6–5   Formation of the A antigen.

■ FIGURE 6–6   Formation of the B antigen.

for the H substance than the A enzyme (α-3-N-acetylgalactosaminyltransferase). Therefore, the average number of A antigens on an AB adult cell is approximately 600,000 sites, compared with an average of 720,000 B antigen sites. Glycosyltransferases and immunodominant sugars responsible for H, A, and B antigen specificities are presented in Table 6–8. Interaction of the *Hh* and ABO genes is reviewed in Figure 6–7.

Molecular Genetics of *ABO*

Advanced Concepts (SBB Level)

The *ABO* gene that codes for the production of glycosyltransferases that convert H substance to blood group A and B is located on chromosome 9 and consists of seven exons.[16] The last two exons (6 and 7) encode for the catalytic domain of the ABO glycosyltransferases.[15] Amino acid substitutions, resulting from deletions, mutations, or gene recombination within these two exons of the coding DNA of variant ABO glycosyltransferases, are responsible for the less efficient transfer of the immunodominant sugar to H substance, resulting in weak serologic reactions.[14] There are only a few base positions that differentiate the common A, B, and O alleles (ABO*A101, ABO*B101 and ABO*O01) from one another.[11] Seven nucleotide positions differentiate ABO*B101 from ABO*A101.[17] In addition, the ABO*O01 O gene is identical to ABO*A101, with the exception of a nucleotide deletion in the coding region at nucleotide position 261.[18] This deletion of a single DNA base pair creates a premature stop codon (three

adjacent bases), resulting in an *O*-transferase, which is functionally inactive and incapable of modifying the H antigen.[18] It is unlikely, therefore, that O individuals would express a protein that is immunologically related to that produced by either A or B transferases. Ongoing research will continue to uncover new alleles and expand the current body of knowledge on the molecular genetics of ABO.

Formation of A, B, and H Soluble Antigens

ABH antigens are integral parts of the membranes of RBCs, endothelial cells, platelets, lymphocytes, and epithelial cells.[8] ABH-soluble antigens can also be found in all body secretions. Their presence is dependent on the ABO genes inherited as well as the inheritance of another set of genes (secretor genes) that regulate their formation. Eighty percent of the random U.S. population are known as secretors because they have inherited a secretor gene (*SeSe* or *Sese*). The inheritance of an *Se* gene codes for the production of a transferase (α-2-L-fucosyltransferase) that results in the modification of the type 1 precursor substance in secretions to express H substance.[19] This H substance can then be modified to express A and B substance (if the corresponding gene is present) in secretions such as saliva.[20] For example, a group A individual who is a secretor (*SeSe* or *Sese*) will secrete glycoproteins carrying A and H antigens. The Se gene does not, however, affect the formation of A, B, or H antigens on the RBC. It is the presence of the *Se*-gene–specified α-2-L-fucosyltransferase that determines whether ABH-soluble substances will be secreted

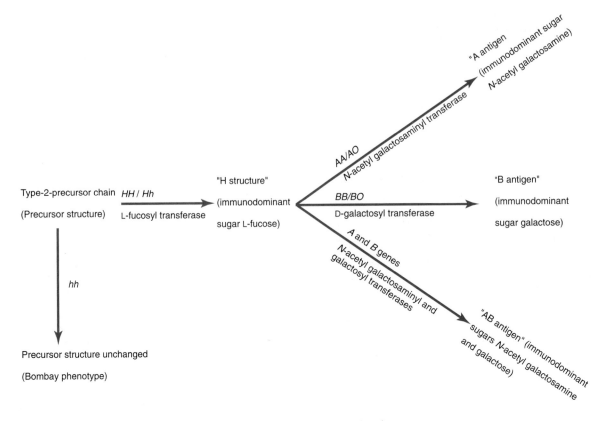

■ FIGURE 6-7   Interaction of the *Hh* and *ABO* genes.

(Fig. 6–8).[21] People who inherit the *sese* genotype are termed nonsecretors.

Comparison of A, B, and H Antigens on RBCs and A, B, and H Soluble Substances

The formation of soluble A, B, and H substances is the same as that described for the formation of A, B, and H antigens on the RBCs, except for a few minor distinctions that are compared in **Table 6–9.**

Tests for ABH secretion may establish the true ABO group of an individual whose RBC antigens are poorly developed. The demonstration of A, B, and H substances in saliva is evidence for the inheritance of an *A* gene, a *B* gene, an *H* gene, and an *Se* gene. The term "secretor" refers only to secretion of A, B, and H soluble antigens in body fluids. The glycoprotein-soluble substances (or antigens) normally found in the saliva of secretors are listed in **Table 6–10. Box 6–1** summarizes the body fluids in which ABH-soluble substances can be found. The procedure for determination of the secretor status (saliva studies) can be found in the appendix at the end of the chapter.

ABO Subgroups

A Subgroups

Basic Concepts

In 1911 von Dungern described two different A antigens based on reactions between group A RBCs and anti-A and anti-A₁. Group A RBCs that react with both anti-A and anti-A₁ are clas-

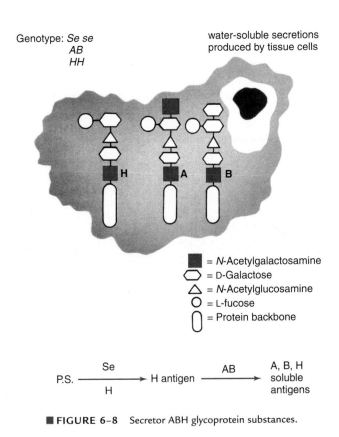

■ FIGURE 6-8   Secretor ABH glycoprotein substances.

TABLE 6–9   Comparison of ABH Antigens on RBCs and in Secretions

ABH Antigens on Red Cells	A, B, and H Soluble Substances
• RBC antigens can be glycolipids, glycoproteins, or glycosphingolipids	• Secreted substances are glycoproteins
• RBC antigens are only synthesized on type 2 precursor chains	• Secreted substances are primarily synthesized on type 1 precursor chains[12]
• Type 2 chain refers to a beta-1→4 linkage in which the number one carbon of the galactose is attached to the number three carbon of the N-acetylglucosamine sugar of the precursor substance	• Type 1 chain refers to a beta-1→3 linkage in which the number one carbon of the galactose is attached to the number three carbon of the N-acetylglucosamine sugar of the precursor substance
• The enzyme produced by the H gene (α-2-L-fucosyltransferase) acts primarily on type 2 chains, which are prevalent on the RBC membrane	• The enzyme produced by the Se gene (α-2-L-fucosyltransferase) preferentially acts on type 1 chains in secretory tissues

BOX 6–1
Fluids in which A, B, and H Substances Can Be Detected in Secretors

- Saliva
- Tears
- Urine
- Digestive juices
- Bile
- Milk
- Amniotic fluid
- Pathologic fluids: pleural, peritoneal, pericardial, ovarian cyst

sified as A_1 whereas those that react with anti-A and not anti-A_1 are classified as A_2 (**Table 6–11**). RBCs from A_1 and A_2 individuals react equally strong with reagent anti-A in ABO forward typing tests.[3]

Classification into A_1 and A_2 phenotypes accounts for 99 percent of all group A individuals. The cells of approximately 80 percent of all group A (or AB) individuals are A_1 (or A_1B), and the remaining 20 percent are A_2 (or A_2B) or weaker subgroups. The difference between A_1 and A_2 is both quantitative and qualitative. **Table 6–12** summarizes the general quantitative and qualitative differences of the subgroups of A.

The production of both types of antigens is a result of an inherited gene at the ABO locus. Inheritance of an A_1 gene elicits production of high concentrations of the enzyme α-3-N-acetylgalactosaminyltransferase, which converts almost all of the H precursor structure to A_1 antigens on the RBCs. A_1 is a very potent gene that creates from 810,000 to 1,170,000 antigen sites on the adult RBC, whereas inheritance of an A_2 gene results in the production of only 240,000 to 290,000 antigen sites on the adult A_2 RBC. The immunodominant sugar on both A_1 and A_2 RBCs is N-acetyl-D-galactosamine.

Qualitative differences also exist, inasmuch as 1 to 8 percent of A_2 individuals produce anti-A_1 in their serum, and 22 to 35 percent of A_2B individuals produce anti-A_1. This antibody can cause discrepancies in ABO testing and incompatibilities in crossmatches with A_1 or A_1B cells. Because anti-A_1 is a naturally occurring IgM cold antibody, it is unlikely to cause a transfusion reaction because it usually reacts better or only at temperatures well below 37° C. It is to be considered clinically significant if it is reactive at 37°C. There must be some difference between the antigenic structure of A_1 and A_2 because, even though the same immunodominant sugar (N-acetyl-D-galactosamine) is attached by the same transferase (α-3-N-acetylgalactosaminyltransferase), A_2 and A_2B individuals cannot recognize the A_1 antigen as being part of their own RBC makeup and are immunologically stimulated to produce a specific A_1 antibody that does not cross-react with A_2 RBCs.

The antigens present on the RBCs of A_1 and A_2 individuals can be represented in two ways. It is generally presented that A_1 has both the A and A_1 antigen on the RBC, whereas A_2 has only A antigen on its surface (**Fig. 6–9**). However, to simplify the concept, one can think of A_1 as having only A_1 antigen sites and A_2 as having only A antigen sites (**Fig. 6–10**). Serum from group B individuals contains two antibodies, anti-A and anti-A_1; therefore, this antibody mixture reacts with both A_1 and A_2 RBCs because both cells have the A antigen. If serum from a group B individual (which contains anti-A and anti-A_1) is adsorbed with A_2 cells (which contain only the A antigen), anti-A will bind to the RBC. The serum left after the cells and attached anti-A are removed by centrifugation is referred to as "absorbed serum" and contains anti-A_1. This absorbed serum

TABLE 6–10   ABH Substance in the Saliva of Secretors (*SeSe* or *Sese*)*

	Substances in Saliva		
ABO Group	**A**	**B**	**H**
O	None	None	↑↑
A	↑↑	None	↑
B	None	↑↑	↑
AB	↑↑	↑↑	↑

* Nonsecretors (*sese*) have no ABH substances in saliva.
↑↑ and ↑, respectively, represent the concentration of ABH substances in saliva.

TABLE 6–11 A_1 Versus A_2 Phenotypes

	Reactions of Patient's RBCs with	
Blood Group	**Anti-A Reagent (anti-A plus anti-A_1)**	**Anti-A_1 Lectin Reagent**
A_1	+	+
A_2	+	0

+ = positive (agglutination)
0 = negative (no agglutination)

TABLE 6–12   Quantitative and Qualitative Differences of Subgroups of A

Quantitative	Qualitative
• ↓ Number of antigen sites	Differences in antigenic structure
• ↓ Amount of transferase enzyme	Subtle differences in transferase enzymes
• ↓ Amount of branching	Formation of anti-A_1, in a percentage of some subgroups

will react only with A_1 antigen sites. The seed of the plant *Dolichos biflorus,* which serve as another source of anti-A_1, is known as anti-A_1 lectin. Lectins are seed extracts that agglutinate human cells with some degree of specificity. This reagent agglutinates A_1 (or A_1B) cells but does not agglutinate A_2 (or A_2B cells). The characteristics of the A_1 and A_2 phenotypes are presented in **Table 6–13.**

H antigen is found in greatest concentration on the RBCs of group O individuals. Group A_1 individuals will not possess a great deal of H antigen because, in the presence of the A_1 gene, almost all of the H antigen is converted to A_1 antigen by placing the large *N*-acetyl-D-galactosamine sugar on the H substance. Because of the presence of so many A_1 antigens, the H antigen on A_1 and A_1B RBCs may be hidden and therefore may not be available to react with anti-H antisera. In the presence of an A_2 gene, only some of the H antigen is converted to A antigens, and the remaining H antigen is detectable on the cell. Weak subgroups of the A antigen will often have a reciprocal relationship between the amount of H antigen on the RBC and the amount of A antigens formed (i.e., more A antigen formed, less H antigen expressed on the RBC). The H antigen on the RBCs of A_1 and A_1B individuals is so well hidden by *N*-acetyl-D-galactosamine that anti-H is occasionally found in the serum. This anti-H is a naturally occurring IgM cold agglutinin that reacts best below room temperature. As can be expected, this antibody is formed in response to a natural substance and reacts most strongly with cells of group O individuals (which have the greatest amount

of H substance on their RBCs) and weakly with the RBCs of A_1B individuals (which contain small amounts of H substance). It is an insignificant antibody in terms of transfusion purposes because it has no reactivity at body temperature, 37°C. However, high-titered anti-H may react at room temperature and present a problem in antibody screening procedures because reagent screening cells are group O (see Chapter 12). This high-titered anti-H may also present a problem with compatibility testing (see Chapter 13). Anti-H lectin from the extract of *Ulex europaeus* closely parallels the reactions of human anti-H. Both antisera agglutinate RBCs of group O and A_2 and react very weakly or not at all with groups A_1 and A_1B. Group B cells give reactions of variable strength **(Fig. 6–11)**.

Advanced Concepts (SBB Level)

The discussion thus far has presented a basic overview of the two major ABO subgroups, A_1 and A_2. A more plausible, yet more detailed, theory of ABO subgroups has been proposed by the identification of four different forms of H antigens, two of which are unbranched straight chains (H_1, H_2) and two of which are complex branched chains (H_3, H_4) **(Fig. 6–12)**.[22] H_1 through H_4 correspond to the precursor structures on which the A enzyme can act to convert H antigen to blood group A active glycolipids. Although the chains differ in length and complexity of branching, the terminal sugars giving rise to their antigenic specificity are identical. Studies on the chemical and physical characteristics of the A_1 and A_2 enzyme transferases have demonstrated that these two enzymes are different qualitatively.[12,13] Straight chain H_1 and H_2 glycolipids can be converted to A^a and A^b antigens, respectively, by both A_1 and A_2 enzymes, with the A_2 enzyme being less efficient. The more complex branched H_3 and H_4 structures can be converted to A^c and A^d antigens by A_1 enzyme and only very poorly by A_2 enzyme. As a result, more unconverted H antigens (specifically H_3 and H_4) are available on group A_2 RBCs, and only A^a and A^b determinants are formed from H_1 and H_2 structures. On the RBCs of some A_2 individuals, A^c is extremely low and A^d is completely lacking **(Box 6–2)**. It is feasible to expect that these are the indi-

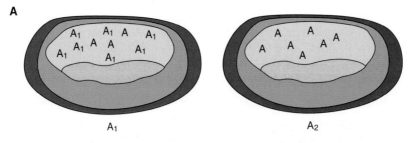

Reactions of Patients Red Cells with

Blood Group	Antigen Present	Anti-A (Anti-A plus Anti-A_1)	Anti-A_1 lectin
A_1	A_1 A	+	+
A_2	A	+	0

■ **FIGURE 6–9** A_1 versus A_2 phenotypes.

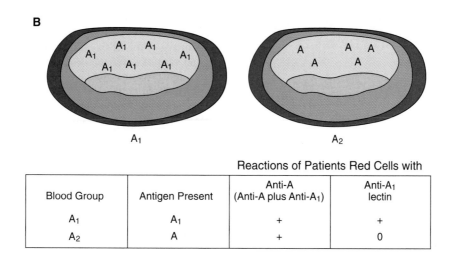

Reactions of Patients Red Cells with

Blood Group	Antigen Present	Anti-A (Anti-A plus Anti-A$_1$)	Anti-A$_1$ lectin
A$_1$	A$_1$	+	+
A$_2$	A	+	0

■ **FIGURE 6–10**   A$_1$ versus A$_2$ phenotypes (alternative conceptual presentation).

viduals in whom one would find anti-A$_1$ in the serum. This anti-A$_1$ antibody could really be an antibody to A^c and A^d determinants, which these A$_2$ individuals lack. Also, in 22 to 35 percent of A$_2$B individuals, anti-A$_1$ can be found in the serum. Inasmuch as the B enzyme transferase is usually more efficient than the A enzyme in converting H structures to the appropriate antigen, A$_2$ enzymes would probably fail completely when paired with a B enzyme. As a result, A$_2$B individuals would be far more likely to lack A^c and A^d components with subsequent production of anti-A^c and anti-A^d (anti-A$_1$).

As stated previously, most group A infants appear to be A$_2$ at birth, with subsequent development to A$_1$ a few months later. Newborn infants have been found to have a deficiency of the branched H$_3$ and H$_4$ antigens and, therefore, also the A^c and A^d antigens, possibly accounting for the A$_2$ phenotype. Adult cells contain a higher concentration of branched H$_3$ and H$_4$ structures and, therefore, A^c and A^d determinants of the A antigen in A$_1$ individuals.

Weak A Subgroups

Basic Concepts

Subgroups weaker than A$_2$ occur infrequently and are most often recognized through an ABO discrepancy. These subgroups of A make up 1 percent of those encountered in the laboratory and therefore are mainly of academic interest. Characteristics of weak ABO subgroups include:

1. Decreased number of A antigen sites per RBC (resulting in weak or no agglutination with anti-A)
2. Varying degrees of agglutination by human anti-A,B[8]
3. Increased variability in the detectability of H antigen, resulting in strong reactions with anti-H
4. Presence or absence of anti-A$_1$ in the serum

Secretor studies and adsorption-elution tests can be utilized to subdivide A individuals into A$_3$, A$_x$, A$_{end}$, etc. **(Table 6–14).**

Occasionally, weak subgroups of A may present practical problems if, for example, an A$_x$ donor that was mistyped as a group O was transfused to a group O transfusion recipient. This is potentially dangerous because the group O patient possesses anti-A,B, which agglutinates and lyses A$_x$ RBCs, causing rapid intravascular hemolysis.

Advanced Concepts (SBB Level)

Weak A phenotypes can be serologically differentiated using the following techniques:

Forward grouping of A and H antigens with anti-A, anti-A,B, and anti-H

Reverse grouping of ABO isoagglutinins and the presence of anti-A$_1$

Adsorption-elution tests with anti-A

Saliva studies to detect the presence of A and H substances

TABLE 6–13	Characteristics of A$_1$ and A$_2$ Phenotypes							
	RBCs with				Naturally Occurring Antibodies in Serum			
Phenotypes	**Anti-A**	**Anti-B**	**Anti-A,B**	**Anti-A$_1$**	**Common**	**Unexpected**	**Substances Present in Saliva of Secretors**	**Number of Antigen Sites RBC × 10^3**
A$_1$	4+	0	4+	4+	Anti-B	None	A, H	810–1170
A$_2$	4+	0	4+	0	Anti-B	Anti-A$_1$ (1%–8% of cases)	A, H	240–290

$$O > A_2 > B > A_2B > A_1 > A_1B$$

greatest
amount of
H

least
amount of
H

■ **FIGURE 6–11**　Reactivity of anti-H antisera or anti-H lectin with ABO blood groups.

Additional special procedures such as serum glycosyltransferase studies for detection of the A enzyme can be performed for differentiation of weak subgroups. Absence of a disease process should be confirmed before subgroup investigation, because ABH antigens are altered in various malignancies and other hematologic disorders. (A discussion of ABO discrepancies due to ABH antigens/antibodies in disease occurs later in this chapter).

Weak A subgroups can be distinguished as A_3, A_x, A_{end}, A_m, A_y, and A_{el}, using the serologic techniques mentioned previously (see **Table 6–14**). The characteristics of each weak A subgroup are presented in the following paragraphs.

A_3. A_3 RBCs characteristically demonstrate a mixed-field pattern of agglutination with anti-A and most anti-A,B reagents.[6] Mixed-field can be defined as small agglutinates within predominantly unagglutinated cells. The estimated number of A antigen sites is approximately 35,000 per RBC.[6] Weak α-3-N-acetylgalactosaminyltransferase activity is detectable in the serum. However, there appears to be a heterogeneity in the A_3 glycosyltransferases isolated from various A_3 phenotypes. Individuals tested were divided into three groups.[23] Group 1 consisted of A_3 phenotypes with an enzyme that had an optimal pH of approximately 7.0 and very low activity. Group 2 consisted of A_3 individuals with no detectable A transferase. Group 3 consisted of an A_3 phenotype demonstrating a serum A enzyme with an activity equivalent to one-third of that normally found in group A_1 serum and an optimal pH activity of 6.0. Additionally, in optimum conditions, serum from this A_3 individual in Group 3 was capable of converting O RBCs into A RBCs that did not show the mixed-field agglutination pattern characteristic of A_3.[6] A_3 enzyme is a product of an allele at the ABO locus inherited in a dominant manner; however, the A_3 blood group has been reported to be very heterogeneous at the molecular level.[24] Anti-A_1 may be present in serum of A_3 individuals, and A substance is detected in the saliva of A_3 secretors.

A_x. A_x RBCs characteristically are not agglutinated by anti-A reagent but do agglutinate with most examples of anti-A,B.[6] The estimated number of A antigen sites is approximately 4000 per RBC.[25] Anti-A can be adsorbed and then eluted from A_x cells without difficulty. A transferase is not usually detectable in the serum or in the RBC membranes of A_x individuals. The molecular genetics of A_x reflects the considerable heterogeneity of the serologic phenotypes.[26] A_x individuals almost always produce anti-A_1 in their serum. Routine secretor studies detect the presence of only H substance in A_x secretors. However, A_x secretors contain A substance detectable only by agglutination/inhibition studies using A_x RBCs as indicators.[25] Caution should be used in interpreting results of secretor studies using A_x indicator cells and anti-A, because not all A_x cells are agglutinated by anti-A.

A_{end}. A_{end} RBCs charateristically demonstrate mixed-field agglutination with anti-A and anti-A,B, but only a very small percentage of the RBCs ($\leq$10 percent) agglutinate.[26] The estimated number of A antigen sites on the few agglutinable RBCs is approximately 3500, whereas no detectable A antigens are demonstrated on RBCs that do not agglutinate.[25] No A glycosyltransferase is detectable in the serum or in the RBC membranes of A_{end} individuals. A_{end} is inherited as an allele at the ABO locus.[4] Secretor studies detect the presence of only H substance in the saliva of A_{end} secretors. Anti-A_1 is found in some A_{end} sera.[4] The phenotypes of A_{finn} and A_{bantu} are considered by some investigators to represent variants of the A_{end} subgroup.[25]

A_m. A_m RBCs are characteristically not agglutinated, or agglutinated only weakly, by anti-A or anti-A,B.[27] A strongly positive adsorption/elution of anti-A confirms the presence of A antigen sites. The estimated number of A antigen sites varies from 200 to 1900 per RBC in A_m individuals.[25] An A enzyme of either the A_1 or A_2 type previously described is detectable in the serum of A_m subgroups.[27] A_m is inherited as a rare allele at the ABO locus.[28] These individuals usually do not produce anti-A_1 in their sera. Normal quantities of A and H substance are found in the saliva of A_m secretors.[27]

A_y. A_y RBCs are not agglutinated by anti-A or anti-A,B. Adsorption and elution of anti-A is the method used to confirm the presence of A antigens. Activity of eluates from A_y RBCs is characteristically weaker than that of eluates from A_m RBCs. Trace amounts of A glycosyltransferase is detectable in the serum of A_y individuals, and saliva secretor studies demonstrate H and A substance, with A substance present in below-normal quantities.[23] A_y individuals usually do not produce anti-A_1. The A_y phenotype can be observed in siblings, implicating a recessive mode of inheritance. This phenotype does not represent expression of an alternate allele at the ABO locus but rather as a germline mutation of an A gene within a family.[4]

A_{el}. A_{el} RBCs typically are unagglutinated by anti-A or anti-A,B; however, adsorption and elution can be used to demonstrate the presence of the A antigen. No detectable A enzyme activity can be demonstrated in the serum or in the RBC membranes of A_{el} individuals by glycosyltransferase studies.[23] The A_{el} phenotype is inherited as a rare gene at the ABO locus.[11] A_{el} individuals usually produce an anti-A_1 that is reactive with A_1 cells and sometimes produce anti-A, which agglutinates A_2 RBCs.[25] Secretor studies demonstrate the presence of only H substance in the saliva of A_{el} secretors.

It should be noted that there are still some reported A variants that do not fit into any of the weak subgroups described, alluding to existence of new alternate alleles or regulation by modifier genes.[11]

A general flowchart for the process of elimination and identification of various subgroups is presented in **Figure 6–13**, with the assumption that the patient's medical history (e.g., recent transfusion, disease states) has been investigated and excluded as a source of discrepancy.

B Subgroups

Subgroups of B are very rare and less frequent than A subgroups.

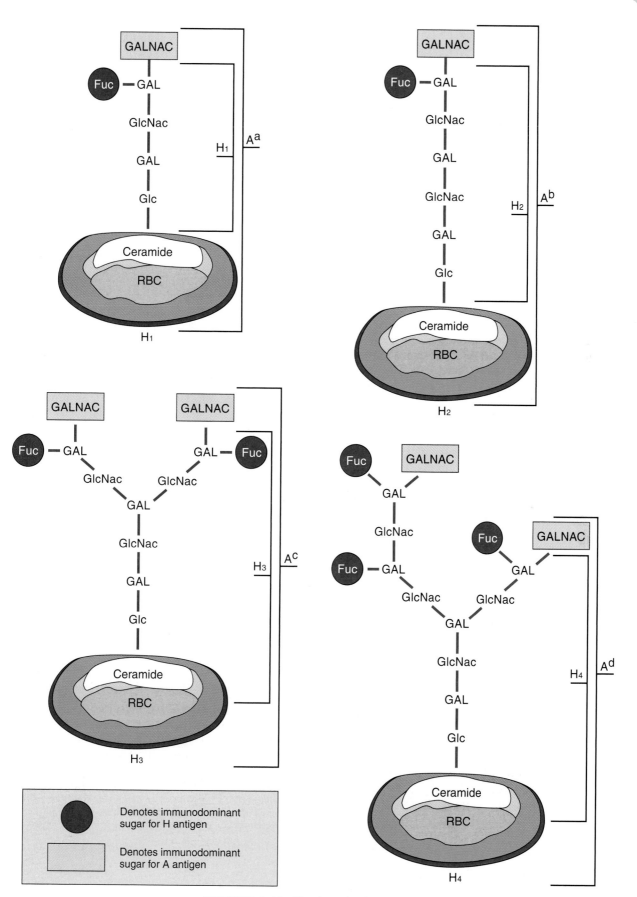

■ FIGURE 6–12 H-active antigenic structures.

BOX 6–2
Structural Characteristics of A_1 and A_2 RBCs

- A_2 RBCs: Predominantly A^a and A^b and unconverted H_3 and H_4 antigen sites
- A_1 red cells: A^a, A^b, A^c, and A^d determinants and no unconverted H_3 and H_4 antigen sites

---

Weak B Subgroups

Advanced Concepts (SBB Level)

RBCs demonstrating serologic activity that is weaker than normal are designated weak B phenotypes or B subgroups and include B_3, B_x, B_m, and B_{el} phenotypes[25] (**Table 6–15**). There are no B subgroups reported that are equivalent to A_{end} or A_y. A classification system similar to A subgroups has been used because of common serologic characteristics. Subgroups of B are usually recognized by variations in the strength of the reaction using anti-B and anti-A,B.

Inheritance of B subgroups, similar to that of the majority of A subgroups, is considered to be a result of alternate alleles at the B locus. Criteria used for differentiation of weak B phenotypes include the following:

1. Strength/type of agglutination with anti-B, anti-A,B, and anti-H
2. Presence or absence of ABO isoagglutinins in the serum
3. Adsorption-elution studies with anti-B
4. Presence of B substance in saliva

These serologic techniques can be used to characterize B subgroups in the following manner.

B_3. This phenotype generally results from the inheritance of a rare gene at the ABO locus and is characterized by a mixed-field pattern of agglutination with anti-B and anti-A,B.[29] B glycosyltransferase is present in the serum but not in the RBC membranes of these individuals. Anti-B is absent in the serum of B_3 phenotypes, but B substance is present in normal amounts in the saliva of secretors. The B_3 subgroup is the most frequent weak B phenotype.[25]

B_x. B_x RBCs typically demonstrate weak agglutination with anti-B and anti-A,B antisera.[4] B glycosyltransferase has not been detected in the serum or in the RBC membranes of B_x phenotypes, but a weakly reactive anti-B usually is produced.[25] B_x RBCs readily adsorb and elute anti-B. Secretor studies demonstrate large amounts of H substance as well as some B substance that can often be detected only by inhibition of agglutination of B_x cells with anti-B.[4] Family studies suggest that B_x is a rare allele at the ABO locus.

B_m. B_m RBCs are characteristically unagglutinated by anti-B or anti-A,B. The B_m RBCs easily adsorb and elute anti-B. B glycosyltransferase is present in the serum of B_m phenotypes but is usually lower in activity and varies from individual to individual.[30] Only very small amounts of B transferase activity is demonstrated in B_m RBC membranes. Reduced activity of B enzyme in hematopoietic tissue is clearly the defect causing the formation of the B_m subgroup, inasmuch as normal B plasma incubated with B_m RBCs and UDP-galactose transforms this subgroup into a normal group B phenotype. Anti-B is not characteristically present in the serum of B_m individuals. Normal quantities of H and B substance are found in the saliva of B_m secretors.

The B_m phenotype is usually the result of inheritance of a rare allele at the ABO locus, although the subgroup B_m may be the product of an interacting modifying gene linked closely to the ABO locus. This modifier gene may depress expression of the B gene, resulting in decreased B enzyme activity.[30] The B_m subgroup is reported to be more frequent in Japan.[25]

B_{el}. B_{el} RBCs are unagglutinated by anti-B or anti-A,B. This extremely rare phenotype must be determined by adsorption and elution of anti-B. No B glycosyltransferase has been identified in the serum or RBC membrane of B_{el} individuals. B_{el} is inherited as a rare gene at the ABO locus. A weak anti-B may be present in the serum of this subgroup. Only H substance is demonstrated in saliva of B_{el} secretors.[31]

Other weak B phenotypes have been reported that do not possess the appropriate characteristics for classification into one of the groups previously discussed.[32] These may represent new classifications and new representations of ABO polymorphism.

TABLE 6–14   Characteristics of Weak ABO Phenotypes

| Phenotypes | RBCs with | | | | Antibodies in Serum | | | Substances present in saliva of secretors | Presence of A transferase in serum | Number of antigen sites RBC $\times 10^3$ |
	Anti-A	Anti-B	Anti-A,B	Anti-H	Anti-A	Anti-B	Anti-A_1			
A_3	++mf	0	++mf	3+	no	yes	sometimes	A, H	sometimes	35
A_x	wk/0	0	2+	4+	+/−	yes	almost always	A(trace), H	rarely	5
A_{end}	wk mf	0	wk mf	4+	no	yes	sometimes	H	no	3.5
A_m*	0/wk	0	0/+	4+	no	yes	no	A, H	yes	1
A_y*	0	0	0	4+	no	yes	no	A, H	trace	1
A_{el}*	0	0	0	4+	some	yes	yes	H	no	.7

*A specificity demonstrated only by absorption/elution procedures
mf = mixed-field agglutination; wk = weak; 0 = negative

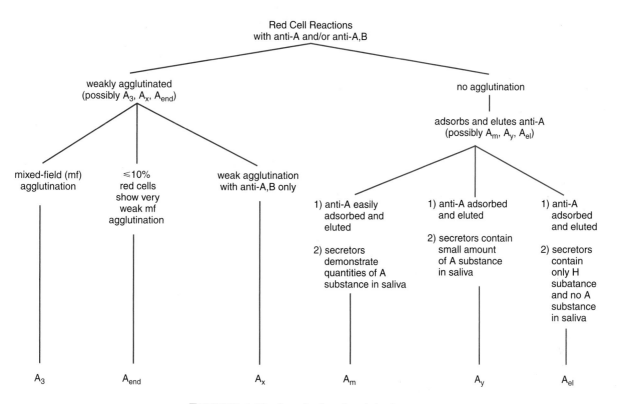

FIGURE 6–13   Investigation of weak A subgroups.

The Bombay Phenotypes (O$_h$)

The Bombay phenotype was first reported by Bhende in 1952 in Bombay, India. It represents the inheritance of a double dose of the h gene producing the very rare genotype hh. As a result, the ABO genes cannot be expressed, and ABH antigens cannot be formed as there is no H antigen made in the Bombay phenotype **(Box 6–3)**. More than 130 Bombay phenotypes have been reported in various parts of the world. These RBCs are devoid of normal ABH antigens and therefore fail to react with anti-A, anti-B, and anti-H. In RBC testing using anti-A and anti-B, the Bombay would phenotype as an O blood group. However, the RBCs of the Bombay phenotype (Oh) do not react with the anti-H lectin (Ulex europaeus), unlike those of the normal group O individual, which react strongly with anti-H lectin.[33] Bombay serum contains anti-A, anti-B, anti-A,B, and anti-H. Unlike the anti-H found occasionally in the serum of A1 and A1B individuals, the Bombay anti-H can often be potent and reacts strongly at 378C. It is an IgM antibody that can bind complement and cause RBC lysis. Transfusing normal group O blood (with the highest concentration of H antigen) to a Bombay recipient (anti-H in the serum) would cause immediate cell lysis. Therefore, only blood from another Bombay individual will be compatible and can be transfused to a Bombay recipient. ABH substance is absent in saliva.[34] **Box 6–4** summarizes the general characteristics of Bombay phenotypes. When family studies demonstrate which ABO genes are inherited in the Bombay phenotype, the genes are written as superscripts (OhA, OhB, OhAB).

TABLE 6–15	Characteristics of B Phenotypes							
	Testing of RBCs				*Naturally Occurring Antibodies in Serum*			
Phenotypes	**Anti-A**	**Anti-B**	**Anti-A,B**	**Anti-H**	**Common**	**Unexpected**	**Substances Present in Saliva of Secretors**	**Presence of a B Transferase in Serum**
B	0	4+	4+	2+	Anti-A	None	B,H	yes
B$_3$	0	++mf	++mf	3+	Anti-A	None	B,H	yes(wk pos)
B$_x$	0	wk	wk	3+	Anti-A	Weak anti-B	H	no
B$_m$*	0	0/wk	0/wk	3+	Anti-A	None	B,H	Yes (wk pos)
B$_{el}$*	0	0	0	3+	Anti-A	Sometimes a weak anti-B	H	no

*B specificity demonstrated only by absorption/elution procedures.
mf = mixed-field; wk= weak; 0=negative.

BOX 6–3
The Bombay Phenotype (O$_h$)

- *hh* genotype
- No H antigens formed; therefore, no A or B antigens formed
- Phenotypes as blood group O
- Anti-A, anti-B, anti-A,B and anti-H present in the serum
- Can only be transfused with blood from another Bombay (O$_h$)

H-Deficient Phenotypes

Basic Concepts

H-deficient phenotypes are those rare phenotypes in which the RBCs are completely devoid of H antigens or that have small amounts of H antigen present. These phenotypes have been classified into the three categories discussed in the following paragraphs.

Category 1: RBC H-Deficient, Nonsecretor; Bombay Phenotype *(hh sese)*. The H gene is very common; 99.99 percent of all individuals have an *HH* or *Hh* genotype. Conversely, the h allele is very rare and does not produce the α-2-L-fucosyltransferase necessary for formation of the H structure. The Bombay phenotype, or O$_h$, inherits the *hh* genotype and therefore lacks normal expression of ABH antigens.

Advanced Concepts

Category 2: RBC H–Partially Deficient, Nonsecretor RBCs of these individuals express weak forms of A and B, which are primarily detected by adsorption and elution studies. If a person is genetically *A* or *B*, the respective enzymes can be detected, but no H enzyme is detectable, even though it has been shown that there is limited production of H antigen on the RBC.[35,36] The notations A$_h$ and B$_h$, respectively, have been used to describe these individuals. AB$_h$ individuals have also been reported. A$_h$, B$_h$, and AB$_h$ have been reported mainly in individuals of European origin.[4] No H, A, or B antigen is present in the saliva, and anti-H is present in the serum. The serum of A$_h$ individuals contains anti-B and no anti-A, although anti-A$_1$ is usually present. In B$_h$ serum, anti-A is always present, and anti-B may be detected.[4] It is postulated that homozygous inheritance of a mutant H (FUT 1) gene codes for the production of low levels of H transferase activity. The small amount of H substance on the RBC is completely used by the A and/or B transferase present. This results in small quantities of A and/or B antigen being present on the RBC with no detectable H antigen. The anti-H present in the serum is weaker in reactivity than the anti-H found in the Bombay phenotype, although it may be active at 37°C.[35] These individuals are designated A$_h$, B$_h$, or AB$_h$.[35,37]

Category 3: RBC H-Deficient, Secretor *(hh Se)*. This category is also known as the para-Bombay phenotype.[38] H-deficient secretors have been found in a variety of ethnic groups and nationalities.[39] RBCs have little or no A, B, and H antigens. RBCs of O$_h$ secretors are not agglutinated by most examples of anti-H but may be agglutinated by strong anti-H reagents. Adsorption and elution of anti-H may reveal the presence of H antigen on the RBC.[4] Cells are not usually agglutinated by anti-A and anti-B; however, some O$_h$^{A} RBCs can mimic the behavior of A$_x$ cells and can agglutinate anti-A,B and potent examples of anti-A. The same reactions with anti-A,B and potent examples of anti-B can be seen with O$_h$^{B} RBCs.[4] A weak H-like antibody, called anti-IH, that is reactive at low temperature is almost always present in the serum. This antibody is nonreactive with cord cells and is not inhibited by secretor saliva. Because of their secretor status, normal levels of H substances are present in the saliva. A and B substances are present in the secretions when *A* and *B* genes are present.[4] Table 6–16 summarizes the characteristics of the various H-deficient categories.

ABO Discrepancies

ABO discrepancies occur when unexpected reactions occur in the forward and reverse grouping. Some of the more common causes of technical errors leading to ABO discrepancies in the forward and reverse groupings are listed in **Box 6–5**. ABO discrepancies can usually be resolved by repeating the test on the same sample by using a saline suspension of RBCs if the initial test was performed using RBCs suspended in serum or plasma. It is important to make sure that any and all technical factors that may have given rise to the ABO discrepancy are reviewed and corrected. It is also essential to acquire information regarding the patient's age, diagnosis, transfusion history, medications, and history of pregnancy. If the discrepancy persists and appears to be due to an error in specimen collection or identification, a new sample should be drawn from the patient and the RBC and serum grouping repeated. When a discrepancy is encountered, results must be recorded, but interpretation of the ABO type must be delayed until the discrepancy is resolved. If blood is from a potential transfusion recipient, it may be necessary to administer group

BOX 6–4
General Characteristics of Bombay O$_{h+}$ (H$_{null}$) Phenotypes

- Absence of H, A, and B, antigens; no agglutination with anti-A, anti-B, or anti-H lectin
- Presence of anti-A, anti-B, anti-A,B and a potent wide thermal range of anti-H in the serum
- A, B, H nonsecretor (no A, B, or H substances present in saliva)
- Absence of α-2-L-fucosyltransferase (H-enzyme) in serum and H antigen on red cells
- Presence of A or B enzymes in serum (depending on ABO genotype)
- A recessive mode of inheritance (identical phenotypes in children but not in parents)
- RBCs of the Bombay phenotype (O$_h$) will not react with the anti-H lectin (*Ulex europaeus*)
- RBCs of the Bombay phenotype (O$_h$) are compatible *only* with the serum from another Bombay individual

TABLE 6–16   Characteristics Reported or Postulated for Categories of H-Deficient Phenotypes (Bombays)

Classification	Proposed Genes Inherited	Glycosyltransferase¶	Red Cell Antigens: A,B, and H Detected	A, B, and H Soluble Substances in Secretions	Antibodies in Serum
1. Red cell H-deficient, non-secretor Bombay phenotype O_h, $O_h{}^B$, $O_h{}^A$, $O_h{}^{AB}$	*hh sese*	None or A and/or B† in serum or RBC stroma	None detectable	None detectable	Anti-A, anti-B, anti-H
2. Red cell H-partially deficient, non-secretor O_h, A_h, B_h, AB_h	A and/or B† *hh* sese*	A and/or B† in serum and RBC stroma	Weak A/B† Residual H when A or B immunodominant sugar is removed with appropriate enzymes	None detectable	Anti-H, Anti-A/anti-B†
3. Red cell H-deficient, secretor $O_h{}^O$, $O_h{}^A$, $O_h{}^B$, $O_h{}^{AB}$	Se	A and/or B† in serum/RBCs, H in serum (weak)	Weak A/B† and H	H substance (normal amounts) A/B† (all normal amounts)	Weak IH Anti-A/anti-B†

* = weak variant present at the *Hh* locus
† = dependent on ABO genotype
¶ = refer to Figure 6–7

O, Rh-compatible RBCs before the discrepancy is resolved. ABO discrepancies may be arbitrarily divided into four major categories.

Group I Discrepancies

Group I discrepancies are associated with unexpected reactions in the reverse grouping due to weakly reacting or missing antibodies. These discrepancies are more common than those in the other groups listed. When a reaction in the serum grouping is weak or missing, a group I discrepancy should be suspected because, normally, RBC and serum grouping reactions are very strong (4+). The reason for the missing or weak isoagglutinins is that the patient has depressed antibody production or cannot produce the ABO antibodies. Some of the more common populations with discrepancies in this group are:

BOX 6–5
Common Sources of Technical Errors Resulting in ABO Discrepancies

- Inadequate identification of blood specimens, test tubes, or slides
- Cell suspension either too heavy or too light
- Clerical errors
- A mix-up in samples
- Missed observation of hemolysis
- Failure to add reagents
- Failure to follow manufacturer's instructions
- Uncalibrated centrifuge
- Contaminated reagents
- Warming during centrifugation

- Newborns
  - The production of ABO antibodies is not detectable until 3 to 6 months of age.
- Elderly patients
  - Production of ABO antibodies is depressed.
- Patients with leukemias (e.g., chronic lymphocytic leukemia) demonstrating hypogammaglobulinemia or lymphomas (e.g., malignant lymphoma) demonstrating hypogammaglobulinemia
- Patients using immunosuppressive drugs that yield hypogammaglobulinemia
- Patients with congenital agammaglobulinemia or immunodeficiency diseases
- Patients with bone marrow transplantations (patients develop hypogammaglobulinemia from therapy and start producing a different RBC population from that of the transplanted bone marrow)
- Patients whose existing ABO antibodies may have been diluted by plasma transfusion or exchange
- ABO subgroups

Resolution of Common Group I Discrepancies

The best way to resolve this discrepancy is to enhance the weak or missing reaction in the serum by incubating the patient serum with reagent A_1 and B cells at room temperature for approximately 15 to 30 minutes. If there is still no reaction after centrifugation, the serum-cell mixtures can be incubated at 4°C for 15 to 30 minutes. An auto control and O cell control must always be tested concurrently with the reverse typing when trying to solve the discrepancy, because the lower temperature of testing will most likely enhance the reactivity of other commonly occurring cold agglutinins, such as anti-I, that react with all adult RBCs. **Table 6–17**

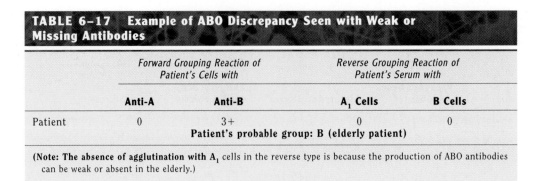

TABLE 6–17   Example of ABO Discrepancy Seen with Weak or Missing Antibodies

| | Forward Grouping Reaction of Patient's Cells with | | Reverse Grouping Reaction of Patient's Serum with | |
	Anti-A	Anti-B	A_1 Cells	B Cells
Patient	0	3+	0	0
	Patient's probable group: B (elderly patient)			

(Note: The absence of agglutination with A_1 cells in the reverse type is because the production of ABO antibodies can be weak or absent in the elderly.)

shows a type of discrepancy that may be seen with weak or missing antibodies.

Advanced Concepts

Rare Group I Discrepancies

Chimerism, as illustrated in Table 6–18, is a rare cause of a weak or missing ABO isoagglutinin. *Chimerism* is defined as the presence of two cell populations in a single individual. Detecting a separate cell population may be easy or difficult, depending on what percentage of cells of the minor population is present. Reactions from chimerism are typically mixed-field. True chimerism is rarely found and occurs in twins, in whom two cell populations will exist through the life of the individual. In utero exchange of blood occurs because of vascular anastomosis. As a result, two cell populations emerge, both of which are recognized as self, and the individuals do not make anti-A or anti-B. Therefore, no detectable isoagglutinins are present in the reverse grouping. If the patient or donor has no history of a twin, then the chimera may be due to dispermy (two sperm fertilizing one egg) and indicates mosaicism. More commonly, artificial chimeras occur, which yield mixed cell populations as a result of:

1. Blood transfusions (e.g., group O cells given to an A or B patient)
2. Transplanted bone marrows or peripheral blood stem cells
3. Exchange transfusions
4. Fetal-maternal bleeding

Group II Discrepancies

Group II discrepancies are associated with unexpected reactions in the forward grouping due to weakly reacting or missing antigens. This group of discrepancies is probably the least frequently encountered. Some of the causes of discrepancies in this group include:

- Subgroups of A (or B) may be present (see the section on ABO subgroups)
- Leukemias may yield weakened A or B antigens (Table 6–19)
- Hodgkin's disease has been reported in some cases to mimic the depression of antigens found in leukemia
- "Acquired B" phenomenon is most often associated with diseases of the digestive tract (e.g., cancer of the colon) (Table 6–20)

Resolution of Group II Discrepancies

The reaction of weakly reactive antigens with their respective antisera can be enhanced by incubating the test mixture at room temperature for up to 30 minutes to increase the association of antibody with antigen. If negative, incubate the text mixture at 4°C for 15 to 30 minutes. Include group O and autologous cells as controls. RBCs can also be pretreated with enzymes and retested with reagent antisera.

The acquired B antigen arises when bacterial enzymes modify the immunodominant blood group A sugar (N-acetyl-D-galactosamine) into D-galactosamine, which is sufficiently similar to the immunodominant blood group B sugar (D-galactose) to cross-react with anti-B antisera. This pseudo-B antigen is formed at the expense of the A_1 antigen and disappears after recovery.[40] The reaction of the appropriate antiserum with these acquired antigens demonstrates a weak reaction, often yielding a mixed-field appearance. Blood group reagents of a monoclonal anti-B clone (ES4) strongly agglutinate cells with the acquired B antigen. The pH of reagents containing ES4 has been lowered and, as a result, only those cells with the strongest examples of acquired B antigen react with the antisera. It should be noted that when the RBCs of

TABLE 6–18   ABO Grouping in Chimera Twins

	Anti-A	Anti-B	Anti-A,B	A_1 Cells	B Cells	RBC %
Twin 1	0	2+mf	2+mf	4+	0	70% B; 30% 0
Twin 2	0	+wk	+wk	4+	0	30% B; 70% 0

0 = negative, mf = mixed field; wk = weak

TABLE 6–19   Serologic Reactions Typical of Leukemia

Patient Phenotype	Forward Grouping Reaction of Patient Cells with		Reverse Grouping Reaction of Patient Serum with	
	Anti-A	Anti-B	A$_1$ Cells	B Cells
A	+mf	0	0	3+
B	0	±/+	4+	0
	Patient diagnosis: Leukemia			

(Note: Weak reactivity with anti-A and anti-B is because the disease, leukemia, has resulted in the weakened expression of the corresponding antigen.)

TABLE 6–21   Example of ABO Discrepancy Caused by Low-Incidence Antibodies in the Reagent Antisera

	Forward Grouping Reaction of Patient Cells with		Reverse Grouping Reaction of Patient Serum with	
	Anti-A	Anti-B	A$_1$ Cells	B Cells
Patient	4+	1+	0	4+
	Patient's probable group: A			

(Note: Reaction with anti-B in the forward type is due to agglutination between a low-incidence antibody in reagent anti-B and the corresponding antigen on the patient's cells.)

blood donors were reacted with this reagent, 1 in 500 were found to have pH-dependent autoagglutinins.[4]

Testing the patient's serum or plasma against autologous RBCs gives a negative reaction because the anti-B in the serum does not agglutinate autologous RBCs with the acquired-B antigen. The acquired-B antigen is also not agglutinated when reacted with anti-B that has a pH greater than 8.5 or less than 6.0.[41] Secretor studies can be performed when trying to characterize the acquired-B phenomenon. If the patient is in fact a secretor, only the A substance is secreted in the acquired-B phenomenon.

Treating RBCs with acetic anhydride reacetylates the surface molecules, then markedly decreases the reactivity of the cells when tested against anti-B. The reactivity of normal B cells is not affected by treatment with acetic anhydride.[25]

Advanced Concepts

Rare Group II Discrepancies

Weakly reactive or missing reactions in RBC grouping may be due to excess amounts of blood group–specific soluble (BGSS) substances present in the plasma in association with certain diseases, such as carcinoma of the stomach and pancreas. Excess amounts of BGSS substances will neutralize the reagent anti-A or anti-B, leaving no unbound antibody to react with the patient cells. This yields a false-negative or weak reaction in the forward grouping. Washing the patient

cells free of the BGSS substances with saline should alleviate the problem, resulting in correlating forward and reverse groupings.

Antibodies to low-incidence antigens in reagent anti-A or anti-B may also result in weakly reactive or missing reactions in RBC grouping (Table 6–21). It is impossible for manufacturers to screen reagent antisera against all known RBC antigens. It has been reported (although rarely) that this additional antibody in the reagent antisera has reacted with the corresponding low-incidence antigen present on the patient's RBCs. This gives an unexpected reaction of the patient's cells with anti-A or anti-B, or both, mimicking the presence of a weak antigen. The best way to resolve this discrepancy is by repeating the forward type, using antisera with a different lot number. If the cause of the discrepancy is a low-incidence antibody in the reagent antisera reacting with a low-incidence antigen on the patient's cells, the chances are that the antibody will not be present in a different lot number of reagent.

In addition, chimerism could cause unexpected reactions in the forward grouping due to the presence of two cell populations and depending on the percentage of the minor populations of cells (see previous discussion).

Group III Discrepancies

These discrepancies are between forward and reverse groupings caused by protein or plasma abnormalities and result in rouleaux formation (Table 6–22), or pseudoagglutination, attributable to:

TABLE 6–20   Example of ABO Discrepancy Caused by an Acquired B Antigen

	Forward Grouping Reaction of Patient Cells with		Reverse Grouping Reaction of Patient Serum with	
	Anti-A	Anti-B	A$_1$Cells	B Cells
Patient	4+	2+	0	4+
	Patient's probable group: A			

(Note: Patient RBCs have acquired a B-like antigen that reacts with reagent anti-B and is associated with cancer of the colon or other diseases of the digestive tract.)

TABLE 6–22   Example of ABO Discrepancy Caused by Rouleaux Formation

	Forward Grouping Reaction of Patient Cells with		Reverse Grouping Reaction of Patient Serum with	
	Anti-A	Anti-B	A$_1$ Cells	B Cells
Patient	4+	2+	2+	4+
	Patient's probable group: A			

(Note: Agglutination with anti-B in forward type and A$_1$ cells in reverse type is due to rouleaux formation as a result of increased serum protein or plasma abnormalities.)

- Elevated levels of globulin from certain disease states, such as multiple myeloma, Waldenström's macroglobulinemia, other plasma cell dyscrasias, and certain moderately advanced cases of Hodgkin's lymphomas
- Elevated levels of fibrinogen
- Plasma expanders, such as dextran and polyvinylpyrrolidone
- Wharton's jelly in cord blood samples

Resolution of Group III Discrepancies

Rouleaux, or a stacking of erythrocytes that adhere in a coin-like fashion giving the appearance of agglutination, can be observed on microscopic examination **(Color Plate 2)**. Cell grouping can usually be accomplished by washing the patient's RBCs several times with saline. Performing a saline dilution or saline replacement technique will free the cells in the case of rouleaux formation in the reverse type. In true agglutination, RBC clumping will still remain after the addition of saline.

Washing cord cells six to eight times with saline should alleviate spontaneous rouleaux due to Wharton's jelly, a viscous mucopolysaccharide material present on cord blood cells, and should result in an accurate RBC grouping. However, because testing is usually not performed on cord serum because the antibodies detected are usually of maternal origin, reverse grouping may still not correlate with the RBC forward grouping.

Group IV Discrepancies

These discrepancies between forward and reverse groupings are due to miscellaneous problems and have the following causes:

- Cold reactive autoantibodies in which RBCs are so heavily coated with antibody that they spontaneously agglutinate, independent of the specificity of the reagent antibody **(Table 6–23)**
- Patient has circulating RBCs of more than one ABO group due to RBC transfusion or marrow transplant
- Unexpected ABO isoagglutinins
- Unexpected non-ABO alloantibodies **(Table 6–24)**

Resolution of Group IV Discrepancies

Potent cold autoantibodies can cause spontaneous agglutination of the patient's cells. These cells often yield a positive

TABLE 6–23   Example of ABO Discrepancy Caused by Cold Autoantibodies

	Forward Grouping Reaction of Patient Cells with		Reverse Grouping Reaction of Patient Serum with	
	Anti-A	**Anti-B**	**A₁ Cells**	**B Cells**
Patient	2+	4+	4+	3+
		Patient's probable group: A		

(Note: Reaction with anti-A in forward type is due to spontaneous agglutination of antibody coated cells; reaction with B cells in reverse type is due to cold autoantibody [e.g., anti -I] reacting with I antigen on B cells.)

TABLE 6–24   Example of ABO Discrepancy Caused by an Unexpected Non-ABO Alloantibody

	Forward Grouping Reaction of Patient Cells with		Reverse Grouping Reaction of Patient Serum with	
	Anti-A	**Anti-B**	**A₁ Cells**	**B Cells**
Patient	4+	4+	1+	1+
		Patient's probable group: AB		

(Note: Reactions with patient serum are due to non-ABO alloantibody agglutinating an antigen other than A₁ and B on reagent red cells.)

direct Coombs' or antiglobulin test (see Chapter 21). If the antibody in the serum reacts with all adult cells, for example anti-I (see I Blood Group System in Chapter 9), the reagent A₁ and B cells used in the reverse grouping also agglutinate.

To resolve this discrepancy, the patient's RBCs could be incubated at 37°C for a short period, then washed with saline at 37°C three times and retyped. If this is not successful in resolving the forward type, the patient's RBCs can be treated with 0.01 M dithiothreitol (DTT) to disperse IgM-related agglutination. As for the serum, the reagent RBCs and serum can be warmed to 37°C, then mixed, tested, and read at 37°C. The test can be converted to the antihuman globulin phase if necessary. Weakly reactive anti-A and/or anti-B may not react at 37°C, which is outside their optimum thermal range. If the reverse typing is negative (and a positive result was expected), an autoabsorption could be performed to remove the autoantibody from the serum, and the absorbed serum can then be used to repeat the serum typing at room temperature.

Unexpected ABO isoagglutinins in the patient's serum react at room temperature with the corresponding antigen present on the reagent cells. Examples of this type of ABO discrepancy include A₂ and A₂B individuals who can produce naturally occurring anti-A₁, or A₁ and A₁B, individuals who may produce naturally occurring anti-H. (Refer to the previous sections on ABO subgroups.) Serum grouping can be repeated using at least three examples of A₁, A₂, B cells, O cells, and an autologous control (patient's serum mixed with patient's RBCs).[3] The specificity of the antibody can be determined by examining the pattern of reactivity (e.g., if the antibody agglutinates only A₁ cells, it can most likely be identified as anti-A₁). The patient's RBCs can be tested with *Dolichos biflorus* to confirm the presence of the ABO subgroup. *Dolichos biflorus* will agglutinate cells of the A₁, but not the A₂ phenotype.

Unexpected alloantibodies in the patient's serum other than ABO isoagglutinins (e.g., anti-M) may cause a discrepancy in the reverse grouping. Reverse grouping cells possess other antigens in addition to A₁ and B, and it is possible that other unexpected antibodies present in the patient's serum will react with these cells. In this situation, a panel could be performed with the patient's serum. Once the unexpected alloantibody(ies) is (are) identified, A₁ and B cells negative for the corresponding antigen can be used in the reverse typing or, once again, the reverse typing can be repeated at 37°C if the ABO isoagglutinins react at this temperature and there is no interference from the unexpected alloantibody.

Advanced Concepts

Rare Group IV Discrepancies

Antibodies other than anti-A and anti-B may react to form antigen-antibody complexes that may then adsorb onto patient's RBCs (e.g., some individuals have antibodies against acriflavine, the yellow dye used in some commercial anti-B reagents; the acriflavin-antiacriflavin complex attaches to the patient's RBCs, causing agglutination in the forward type). Some individuals have antibodies against acriflavin in their serum. The patient's antibody combines with the dye and attaches to the patient's RBCs, resulting in agglutination in the forward grouping. Washing the patient's cells three times with saline and then retyping them should resolve this discrepancy.

Cis-AB

Cis-AB refers to the inheritance of both AB genes from one parent carried on one chromosome and an O gene inherited from the other parent. This results in the offspring inheriting three ABO genes instead of two **(Fig. 6–14)**. The designation cis-AB is used to distinguish this mode of inheritance from the more usual AB phenotype in which the alleles are located on different chromosomes. RBCs with the cis AB phenotype (a rare occurrence) express a weakly reactive A antigen (analogous to A_2 cells) and a weak B antigen.[4] The B antigen usually yields a weaker reaction with the anti-B from random donors, with mixed-field agglutination typical of subgroup B_3 reported in several cases. Weak anti-B (present in the serum of most cis-AB individuals) leads to an ABO discrepancy in the reverse grouping. The serum of most cis-AB individuals contains a weak anti-B, which reacts with all ordinary B RBCs, yet not with cis-AB RBCs. A and B transferase levels are lower than those found in ordinary group AB sera.[4] Some investigators have suggested that the B antigen in the cis-AB represents only a piece of the normal B antigen. Cis-AB blood can be classified into four categories: A_2B_3, A_1B_3, A_2B, and A_2B_x. Various hypotheses have been offered to explain the cis-AB phenotype. Many favor a crossing over of a portion of a gene, resulting in unequal expression by the recombinant. However, the banding pattern of the distal end of the long arm of chromosome 9 representing the ABO locus is normal.

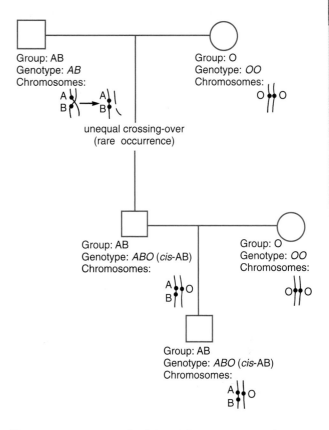

■ FIGURE 6–14   Example of cis-AB inheritance to unequal crossing-over. □ = male; ○ = female. (From Harmening-Pittiglio,[27] p 7 with permission.)

There have been other examples of cis-ABs that do not fit the above scenario. In these examples, there was a mutation at the ABO locus, and an enzyme was produced that was capable of transferring both A-specific and B-specific sugars to the precursor molecule.[42]

Some examples of serologic reactions involving ABO discrepancies have been provided with answers for review and self-evaluation **(Table 6–25)**. Finally, you have been briefly introduced to ABO, the first and "simplest" blood group system known.

TABLE 6–25   ABO Discrepancies Between Forward and Reverse Grouping

	Forward Grouping		Reverse Grouping					
Patient	Anti-A	Anti-B	A_1 Cells	B Cells	O Cells	Auto-Control	Possible Cause	Resolution Steps
1	0	0	0	0	0	0	Group O newborn or elderly patient; patient may have hypogammaglobulinemia or agammaglobulinemia, or may be taking immunosuppressive drugs	Check age and diagnosis of patient and immunoglobulin levels if possible; incubate at RT for 30 min or at 4°C for 15 min; include group O and autologous cells at 4°C
2	4+	0	1+	4+	0	0	Subgroup of A: probable A_2 with anti-A_1	React patient cells with anti-A_1 lectin, test serum against additional A_1, A_2, and O cells

(continued)

TABLE 6–25.   ABO Discrepancies Between Forward and Reverse Grouping (continued)

	Forward Grouping		Reverse Grouping					
Patient	Anti-A	Anti-B	A_1 Cells	B Cells	O Cells	Auto-Control	Possible Cause	Resolution Steps
3	4+	4+	2+	2+	2+	2+	(1) Rouleaux (multiple myeloma patient; any patient with reversed albumin-to-globulin ratio or patients given plasma expanders) (2) Cold autoantibody (probable group AB with an auto anti-I) (3) Cold autoantibody with underlying cold or RT reacting alloantibody (probable group AB with an auto anti-I and a high-frequency cold antibody, (e.g., anti-P_1, anti-M, anti-Le^b)	(1) Wash RBCs; use saline dilution or saline replacement technique (2) Perform cold panel and autoabsorb or rabbit erythrocyte stroma (REST) absorb (see Chapter 12) or reverse type at 37°C (3) Perform cold panel autoabsorb or REST, and run panel on absorbed serum; select reverse cells lacking antigen for identified alloantibody; repeat reverse group on absorbed serum to determine true ABO group or at 37°C
4	4+	4+	1+	0	0	0	Subgroup of AB; probable A_2B with anti-A_1	Use anti-A_1 lectin, test serum against additional A_1, A_2, and O cells
5	4+	0	0	4+	3+	0	A_1 with potent anti-H	Confirm A_1 group with anti-A_1 lectin; test additional A_2, O, and A_1 cells and an O_h if available
6	0	0	4+	4+	4+	0	O_h Bombay	Test with anti-H lectin; test O_h cells if available; send to reference laboratory for confirmation
7	0	0	2+	4+	0	0	Subgroup of A; probable A_x with anti-A_1	Perform saliva studies or absorption/elution
8	4+	2+	0	4+	0	0	Group A with an acquired B antigen	Check history of patient for lower gastrointestinal problem or septicemia; acidify anti-B typing reagent to pH 6.0 by adding 1 or 2 drops of $1N$ HCl to 1 mL of anti-B anti-sera, and measure with a pH meter (this acidified anti-B antisera would agglutinate only true B antigens *not* acquired B antigens), test serum against autologous cells
9	4+	4+	2+	0	2+	0	Group AB with alloantibody	Perform antibody screen and panel, identify room temperature antibody, repeat serum type with antigen negative *reagent* cells or perform serum type at 37°C
10	0	4+	4+	1+	1+	1+	Group B with cold autoantibody	Enzyme-treat RBCs and perform autoabsorption at 4°C or perform prewarmed testing

*AutoAbsorption should not be performed on patient's cells that have been transfused within the last 3 months.
RT = room temperature

CASE STUDY

A 45-year old woman, para 3 gravida 3, with a history of five cases of dilation and curettage, is scheduled for a partial hysterectomy at a community hospital. Preoperation laboratory tests include a type and screen. There is no history of transfusions.

ABO and Rh Typing

(handwritten: Anti A, Anti B, D pos)

Anti-A	Anti-B	Anti-A,B	A1C	BC	Anti-D
3+	0	3+	2+	4+	3+

Antibody Screen

	37°C	AHG	CC
SCI	0	0	√
SCII	0	0	√
SCIII	0	0	√

The results indicate an ABO discrepancy in the reverse grouping with a negative antibody screen. The blood bank technologist proceeded to type the patient RBCs with anti-A_1 lectin, *Dolichos biflorus*. This was decided because, based on the negative antibody screen and patient history, an alloantibody was most likely not causing the ABO discrepancy.

Anti-A_1 lectin

	Anti-A_1 lectin
Patient RBCs	0

The patient's serum was then tested with A_2 cells and O cells.

	A_2 Cells	O Cells
Patient serum	0	0

The reaction with anti-A_1 lectin indicates the patient's cells are not type A_1, and the additional serum studies show that the antibody is not directed toward a possible alloantibody reacting at room temperature and that the antibody is not anti-A, in that only anti-A would react with A_2 cells. If a cold autoantibody or alloantibody was causing the discrepancy, serum would likely react with the O cells.

Results indicate the patient is a likely type A_2 who has formed an anti-A_1. During surgery, the OR ordered two units of packed RBCs.

Two type O-positive packed RBCs were crossmatched with the patient serum and found to be compatible. Only one unit was transfused without episode. The patient was discharged 4 days later.

In this case, there was an ABO discrepancy caused by anti-A_1 in the reverse grouping. Although, anti-A_1 is considered to be nonreactive at 37°C, it was decided to transfuse type O positive cells to this patient.

➤ ABO frequencies: group O, 45%; group A, 40%; group B, 11%; group AB, 4%.

➤ ABO blood group system has naturally occurring antibodies that are primarily IgM.

➤ *ABO* genes, like those of most other blood groups, are inherited in a codominant manner.

➤ ABH-soluble antigens are secreted by tissue cells and are found in all body secretions. The antigens secreted depend on the person's ABO group.

➤ ABO reverse grouping is omitted from cord blood testing on newborns because their antibody titer levels are generally too low for detection.

➤ ABO RBC antigens can be glycolipids, glycoproteins, or glycosphingolipids; ABO-secreted substances are glycoproteins.

➤ L-fucose is the immunodominant sugar responsible for H specificity.

➤ *N*-acetylgalactosamine is the immunodominant sugar responsible for A specificity.

➤ D-galactose is the immunodominant sugar responsible for B specificity.

➤ The *hh* genotype is known as the Bombay phenotype, or O_h, and lacks normal expression of the ABH antigens.

➤ Group O persons contain the greatest amount of H substance; group A_1B persons contain the least amount of H substance.

➤ Approximately 80% of A persons inherit the A gene phenotype as A_1; the remaining 20% phenotype as A_2 or weaker subgroups.

➤ Approximately 1% to 8% of A_2 persons produce anti-A_1 in their serum.

➤ Glycoproteins in secretions are formed on type 1 precursor chains.

➤ The ABH antigens on RBCs are formed on type 2 precursor chains.

➤ Forward and reverse grouping normally yield strong (4+) reactions.

➤ Group A persons contain anti-B in their serum; group B persons contain anti-A in their serum; group AB persons contains neither anti-A nor anti-B in their serum; group O persons contain both anti-A and anti-B in their serum.

➤ Approximately 78% of the random population inherit the *Se* gene and are termed *secretors*; the remaining 22% inherit the *se* gene and are termed *nonsecretors*.

➤ The *Se* gene codes for the production of L-fucosyltransferase.

REVIEW QUESTIONS

1. An ABO type on a patient gives the following reactions:

Patient Cells With		Patient Serum With	
Anti-A	Anti-B	A_1 cells	B cells
4+	4+	Neg	Neg

What is the patient's blood type?
a. O
b. A
c. B
d. AB

2. The major immunoglobulin class(es) of anti-B in a group A individual is (are):
a. IgM
b. IgG
c. IgM and IgG
d. IgM and IgA

3. What are the possible ABO phenotypes of the offspring from the mating of a group A to a group B individual?
a. O, A, B
b. A, B
c. A, B, AB
d. O, A, B, AB

4. The immunodominant sugar responsible for blood group A specificity is:
a. L-fucose
b. N-acetyl-D-galactosamine
c. D-galactose
d. Uridine diphosphate-N-acetyl-D-galactose

5. What ABH substance(s) would be found in the saliva of a group B secretor?
a. H
b. H and A
c. H and B
d. H, A, and B

6. An ABO type on a patient gives the following reactions:

Patient Cells With			Patient Serum With	
Anti-A	Anti-B	Anti-A_1	A_1 cells	B cells
4+	4+	Neg	2+	Neg

The reactions above may be seen in a patient who is:
a. A_1 with acquired B
b. A_2B with anti-A_1
c. AB with increased concentrations of protein in the serum
d. AB with an autoantibody

7. Which of the following ABO blood groups contains the least amount of H substance?
a. A_1B
b. A_2
c. B
d. O

8. You are working on a specimen in the laboratory that you believe to be a Bombay phenotype. Which of the following reactions would you expect to see?
a. Patient's cells + *Ulex europaeus* = no agglutination
b. Patient's cells + *Ulex europaeus* = agglutination
c. Patient's serum + group O donor RBCs = no agglutination
d. Patient's serum + A_1 and B cells = no agglutination

9. An example of a technical error that can result in an ABO discrepancy is:
a. Acquired-B phenomenon
b. Missing isoagglutinins
c. Cell suspension that is too heavy
d. Acriflavin antibodies

10. An ABO type on a patient gives the following reactions:

Patient Cells With		Patient Serum With			
Anti-A	Anti-B	A_1 cells	B cells	O cells	Autocontrol
4+	Neg	2+	4+	2+	Neg

These results are most likely due to:
a. ABO alloantibody
b. Non-ABO alloantibody
c. Rouleaux
d. Cold autoantibody

REFERENCES

1. Zik, D. Walter H. Emily Cooley Lecture 2002: Transfusion Safety in the Hospital. Transfusion 43:1190–1199, 2003.
2. Kruskall, MS, et al: Transfusion to blood group A and O patients of group B RBCs that have been enzymatically converted to group O. Transfusion 40:1290–1298, 2000.
3. Brecher, M: Technical Manual. American Association of Blood Banks, Bethesda, MD, 2002.
4. Watkins, WM: The ABO blood group system: Historical background. Transfus Med 11:243–265, 2001.
5. Garratty, G, Glynn, SA, and McEntire, R: ABO and Rh (D) phenotype frequencies of different racial/ethnic groups in the United States. Transfusion 44:703–706, 2004.
6. Daniels, G: Human Blood Groups, ed 2. Blackwell Science, Malden, MA, 2002.
7. Landsteiner, K, and Witt, DH: Observations on the human blood groups: Irregular reactions. Isoagglutinin in sera of group 4. The fact A_1. J Immunol 2:221, 1967.
8. Dodd, BE, et al: The cross-reacting antibodies of group O sera: Immunological studies and a possible explanation of the observed facts. Immunology 12:39, 1967.
9. Olsson, ML, and Chester, MA: Polymorphism and recombination events at the ABO locus: A major challenge for genomic ABO blood grouping strategies. Transfus Med 11:295–313, 2001.
10. Chester, MA, and Olsson, ML: The ABO blood group gene: A locus of considerable genetic diversity. Transfus Med Rev 15:177–200, 2001.
11. Seltsam, A, et al: Systematic analysis of ABO gene diversity within exons 6 and 7 by PCR screening reveals new ABO alleles. Transfusion 43:428–439, 2003.
12. Yamamoto, F: Cloning and regulation of the ABO genes. Transfus Med 11:281–294, 2001.
13. Hosoi, E, Hirose, M, and Hamano, S: Expression levels of H-type alpha (1,2)-fucosyltransferase gene and histo-blood group ABO gene corresponding to hematopoietic cell differentiation. Transfusion 43:65–71, 2003.
14. Yamamoto, F: Molecular genetics of ABO. Vox Sang 78:91–103, 2000.
15. Lee, AH, and Reid, ME: ABO blood group system: A review of molecular aspects. Immunohematology 16:1–6, 2000.
16. Olsson, ML, and Chester, MA: Polymorphism and recombination events at the ABO locus: A major challenge for genomic ABO blood grouping strategies. Transfus Med 11:295–313, 2001.
17. Ogasawara, K, et al: Recombination and gene conversion-like events may contribute to ABO gene diversity causing various phenotypes. Immunogenetics 53:190–199, 2001.
18. Oriol, R, et al: Molecular genetics of H. Vox Sang 78:105–108, 2000.
19. Svensson, L, Pettersson, A, and Henry, SM: Secretor genotyping for A385T, G428A, C571T, 685delTGG, G849A, and other mutations from a single PCR: Transfusion 40:856–860, 2000.

20. Oriol R, et al: Molecular genetics of H. Vox Sang 78:105–108, 2000.

21. Pang H, et al: Two distinct Alu-mediated deletions of the human ABO-secretor (FUT2) locus in Samoan and Bangladeshi populations. Hum Mutat 16:274, 2000.

22. Fujitani N, et al: Expression of H type 1 antigen of ABO histo–blood group in normal colon and aberrant expressions of H type 2 and H type 3/4 antigens in colon cancer. Glycoconj J 17:331–338, 2000.

23. Seltsam, A, et al: Systematic analysis of the ABO gene diversity within exons 6 and 7 by PCR screening reveals new ABO alleles. Transfusion 43:428–439, 2003.

24. Barjas-Castro, ML, et al: Molecular heterogeneity of the A3 group. Clin Lab Haematol 22:73–78, 2000.

25. Beattie, KM: Perspectives on some usual and unusual ABO phenotypes. In Bell, CA (ed): A Seminar on Antigens on Blood Cells and Body Fluids. American Association of Blood Banks, Washington, DC, 97–149, 1980.

26. Lopez, M, et al: Activity of IgG and IgM ABO antibodies against some weak A (A3, Ax, Aend) and weak B (B3, Bx) red cells. Vox Sang 37:281–285, 1979.

27. Catron JP, et al: Assay of alpha-N-acetylgalactosaminyltransferase in human sera: Further evidence for several types of Am individuals. Vox Sang 28:347–365, 1975.

28. Asamura, H, et al. Molecular genetic analysis of the AM phenotype of the ABO blood group system. Vox Sang 83:263–267, 2002.

29. Marcus, SL, et al: A single point mutation reverses the donor specificity of human blood group B–synthesizing galactosyltransferase. J Biol Chem 278:12403–12405, 2003.

30. Koscielak, J, Pacuszka, T, and Dzierkowa-Borodej, W: Activity of B-gene-specified galactosyltransferase in individuals with Bm phenotypes. Vox Sang 30:58–67, 1976.

31. Lin, PH, et al: A unique 502C>T mutation in exon 7 of ABO gene associated with the Bel phenotype in Taiwan. Transfusion 43:1254–1259, 2003.

32. Boose, GM, Issitt, C, and Issitt, PD: Weak B antigen in a family. Transfusion 18:570–571, 1978.

33. Thomas, CJ, and Surolia, A: Kinetic analysis of the binding of Ulex Europaeus agglutinin 1 (UEA 1) to H-antigenic fucolipid. Arch Biochem Biophys 374:8–12, 2000.

34. Koda, Y, et al: An Alu-mediated large deletion of the FUT2 gene in individuals with the ABO-Bombay phenotype. Hum Gen 106:80–85, 2000.

35. Mak, KH, et al: Serologic characteristics of H-deficient phenotypes among Chinese in Hong Kong. Transfusion 36:994–999, 1986.

36. Watkins, WM: Changes in the specificity of blood-group induced by enzymes from *Trichomonas foetus*. Immunology 5:245–266, 1962.

37. Salmon, C, et al: H-deficient phenotypes: A proposed practical classification of Bombay Ah, H2, Hm. Blood Transfus Immunohaematol 23:233–248, 1980.

38. Yip, SP, et al: Molecular genetic analysis of para-Bombay phenotypes in Chinese: A novel non-functional FUT1 allele is identified. Vox Sang 83:258–262, 2002.

39. Sun, CF, et al: Novel mutations, including a novel G659A missense mutation, of the FUT1 gene are responsible for the para-Bombay phenotype. Ann Clin Lab Sci 30:387–390, 2000.

40. Judd, WJ, and Annesley, TM: The acquired-B phenomenon. Transfus Med Rev 10:111–117, 1996.

41. Mallory, D: Immunohematology Methods and Procedures. American Red Cross, Rockville, MD, 1993.

42. Harmening-Pittiglio, D: Genetics and biochemistry of A, B, H and Lewis antigens. In Wallace, ME, and Gibbs, FL (eds): Blood Group System: ABH and Lewis. American Association of Blood Banks, Arlington, VA, 1986.

BIBLIOGRAPHY

Abe, K, Levery, SB, and Hakomori, S: The antibody specific to type 1 chain blood group A determinant. J Immunol 132(4):1951, 1984.

Adatia, A, et al: Comparison of the absorption of allo-anti-B by red cells and by a synthetic immunoabsorbent using the autoanalyzer. Rev Fr Transfus Immunohematol 26(6):585, 1983.

Anderson, DE, and Haas, C: Blood type A and familial breast cancer. Cancer 54(9):1845, 1984.

Atichartakarn, V, et al: Autoimmune hemolytic anemia due to anti-B autoantibody. Vox Sang 49(4):301, 1985.

Baechtel, FS: Secreted blood group substances: Distributions in semen and stabilities in dried semen stains. J Forensic Sci 30(4):1119, 1985.

Bakacs, T, Ringwald, G, and Jokuti, I: Direct ADCC lysis of O, Rh-positive (R 1 R2) erythrocytes by lymphocytes of individuals sensitized against antigen D. Immunol Lett 4(1):53, 1982.

Beattie, KM, et al: Blood group chimerism as a clue to generalized tissue mosaicism. Transfusion 4:77, 1964.

Beattie, KM, et al: Two chimeras detected during routine grouping test by autoanalyzer. Transfusion 17:681, 1977.

Bensinger, WI, Buckner, CD, and Clift, RA: Whole blood immunoadsorption of anti-A or anti-B antibodies. Vox Sang 48(6):357, 1985.

Bensinger, WI, et al: Immune adsorption of anti-A and anti-B antibodies. Prog Clin Biol Res 88:295, 1982.

Bernoco, M, et al: Detection of combined ABH and Lewis glycosphingolipids in sera of H-deficient donors. Vox Sang 49(1):58:1985.

Bolton, S, and Thorpe, JW: Enzyme-linked immunoabsorbent assay for A and B water-soluble blood group substances. J Forensic Sci 31(1):27, 1986.

Boose, GM, Issitt, C, and Issitt, P: Weak B antigen in a family. Transfusion 18:570, 1978.

Bracey, AW, and Van-Buren, C: Immune anti-A1 in A2 recipients of kidneys from group O donors. Transfusion 26(3):282, 1986.

Brand, A, et al: ABH antibodies causing platelet transfusion refractoriness. Transfusion 26(5):463, 1986.

Breimer, ME, and Karlsson, KA: Chemical and immunological identification of glycolipid-based blood group ABH and Lewis antigens in human and kidney. Biochem Biophys Acta 755(2):170, 1983.

Brouwers, HA, et al: Sensitive methods for determining subclasses of IgG anti-A and anti-B in sera of blood-group O women with a blood-group A or B child. Br J Haematol 66(2):267, 1987.

Cartron, J, et al: Assay of alpha-N-acetylgalactosaminyl-transferases in human sera: Further evidence for several types of Am individuals. Vox Sang 28:347, 1975.

Cartron, J, et al: Study of the alpha-N-acetylgalactsaminyl-transferase in sera and red cell membranes of human A subgroups. J Immunogenet 5:107, 1978.

Cartron, J, et al: "Weak A" phenotypes: Relationship between red cell agglutinability and antigen site density. Immunology 27:723, 1974.

Cheng, MS: Two similar cases of weak agglutination with anti-B reagent. Lab Med 12:506, 1981.

Clausen, H, Holmes, E, and Hakomori, S: Novel blood group H glycolipid antigens exclusively expressed in blood group A and AB erythrocytes (type 3 chain H). II. Differential conversion of different H substrates by A1 and A2 enzymes and type 3 chain H expression in relation to secretor status. J Biol Chem 261(3):1388, 1986.

Clausen, H, et al: Blood group A glycolipid (Ax) with globo-series structure which is specific for blood group A1 erythrocytes: One of chemical bases for A1 and A2 distinction. Biochem Biophys Res Commun 124(2):523, 1984.

Clausen, H, et al: Further characterization of type 2 and type 3 chain blood group A glycosphingolipids from human erythrocyte membranes. Biochemistry 25(22):7075, 1986.

Cohen, F, and Zuelzer, WW: Interrelationship of the various subgroups of the blood group A: Study with immunofluorescence. Transfusion 5:223, 1965.

Dodd, BE, and Lincoln, PJ: Serological studies of the H activity of Oh red cells with various anti-H reagents. Vox Sang 35:168, 1978.

Dodd, BE, and Wood, NJ: Elution of group-specific substance A from RBC of various subgroups of A and its effect on the agglutination of AX RBC. Vox Sang 43(5):248, 1982.

Dunstan, RA: Status of major red cell blood group antigens on neutrophils, lymphocytes and monocytes. Br J Haematol 62(2):301, 1986.

Economidou, J, Hughes-Jones, N, and Gardner, B: Quantitative measurements concerning A and B antigen sites. Vox Sang 12:321, 1967.

Feng, CS, et al: Variant of type B blood in an El Salvador family: Expression of a variant B gene enhanced by the presence of an A2 gene. Transfusion 24(3):264, 1984.

Finne, J: Identification of the blood group ABH-active glycoprotein components of human erythrocyte membrane. Eur J Biochem 104:181, 1980.

Fukuda, MN, and Hakomori, S: Structures of branched blood group A–active glycosphingolipids in human erythrocytes and polymorphism of A- and H-glycolipids in A1 and A2 subgroups. J Biol Chem 257(1):446, 1982.

Furukawa, K, Mattes, MJ, and Lloyd, KO: A1 and A2 erythrocytes can be distinguished by reagents that do not detect structural differences between the two cell types. J Immunol 135(6):4090, 1985.

Gardas, A, and Koscielak, J: A, B and H blood group specificities in glycoprotein and glycolipid fractions of human erythrocyte membrane: Absence of blood group active glyco-proteins in the membrane of non-secretors. Vox Sang 20:137, 1971.

Gart, JJ, and Nam, JM: A score test for the possible presence of recessive alleles in generalized ABO-like genetic systems. Biometrics 40(4):887, 1984.

Gemke, RJ, et al: ABO and Rhesus phenotyping of fetal erythrocytes in the first trimester of pregnancy. Br J Haematol 64(4):689, 1986.

Greenwell, P, et al: Fucosyltransferase activities in human lymphocytes and granulocytes: Blood group H gene-specified alpha-2-L-fucosyltransferase is a discriminatory marker of peripheral blood lymphocytes. FEBS Lett 164(2):314, 1983.

Hakomori, S, Stellner, K, and Watanabe, K: Four antigen variants of blood group A glycolipid: Examples of highly complex, branched chain glycolipid of animal cell membrane. Biochem Biophys Res Commun 49:1061, 1972.

Handa, V, et al: The Oh (Bombay group) phenotype. J Indian Med Assoc 82(12):446, 1984.

Hanfland, P: Characterization of B and H blood group active glycosphingolipids from human B erythrocyte membranes. Chem Phys Lipids 15:105, 1975.

Herron, R, et al: A specific antibody for cells with acquired B antigen. Transfusion 22(6):525, 1982.

Hirschfeld, J: Conceptual framework shifts in immunogenetics. I. A new look at cis-AB antigens in the ABO system. Vox Sang 33:286, 1977.

Hummell, K, et al: Inheritance of cis-AB in three generations (family Lam). Vox Sang 33:290, 1977.

Kannagi, R, Levery, SB, and Hakomori, S: Blood group H antigen with globo-series structure: Isolation and characterization from human blood group O erythrocytes. FEBS Lett 175(2):397, 1984.

Knowles, RW, et al: Monoclonal anti-type 2 H: An antibody detecting a precursor of the A and B blood group antigens. J Immunogenet 9(2):69, 1982.

Kogure, T, and Furukawa, K: Enzymatic conversion of human group O red cells into group B-active cells by alpha-N-galactosyltransferase of sera and salivas from group B and its variant types. J Immunogenet 3:147, 1976.

Koscielak, J, et al: Structures of fucose containing glycolipids with H and B blood group activity and of sialic acid and glucosamine containing glycolipid of human erythrocyte membrane. Eur J Biochem 37:214, 1973.

Koscielak, J, et al: Weak A phenotypes possibly caused by mutation. Vox Sang 50(3):187, 1986.

Le-Pendu, J, et al: Alpha-2-L-fucosyl-transferase activity in sera of individuals with H-deficient red cells and normal H antigen in secretions. Vox Sang 44(6):360, 1983.

Levine, P, et al: A_h, an incomplete suppression of A resembling O_h. Vox Sang 6:561, 1961.

Lin-Chu, M, et al: The para-Bombay phenotype in Chinese persons. Transfusion 27(5):388, 1987.

Lopez, M, et al: Activity of IgG and IgM ABO antibodies against some weak A (A_3, A_x, A_{end}) and weak B (B_3, B_x) red cells. Vox Sang 37:281, 1979.

Madsen, G, and Heisto, H: A Korean family showing inheritance of A and B on the same chromosome. Vox Sang 14:211, 1968.

Makela, O, Ruoslahti, E, and Ehnholm, C: Subtypes of human ABO blood groups and subtype-specific antibodies. J Immunol 3:763, 1969.

Marsh, WL, et al: Inherited mosaicism affecting the blood groups. Transfusion 15:589, 1975.

Mohn, JF, et al: An inherited blood group A variant in the Finnish population. I. Basic characteristics. Vox Sang 25:193, 1973.

Mollison, PL, Engelfriet, CP, and Contreras, M. Blood Transfusion in Clinical Medicine. Blackwell Scientific, London, 1993.

Moores, PP, et al: Some observations on "Bombay" bloods, with comments on evidence for the existence of two different O_h phenotypes. Transfusion 15:237, 1975.

Oriol, R, Le Pendu, J, and Mollicone, R. Genetics of ABO, H, Lewis, X and related antigens. Vox Sang 51:161–171, 1986.

Pacuszka, T, et al: Biochemical serological and family studies in individuals with cis-AB phenotypes. Vox Sang 29:292, 1975.

Poretz, RD, and Watkins, WM: Galactosyltransferases in human submaxillary glands and stomach mucosa associated with the biosynthesis of blood group specific glycoproteins. Eur J Biochem 25:455, 1972.

Race, C, and Watkins, WM: The action of the blood group B gene-specified alpha-galactosyltransferase from human serum and stomach mucosal extracts on group O and "Bombay" O_h erythrocytes. Vox Sang 23:385, 1972.

Race, RR, and Sanger, R: Blood Groups in Man, ed 6. Blackwell Scientific, Oxford, 1975, pp 522–524, 531–535.

Rawson, AJ, and Abelson, N: Studies in blood group antibodies. III. Observations on the physiochemical properties of isohemagglutinins and isohemolysins. J Immunol 85:636, 1960.

Reed, ME, and Lomas-Francis, C: The Blood Group Antigen Facts Book. Academic Press, New York, 1997, pp 3–26.

Reed, TE, and Moore, BPL: A new variant of blood group A. Vox Sang 9:363, 1964.

Renkonen, KO: Blood-group–specific haemagglutinins in seed extracts. Vox Sang 45(5):397, 1983.

Roath, S, et al: Transient acquired blood group B antigen associated with diverticular bowel disease. Acta Haematol (Basel) 77(3):188, 1987.

Romano, EL, Mollison, PL, and Linares, J: Number of B sites generated on group O red cells from adults and newborn infants. Vox Sang 34:14, 1978.

Romans, DG, Tilley, CA, and Dorrington, KJ: Monogamous bivalency of IgG antibodies. I. Deficiency of branched ABHI-active oligosaccharide chains on red cells of infants causes the weak antiglobulin reactions in hemolytic disease of the newborn due to ABO incompatibility. J Immunol 124:2807, 1980.

Rubinstein, P, et al: A dominant suppressor of A and B. Vox Sang 25:377, 1973.

Rudmann, SV: Textbook of Blood Banking and Transfusion Medicine. WB Saunders, Philadelphia, 1995.

Sabo, B, et al: The cis-AB phenotype in three generations of one family: Serological enzymatic and cytogenetic studies. J Immunogenet 5:87, 1978.

Salmon, C, et al: Quantitative and thermodynamic studies of erythrocytic ABO antigens. Transfusion 16:580, 1976.

Sathe, MS, Gorakshakar, AC, and Bhatia, HM: Blood group specific transferases in Bombay (O_h) para-Bombay and weaker A and B variants. Indian J Med Res 81:53, 1985.

Schenkel-Brunner, H: Blood-group ABH antigens of human erythrocytes. Eur J Biochem 104:529, 1980.

Schenkel-Brunner, H, Chester, MA, and Watkins, WM: Alpha-L-fucosyl-transferases in human serum from donors of different ABO, secretor and Lewis blood group phenotypes. Eur J Biochem 30:269, 1972.

Schenkel-Brunner, H, Prohaska, R, and Tuppy, H: Action of glycosyltransferases upon "Bombay" (O_h) erythrocytes: Conversion to cells showing blood group H and A specificities. Eur J Biochem 56:591, 1975.

Schenkel-Brunner, H, and Tuppy, H: Enzymatic conversion of human blood group O erythrocytes into A_2 and A_1 cells by alpha-N-acetyl-D-galacto-saminyltransferases of blood group A individuals. Eur J Biochem 34:125, 1973.

Schenkel-Brunner, H, and Tuppy, H: Enzymatic conversion of human O into A erythrocytes and of B into AB erythrocytes. Nature 223:1272, 1969.

Schmidt, P, et al: A hemolytic transfusion reaction due to the transfusion of A_x blood. J Lab Clin Med 54:38, 1959.

Seyfried, H, Waleska, I, and Werblinska, B: Unusual inheritance of ABO group in a family with weak B antigens. Vox Sang 3:268, 1964.

Smalley, CE, and Tucker, EM: Blood group A antigen site distribution and immunoglobulin binding in relation to red cell age. Br J Haematol 54(2):209, 1983.

Solomon, J, Waggoner, R, and Leyshon, CW: A quantitative immunogenetic study of gene suppression involving A_1 and H antigens of the erythrocyte without affecting secreted blood group substances: The ABH phenotypes A_h and O_h. Blood 25:470, 1965.

Stayboldt, C, Rearden, A, and Lane, TA: B antigen acquired by normal A_1 red cells exposed to a patient's serum. Transfusion 27(1):41, 1987.

Sturgeon, P, Moore, BPL, and Weiner, W: Notations for two weak A variants: A_{end} and A_{el}. Vox Sang 9:214, 1964.

Takasaki, S, and Kobata, A: Chemical characterization and distribution of ABO blood group active glycoprotein in human erythrocyte membrane. J Biol Chem 251:3610, 1976.

Takasaki, S, Yamashita, K, and Kobata, A: The sugar chain structures of ABO blood group active glycoproteins obtained from human erythrocyte membrane. J Biol Chem 253:6086, 1978.

Topping, MD, and Watkins, WM: Isoelectric points of the human blood group A_1, A_2 and B gene–associated glycosyltransferases in ovarian cyst fluids and serum. Biochem Biophys Res Commun 34:89, 1975.

Tuppy, H, and Schenkel-Brunner, H: Occurrence and assay of alpha-H-acetyl-galactosaminyltransferase in the gastric mucosa of humans belonging to blood group A. Vox Sang 17:139, 1969.

Viitala, J, Finne, J, and Krusius, T: Blood group A and H determinants in polyglycosyl peptides of A1 and A2 erythrocytes. Eur J Biochem 126(2):401, 1982.

Watanabe, K, Laine, RA, and Hakomori, S: On neutral fucoglycolipids having long branched carbohydrate chains: H-active I-active glycosphingolipids of human erythrocyte membranes. Biochemistry 14:2725, 1975.

Watkins, WM: Blood group substances: Their nature and genetics. In Surgenor, D (ed): The Red Blood Cell. Academic Press, New York, 1974, p 303.

Watkins, WM: Glycoproteins: Their composition, structure and function. In Gottschalk, A (ed): Glycoproteins, ed 2. Elsevier, Amsterdam, 1972, pp 830–891.

Westerveld, A, et al: Assignment of the AK_1:Np:ABO linkage group to human chromosome 9. Proc Natl Acad Sci 73:895, 1976.

Wheeler, DA, et al: Serologic and biochemical studies of a previously unclassified blood type B variant. 63(3):711, 1984.

Wiener, AS, and Cioffi, AF: A group B analogue of subgroup A3. Am J Clin Pathol 58:693, 1972.

Wiener, AS, and Socha, WW: Macro- and microdifferences in blood group antigens and antibodies. Int Arch Allergy Appl Immunol 47:946, 1974.

Wittemore, NB, et al: Solubilized glycoprotein from human erythrocyte membranes possessing blood group A, B and H activity. Vox Sang 17:289, 1969.

Wrobel, DM, et al: "True" genotypes of chimeric twins revealed by blood group gene products in plasma. Vox Sang 27:395, 1974.

Wu, AM, et al: Immunochemical studies on blood groups: The internal structure and immunological properties of water-soluble human blood group A substance studied by Smith degradation, liberation, and fractionation of oligosaccharides and reaction with lectins. Arch Biochem Biophys 215(2):390, 1982.

Yamaguchi, H: A review of cis-AB blood. Jinrui Idengaku Zasshi 18:1, 1973.

Yamaguchi, H, Okubo, Y, and Hazama, F: Another Japanese A_2B_3 blood group family with the propositus having O group father. Proc Jpn Acad 42:517, 1966.

Yamaguchi, H, Okubo, Y, and Tanaka, M: Cis-AB bloods found in Japanese families. Jinrui Idengaku Zasshi 15:198, 1970.

Yokoyama, M, Stacey, SM, and Dunsford, I: B_x: A new subgroup of the blood group B. Vox Sang 2:348, 1957.

Yoshida, A, et al: A case of weak blood group B expression (Bm) associated with abnormal blood group galactosyltransferase. Blood 59(2):323, 1982.

Yoshida, A, et al: An enzyme basis for blood type A intermediate status. Am J Hum Genet 34(6):919, 1982.

Yoshida, A, Yamaguchi, YF, and Dave, V: Immunologic homology of human blood group glycosyltransferases and genetic background of blood group (ABO) determination. Blood 54:344, 1979.

PROCEDURAL APPENDIX

Determination of the Secretor Property

Principle

Certain blood group substances occur in soluble form in a large proportion (78%) of individuals in secretions such as saliva and gastric juice (see **Table 6–11**). These individuals are termed "secretors" (they possess the *Se* gene) and secrete ABH-soluble antigens. These water-soluble blood group substances are readily detected in very minute quantities because they have the property of reacting with their corresponding antibodies and thereby neutralizing or inhibiting the capacity of the antibody to agglutinate erythrocytes possessing the corresponding antigen. The reaction is termed *hemagglutination inhibition* and provides a means of assaying the relative activity or potency of these water-soluble blood group substances.

Materials

Saliva
Human polyclonal anti-A and anti-B serum
Anti-H lectin from *Ulex europaeus*
Test tubes
Pipettes
Saline
2% to 5 % washed group A, B, and O cells

Procedure

1. Collect about 2 to 3 mL of saliva in a test tube.
2. Centrifuge at 900 to 1000 × g for 8 to 10 minutes.
3. Transfer supernatant to a clean test tube, and place stoppered tube in a boiling water bath for 10 minutes. This inactivates enzymes that might otherwise destroy blood group substances.
4. Recentrifuge at 900 to 1000 × g for 8 to 10 minutes.
5. Collect clear supernatant into a clean tube.
6. Dilute saliva with an equal volume of saline (undiluted saliva contains nonspecific glycoproteins that can inhibit antisera and lead to incorrect results).
7. Add one drop of diluted antiserum to an appropriately labeled tube (anti-A, anti-B, anti-H). For dilution, titrate anti-H, anti-A, and anti-B, testing against appropriate cells at immediate spin. Select the dilution giving 2+

agglutination, and prepare a sufficient quantity to complete the test.
8. Add one drop of supernatant saliva to each tube. Mix and incubate at room temperature for 8 to 10 minutes.
9. Add one drop of the appropriate indicator cells (A, B, or O cells) to the properly labeled tube.
10. Mix and incubate at room temperature for 30 to 60 minutes.
11. Centrifuge.
12. Observe for macroscopic agglutination.

Control

1. One drop of saline is used in place of dilute saliva. Test in parallel with the saliva.
2. Test saliva from a known secretor and a nonsecretor in parallel with test saliva.

Interpretations

1. Nonsecretor: Agglutination of RBCs by antiserum-saliva mixture; control tube positive.
2. Secretor: No agglutination of RBCs by antiserum and saliva mixture; control tube positive. The antiserum has been neutralized by the soluble blood group substances or antigens in the saliva, which react with their corresponding antibody. Therefore, no free antibody is available to react with the antigens on the reagent RBCs used in the testing. This negative reaction is a positive test for the presence of ABH-soluble antigens and indicates that the individual is a secretor.

ABH Substances in Saliva

ABH Substances in Saliva			
ABO Group	**A**	**B**	**H**
Secretors			
A	Much	None	Some
B	None	Much	Some
O	None	None	Much
AB	Much	Much	Some
Nonsecretors			
A, B, O, and AB	None	None	None

seven

The Rh Blood Group System

Merilyn Wiler, MA Ed, MT(ASCP)SBB

OBJECTIVES

On completion of this chapter, the learner should be able to:

1. Explain the derivation of the term Rh.
2. Differentiate Rh from LW.
3. Compare and contrast the Fisher-Race and Wiener theories of Rh inheritance.
4. Translate the five major Rh antigens, genotypes, and haplotypes from one nomenclature to another, including Fisher-Race, Wiener, Rosenfield, and ISBT nomenclatures.
5. Define the basic biochemical structure of Rh.
6. Compare and contrast the genetic pathways for the regulator type of Rh_null and the amorphic Rh_null.
7. Describe and differentiate three mechanisms that result in weak-D expression on red blood cells.
8. List three instances in which the weak-D status of an individual must be determined.
9. List and differentiate four types of Rh typing reagents. Give two advantages of each type.
10. Define three characteristics of Rh antibodies.
11. Describe three symptoms associated with an Rh hemolytic transfusion reaction.
12. Compare and contrast Rh_null and Rh_mod.
13. List four Rh antigens (excluding DCcEe), and give two classic characteristics of each antigen.
14. Determine the most probable genotype of an individual when given the individual's red blood cell typing results, haplotype frequencies, and race.

Introduction

The term *Rh* refers not only to a specific red blood cell (RBC) antigen but also to a complex blood group system that is currently composed of nearly 50 different antigenic specificities. Although the Rh antibodies were among the first to be described, scientists have spent years unraveling the complexities of the Rh system and its mode of inheritance, the genetic control of the Rh system, and the biochemical structure of the Rh antigens.

History of the Rh System

Before 1939, the only significant blood group antigens recognized were those of the ABO system. Transfusion medicine was thus based on matching ABO groups. Despite ABO matching, blood transfusions continued to result in morbidity and mortality.

As the 1930s ended, two significant discoveries were made that would further the safety of blood transfusion and eventually result in defining the most extensive blood group system known. It began when Levine and Stetson[1] described a hemolytic transfusion reaction in an obstetrical patient. After delivery of a stillborn infant, a woman required transfusions. Her husband, who had the same ABO type, was selected as her donor. After transfusion, the recipient demonstrated the classic symptoms of an acute hemolytic transfusion reaction. Subsequently, an antibody was isolated from the mother's serum that reacted both at 37°C and at 20°C with the father's RBCs. It was postulated that the fetus and the father possessed a common factor that the mother lacked. While the mother carried the fetus, she was exposed to this factor and subsequently built an antibody that reacted against the transfused RBCs from the father, which resulted in the hemolytic transfusion reaction.

A year later, Landsteiner and Wiener[2] reported on an antibody made by guinea pigs and rabbits when they were transfused with rhesus monkey RBCs. This antibody, which agglutinated 85 percent of human RBCs, was named Rh. Another investigation by Levine and coworkers[3] demonstrated that the agglutinin that had caused the hemolytic transfusion reaction and the antibody described by Landsteiner and Wiener appeared to define the same blood group. Many years later it was recognized that the two antibodies were different. However, the name Rh was retained for the human-produced antibody, and the anti-rhesus antibody formed by the animals was renamed anti-LW in honor of those first reporting it (Landsteiner and Wiener).

Further research resulted in defining Rh as a primary cause of hemolytic disease of the newborn (HDN, also called erythroblastosis fetalis) and a significant cause of hemolytic transfusion reactions. Continued investigation[4–7] showed additional blood group factors associated with the original agglutinin. By the mid-1940s, five antigens made up the Rh system. Today the Rh blood group system is made up of nearly 50 different specificities.

Nomenclatures of the Rh System

The terminologies used to describe the Rh system are derived from four sets of investigators. Two of the terminologies are based on the postulated genetic mechanisms of the Rh system. The third terminology describes only the presence or absence of a given antigen. The fourth is the result of the combined efforts of the International Society of Blood Transfusion (ISBT) Working Party on Terminology for Red Cell Surface Antigens. The genetic pathways are described in detail after the discussion of the nomenclatures, although reference to the former may be included here.

Fisher-Race: The DCE Terminology

In the early 1940s, Fisher and Race[8] were investigating the antigens found on human RBCs, including the newly defined Rh antigen. They postulated that the antigens of the system were produced by three closely linked sets of alleles (**Fig. 7–1**). Each gene was responsible for producing a product (or antigen) on the RBC surface. Each antigen and corresponding gene were given the same letter designation (when referring to the gene, the letter is italicized).

Fisher and Race named the antigens of the system D, d, C, c, and E and e. Now it is known that "d" represents the absence of D antigen. The phenotype (blood type observed during testing) of a given RBC is defined by the presence of *D*, *C, c, E,* and *e* expression. The gene frequency for each Rh antigen is given in **Table 7–1**, and the Rh haplotype (the complement of genes inherited from either parent) frequencies are given in **Table 7–2**. Notice how the frequencies vary with race.

According to the Fisher-Race proposal, each person inherits a set of *Rh* genes from each parent (i.e., one *D* or *d,* one *C* or *c,* and one *E* or *e*) (see **Fig. 7–1**). Because *Rh* genes are codominant, each inherited gene expresses its corresponding antigen on the RBC. The combination of maternal and paternal haplotypes determines one's genotype (the *Rh* genes inherited from each parent) and dictates one's phenotype (the antigens expressed on the RBC that can be detected serologically). An individual's Rh phenotype is reported as DCE rather than CDE because Fisher postulated that the *C/c* locus lies between *D/d* and *E/e* loci. This information is based on frequencies of the various gene combinations.

It is essential to remember that d does not represent an antigen but simply represents the absence of the D antigen. C, c, E, and e represent actual antigens recognized by specific antibodies. For many students, the Fisher-Race nomenclature represents the easiest way to think about the five major Rh system antigens, but it has shortcomings in that many of the newer Rh antigens are not assigned names using the Fisher-Race nomenclature.

In very rare instances, an individual may fail to express any allelic antigen at one or both Rh loci; that is, a person may express neither C or c, E or e, nor CcEe. The genotype for the

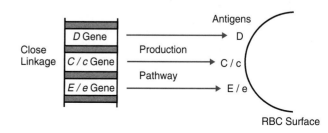

■ **FIGURE 7–1**   Fisher-Race concept of Rh (simplified). Each gene produces one product.

TABLE 7-1   Gene Frequency of Rh Antigens

Gene	Frequency (%)
D	85
d	15
(absence of D)	
C	70
E	30
c	80
e	98

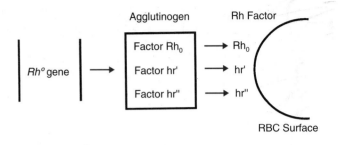

FIGURE 7-2 Wiener's agglutinogen theory. Antibody will recognize each factor within the agglutinogen.

Rh-positive person exhibiting a deletion phenotype such as these is written -De or -DE, CD- or cD-, or -D-, respectively. The last is sometimes referred to as a double deletion. The person expressing no Rh antigens on the RBC is said to be Rh$_{null}$, and the phenotype may be written as ——/——. Weakened expression of all Rh antigens of an individual has also been reported. These individuals are said to have the Rh$_{mod}$ phenotype, and there is no unique way of indicating this using the Fisher-Race terminology.

Wiener: The Rh-Hr Terminology

In his early work defining the Rh antigens, Wiener[10] believed that the gene responsible for defining Rh actually produced an agglutinogen that contained a series of blood factors. According to Rh-Hr terminology, this *Rh* gene produces at least three factors within an agglutinogen **(Fig. 7–2)**. The agglutinogen may be considered the phenotypic expression of the haplotype. Each factor is an antigen recognized by an antibody. Antibodies can recognize single or multiple factors (antigens).

Table 7–3 lists the major agglutinogens and their respective factors, along with the shorthand term that has come to represent each agglutinogen. The Wiener terminology is complex and unwieldy; nevertheless, it is used by many blood bankers interchangeably with the other nomenclatures.

Fisher-Race nomenclature may be converted to Wiener nomenclature and vice versa. It is important to remember that an agglutinogen in the Wiener nomenclature actually represents the presence of a single haplotype capable of expressing three different antigens (see **Table 7–3**). When describing an agglutinogen, the uppercase R denotes the presence of the original factor, the D antigen. The lowercase r indicates the absence of the D antigen. The presence of uppercase C is indicated by a one (1) or single prime ('). Lowercase c is implied when there is no 1 or ' indicated. That is, R_1 is the same as *DCe; r'* denotes *dCe;* and R_0 is equivalent to *Dce*. The presence of E is indicated by the Arabic number two (2) or double prime ("). Lowercase e is implied when there is no 2 or " indicated. That is, R_2 is the same as *DcE; r"* denotes *dcE;* and r is equivalent to *dce*. When both C and E are uppercase, the letter z or y is used. R_z denotes *DCE*, whereas r^y represents *dCE*. Italics and superscripts are used when describing the Rh genes in the Wiener nomenclature. Standard type is used to describe the gene product or agglutinogen. Subscripts are used with the uppercase R and superscripts with the lowercase r. The phenotypes of Rh$_{null}$ and Rh$_{mod}$ are written as stated. The genotype for the Rh$_{null}$ that arises from an amorphic gene at both Rh loci is written as $\overline{\overline{rr}}$ and pronounced "little r double bar"

When referring to the Rh antigens (or factors) in Wiener nomenclature, the single prime (') refers to either C or c, and the double prime (") to either E or e. If the r precedes the h (i.e., rh' or rh"), this refers to the C or E antigens, respectively. When the h precedes the r, this refers to either the c (hr') or e (hr") antigen. Rh$_0$ is equivalent to D. In the Wiener nomenclature, there is no designation for the absence of D antigen. By using these designations, the researcher should be able to recognize immediately which factors are present on the RBCs described. However, it is difficult to use the Wiener nomenclature to adequately describe additional alleles within an agglutinogen. Because of this, many of the more recently described antigens of the *Rh* system have not been given Rh-Hr designations.

Rosenfield and Coworkers: Alpha/Numeric Terminology

As the Rh blood group system expanded, it became more difficult to assign names to new antigens using existing terminologies. In the early 1960s Rosenfield and associates[11] proposed a system that assigns a number to each antigen of the Rh system in order of its discovery or recognized relationship to the Rh system **(Table 7–4)**. This system has no genetic basis, but simply demonstrates the presence or absence of the antigen on the RBC. A minus sign preceding a number designates absence of the antigen. If an antigen has not been typed, its number will not appear in the sequence.

TABLE 7-2   Fisher-Race Phenotypes of the Rh System: Frequencies in the United States

Gene combination	Frequency (%)			
	White	Black	Native American	Asian
DCe	42	17	44	70
dce	37	26	11	3
DcE	14	11	34	21
Dce	4	44	2	3
dCe	2	2	2	2
dcE	1	0	6	0
DCE	0	0	6	1
dCE*	0	0	0	0

Widmann,[9] p 130, with permission. *Frequency less than 1%, but phenotype has been found.

TABLE 7–3   Rh-Hr Terminology of Wiener

Gene	Agglutinogen	Blood Factors	Shorthand Designation	Fisher-Race Antigens
Rh^0	Rh_0	$Rh_0hr'hr''$	R_0	Dce
Rh^1	Rh_1	$Rh_0rh'hr''$	R_1	DCe
Rh^2	Rh_2	$Rh_0hr'rh''$	R_2	DcE
Rh^z	Rh_z	$Rh_0rh'rh''$	R_z	DCE
rh	rh	$hr'hr''$	r	dce
rh'	rh'	$rh'hr''$	r'	dCe
rh''	rh''	$hr'rh''$	r''	dcE
rh^y	rh_y	$rh'rh''$	r^y	dCE

An advantage of this nomenclature is that the RBC phenotype is thus succinctly described.

For the five major antigens, D is assigned Rh1, C is Rh2, E is Rh3, c is Rh4, and e is Rh5. For RBCs that type D + C + E + c negative, e negative, the Rosenfield designation is Rh: 1, 2, 3, −4, −5. If the sample was not tested for e, the designation would be Rh: 1, 2, 3, −4. All Rh system antigens have been assigned a number.

The numeric system is well suited to electronic data processing. Its use expedites data entry and retrieval. Its primary limiting factor is that there is a similar nomenclature for numerous other blood groups such as Kell, Duffy, Kidd, Lutheran, Scianna, and more. K:1,2 refers to the K and k antigens of the Kell blood group system. Therefore, when using the Rosenfield nomenclature on the computer, one must use both the alpha (Rh:, K:) and the numeric (1, 2, −3, etc.) to denote a phenotype.

International Society of Blood Transfusion: Numeric Terminology

As the world of blood transfusion began to cooperate and share data, it became apparent that there was a need for a universal language. The ISBT formed the Working Party on Terminology for Red Cell Surface Antigens. Its mandate was to establish a uniform nomenclature that is both eye- and machine-readable and is in keeping with the genetic basis of blood groups.[12] The ISBT adopted a six-digit number for each authenticated blood group specificity. The first three numbers represent the system and the remaining three the antigenic specificity. The number 004 was assigned to the Rh blood group system, and then each antigen assigned to the Rh system was given a unique number to complete the six-digit computer number. **Table 7–5** provides a listing of these numbers.

When referring to individual antigens, an alphanumeric designation similar to the Rosenfield nomenclature may be used. The alphabetic names formerly used (e.g., Rh, Kell) were left unchanged but were converted to all uppercase letters (i.e., RH, KELL). Therefore, D is RH1, C is RH2, and so forth. (*Note:* There is no space between the RH and the assigned number.)

The phenotype designation includes the alphabetical symbol that denotes the blood group, followed by a colon and then the specificity numbers of the antigens defined. A minus sign preceding the number indicates that the antigen was tested for but was not present. The phenotype D+ C− E+ c+ e+ or DccEe or R_2y would be written RH:1,−2,3,4,5.

When referring to a gene, an allele, or a haplotype, the symbols are italicized, followed by a space or asterisk, and then the numbers of the specificities are separated by commas. R^1 or *DCe* would be *RH 1,2,5.*

TABLE 7–4   Common Rh Types by Three Nomenclatures

	Genotype			
	Wiener	**Fisher-Race**	**Rosenfield**	**Frequency (%) (approx., White)**
Common genotypes	R^1r	*DCe/dce*	*Rh:1,2,−3,4,5*	33
	R^1R^1	*DCe/DCe*	*Rh:1,2,−3,−4,5*	18
	rr	*dce/dce*	*Rh:−1,−2,−3,4,5*	15
	R^1R^2	*DCe/DcE*	*Rh:1,2,3,4,5*	11
	R^2r	*DcE/dce*	*Rh:1,−2,3,4,5*	9
	R^2R^2	*DcE/DcE*	*Rh:1,−2,3,4,−5*	2
Rarer genotypes	$r'r$	*dCe/dce*	*Rh:−1,2,−3,4,5*	1
	$r'r'$	*dCe/dCe*	*Rh:−1,2,−3,−4,5*	0.01
	$r''r$	*dcE/dce*	*Rh:−1,−2,3,4,5*	1
	$r''r''$	*dcE/dcE*	*Rh:−1,−2,3,4,−5*	0.03
	R^0r	*Dce/dce*	*Rh:1,−2,−3,4,5*	2
	R^0R^0	*Dce/Dce*	*Rh:1,−2,−3,4,5*	0.1
	r^yr	*dCE/dce*	*Rh:−1,2,3,4,5*	rare

Handbook of Clinical Laboratory Science. CRC Press, Boca Raton, FL, 1977, p 342, with permission.

TABLE 7–5   The Antigens of the Rh Blood Group System in Four Nomenclatures

Numeric	Fisher-race	Weiner	ISBT Number	Other Names or Comment
Rh1	D	Rh_0	004001	
Rh2	C	rh'	004002	
Rh3	E	rh''	004003	
Rh4	c	hr'	004004	
Rh5	e	hr''	004005	
Rh6	ce	hr	004006	f
Rh7	Ce	rh_i	004007	
Rh8	C^w	rh^{w1}	004008	
Rh9	C^x	rh^x	004009	
Rh10	ce^s	hr^v	004010	V
Rh11	E^w	rh^{w2}	004011	
Rh12	G	rh^G	004012	
Rh13		Rh^A	004013	
Rh14		Rh^B	004014	
Rh15		Rh^C	004015	
Rh16		Rh^D	004016	
Rh17		Hr_0	004017	
Rh18		Hr	004018	
Rh19		hr^s	004019	
Rh20	e^s		004020	VS
Rh21	C^G		004021	
Rh22	CE	rh	004022	Jarvis
Rh23	D^w		004023	Wiel
Rh24	E^T		004024	
Rh25*/†			004025	
Rh26	c-like		004026	Deal
Rh27	cE	rh_{ii}	004027	
Rh28		hr^H	004028	Hernandez
Rh29			004029	total Rh
Rh30	D^{cor}		004030	Go^a
Rh31		hr^B	004031	
Rh32		$\bar{\bar{R}}^N$	004032	Troll
Rh33		R_0^{Har}	004033	Hill
Rh34		Hr^B	004034	Bastiaan
Rh35			004035	1114
Rh36			004036	Be^a (Berrens)
Rh37			004037	Evans
Rh38†			004038	Duclos
Rh39			004039	
Rh40	C-like		004040	Targett
Rh41	Tar		004041	
Rh42	Ce-like		004042	Thornton
Rh43	Ce^S	rh_i^s	004043	Crawford
Rh44			004044	Nou
Rh45			004045	Riv
Rh46			004046	Sec
Rh47	"Allelic"	to $\bar{\bar{R}}^N$	004047	Dav
Rh48			004048	JAL
Rh49			004049	Stem
Rh50			004050	FPTT
Rh51			004051	MAR
Rh52			004052	BARC
Rh53			004053	JAHK

*Rh25 was formerly assigned to the LW antigen. LW is now known as LW^a and is no longer considered a member of the Rh system.
†Obsolete names: Rh25 formerly LW, Rh38 formerly Duclos.

Summary: Rh Terminologies

Blood bankers must be familiar with the Fisher-Race, Wiener, Rosenfield, and ISBT nomenclatures and must be able to translate among them when reading about, writing about, or discussing the Rh system.

Tables 7–4 and **7–6** summarize the data presented in this section. These tables also include probable genotypes based on the antigens found in selected RBC populations.

Table 7–6 correlates Rh phenotypes with the most probable genotype in a designated population. Results of typing do not define genotype, only phenotype. Other genotypes that can occur with the given test results are also listed, but they are not commonly seen.

Determining probable genotypes is useful for parentage studies as well as for population studies. Probable genotypes also may be useful in predicting the potential for HDN in offspring of an Rh-negative woman with an Rh antibody.

TABLE 7–6 Eighteen Possible Reaction Patterns with Five Antisera*

D	C	E	c	e	Whites (%)	Blacks (%)	Whites	Blacks	Other Possibilities (Both Groups)
+	+	−	+	+	31	15 9	DCe/dce	DCe/Dce or DCe/dce	dCe/Dce
+	+	−	−	+	18	3	DCe/DCe	DCe/DCe	DCe/dCe
+	+	+	+	+	12	4	DCe/DcE	DCe/DcE	DCe/dcE, dCe/DcE, DCE/dce, DCE/Dce, or dCE/Dce
+	−	+	+	+	11	10 6	DcE/dce	DcE/Dce or DcE/dce	dcE/Dce
+	−	+	+	−	2	1	DcE/DcE	DcE/DcE	DcE/dcE
+	−	−	+	+	3	19 23	Dce/dce	Dce/Dce, or Dce/dce	----
−	−	−	+	+	15	7	dce/dce	dce/dce	----
−	+	−	+	+	1	1	dCe/dce	dCe/dce	----
−	−	+	+	+	1	rare	dcE/dce	dcE/dce	----
−	+	+	+	+	Each of these pheno- types occur with a frequency of less than 0.2% in both racial groups.			dCe/dcE	dCE/dce
−	+	−	−	+				dCe/dCe	----
−	−	+	+	−				dcE/dcE	----
+	+	+	−	+				DCE/DCe	DCE/dCe
+	+	+	+	−				DCE/DcE	DCE/dcE
+	+	+	−	−				DCE/DCE	DCE/dCE
−	+	+	−	+				dCE/dCe	----
−	+	+	+	−				dCE/dcE	----
−	+	+	−	−				dCE/dCE	----

*Percentages are rounded off.

There are substantial differences in the probable genotypes of various populations. These differences must be remembered when trying to locate compatible blood for recipients with unusual or multiple Rh antibodies.

To further emphasize the interchangeable use of the terminologies for the basic antigens, see **Table 7–4**, which defines common genotypes using the Fisher-Race, Wiener, and Rosenfield nomenclatures. The frequencies listed are for those found in the white population.

Proposed Genetic Pathways

Mechanisms of Antigen Production

Many theories have been proposed to explain genetically the results of serologic and biochemical studies in the Rh system. Two theories of Rh genetic control were initially postulated. Wiener postulated that a single gene produces a single product that contains separately recognizable factors (see **Fig. 7–2**). In contrast, Fisher and Race proposed that the Rh locus contains three distinct genes that control the production of their respective antigens (see **Fig. 7–1**).

It is currently accepted that only two closely linked genes located on chromosome 1 control the expression of Rh; one gene (*RHD*) codes for the presence or absence of the D polypeptides and the second gene (*RHCE*) for either RHCe, RHcE, RHce, or RHCE polypeptides[13,14] (**Fig. 7–3**). Another gene (*RHAG*), which resides on chromosome 6, produces a Rh-associated glycoprotein that is very similar in structure to the Rh proteins and within the RBC membrane forms complexes with the Rh polypeptides. RHAG is called a coexpressor and must be present for the successful expression of the Rh antigens but by itself does not express any of the Rh antigens. The genes for elliptocytosis, 6-phosphogluconate dehydroge-

nase (PGD), phosphoglucomutase (PGM), and phosphopyruvate hydratase (PPH)[15] also reside on chromosome 1.

The Rh genes are inherited as codominant alleles. Offspring inherit one Rh haplotype from each parent. **Figure 7–4** is an example of a normal Rh inheritance pattern. In rare instances, individuals express no Rh antigens on their RBCs. These individuals are said to have the Rh_{null} phenotype and are discussed in more detail later in this chapter.

Biochemistry of the Rh Antigens

The final result of gene action in RBC groups is the production of a biochemical structure; in the Rh system it is a non-glycosylated protein. This means that there are no carbohydrates attached to the protein.

The Rh antigens are transmembrane polypeptides and are an integral part of the RBC membrane.[16] The gene products of RHD and RHCE are remarkably similar in that both encode for proteins composed of 417 amino acids that traverse the

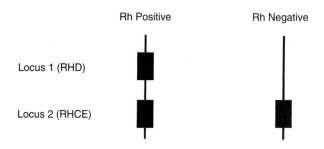

■ **FIGURE 7–3** Rh inheritance: two-loci theory. Locus 1 codes for the presence or absence of *D/d*. Locus 2 codes for the presence of *Ce, cE, ce,* or *CE.*

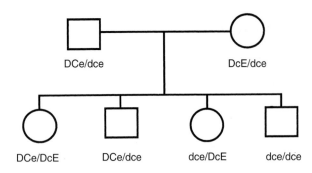

FIGURE 7-4   Example of a normal pattern of Rh inheritance.

TABLE 7-7   Number of D Antigen Sites of Cells with Various Phenotypes

Rh Phenotype	Number of D Antigen Sites
R_1r	9,900–14,600
R_0r	12,000–20,000
R_2r	14,000–16,600
R_1R_1	14,500–19,300
R_1R_2	23,000–31,000
R_2R_2	15,800–33,300
D--	110,000–202,000

cell membrane 12 times and that their sequence differs by only 44 base pairs.[17] The gene products of *RHCE, RHCe, RHce,* and *RHcE* are even more similar. C and c differ from one another in four amino acid positions, and one amino acid differentiates E from e **(Fig. 7–5)**. Only small loops of the Rh proteins are exposed on the surface of the RBC and provide the conformational requirements for the serologic differences between the Rh blood types.

As part of the research on the biochemistry of the Rh antigens, investigations have been performed to determine the quantity of antigen sites on RBCs of various Rh phenotypes. In comparison with ABO and Kell (K) blood groups, A_1 cells possess approximately 1.0×10^6 A antigens, whereas homozygous Kell cells have 6000 K sites. The number of D antigen sites were measured on a variety of Rh phenotypes by Hughes-Jones and coworkers, and the results are summarized in **Table 7–7**.[13] The greatest number of D antigen sites are on cells of the rare Rh phenotype D--. (D-- cells carry only D antigen and completely lack Cc and Ee.) However, of the commonly encountered Rh genotypes, R^2R^2 cells possess the largest number of D antigen sites.

Weak D: Variations of the Rh₀ (D) Antigen Expression

When Rh-positive RBC samples are typed for the D antigen, they are expected to react strongly (macroscopically) with anti-D reagents. However, with certain RBCs the testing must be carried through the antiglobulin phase of testing to demonstrate the presence of the D antigen. RBCs carrying the weaker D antigen have historically been referred to as having

the Du type. Now they are referred to as expressing weak D and are considered Rh-positive. Three different mechanisms have been described that can explain the weakened expression of the D antigen.[18]

Genetic Weak D

The first mechanism results from inheritance of *D* genes that code for a weakened expression of the D antigen.[19] The D antigens expressed appear to be complete but few in number. On a molecular level, these quantitative differences in D expression are attributed to mutations of the Rh polypeptide.[18] Inheritance of these genes can be tracked vertically from one generation to the next and are seen most frequently in blacks. The genetic weak D is rare and seldom found in whites.

C Trans

The second mechanism that may result in weakened expression of the D antigen is described as a position effect or gene interaction effect.[20] In individuals showing the gene interaction weak D, the allele carrying *D* is trans (or in the opposite haplotype) to the allele carrying *C,* for example, *Dce/dCe.* The Rh antigen on the RBC is normal, but the steric arrangement of the C antigen in relationship to the D antigen appears to interfere with the expression of the D antigen. This interference with D expression does not occur when the *C* gene is inherited in the cis position to *D,* such as *DCe/dce.* It is not possible to distinguish the genetic weak D from the position effect weak D serologically. Family studies are necessary to distinguish which type of weakened D antigen is being demonstrated. Practically speaking, this is unnecessary because the D antigen is structurally complete. These individuals can receive D-positive RBCs with no adverse effects.

Partial D (D Mosaic)

The third instance in which the D antigen expression can be weakened is when one or more of the D epitopes within the entire D protein is either missing and/or is altered.[21] Cells with a partial-D antigen usually type weaker than expected or may not react at all when routine procedures are used with most commercial anti-D reagents.

In the early 1950s, several reports[22,23] described individuals who were typed D-positive but who produced an anti-D that reacted with all D-positive samples except their own. The formation of alloanti-D by D-positive individuals required explanation.

Wiener and Unger[24] postulated that the D antigen is made of antigenic subparts, genetically determined, that could be

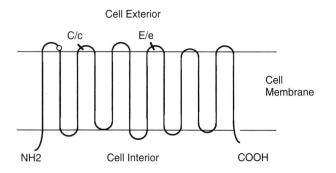

FIGURE 7-5   Model of Rh polypeptide. "o" denotes where the sequence of D diverges from C/c or E/e. The C/c and E/e respectively denote the region responsible for the serologic difference between C/c and E/e.

absent in rare instances. If an individual lacked one (or more) pieces, or epitopes, of the total D antigen, alloantibody can be made to the missing fraction(s) if exposed to RBCs that possess the complete D antigen. This theory has become well accepted.

Tippett and Sanger[25] worked with RBCs and sera of partial-D individuals to classify these antigens. Their work, which was based on the reactivity of anti-D sera from D-positive people, with RBCs from D-positive people who also made anti-D has led to a method of categorizing the partial D. Seven categories were recognized, designated by Roman numbers I through VII. Category I is now obsolete, and a few of the categories have been further subdivided.

Today, the partial-D antigens can be classified on a molecular level and are attributed to the transfer of either whole exons or partial (or patched exon) transfers that range from single nucleotide to multiple exons.[26]

With the advent of monoclonal antibodies and the depletion and deterioration of the available anti-D made by persons with partial-D genotype, Tippett and coworkers[27] pursued the classification of partial-D antigens using monoclonal anti-D (MAb-D). Table 7–8 presents a summary of the partial-D categories. Today the molecular basis of partial-D antigens has been determined.

Although understanding the difference between the genetic weak D, weak D caused by C trans, and the partial D helps explain why some persons with the weak-D phenotype develop anti-D and others do not, no differentiation in weak status is made in the routine blood bank. The donors and patients are classified simply as Rh-positive or Rh-negative. The anti-D made by individuals expressing partial D can cause HDN or transfusion reactions, or both. Once anti-D is identified, Rh-negative blood should be used for transfusion. The identification of a person with a partial-D gene routinely occurs after the person begins producing anti-D. This discovery should prompt collection of additional samples to be sent to a reference laboratory for $Rh_0(D)$ classification.

Determination of D Status

Determining the D status of an RBC sample is required when testing donor bloods. Blood for transfusion is considered Rh-positive if either the D or the weak-D test is positive. Any donor blood sample that is typed $Rh_0(D)$-negative by the slide or rapid tube method must be tested further by an indirect antihuman globulin technique. If both tests are negative, the donor sample is considered Rh-negative. If the donor sample tests positive in any phase of $Rh_0(D)$ testing, the sample is considered Rh-positive.

For transfusion recipients, the application of the test for weak D is controversial. Because blood recipients with the C trans weak D and those with the genetic weak D clearly have the complete D antigen and cannot produce alloanti-D, Rh-positive blood may be transfused. The very rare individuals with a partial-D phenotype can form alloanti-D when exposed to D-positive RBCs. However, many workers believe that the number of individuals homozygous for the partial-D gene is so low, the risk of sensitizing a partial-D individual so low, and the supply of Rh-negative blood so precious that an intended blood recipient who types weak D–positive should be given Rh-positive blood. Policy regarding transfusion of weak-D recipients is established individually within each transfusion service. Regulatory agencies do not require routine testing for weak D in blood recipients unless the intended recipient has, or in the past has had, anti-D in his or her serum.

Determining the $Rh_0(D)$ status (including weak-D status) of obstetric patients is critical. All Rh-negative, weak D–negative obstetric patients are candidates for Rh immune globulin (RhIg) (a drug injected to prevent Rh-negative individuals who are exposed to Rh-positive RBCs from developing anti-D). Likewise, when the mother is Rh-negative and the newborn is typed Rh-negative, the weak-D status of the newborn must be determined to assess the likelihood of maternal sensitization and the need for Rh immune globulin prophylaxis for the mother.

There are instances when an accurate Rh type cannot be determined through routine testing. If a newborn's cells are coated with maternal IgG anti-D in utero, very few D antigen sites are available to react with reagent anti-D (termed "blocking phenomena"). Elution of the sensitizing antibody (removing the antibody) and identifying it as anti-D will verify that the infant's RBCs are D-positive. Other complex Rh typing difficulties arise in persons suffering from warm autoimmune hemolytic anemia. Many of the antibodies produced in this

TABLE 7–8   Epitope Profiles of Partial D Antigens

	Reactions with Monoclonal Anti-D Antibodies							
Cells	epD1	epD2	epD3	epD4	epD5	epD6/7	epD8	epD9
I	+		+	0	+	+	+	0
IIIa	+	+	+	+	+	+	+	+
IIIb	+	+	+	+	+	+	+	+
IIIc	+	+	+	+	+	+	+	+
IVa	0	0	0	+	+	+	+	0
IVb	0	0	0	0	+	+	+	0
Va	0	+	+	+	0	+	+	+
VI	0	0	+	+	0	0	0	+
VII	+	+	+	+	+	+	0	+
DFR	:	:	+	+	:	:	0	+
DBT	0	0	0	0	0	:	+	0
R_0^{Har}	0	0	0	0	:	:	0	0

+ = positive reaction   0 = negative reaction   : = positive with some antibodies and negative with other antibodies.

disorder are directed against the patient's own RBCs and react as though they were Rh-specific. Resolution of these anomalies is beyond the scope of this chapter and frequently requires referral to reference laboratories for resolution or confirmation.

Detection of Rh Antibodies and Antigens

Rh Antibodies

Although the Rh system was first recognized by saline tests used to detect IgM antibodies, most Rh antibodies are IgG immunoglobulins and react optimally at 37°C or after antiglobulin testing. Rh antibodies are usually produced following exposure of the individual's immune system to foreign RBCs, through either transfusion or pregnancy. Rh antigens are highly immunogenic; the D antigen is the most potent.[28] A comparison of the immunogenicity of the common Rh antigens is described in **Figure 7–6**. Exposure to less than 0.1 mL of Rh-positive RBCs can stimulate antibody production in an Rh-negative person.

IgG_1, IgG_2, IgG_3, and IgG_4 subclasses of Rh antibodies have been reported. IgG_1 and IgG_3 are of the greatest clinical significance because the reticuloendothelial system rapidly clears RBCs coated with IgG_1 and IgG_3 from the circulation. IgA Rh antibodies have also been reported but are not routinely tested for in the blood bank.[25]

As with most blood group antigen sensitization, IgM Rh antibodies are formed initially, followed by a transition to IgG. Rh antibodies often persist in the circulation for years. An individual with low-titer Rh antibody may experience an anamnestic (secondary) antibody response if exposed to the same sensitizing antigen. Therefore, in the clinical setting, accuracy of D typing is essential, as is the careful checking of patient history to determine whether an Rh antibody has been identified previously. Most commonly found Rh antibodies are considered clinically significant. Therefore, antigen-negative blood must be provided to any patient with a history of Rh antibody sensitization, whether the antibody is currently demonstrable or not.

Rh antibodies do not bind complement. For complement to be fixed (or the complement cascade activated), two IgG immunoglobulins must attach to an RBC in close proximity. Rh antigens (to which the antibody would attach) are not situated on the RBC surface this closely. Therefore, when an Rh antibody coats the RBCs, intravascular, complement-mediated hemolysis does not occur. RBC destruction resulting from Rh antibodies is primarily extravascular.

Because Rh antibodies are primarily IgG and can traverse the placenta and because Rh antigens are well developed early in fetal life, Rh antibodies formed by Rh-negative pregnant women do cross the placenta and may coat fetal RBCs that carry the corresponding antigen. This results in the fetal cells testing positive by the direct antiglobulin test and in HDN, the coated fetal cells are removed prematurely from the fetal circulation (see Chapter 20). Until the discovery of Rh immune globulin, anti-D was the most frequent cause of HDN.

Rh Antigen Typing Reagents

The reagents used to type for D and for the other Rh antigens may be derived from a variety of sources. The reagents may be high-protein–based or low-protein–based, saline-based, chemically modified, monoclonal, or blends of monoclonals.

Saline reactive reagents, which contain IgM immunoglobulin, were the first typing reagents available to test for the D antigen. Saline anti-D has the advantage of being low-protein–based and can be used to test cells that are coated with IgG antibody. The primary disadvantages of saline typing reagents are their limited availability, cost of production, and lengthy incubation time. Because saline anti-D is an IgM immunoglobulin, it cannot be used for weak-D typing.

In the 1940s, high-protein anti-D reagents were developed. Human plasma containing high-titer D-specific antibody is used as the raw material. Potentiators of bovine albumin and macromolecular additives such as dextran or polyvinylpyrrolidone are added to the source material to optimize reactivity in the standard slide and rapid tube tests.[29] These reagents are commonly referred to as high-protein reagents. The presence of potentiators and the higher protein concentration, however, increase the likelihood of false-positive reactions. To assess the validity of the high-protein Rh typing results, a control reagent was manufactured and had to be tested in parallel with each Rh test. If the control reacted, the test result was invalid and had to be repeated using a different technique or reagent anti-D. The major advantages of high-protein anti-D reagents are reduced incubation time and the ability to perform weak-D testing and slide typing with the same reagent.

In the late 1970s, scientists chemically modified the IgG anti-D molecule by breaking the disulfide bonds that maintain the antibody's rigid shape.[30] This allows the antibody to relax and to span the distance between RBCs in a low-protein medium. The chemically modified reagents can be used for both slide and tube testing and do not require a separate, manufactured Rh control as long as the samples type as A, B, or O. When samples test AB Rh-positive or when the Rh test is performed by itself, a separate saline control must be used to ensure that the observed reactions are true agglutination and not a result of spontaneous agglutination. Fewer false-positive test reactions are obtained because of the lower-protein suspending medium. Because of its lower-protein base and ready availability, the chemically modified anti-D replaced the need for saline anti-D reagents.

Monoclonal antibody reagents have become available more recently. These reagents are derived from single clones of antibody-producing cells. The antibody-producing cells are hybridized with myeloma cells to increase their reproduction rate and thereby to maximize their antibody-producing capabilities. Because the D antigen appears to be a mosaic and the monoclonal Rh antibodies have a narrow specificity, monoclonal anti-D reagents are usually a combination of monoclonal anti-D reagents from several different clones to ensure reactivity with a broad spectrum of Rh-positive RBCs. Some companies also blend anti-IgM and anti-IgG anti-D to maximize visualization of reactions at immediate spin testing and

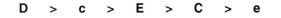

D > c > E > C > e

■ **FIGURE 7–6** Immunogenicity of common Rh antigens. (For a detailed discussion, refer to Mollison.[28])

to allow indirect antiglobulin testing for weak D with the same reagent. The monoclonal blends can be used for slide, tube, microwell, and most automated Rh testing. Because these reagents are not human-derived, they lack all potential for transmitting infectious disease.

As with all commercial typing reagents, Rh antigen typing must be performed with strict adherence to manufacturer's directions, use of proper controls, and accurate interpretation of test and control results. **Table 7–9** summarizes several common causes of false Rh typing results and suggests corrective actions that may be taken to obtain an accurate Rh type.

Clinical Considerations

Transfusion Reactions

Rh antigens are highly immunogenic. The D antigen is the most immunogenic antigen outside the ABO system. When anti-D is detected, a careful medical history will reveal RBC exposure through pregnancy or transfusion of products containing RBCs. Circulating antibody appears within 120 days of a primary exposure and within 2 to 7 days after a secondary exposure.

Rh-mediated hemolytic transfusion reactions, whether caused by primary sensitization or secondary immunization, usually result in extravascular destruction of immunoglobulin-coated RBCs. The transfusion recipient may have an unexplained fever, a mild bilirubin elevation, and a decrease in hemoglobin and haptoglobin. The direct antihuman globulin test is usually positive, and the antibody screen may or may not demonstrate circulating antibody. When the direct antiglobulin test indicates that the recipient's RBCs are coated with IgG, elution studies may be helpful in defining the offending antibody specificity. If antibody is detected in either the serum or eluate, subsequent transfusions should lack the implicated antigen. It is not unusual for a person with a single Rh antibody to produce additional Rh antibodies if further stimulated.[28]

Hemolytic Disease of the Newborn (HDN)

HDN is briefly described here because of the historic significance of the discovery of the Rh system in elucidating its cause. As stated previously, anti-D was discovered in a woman after delivery of a stillborn fetus. The mother required transfusion. The father's blood was transfused, and the mother subsequently experienced a severe hemolytic transfusion reaction. Levine and Stetson[1] postulated that the antibody causing the transfusion reaction also crossed the placenta and destroyed the RBCs of the fetus, causing its death. The offending antibody was subsequently identified as anti-D.[3]

HDN caused by Rh antibodies is often severe because the Rh antigens are well developed on fetal cells, and Rh antibodies are primarily IgG, which readily cross the placenta.

After years of research, a method was developed to prevent susceptible (Rh_0 D-negative) mothers from forming anti-D, thus preventing $Rh_0(D)$ HDN. Rh-immune globulin, a purified preparation of IgG anti-D, is given to a D-negative woman during pregnancy and following delivery of a D-positive fetus.[31] Rh-immune globulin is effective only in preventing anti-D HDN. No effort has been made to develop immune globulin products for other Rh antigens (e.g., C, c, E, e). When present, Rh HDN may be severe and may require aggressive treatment. Refer to Chapter 20 for a more detailed discussion of HDN—its etiology, serology, and treatment.

Rh Deficiency Syndrome: Rh_{null} and Rh_{mod}

It is the rare individual who fails to express any Rh antigens on the RBC surface or exhibits a severely reduced expression

TABLE 7–9 False Reactions with Rh Typing Reagents

False-Positives		False-Negatives	
Likely Cause	**Corrective Action**	**Likely Cause**	**Corrective Action**
1. Cell suspension too heavy	1. Adjust suspension, retype	1. Immunoglobulin-coated cells (in vivo)	1. Use saline-active typing reagent
2. Cold agglutinins	2. Wash with warm saline, retype	2. Saline-suspended cells (slide)	2. Use unwashed cells
3. Test incubated too long or drying (slide)	3. Follow manufacturer's instructions precisely	3. Failure to follow manufacturer's directions precisely	3. Review directions; repeat test
4. Rouleaux	4. Use saline-washed cells, retype	4. Omission of reagent manufacturer's directions	4. Always add reagent first and check before adding cells
5. Fibrin interference	5. Use saline-washed cells, retype	5. Resuspension too vigorous	5. Resuspend all tube tests gently
6. Contaminating low-incidence antibody in reagent	6. Try another manufacturer's reagent or use a known serum antibody	6. Incorrect reagent selected	6. Read vial label carefully; repeat
7. Polyagglutination	7. See chapter on polyagglutination	7. Variant antigen	7. Refer sample for further investigation
8. Bacterial contamination of reagent vial	8. Open new vial of reagent, retype	8. Reagent deterioration	8. Open new vial
9. Incorrect reagent selected	9. Repeat test; read vial label carefully		

of all Rh antigens. The individuals who lack all Rh antigens on their RBCs are said to have the Rh$_{null}$ syndrome, which can be produced by two different genetic mechanisms.[26]

In the regulator-type Rh$_{null}$ syndrome, there is a mutation in the *RHAG* gene. This results in no Rh polypeptides or RHAG antigen expression on the RBCs, even though these individuals usually have a normal complement of *RHD* and *RHCE* genes. These individuals can pass the normal *RHD* and *RHCE* genes to their children.

In the second type of Rh$_{null}$ syndrome (the amorphic type), there is a mutation in each of the *RHCE* genes and a deletion of the *RHD* gene. The *RHAG* gene is normal.

Individuals with the Rh$_{null}$ syndrome demonstrate a mild compensated hemolytic anemia,[32] reticulocytosis, stomatocytosis, a slight-to-moderate decrease in hemoglobin and hematocrit levels, an increase in hemoglobin F, a decrease in serum haptoglobin, and possibly an elevated bilirubin level. The severity of the syndrome is highly variable from individual to individual, even within one family. When transfusion of individuals with Rh$_{null}$ syndrome is necessary, only Rh$_{null}$ blood can be given.

Individuals of the Rh$_{mod}$ phenotype have a partial suppression of Rh gene expression and exhibit features similar to those with the Rh$_{null}$ syndrome; however, the clinical symptoms are usually less severe and rarely clinically remarkable.[33] RBCs classified as Rh$_{mod}$ do not completely lack Rh or LW antigens. Rh$_{null}$ and Rh$_{mod}$ RBCs exhibit other blood group antigens; however, S, s, and U antigen expression may be depressed.[34] Rh$_{null}$ RBCs are negative for FY5.

Unusual Phenotypes and Rare Alleles

Some of the less frequently encountered Rh antigens are discussed briefly in the following paragraphs. Refer to other textbooks for in-depth discussions.[15,16]

C^w

C^w was originally considered an allele at the *C/c* locus.[35] Later studies showed that it can be expressed in combination with both *C* and *c* and in the absence of either allele. It is now known that the relationship between C/c and C^w is only phenotypic and that C^w is antithetical to the high-incidence antigen MAR.[36] C^w is found in about 2 percent of whites and is very rare in blacks. Anti-C^w has been identified in individuals without known exposure to foreign RBCs as well as after transfusion or pregnancy. Anti-C^w may show dosage (i.e., reacting more strongly with cells from individuals who are homozygous for C^w). Because of the low incidence of C^w, C^w antigen–negative blood is readily available.

f (ce)

The f antigen is expressed on the RBC when both *c* and *e* are present on the same haplotype (i.e., cis position); it has been called a *compound* antigen.[37] However, f is a single entity. Phenotypically, the following samples appear the same when tested with the five major Rh antisera: *Dce/DCE* and *DcE/DCe*. However, when tested with anti-f, only the former reacts. Anti-f has been reported to cause HDN and transfusion reactions.

rh$_i$ (Ce)

Similar to f, rh$_i$ is present when *C* and *e* are in the cis configuration, has been called a compound antigen, and is a single entity.[37] A sample with the phenotype D + C + E + c + e + can be either *DcE/DCe* or *Dce/DCE*. Anti-rh$_i$ reacts only with *Dce/DCe* RBCs.

G

G is an antigen that is present on most D-positive and all C-positive RBCs. In the test tube, anti-G reacts as though it were a combination of anti-C plus anti-D.[38] G was originally described in an rr person who received Dccee RBCs. Subsequently, the recipient produced an antibody that appeared to be anti-D plus anti-C, which should be impossible because the C antigen was not on the transfused RBCs. Further investigation showed that the antibody was directed toward D + G.

Rh:13, Rh:14, Rh:15, Rh:16

Rh:13, Rh:14, Rh:15, and Rh:16 define four different parts of the D mosaic, as it was originally described. Although these parts are included in the partial-D categories II to VII as defined by Tippett and Sanger,[25,27] they are not directly comparable.

Hr$_0$

Hr$_0$ is an antigen present on all RBCs with the "common" Rh phenotypes (e.g., R$_1$R$_1$, R$_2$R$_2$, rr).[40] When RBCs phenotype as D--, the most potent antibody they make is often one directed against Hr$_0$.

Rh:23, Rh:30, Rh:40

Rh:23, Rh:30, and Rh:40 are all low-frequency antigens associated with a specific category of partial-D. Rh:23 (also known as Wiel and D^w) is an antigenic marker for category Va partial-D.[41] Rh:30 (also known as Go^a or D^{cor}) is a marker for category IVa partial-D.[42] Rh:40 (also known as Tar or Targett) is a marker for category VII.[43]

Rh:33

The low-incidence antigen Rh:33 is associated with a rare variant of the $R^0(Dce)$ gene called R_0^{Har}.[44] R_0^{Har} gene codes for normal amounts of c, reduced amounts of e, reduced f, reduced Hr$_0$, and reduced amounts of D antigen. The D reactions are frequently so weak that the cells are frequently mistakenly typed as Rh negative. To denote the weakened expression of an antigen in Fisher-Race nomenclature the letter is placed in parentheses. The R_0^{Har} gene expresses (D)c(e) and has been found in whites.

Rh:32

Rh:32 is a low-frequency antigen associated with a variant of the $R^1[D(C)(e)]$ gene that is called $\overline{\overline{R}}^N$.[45] The C antigen and e antigen are expressed weakly. The D antigen expression is exaggerated or exalted. This gene has been found primarily in blacks.

e Variants

It appears, especially in the black population, that the e antigen may exhibit the same mosaic quality described for D. Because of these variations, e typings can be unreliable.[17,46]

Among the variants at the e locus are hr^S, hr^B, and $VS(e^s)$, with a variant R^0 or r gene making e plus one or the other of these pieces. Such variants are usually recognized when they make antibodies that behave as anti-e, even though their RBCs type as e-positive with routine Rh typing reagents.

V, VS

The $V(ce^S)$ antigen is found in about 30 percent of randomly selected American blacks. In selected individuals, it appears to be the serologic counterpart of f because it is present when c is cis with e^S.[47] (The $VS(e^s)$ antigen is also relatively common in blacks with the VS antibody, reacting with all V-positive RBCs and additionally with $r's$ RBCs.[48]) Although the relationship of V to VS remains somewhat less than clear, both are markers associated with the black population.

Deletions

There are very uncommon phenotypes that demonstrate no Cc and/or Ee reactivity. Many examples lacking all Cc or Ee often have an unusually strong D antigen expression, frequently called exalted D. The deletion phenotype is indicated by the use of a dash (–), as in the following examples: DC–, Dc–, D–E, D––. The antibody made by D–– people is called anti–Rh 17 or anti-Hr$_0$.

A variation has been recognized within the deletion D––, called D••. The D antigen in the D•• is stronger than that in DC–, D–E, Dc–, or D–e samples but weaker than that of D–– samples. A low-incidence antigen called Evans (Rh:37) accompanies the Rh structure of D•• cells.[49]

Transfusion of individuals with a Rh deletion or D•• phenotype is difficult if multiple antibodies are present; blood of a similar phenotype would be required.

THE LW ANTIGEN

A discussion of the LW antigen begins with the time when Rh antigens were first recognized. The antibody produced by injecting rhesus monkey RBCs into guinea pigs and rabbits was identified as having the same specificity as the antibody Levine and Stetson[1] described earlier. The antibody was given the name anti-Rh, for anti-rhesus, and the blood group system was established. Many years later, it was recognized that the two antibodies were not identical; the anti-rhesus described by Landsteiner and Wiener[2] was renamed anti-LW in their honor.

Phenotypically, there is a similarity between the Rh and LW systems. Anti-LW reacts strongly with most D-positive RBCs, weakly (sometimes not at all) with Rh-negative RBCs, and never with Rh$_{null}$ cells. The independent segregation of LW from the Rh blood group genes was established by a family study on a D-positive LW-negative woman; other family studies support this point.[45,50]

The nomenclature describing the various expressions of the LW antigen has evolved.[51] An excellent description of this is found in other reference texts.[46]

There are three alleles at the LW locus: LW^a, LW^b, and LW

TABLE 7–10 LW Phenotypes and Genotypes

Phenotype	Genotype
LW(a+b−)	LW^a LW^a or LW^a LW
LW(a+b+)	LW^a LW^b
LW(a−b+)	LW^b LW^b or LW^b LW
LW(a−b−)	LW LW

Sistonen and Tippett, p 252, with permission.
Note: Rh$_{null}$ individuals are phenotypically LW(a−b−) because of the genetic mechanism causing the Rh$_{null}$ status. The LW genotype of Rh$_{null}$ may be determined by family studies.

(a silent allele). Persons lacking LW antigen altogether are LW/LW and express no LW on the RBCs. **Table 7–10** is a summary of LW phenotypes and genotypes. LW^a is very common, and LW^b is rare. When the Rh$_{null}$ is present due to the suppression mechanism, the Rh and LW genes are not expressed on the RBC; however, the Rh and LW genes are normal and, when passed to offspring, can be expressed normally. The amorphic Rh$_{null}$ individual inherits the $\overline{\overline{rr}}$ genes, which do not express Rh antigens; therefore, LW genes cannot be expressed.

Anti-LW usually reacts more strongly with D-positive RBCs than with D-negative adult RBCs. A weak anti-LW may react only with D-positive RBCs, and enhancement techniques may be required to demonstrate its reactivity with D-negative cells. Anti-LW reacts equally well with cord cells regardless of their D type.[15] This is an important characteristic to remember when trying to differentiate anti-LW from anti-D. Also, anti-LW more frequently appears as an autoantibody, which does not present clinical problems.

Because of the complexity of the Rh blood group system, a tremendous amount of literature exists. The inquisitive reader can continue to piece together the puzzle by consulting the sources included in the references.

SUMMARY CHART:
Important Points to Remember (MT/MLT)

➤ The Rh antibody was so named on the basis of antibody production by guinea pigs and rabbits when transfused with rhesus monkey RBCs.

➤ Historically, Rh was a primary cause of HDN, erythroblastosis fetalis, and a significant cause of hemolytic transfusion reactions.

➤ Fisher-Race DCE terminology is based on the theory that antigens of the system are produced by three closely linked sets of alleles and that each gene is responsible for producing a product (or antigen) on the RBC surface.

➤ A person who expresses no Rh antigens on the RBC is said to be Rh$_{null}$, and the phenotype may be written as ——/——.

➤ In the Wiener Rh-Hr nomenclature, it is postulated that the gene responsible for defining Rh actually produces an agglutinogen that contains a series of blood factors, in which each factor is an antigen recognized by an antibody.

➤ It is currently accepted that two closely linked genes control the expression of Rh; one gene (RHD) codes for the presence or absence of D, and a second gene (RHCE) codes for the expression of CcEe antigens.

➤ In the Rosenfield alpha/numeric terminology, a number is assigned to each antigen of the Rh system in order of its discovery (Rh1 = D, Rh2 = C, Rh3 = E, Rh4 = c, Rh5 = e).

➤ Rh antigens are characterized as nonglycosylated proteins in the RBC membrane.

➤ The most common genotype in whites is R^1r (31%); the most common genotype in blacks is R^0r (23%), followed by R^0R^0 at 19%.

➤ The Rh antigens are inherited as codominant alleles.

➤ A partial-D individual is characterized as lacking one or more pieces or epitopes of the total D antigen and may produce alloantibody to the missing fraction if exposed to RBCs with the complete D antigen.

➤ Blood for transfusion is considered Rh-positive if either the D or weak-D test is positive; if both the D and weak-D tests are negative, blood for transfusion is considered Rh-negative.

➤ Most Rh antibodies are IgG immunoglobulins and react optimally at 37°C or following antiglobulin testing; exposure to less than 0.1 mL of Rh-positive RBCs can stimulate antibody production in an Rh-negative person.

➤ Rh-mediated hemolytic transfusion reactions usually result in extravascular hemolysis.

➤ Rh antibodies are IgG and can cross the placenta to coat fetal (Rh-positive) RBCs.

REVIEW QUESTIONS

1. The Rh system was first recognized in a case report about what disorder?
   a. A hemolytic transfusion reaction
   b. Hemolytic disease of the newborn
   c. Circulatory overload
   d. Autoimmune hemolytic anemia

2. What antigen is found in 85% of the white population and is always significant for transfusion purposes?
   a. d
   b. c
   c. D
   d. E
   e. e

3. How are weaker-than-expected reactions with anti-D typing reagents categorized?
   a. Rh_{mod}
   b. Partial D
   c. DAT positive
   d. D^w

4. Cells carrying a weak-D antigen require the use of what test to demonstrate its presence?
   a. Indirect antiglobulin test
   b. Direct antiglobulin test
   c. Microplate test
   d. Warm auto-absorption test

5. How are Rh antigens inherited?
   a. Autosomal recessive alleles
   b. Sex-linked genes
   c. Codominant alleles
   d. X-linked

6. Biochemically speaking, what type of molecules are Rh antigens?
   a. Glycophorins
   b. Simple sugars
   c. Proteins
   d. Lipids

7. Rh antibodies react best at what temperature (°C)?
   a. 22
   b. 18
   c. 15
   d. 37

8. Rh antibodies are primarily of which immunoglobulin class?
   a. IgA
   b. IgM
   c. IgG
   d. IgD
   e. IgE

9. Rh antibodies have been associated with which of the following clinical conditions?
   a. Erythroblastosis fetalis
   b. Thrombocytopenia
   c. Hemolytic transfusion reactions
   d. Hemophilia A
   e. Both A and C

10. What do Rh_{null} cells lack?
    a. Lewis antigens
    b. Normal oxygen-carrying capacity
    c. Rh antigens
    d. MNSs antigens

11. What antigen system is closely associated phenotypically with Rh?
    a. McCoy
    b. Lutheran
    c. Duffy
    d. LW

12. Anti-LW will not react with which of the following?
    a. Rh-positive RBCs
    b. Rh-negative RBCs
    c. Rh_{null} RBCs
    d. Rh:33 RBCs

13. Convert the following genotypes from Wiener nomenclature to Fisher-Race and Rosenfield nomenclatures, and list the antigens present in each haplotype.
    a. R_1r
    b. R_2R_0

c. R_zR_1

d. r^yr

14. Which Rh phenotype has the strongest expression of D?

a. R_1r

b. R_1R_2

c. R_2r

d. R_2R_2

e. D--

REFERENCES

1. Levine, P, and Stetson, RE: An unusual case of intragroup agglutination. JAMA 113:126, 1939.
2. Landsteiner, K, and Wiener, AS: An agglutinable factor in human blood recognized by immune sera for rhesus blood. Proc Soc Exp Biol (NY) 43:223, 1940.
3. Levine, P, et al: The role of isoimmunization in the pathogenesis of erythroblastosis fetalis. Am J Obstet Gynecol 42:925, 1941.
4. Race, RR, et al: Recognition of a further common Rh genotype in man. Nature 153:52, 1944.
5. Mourant, AE: A new rhesus antibody. Nature 155:542, 1945.
6. Stratton, F: A new Rh allelomorph. Nature 158:25, 1946.
7. Levine, P: On Hr factor and Rh genetic theory. Science 102:1, 1945.
8. Race, RR: The Rh genotypes and Fisher's theory. Blood 3 (Suppl 2): 27, 1948.
9. Widmann, FK (ed): Technical Manual of the American Association of Blood Banks, ed 9. American Association of Blood Banks, Arlington, VA, 1985.
10. Wiener, AS: Genetic theory of the Rh blood types. Proc Soc Exp Biol (NY) 54:316, 1943.
11. Rosenfield, RE, et al: A review of Rh serology and presentation of a new terminology. Transfusion 2:287, 1962.
12. Lewis, M: Blood group terminology 1990. Vox Sang 58:152, 1990.
13. Hughes-Jones, NC, Gardner, B, and Lincoln, PJ: Observations of the number of available c, D, and E antigen sites on red cells. Vox Sang 21:210, 1971.
14. Tippett, PA: A speculative model for the Rh blood groups. Ann Hum Genet 50:241, 1986.
15. Race, RR, and Sanger, R: Blood Groups in Man, ed 6. Blackwell Scientific, Oxford, 1975.
16. Issitt, PD: Serology and Genetics of the Rh Blood Group System. Montgomery Scientific Publications, Cincinnati, 1985.
17. Vengelen-Tyler, V (ed): Technical Manual, ed 12. American Association of Blood Banks, Bethesda, MD, 1996.
18. Wagner, FF, et al: Molecular basis of weak D phenotype. Blood 93:385–393, 1999.
19. Race, RR, Sanger, R, and Lawler, SD: The Rh antigen Du. Ann Eugen Lond 14:171, 1948.
20. Capellini, R, Dunn, LC, and Turri, M: An interaction between alleles at the Rh locus in man which weakens the reactivity of the Rh₀ factor (D₀). Proc Natl Acad Sci 41:283, 1955.
21. Tippett, P, Lomas-Francis, C, and Wallace, M: The Rh antigen D: Partial D antigens and associated low incidence antigens. Vox Sang 70:123–131, 1996.
22. Shapiro, M: The ABO, MN, P and Rh blood group systems in South African Bantu: A genetic study. South Afr Med J 25:187, 1951.
23. Argall, CI, Ball, JM, and Trentelman, E: Presence of anti-D antibody in the serum of Du patient. J Clin Lab Med 41:895, 1953.
24. Wiener, AS, and Unger, LJ: Rh factors related to the Rh₀ factor as a source of clinical problems. JAMA 169:696, 1959.
25. Tippett, P, and Sanger, R: Observations on subdivisions of the Rh antigen D. Vox Sang 7:9, 1962.
26. Huang, CH, Liu, P and Cheng, JG: Molecular biology and genetics of the Rh blood group system. Semin Hematol 37:150–165, 2000.
27. Tippett, P, Lomas-Francis, C, and Wallace, M. The Rh antigen D: Partial D antigens and associated low incidence antigens. Vox Sang 70:123–131, 1996.
28. Mollison, PL: Blood Transfusion in Clinical Medicine, ed 6. Blackwell Scientific Publications, Oxford, 1988.
29. Diamond, LK, and Denton, RC: Rh agglutination in various media with particular reference to the value of albumin. J Clin Lab Med 30:821, 1945.
30. Romans, DG, et al: Conversion of incomplete antibodies to direct agglutinins by mild reduction. Proc Natl Acad Sci USA 74:2531, 1977.
31. Queenan, JT: Modern Management of the Rh Problem, ed 2. Harper & Row, New York, 1977.
32. Schmidt, PJ, and Vos, GH: Multiple phenotypic abnormalities associated with Rhnull (—/—). Vox Sang 13:18, 1967.
33. Chown, B, et al: An unlinked modifier of Rh blood groups: Effects when heterozygous and when homozygous. Am J Hum Genet 24:623, 1972.
34. Schmidt, PJ, et al: Aberrant U blood group accompany Rh$_{null}$. Transfusion 7:33, 1967.
35. Callendar, ST, and Race, RR: A serological and genetic study of multiple antibodies formed in response to blood transfusion by a patient with lupus erythematosus diffuses. Ann Eugen Lond 13:102, 1946.
36. Sistonen, P, et al: MAR, a novel high-incidence Rh antigen revealing the existence of an allele sub-system including Cʷ (Rh8) and Cˣ (Rh9) with exceptional distribution in the Finnish population. Vox Sang 66:287–292, 1994.
37. Rosenfield, RE, and Haber, GV: An Rh blood factor, Rh1 (Ce) and its relationship to hr (ce). Am J Hum Genet 10:474, 1958.
38. Allen, FH, and Tippett, PA: A new Rh blood type which reveals the Rh antigen G. Vox Sang 3:321, 1958.
39. Wiener, AS, and Unger, LJ: Further observations on the blood factors RhA, RhB, RhC, RhD. Transfusion 2:230, 1962.
40. Allen, FH, Jr, and Corcoran, PA: Proc 11th Ann Mtg. AABB, Cincinnati, Abstract, 1958.
41. Chown, B, et al: The Rh antigen Dw (Wiel). Transfusion 4:169, 1964.
42. Lewis, M, et al: Blood group antigen Goa and the Rh system. Transfusion 7:440, 1967.
43. Lewis, M, et al: Assignment of the red cell antigen Targett (Rh 40) to the Rh blood group systems. Am J Hum Genet 31:630, 1979.
44. Giles, CM, et al: An Rh gene complex which results in a "new" antigen detectable by a specific antibody, anti-Rh 33. Vox Sang 21:289, 1971.
45. Rosenfield, RE, et al: Problems in Rh typing as revealed by a single Negro family. Am J Hum Genet 12:147, 1960.
46. Issitt, PD: Applied Blood Group Serology, ed 3. Montgomery Scientific Publication, Miami, FL, 1985.
47. DeNatale, A, et al: A "new" Rh antigen, common in Negroes, rare in white people. JAMA 159:247, 1955.
48. Sanger, R, et al: An Rh antibody specific for V and Rs. Nature (Lond) 186:171, 1960.
49. Contreras, M, et al: The Rh antigen Evans. Vox Sang 34:208, 1978.
50. Vos, GH, et al: A sample of blood with no detectable Rh antigens. Lancet i:14, 1961.
51. Sistonen, P, and Tippett, P: A "new" allele giving further insight into the LW blood group system. Vox Sang 42:252, 1982.

eight

The Lewis System and the Biological Significance

**Denise M. Harmening, PhD, MT (ASCP), CLS (NCA), and
Mitra Taghizadeh, MS, MT (ASCP)**

OBJECTIVES

On completion of this chapter, the learner should be able to:

1. Describe the formation and secretion of Lewis antigens and their adsorption onto the red cells.
2. Discuss the inheritance of the Lewis genes and their interactions with the other blood group genes.
3. List substances present in secretions and the Lewis phenotypes based on a given genotype.
4. Define the role of secretor genes in formation of Lewis antigens.
5. List the Lewis phenotypes and their frequencies in the white and black populations.
6. Indicate the process of development of the Lewis antigens after birth.
7. Describe the changes in the Lewis phenotypes during pregnancy.
8. List the characteristics of the Lewis antigens.
9. List the characteristics of the Lewis antibodies.
10. Discuss the significance of Lewis antibodies.
11. Discuss the biologic significance of the Lewis antigens.

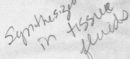

Introduction

The Lewis blood group system is unique in that it is believed to be the only system that is not manufactured by the red blood cell (RBC). Lewis antigens are not synthesized by the RBCs and incorporated into the RBC membrane structure. Instead, these antigens are manufactured by tissue cells and secreted into body fluids. These antigens, therefore, have been referred to as a system rather than as a blood group because they are found primarily in the secretions and the plasma. These antigens are then adsorbed onto the RBC membrane from plasma, but they are not really an integral part of the membrane structure. <u>Because Lewis-soluble antigens are manufactured by tissue cells, antigen production depends not only on the inheritance of Lewis genes but also on the inheritance of the secretor gene.</u> Genetic interaction also exists between the Lewis and *ABO* genes because the amount of Lewis antigen detectable on the RBC is influenced by the *ABO* genes inherited.

This chapter is divided into basic concepts and advanced concepts. Students at MT and MLT levels should focus on understanding the topics marked by asterisks in the chapter outline above. Additional concepts are included for advanced learning.

Inheritance

Similar to *ABO* genes, Lewis genes (*Le*) do not code for the production of Lewis antigens but rather produce a specific glycosyltransferase, L-fucosyltransferase. This enzyme adds L-fucose to the basic precursor substance. The *Le* gene is located on the short arm of chromosome 19 and is <u>distantly linked to *Se* and *H* genes</u>, which are located on the same chromosome.[1,2] In whites, 90 percent of the population possesses *Le* gene. This gene codes for a specific glycosyltransferase, α-4-L-fucosyltransferase, which transfers L-fucose to type 1 chain oligosaccharide on glycoprotein or glycolipid structures. Type 1 chain refers to the beta linkage of the number 1 carbon of galactose to the number 3 carbon of *N*-acetylglucosamine (GlcNAc) residue of the precursor structure **(Fig. 8–1)**. The inheritance of the *Le* gene acts in competition with ABO genes, adding L-fucose to the GlcNAc sugar of the common precursor structure manufactured by tissue cells **(Fig. 8–2)**. The structure formed is known as Le^a-soluble antigen. It is then secreted and adsorbed onto the RBCs, lymphocytes, and platelet membranes from plasma.[1,3] Lewis antigen is also found on other tissues, such as the pancreas, stomach, intestine, skeletal muscle, renal cortex, and adrenal glands.[3] In the addition of L-fucose to type 1 chain catalyzed by Lewis enzyme, the number 1 carbon of L-fucose is attached to the number 4 carbon of GlcNAc. This transfer reaction can occur only in type 1 precursor structures. Addition of L-fucose cannot occur with type 2 precursor structures because, in type 2 structures, the number 4 carbon of GlcNAc is already linked to galactose (see **Fig. 8–1**).

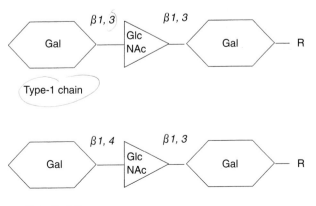

■ FIGURE 8–1   Structure of type-1 and type-2 chains. Gal = D-galactose; GlcNAc= *N*-acetyl-D-glucosamine; R = other biochemical residues.

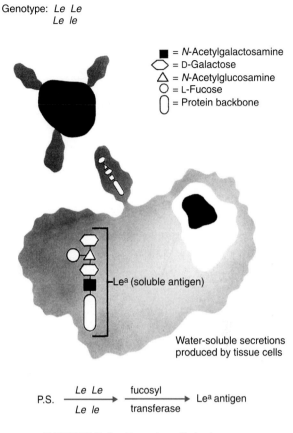

Genotype: *Le Le*
          Le le

■ = *N*-Acetylgalactosamine
◇ = D-Galactose
△ = *N*-Acetylglucosamine
○ = L-Fucose
▯ = Protein backbone

Le^a (soluble antigen)

Water-soluble secretions produced by tissue cells

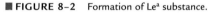

$$\text{P.S.} \xrightarrow[\text{\small *Le le*}]{\text{\small *Le Le*}} \xrightarrow[\text{transferase}]{\text{fucosyl}} \text{Le}^a \text{ antigen}$$

■ FIGURE 8–2   Formation of Le^a substance.

Basic Concepts: The Lewis (Le) Phenotypes

The Lewis (a+b−) Phenotype: Nonsecretors (LE1-007.001)

Le^a substance is secreted regardless of the secretor status. The term "secretor" refers only to the presence of water-soluble ABH antigen substances in the body fluids, which are influenced by the independently inherited secretor genes *Se* and *se* (for a review of secretors, see Chapter 6). <u>Therefore, an individual can be a nonsecretor (*sese*) of ABH and still secrete Le^a into the body fluids, producing the phenotype Lewis a-positive b-negative on the RBCs. This is written Le (a+b−). All Le (a+b−) individuals are nonsecretors of ABH substances.</u>[4] Lewis enzyme has been detected in saliva, milk, submaxillary glands, gastric mucosa, and kidney and cyst fluids.[5] Lewis fucosyltransferase has not been detected in plasma or in RBC stroma. Lewis antigens produced in saliva and other secretions are glycoproteins, but Lewis cell-bound antigens absorbed from plasma onto the RBC membranes are glycolipids. The phenotype Lewis a results from the transfer of fucose to a type 1 chain by the action of enzyme L-fucosyl transferase.[2] Formation of Le^a from the type 1 precursor structure is depicted in **Figures 8–3 and 8–4**.

The Lewis (a−b+) Phenotype: Secretors (LE2-007.002)

The genetically independent *Sese*, *ABO*, *Hh*, and Lewis genes are intimately associated in the formation of the Le^b antigen.

Le^a secreted independently of the Se gene

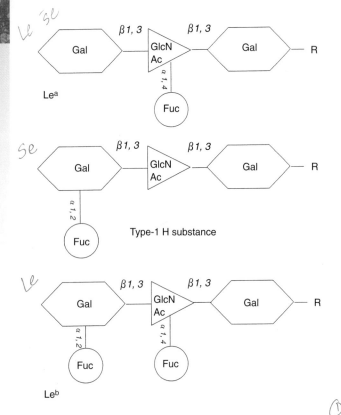

(handwritten margin notes:) Le 'Se', Se, Le

■ **FIGURE 8–3** Action of Le gene transferase enzyme. Le^a = gene codes for L-fucosyltransferase, which adds L-fucose (FUC) to the carbon number 4 of *N*-acetylglucosamine of type-1 precursor structure. Type-1 H substance = *Se* gene codes for L-fucosyl transferase, which adds L-fucose to the carbon number 2 of terminal galactose. Le^b = in the presence of Le, Se, a second fucose is added to the carbon number 4 of the subterminal *N*-acetylglucosamine of type-1 H substance. Gal = D-galactose; GlcNAc = *N*-acetyl-*D*-glucosamine; Fuc = L-fucose; R = other biochemical residues.

Le^a and Le^b are not alleles. The phenotype Le (a−b+) is the result of the genetic interaction of *Lele* and *Sese* genes. Le^b antigen represents the product of genetic interaction between *Le(FUT3)* and *Se(FUT2)* genes.[6] The *Se* gene does not control the expression of the *H* gene. Lewis and secretor genes are two independent genes that code for different but related α-2-L-fucosyltransferases.[1,7] The inheritance of the *Se* gene codes for the enzyme α-2-L-fucosyltransferase, which adds L-fucose to type 1 precursor substance and thus forms type 1 H.[2,6] The inheritance of the *Le* gene codes for the addition of another L-fucose that is added to the subterminal *N*-acetylglucosamine and thus forms Le^b antigen[2,6] (see **Figs. 8–3** and **8–4**; **Fig. 8–5**). Some precursor chains are not acted on by the Se fucosyltransferase but may accept L-fucose from the Lewis fucosyltranferase forming Le^a (see **Fig. 8–2**). Therefore, both Le^a-soluble and Le^b-soluble antigens can be found in the secretions. However, only Le^b adsorbs onto the RBC from plasma.[6] This is probably because higher concentrations of Le^b in plasma allow Le^b-soluble antigen to compete more successfully for sites of adsorption onto the RBC membrane. As a result, the RBCs of these individuals always phenotype as Le(a−b+), even though both Le^a- and Le^b-soluble antigens are present in the secretions and plasma. In secretors, biochemical studies indicate that Le and Se fucosyltransferases compete for the type 1 chain precursor.[8] Se glycosyltrans-

(handwritten margin note:) With a Se Le^a is found in secretins but only Le^b on RBCs

ferase catalyzes the synthesis of H on type 1 chain precursor structures. The respective amounts of Le^a and type 1 H substances formed in secretions are determined by the ratio of these two fucosyltransferases. In nonsecretors (*sese*), only Le^a antigens are formed in secretions, inasmuch as no Se enzyme is present in secretory cells. As a result, all type 1 chain precursor glycoproteins are available for the Le enzyme α-4-L-fucosyltransferase. The *H* gene functions by adding L-fucose to D-galactose of the type 2 chain on the RBC membrane paragloboside structure, forming the H antigen as described for formation of ABH antigens (see Chapter 6). Therefore, only Le^a antigen is secreted by the tissue cells and subsequently adsorbed onto the erythrocyte from plasma, yielding the phenotype Le(a+b−). Lewis antigens have also been detected on the surface of platelets and lymphocytes, regardless of the secretor status, but not on the surface of granulocytes or monocytes.[1,9,10]

The Lewis (a−b−) Phenotype: Secretors or Nonsecretors

A third type of RBC phenotype is the Lewis a-negative b-negative, written Le(a−b−) **(Fig. 8–6)**. The lack of the Lewis antigens on the RBCs of this group is not caused by the absence of the Lewis gene (*FUT3*) but rather by specific point mutations in the *Le* gene. These mutations give rise to a nonfunctional or partially active Lewis transferase (Le^w) causing the negative expression of the Lewis antigen on the RBCs.[7,11,12] According to this finding, the Lewis antigen is absent only on the RBCs tested serologically with the Lewis antisera; however, the Lewis antigen (less than 5 percent compared with that made by the Lewis-positive individuals)[1] is present in the tissues and secretions of the Le(a−b−) secretors.[7,11] The main substances found in the secretions of Le(a−b−) individuals depend on the secretor status and the ABO genotype of the person. The Le(a−b−) nonsecretors express type 1 precursor, whereas the Le(a−b−) secretors express H type 1 substances plus ABH antigens associated with the related ABO genes inherited.

The *lele* genotype is much more common in blacks than in whites. The frequencies of these Lewis RBC phenotypes in the white population are as follows: Le(a−b+), 72 percent; Le(a+b−), 22 percent; and Le(a−b−), 6 percent. In the black population, the frequencies are Le(a−b+), 55 percent; Le(a+b−), 23 percent; and Le(a−b−), 22 percent **(Table 8–1)**. All Le(a−b+) individuals are ABH secretors and also secrete Le^a and Le^b. All Le(a+b−) individuals are ABH nonsecretors, yet all secrete Le^a. It is no surprise, then, that the frequencies of these Lewis phenotypes parallel the frequency of the secretor gene. Approximately 78 to 80 percent of whites are secretors, and 20 percent are nonsecretors. In terms of Le(a−b−) individuals, 80 percent are ABH secretors, and 20 percent ABH nonsecretors. The antigen expressed by Le(a−b−) secretors is type 1 H (Le^d) substance, whereas the antigen expressed by Le(a−b−) nonsecretors is type 1 precursor substance (Le^c)[1] (see **Figs. 8–1, 8–3,** and **8–6**).

Advanced Concepts: Biochemistry of Lewis Antigens

The Lewis antigens or substances found in the secretions are glycoproteins, as are the ABH substances from secretors. The glycoproteins are composed of 80 percent carbohydrates and

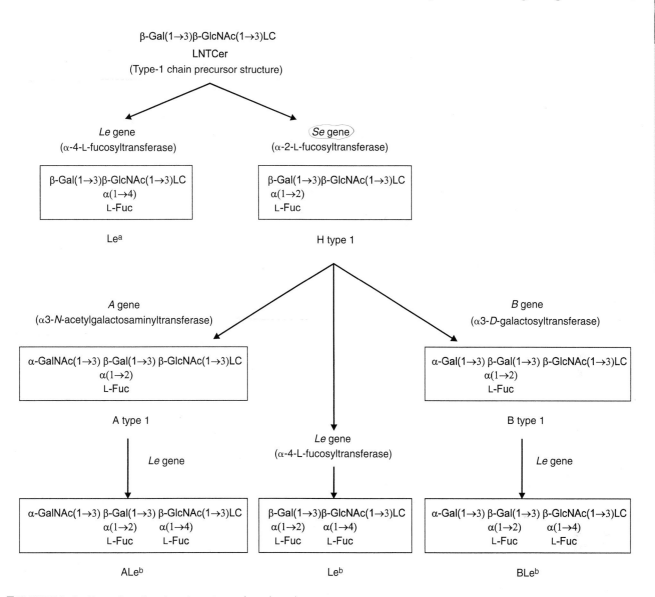

■ FIGURE 8–4 Formation of Lewis antigens (Le^a, Le^b, ALe^b, BLe^b) adsorbed from plasma. LC (lactosylceramide) = β-Gal (1→4) β-Glc(1→1) Cer; LNTCer = lacto-N-tetraosylceramide; Gal = galactose; GlcNAc = N-acetylglucosamine; Fuc = fucose; GalNAc = N-acetylgalactosamine.

15 percent amino acids.[13] In plasma, Lewis antigens are gly-colipids (glycosphingolipids).[2] These antigens are carried by lipoproteins present in plasma that adhere to RBC membranes, forming glycosylceramides. All of the Lewis antigens found on RBCs have been absorbed from plasma. The exact site for the synthesis of Lewis glycolipids in the plasma is not known; however, it has been postulated that they may originate mainly from the intestinal tract epithelial cells. Other exocrine organs such as the liver, kidney, and pancreas also contribute to the plasma glycolipids.[1,7,14] About one-third of the total Lewis glycolipids in blood are bound to the RBCs, and the rest are in plasma.[1] Using plasma as a source of Lewis glycosphingolipids, Le(a–b–) RBCs incubated with Le^a-positive or Le^b-positive plasma can be converted to Le(a+b–) or Le(a–b+), depending on the substance present in the plasma. With saliva as a source of Lewis substances, Le(a–b–) RBCs cannot be converted into Lewis-positive phenotypes because Lewis substances in saliva, being glycoproteins, are not adsorbed onto the RBC membranes. The Lewis specificity, similar to that of ABH antigens, resides in the carbohydrate

portion of the molecule. Both Le^a and Le^b are formed by the addition of a fucose molecule to the precursor structure of a type 1 chain in secretions (see Figs. 8–2 and 8–5). In addition, A or B enzymes (N-acetylgalactosaminyltransferase or D-galactosyltransferase) in secretor individuals can form A or B antigens in secretions by adding the appropriate sugar residue to type 1 or type 2 H substances. The substances present in secretions and antigens present on RBCs, depending on Lele, Sese, and ABO genes inherited, are listed in Table 8–2. The Lewis gene-specified fucosyltransferase competes with A and B gene-specified enzymes for the same type 1 H substrate. As a result, individuals who inherit Le and Se genes have more Lewis and fewer A or B plasma glycolipids than Se, lele individuals. Le^a and Le^b antigens, once formed in secretions, can no longer be used as substrates for H and A or B enzymes, owing to chain termination signaled by the Lewis transferase. As a result, presence or absence of the Le gene affects the concentration of H, A, and B type 1 chain substances found in secretions. Le gene does not affect synthesis of type 2 chain H-, A-, and B-soluble antigens found in secretions. Antigens

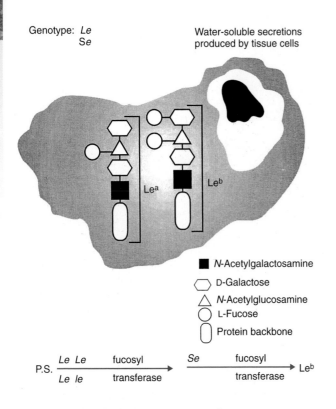

Genotype: *Le*
Se

Water-soluble secretions produced by tissue cells

Le^a

Le^b

■ *N*-Acetylgalactosamine
⬡ D-Galactose
△ *N*-Acetylglucosamine
○ L-Fucose
▢ Protein backbone

P.S. $\dfrac{Le\ Le}{Le\ le}$ $\xrightarrow[\text{transferase}]{\text{fucosyl}}$ $\xrightarrow[\text{transferase}]{Se\quad\text{fucosyl}}$ Le^b

■ **FIGURE 8–5**   Formation of Le^b substance.

of all other blood group systems are built on type 2 precursor chains found on the RBC membrane because these determinants are manufactured by the RBC.[2] Characteristics of Lewis and ABH substances found in secretions are compared in Table 8–3.

Development and Changes of Lewis Antigens After Birth

Depending on the genes inherited, Le^a and Le^b glycoproteins as well as ABH substances will be present in the saliva of newborn infants. In plasma there are no detectable Lewis glycosphingolipids at birth.[15] Therefore, cord blood and RBCs from newborn infants phenotype as Le(a−b−). It is the low level of plasma Lewis antigens that accounts for this fact, because the plasma of newborn infants has been demonstrated to be incapable of transforming Le(a−b−) adult cells into Lewis-positive phenotype. However, Le(a−b−) erythrocytes from infants can be transformed into the Le(a+b−) phenotype by incubation with plasma from an Le(a+b−) adult.[16] When the genotypes *Le* and *sese* are inherited, Lewis antigens (Le^a and Le^b) are not detectable on cord RBCs, but these infants do secrete Le^a substance in their saliva. Lewis glycosphingolipids become detectable in plasma after approximately 10 days of life. In individuals who inherit *Le* and *Se* genes, a transformation can be followed from the Le(a−b−) phenotype at birth to Le(a+b−) after 10 days, to Le(a+b+), and finally to Le(a−b+), the true Lewis phenotype after 6 to

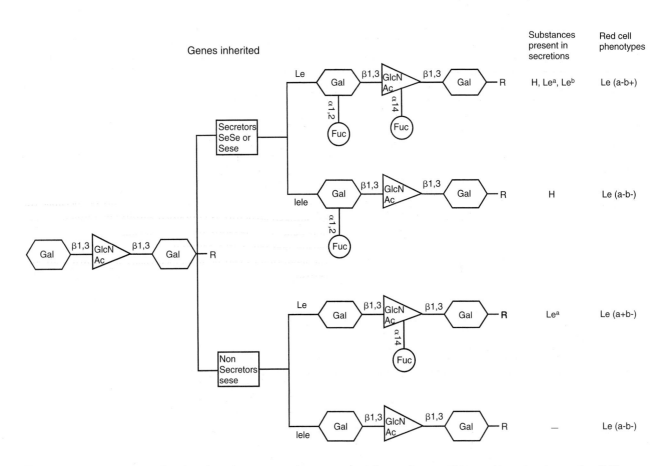

■ **FIGURE 8–6**   Formation of Lewis antigens in secretors and nonsecretors. Gal = D-galactose; GlcNAc = *N*-acetyl-D-glucosamine; FUC = L-fucose; R = other biochemical residues.

TABLE 8-1   Phenotypes and Frequencies in the Lewis System

	Adult Phenotype Frequency (%)	
Phenotype	Whites	Blacks
Le(a+b−)	22	23
Le(a−b+)	72	55
Le(a−b−)	6	22

7 years.[17,18] In contrast, individuals who inherit *Le* and *sese* genes phenotype as Le(a−b−) at birth and transform to Le(a+b−) after 10 days. The Le(a+b−) phenotype persists throughout life. Individuals with *lele* genes phenotype as Le(a−b−) at birth and for the rest of their lives.

Changes in Lewis Phenotype

A decrease in expression of Lewis antigens has been demonstrated on RBCs from many pregnant women, resulting in Le(a−b−) phenotypes during gestation.[3,19] The mechanism causing production of this phenotype during pregnancy is uncertain. It has been suggested that physiologic changes in the composition of blood that affect the distribution of Lewis glycolipid between plasma and RBCs are responsible for this phenomenon. Of the total Lewis glycolipids in whole blood, approximately one-third of Le^b is associated with RBCs, and the rest is bound to plasma lipoproteins.[19] Other investigators have proposed that the large increase in the ratio of plasma lipoproteins to RBC mass that occurs during pregnancy is responsible for Le(a−b−) phenotypes.[3,20] In this instance, a greater amount of Le^b glycolipids would be bound to plasma lipoproteins instead of adsorbing onto the RBCs.[17] Lack of expression of Lewis antigens (Le^a and Le^b) has been demonstrated on the RBCs of patients with cancer, alcoholic cirrhosis, and viral and parasitic infections. This transformation of Lewis-positive phenotypes to Lewis-negative phenotypes is caused by abnormal lipid metabolism, changes in triglycerides and high-density lipoproteins,[1] and/or other neoplastic changes occurring in cancer patients.[21,22] Other factors involved in the expression of the Lewis phenotype may be genetic, such as a single-point mutation caused by leucine to arginine substitution in the Lewis fucosyltransferase.[1] This mutation causes a decrease in adsorption of Lewis antigen onto RBCs from plasma, resulting in Le(a−b−) phenotype in individuals who have Le^a and Le^b in their saliva.[1] A summary of Lewis antigen characteristics can be found in **Box 8–1**.

Lewis Antibodies

Basic Concepts

Antibodies to Lewis blood group antigens (anti-Le^a and anti-Le^b) are frequently detected in antibody screening procedures. Lewis antibodies are generally produced by Le(a−b−) persons. Lewis antibodies are considered naturally occurring because they are present without previous exposure to the antigen-positive RBCs. They are generally immunoglobulin M (IgM) in nature and do not cross the placenta to cause hemolytic disease of the newborn (HDN). However, because they are IgM antibodies, these hemolysins can activate complement and therefore can occasionally cause in vivo and in vitro hemolysis. An interesting aspect of Lewis antibodies is that they occur quite frequently in the sera of pregnant women.[23] Lewis antibodies are more reactive with enzyme-treated cells than with untreated cells and more reactive with group O cells than with group A or B cells. Anti-Le^a and anti-Le^b may occur together and can be neutralized by the Lewis substances present in plasma or saliva.

Anti-Le^a

Anti-Le^a is the most commonly encountered antibody of the Lewis system produced in 20 percent of individuals with Le(a−b−) phenotypes. The antibody is often of the IgM class; however, some may have IgG components or may be entirely IgG.[24] The IgG form of anti-Le^a does not bind to the RBCs as efficiently as does the IgM form and thereby is not generally detected in routine blood bank procedures. However, IgG anti-Le^a has been detected on RBCs using enzyme-linked immunosorbent assay.[24] The IgG Lewis antibodies can be formed after massive transfusions of Lewis-positive antigens in individuals whose serum lacked Lewis antibodies before receiving the transfusions.[23,25] The IgM form of Le^a antibody binds complement and therefore can cause in vivo and in vitro hemolysis. The antibody reactivity is enhanced by enzyme-treated RBCs. The Le^a antibody is frequently detected with saline-suspended cells at room temperature. However, it sometimes reacts at 37°C and Coombs phase and therefore can cause hemolytic transfusion reactions.[17] Anti-Le^a is easily neutralized with plasma or saliva that contains Le^a substance. Persons who are Le(a−b+) do not make anti-Le^a because the Le^a antigen structure is contained within Le^b antigen epitope and Le(a−b+) persons have Le^a substance present in their plasma and saliva.[1,17] Caution must be used, however, because the agglutinates can be dispersed easily if the RBCs are not resuspended gently.

TABLE 8-2   Substances Present in Secretions and Antigens Present on Red Cells, Depending on the Lewis, Hh, Se, and ABH Genes Inherited

Gene Inherited	Substances Present in Secretions	Red Cell Phenotype
Le, Se, A/B/H	Le^a, Le^b, A, B, H	A, B, H, Le(a−b+)
lele, Se, A/B/H	A, B, H	A, B, H, Le(a−b−)
Le, sese, A/B/H	Le^a	A, B, H, Le(a+b−)
lele, sese, A/B/H	—	A, B, H, Le(a−b−)
Le, sese, hh, A/B	Le^a	O$_h$, Le(a+b−)
Le, Se, hh, A/B	Le^a, Le^b, A, B, H	A, B, Le(a−b+)*

* = para-Bombay phenotype

TABLE 8–3   Characteristics of Lewis, A, B, and H Substances Found in Secretions

	Lewis Substances in Secretion	ABH Substances in Secretion
Genetic control	*Le* gene (Le[a] formation is not dependent or controlled by Se gene)	*Se* gene
Glycosyltransferase	α-4-L-fucosyltransferase (Le)	α-4-L-fucosyltransferase (H) α-3-*N*-acetylgalactosaminyltransferase (A) α-3-D-galactosyltransferase (B)
Substrate precursor structure Factors affecting formation	Type 1 chains 1. Once formed, Le[a] and Le[b] are no longer substrates for H or AB enzymes, respectively. 2. Lewis and H fucosyltransferases compete for type 1 chain precursor structure. 3. Lewis and AB enzymes compete for type 1 H substance.	Type 1 or type 2 chains 1. Type 2 chain, A, B, and H substance formation is unaffected by the presence of the Lewis enzyme. 2. A or B type 1 substances can act as substrates for Lewis enzyme forming ALe[b] or BLe[b] "compound" antigenic glycoproteins. 3. Formation of type 1 chain, A, B, and H substances is competitively inhibited by the presence of Lewis enzyme.

Anti-Le[b]

Anti-Le[b] is not as common or generally as strong as anti-Le[a]. Although it is usually an IgM agglutinin, it does not fix complement as readily as anti-Le[a]. Anti-Le[b] is usually produced by an Le(a−b−) individual; only occasionally will an Le(a+b−) individual produce an anti-Le[b]. Like anti-Le[a], anti-Le[b] is neutralized by plasma or saliva containing Le[b] substance. A summary of Lewis antibodies and their serologic characteristics can be found in **Box 8–2** and **Table 8–4**, respectively.

Advanced Concepts

Anti-Le[b]

An interesting aspect of anti-Le[b] is that it can be classified into two categories: anti-Le[bH] and anti-Le[bL]. Anti-Le[bH] reacts best when both the Le[b] and the H antigens are present on the RBC, such as group O and A₂ cells.[3] Anti-Le[bH] is probably an antibody to a compound antigen. In phenotyping RBCs, especially A₁ and A₁B cells, the antiserum being used is not anti-Le[bH]. Anti-Le[bL] is the Le[b] antibody that recognizes any Le[b] antigen regardless of the ABO type. Anti-Le[bH] can be neutralized by either H or combined H and Le[b] substance. Anti-Le[bL] is the antibody of choice for phenotyping RBCs.

Neither anti-Le[bH] nor anti-Le[bL] is frequently implicated in

hemolytic transfusion reactions, and the lack of reports in the literature suggests that anti-Le[b] in general has no clinical significance.[23] Formation of possible Lewis antibodies in different RBC phenotypes is summarized in **Table 8–5**.

Anti-Le[x]

Anti-Le[x] agglutinates all Le(a+b−) and Le(a−b+) RBCs and is formed by all individuals who are phenotyped as Le(a−b−). Anti-Le[x] also agglutinates approximately 90 percent of all white cord blood initially phenotyping as Le(a−b−). In 1981 Schenkel-Brunner and Hanfland[26] defined the binding site of Le[x] antibodies by immunoadsorption studies. The binding site of Le[x] antibodies was found to be the smaller disaccharide structure of fucose-α(1→4)GlcNAc-R.[15,26] The reactivity of the Le[x] determinant as defined by these authors is inhibited by the Le[a] glycolipid similar to the inhibition of normal anti-Le[a]. This occurs because the specificities of both antibodies are determined by a fucose-α(1→4)GlcNAc linkage, which is present in both the Le[x] determinant and Le[a] antigen as a product of the Lewis α-4-L-fucosyltransferase.

Le(a−b−x+) cord cells do not react with anti-Le[a] or anti-Le[b]. This may be a result of the hidden nature of the Le[x] determinant **(Fig. 8–7)**, which is covered by the addition of many more carbohydrates to the disaccharide chain. A somewhat similar analogy can be made with the A, B, and H antibodies and antigens. H-positive O cells, analogous to Lewis

BOX 8–1
Lewis Antigens

● Poorly developed at birth
● Reversibly adsorbed onto red cells from plasma
● Not found on cord blood or newborn red cells Le(a−b−)
● Lewis glycolipids detectable in plasma after approximately 10 days of life
● Transformation of Lewis phenotype after birth seen in individuals who inherit *Le* and *Se* genes: Le(a−b−) to Le(a+b−) to Le(a+b+) to Le(a−b+) (the true phenotype)
● Decrease in expression demonstrated in red cells from many pregnant women, resulting in Le(a−b−) phenotype during gestation
● Do not show dosage in serologic reactions

BOX 8–2
Lewis Antibodies

● Usually naturally occurring
● Predominantly IgM
● May cause in vivo hemolysis of red cells
● Sometimes reacts at 37°C and Coombs phase more weakly than at room temperature
● Enhanced by enzymes
● Readily neutralized by Lewis blood group substances
● Rarely causes in vitro hemolysis; however, in vivo posttransfusion hemolysis reported in cases in which Lewis Ab strongly reacts in Coombs phase

TABLE 8-4   Serologic Characteristics of Anti-Leᵃ and Anti-Leᵇ Antibodies in Vitro

	Anti-Leᵃ	Anti-Leᵇ
Saline 4–22°C	Most	Most
Albumin 37°C	Few	Few
AHG	Many	Few
Enzymes	Many	Few
Hemolysis	Some	Occasional

(a−b−x+) cells, do not react with anti-A or anti-B, but anti-H (analogous to anti-Leˣ) does agglutinate selected A and B cells. The fact that the reactivity of anti-Leˣ cannot be separated using Le(a+b−) or cord RBCs indicates that this antibody is detecting a Lewis precursor antigen present in the biochemical structure of Leᵃ and Leᵇ.[1,17,27]

Clinical Significance of Lewis Antibodies

Although some cases of hemolytic transfusion reactions caused by anti-Leᵃ have been reported and there have been cases of in vivo RBC destruction due to anti-Leᵇ, Lewis antibodies are generally considered insignificant in blood transfusion practices. This is because:

1. Lewis antibodies can be neutralized by the Lewis substances present in the plasma and can thereby be decreased in quantity.
2. The Lewis antigens dissociate from the RBCs as readily as they bind to the RBCs. In other words, the Lewis-positive donor RBCs can become Lewis-negative RBCs following transfusion into an individual with a Lewis-negative phenotype. These antigens released into the plasma can further neutralize any Lewis antibodies present in the recipient plasma.
3. Lewis antibodies are generally IgM and therefore cannot cross the placenta and cause HDN. In addition, Lewis antigens are not fully developed at birth (Box 8–3).

For these reasons, the presence of Lewis antibodies in a patient's serum does *not* require transfusions of Lewis-negative RBCs, as long as pretransfusion tests performed at 37°C and Coombs phase are compatible and there is no evidence of in vitro hemolysis. The Lewis antibodies reactive at 37°C and antihuman globulin phase, however, should not be ignored because these antibodies can cause in vivo RBC destruction. In the presence of multiple antibodies, Lewis antibodies often complicate antibody identification, but they can be easily inhibited with saliva from secretors or with commercially available Lewis substance.[3]

TABLE 8-5   Lewis Antigen on the RBCs and Possible Antibodies Produced in the Plasma

Red Cell Phenotype	Possible Antibodies Produced
Le(a−b−)	Anti-Leᵇ
Le(a−b+)	—
Le(a−b−)	Anti-Leᵃ, Anti-Leᵇ
Leˣ	—

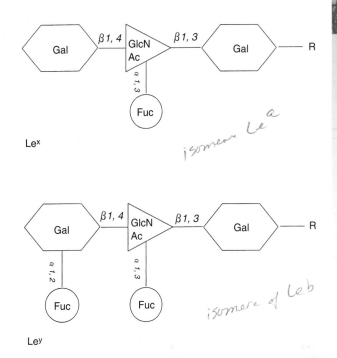

■ **FIGURE 8-7**   Structure of Leˣ and Leʸ from type-2 chains. Gal = D-galactose; GlcNAc = N-acetyl-D-glucosamine; R = other biochemical residues.

Advanced Concepts: Other Lewis Antigens

The Lewis (a+b+) Phenotype: Partial Secretors

It is postulated that a weak variant of the secretory gene (*Se*) referred to as *Seʷ* is responsible for the expression of Le(a+b+) phenotype. The *Seʷ* allele is rare or absent in whites and should not be confused with the occasional expression of Leᵃ antigen in Le(a−b+) individuals. The Le(a+b+) phenotype is referred to as *partial secretory phenotype* and is frequently found in Polynesians, Australians, and Asians.[2,7,12] Individuals with the *Seʷ* gene have a reduced amount of ABH substances in their secretions because of the competition of Le and Se transferases for type 1 precursors. In non–group O individuals, there is even more competition for H type 1 by the A and B glycosyltransferase, and therefore less Leᵇ is formed.[28] The Lewis(a+b+) phenotype has been reported more in group O than in non–group O individuals. Detection of the Le(a+b+) phenotype is also dependent on the potency and type of the antisera used.[1,7]

BOX 8-3
Factors Contributing to Clinical Insignificance of Lewis Antibodies

- Neutralization of Lewis antibodies by Lewis substances present in the plasma
- Loss of red cell Lewis antigen(s) into the plasma
- Lack of reactivity at 37°C and antihuman globulin phase
- Generally IgM in nature and incapable of crossing placenta
- Lewis antigens poorly developed in newborn infants

It is worth noting that the Se^w allele has been cloned, and it is suggested that the weak expression of secretor transferase (Se^w) is caused by point mutations in the coding region of *FUT2*.[7] In addition, the occurrence of the nonsecretor gene (*se*) has been found to be uncommon in Polynesians.[4]

Le^c and Le^d (Type 1 Precursor and Type 1 H Structure)

Le^d antigen was first described by Potapov,[29] who reported an antibody in the serum that reacted with RBCs from Le(a−b−) ABH-secretor individuals. In his report, he predicted another hypothetical antibody, anti-Le^c, which would detect the Lewis antigen on RBCs of Lewis (a−b−) ABH nonsecretors. In 1972, Gunson and Latham reported such an antibody that defined the Le^c antigen.[30]

Le^c and Le^d type 1 chain structures have also been proposed by Graham[31] and Hanfland[32] and their coworkers, who obtained anti-Le^c and anti-Le^d antibodies following immunization of goats with human saliva. In their investigation, anti-Le^d was strongly inhibited by a fucose containing saccharide of the type 1 H chain structure. These investigators suggest that neither Le^c nor Le^d antigens are associated with the Lewis system. Le^c represents type 1 precursor structure, and Le^d is type 1 H structure (**Fig. 8–8**). More recent findings suggest that there are two types of Le^c substances referred to as single Le^c and branched Le^c.[1,33,34]

Le^c present in saliva, plasma, and on RBCs is a combination of a branched structure and unbranched forms.[1,34] The branched structures are the main glycolipids on RBCs in Le(a−b−) nonsecretors and cause agglutination using polyclonal antibodies. The branched structures are either absent or poorly detected on Le(a−b−) cord cells because of the lack of specificity of anti-Le^c antibodies for the cord cells. Le^c in its unbranched single form (lactotetraosylceramide) does not cause agglutination of the RBCs with polyclonal antibodies. Single Le^c is the precursor to Le^a and Le^d (type 1 H). Le^d is formed by the action of the Se transferase on type 1 precursor substance (Le^c).[1]

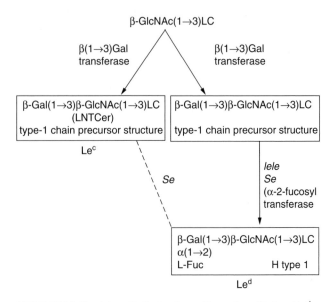

■ **FIGURE 8–8**   A hypothetical pathway. Formation of Le^c and Le^d. Based on the work of Graham, Hanfland, and associates.[28,29]

Formation of Lewis antigens in secretions and through their adsorption onto RBCs depends on the genetic makeup of the individual (**Table 8–6**).

The Le^c and Le^d antigens are found in Lewis-negative individuals (*lele*) who have the Le(a−b−) phenotypes. Le^c antigen is found only in Le(a−b−) individuals who are ABH nonsecretors. Le^d antigen is found only in Le(a−b−) individuals who are ABH secretors. In view of these findings, perhaps Lewis phenotypes would be correctly written as Le(a−b−c+d−) and Le(a−b−c−d+), similar to the two new phenotypes previously described. Le^c is analogous to Le^a; they are very similar biochemically and secreted only by ABH nonsecretors (*sese*). Similarly, Le^c is adsorbed onto the RBC only after exposure to the plasma or secretions containing the soluble antigen. This close similarity between Le^a and Le^c accounts for the observation that the Le(a−b−) individuals

TABLE 8–6 Review of the Genetic Interaction Among Lewis, *Hh*, Secretor, and ABH Genes		
Hypothetical Genotype	**Substances Present in Saliva**	**RBC Phenotype**
LeLe HH SeSe AA	A, H, Le^a, Le^b	A Le(a−b+)
lele Hh Sese AO	A, H	A Le(a−b−)
Lele Hh sese AO	Le^a	A Le(a+b−)
lele HH sese AO	Le^c	A Le(a−b−)
lele HH sese AB	Le^c	AB Le(a−b−)
LeLe HH, Sese, AB	A, B, H, Le^a, Le^b	AB Le(a−b+)
lele Hh SeSe AB	A, B, H, Le^c, Le^d	AB Le(a−b−)
Lele Hh sese AB	Le^a	AB Le(a+b−)
Lele HH SeSe OO	H, Le^a, Le^b	O Le(a−b+)
lele Hh SeSe OO	H, Le^c, Le^d	O Le(a−b−)
LeLe HH sese OO	Le^a	O Le(a+b−)
lele Hh sese OO	Le^c	O Le(a−b−)
lele hh Sese AB*	A, B, H	AB Le(a−b−)*
LeLe hh SeSe AB*	Le^a, Le^b, A, B, H	AB Le(a−b+)
Lele hh sese AB	Le^a	O^h Le(a+b−)
lele hh sese AB	Le^c	O^h Le(a−b−)

*para-Bombay phenotype

who produced anti-Le^a are all ABH secretors with an Le(a−b−c−d+) phenotype.[1,34]

The presence of Le^c in Le(a−b−) ABH nonsecretors probably prevents the formation of anti-Le^a, inasmuch as Le^c and Le^a are biochemically very similar. Saliva from these Le(a−b−c+d−) ABH nonsecretors has been found to contain Le^c-soluble antigens.

Le^d antigen is analogous to the Le^b antigen and is found only in Le(a−b−) secretors; its correct phenotype is Le(a−b−c−d+). Le^d is also thought to be biochemically similar to Le^b. The Le^c-soluble and Le^d-soluble antigens subsequently adsorb (as all Lewis antigens do) to the RBC membrane after exposure to plasma containing the soluble antigens.[1,34]

In the rare Bombay phenotype O$_h$ (see Chapter 6), individuals cannot synthesize the H, A, or B antigens on their RBCs because they lack the H structure necessary for formation of these antigens (see **Figs. 8–2** and **8–5**). As a result, all O$_h$ individuals have a phenotype of either Le(a+b−), if the Lewis gene (*Le*) is inherited, or Le(a−b−), if the Lewis genotype is *lele*[2] (**Fig. 8–9**). A more specific phenotype for the O$_h$ individual of the Lewis genetic makeup (*lele*) would be Le(a−b−c+d+) because all O$_h$ individuals are nonsecretors of all ABH substances, yet are capable of secreting Le^c substances in the saliva.

In equally rare para-Bombay individuals, at least one functional *Se* gene is present in addition to two null alleles at the H locus. These individuals have A, B, and H antigens in their secretions, with a weak AB antigen on their RBCs. The weak antigen on their RBCs may be adsorbed from plasma or may be due to the presence of an alternative gene at the H locus.[2,17,27] This alternative gene gives rise to a small amount of H antigen, all of which is transformed into the A and B antigens.

To make the Lewis system even more complicated and intriguing, interaction among *ABO, H, Se,* and *Le* genes results not only in the formation of the Le^a and Le^b substances but also in the compound antigen products ALe^b and BLe^b. This has been confirmed because an anti-A^1 Le^b antibody has been described in the Lewis system. The compound antibody reacts only with RBCs that possess both the A$_1$ and the Le^b antigenic determinants and is believed to be the result of genetic interaction among the A$_1$, *Le, H,* and *Se* genes.[35] For a review of the genetic interaction that occurs between the *Le, H, Se,* and *ABO* genes, which results in the various substances found in secretions as well as RBC phenotypes, refer to **Table 8–6**, which gives various hypothetical genotypes.

Le^x and Le^y

Le^x(X) is referred to as a type 2 isomer of Le^a,[1,7,16] which is formed by the addition of fucose-α (1→3) GlcNAc linkage on

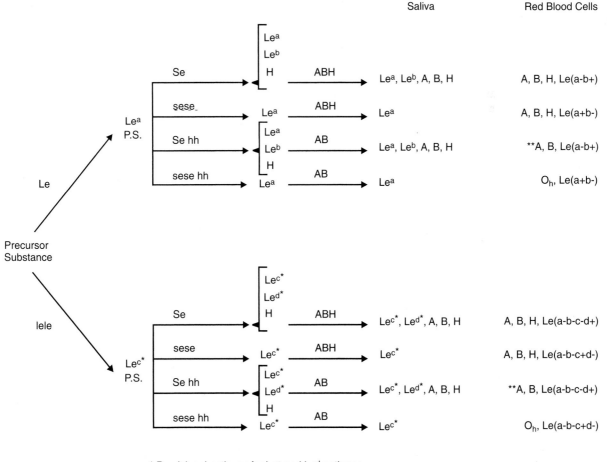

* Provisional pathway for Le^c and Le^d antigens

** Para-Bombay Phenotype

■ **FIGURE 8–9**   Genetic pathway for the production of the A, B, H, Le^a, and Le^b blood group substances.

the type 2 chain (see **Fig. 8–7**). This Le^x is the same antigenic structure called stage-specific embryonic antigen-1 (SSEA-1).[36]

Le^y(Y) is defined as a type 2 isomer of Le^b and is made by addition of fucose-α (1$\rightarrow$3) GlcNAc linkage on type 2 H substance (see **Fig. 8–7**).

Other Lewis-related type 2 structures are ALe^x (AX), ALe^y (AY), and BLe^y (BY). ALe^y and BLe^y are important markers of the cell membrane.[1,7]

Lewis and secretor fucosyltransferases can use type 1 and type 2 precursor substances to form type 1 and type 2 antigens; however, type 2 antigens are primarily made by other α-3-fucosyltransferases, such as FUT4, FUT5, FUT6, and FUT7.[1] In addition, *Se* and *H* genes can both act on the type 2 precursors to form H type 2 and related structures. However, the H type 2 and related structures found in the secretions are formed by the effect of the *Se* gene on type 2 precursor.[7] **Table 8–7** summarizes the Lewis antigens made from type 1 and type 2 precursor substances.

Biologic Significance of the Lewis System

Although the Lewis system is not considered a significant system in transfusion medicine, it has significance at the tissue level for the establishment of a biologic relationship between blood group antigens and diseases.[1,7]

The biologic role of the Lewis system in disease is intricate because of the complexity of the Lewis structure, causing diversity of the cell surface markers. However, it is clearly known that the Lewis system is associated with factors causing certain diseases, such as peptic ulcers, ischemic heart disease, cancer, and kidney transplant rejection[2,3]. In addition, Lewis antigens have receptors to interact with microorganisms expressing a particular lectin. For example, Le^b has receptors for *Helicobacter pylori*.[2,3,37–39] This miroorganism causes a variety of diseases including gastric and duodenal ulcers, mucosa-associated lymphoid tissue lymphoma, atrophic gastritis, and adenocarcinoma.[40] *H. pylori* expresses Lewis antigens as a component in its lipopolysaccharide structure.[40,41] The Lewis antigen expression by this gastric pathogen is considered to be a major factor for causing chronic diseases.[41] The Lewis antigens expressed by *H. pylori* are indicated to be Le^x, Le^y, Le^a, Le^b, and H type 1.[40] The absence of Lewis a and Lewis b in asymptomatic patients suggests that the expression of these antigens is associated with a more severe disease state.[41] There is also a lower expression of Le^x and Le^y in asymptomatic individuals as compared with symptomatic patients, which supports the hypothesis that the expression of these antigens is correlated with pathology of the disease.[41] However, the role of the Lewis antigens in the infectious process is not clear.[41] It has also been postulated that *H. pylori* induces anti-Lewis antibodies that cross-react with the gastric mucosa.[42] In addition, anti-Lewis x and anti-Lewis y have been found in the serum of patients with gastric cancer.[42]

It has been postulated that tumor developments and their metastatic processes are associated with changes in cell surface carbohydrates.[43] These alterations may cause the formation of tumor-associated antigens. Altered expression of Lewis antigens such as sialylated Lewis a and sialylated Lewis x, have been associated with different types of carcinomas and their related prognoses.[39,44] Sialyl Le^x and Le^a antigens are found to serve as ligands mediating adhesion of cancer cells to the endothelium of blood and lymphatic vessels, which contributes to the tumor metastatic process.[39,43,44] Increased sialyl Le^x and sialyl Le^a have been found in gastric cancer tissue and reported to correlate with poor prognoses in patients with gastric cancer.[43,44] It has also been postulated that there is an association between sialyl Lewis x antigen and poor prognosis in patients with breast cancer.[45]

In addition, it has been reported that H type 2 and Le^y have angiogenic and procoagulant activities that may contribute to tumor growth and metastasis.[39] Increased Lewis Y antigen has been found on synovial fluid granulocytes of patients with arthritic diseases, which suggests a role for this antigen in inflammatory responses.[46]

Furthermore, the lack of *Le* and *Se* genes in the Le(a$-$b$-$) phenotype is associated with an increased risk for coronary heart disease. However the underlying mechanisms are not yet established.[47,48] Le^x and Le^y are associated with gastrointestinal, colorectal, and lung cancers.[17] Le^x antigen is a marker for Reed-Sternberg cells of Hodgkin's disease.[17]

It has also been reported that the presence of Lewis antibodies in Lewis-negative individuals is associated with a higher renal allograft rejection than in Lewis-positive people.[3,7] Anti-Le^a has been reported to be associated with renal failure in Lewis-negative bone marrow transplant patients. Some Lewis antibodies occur in patients with cancer, such as anti-ALe^d in patients with cancer of the stomach, anti-Le^c in patients with bronchogenic carcinoma, anti-Le^{bH} in patients with metastatic carcinoma of the bladder, and auto-anti-Le^a in Le(a$-$b$+$) individuals with carcinoma of esophagus. The presence of some Lewis antibodies is found to be beneficial to patients. For example, anti-Le^c may cause regression of some tumors, and monoclonal antibodies to type 1 Lewis substance have an antitumor effect both in vivo and in vitro.[1] The biologic significance of the Lewis system needs more research because of controversial findings in some areas.

Summary

Traditionally, six antigens have been associated with the Lewis system: Le^a, Le^b, Le^c, Le^d, Le^x, and Le^y. All these antigens can be detected in secretions and on RBCs (after adsorption from plasma). The Lewis system represents a tissue group, inasmuch as Lewis antigens are not synthesized by RBCs but rather are adsorbed from plasma. In secretions, these antigens exist as glycoproteins. In plasma and on RBCs, they are glycolipids. The structure of the Le^a and Le^b glycosphingolipids from human plasma and RBCs has been defined biochemically. Le^a represents a lacto-*N*-fucopentaosyl[7] ceramide, depicted here:

TABLE 8–7	Type 1 and Type 2 Antigens

Type 1	Type 2
Le^c	Type 2 precursor
Le^d	H type 2
Le^a	Le^x
Le^b	Le^y
A type 1	A type 2
A Le^b	A Le^y

β-Gal(1→3) β-GlcNAc(1→3)LC β-Gal(1→4) β-Glc(1→1)Cer

$\qquad\qquad$ |

$\qquad\qquad$ α(1→4)

$\qquad\qquad$ |

$\qquad\qquad$ Fuc $\qquad\qquad\qquad\qquad\qquad$ Type 1 chain

Le^b represents a lacto-*N*-difucohexaosyl (1) ceramide, depicted here:

β-Gal(1→3) β-GlcNAc(1→3)LC β-Gal(1→4) β-Glc(1→1)Cer

$\quad$ | $\qquad\qquad$ |

$\quad$ α(1→2) $\qquad$ α(1→4)

$\quad$ | $\qquad\qquad$ |

$\quad$ Fuc $\qquad\qquad$ Fuc

Le^c is found in the Lewis-negative (*lele*) nonsecretors, Le^d in *lele* secretors. The biochemical structure of Le^c and Le^d are type 1 precursor and type 1 H substance, respectively (see **Fig. 8–8**). Le^c as a compound structure (type 1 and type 2) has also been demonstrated. Le^x antigen is defined as a type 2 isomer of Le^a, and Le^y antigen is defined as a type 2 isomer of Le^b.

CASE STUDY

A 35-year-old woman was seen by her obstetrician for a prenatal care examination. A blood test for prenatal type and screen showed the following:

ABO-Rh Typing					
Anti-A	Anti-B	Anti-D	Rh Control	A$_1$ Cell	B Cell
0	4 +	4 +	0	4 +	0

Antibody Screen				
		IS	37°C	Antihuman Globulin
I	R$_1$R$_1$	1 +	1 +	1 +
II	R$_2$R$_2$	1 +	1 +	0

The results of a 10-RBC panel indicate that anti-Le^a and anti-Le^b are present in the patient's serum. The anti-Le^b reactivity is seen only at IS and 37°C, with the 37°C reactivity most likely a carryover from the IS reading. Therefore, anti-Le^b is not clinically significant because it does not react at antihuman globulin.

The anti-Le^a reactivity is present at all phases—IS, 37°C, and antihuman globulin. A prewarmed antibody screen should be performed before considering the anti-Le^a to be clinically significant. The majority of the anti-Le^a antibodies are nonreactive at antihuman globulin using the prewarmed technique.

The results in this case illustrate that:
1. Lewis antibodies are present in the serum of pregnant women.
2. The antibodies are insignificant or are not associated with HDN, HTR, or both, because newborn infants lack the Lewis antigens and IgM antibodies do not cross the placenta.

SUMMARY CHART:
Important Points to Remember
(MT/MLT/SBB)

➤ Lewis blood group antigens are not synthesized by the RBCs. These antigens are made by tissue cells, secreted into body fluids and plasma, and adsorbed onto the RBC membrane.

➤ Lewis antigens present in secretions are glycoproteins; Lewis cell-bound antigens absorbed from plasma onto RBC membranes are glycolipids.

➤ The *Le* gene codes for L-fucosyltransferase, which adds L-fucose to the type 1 chain.

➤ *Le* gene is needed for the expression of Le^a substance, and *Le* and *Se* genes are needed to form Le^b substance.

➤ Le^a antigen is formed by the addition of L-fucose to the number 4 carbon of *N*-acetylglucosamine of type 1 precursor structure.

➤ All Le(a+b−) persons are ABH nonsecretors and have only Le^a substance in secretions.

➤ Le^b antigen is formed when a second L-fucose is added to the number 4 carbon of the subterminal *N*-acetyl-D-glucosamine of type 1 H.

➤ All Le(a−b+) persons are ABH secretors and have both Le^a and Le^b substances in secretions.

➤ The most common Lewis phenotype in both whites and blacks is Le(a−b+).

➤ The *lele* genotype is more common among blacks than in whites and will phenotype as Le(a−b−).

➤ Lewis antigens are poorly expressed at birth.

➤ Lewis antigens do not demonstrate dosage in serologic reactions.

➤ Lewis antibodies are generally IgM (naturally occurring); antibodies are capable of binding complement and are enhanced by enzymes; Lewis substance in secretions can neutralize Lewis antibodies.

➤ Lewis antibodies are frequently encountered in pregnant women.

➤ Lewis antibodies are not considered significant in transfusion medicine.

REVIEW QUESTIONS

1. Where are the Lewis antigens produced?
   a. Platelets
   b. RBCs
   c. White blood cells
   d. Tissue cells
   e. All of the above

2. Biochemically, Lewis antigens are classified as what in secretions?
   a. Glycoproteins
   b. Glycolipids

c. Polyproteins

d. Glycophorins

3. Biochemically, Lewis antigens are classified as what in plasma and on RBCs? (Use answer choices for Question 2.)

4. Which of the following characteristics best describes Lewis antibodies?
   a. IgM, naturally occurring, cause HDN
   b. IgM, naturally occurring, do not cause HDN
   c. IgG, in vitro hemolysis, cause hemolytic transfusion reactions
   d. IgG, in vitro hemolysis, do not cause hemolytic transfusion reactions

5. The *Le* gene codes for a specific glycosyltransferase that transfers an L-fucose to the *N*-acetylglucosamine on:
   a. Type 1 precursor chain
   b. Type 2 precursor chain
   c. Types 1 and 2 precursor chain
   d. Either type 1 or type 2 in any one individual but not in both

6. Secretions of a person with the genes *B, Se,* and *Le* contain which of the following?
   a. B substance, H substance, Le^a and Le^b substances
   b. B substance, Le^a substance
   c. H substance, Le^a and Le^b substances
   d. H substance, Le^a substance

7. Secretions of a person with the genes *B, sese,* and *Le* contain which of the following?
   a. B substance, Le^a substance
   b. H substance, Le^a substance
   c. H substance, Le^a and Le^b substance
   d. Le^a substance

8. An individual with genes *A, H, Se,* and *lele* has which of the following phenotypes?
   a. ABH, Le(a−b−)
   b. ABH, Le(a+b−)
   c. AH, Le(a−b−)
   d. AH, Le(a+b−)

9. Transformation to Le^b phenotype after birth may be as follows:
   a. Le(a−b−) to Le(a+b−) to Le(a+b+) to Le(a−b+)
   b. Le(a+b−) to Le(a−b−) to Le(a−b+) to Le(a+b+)
   c. Le(a−b+) to Le(a+b+) to Le(a+b+) to Le(a−b−)
   d. Le(a+b+) to Le(a+b−) to Le(a−b−) to Le(a−b+)

10. In what way do the Lewis antigens change during pregnancy?
    a. Le^a antigen increases only
    b. Le^b antigen increases only
    c. Le^a and Le^b both increase
    d. Le^a and Le^b both decrease

11. Le^c and Le^d antigens are found in individuals with the phenotype of:
    a. Le(a−b−)
    b. Le(a+b−)

c. Le(a−b+)

d. Le(a+b−)

12. Anti-Le^x agglutinates which of the following antigens?
    a. All Le(a+b−) RBCs
    b. All Le(a−b+) RBCs
    c. All Le(a−b−) RBCs
    d. Two of the above

13. The Lewis phenotype that is most commonly associated with *H. pylori* infection is:
    a. Le(a+b−)
    b. Le(a−b+)
    c. Le(a−b−)
    d. Le(a−x+)

REFERENCES

1. Henry, S, et al: Lewis histo-blood group system and associated secretory phenotypes. Vox Sang 69:166, 1995.
2. Simon, TL, et al: Rossi's Principles of Transfusion Medicine, ed 3. Lippincott Williams & Wilkins, Philadelphia, 2002, pp 102–104.
3. Hillyer, CD, et al: Blood Banking and Transfusion Medicine: Basic Principles and Practice. Churchill Livingstone, Philadelphia, 2003, pp 26–27.
4. Henry, S, et al: A second nonsecretor allele of the blood group a(1,2) fucosyltransferase gene (FUT2). Vox Sang 70:21, 1996.
5. Salmon, C, et al: The Human Blood Groups. Masson Pub, New York, 1984, p 162.
6. Hillyer, CD, et al: Handbook of Transfusion Medicine. American Press, San Diego, 2001, pp 98–99.
7. Henry, SM: Immunohematology: Journal of blood group serology and education. American Red Cross 13(2):51, 1996.
8. Watkins, WM, et al: Regulation of expression of carbohydrate blood group antigens. Biochimie 70:1597, 1988.
9. Dunstan, RA: Status of major red cell blood group antigens on neutrophils, lymphocytes, and monocytes. Br J Haematol 62: 301, 1986.
10. Dunstan, RA: The expression of ABH antigens during in vitro megakaryocyte maturation: Origin of heterogeneity of antigen density. Br J Haematol 62:587, 1986.
11. Elmgren, A, et al: DNA sequencing and screening for point mutations in the human Lewis (FUT3) gene enables molecular genotyping of the human Lewis blood group system. Vox Sang 70:97, 1996.
12. Anderson, KC, and Ness, PM: Scientific Basis of Transfusion Medicine: Implications for Clinical Practice, ed 2. WB Saunders, Philadelphia, 2000, p 147.
13. Watkins, WM: Blood group substances: In the ABO system the genes control the arrangement of sugar residues that determines blood group specificity. Science 152:172, 1966.
14. Hauser, R: Le^a and Le^b tissue glycosphingolipids. Transfusion 53:577, 1995.
15. Wendell, RF: Clinical Immunohematology: Basic Concept and Clinical Applications. Blackwell Scientific, Oxford, England, 1990, pp 187–199.
16. Hanfland, P, and Graham, HA: Immunochemistry of the Lewis blood-group system: Partial characterization of Le^a, Le^b, and H-type 1 (Le^{dH}) blood group active glycosphingolipids from human plasma. Arch Biochem Biophys 210:383, 1981.
17. Petz, LD, et al: Clinical Practice of Transfusion Medicine, ed 3. Churchill Livingstone, New York, 1995, pp 81–89.
18. Walker, RH: Technical Manual, ed 13. American Association of Blood Banks, Bethesda, MD, 1999, pp 286–288.
19. Churchill, WH, and Kutz, SR: Transfusion Medicine. Blackwell Scientific, Oxford, England, 1988, p 57.
20. Hammar, L, et al: Lewis phenotype of erythrocytes and Le^b active glycolipid in serum of pregnant women. Vox Sang 40:27, 1981.
21. Langkilde, NC, et al: Lewis negative phenotype and bladder cancer. Lancet 335:926, 1990.
22. Idikio, HA, and Manickavel, V: Lewis blood group antigens (a and b) in human breast tissues: Loss of Lewis-b in breast cancer cells and correlation with tumor grade. Cancer 68(6): 1303, 1991.
23. Mollison, PL, et al: Blood Transfusion in Clinical Medicine, ed 10. Blackwell Science, Oxford, England, 1997, pp 132–148.
24. Cowles, JW, et al: The fine specificity of Lewis blood group antibodies: Evidence for maturation of immune response. Vox Sang 56:107, 1989.
25. Cheng, MS, and Lukomskyj, L: Lewis antibody following a massive blood transfusion. Vox Sang 57:155, 1989.
26. Schenkel-Brunner, H, and Hanfland, P: Immunochemistry of the Lewis blood group system. III. Studies on the molecular basis of the Le^x property. Vox Sang 40:358, 1981.
27. Bryant, NJ: An Introduction to Immunohematology, ed 3. WB Saunders, Philadelphia, 1994, pp 110–111, 129–136.
28. Turgeon, ML: Fundamentals of Immunohematology: Theory and Technique, ed 2. Williams & Wilkins, Philadelphia, 1995, pp 120–124.
29. Potapov, MI: Detection of the antigen of the Lewis system, characteristic of the

erythrocytes of the secretor group Le(a−b−). Probl Hematol Blood Transfus (USSR) 1970, pp 11–45.

30. Gunson HH, and Latham, V: An agglutinin in human serum reacting with cells from Le (a−b−) nonsecretor individual. Vox Sang 22:344, 1972.

31. Graham, HA: Genetic and immunochemical relationships between soluble and cell-bound antigens of the Lewis system. In Mohn, JF, et al (eds): Human Blood Groups. Proc Fifth Intern Conv Immunology. Karger, Basel, 1977, pp 257–267.

32. Hanfland, P, et al: Immunochemistry of the Lewis blood-group system. FEBS Lett 142:77, 1982.

33. Hanfland, P, et al: Immunochemistry of the Lewis blood-group system: Isolation and structures of Lewis-c active and related glycosphingolipids from the plasma of blood group O Le(a−b−) nonsecretors. Arch Biochem Biophys 246:655, 1986.

34. Oriol, R: Genetic control of the fucosylation of ABH precursor chains: Evidence for new epistatic interactions in different cells and tissues. J Immunogenet 17:235, 1990.

35. Seaman, MJ, et al: Siedler: An antibody which reacts with A, (Le(a−b−) red cells. Vox Sang 15:25, 1968.

36. Oriol, R, et al: Genetics of ABO, H, Lewis, X and related antigens. Vox Sang 51:161, 1986.

37. Reid, ME, and Lomas-Francis, C: The Blood Group Antigen Facts Book. Academic Press, San Diego, 1997, pp 210–215.

38. Silberstein, LE: Molecular and Functional Aspects of Blood Group Antigens. American Association of Blood Banks, Bethesda, MD, 1995, pp 52, 181–182.

39. Severine, M, et al: ABH and Lewis histo-blood group antigens, a model for the meaning of oligosaccharide diversity in the face of a changing world. Biochimie 83(7): 565, 2001.

40. Appelmelk, BJ, et al: Why *Helicobacter pylori* has Lewis antigens. Trends Microbiol 8(12):565, 2000.

41. Rasco, DA, et al: Lewis antigen expression by *Helicobacter pylori*. J Infect Dis 184:315, 2001.

42. Heneghan, MA, et al: Relationship of anti-Lewis X and anti-Lewis y antibodies in serum samples from gastric cancer and chronic gastritis patients to *Helicobacter pylori*-mediated autoimmunity. Infect Immun 69(8):4774, 2001.

43. Nakagoe, T, et al: Increased expression of sialyl Lewis(X) antigen as a prognostic factor in patients with stage 0, I, and II gastric cancer. Cancer Lett 175(2):213, 2002.

44. Kim, MJ, et al: Altered expression of Lewis antigen on tissue and erythrocytes in gastric cancer patients. Yonsei Med J 43(4):427, 2002.

45. Nakagoe, T, et al: Expression of ABH/Lewis-related antigens as prognostic factors in patients with breast cancer. J Cancer Res Clin Oncol 128(5):257, 2002.

46. Dettke M, et al: Increased expression of the blood group-related Lewis Y antigen on synovial fluid granulocytes of patients with arthritic joint diseases. Rheumatol 40(9):1033, 2001.

47. Ellison, RC, et al: Lewis blood group phenotype as an independent risk factor for coronary heart disease (the NHLBI Family Heart Study). Am J Cardiol 83(3):345, 1999.

48. Salomaa, V, et al: Genetic background of Lewis negative blood group phenotype and its association with atherosclerotic disease in the NHLBI family heart study. J Int Med 247(6):689, 2000.

BIBLIOGRAPHY

Abhyankar, S, et al: Positive cord blood "DAT" due to anti-Le^a: Absence of hemolytic disease of the newborn. Am J Pediatr Hematol Oncol 11(2):185, 1989.

Blaney, KD, and Howard, PR: Basic and Applied Concepts of Immunohematology. Mosby, St. Louis, 2000, pp 137–139.

Bernoco, M, et al: Detection of combined ABH and Lewis glycosphingolipids in sera of deficient donors. Vox Sang 49(1):58, 1985.

Boorman, KE, et al: Blood Group Serology, ed 6. Churchill Livingstone, New York, 1988, pp 69–80.

Boren, T, et al: Attachment of *Helicobacter pylori* to human gastric epithelium mediated by blood group antigens. Science 262:1892, 1993.

Caillard, T, et al: Failure of expression of α-3-fucosyltransferase in human serum is coincident with the absence of the X (or Le(x)) antigen in the kidney but not on leukocytes. Exp Clin Immunogenet 5(1):15, 1988.

Clausen, H, and Hakomori, S: ABH and related histo-blood group antigens: Immunochemical differences in carrier isotypes and their distribution. Vox Sang 56:1, 1989.

Cowels, JW, et al: Comparison of monoclonal antisera with conventional antisera for Lewis blood group antigen determination. Vox Sang 52(1–2): 83, 1987.

Hanfland, P, et al: Immunochemistry of the Lewis blood group system: Isolation and structures of Lewis-c active and related glycosphingolipids from the plasma of blood group Le(a−b−) nonsecretors. Arch Biochem Biophys 246(2):655, 1986.

Issitt, PD, and Anstee, DJ: Applied Blood Group Serology, ed 4. Montgomery Scientific, Durham, NC, 1998, pp 247–271.

Le-Pendu, J, et al: Expression of ABH and X (Le^x) antigens in various cells. Biochimie 70(11):1613, 1988.

Mollicone, R, et al: Acceptor specificity and tissue distribution of three human α-3-fucosyltransferase. Eur J Biochem 191(1):169, 1990.

Mollison, PL, et al: Blood Transfusion in Clinical Medicine, ed 10. Blackwell Science, Oxford, England, 1997, pp 132–148.

Mc Cullough, J,: Transfusion Medicine. McGraw-Hill, 1998, pp 184–185.

Murphy, MF, and Pamphilon, DH: Practical Transfusion Medicine. Blackwell Science, Oxford, England, 2001, p 28.

Oriol, R: Genetic regulation of the expression of ABH and Lewis antigens in tissues. APMIS Suppl 27:28, 1992.

Rossi, EC, et al: Principles of Transfusion Medicine. Williams & Wilkins, Baltimore, 1992, p 70.

Shulman, IA: Problem Solving in Immunohematology, ed 4. ASCP Press, Chicago, 1992, pp 62–64.

Turgeon, ML: Fundamentals of Immunohematology: Theory and Technique. Lea & Febiger, Philadelphia, 1989, pp 137–159.

Ura, Y, et al: Quantitative dot blot analyses of blood group-related antigens in paired normal and malignant human breast tissues. Int J Cancer 50(1):57, 1992.

Walker, RH: Technical Manual, ed 12. American Association of Blood Banks, Bethesda, MD, 1996, pp 246–248.

Watkins, WM: Regulation of expression of carbohydrate blood group antigens. Biochimie 70(11):1597, 1988.

Whitlock, SA: The Clinical Laboratory Manual Series: Immunohematology. Delmar, Albany, NY, 1997, pp 79–80.

nine

Other Major Blood Group Systems

Regina M. Leger, MSQA, MT(ASCP)SBB, CQMgr(ASQ), and
Loni Calhoun, MT(ASCP)SBB

OBJECTIVES

On completion of this chapter, the learner should be able to:

Antigen Characteristics

1. List the antigen frequencies for the common antigens K, M, S, s, Fy^a, Fy^b, Jk^a, Jk^b, and P_1.
2. Define Kp^a, Js^a, and Lu^a as low-incidence antigens and Kp^b, Js^b, Lu^b, and I as high-incidence antigens.
3. Associate the antigen phenotypes S−s−U−, Js(a+), and Fy(a−b−) with blacks.
4. Define the null phenotypes M^k, p, K_o, Fy(a−b−), Jk(a−b−), and Lu(a−b−) and describe their role in problem-solving.
5. Compare both dominant and recessive forms of the Lu(a−b−) and Jk(a−b−) phenotypes.
6. Describe the reciprocal relationship of I antigen to i antigen.
7. Associate I, P_1, and Lutheran antigens as being poorly expressed on cord red blood cells (RBCs).
8. Define the association of M and N with glycophorin A (GPA) and S and s with glycophorin B (GPB).

Antibody Characteristics

1. Define antibodies to M, N, I, and P_1 as being typically non–RBC-induced ("naturally occurring"), cold-reacting agglutinins that are usually clinically insignificant.

2. Describe antibodies to K, k, S, s, Fy^a, Fy^b, Jk^a, and Jk^b as usually induced by exposure to foreign RBCs ("immune"), antiglobulin-reactive antibodies that are clinically significant.
3. List the antibody specificities that commonly show dosage (anti-M, -N, -S, -s, -Fy^a, -Fy^b, -Jk^a and -Jk^b).
4. Differentiate antigens that are denatured by routine blood bank enzymes (M, N, S, s, Fy^a, Fy^b) from antigens whose reactivity with antibody is enhanced (I, i, P_1, Jk^a, Jk^b).
5. Identify which of the Kell, Kx, Duffy, and Lutheran blood group systems have antigens destroyed by treatment with 2-aminoethylisothiouronium (AET) or dithiothreitol (DTT) and which of the Kell, MNS, and Duffy antigens that are destroyed by treatment with ZZAP.

Clinical Significance and Disease Association

1. Identify or correlate the common 37°C antihuman globulin-reactive antibodies K, k, S, s, Fy^a, Fy^b, Jk^a, and Jk^b with transfusion reactions and hemolytic disease of the newborn (HDN).

2. Describe why the Kidd antibodies are a common cause of delayed hemolytic transfusion reactions.
3. Correlate autoanti-I with *Mycoplasma pneumoniae* infections and autoanti-i with infectious mononucleosis.
4. Describe the common characteristics of the McLeod syndrome, including very weak Kell antigen expression, acanthocytosis, and late onset of muscular and neurological abnormalities.
5. Describe the association of the Fy(a−b−) phenotype with *Plasmodium vivax* resistance.
6. Identify Jk(a−b−) RBCs with a resistance to lysis that normally occurs in 2M urea, a common diluting fluid used for automated platelet counters.

Introduction

This chapter contains more information than blood bank technologists or technicians need to know to work capably at the bench. It is hoped that the extra details will challenge the reader to learn more and will serve as a reference when antigens and antibodies are encountered in real-life situations.

Antigen and antibody characteristics are summarized on the front and back cover of this book so that students can easily access pertinent information when performing antibody identification. Students should review this chapter's objectives, read the material, and then refer to the antigen-antibody characteristic chart to see how much they really know.

Terminology

A blood group system is a group of antigens produced by alleles at a single gene locus or at loci so closely linked that crossing over does not occur or is very rare.[1] With a few notable exceptions, most blood group genes are located on the autosomal chromosomes and demonstrate straightforward mendelian inheritance.

Most blood group alleles are codominant and express a corresponding antigen. For example, a person who inherits alleles *K* and *k* expresses both K and k antigens on his or her RBCs. Some genes code for complex structures that carry more than one antigen (e.g., the glycophorin B structure, which carries S or s antigen, also carries 'N' and U determinants).

Silent or amorphic alleles exist that make no antigen, but they are rare. When paired chromosomes carry the same silent allele, a null phenotype results. Null phenotype RBCs can be very helpful when evaluating antibodies to unknown high-incidence antigens. For example, an antibody reacting with all test cells except those with the phenotype Lu(a−b−) may be directed against the antigens in the Lutheran system or an antigen phenotypically related to the Lutheran system.

In some blood group systems, the null phenotype results in RBC abnormalities.

Some blood group systems have regulator or modifying genes, which alter antigen expression. These are not necessarily located at the same locus as the blood group genes they affect and may segregate independently. One such modifying gene is *In(Lu)*, which inhibits or suppresses the expression of all the antigens in the Lutheran blood group system as well as many other antigens, including P₁ and i. It is a rare dominant gene inherited independently of the genes coding for Lutheran, P₁, and i antigens.

Although gene and antigen names seem confusing at first, certain conventions are followed when writing alleles, antigens, and phenotypes.[1] Some examples are given in **Table 9–1**. Genes are underlined or written in italics, and their allele number or letter is always superscript. Antigen names are not italicized and are most easily learned by everyday use. Phenotype designation depends on the antigen nomenclature and whether letters or numbers are used. These are also best learned through use. One must remember that serologic tests determine only RBC phenotype, not genotype. Genotype is determined by family or DNA studies.

Antibodies are described by their antigen notation with the prefix "anti-." Use of correct blood group terminology, especially for antibodies identified in a patient's serum, is very important so that correct information is conveyed for patient care.

To help standardize blood group system and antigen names and devise a nomenclature that was both eye- and machine-readable, the International Society of Blood Transfusion (ISBT) formed a Working Party on Terminology for Red Cell Surface Antigens in 1980.[2] The numeric system proposed by this group was not intended to replace traditional terminology but rather to enable communication on computer systems where numbers are necessary. Each known system is given a number and letter designation, and each antigen within the system is numbered sequentially in order of discovery. For example, using the ISBT terminology, the

TABLE 9–1   Examples of Correct Blood Group Terminology

	Antigen				Phenotype	
System	**Gene**	**Conventional**	**ISBT**	**Antibody**	**Antigen Positive**	**Antigen Negative**
Kell	*K*	K	K1	Anti-K	K+	K−
Kidd	*Jkᵃ*	Jkᵃ	JK1	Anti-Jkᵃ	Jk(a+)	Jk(a−)
P	*P¹*	P₁	P1	Anti-P₁	P₁+	P₁−
Lutheran	*Lu⁴*	Lu4	LU4	Anti-Lu4	Lu:4	Lu:−4

Kell blood group system (KEL) is 006; the K antigen is 006001. This committee's work is ongoing, and the assignment of RBC antigens to blood group systems is periodically updated.[3]

As described in the next chapter, RBC antigens are assigned by the ISBT to a system, collection, or low- or high-incidence series. In this chapter, traditional terminology is used, but the ISBT symbol and number are indicated for the blood group systems and collections discussed.

Biochemistry of RBC Antigens

Although blood bank personnel use routine serologic tests to detect RBC antigens, researchers use more sophisticated techniques to analyze their biochemistry and structure. Because these methods contribute so greatly to the knowledge of antigen function and expression, students should understand the principles behind some of the basic research tools.

RBC proteins can be studied by staining intact membranes from osmotically lysed "ghost" RBCs, but more often the membranes are dissociated first into lipid and protein components. Lipids are separated with organic solvents, loosely bound proteins are solubilized by changing pH or ionic strength or by using chelating agents, and tightly bound proteins are solubilized with detergents such as sodium dodecyl sulfate (SDS).

Solubilized proteins can be separated from one another by using polyacrylamide gel electrophoresis (PAGE), wherein protein migration depends on molecular size and charge. When SDS and PAGE are used together, the negative charge of the detergent overpowers the charge of the protein, and separation occurs by size alone. By comparing relative electrophoresis mobilities with SDS-PAGE, the relative molecular mass of a protein is determined. This value relates to, but is not quite the same as, the actual molecular weight of the protein or the molecular weight calculated from amino acid sequencing studies.

After proteins are separated, the electrophoretic bands can be stained with Coomassie blue, which stains protein, or periodic acid–Schiff (PAS), which stains sialic acid–rich proteins. Bands detected with PAS represent glycoprotein.

Membrane proteins can also be separated according to their biologic activity by passing them through affinity chromatography columns. The support media in a column can be coupled with specific antibodies, lectins, membrane receptors, or special enzymes. Only high-affinity proteins bind; others can be washed away. Once isolated, the bound protein can be eluted and its amino acid sequence determined. **Table 9–2** lists the amino acids found in protein sequences and the three-letter abbreviation used to identify them.

The carbohydrates attached to proteins and lipids can also be studied. Glycopeptide linkages, the attachment of sugars to proteins, are categorized as *N*-glycosidic (*N*-acetylglucosamine [GlcNAc] attached to asparagine [Asn]) or *O*-glycosidic (sugars, usually *N*-acetylgalactosamine [GalNAc] or galactose [Gal], attached to serine [Ser] or threonine [Thr]). The sugars with a carbohydrate chain itself are studied by sequentially removing them with specific glycosidase enzymes.

Deoxyribonucleic acid (DNA) technology has also enhanced our knowledge of RBC antigens.[4,5] When isolated from cells or obtained by the reverse transcription of mRNA,

TABLE 9–2   Amino Acids and Their Three-Letter Abbreviations

Amino Acid	Abbreviation
Alanine	Ala
Arginine	Arg
Asparagine	Asn
Aspartic acid	Asp
Cysteine	Cys
Glutamine	Gln
Glutamic acid	Glu
Glycine	Gly
Histidine	His
Isoleucine	Ile
Leucine	Leu
Lysine	Lys
Methionine	Met
Phenylalanine	Phe
Proline	Pro
Serine	Ser
Threonine	Thr
Tryptophan	Trp
Tyrosine	Tyr
Valine	Val

DNA can be amplified by polymerase chain reaction and cloned and sequenced for amino acid configuration and tertiary structure. Recent technological advances enable us to learn more about the biologic function of the structures that carry the RBC antigens.

The MNS (002) Blood Group System

Following the discovery of the ABO blood group system, Landsteiner and Levine began immunizing rabbits with human RBCs, hoping to find new antigen specificities. Among the antibodies recovered from these rabbit sera were anti-M and anti-N, both of which were reported in 1927.[6,7] Data from family studies suggested that M and N were antithetical antigens. In 1947, after the implementation of the antiglobulin test, Walsh and Montgomery[8] discovered S, a distinct antigen that appeared to be genetically linked to M and N. Its antithetical partner, s, was discovered in 1951.[9] Family studies (and later, molecular genetics) demonstrated the close linkage between the genes controlling M, N and S, s antigens. The frequencies of the common MN and Ss phenotypes are listed in **(Table 9–3)**. There is a disequilibrium in the expression of S and s with M and N. In whites, the common haplotypes were calculated to appear in the following order of relative frequency: $Ns > Ms > MS > NS$.[1,10]

In 1953, an antibody to a high-incidence antigen, U, was reported by Weiner.[11] The observation by Greenwalt et al[12]

TABLE 9–3   Frequency of MNS Phenotypes

Phenotype	Whites (%)	Blacks (%)
M+N−	28	26
M+N+	50	44
M−N+	22	30
S+s−	11	3
S+s+	44	28
S−s+	45	69
S−s−U−	0	<1

that all U− RBCs were also S−s− resulted in the inclusion of U into the system.

Forty-three antigens have been included in the MNS system, making it almost equal to Rh in size and complexity **(Table 9–4)**. Most of these antigens are of low incidence and were discovered in cases of HDN or incompatible crossmatch. Others are high-incidence antigens. Antibodies to these low- and high-incidence antigens are not commonly encountered in the blood bank.

The MNS system (also referred to as the MN or MNSs system) has been assigned the ISBT numeric designation 002, second after ABO.

Basic Concepts

M and N Antigens

The M and N antigens are found on a well-characterized glycoprotein called glycophorin A (GPA), the major RBC sialic acid–rich glycoprotein (sialoglycoprotein, SGP). The antigens

are defined by the first and fifth amino acids on this structure (see Biochemistry section and Figure 9–1), but antibody reactivity may also be dependent on adjacent carbohydrate chains, which are rich in sialic acid.

There are about 10^6 copies of GPA per RBC.[13] The antigens are well developed at birth.

Because M and N are located at the outer end of GPA, they are easily destroyed or removed by the routine blood bank enzymes ficin, papain, and bromelin and by the less common enzymes trypsin and pronase. The antigens are also destroyed by ZZAP, a solution of dithiothreitol (DTT) and papain or ficin, but they are not affected by DTT alone, AET, α-chymotrypsin, chloroquine, or glycine-acid-EDTA treatment. Treating RBCs with neuraminidase, which cleaves sialic acid (also known as neuraminic acid or NeuNAc), abolishes reactivity with only some examples of antibody. M and N antibodies are heterogeneous; some may recognize only specific amino acids, but others recognize both amino acids and carbohydrate chains.

M and N have not been detected on lymphocytes, mono-

TABLE 9–4	Summary of MNS Antigens		
ISBT NUMBER	**ANTIGEN NAME**	**FREQUENCY (%)**	**YEAR DISCOVERED**
MNS1	M	78	1927
MNS2	N	72	1927
MNS3	S	55	1947
MNS4	s	89	1951
MNS5	U	>99.9	1953
MNS6	He	0.8	1951
MNS7	Mi^a	<1	1951
MNS8	M^c	<0.1	1953
MNS9	Vw	<1	1954
MNS10	Mur	<0.1	1961
MNS11	M^g	<0.01	1958
MNS12	Vr	<0.1	1958
MNS13	M^e	<1	1961
MNS14	Mt^a	0.25	1962
MNS15	St^a	<0.1	1962
MNS16	Ri^a	<0.1	1962
MNS17	Cl^a	<0.1	1963
MNS18	Ny^a	<0.1	1964
MNS19	Hut	<0.1	1966
MNS20	Hil	<0.1	1966
MNS21	M^v	<0.6	1966
MNS22	Far	<0.1	1968
MNS23	S^D	<0.01	1978
MNS24	Mit	0.12	1980
MNS25	Dantu	<0.1	1982
MNS26	Hop	<0.1	1977
MNS27	Nob	<0.1	1977
MNS28	En^a	>99.9	1969
MNS29	EnKT	>99.9	1986
MNS30	'N'	>99.9	1977
MNS31	Or	<0.1	1964
MNS32	DANE	(low)	1991
MNS33	TSEN	(low)	1992
MNS34	MINY	(low)	1992
MNS35	MUT	<0.1	1992
MNS36	SAT	(low)	1991
MNS37	ERIK	(low)	1993
MNS38	Os^a	(low)	1983
MNS39	ENEP	>99.9	1995
MNS40	ENEH	>99.9	1993
MNS41	HAG	(low)	1995
MNS42	ENAV	>99.9	1996
MNS43	MARS	(low)	1992

cytes, or granulocytes by immunofluorescence flow cytometry, nor have they been detected on platelets.[14] GPA and M and N have been detected on renal capillary endothelium and epithelium.[15]

S and s Antigens

S and s antigens are located on a smaller glycoprotein called GPB that is very similar to GPA (see Biochemistry and **Figure 9–1**). S and s are differentiated by the amino acids at position 29 on GPB. S has methionine, whereas s has threonine. The epitope may also include the amino acid residues at position 34 and 35 and the carbohydrate chain attached to threonine at position 25.[10] There are fewer copies (about $1.7–2.4 \times 10^5$) of GPB than GPA per RBC.[10] In addition, there is about 1.5 times more GPB produced by the *S* gene than by the *s* gene.[1] S and s also are well developed at birth.

S and s antigens are less easily degraded by enzymes because the antigens are located farther down the glycoprotein, and enzyme-sensitive sites are less accessible. Ficin, papain, bromelin, pronase, and chymotrypsin can destroy S and s activity, but the amount of degradation may depend on the strength of the enzyme solution, length of treatment, and enzyme-to-cell ratio. Trypsin does not destroy the S and s antigens; neither does DTT, AET, chloroquine, nor glycine-acid-EDTA treatment. Like M and N, S and s are considered RBC antigens; they are not found on platelets, lymphocytes, monocytes, and granulocytes.[14]

Anti-M

Many examples of anti-M are naturally occurring saline agglutinins that react below 37°C. Although we may think of agglutinating anti-M as IgM, 50 percent to 80 percent are IgG or have an IgG component.[1] They usually do not bind complement, regardless of their immunoglobulin class, and they do not react with enzyme-treated RBCs. The frequency of saline-reactive anti-M in routine blood donors is 1 in 2500 to 5000.[14] It appears to be more common in children than in adults and is particularly common in patients with burns.[13]

Because of antigen dosage, many examples of anti-M may react better with M+N− RBCs (genotype *MM*) than with M+N+ RBCs (genotype *MN*). Very weak anti-M may not react with M+N+ RBCs at all, making antibody identification difficult. Antibody reactivity can be enhanced by increasing the serum-to-cell ratio or incubation time, or both, by decreasing incubation temperature or by adding a potentiating medium such as albumin, low ionic strength solution (LISS), or polyethylene glycol (PEG).

Some examples of anti-M are pH-dependent, reacting best at pH 6.5. These antibodies may be detected in plasma, which is slightly acidic from the anticoagulant but not in unacidified serum.[1] Other examples of anti-M react only with RBCs exposed to glucose solutions. Such antibodies react with M+ reagent RBCs or donor RBCs stored in preservative solutions containing glucose but do not react with freshly collected M+ RBCs. The significance of both pH-dependent and glucose-dependent antibodies in transfusion is questionable.

As long as anti-M does not react at 37°C, it is not clinically significant in transfusion. It is sufficient to provide units that are crossmatch-compatible at 37°C and the antiglobulin phase without typing for M antigen. Sometimes, compatible units carry the M antigen; for example, M+N+ RBCs, which do not react with weak anti-M. Only rarely do such units stimulate a change in the antibody's thermal range.

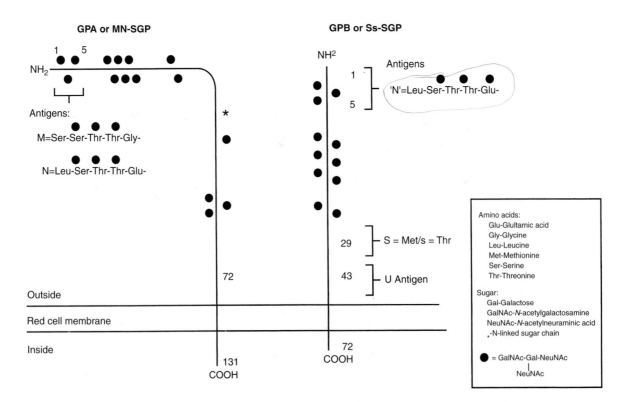

■ **FIGURE 9–1**   Comparison of GPA and GPB.

Anti-M rarely causes hemolytic transfusion reactions, decreased cell survival, or HDN. However, when 37°C-reactive IgG anti-M is found in a pregnant woman, the physician should be forewarned; some HDN cases have been severe.[1]

Anti-N

The serologic characteristics of the common anti-N (made by individuals whose RBCs type M+N− and S+ or s+) are similar to those of anti-M: a cold-reactive IgM or IgG saline agglutinin that does not bind complement or react with enzyme-treated RBCs. Anti-N can demonstrate dosage, reacting better with M−N+ (NN) RBCs than with M+N+ (MN) RBCs. Rare examples are pH- or glucose-dependent (see the preceding section on anti-M).

Also like anti-M, anti-N is not clinically significant unless it reacts at 37°C. It has been implicated only with rare cases of mild HDN.[1]

Anti-N is rarer than anti-M because the terminal end of GPB carries the same amino acid sequence and sugars as GPA when N is expressed (GPA^N). This N-like structure, called 'N', may prevent N-individuals from recognizing N as a foreign antigen. The most potent antibodies are found in rare individuals who type M+N−S−s− and lack N and 'N'.

Anti-N is also seen in renal patients, regardless of their MN type, who are dialyzed on equipment sterilized with formaldehyde. Dialysis-associated anti-N reacts with any N+ or N− RBC treated with formaldehyde and is called anti-N^f. Formaldehyde may alter the M and N antigens so that they are recognized as foreign. The antibody titer decreases when dialysis treatment and exposure to formaldehyde stop. Because anti-N^f does not react at 37°C, it is clinically insignificant in transfusion. However, it has been associated with the rejection of a chilled transplanted kidney.[16]

Anti-S and Anti-s

Most examples of anti-S and anti-s are IgG, reactive at 37°C and the antiglobulin test phase. A few express optimal reactivity between 10° and 22°C by saline indirect antiglobulin test. If anti-S or anti-s specificity is suspected, incubating tests at room temperature and performing the antiglobulin test without incubating at 37°C may help in its identification. Dosage effect can be exhibited by many examples of anti-S and anti-s, although it may not be as dramatic as seen with anti-M and anti-N.[1]

The antibodies may or may not react with enzyme-treated RBCs, depending on the extent of treatment. Treated RBCs should be tested for S or s antigen expression with known antisera before enzyme reactions are interpreted. Although seen less often than anti-M, anti-S and anti-s are more likely to be clinically significant. They may bind complement, and they have been implicated in severe hemolytic transfusion reactions with hemoglobinuria. They have also caused HDN.

Units selected for transfusion must be antigen-negative and crossmatch-compatible. Because only 11 percent of whites and 3 percent of blacks are s−, it can be difficult providing blood for a patient with anti-s. S− units are much easier to find (45 percent of whites and 69 percent of blacks are

S−). Antibodies to low-incidence antigens are commonly found in reagent anti-S, and these can cause discrepant antigen typing results.

Advanced Concepts

Biochemistry

GPA, the structure carrying the M and N antigens, has a molecular weight of 36 kD and consists of 131 amino acids. The hydrophilic NH₂ terminal end, which lies outside the RBC membrane, has 72 amino acid residues, 15 O-glycosidically linked oligosaccharide chains (GalNAc-serine/threonine), and 1 N-glycosidic chain (sugar-asparagine). The portion that traverses the membrane is hydrophobic and contains 23 amino acids.[13] The hydrophilic COOH end, which contains 36 amino acids and no carbohydrates, lies inside the membrane and interacts weakly with the membrane cytoskeleton. M and N antigens differ in their amino acid residues at positions 1 and 5 (see Fig. 9–1). M has serine and glycine at these positions, whereas N has leucine and glutamic acid.

GPB, the structure carrying S, s, and U antigens, has a molecular weight of 20 kD and contains 72 amino acids and 11 O-linked oligosaccharide chains and no N-glycans. It has an outer glycosylated portion of 44 amino acids, a hydrophobic portion of 20 amino acids that traverses the RBC membrane, and a short cytoplasmic "tail" of 8 amino acids.

The first 26 amino acids on GPB are identical to the first 26 amino acids on the N form of GPA (GPA^N). This N activity of GPB is denoted as 'N' (N-quotes) to distinguish it from the N activity of GPA^N. Anti-N reagents do not recognize the 'N' structure. The U antigen, expressed when normal GPB is present, is located very close to the RBC membrane (see the later section on the U–phenotype).

Most O-linked carbohydrate structures on GPA and GPB are branched tetrasaccharides containing one GalNAc, one Gal, and two NeuNAc (sialic acid). Heterogeneity does occur within these chains (they can lack a sugar or have sugar substitutions), but their significant feature is NeuNAc, which helps give the RBC its negative charge. About 70 percent of the RBC NeuNAc is carried by GPA, and about 16 percent is carried by GPB.

GPA associates with protein band 3, which affects the expression of the antigen Wr^b of the Diego blood group system (located on protein band 3). GPB appears to be associated with the Rh protein and Rh-associated glycoprotein complex as evidenced by the greatly reduced S and s expression on Rh_null RBCs.[10]

Other antigens within the MNS system have been evaluated biochemically and at the molecular level. Some are associated with altered GPA because of amino acid substitutions and/or changes in carbohydrate chains. Others are expressed on variants of GPA or GPB. Still others result from a genetic event that encodes a hybrid glycophorin that has parts of both GPA and GPB. The altered glycophorins are associated with changes in glycosylation, changes in molecular weight, loss of high-incidence antigens or the appearance of novel low-incidence antigens, and/or alterations in the expression of MNS antigens.[1,10,13]

The heterogeneity of GPA and GPB leads to speculation about their physiologic function. RBCs that lack GPA and/or

GPB are not associated with disease or decreased RBC survival (see the later section on Disease Associations).

Genetics

The genes *GYPA* and *GYPB,* which code for GPA and GPB, respectively, are located on chromosome 4 at 4q28–q31. The known alleles for *GYPA (M/N)* and *GYPB (S/s)* are codominant. Because of their many similarities and primate antigen studies, some suggest that *GYPB* arose from a duplication of an ancestral *GYPA* gene and that the other alleles arose by further mutations.[1,17]

GYPA is organized into seven exons (portions that are translated into functional protein; the unused portions or introns are spliced out): exon A1 encodes a leader protein that helps insert the structure into the membrane during formation; exon A2 encodes the first 26 amino acids; exon A3 has inverted repeat sequences known to be sites for DNA recombination; exon A4 encodes the remaining extracellular portion; exon A5, the transmembrane protein; and exons A6 and A7, the cytoplasmic portion. Exon A7 also contains the stop codon.[17]

GYPB has a size and arrangement similar to those of *GYPA* but only five exons: exons B1 and B2, which are nearly identical to exons A1 and A2, encode a leader protein and amino acids 1 through 26; exon B3 is analogous to exon A4, encoding the portion of the molecule that carries S and s; exon B4, similar to exon A5, encodes a larger transmembrane portion because of a mutation that affects an mRNA splice site; and exon B5 encodes the cytoplasmic portion and final stop codon. There is no counterpart to exon A3 because of another splice site mutation, nor is there an exon A6 or A7 counterpart.

A third highly homologous gene, *GYPE,* does not appear to make a glycoprotein that has been definitively recognized on the RBC surface.

Misalignment of *GYPA* and *GYPB* during meiosis, followed by an unequal crossing over appears to provide an explanation for some of the variant glycophorins observed in the MNS system. The resulting new reciprocal *GYP(A-B)* and *GYP(B-A)* genes encode GP(A-B) and GP(B-A) hybrid glycophorins, respectively **(Fig. 9–2)**.[10,17]

For more complex variant glycophorins, a gene conversion event probably occurs. Gene conversion is not completely understood; it involves a nonreciprocal exchange of genetic material from one gene to another homologous gene **(Fig. 9–3)**.[10] The point of fusion between the GPA and GPB part in the hybrid glycophorin can give rise to novel antigens, e.g., antigen of low incidence. Also, expected antigens may be missing if the coding exons are replaced by the inserted genetic material.

M and N Lectins

A number of plant lectins have proved useful in studying GPA biochemistry, some with practical application.[10] Those having N reactivity include *Bauhinia variegata, Bauhinia purpura,* and *Vicia graminea.* When diluted, *V. graminea* lectin behaves as anti-N and so makes an appropriate typing reagent.[1,10]

When antigen typing RBCs with lectins, remember that only specific carbohydrate structures are recognized by these reagents. Results may not parallel those obtained with human antibody or other lectins, especially when RBCs with altered or variant SGPs are tested.

GPA- and GPB-Deficient Phenotypes

RBCs of three rare phenotypes lack either GPA or GPB or both GPA and GPB and, consequently, all MNS antigens that are normally expressed on those structures.

U-Phenotype. The U (for *universal*) antigen is located on GPB very close to the RBC membrane between amino acids 33 and 39. This high-incidence antigen is found on RBCs of all individuals except about 1 percent of American blacks (and 1 to 35 percent of African blacks),[17] who lack GPB because of a partial or complete deletion of *GYPB.* They usually type S−s−U− and make anti-U in response to transfusion or pregnancy. Anti-U is typically IgG and has been reported to cause hemolytic transfusion reactions and HDN.

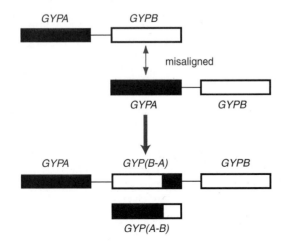

■ **FIGURE 9–2**   How misalignment during meiosis can lead to a crossover and reciprocal *GYP(B-A) and GYP(A −B)* hybrids.

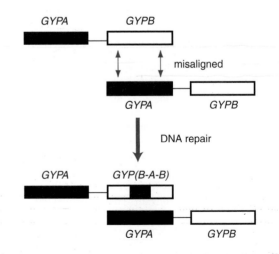

■ **FIGURE 9–3**   In a gene conversion event, nucleotides from one strand of DNA are transferred to the misaligned homologous gene. If this is the coding strand, a hybrid glycophorin will be formed; the partner chromosome will be repaired and carry the naïve (unaltered) *GYPA* and *GYPB* genes.

The U antigen is resistant to enzyme treatment; thus, most examples of anti-U react equally well with untreated and enzyme-treated RBCs; there are rare examples of broadly reactive anti-U, however, that do not react with papain-treated RBCs.[1]

Some examples of anti-U react with apparent U− RBCs, although weakly, by adsorption and elution.[10] Such RBCs are said to be U variant (Uvar). Uvar RBCs have an altered GPB that does not express S or s. There is a strong correlation between the low-incidence antigen He (MNS6), found in about 3 percent of African-Americans, and Uvar expression.[10]

Because examples of anti-U are heterogeneous, U− units selected for transfusion must be crossmatched to determine compatibility. Some patients may tolerate Uvar units; others may not. If the patient is U− and N−, the antibody may actually be a potent anti-N plus anti-U, making the search for compatible blood even more difficult.

En(a−) Phenotype. In 1969 Darnborough et al[18] and Furuhjelm et al[19] described an antibody to the same high-incidence antigen, called Ena (for *envelope*), which reacted with all RBCs except those of the propositi. Both En(a−) individuals appeared to be M−N− with reduced NeuNAc on their RBCs. The RBCs of the two individuals were mutually compatible.

Most En(a−) individuals produce anti-Ena, which is an umbrella term for reactivity against various portions of GPA unrelated to M or N, but not all antibodies detect the same portion. Anti-EnaTS recognizes a trypsin-sensitive (TS) area on GPA between amino acids 20 and 39. Anti-EnaFS reacts with a ficin-sensitive (FS) area between amino acids 46 and 56, and anti-EnaFR reacts with a ficin-resistant (FR) area around amino acids 62 to 72.[1,10]

Although the gene responsible for this phenotype has been termed *En*, it is now known that the En(a−) phenotype has more than one origin. Typically, the En(a−) phenotype results from homozygosity for a gene deletion at the *GYPA* locus; consequently, no GPA is produced, but GPB is not affected. This type of En(a−) inheritance is called En(a−)Fin. The En(a−) phenotype in the English report, however, probably represents heterozygosity for a hybrid gene

along with the rare *Mk* gene; this type is often called En(a−)UK.

Mk Phenotype. The rare silent gene *Mk* was identified in 1964 by Metaxas and Metaxas-Buhler[20] when they studied an M−N+ (*NMk*) mother who had an M+N− (*MMk*) child. The RBCs of these rare individuals expressed half the amount of normal MN and Ss on SDS-PAGE analysis. In 1979 Tokunaga et al[21] reported finding two related *MkMk* blood donors in Japan. The RBCs of these individuals typed M−N−S−s−U−, but they had a normal hematologic picture. More individuals have since been identified, and it is now known that the *Mk* gene represents a single, near-complete deletion of both *GYPA* and *GYPB*[10]; thus, Mk is the null phenotype in the MNS system. The *MkMk* genotype is associated with decreased RBC sialic acid content but increased glycosylation of RBC membrane bands 3 and 4.1.

The Miltenberger Series

The Miltenberger series of low-incidence antigens was developed to bring order to a group of specificities that appeared to be related to one another. This relationship, however, is purely serologic. The Miltenberger classification still appears in the literature, although it is no longer feasible to continue expansion of the original series.

After the first five antigens were defined, Cleghorn performed a series of cross tests with their respective antibodies and separated the RBCs into five phenotypes: MiI, MiII, MiIII, MiIV, and MiV. These phenotypes have been redefined and expanded to 11 with the discovery of additional antigens (**Table 9–5**).[10]

Biochemical and molecular studies have simplified understanding of the Miltenberger series. Each phenotype represents a distinct variant GP or hybrid molecule. Tippett et al[22] proposed that the Miltenberger terminology be dropped in favor of one that recognized the glycoprotein variant and the name of the first propositus. The associated GP variants are listed in **Table 9–5**. Many other variant MN glycoproteins associated with the Miltenberger phenotypes are described elsewhere.[1,10]

TABLE 9–5   The Miltenberger Series

Current Class	Proposed# Terminology	Vw	Mur	Hil	Hut	Hop	Nob	DANE	MUT	TSEN	MINY	Biochemistry*	
Mi.I	GP.Vw	+	0	0	0	0	0	0	0	0	0	GP ABA	aa28 Thr→Ser
Mi.II	GP.Hut	0	0	0	+	0	0	0	+	0	0	GP ABA	aa28 Thr→Lys
Mi.III	GP.Mur	0	+	+	0	0	0	0	+	0	+	GP BAB	
Mi.IV	GP.Hop	0	+	0	0	+	0	0	+	+	+	GP BAB	
Mi.V	GP.Hil	0	0	+	0	0	0	0	0	0	+	GP AB	
Mi.VI	GP.Bun	0	+	+	0	+	0	0	+	0	+	GP BAB	
Mi.VII	GP.Nob	0	0	0	0	0	+	0	0	0	0	GP ABA	aa49 Arg→Thr aa52 Thr→Ser
Mi.VIII	GP.Joh	0	0	0	0	+	+	0	0	NT	0	GP ABA	
Mi.IX	GP.Dane	0	+	0	0	0	0	+	0	0	0	GP ABA	
Mi.X	GP.HF	0	0	+	0	0	0	0	+	0	+	GP BAB	
Mi.XI	GP.JL	0	0	0	0	0	0	0	NT	+	+	GP ABs	

Reid, MD, and Lomas-Francis, C: The Blood Group Antigen Facts Book. Academic Press, New York, 1997. NT = not tested.

Other Antibodies in the MNS System

Antibodies to antigens other than M, N, S, and s are rarely encountered and can usually be grouped into two categories: those directed against low-incidence antigens and those directed against high-incidence antigens.

Antibodies to high-incidence antigens are easily detected with antibody detection RBCs. Antibodies to low-incidence antigens are rarely detected by the antibody screen but are seen as an unexpected incompatible crossmatch or an unexplained case of HDN. Few hospital blood banks have the test cells available to identify the specificity, but enzyme reactivity and MNS antigen typing may offer clues.

It is common practice to transfuse units that are crossmatch-compatible at 37°C and in the antiglobulin phase when antibodies to antigens of low incidence are present. Typing sera for MNS antigens other than M and N and S and s are not generally available, so the antigen status of compatible RBCs can seldom be confirmed. If the antibody is directed to an antigen of high incidence, the assistance of an immunohematology reference laboratory may be needed for antibody identification and obtaining appropriate antigen negative units.

Autoantibodies

Autoantibodies to M and N have been reported.[1] Not all examples of anti-M in M+ individuals or anti-N in N+ individuals are autoantibodies. Many fail to react with the patient's own RBCs. It may be that these individuals have altered GPA and that their antibody is specific for a portion of the common antigen they lack.

Autoantibodies to U and En[a] are more common and may be associated with warm-type autoimmune hemolytic anemia.

Disease Associations

GPA[M] may serve as the receptor by which certain pyelonephritogenic strains of *Escherichia coli* gain entry to the urinary tract.

The malaria parasite *Plasmodium falciparum* appears to use alternative receptors, including GPA, GPB, and GPC[23] for cell invasion; some of these receptors also involve NeuNAc. In an attempt to identify the receptor, the invasion rate into cells with normal and rare phenotypes was studied. Reduced invasion is seen with En(a−), U−, M^kM^k, Tn and Cad RBCs (which have altered oligosaccharides on glycophorins), Ge−, and normal RBCs treated with neuraminidase and trypsin.[10]

The P Blood Group: P (003) and Globoside (028) Blood Group Systems and Related Antigens

Traditionally, the P Blood Group comprised the P, P_1, and P^k antigens and, later, Luke. The biochemistry and molecular genetics, although not completely understood as yet, make it clear that at least two biosynthetic pathways and genes at different loci are involved in the development and expression of these antigens. Consequently, these antigens cannot be considered a single blood group system. Currently, in ISBT nomenclature P_1 is assigned to the P Blood Group System (003), P to the new Globoside Blood Group System (028)[3], and P^k and LKE are assigned to the Globoside Collection (209). For simplicity in this chapter, these antigens will be referred to as the P blood group.

The P blood group was introduced in 1927 by Landsteiner and Levine.[7] In their search for new antigens, they injected rabbits with human RBCs and produced an antibody, initially called anti-P, that divided human RBCs into two groups: P+ and P−.

In 1951 Levine et al[24] described anti-Tj[a] (now known as anti-PP₁P[k]), an antibody to a high-incidence antigen that Sanger[25] later showed was related to the P blood group. Because anti-Tj[a] defined an antigen common to P+ and P− cells and was made by an apparent P null individual, the original antigen and phenotypes were renamed. Anti-P became anti-P_1; the P+ phenotype became P_1; the P− phenotype became P_2; and the rare P null individual became p.

The P blood group became more complex in 1959 when Matson et al[26] described a new antigen, P^k. P^k is expressed on all RBCs except those of the very rare p phenotype, but it is not readily detected unless P is absent, i.e., in the P_1^k and P_2^k phenotypes.

The antigens and phenotypes associated with the P blood group are summarized in **Table 9–6**. There are two common phenotypes: P_1 and P_2, and three rare phenotypes: p, P_1^k, and P_2^k. The P_1 phenotype describes RBCs that react with anti-P_1 and anti-P; the P_2 phenotype describes RBCs that do not react with anti-P_1 but do react with anti-P. When RBCs are tested only with anti-P_1 and not with anti-P, the phenotype should be written as P_1+ or $P_1−$. RBCs of the p phenotype do not react with anti-P_1, anti-P, or anti-P^k. RBCs of the P_1^k phenotype react with anti-P_1 and anti-P^k but not with anti-P. RBCs of the P_2^k phenotype react with anti-P^k but not with anti-P_1 or anti-P.

Individuals with the p phenotype (P null) are very rare: 5.8 in a million. P nulls are slightly more common in Japan, North Sweden, and in an Amish group in Ohio.[1]

TABLE 9–6	**P Blood Group: Phenotypes, Antigens and Antibodies**			
			Frequency	
Phenotype	Antigens Present	Possible Antibodies	Whites	Blacks
P_1	P_1, P, (P^k)	None	79%	94%
P_2	P, (P^k)	Anti-P_1	21%	6%
p	None	Anti-PP₁P[k]	Rare	Rare
P_1^k	P_1, P^k	Anti-P	Very rare	Very rare
P_2^k	P^k	Anti-P, Anti-P_1	Very rare	Very rare

The antibodies generally fall into two categories: clinically insignificant or potently hemolytic.

Basic Concepts

The P blood group antigens, like the ABH antigens, are synthesized by sequential action of glycosyltransferases, which add sugars to precursor substances. The precursor of P_1 can also be glycosylated to type 2H chains, which carry ABH antigens. P_1, P, or P^k may be found on RBCs, lymphocytes, granulocytes, and monocytes; P can be found on platelets, epithelial cells, and fibroblasts. P and P^k have also been found in plasma as glycosphingolipids and as glycoproteins in hydatid cyst fluid.[10] The antigens have not been identified in secretions.[14] RBCs carry approximately 14×10^6 copies of globoside, the P structure, per adult RBC and about 5×10^5 copies of P_1.[13]

The P_1 Antigen

The expression of P_1 changes during fetal development. The antigen is found on fetal RBCs as early as 12 weeks, but it weakens with gestational age. Ikin et al[27] found that young fetuses were more frequently and more strongly P_1+ than older fetuses. The antigen is poorly expressed at birth and may take up to 7 years to be fully expressed.[10]

Antigen strength in adults varies from one individual to another, a fact first noted by Landsteiner and Levine,[7] who found that some P_1+ people were P_1 strong (P_1+^s) and others were P_1 weak (P_1+^w). These differences appear to be quantitative, not qualitative, and may either be controlled genetically or represent homozygous versus heterozygous inheritance of the gene coding for P_1. The strength of P_1 can also vary with race. Blacks have a stronger expression of P_1 than whites. The rare dominant gene *In(Lu)*, discussed in the Lutheran section, inhibits the expression of P_1 so that P_1 individuals who inherit this modifier gene may type serologically as P_1-.

The P_1 antigen deteriorates rapidly on storage. When old cells are typed or used as controls for typing reagents or when older cells are used to detect anti-P_1 in serum, false-negative reactions may result.

Anti-P_1

Anti-P_1 is a common, naturally occurring IgM antibody in the sera of P_1- individuals. Anti-P_1 is typically a weak, cold-reactive saline agglutinin optimally reactive at 4°C and not seen in routine testing. Stronger examples react at room temperature, and rare examples react at 37°C and bind complement, which is detected in the antiglobulin test when polyspecific reagents are used. Antibody activity can be neutralized or inhibited with soluble P_1 substance or bypassed using prewarm test methods.

Examples of anti-P_1 that react only at temperatures below 37°C can be considered clinically insignificant. For the examples of anti-P_1, which are stronger at room temperature, setting up tests using a prewarm technique (which avoids carryover agglutination from room temperature reactivity) may be necessary to determine if the antibody is reactive at 37°C.

Because P_1 antigen expression on RBCs varies and deteriorates during storage, antibodies may react only with RBCs having the strongest expression and give inconclusive patterns of reactivity when antibody identification is performed.

Incubating tests at room temperature or lower or pretreating test cells with enzymes can enhance reactions to confirm specificity. Providing units that are crossmatch-compatible at 37°C and the antiglobulin phase, without typing for P_1, is an acceptable approach to transfusion. Giving P_1+ units under these circumstances does not cause a rise in antibody titer or a change in its thermal range of reactivity.[14]

Rare examples of anti-P_1 that react at 37°C can cause in vivo RBC destruction; both immediate and delayed hemolytic transfusion reactions have been reported.[14,28] These rare antibodies react well in the antiglobulin phase, bind complement, and may lyse test cells, especially if they are enzyme-treated. Although it is tempting to assume that such antibodies are IgG, many have been identified as IgM; IgG forms are rare. HDN is not associated with anti-P_1, presumably because the antibody is usually IgM and the antigen is so poorly developed on fetal cells.

Advanced Concepts

Biochemistry

The RBC antigens of the P blood group exist as glycosphingolipids. As with ABH, the antigens result from the sugars added sequentially to precursor structures. Biochemical analyses have shown that the precursor substance for P_1 is also a precursor for type 2H chains that carry ABH antigens. However, the genes responsible for the formation of the P_1 and ABH antigens are independent. As with ABH, P blood group antigens are resistant to enzyme, DTT, chloroquine, or glycine-acid-EDTA degradation.

There are two distinct pathways for the synthesis of the P blood group antigens, as shown in **Figure 9–4**. The common precursor is lactosylceramide (or Gb2, also known as ceramide dihexose or CDH). The pathway on the left results in the formation of paragloboside and P_1. Paragloboside is also the type 2 precursor for ABH.

The pathway shown on the right side of **Figure 9–4** leads to the production of the globoside series: P^k, P, and Luke (LKE). P^k (globotriosylceramide or Gb3) is synthesized by the addition of galactose to lactosylceramide; P^k is subsequently converted to P (globoside or Gb4) by the addition of N-acetylgalactosamine. The Luke or LKE antigen is formed by the addition of galactose and sialic acid to globoside (or P antigen).

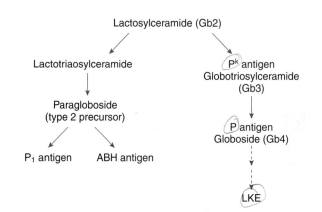

FIGURE 9–4 Biosynthetic pathways of the P blood group antigens.

Genetics

The gene encoding the enzyme responsible for the synthesis of P^k from lactosylceramide, a 4-α-galactosyltransferase (Gb3 or P^k synthase), was cloned independently by three research groups in 2000.[3,29] The gene encoding the 3-β-N-acetylgalactosaminyl-transferase (Gb4 synthase) that is responsible for converting P^k to P was also cloned in 2000.[3,29] Several mutations in both genes have been identified that result in the p and P^k phenotypes.[29–31]

The genetic relationship of P_1 to P and P^k is not yet understood. RBCs of the p phenotype are P_1- in addition to P$-$ and P^k- (the P_1- status of p RBCs cannot be explained). It is still unclear if another gene is involved in the synthesis of P_1 or if another mechanism exists.[29] The P_1 gene (located on chromosome 22) and the P gene (located on chromosome 3) are inherited independently.

The gene for the synthesis of LKE has not yet been cloned.

Other Sources of P_1 Antigen and Antibody

The discovery of strong anti-P_1 in two P_1- individuals infected with *Echinococcus granulosus* tapeworms led to the identification of P_1 and P^k substance in hydatid cyst fluid.[32] This fluid was subsequently used in many of the studies that identified the biochemical structures of the P blood group.

A P_1-like antigen has also been found on RBCs, in plasma, in droppings of pigeons and turtledoves, and in the egg white of turtledoves. Exposure to these birds may place P_1- bird handlers at risk of making strong, clinically significant anti-P_1. The P_1 antigen in bird droppings may be attributed to certain gram-negative avian bacteria rather than to the birds themselves.[33]

Strong antibodies to P_1 have also been associated with fascioliasis (bovine liver fluke disease), *Clonorchis sinensis,* and *Opisthorchis viverrini* infections. P_1 substance has been identified in extracts of *Lumbricoides terrestris* (the common earthworm) and *Ascaris suum.*[10]

Soluble P_1 substances have potential use in the blood bank and are commercially available. When it is necessary to confirm antibody specificity or to identify underlying antibodies, these substances can be used to neutralize anti-P_1 if prewarmed methods do not eliminate reactivity.

Anti-PP_1P^k

Originally called anti-Tj^a, anti-PP_1P^k was first described in the serum of Mrs. Jay, a p individual with adenocarcinoma of the stomach.[24] Her tumor cells carried P system antigens, and the antibody was credited as having cytotoxic properties that may have helped prevent metastatic growth postsurgery (the T in the Tj^a refers to *tumor*).

Anti-PP_1P^k is produced by all p individuals early in life without RBC sensitization and reacts with all RBCs except those of the p phenotype. Unlike antibodies made by other blood group null phenotypes, the anti-P, anti-P_1, and anti-P^k components of anti-PP_1P^k are separable through adsorption.[10] Components of anti-PP_1P^k have been shown to be IgM and IgG.[10] They react over a wide thermal range and efficiently bind complement, which makes them potent hemolysins. Anti-PP_1P^k has the potential to cause severe hemolytic transfusion reactions and HDN.

The antibody is also associated with an increased incidence of spontaneous abortions in early pregnancy. Although the reason for this is not fully known, it has been suggested that having an IgG anti-P component is an important factor.[34] Women with anti-P and anti-PP_1P^k and a history of multiple abortions have successfully delivered infants after multiple plasmaphereses to reduce their antibody level during pregnancy.[35,36]

Alloanti-P

In addition to being a component of the anti-PP_1P^k in p individuals (see above), anti-P is found as a naturally occurring alloantibody in the sera of all P^k individuals. Its reactivity is similar to that of anti-PP_1P^k in that it is usually a potent hemolysin reacting with all cells except the autocontrol and those with the p phenotype. However, it differs from anti-PP_1P^k in that it does not react with cells having the extremely rare P^k phenotype, and the individual making the antibody may type P_1+. Alloanti-P is rarely seen, but because it is hemolytic with a wide thermal range of reactivity it is very significant in transfusion. IgG class anti-P may occur and has been associated with habitual early abortion.

Autoanti-P Associated with Paroxysmal Cold Hemoglobinuria

Anti-P specificity is also associated with the cold-reactive IgG autoantibody in patients with paroxysmal cold hemoglobinuria (PCH). Historically, this rare autoimmune disorder was seen in patients with tertiary syphilis; it now more commonly presents as a transient, acute condition secondary to viral infection, especially in young children. The IgG autoantibody in PCH is described as a biphasic hemolysin: in vitro the antibody binds to RBCs in the cold and, via complement activation, the coated RBCs lyse as they are warmed to 37°C. The autoantibody typically does not react in routine test systems but is demonstrable only by the Donath-Landsteiner test. The etiology and diagnosis of PCH are more fully discussed in Chapter 21.

Anti-P^k

Anti-P^k has been isolated from some examples of anti-PP_1P^k by selective adsorption with P_1 cells. Autoanti-P^k has been reported in the serum of P_1 individuals with biliary cirrhosis and autoimmune hemolytic anemia.[10] Anti-P^k activity can be inhibited with hydatid cyst fluid.

Antibodies to Compound Antigens

Considering the biochemical relationship of the P blood group antigens to ABH and I, it is not surprising that antibodies requiring more than one antigenic determinant have been described, including anti-IP_1, -iP_1, -I^TP_1, and -IP. Most examples are cold-reactive agglutinins.

Luke (LKE) Antigen and Antibody

In 1965 Tippett et al[37] described an antibody in the serum of a patient with Hodgkin's lymphoma that divided the population into three phenotypes: 84 percent tested Luke+, 14 percent were weakly positive or Luke(w), and 2 percent were

Luke−. Although this mendelian dominant character segregated independently of the P blood group, it was thought to be phenotypically related because the antibody reacted with all RBCs except 2 percent of P_1 and P_2 phenotypes and those having the rare p and P^k phenotypes. All individuals with the p and P^k phenotype are Luke− (or LKE−). Using the original antibody, the Luke(w) phenotype was more commonly found with P_2 than P_1 and more common with A_1 and A_1B than with A_2, B, or O phenotypes, although subsequent examples did not parallel these findings.

LKE− individuals may be either P_1 or P_2. The P^k antigen is more strongly expressed on LKE− RBCs than on LKE+ RBCs.

Only five examples of human alloanti-LKE are known.[10] The original was a saline agglutinin that reacted best at 4°C. Using enzyme methods and additional complement, it became a potent hemolysin. The other examples were much weaker and clinically insignificant.

Disease Associations

Several pathologic conditions associated with the P blood group antigens have been described: parasitic infections are associated with anti-P_1, early abortions with anti-PP_1P^k or anti-P, and PCH with autoanti-P.

The P system antigens may also be associated with urinary tract infections. Some pyelonephritogenic strains of *E. coli* ascend the urinary tract in ladderlike fashion by adhering to P_1 and/or P^k glycolipids on uroepithelial cells. The fimbriae or pili of such organisms have receptor sites for structures involving Gal(α1-4)Gal(β1-4), the terminal sugars for P_1 and P^k. Other globoside associations have been identified with infection. *Streptococcus suis,* which occasionally causes meningitis and septicemia in humans, binds exclusively to P^k antigen. A class of toxins secreted by *Shigella dysenteriae, Vibrio cholerae, Vibrio parahaemolyticus,* and some pathogenic strains of *E. coli* also have binding specificity for a Gal(α1-4)Gal(β1-4) moiety. In addition, globoside is the receptor of human parvovirus B19.[10]

The I (027) Blood Group System and i Antigen

The existence of cold agglutinins in the serum of normal individuals and in patients with acquired hemolytic anemia has long been recognized. In 1956 Wiener et al[38] gave a name to one such agglutinin, calling its antigen "I" for *individuality.* The antibody reacted with all but 5 of 22,000 blood specimens tested (i.e., most were I+). The nonreactive I− specimens were thought to be from homozygotes for a rare gene producing the "i" antigen; the I− phenotype in adults is now called adult i. In 1960, Marsh and Jenkins[39] reported finding anti-i, and the unique relationship between I and i began to unfold.

The I antigen together with the i antigen used to comprise the Ii Blood Group Collection (207). I and i are not antithetical antigens. Rather, they are branched and linear carbohydrate structures, respectively, that are formed by the action of glycosyl transferases. However, the gene encoding the transferase that converts i active straight chains into I active branched chains has been cloned, and several mutations responsible for the rare adult i phenotype have been identified.[40] Consequently, I has been raised to Blood Group System

status; the new I System (027) has only one antigen, I.[3] The i antigen remains in the Ii collection (207).

Basic Concepts

The I and i Antigens

The antigens are best introduced by classic serologic facts. Both I and i are high-incidence antigens, but they are expressed in a reciprocal relationship that is developmentally regulated. At birth, infant RBCs are rich in i; I is almost undetectable. During the first 18 months of life, the quantity of i slowly decreases as I increases until adult proportions are reached; adult RBCs are rich in I and have only trace amounts of i antigen.

There is no true I− or i− phenotype. The number of I copies per adult RBC varies $0.3-5.0 \times 10^5$.[14] The estimated number of i antigen varies $0.2-0.65 \times 10^5$ on cord RBCs and $0.3-0.7 \times 10^5$ on adult i RBCs.[10,14] The strength of I and i varies from individual to individual, and the relative amount detected will depend on the example of anti-I or anti-i used. A wide normal range of reactivity can be observed with both anti-I and anti-i. Data suggest that an RBC's i reactivity is inversely proportional to marrow transit time and RBC age in circulation.

Some people appear not to change their i status after birth. They become the rare adult i. Adult i RBCs generally express more i antigen than do cord RBCs. A spectrum of Ii phenotypes and their characteristics are listed in **Table 9–7**.

Treatment of RBCs with enzymes enhances the I and i antigens.

Anti-I

Anti-I is a common autoantibody that can be found in virtually all sera, although testing at 4°C and/or against enzyme-treated RBCs may be required to detect the reactivity.[1] Consistently strong agglutination with adult RBCs and weak or no agglutination with cord RBCs define its classic activity. Common reactivity patterns are in **Table 9–7**.

Autoanti-I, found in the serum of many normal healthy individuals, is benign, i.e., not associated with in-vivo RBC destruction. It is usually a weak, naturally occurring, saline-reactive IgM agglutinin with a titer level less than 64 at 4°C. Stronger examples agglutinate test cells at room temperature and/or bind complement, which can be detected in the antiglobulin test if polyspecific reagents are used. Some may react only with the strongest I+ RBCs and give inconsistent reactions with panel RBCs.

Incubating tests in the cold enhances anti-I reactivity and helps confirm its identity; albumin and enzyme methods also enhance anti-I reactivity. Testing enzyme-treated RBCs with

TABLE 9–7	I and i Antigens		
	Strength of Reactivity With:		
Phenotype	Anti-I	Anti-i	Anti-I^T
Adult I	Strong	Weak	Weak
Cord	Weak	Strong	Strong
Adult i	Weak	Strong	Weakest

slightly acidified serum may even promote hemolysis. Occasionally, benign cold autoanti-I can cause problems in pretransfusion testing. Usually, avoiding room temperature testing and using anti-IgG instead of a polyspecific anti-human globulin help to eliminate detection of cold reactive antibodies that may bind complement at lower temperatures. Cold autoadsorption to remove the autoantibody from the serum may be necessary for stronger examples; cold autoadsorbed plasma or serum can also be used in ABO typing. A prewarm technique can also be used to avoid antibody binding at lower temperatures once the reactivity has been confirmed as autoantibody.

Pathogenic autoanti-I, e.g., the type associated with cold agglutinin syndrome, typically consists of strong IgM agglutinins with higher titers and a broad thermal range of activity, reacting up to 30° or 32°C. When peripheral circulation cools in response to low ambient temperatures, these antibodies attach in vivo and cause autoagglutination and vascular occlusion (acrocyanosis) or hemolytic anemia. Refer to Chapter 21 for more information.

Pathogenic anti-I typically reacts with adult and cord RBCs equally well at room temperature and at 4°C, and antibody specificity may not be apparent unless the serum is diluted or warmed to 30° or 37°C. Potent cold autoantibodies can also mask clinically significant underlying alloantibodies and complicate pretransfusion testing. Procedures to deal with these problems are discussed in other chapters.

The production of autoanti-I may be stimulated by microorganisms carrying I-like antigen on their surface. Patients with *M. pneumoniae* often develop strong cold agglutinins with I specificity as a cross-reactive response to mycoplasma antigen[41] and can experience a transient episode of acute abrupt hemolysis just as the infection begins to resolve. A *Listeria monocytogenes* organism from a patient with cold autoimmune hemolytic anemia has been reported to adsorb anti-I and stimulate its production in rabbits.

Alloanti-I exists as an IgM or IgG antibody in the serum of most individuals with the adult i phenotype. Although adult i RBCs are not totally devoid of I, the anti-I in these cases does not react with autologous RBCs. It has been traditional to transfuse compatible adult i units to these people, although such practice may be unnecessary, especially when the antibody is not reactive at 37°C.[1] Technologists must be aware that strong autoanti-I can mimic alloanti-I: if enough autoantibody and complement are bound to a patient's RBCs, blocking the antigenic sites, they may falsely type I-negative.

Anti-I is not associated with HDN because the antibody is IgM, and antigen is poorly expressed on infant RBCs.

Anti-i

Alloanti-i has never been described. Autoanti-i is a fairly rare antibody that gives strong reactions with cord RBCs and adult i RBCs and weaker reactions with adult I RBCs. Most examples of autoanti-i are IgM and react best with saline-suspended cells at 4°C. Only very strong examples of autoanti-i are detected in routine testing because standard test cells (except cord RBCs) have poor i expression. See **Table 9–7.**

Unlike anti-I, autoanti-i is not seen as a common antibody in healthy individuals. Potent examples are associated with infectious mononucleosis (Epstein-Barr virus infections), reticuloses, myeloid leukemias, and alcoholic cirrhosis. High-titer autoantibodies with a wide thermal range may contribute to hemolysis, but because i expression is generally weak they seldom cause significant hemolysis. IgG anti-i has also been described and has been associated with HDN.[1]

Advanced Concepts

Biochemistry and Genetics

An early association of I and i to ABH was demonstrated by complex antibodies involving both ABH and Ii specificity (see the subsequent section on Antibodies to Compound Antigens). It was also known that I activity increased when ABH sugars were removed with specific enzymes and that adults with the Bombay phenotype (O_h) had the greatest amount of I antigen on their RBCs.[42] Thanks to these observations and work by Feizi, Hakomori, Watanabe, and others (reviewed elsewhere[1,10]), we now know that I and i antigens are defined by a series of carbohydrates on the inner portion of ABH oligosaccharide chains.

ABH and Ii determinants on the RBC membrane are carried on type 2 chains that attach either to proteins or to lipids. See **Figure 9–5** for examples of glycolipid structures for i and I antigens. The i antigen activity is defined by at least two repeating N-acetyllactosamine [Gal(β1-4)GlcNAc(β1-3)] units in linear form. I antigen activity is associated with a branched form of i antigen. The *IGnT* (also known as *GCNT2*) gene on chromosome 6p24 encodes the N-acetylglucosaminyltransferase, which adds GlcNAc in a β1-6 linkage to form the branches.[40,43]

In summary, fetal, cord, and adult i RBCs carry predominantly unbranched chains and have the i phenotype. Normal adult cells have more branched structures and express I antigen. The gene responsible for I antigen (*IGnT*) codes for the branching enzyme. Family studies show that the adult i phenotype is recessive. Heterozygotes, e.g., children inheriting I from one parent and i from the other parent, have intermediate I expression. Several gene mutations have been identified that result in the adult i phenotype.[40,43]

Other Sources of I and i Antigen

I and i antigens are found on the membranes of leukocytes and platelets in addition to RBCs. Some anti-I and anti-i are cytotoxic.[10] It is quite likely that the antigens exist on

Antigen	Structure
(none)	Gal(β1-4)GlcNAc(β1-3)Gal(β1-3)Gal(β1-4)Glc-Cer
i	Gal(β1-4)GlcNAc(β1-3)Gal(β1-4)GlcNAc(β1-3)Gal(β1-4)Glc-Cer
I	Gal(β1-4)GlcNAc(β1-3) $\quad\quad\quad\quad\quad\quad\quad\quad\quad$>Gal($\beta$1-4)GlcNAc($\beta$1-3)Gal($\beta$1-4)Glc-Cer Gal($\beta$1-4)GlcNAc($\beta$1-6)

■ **FIGURE 9–5** The linear and branched structures carrying i and I activity.

other tissue cells, much like ABH, but this has not been confirmed.

I and i have also been found in the plasma and serum of adults and newborns and in saliva, human milk, amniotic fluid, urine, and ovarian cyst fluid. The antigens in secretions do not correlate with RBC expression and are thought to develop under separate genetic control. For example, the quantity of I antigen in the saliva of adult i individuals and newborns is quite high.

The I antigen has been found on the RBCs or in body fluids of other animal species, including rabbits, sheep, and cattle.[14] The RBCs from most adult primates express i antigen and mimic those from newborn or i adults.

The I^T Antigen and Antibody

In 1965 Curtain et al[44] reported a cold agglutinin in Melanesians that did not demonstrate classical I or i specificity. In 1966 Booth and colleagues[45] confirmed these observations and carefully described the agglutinin's reactivity. This agglutinin reacted strongly with cord RBCs, weakly with normal adult RBCs, and most weakly with adult i RBCs. They concluded that the agglutinin recognizes a transition state of i into I and designated the specificity I^T (T for *transition*). Detection of I^T on fetal RBCs ranging in age from 11 to 16 weeks, however, does not support this hypothesis.[46]

This benign IgM anti-I^T was frequently found in two populations: Melanesians and the Yanomama Indians in Venezuela. Whether it is associated with an organism or parasite in these regions is unknown.

Examples of IgG anti-I^T reacting preferentially at 37°C have also been found; the first four cases were in patients with hemolytic anemia and Hodgkin's lymphoma.[46,47] Additional examples of IgM and IgG anti-I^T in patients with warm autoimmune hemolytic anemia, but not with Hodgkin's lymphoma, have also been reported.[1]

Antibodies to Compound Antigens

Many other I-related antibodies have been described: anti-IA, -IB, -IAB, -IH, -iH, -IP$_1$, -I^{T}P$_1$, -IHLe^b, and -iHLe^b. Bearing in mind the close relationship of I to the biochemical structures of ABH, Lewis, and P antigens, one should not be surprised to find antibodies that recognize compound antigens. These specificities are not mixtures of separable antibodies; rather, both antigens must be present on the RBCs for the antibody to react. For example, anti-IA reacts with RBCs that carry both I and A but will not react with group O, I+, or group A adult i RBCs. Table 9–8 summarizes some common cold autoantibodies.

Disease Associations

Well-known associations between strong autoantibodies and disease or microorganisms have already been discussed: anti-I and cold agglutinin syndrome and *M. pneumoniae*, anti-i and infectious mononucleosis, and anti-I^T and Hodgkin's lymphoma. Cold autoantibodies have also been reported in influenza infections, but other associations are rare.

Diseases can also alter the expression of I and i antigens on RBCs. Conditions associated with increased i antigen on RBCs include those with shortened marrow maturation time or dyserythropoiesis: acute leukemia, hypoplastic anemia, megaloblastic anemia, sideroblastic anemia, thalassemia, sickle cell disease, paroxysmal nocturnal hemoglobinuria (PNH), and chronic hemolytic anemia.[1,10] Except in some cases of leukemia, the increase in i on RBCs is not usually associated with a decrease in I antigen; the expression of I antigen can appear normal or sometimes enhanced. Reactive lymphocytes in infectious mononucleosis are reported to have increased i antigen. Those from patients with chronic lymphocytic leukemia have less lymphocyte i antigen than normal control subjects.[10]

Chronic dyserythropoietic anemia type II or hereditary erythroblastic multinuclearity with a positive acidified serum test (HEMPAS) is associated with much greater i activity on RBCs than control cord RBCs. HEMPAS RBCs are very susceptible to lysis with both anti-i and anti-I, and lysis by anti-I appears to be the result of increased antibody uptake and increased sensitivity to complement.[1]

I antigen may be involved in binding immune complexes consisting of drug and drug antibodies. Immune complexes involving rifampin, nitrofurantoin, dexchlorphenyramine, and thiopental have been associated with binding to I antigens on RBCs and subsequent complement activation and hemolysis.[4]

In Asians, the adult i phenotype has been associated with congenital cataracts. Mutations at the *I* locus have been identified in three Taiwanese families with the adult i phenotype, which suggests a molecular genetic mechanism for this condition in this population.[43]

The Kell (006) and Kx (019) Blood Group Systems

The Kell blood group system consists of 24 high-incidence and low-incidence antigens; it was the first blood group system discovered after the introduction of antiglobulin testing. Anti-K (originally called Kell) was identified in 1946 in the serum of Mrs. Kellaher. The antibody reacted with the RBCs of her newborn infant, her older daughter, her husband, and

TABLE 9–8	Typical Reactions of Some Cold Autoantibodies*							
Antibody	A$_1$ Adult	A$_2$ Adult	B Adult	O Adult	O Cord	A Cord	O$_h$ Adult	O$_i$ Adult
Anti-I	++++	++++	++++	++++	0/+	0/+	++++	(0)
Anti-i	0/+	0/+	0/+	0/+	++++	++++	0/+	++++
Anti-H	0/+	++	+++	++++	+++	0/+	(0)	+++
Anti-IH	0/+	++	+++	++++	0/+	0/+	(0)	(0)
Anti-IA	++++	+++	0/+	0/+	0/+	0/+	(0)	(0)

*Reactions vary with antibody strength; very potent examples may need to be diluted before specificity can be determined.
0 = negative; + = positive.

about 7 percent of the random population.[10] In 1949 Levine et al[48] described anti-k (Cellano), the high-incidence antithetical partner to K.

Kell remained a two-antigen system until Allen and Lewis[49] and Allen et al[50] described the antithetical antigens Kpa and Kpb in 1957 and 1958, respectively. Inheritance patterns and statistics confirmed their relationship to the Kell system. Likewise, Jsa, described in 1958 by Giblett,[51] and Jsb, described by Walker et al in 1963,[52] were found to be antithetical and related to the Kell system.

The discovery of the null phenotype in 1957,[53] designated K_o, helped associate many other antigens with the Kell system. Antibodies that reacted with all RBCs except those with the K_o phenotype recognized high-incidence antigens that were phenotypically related. More discoveries followed, including the description of the McLeod phenotype by Allen et al in 1961.[54] This phenotype, with its weakened expression of Kell antigens and pathologic syndrome, brought into focus another antigen, Kx, made by a gene on the X chromosome.

The 24 antigens now included in the Kell blood group system, designated by the symbol KEL or 006 by the ISBT, are listed in Table 9–9. The associated antigen Kx is the only antigen in the Kx system, ISBT number 019.

Basic Concepts

For many years it was believed that Kell blood group antigens are found only on RBCs. They have not been found on platelets or on lymphocytes, granulocytes, or monocytes by means of using immunofluorescent flow cytometry. There is recent evidence, however, that Kell glycoprotein is abundantly present in testes and, to a lesser extent, in other tissues.[10]

The K antigen can be detected on fetal RBCs as early as 10 weeks (k at 7 weeks) and is well developed at birth. The total number of K antigen sites per RBC is quite low: Hughes-Jones and Gardner[55] found about 6000 sites on K+k– RBCs and only 3500 sites on K+k+ RBCs, although others have found up to 18,000 sites per RBC. Despite its lower quantity, K is very immunogenic.

The antigens are not denatured by routine blood bank enzymes ficin and papain but are destroyed by trypsin and chymotrypsin when used in combination.[4] Thiol-reducing agents, such as 100–200 mM DTT, 2-mercaptoethanol, AET, and ZZAP (which contains DTT in addition to enzyme), destroy Kell antigens but not Kx. Glycine acid-EDTA (an IgG removal agent) also destroys Kell antigens.

The frequencies of common Kell phenotypes are listed in Table 9–10. There are five sets of antithetical antigens; antithetical relationships have not been established for the other high- and low-incidence antigens. Some of the Kell antigens, e.g., Jsb, are more prevalent in certain populations.

K and k Antigens

Excluding ABO, K is rated second only to D in immunogenicity. When K– people are transfused with a unit of K+ blood, the probability of their developing anti-K may be as high as 10 percent.[55] Fortunately, the incidence of K antigen is low, and the chance of receiving a K+ unit is small. If anti-K develops, compatible units are easy to find.

TABLE 9–9   Kell System Antigens

Number	Name	Frequency (%)	Antithetical Partner	Comments
1	K	9.0	k	aa 193: Met
2	k	99.8	K	aa 193: Thr
3	Kpa	2 (whites)	Kpb, Kpc	aa 281: Trp
4	Kpb	>99.9	Kpa, Kpc	aa 281: Arg
5	Ku	>99.9		
6	Jsa	<0.1 whites 20 blacks	Jsb	aa 597: Pro
7	Jsb	>99.9 whites 99 blacks	Jsa	aa 597: Leu
10	Ula	<3 Finns		aa 494: Val
11	Côté	>99.9	K17	aa 302: Val
12	Boc	>99.9		aa 548: His
13	SGRO	>99.9		
14	San	>99.9	K24	aa 180: Arg
16	k-like	99.8		
17	Wka	0.3	K11	aa 302: Ala
18	VM	>99.9		aa 130: Arg
19	Sub	>99.9		aa 492: Arg
20	Km	>99.9		Absent from McLeod RBCs
21	Kpc	<0.1	Kpa, Kpb	aa 281: Gln
22	Ikar	>99.9		aa 322: Ala
23	Centauro	<0.5		aa 382: Arg
24	CL	<2.0	K14	aa 180: Pro
25	VLAN	<0.1		aa 248: Arg
26	TOU	>99.9		aa 406: Arg
27	RAZ	>99.9		aa 299: Glu

Obsolete: K8, K9, K15

Compiled from Reid, MD, and Lomas-Francis, C: The Blood Group Antigen Facts Book. Academic Press, New York, 1997; and Daniels, G: Human Blood Groups. Blackwell Science, Oxford, 2002.

TABLE 9–10   Kell System Phenotype Frequencies

Phenotype	Whites (%)	Blacks (%)
K−k+	91.0	96.5
K+k+	8.8	3.5
K+k−	0.2	<0.1
Kp(a+b−)	<0.1	0
Kp(a+b+)	2.3	Rare
Kp(a−b+)	97.7	100
Js(a+b−)	0	1
Js(a+b+)	Rare	19
Js(a−b+)	100	80

Antibodies to k antigen are seldom encountered. Only 2 in 1000 individuals lack k and are capable of developing the antibody. The likelihood that these few individuals receive transfusions and become immunized is even less.

Kp^a, Kp^b, and Kp^c Antigens

Alleles Kp^a and Kp^c are low-incidence mutations of their high-incidence partner Kp^b. The Kp^a antigen is found in about 2 percent of whites. The Kp^a gene is associated with suppression of other Kell antigens on the same molecule, including k and Js^b.[10] The effect appears to result from a reduced amount of the Kell glycoprotein (produced by the Kp^a allele) inserted in the RBC membrane.[10]

The Kp^c antigen is even more rare. In 1979 Yamaguchi et al[56] discovered several siblings from a consanguineous married couple in Japan who typed Kp(a−b−) but otherwise had normal Kell antigens. The researchers concluded that both parents carried a new allele, Kp^c, for which the children were homozygous. Gavin et al[57] then showed that Kp^c and Levay, the first low-incidence antigen ever described, were identical. (The Kell system had not yet been discovered when anti-Levay was first reported.)

Js^a and Js^b Antigens

The Js^a antigen, antithetical to the high-incidence antigen Js^b, is found in about 20 percent of blacks but in fewer than 0.1 percent of whites. The incidence of Js^a in blacks is almost 10 times greater than the incidence of the K antigen in blacks.[14] Js^a and Js^b were linked to the Kell system when it was discovered that K_o RBCs were Js(a−b−).

Anti-K

Outside the ABO and Rh antibodies, anti-K is the most common antibody seen in the blood bank. Anti-K is usually IgG and reactive in the antiglobulin phase, but some examples agglutinate saline-suspended RBCs. About 20 percent bind complement, but they are seldom lytic. The antibody is usually made in response to antigen exposure through pregnancy and transfusion and can persist for many years.

Naturally occurring IgM examples of anti-K are rare and have been associated with bacterial infections. Marsh et al[58] studied an IgM anti-K in an untransfused 20-day-old infant with an *E. coli* O125:B15 infection whose mother did not make anti-K. The organism was shown to have a somatic K-like antigen that reacted with the infant's antibody, so the bacterial antigen was thought to have been the stimulus. The antibody

disappeared after recovery. Other organisms implicated with naturally occurring anti-K or known to react with anti-K include mycobacteria, *Enterococcus faecalis*, *Morganella morganii*, *Campylobacter jejuni*, and *Campylobacter coli*.[10,14]

Some examples of anti-K react poorly in methods incorporating low-ionic media, such as LISS, and in some automated systems. The most reliable method of detection is the indirect antiglobulin test. Routine blood bank albumin or enzyme methods do not affect antibody reactivity, but DTT, ZZAP, 2ME, AET and glycine-acid-EDTA treatments destroy Kell antigens. The potentiating medium, PEG, may increase reactivity.

Anti-K has been implicated in severe hemolytic transfusion reactions. Although some examples of anti-K bind complement, in-vivo RBC destruction is usually extravascular via the macrophages in the spleen. Anti-K is also associated with severe HDN. The antibody titer does not always accurately predict the severity of disease; stillbirth has been seen with anti-K titers as low as 64. Fetal anemia in anti-K HDN may be associated with suppression of erythropoiesis due to destruction of erythroid precursor cells rather than destruction of circulating antigen-positive RBCs; Kell glycoprotein is expressed early on fetal RBCs.[10] When a pregnant woman is identified as making anti-K, it is prudent to type the father for the K antigen, and if K+, monitor the fetus carefully for signs of HDN.

Antibodies to Kp^a, Js^a, and Other Low-Incidence Kell Antigens

Antibodies to the low-incidence Kell antigens are rare because so few people are exposed to these antigens. Because routine antibody detection RBCs do not carry low-incidence antigens, the antibodies are most often detected through unexpected incompatible crossmatches or cases of HDN.

The serologic characteristics and clinical significance of these antibodies parallel anti-K. The original anti-Kp^a was naturally occurring, but most antibodies are "immune."

Antibodies to k, Kp^b, Js^b, and Other High-Incidence Kell Antigens

Antibodies to high-incidence Kell system antigens are rare because so few people lack these antigens. They also parallel anti-K in serologic characteristics and clinical significance.

The high-incidence antibodies are easy to detect but difficult to work with because most blood banks do not have the antigen-negative panel cells needed to rule out other alloantibodies nor do they have typing reagents to phenotype the patient's RBCs. Testing an unidentified high-incidence antibody against DTT- or AET-treated RBCs is a helpful technique: reactivity that is abolished with DTT or AET treatment suggests that the antibody may be related to the Kell system and enables the technologist to exclude common alloantibodies. Caution is needed before assigning Kell system specificity until antigen-negative RBCs are tested because DTT and AET also denature JMH and high-incidence antigens in the LW, Lutheran, Dombrock, Cromer, and Knops systems. Finding compatible units for transfusion can be difficult; siblings and rare-donor inventories are the most likely sources. Patients with antibodies to high-incidence antigens should be encouraged to donate autologous units and, if possible, to participate in a rare-donor program.

Advanced Concepts

Biochemistry

The Kell antigens are located on a 93-kD RBC membrane glycoprotein that consists of 731 amino acids and spans the membrane once. The N-terminal domain is intracellular, and the large external C-terminal domain is highly folded by disulfide linkages **(Fig. 9–6)**. The Kell glycoprotein is covalently linked with another protein, called Kx, by a single disulfide bond. The Kx protein (440 amino acids and 37 kD) is predicted to span the RBC membrane ten times.[59]

The Kell glycoprotein is a member of the M13 (neprilysin) family of zinc endopeptidases and has been shown to cleave big endothelins, but how this relates to the physiologic role of the Kell glycoprotein remains unclear.[59] The amino acid sequence of the Kx protein is similar to that of an Na^+-dependent glutamate transporter in rabbits.[10]

Genetics

The *KEL* gene, located on chromosome 7 (at 7q33), is organized into 19 exons of coding sequence. Single base mutations encoding amino acid substitutions are responsible for the different Kell antigens. **Table 9–9** summarizes known amino acid (aa) differences and their positions on the glycoprotein. A rare silent allele at the *KEL* locus has been designated K^o.

No *KEL* haplotype has been shown to code for more than one low-incidence antigen. People who test positive for two low-incidence Kell antigens have always been found to carry the encoding alleles on opposite chromosomes. For example, someone who types Kp(a+) and Js(a+) is genetically *kKp^{a}Js^b* on one chromosome and *kKp^{b}Js^a* on the other.

The *XK* gene, which encodes the Kx antigen, is independent of *KEL* and is located on the X chromosome at position Xp21.1.[10]

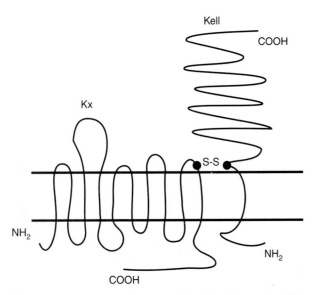

■ FIGURE 9–6 Proposed structures for Kell and Kx proteins. The two proteins are linked through one disulfide bond. The conformation of the large external domain of the Kell glycoprotein is unknown; 15 cysteine residues suggest the presence of disulfide bonds and extensive folding.

The Kx Antigen

Kx is present on all RBCs except those of the rare McLeod phenotype (see below). When Kell antigens are denatured with AET or DTT, the expression of Kx increases. Because of this inverse relationship, it was initially suggested that Kx might be a precursor or backbone for Kell, and Kx was given the designation K15. However, it is now known that Kx is carried on a separate protein that is encoded by a gene on the X chromosome. Kx has been placed in its own blood group system, called XK, and the number K15 is obsolete.

The K$_o$ Phenotype and Anti-Ku(K5)

K^o is a silent Kell allele. Inheriting two K^o genes results in the recessive null phenotype. K$_o$ RBCs lack expression of all Kell antigens. Several mutations responsible for the K$_o$ phenotype have been identified in unrelated propositi.[10] K$_o$ cells have no membrane abnormality and survive normally in circulation. The phenotype is rare; data suggest a frequency of 1:25,000 in whites.[10]

Immunized individuals with the K$_o$ phenotype typically make an antibody called anti-Ku (K5) that recognizes the "universal" Kell antigen (Ku) present on all cells except K$_o$. Anti-Ku appears to be a single specificity and cannot be separated into components. Anti-Ku has caused both HDN and hemolytic transfusion reactions.[10]

Because K$_o$ RBCs are negative for k, Kp^b, Js^b, and so forth, they are very useful in investigating complex antibody problems. They can help confirm a Kell system specificity or rule out other underlying specificities. When K$_o$ cells are not available, they can be made artificially by treating normal cells with DTT, AET or glycine-acid-EDTA.

Other Kell Antigens

K11 and K17. In 1971 Guévin et al[60] described anti-Côté (now called anti-K11), which reacted with all RBCs tested except those of the propositus, two of her eight siblings, and K$_o$ RBCs. The antigen appeared to be phenotypically related to the Kell system. Three years later, Strange et al[61] noticed through family studies of K+Wk(a+) individuals that the low-incidence antigen Wk^a was always inherited with k and not with K. Wk^a and K11 were subsequently confirmed to be alleles by Sabo et al.[62] Wk^a was given the name K17 to show its placement into the Kell system.

K14 and K24. K14, like K11, is a high-incidence antigen phenotypically related to the Kell system. In 1985 its antithetical low-incidence antigen, K24, was described.[63]

Low-Incidence Antigens with No Known Antithetical Partners: K10 (Ul^a), K23, and K25 (VLAN). K10 (Ul^a) is found in about 3 percent of random Finns, 0.46 percent of Japanese, and 1 of 12 Chinese.[10] Three informative Finnish families helped place Ul^a into the Kell system. A high-incidence antithetical antigen has not yet been described.

K23 was detected in a maternal serum associated with a positive DAT on the RBCs of the woman's third child. The antibody was no longer reactive when the paternal RBCs were treated with AET. Immunoprecipitation studies demonstrated the antigen was carried on the Kell glycoprotein. Although the antibody in this case caused a strong positive DAT, it did not cause clinical HDN.[1]

K25 (VLAN) was initially identified through an incompatible crossmatch. Because the antibody-antigen reactivity was abolished after the RBCs were treated with AET, a new Kell system antibody was suspected. VLAN was shown to be part of the Kell system through the monoclonal antibody-specific immobilization of erythrocyte antigens (MAIEA) assay.

High-Incidence Antigens with No Known Antithetical Partners: K12, K13, K18, K19, K22, K26, and K27. These discrete, very high-incidence antigens have all been shown to be governed by the KEL locus and/or expressed on the Kell glycoprotein. None of the antigens are found on K_o RBCs, and they are weakly expressed on McLeod phenotype RBCs. K:−18 is the only Kell antigen that has not been shown to be inherited; there are only two known K:−18 individuals.[10] Known molecular bases for these antigens are shown in **Table 9–9**.

Miscellaneous Kell Antigen Assignments. The antigen designations K8 (also called K^W), K9 (KL), and K15 (Kx) are obsolete (Kx, as previously mentioned, was moved to the Kx system). The specificities KL, Kx, and Km (K20) are related: a young boy named Claas with both the McLeod phenotype (see next section) and probable chronic granulomatous disease (CGD) made an antibody called anti-KL, which was found to be two separable antibodies to Kx and Km.[64] Kx and Km are high-incidence antigens present on all RBCs with two exceptions: RBCs with the McLeod phenotype lack Kx and Km; K_o RBCs lack Km but strongly express Kx. The expression of Kell antigens on RBCs with common, McLeod, and K_o phenotypes is summarized in **Table 9–11**.

K16 is a high-incidence k-like antigen seen on k+ RBCs but not expressed on McLeod RBCs; it is unclear if this effect is qualitative or quantitative.

The McLeod Phenotype and Syndrome

In 1961 Allen et al[54] described a young male blood donor who initially appeared to be Kell null but who demonstrated weak expression of k, Kp^b, and Js^b detectable by adsorption-elution methods. This unusual phenotype was called McLeod, after the donor.

The McLeod phenotype is very rare (occurrence has been reported in fewer than 100 families). All who have it are male, and inheritance is X-linked through a carrier mother. McLeod phenotype RBCs lack Kx and Km and have marked depression of all other Kell antigens. The weakened expression of the Kell antigens is designated by a superscript "w" for weak, e.g., $K-k+^w Kp(a-b+^w)$. The McLeod phenotype has been associated with several mutations and deletions at the XK locus.[65]

A significant proportion of the RBCs in individuals with the McLeod phenotype are acanthocytic (having irregular shapes and protrusions) with decreased deformability and reduced in-vivo survival. As a result, people with the McLeod phenotype have a chronic but often well-compensated hemolytic anemia characterized by reticulocytosis, bilirubinemia, splenomegaly, and reduced serum haptoglobin levels.

Individuals with the McLeod phenotype have a variety of muscle and nerve disorders that, together with the serologic and hematologic picture, are collectively known as the McLeod syndrome. McLeod individuals develop a slow, progressive form of muscular dystrophy between ages 40 and 50 years and cardiomegaly (leading to cardiomyopathy). The associated neurologic disorder presents initially as areflexia (a lack of deep tendon reflexes) and progresses to choreiform movements (well-coordinated but involuntary movements). These individuals also have elevated serum creatinine phosphokinase levels of the MM type (cardiac/skeletal muscle) and carbonic anhydrase III levels.

An association between the rare Kell phenotypes, including the McLeod phenotype, and the rare X-linked CGD was made by Giblett et al in 1971.[66] CGD is characterized by the inability of phagocytes to make NADH-oxidase, an enzyme important in generating H_2O_2, which is used to kill ingested bacteria.[67] Afflicted children die at an early age from overwhelming infections. Not all males with the McLeod phenotype have CGD, nor do all patients with CGD have the McLeod phenotype.

At one time it was suggested that CGD was caused by a lack of Kx on white blood cells, and several alleles at the XK locus were proposed to explain Kx expression on McLeod RBCs and CGD white blood cells. More recent data have shown that this theory is not valid. The XK gene resides on the X chromosome near deletions associated with CGD, Duchenne muscular dystrophy, and retinitis pigmentosa, in the Xp21 region.[65]

The expression of Kx in women who are carriers of the McLeod phenotype follows the Lyon hypothesis, which states that in early embryo development, one X chromosome randomly shuts down in female cells that have two. All cells descending from the resulting cell line express only the allele on the active chromosome. Hence, McLeod carriers exhibit two RBC populations: one having Kx and normal Kell antigens, the other having the McLeod phenotype and acanthocytosis. The percentage of McLeod phenotype RBCs in carriers varies from 5 percent to 85 percent.[1]

Altered Expressions of Kell Antigens

Weaker-than-normal Kell antigen expression is associated with the McLeod phenotype and the suppression by the Kp^a gene (cis-modified effect) on Kell antigens (most obvious when there is a K^o gene in trans). Weak expression of Kell antigens on RBCs of K:−13 individuals may be due to the cis

TABLE 9–11   Summary of Kell Antigens on RBCs Having Common, K_o, and McLeod Phenotypes

| Phenotype | RBC Antigen Expression | | |
	Kell Antigens	Km	Kx
common	k, Kp^b, Js^b, K11...	Strong	Weak
K_o	none	None	Strong
McLeod	trace k, Kp^a, Js^b, K11...	None	None

effect, similar to Kp^a, but the antithetical low incidence partner has not yet been identified.

Depressed Kell antigens are also seen on RBCs with the rare Gerbich-negative phenotypes Ge: −2, −3 and Ge: −2, −3, −4. The phenotypic relationship between Gerbich and Kell is not understood. Marsh and Redman[68] proposed the umbrella term K_{mod} to describe other phenotypes with very weak Kell expression, often requiring adsorption-elution tests for detection. As a group, these RBCs have a reduced amount of Kell glycoprotein and enhanced Kx expression. Some K_{mod} individuals make an antibody that resembles anti-Ku, but that does not react with other K_{mod} RBCs (unlike anti-Ku made by K_o individuals).

Patients with autoimmune hemolytic anemia, in which the autoantibody is directed against a Kell antigen, may have depressed expression of that antigen. Antigen strength returns to normal when the anemia resolves and the DAT becomes negative. This phenomenon appears to be more common in the Kell system than in others.[1]

Finally, RBCs may appear to acquire Kell antigens. McGinnis et al[69] described a K− patient who acquired a K-like antigen during a *Streptococcus faecium* infection. Cultures containing the disrupted organism converted K− cells to K+ but bacteria-free filtrates did not.

Autoantibodies

Marsh et al[70] reported that 1 in 250 autoantibodies do not react with K_o RBCs and are therefore related to the Kell system. The actual frequency of these antibodies could be much higher, because the study detected autoantibody with pure Kell specificity, not mixtures of Kell with other autoantibodies.[1] They may be benign or hemolytic.

Most Kell autoantibodies are directed against undefined high-incidence Kell antigens, but identifiable autoantibodies to K, Kp^b, and K13 have been reported. Issitt noted a possible association between autoanti-K and head injuries or brain tumors.[1]

Mimicking specificities have been reported, such as when an apparent anti-K is eluted from DAT+ K− RBCs and the anti-K in the eluate can be adsorbed onto K− RBCs.

The Duffy (008) Blood Group System

The Duffy blood group system was named for Mr. Duffy, a multiply transfused hemophiliac who in 1950 was found to have the first described example of anti-Fy^a.[71] One year later the antibody defining its antithetical antigen, Fy^b, was described by Ikin et al[72] in the serum of a woman who had had three pregnancies.

In 1955 Sanger et al[73] reported that the majority of African Americans tested were Fy(a−b−). The gene responsible for this null phenotype was called *Fy. FyFy* appeared to be a common genotype in blacks, especially in Africa; the gene is exceedingly rare in whites.

In 1975 Miller et al[74] made the observation that Fy(a−b−) RBCs resist infection in vitro by the monkey malaria organism *Plasmodium knowlesi*. It was later shown that Fy(a−b−) RBCs also resist infection by *P. vivax* (one of the organisms causing malaria in humans).[75]

Antibodies to the four additional antigens assigned to the Duffy blood group system, Fy3, Fy4, Fy5, and Fy6, are rarely encountered. RBCs that are Fy(a−b−) are also Fy: −3, −5, −6. Fy5 is also not present on Rh_{null} RBCs, regardless of the Fy^a or Fy^b status of those RBCs. The Duffy blood group system is designated by the symbol FY or 008 by the ISBT.

Basic Concepts

Fy^a and Fy^b Antigens

The Duffy antigens most important in routine blood bank serology are Fy^a and Fy^b. They can be identified on fetal RBCs as early as 6 weeks gestational age and are well developed at birth. There are about 13,000 to 14,000 Fy^a or Fy^b sites on Fy(a+b−) and Fy(a−b+) RBCs, respectively; there are half that number of Fy^a sites on Fy(a+b+) RBCs.[10] The antigens have not been found on platelets, lymphocytes, monocytes, or granulocytes, but they have been identified in other body tissues, including brain, colon, endothelium, lung, spleen, thyroid, thymus, and kidney cells.[4]

The frequencies of the common phenotypes in the Duffy system are given in **Table 9–12**. The disparity in distribution in different races is notable.

Fy^a and Fy^b antigens do not store well in saline suspension and tend to elute from RBCs stored in a medium with low pH or low ionic strength. This can lead to inhibitory substances in the supernatant fluid, which can weaken the reactivity of an anti-Fy^a or anti-Fy^b.[14] These changes are not seen in RBCs stored in licensed anticoagulants, e.g., ACD, CPD, CPD-A1, or the reagent solutions used by commercial manufacturers for reagent RBCs.[1]

Fy^a and Fy^b antigens are destroyed by common proteolytic enzymes, such as ficin, papain, bromelin, and chymotrypsin, and by ZZAP (which contains either papain or ficin in addition to DTT); they are not affected by AET or glycine-acid-EDTA treatment. Neuraminidase may reduce the molecular weight of Fy^a and Fy^b, but it does not destroy antigenic activity; neither does purified trypsin.

Anti-Fy^a and Anti-Fy^b

Anti-Fy^a is a common antibody and is found as a single specificity or in a mixture of antibodies. Anti-Fy^a occurs three times less frequently than anti-K. Anti-Fy^b is 20 times less

TABLE 9–12	Frequency of Duffy Phenotypes		
Phenotype	**Whites (%)**	**American Blacks (%)**	**Chinese (%)[76]**
Fy(a+b−)	17	9	90.8
Fy(a+b+)	49	1	8.9
Fy(a−b+)	34	22	0.3
Fy(a−b−)	Very rare	68	0

common than anti-Fy^a and often occurs in combination with other antibodies. [The Fy^a antigen appears to be more immunogenic in Fy(a−b+) whites than in Fy(a−b−) blacks, since in two studies, only 25 of 130 patients who produced anti-Fy^a were Fy(a−b−) blacks.[14]]

The antibodies are usually IgG and react best at the antiglobulin phase. Some examples of anti-Fy^a and anti-Fy^b bind complement. A few examples are saline agglutinins. Antibody activity is enhanced in a low ionic strength medium. Because anti-Fy^a and anti-Fy^b do not react with enzyme-treated RBCs, this is a helpful technique when multiple antibodies are present.

Some examples of anti-Fy^a and anti-Fy^b show dosage, which may be more obvious with examples of saline agglutinins. This is significant because some reagent RBCs that appear to be from homozygotes (and have a double dose of either Fy^a or Fy^b) may actually be from heterozygotes if they are from black donors; a silent allele, *Fy*, is commonly found in blacks. For example, Fy(a+b−) RBCs will have a double dose of Fy^a if they are from a white *Fy^{a}Fy^a* donor but will have a single dose of Fy^a if they are from a black donor who is genetically *Fy^{a}Fy*. Additional phenotypic markers commonly found in black donors can give a clue to the possible presence of the silent *Fy* allele: R$_o$, S−s−, V+VS+, Js(a+), Le(a−b−).

Anti-Fy^a and anti-Fy^b have been associated with acute and delayed hemolytic transfusion reactions. Once the antibody is identified, Fy(a−) or Fy(b−) blood must be given; finding such units in a random population is not difficult. Anti-Fy^a and anti-Fy^b are associated with HDN ranging from mild to severe.

Rare autoantibodies with mimicking Fy^a and Fy^b specificity have been reported, e.g., anti-Fy^b that can be adsorbed onto and eluted from Fy(a+b−) RBCs. Issitt and Anstee[1] suggest that these may represent alloantibodies with "sloppy" specificity made early in an immune response.

Advanced Concepts

Biochemistry

Enzymes, membrane solubilization methods, immunoblotting, radiolabeling, and amino acid sequencing have all been used to study the biochemistry of Duffy antigens.[1] Duffy antigens reside on a glycoprotein of 336 amino acids that has a relative mass of 36 kD and two *N*-glycosylation sites (Fig. 9–7).[75] The glycoprotein is predicted to traverse the cell membrane seven times and has two predicted disulfide bridges.

The amino acid at position 42 on the Duffy glycoprotein defines the Fy^a and Fy^b polymorphism: Fy^a has glycine, and Fy^b has aspartic acid. The Fy3 epitope, as defined by monoclonal antibody, is on the third extracellular loop, and Fy6 appears to involve amino acids 19 through 25.[75]

The Duffy glycoprotein is a member of the superfamily of chemokine receptors and is known as the Duffy antigen receptor for chemokines.

Genetics

In 1968 the Duffy gene was linked to a visible inherited abnormality of chromosome 1, thus becoming the first human gene to be assigned to a specific chromosome.[77] The gene is located near the centromere on the long arm of the chromosome

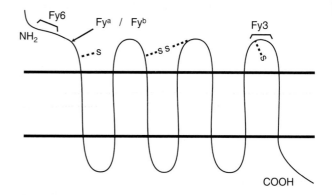

■ **FIGURE 9–7**   Proposed structure for the Duffy protein. Disulfide bonds probably link the NH$_2$ terminal domain and the third loop and the first and second loop.

at position 1q22-23. The *Fy* locus is syntenic to *Rh*, which is located near the tip of the short arm; that is, they are on the same chromosome, but they are far enough apart that linkage cannot be demonstrated and serologically they appear to segregate independently.

There are three common alleles at the *Fy* locus: *Fy^a* and *Fy^b* that encode the antithetical antigens Fy^a and Fy^b, respectively, and a silent allele, *Fy*, that is the major allele in blacks. The *Fy* gene in Fy(a−b−) blacks has been found to be an *Fy^b* variant with a change in the promoter region of the gene, which disrupts the binding site for mRNA transcription in the RBC.[13] Consequently, Fy(a−b−) blacks do not express Fy^b on their RBCs but express Fy^b in other tissue. The presence of Fy^b in tissues presumably precludes the recognition of Fy^b as foreign; thus, no anti-Fy^b is made by these individuals. A molecular analysis of Fy(a−b−) whites revealed a 14 base pair deletion in the *Fy* gene, resulting in a reading frame shift and the introduction of a translation stop codon.[10] These individuals carry no Duffy protein on their RBCs or on other tissues and thus can form anti-Fy^b and anti-Fy3.

Typing for Duffy antigens has been performed on the RBCs of chimpanzees, gorillas, and old and new world monkeys. The results suggest that *Fy3* developed first, then *Fy^b*, and that *Fy^a* arose during human evolution.

Fy^x

Fy^x was described in 1965 by Chown et al[78] as a new allele at the *Fy* locus. It does not produce a distinct antigen but, rather, an inherited weak form of Fy^b that reacts with some but not all examples of anti-Fy^b. Fy^x has been described in white populations. Individuals with *Fy^x* may type Fy(b−), but their RBCs adsorb and elute anti-Fy^b. They also have depressed expression of their Fy3 and Fy5 antigens. There is no anti-Fy^x.

The decreased expression of Fy^b due to *Fy^x* appears to be related to a reduced amount of Duffy glycoprotein on the surface of RBCs.[79]

Fy3 Antigen and Antibody

In 1971 Albrey et al[80] reported finding anti-Fy3 in the serum of an Fy(a−b−) white Australian female. It reacted with all RBCs tested except those of the Fy(a−b−) phenotype.

Because it was an inseparable anti-Fy^{a}Fy^b, it was thought to react with an antigenic determinant or precursor common to both Fy^a and Fy^b and was called Fy3. Unlike Fy^a and Fy^b, the Fy3 antigen is not destroyed by enzymes.

Anti-Fy3 is a rare antibody made by Fy(a−b−) individuals who lack the Duffy glycoprotein. The Fy(a−b−) phenotype has been found in white, black, and Cree Indian families.[1] Blacks with the Fy(a−b−) phenotype rarely make anti-Fy3. Examples of anti-Fy3 produced by non-blacks appear to react with all Duffy positive cells equally well. Those made by blacks are similar, but they react weakly or not at all with Duffy positive cord RBCs. There may be a subtle difference in the Duffy glycoprotein expressed on tissue that is recognized as foreign.[10] Some patients who make anti-Fy3 initially make anti-Fy^a.

Fy4 Antigen and Antibody

In 1973 Behzad et al[81] described anti-Fy4 in the serum of a young Fy(a+b+) black female with sickle cell anemia. The antibody reacted with RBCs from all Fy(a−b−) blacks, many Fy(a+b−) and Fy(a−b+) blacks, but not usually with Fy(a+b+) blacks, and not with whites of any Duffy type. It was concluded that most Fy(a−b−) blacks carry an Fy4 antigen, perhaps in place of Fy^a, Fy^b, and Fy3, and are genetically *Fy^{4}Fy^4*. The Fy4 antigen, like Fy3, is not destroyed by enzymes.

No other example of anti-Fy4 has been reported; it is now thought unlikely that Fy4 is located on the Duffy glycoprotein.[10]

Fy5 Antigen and Antibody

Anti-Fy5 was discovered by Colledge et al[82] in 1973 in the serum of an Fy(a−b−) black child who later died of leukemia. Initially it was thought to be a second example of anti-Fy3 because it reacted with all Fy(a+) or Fy(b+) RBCs but not with Fy(a−b−) cells. The antibody differed in that it reacted with the cells from an [Fy(a−b−)Fy:-3 white female,] but it did not react with Fy(a+) or Fy(b+) Rh$_{null}$ RBCs and reacted only weakly with Fy(a+) or Fy(b+) D−− RBCs.

Sometimes, sera containing anti-Fy5 also contain anti-Fy^a. Several examples of anti-Fy5 have been reported in multiply transfused Fy(a−b−) sickle cell patients with a mixture of other antibodies.

The molecular structure of Fy5 is not known, but it appears to be the result of interaction between the Rh complex and the Duffy glycoprotein. People who are Fy(a−b−) and/or Rh$_{null}$ do not make Fy5 antigen and are at risk of making the antibody, although few do. Like Fy3, Fy5 is not destroyed by enzymes.

Fy6 Antigen and Antibody

In 1987 Nichols et al[83] described a murine monoclonal antibody that reacted much like anti-Fy3, except that its reactivity was destroyed by ficin, papain, and chymotrypsin. Trypsin enhanced its reactivity. The antibody appeared to define the Duffy receptor used by *P. vivax* to penetrate RBCs. It is now known that Fy6 involves amino acids 19 to 25 on the extracellular domain of the Duffy glycoprotein. No human examples of anti-Fy6 have been reported to date.

The Duffy-Malaria Association

A correlation between the Duffy antigens and malaria infection has long been suspected. Since 1955 it has been known that Africans and black Americans were resistant to infection by *P. vivax* and that these same populations are Fy(a−b−).

Because *P. vivax* could not be grown in culture at that time, Miller et al[74] conducted in-vitro studies with the simian parasite *P. knowlesi*, which could be cultured and would invade human RBCs. Miller and colleagues confirmed that malaria merozoites invaded only RBCs carrying normal Fy^a or Fy^b antigen. When antigen sites were blocked by antibody or denatured with certain enzymes, the RBCs became resistant to invasion. Because the resistance factors for *P. knowlesi* and *P. vivax* were so parallel in West African populations, it was suggested that Fy^a and Fy^b might also be the invasion receptor for *P. vivax*. In-vivo epidemiologic data supported this hypothesis.[84–86]

Close evaluation of the invasion process of *P. knowlesi* suggests that two receptor sites are involved: one for attachment and one for invasion.[87] Initial attachment of the merozoite to the RBC occurs regardless of Duffy type, but the junction and invasion are Duffy antigen–dependent.

Data from human and old and new world monkey RBCs and their susceptibility to invasion by *P. vivax* and *P. knowlesi* indicate that Fy6 is important for invasion for *P. vivax*.[10] The monoclonal anti-Fy6 has been shown to block invasion of RBCs by *P. vivax*.[87]

The Kidd (009) Blood Group System

The Kidd blood group is the simplest and most straightforward system described in this chapter. In 1951 Allen et al[88] reported finding an antibody in the serum of a Mrs. Kidd, whose infant had HDN. The antibody, named anti-Jk^a, reacted with 77 percent of Bostonians. Its antithetical partner, Jk^b, was found 2 years later by Plaut et al[89] The null phenotype Jk(a−b−) was described by Pinkerton et al[90] in 1959. The propositus made an antibody to a high-incidence antigen called Jk3, which is present on any RBC positive for Jk^a or Jk^b. No other antigens associated with the Kidd system have been described.

The Kidd system is designated by the symbol JK or 009 by the ISBT. It has special significance to routine blood banking because of its antibodies, which can be difficult to detect and are a common cause of hemolytic transfusion reactions.

Basic Concepts

Jk^a and Jk^b Antigens

Jk^a and Jk^b are common RBC antigens. **Table 9–13** summarizes the frequencies of the four known phenotypes. There are notable racial differences in antigen frequency: 91 percent of blacks and 77 percent of whites are Jk(a+); 57 percent of blacks and only 28 percent of whites are Jk(b−).

Jk^a and Jk^b antigens are well developed on the RBCs of neonates. Jk^a has been detected on fetal RBCs as early as 11 weeks; Jk^b has been detected at 7 weeks.[10] Although this early development of Kidd antigens contributes to the potential for HDN, anti-Jk^a and anti-Jk^b are only rarely responsible for severe HDN. Jk(a+b−) RBCs carry 14,000 antigen sites per cell.[10] The Kidd antigens are not very immunogenic.

TABLE 9-13	Frequencies of Kidd Phenotypes		
Phenotype	**Whites (%)**	**Blacks (%)**	**Asians (%)**
Jk(a+b−)	28	57	23
Jk(a+b+)	49	34	50
Jk(a−b+)	23	9	27
Jk(a−b−)	Exceedingly rare	Exceedingly rare	0.9−<0.1

Kidd antigens are not denatured by papain or ficin; treatment of RBCs with enzymes generally enhances reactivity with Kidd antibodies. Kidd antigens are also not affected by chloroquine diphosphate, AET, DTT, or glycine-acid-EDTA.

The antigens are not found on platelets, lymphocytes, monocytes, or granulocytes by means of sensitive radioimmunoassay or immunofluorescent techniques.[14]

Anti-Jk^a and Anti-Jk^b

Kidd antibodies have a notorious reputation in the blood bank. They demonstrate dosage, are often weak, and are found in combination with other antibodies, all of which make them difficult to detect.

Anti-Jk^a is more frequently encountered than anti-Jk^b, but neither antibody is common. The antibodies are usually IgG (antiglobulin reactive) but may also be partly IgM and are made in response to pregnancy or transfusion.

The ability of Kidd antibodies to show dosage can confound inexperienced serologists. Many anti-Jk^a and anti-Jk^b react more strongly with RBCs that carry a double dose of the respective antigen and may not react with Jk(a+b+) RBCs. An anti-Jk^a that reacts only with Jk(a+b−) RBCs can give inconclusive panel results and appear compatible with Jk(a+b+) cells. Readers are urged to rule out anti-Jk^a and anti-Jk^b only with Jk(a+b−) and Jk(a−b+) panel cells, respectively, and to type all crossmatch-compatible units with commercial antisera. To ensure that stored antisera can indeed detect weak expressions of the antigen, Jk(a+b+) RBCs should be tested in parallel as the positive control.

Antibody reactivity can also be enhanced by using LISS or PEG (to promote IgG attachment), by using four drops of serum instead of two (to increase the antibody/antigen ratio), or by using enzymes such as ficin or papain. In-vitro hemolysis can sometimes be observed with enzyme-treated RBCs; antigen dose may influence this hemolytic activity.[1]

Many examples of the Kidd antibodies bind complement. Rare examples are detected only by the complement they bind (i.e., they are nonreactive in antiglobulin tests using anti-IgG reagents). Using polyspecific reagents with both anti-IgG and anti-complement can be helpful in these situations.[1]

Kidd antibodies that are complement-dependent do not store well. When anti-Jk^a or anti-Jk^b specificity cannot be confirmed in a stored serum, fresh normal serum (as a source of complement) can be added and tested with polyspecific antiglobulin reagent.[1]

The titer of anti-Jk^a or anti-Jk^b quickly declines in vivo. A strong antibody identified following a transfusion reaction may be undetectable in a few weeks or months.[1] This confirms the need to check blood bank records for previously identified antibodies before a patient is transfused. It is equally important to inform the patient that he or she has such an antibody and to provide a wallet card that notes the specificity in case the patient is transfused elsewhere.

The decline in antibody reactivity and the difficulty in detecting Kidd antibodies are reasons why they are a common cause of hemolytic transfusion reactions, especially of the delayed type. Although intravascular hemolysis has been noted in severe reactions, coated RBCs more often are removed extravascularly. The rate of clearance of incompatible RBCs can vary but is usually rapid.

Contrary to their hemolytic reputation in transfusion, most Kidd antibodies are only rarely associated with severe cases of HDN.

Advanced Concepts

Biochemistry

Heaton and McLoughlin[91] reported in 1982 that Jk(a−b−) RBCs resist lysis in 2M urea, a solution commonly used to lyse RBCs in a sample before it is used in some automated platelet-counting instruments. Urea crosses the RBC membrane, causing an osmotic imbalance and an influx of water, which rapidly lyses normal cells. With Jk(a+) or Jk(b+) RBCs, lysis in 2M urea occurs within 1 minute; with Jk(a−b−) cells, lysis is delayed 30 minutes.[10]

Sinor et al[92] identified the Jk^a protein as a single band with a relative mass of 45 kD that was not affected by reduction and alkylation and appeared not to be glycosylated. A cDNA clone was subsequently isolated that produces the Kidd glycoprotein and RBC urea transporter. The predicted glycoprotein has 389 amino acids with 10 membrane-spanning domains and two N-glycosylation sites, one of which is extracellular **(Fig. 9–8)**.

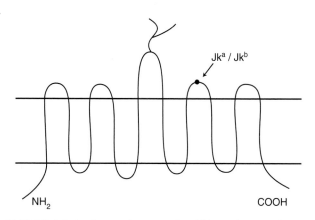

■ **FIGURE 9–8**   Proposed structure for Kidd protein. One of two proposed N-glycans is extracellular and is located on the third extracellular loop; the Jk^a/Jk^b polymorphism is located on the fourth extracellular loop.

Genetics

Jk^a and Jk^b are inherited as codominant alleles. The Jk locus is on chromosome 18 at position 18q11-q12. The gene, a member of the urea transporter gene family, is organized into 11 exons. The Jk^a/Jk^b polymorphism is associated with an amino acid substitution at position 280, predicted to be located on the fourth extracellular loop of the glycoprotein. Molecular studies have demonstrated the silent Jk allele can arise from mutations in both the Jk^a and Jk^b alleles.

Jk(a−b−) Phenotype and the Recessive Allele, Jk

People with the null phenotype lack Jk^a, Jk^b, and the common antigen Jk3. Although very rare, the Jk(a−b−) phenotype is most abundant among Polynesians, and it has also been identified in Filipinos, Indonesians, Chinese, and Japanese.[1] The null phenotype has also been reported in several European families (Finnish, French, Swiss, and English) and in the Mato Grosso Indians of Brazil. The delayed lysis of Jk(a−b−) RBCs in 2M urea has proved an easy way to screen families and/or populations for this rare phenotype.

No clinical abnormalities have been associated with the Jk(a−b−) phenotype to date. Several unrelated Jk(a−b−) individuals have been found to have normal blood urea nitrogen, creatinine, and serum electrolytes, but studies on two individuals show a marked defect in their ability to concentrate urine.[4]

Family studies show that most Jk(a−b−) nulls are homozygous for the rare "silent" allele Jk. Parents of $JkJk$ offspring and children of $JkJk$ parents type Jk(a+b−) or Jk(a−b+) but never Jk(a+b+), because they are genetically Jk^aJk or Jk^bJk. Their RBCs also demonstrate a single dose of Jk^a or Jk^b antigen in titration studies.

Jk(a−b−) Phenotype and the Dominant In(Jk) Allele

Another genetic explanation for the Jk(a−b−) phenotype was reported by Okubo et al.[93] They discovered a dominant pattern of inheritance within a Japanese family and proposed the existence of a dominant inhibitor to the Kidd system, $In(Jk)$, analogous to $In(Lu)$ in the Lutheran blood group system. Dominant type Jk(a−b−) RBCs adsorb and elute anti-Jk3 and anti-Jk^a and/or anti-Jk^b (depending on which genes were inherited), indicating that the antigens are expressed but only very weakly. Individuals with the In(Jk) Jk(a−b−) phenotype do not make anti-Jk3. Family studies show that the $In(Jk)$ gene does not reside at the Jk locus.

Anti-Jk3

Alloanti-Jk3 is an IgG antiglobulin-reactive antibody that looks like an inseparable anti-Jk^aJk^b. Because panel cells are Jk(a+) or Jk(b+), anti-Jk3 reacts with all RBCs tested except the auto-control. Most blood banks do not have the rare cells needed to confirm anti-Jk3; however, they can easily determine its most probable specificity by means of antigen typing. The individual making the antibody will type Jk(a−b−). Like other Kidd antibodies, anti-Jk3 reacts optimally by an antiglobulin test, and the reactivity is enhanced with enzyme pretreatment of the RBCs.

Anti-Jk3 has been associated with severe immediate and delayed hemolytic transfusion reactions and with mild HDN. Compatible units are best found by typing siblings or searching the rare donor files.

Autoantibodies

Autoantibodies with Kidd specificity (anti-Jk^a, anti-Jk^b, and anti-Jk3) are rare, but they have been associated with autoimmune hemolytic anemia.[1] Some examples are drug-related: one was found in a patient taking alpha-methyldopa (Aldomet)[94]; another was chlorpropamide-dependent.[95]

Examples of benign autoanti-Jk^a have been associated with butyl, ethyl, methyl, and propyl esters of parahydroxybenzoate or paraben.[96] These chemicals are used in some commercially prepared LISS, cosmetics, food preservatives, and pharmaceuticals. The antibodies are seen when paraben-containing LISS is used in antibody detection tests with Jk(a+) cells.

As with other blood groups, Kidd autoantibodies may have mimicking specificity or be associated with depressed antigen expression. One pregnant woman with an apparent compensated anemia was found to have mimicking autoanti-Jk^b and -Jk3; the antibodies could be adsorbed by Jk(a+b−) and Jk(a−b−) RBCs.[97] In another report, a woman who was Jk(a+b−) transiently typed as Jk(a−b−) and had anti-Jk3.[98]

Disease Associations

Although Jk^a and Jk^b are thought to be human RBC antigens, three organisms have been associated with Jk^b-like specificity. Two, *Enterococcus faecium* and *Micrococcus*, were able to convert Jk(b−) cells to Jk(b+), and one, *Proteus mirabilis*, may have been the stimulus for an autoanti-Jk^b.[99]

The Lutheran (005) Blood Group System

Lutheran antigens have been recognized since 1945, when the first example of anti-Lu^a was discovered in the serum of a patient with lupus erythematosus diffusus, following the transfusion of a unit of blood carrying the corresponding low-incidence antigen.[100] (This patient also made anti-c, anti-N, the first example of anti-C^W, and anti-Levay, now known as Kp^c!) The new antibody was named Lutheran, a misinterpretation of the donor's name, Luteran. In 1956 Cutbush and Chanarin[101] described anti-Lu^b, which defined the antithetical partner to Lu^a.

The blood group system appeared complete until 1961, when Crawford et al[102] described the first Lu(a−b−) phenotype. Unlike most null phenotypes at the time, this one demonstrated dominant inheritance. In 1963 Darnborough et al[103] found a more traditional Lu(a−b−) phenotype inherited as a recessive silent allele.

Using rare Lu(a−b−) RBCs to test antibodies to unknown high-incidence antigens, some sera showed a phenotypic relationship to Lutheran. That is, they reacted with all RBCs tested except those with the Lu(a−b−) phenotype, even though the antibody producers appeared to have normal Lutheran antigens. These specificities were not identical to one another, and they were given the numeric designations Lu4, Lu5, Lu6, and so on, to represent their association to the system. Within this group, three pairs of antithetical antigens (Lu6 and Lu9, Lu8 and Lu14, and Lu18 and Lu19) have been shown to be inherited at the Lutheran locus; several antigens have been shown to be located on the Lutheran glycoprotein, and three antigens (Lu11, Lu16, Lu17), often referred to as para-Lutheran, have limited evidence that they belong to the Lutheran system.[10] All are summarized in **Table 9–14**.

The ISBT designation of the Lutheran blood group system is LU or 005.

Basic Concepts

Blood bankers seldom deal with the serology of the Lutheran blood group system because the antigens are either very high- or very low-incidence. Either so many people have the antigen, so only a few are capable of making alloantibody, or the antigens are so rare that only a few people are ever exposed. Consequently, the antibodies are seen infrequently. The antigens also have questionable immunogenicity.

Lu^a and Lu^b Antigens

Lu^a and Lu^b are antigens produced by allelic codominant genes. Common phenotypes are listed in **Table 9–15**. Most individuals are Lu(b+); only a few are Lu(a+).

Lutheran antigen expression is variable from one individual to another; antigen expression on one individual's RBCs can also vary. Lu^b antigen strength as measured with a purified monoclonal anti-Lu^b (BRIC 108) confirmed low Lu^b site density and variable expression. The number of Lu^b sites per RBC was estimated to be from 1640 to 4070 on Lu(a−b+) RBCs and 850 to 1820 on Lu(a+b+) RBCs.[10]

Although the antigens have been detected on fetal RBCs as early as 10 to 12 weeks of gestation, they are poorly developed at birth and do not reach adult levels until age 15 years. Lutheran antigens have not been detected on platelets, lymphocytes, monocytes, or granulocytes by means of sensitive radioimmunoassay or immunofluorescent techniques.[14] Lutheran glycoprotein, however, is widely distributed in tissues: brain, lung, pancreas, placenta, skeletal muscle, and hepatocytes (especially fetal hepatic epithelial cells).[10]

Anti-Lu^a

Most examples of anti-Lu^a are IgM naturally occurring saline agglutinins that react better at room temperature than at 37°C. A few react at 37°C by indirect antiglobulin test. Some are capable of binding complement, but invitro hemolysis has not been reported. Lutheran antibodies are unusual in that they may be IgA as well as IgM and IgG.[14]

Anti-Lu^a often goes undetected in routine testing because most reagent cells are Lu(a−). Anti-Lu^a is more likely encountered as an incompatible crossmatch or during an antibody workup for another specificity. Experienced technologists recognize Lutheran antibodies by their characteristic loose, mixed-field reactivity in a test tube. Anti-Lu^a is not profoundly altered with the common blood bank enzymes ficin and papain, but it can be destroyed with trypsin, chymotrypsin, pronase, AET, and DTT. Most Lu^a antibodies are clinically insignificant in transfusion. There is one report of normal or near-normal survival of Lu(a+) RBCs in a patient with anti-Lu^a.[1] There are no documented cases of immediate and only rare and mild delayed transfusion reactions due to anti-Lu^a.[1]

Because Lutheran antigens are poorly expressed on cord RBCs, cases of HDN associated with anti-Lu^a are mild. Infants may exhibit weakly positive or negative direct antiglobulin

TABLE 9–15   Frequencies of Lutheran Phenotypes

Phenotype	Whites (%)
Lu (a+b−)	0.15
Lu (a+b+)	7.5
Lu (a−b+)	92.35
Lu (a−b−)	Very rare

TABLE 9–14   Summary of the Lutheran Antigens

Conventional Name	Frequency (%)	Year Discovered	Molecular Basis	Comments
Lu^a	8.0	1945	aa 77: His	Antithetical to Lu^b
Lu^b	99.8	1956	aa 77: Arg	Antithetical to Lu^a
Lu3	>99.9	1963		
Lu4	>99.9	1971		on Lu glycoprotein
Lu5	>99.9	1972	aa 109: Arg	on Lu glycoprotein
Lu6	>99.9	1972	aa 275: Ser	Antithetical to Lu9
Lu7	>99.9	1972		on Lu glycoprotein
Lu8	>99.9	1972	aa 204: Met	Antithetical to Lu14
Lu9	2.0	1973	aa 275: Phe	Antithetical to Lu6
Lu11	>99.9	1974		Para-Lutheran
Lu12	>99.9	1973		on Lu glycoprotein
Lu13	>99.9	1983	aa 447: Ser	on Lu glycoprotein
Lu14	2.4	1977	aa 204: Lys	Antithetical to Lu8
Lu16	>99.9	1980		Para-Lutheran
Lu17	>99.9	1979		Para-Lutheran
Au^a, Lu18	80.0	1961	aa 539: Thr	Antithetical to Au^b
Au^b, Lu19	50.0	1989	aa 539: Ala	Antithetical to Au^a
Lu20	>99.9	1992	aa 302: Thr	on Lu glycoprotein
Obsolete: Lu10, Lu15				

tests and mild to moderate elevations in bilirubin. Many require no treatment; others respond to simple phototherapy. In one report of mild HDN, the mother's antibody titer rose to 4096.[104]

Anti-Lu^b

Although the first example of anti-Lu^b was a room-temperature agglutinin, and IgM and IgA antibodies have been noted, most anti-Lu^b is IgG and reactive at 37°C at the antiglobulin phase. It is made in response to pregnancy or transfusion.

Alloanti-Lu^b reacts with all cells tested except the autocontrol, and reactions are often weaker with Lu(a+b+) RBCs and cord RBCs. Ficin or papain does not significantly alter reactivity. AET or DTT should destroy Lu^b antigen through disruption of the disulfide bond of the glycoprotein, but this may require optimal conditions. Autologous RBCs will test Lu(a+) if typing sera are available.

Anti-Lu^b has been implicated with shortened survival of transfused cells and post-transfusion jaundice, but severe or acute hemolysis has not been reported. Chromium survival studies demonstrate a rapid initial clearance of some Lu(b+) RBCs but much slower removal of those remaining.[14] Anti-Lu^b may be regarded as clinically significant, but blood should not be withheld in emergency situations just because compatible units cannot be found. Like anti-Lu^a, anti-Lu^b is associated with only mild cases of HDN.

Advanced Concepts

Biochemistry

Using immunoblot methods and a monoclonal antibody (BRIC 108), which initially appeared to have Lu^b-like activity, Parsons et al[105] identified two proteins with molecular weights of 85 and 78 kD. These two glycoproteins, now known as the Lutheran glycoproteins, contain both *N*- and *O*-linked oligosaccharides and intrachain disulfide bonds. Subsequent immunoblotting with human antibodies to Lutheran antigens has demonstrated that Lu^a, Lu^b, Lu3, Lu4, Lu6, Lu8, Lu12,[106] Au^a (Lu18), and Au^b (Lu19)[107] are located on the Lutheran glycoprotein. Parsons et al[108] isolated a cDNA clone that encodes the Lutheran glycoproteins. The predicted 85-kD protein contains 597 amino acids with five potential *N*-glycosylation sites. It traverses the cell membrane just once and has a cytoplasmic domain of 59 amino acids **(Fig. 9–9)**. A smaller isoform (78 kD) lacks part of the cytoplasmic domain. The external portion consists of five disulfide-bonded domains (three are constant, and two are variable). The Lutheran glycoproteins belong to the immunoglobulin superfamily of proteins. This superfamily includes immunoglobulin heavy and light chains, HLA class I and II peptides, T-cell adhesion molecules, CD4 and CD8, immunoglobulin receptors, and the neuronal adhesive molecule N-CAM, among others. Although its biologic role is still uncertain, the Lutheran protein most probably plays some role in adhesion or intracellular signaling.

The molecular basis for the four pairs of antithetical antigens and several of the high-incidence antigens has been determined through the creation of Lutheran glycoprotein mutants.

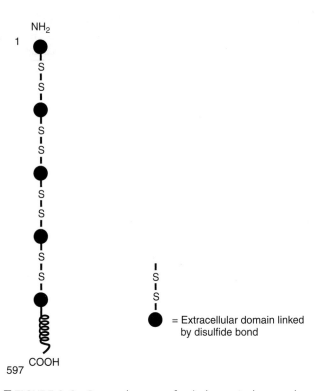

■ **FIGURE 9–9**   Proposed structure for single-pass Lutheran molecule.

Genetics

The *Lu* gene is located on chromosome 19 at position 19q13.2-q13.3, along with genes that govern expression of several blood group antigens (H, Se, Le, LW, Ok^a) and genes for C3, apolipoprotein C-II (APO), and myotonic dystrophy. A linkage between *Lu* and the Se gene (*FUT2*) was the first example of autosomal linkage described in humans.

Lu(a−b−) Phenotypes

Three genetic explanations for the Lu(a−b−) phenotype have been described. These are summarized in **Table 9–16**.

Dominant *In(Lu)* Type. The first Lu(a−b−) family study was reported by the propositus herself.[102] Because the phenotype was seen in successive generations in 50 percent of members in her family and others, and because null individuals passed normal Lutheran genes to their offspring, the expression of Lutheran was thought to be suppressed by a rare dominant regulator gene later called *In(Lu)* for "inhibitor of Lutheran." *In(Lu)* segregates independently from Lutheran. Blood donor screenings have shown the frequency of this type Lutheran null to be 1:3000 to 1:5000.[109]

Dominant-type Lu(a−b−) RBCs carry trace amounts of Lutheran antigens as shown by adsorption-elution studies. For example, a person who inherits two normal *Lu^b* genes plus *In(Lu)* will type Lu(a−b−) with routine methods but will adsorb and elute anti-Lu^b. Individuals with the *In(Lu)* type of Lu(a−b−) RBCs do not make anti-Lu3.

Inheriting just one *In(Lu)* gene prevents normal expression of all Lutheran antigens, as well as P_1, i, and AnWj, which

TABLE 9-16   Summary of Lu(a-b-) Phenotypes

Mode of Inheritance	Gene Responsible	Lu Antigens	Other RBC Antigens Affected	Make Anti-Lu3?
Dominant	*In(Lu)*	Extremely weak	Reduced P_1, i, In^b, AnWj, MER2, CD44	No
Recessive	*Lu*	None	Not affected	Yes
X-linked	*XS2*	Extremely weak	Not affected	No

are genetically independent. The I antigen appears unaffected. Other unrelated antigens that are suppressed include In^b, MER2, epitopes on the common glycoprotein CD44, concanavalin A receptor, and the receptor for horse antilymphocyte globulin. Early evidence that *In(Lu)* RBCs are weak for the Knops system antigens, Kn^a, McC^a, Sl^a, and Yk^a, and for Cs^a antigen has not been confirmed. The expression of CR1, the structure that carries the Knops system antigens, does not appear to be regulated by *In(Lu)*.[10]

In(Lu) may also affect RBC shape and metabolism. Udden and others[110] observed abnormal poikilocytosis and acanthocytosis in some *In(Lu)* individuals, although this was variable within families. RBCs from the original *In(Lu)* propositus appear morphologically normal when first collected but become abnormal during storage more quickly than RBCs with normal Lutheran antigens. These RBCs also hemolyze more during 4°C storage in modified Alsever's solution; this hemolysis could be reduced by the addition of glucose or ATP. The osmotic fragility of *In(Lu)* RBCs is normal, but these cells significantly resist lysis when incubated in plasma at 37°C. *In(Lu)* RBCs appear to lose more K$^+$ than they gain Na$^+$ under these conditions.[10]

Recessive *LuLu* Type. In some families, the Lu(a-b-) phenotype demonstrates recessive inheritance, the result of having two rare silent alleles *LuLu* at the Lutheran locus.[103] The parents and offspring of these nulls may type Lu(a-b-), but dosage studies and titers show them to carry a single dose of Lu^b.

Unlike the *In(Lu)* type, recessive Lu(a-b-) people truly lack all Lutheran antigens (i.e., they have the null phenotype) and can make an inseparable anti-Lu^{ab} called anti-Lu3. They also have normal antigen expression of P_1, i, and the many other antigens that *In(Lu)* affects. This distinction emphasizes the importance of testing an antibody against recessive Lu(a-b-) RBCs before calling its antigen phenotypically related to Lutheran.

Recessive X-Linked Inhibitor Type. In 1986 Norman et al[111] described an Lu(a-b-) phenotype in a large Australian family that fit neither an *In(Lu)* nor a *LuLu* pattern. All Lu(a-b-) family members were male and carried trace amounts of Lu^b detected by adsorption-elution. Although P_1 expression was weak, i was well expressed, but I was depressed. The pattern of inheritance suggested an X-borne inhibitor to Lutheran. The researchers proposed calling the locus *XS*, *XS1* being the common allele and *XS2* the rare inhibitor that suppresses in a hemizygous state. There have been no other families reported with this rare X-linked Lu(a-b-) phenotype.[1]

Lu(w) Phenotype. Several Lu(a-b+^{w}) and Lu(a+^{w}b+^{w}) individuals with weakened Lutheran antigens have been described. Although not proved, this phenotype, also

known as Lu(w), may result from *In(Lu)* with a lesser degree of penetrance or an allele to *In(Lu)* that causes less suppression.

Anti-Lu3

Anti-Lu3 is a rare antibody that reacts with all RBCs except those testing Lu(a-b-). The antibody looks like inseparable anti-Lu^{ab} and recognizes a common antigen, Lu3, that is present whenever Lu^a or Lu^b is present (much like the Jk3 association with Jk^a and Jk^b). Anti-Lu3 is usually antiglobulin-reactive.

This antibody is made only by *LuLu* individuals, i.e., the recessive type of Lu(a-b-). RBCs from dominant and X-linked type Lu(a-b-) individuals can be safely transfused to patients with anti-Lu3.

Lu6/Lu9 and Lu8/Lu14

In 1972 Lu6[112] and Lu8[113] designations were given to two nonidentical antibodies directed against high-incidence antigens related to the Lutheran system. The antibodies reacted with all RBCs except autologous and Lu(a-b-) cells, but they were made by Lu(a-b+) individuals.

In 1973 Molthan et al[114] described anti-Lu9, an antibody that reacted with 2 percent of random donors and that gave very strong reactions with Lu:-6 RBCs. In 1977 Judd et al[115] described anti-Lu14, another antibody to a low-incidence antigen that was strongly expressed on Lu:-8 RBCs.

Au^a (Lu18) and Au^b (Lu19)

Au^a (Auberger) was described in 1961 by Salmon et al[116] as an antigen found in 80 percent of whites. In 1989 its antithetical antigen, Au^b, was reported by Frandson et al.[117] Because the antigens were suppressed by *In(Lu)* and were destroyed by trypsin, chymotrypsin, and pronase, they were closely associated with the Lutheran system except that, in one family study, they were inherited independently. Serologists considered them another set of antigens suppressed by Lutheran inhibitors.

Au^a and Au^b were subsequently shown to be expressed on the Lutheran glycoprotein,[107] and the Au(a-) family members associated with the earlier genetic exclusion were retested and found to test Au(a+). Family linkage studies also demonstrated that the Auberger and Lutheran antigens were controlled by the same gene.[118]

Other Lutheran Antigens

Lu4, Lu5, Lu7, Lu12, Lu13, and Lu20 are antigens of very high incidence that are absent from Lu(a-b-) RBCs, but they have not been shown to be inherited at the *Lu* locus. All have been shown to be located on the Lutheran glycoprotein, and all but Lu20 have been shown to be inherited. Their antibodies parallel the characteristics of anti-Lu6 and anti-Lu8: they do not react with Lu(a−b−) RBCs or autologous cells, which carry otherwise normal Lutheran antigens.

The high-incidence antigens Lu11, Lu16, and Lu17 are phenotypically related to Lutheran. These antigens are absent from Lu(a−b−) RBCs of the recessive and In(Lu) types, but they have not been shown to be located on the Lutheran glycoprotein nor have they been shown to be inherited; evidence that these antigens belong to the Lutheran system is thus very limited.

The An/Wj antigen was once associated with the Lutheran system because it is not expressed or only weakly expressed on In(Lu) Lu(a−b−) RBCs and was given the designation Lu15; this became obsolete when An/Wj was found on *LuLu* RBCs.

Lu10 is another designation no longer used. It was reserved for Singleton, an antigen thought to be the allele of Lu5; the antibody reacted strongly with Lu:-5 RBCs. However, five other examples of Lu:−5 cells were later tested and found to be negative with the Singleton serum.[1]

Applications to Routine Blood Banking

The major blood group systems outside of ABO and Rh become important only after patients develop unexpected antibodies. Then a fundamental knowledge of antibody characteristics, clinical significance, and antigen frequency is needed to help confirm antibody specificity and to select appropriate units for transfusion.

Only a few antibody specificities are commonly seen: M, P_1, and I antibodies react at room temperature and are considered clinically insignificant; K, S, s, Fy^a, Fy^b, Jk^a, and Jk^b antibodies react in the antiglobulin phase and are clinically significant. These and selected others are summarized in **Table 9–17**.

Not all antibody problems are easily solved; panel reactions

TABLE 9–17   Summary of Antibody Characteristics

	Reactivity				Bind Complement	In Vitro Hemolysis	HTR	HDN	Compatible in U.S. Population (%)
Antibody	**≤RT**	**37**	**AHG**	**Enzymes**					
M**	Most	Few	Few	Destroy	(Rare)*	No	Few	Mild—severe	22
N**	Most	Few	Few	Destroy	(Rare)	No	Rare	Moderate	2B
S	Some	Some	Most	Variable effect	Some	No	Yes	Mild	45 W
									69 B
s	Few	Few	Most	Variable effect	Few	No	Yes	Mild—severe	11 W
									3 B
U	Rare	Some	Most	No change	(Rare)	No	Yes	Mild—severe	<1 B
P_1**	Most	Some	Rare	Enhance	Rare	Rare	Rare	(No)	21
$PP_1P^{k\dagger}$	Most	Some	Some	Enhance	Most	Most	(Yes)	Mild	<0.1
$P^\dagger$	Most	Some	Some	Enhance	Most	Some	(Yes)	Mild—severe	<0.1
I‡	Most	Few	Few	Enhance	Most	Few	Rare	(No)	See text
i‡	Most	Few	Few	Enhance	Most	Few	(?)	Mild	See text
K	Some	Some	Most	No change	Some	No	Yes	Mild—severe	91
k	Few	Few	Most	No change	(Some)	No	Yes	Mild	0.2
Kp^a	Some	Some	Most	No change	(Some)	No	Yes	Mild	99.7
Kp^b	Few	Few	Most	No change	(Some)	No	Yes	Mild	<0.1
Js^a	Few	Few	Most	No change	(Some)	No	Yes	Moderate	100 W
									80 B
Js^b	(No)	(No)	Most	No change	(Some)	No	Yes	Mild—moderate	1 B
Fy^a	Rare	Rare	Most	Destroy	Some	No	Yes	Mild—severe	34 W
Fy^b	Rare	Rare	Most	Destroy	Some	No	Yes	(Yes)	17 W
									77 B
$Jk^{a\S}$	Few	Few	Most	Enhance	All	Some	Yes	Mild	23
$Jk^{b\S}$	Few	Few	Most	Enhance	All	Some	Yes	Mild	28 W
									57 B
$Lu^{a\,\S\S}$	Most	Few	Few	Variable effect	Some	No	(?)	Mild	92
$Lu^{b\,\S\S}$	Few	Few	Most	Variable effect	Some	No	Yes	Mild	0.15

B = blacks; HDN = hemolytic disease of the newborn; HTR = hemolytic transfusion reactions; ≤ RT = room temperature or colder; W = whites.
*Comments in parentheses are postulated and not based on reported cases.
**Usually clinically insignificant
†Potent hemolysins may be associated with early abortions
‡Usually autoantibodies clinically insignificant
§Associated with severe delayed HTR
§§IgG4 and IgA antibody classes seen.

are sometimes inconclusive. As described in this chapter, the existence of silent, regulator, and inhibitor genes can affect antigen expression. It is hoped that the reader will find that the information in this chapter provides a starting point for serological problem solving. For further detailed information about the RBC antigens and antibodies described here, the reader is referred to Issitt and Anstee[1] and Daniels.[10] Resolution of antibody problems involving the unusual specificities described here may require the assistance of an immunohematology reference laboratory.

SUMMARY CHART:

Important Points to Remember (MT/MLT/SBB)

The MNS Blood Group System

➤ Anti-M and anti-N are cold-reactive saline agglutinins that do not bind complement or react with enzyme-treated cells; anti-N has been found in renal patients undergoing dialysis treatment; both anti-M and anti-N may demonstrate dosage.

➤ Anti-S and anti-s are IgG antibodies, reactive at 37°C and the antiglobulin phase; they may bind complement and have been associated with HDN and hemolytic transfusion reactions.

➤ The S−s−U− phenotype is found in blacks.

➤ Anti-U is usually an IgG antibody and has been associated with hemolytic transfusion reactions and HDN.

The P Blood Group

➤ The P blood group consists of the biochemically related antigens P, P_1, P^k and LKE; there is also a biochemical relationship between the P blood group antigens and the ABH and I antigens.

➤ P_1 antigen expression is variable; P_1 antigen is poorly developed at birth.

➤ Anti-P_1 is a common naturally occurring IgM antibody in the sera of P_1− individuals; it is usually a weak, cold-reactive saline agglutinin seldom detected in routine testing and can be neutralized with soluble P_1 substance found in hydatid cyst fluid.

➤ Anti-PP_1P^k is produced by all p individuals early in life without RBC sensitization and reacts with all RBCs except those of other p individuals; antibodies may be a mixture of IgM and IgG, efficiently bind complement, and may demonstrate in-vitro hemolysis.

➤ Anti-P is found as a naturally occurring alloantibody in the sera of all P^k individuals.

➤ Paroxysmal cold hemoglobinuria (PCH) is usually caused by autoantibodies that demonstrate anti-P specificity.

➤ PCH autoantibodies are IgG biphasic hemolysins usually demonstrable only by the Donath-Landsteiner test.

The I and i Antigens

➤ I and i antigens are not antithetical; they have a reciprocal relationship.

➤ Most adult RBCs are rich in I and have only trace amounts of i antigen.

➤ At birth, infant RBCs are rich in i; I is almost undetectable; over the next 18 months of development the infant's RBCs will convert from i to I antigen.

➤ Anti-I is typically a benign, weak, naturally occurring, saline-reactive IgM autoagglutinin, usually detectable only at 4°C.

➤ Pathogenic anti-I is typically a strong cold autoagglutinin that demonstrates high titer reactivity at 4°C and reacts over a wide thermal range (up to 30°–32°C).

➤ Potent cold autoantibodies can mask clinically significant underlying alloantibodies and complicate pretransfusion testing.

➤ Patients with *M. pneumoniae* infections may develop strong cold agglutinins with autoanti-I specificity.

➤ Anti-i is a rare IgM agglutinin that reacts optimally at 4°C; potent examples may be associated with infectious mononucleosis.

The Kell Blood Group System

➤ The Kell blood group antigens are well developed at birth and are not destroyed by enzymes.

➤ The Kell blood group antigens are destroyed by DTT, ZZAP, and glycine-acid-EDTA.

➤ Excluding ABO, the K antigen is rated second only to D antigen in immunogenicity.

➤ The k antigen is a high-incidence antigen.

➤ Anti-K is usually an IgG antibody reactive in the AHG phase and is made in response to pregnancy or transfusion of RBCs; it has been implicated in severe hemolytic transfusion reactions and HDN.

➤ The McLeod phenotype, affecting only males, is described as a rare phenotype with decreased Kell system antigen expression. The McLeod syndrome includes the clinical manifestations of abnormal RBC morphology and compensated hemolytic anemia and neurologic and muscular abnormalities. Some males with the McLeod phenotype also have the X-linked chronic granulomatous disease.

The Duffy Blood Group System

➤ Fy^a and Fy^b antigens are destroyed by enzymes and ZZAP; they are well developed at birth. The Fy(a−b−) phenotype is prevalent in blacks but virtually nonexistent in whites.

➤ Fy(a−b−) RBCs were shown to resist infection by the malaria organisms *P. knowlesi* and *P. vivax*.

➤ Anti-Fy^a and anti-Fy^b are usually IgG antibodies and react optimally at the antiglobulin phase of testing; both antibodies have been implicated in delayed hemolytic transfusion reactions and HDN.

The Kidd Blood Group System

➤ Anti-Jk^a and anti-Jk^b may demonstrate dosage, are often weak, and are found in combination with other antibodies; both are typically IgG and antiglobulin-reactive.

➤ Kidd system antibodies may bind complement and are made in response to foreign RBC exposure during pregnancy or transfusion.

➤ Kidd system antibodies are a common cause of delayed hemolytic transfusion reactions.

➤ Kidd system antibody reactivity is enhanced with enzymes, LISS, and PEG.

The Lutheran Blood Group System

➤ Lu^a and Lu^b are antigens produced by allelic codominant genes; they are poorly developed at birth.

➤ Anti-Lu^a may be a naturally occurring saline agglutinin that reacts optimally at room temperature.

➤ Anti-Lu^b is an IgG antibody reactive at the AHG phase; usually produced in response to foreign RBC exposure during pregnancy or transfusion.

➤ The Lu(a−b−) phenotype is rare and may result from three different genetic backgrounds.

REVIEW QUESTIONS

1. Which of the following best describes MN antigens and antibodies?
   a. Well developed at birth, susceptible to enzymes, generally saline-reactive
   b. Not well developed at birth, susceptible to enzymes, generally saline-reactive
   c. Well developed at birth, not susceptible to enzymes, generally saline-reactive
   d. Well developed at birth, susceptible to enzymes, generally antiglobulin-reactive

2. Which autoantibody specificity is found in patients with paroxysmal cold hemoglobinuria?
   a. I
   b. i
   c. P
   d. P$_1$

3. Which of the following is the most common antibody seen in the blood banks after ABO and Rh antibodies?
   a. Anti-Fy^b
   b. Anti-k
   c. Anti-Js^a
   d. Anti-K

4. Which blood group system is associated with resistance to *P. vivax* malaria?
   a. P
   b. Kell
   c. Duffy
   d. Kidd

5. Which antibody does **NOT** fit with the others with respect to optimum phase of reactivity?
   a. Anti-S
   b. Anti-P$_1$
   c. Anti-Fy^a
   d. Anti-Jk^b

6. Which of the following Duffy phenotypes is prevalent in blacks but virtually nonexistent in whites?
   a. Fy(a+b+)
   b. Fy(a−b+)
   c. Fy(a−b−)
   d. Fy(a+b−)

7. Antibody detection cells will **NOT** routinely detect which antibody specificity?
   a. Anti-M
   b. Anti-Kp^a
   c. Anti-Fy^a
   d. Anti-Lu^b

8. About how many donors will need to be antigen-typed to find 3 Fy(a−) units for crossmatch?
   a. 3
   b. 5
   c. 10
   d. 12

9. Which of the following blood group systems is known for showing dosage?
   a. I
   b. P
   c. Kidd
   d. Lutheran

10. Which antibody is most commonly associated with delayed hemolytic transfusion reactions?
    a. Anti-s
    b. Anti-k
    c. Anti-Lu^a
    d. Anti-Jk^a

11. A patient with an *M. pneumoniae* infection will most likely develop a cold autoantibody with specificity to which antigen?
    a. I
    b. i
    c. P
    d. P$_1$

12. Which antigen is routinely destroyed by enzymes?
    a. P$_1$
    b. Js^a
    c. Fy^a
    d. Jk^a

REFERENCES

1. Issitt, PD, and Anstee, DJ: Applied Blood Group Serology, ed 4. Montgomery Scientific, Durham, NC, 1998.
2. Garratty, G, et al: Terminology for blood group antigens and genes: Historical origins and guidelines in the new millennium. Transfusion 40:477, 2000.
3. Daniels, GL, et al: International Sciety of Blood Transfusion Committee on terminology for red cell surface antigens: Vancouver report. Vox Sang 84:244, 2003.
4. Cartron, JP, and Rouger, P (eds): Blood Cell Biochemistry, vol 6: Molecular Basis of Human Blood Group Antigens. Plenum, New York, 1995.
5. Avent, N: Human erythrocyte antigen expression: Its molecular bases. Br J Biomed Sci 54:16, 1997.
6. Landsteiner, K, and Levine, P: A new agglutinable factor differentiating individual human bloods. Proc Soc Exp Biol 24:600, 1927.
7. Landsteiner, K, and Levine, P: Further observations on individual differences of human blood. Proc Soc Exp Biol 24:941, 1927.
8. Walsh, RJ, and Montgomery, C: A new human isoagglutinin subdividing the MN groups. Nature 160:504, 1947.
9. Levine, P, et al: A new blood group factor, s, allelic to S. Proc Soc Exp Biol 78:218, 1951.
10. Daniels, G: The Human Blood Groups, ed 2. Blackwell Science, Oxford, 2002.
11. Wiener, AS, Unger, LJ, and Gordon, EB: Fatal hemolytic transfusion reaction caused by sensitization to a new blood group factor U. JAMA 153:1444, 1953.
12. Greenwalt, TJ, et al: An allele of the S(s) blood group genes. Proc Natl Acad Sci 40:1126, 1954.
13. Reid, MD, and Lomas-Francis, C: The Blood Group Antigen Facts Book. Academic Press, New York, 1997.
14. Mollison, PL, Engelfriet, CP, and Contreras, M: Blood Transfusion in Clinical Medicine, ed 10. Blackwell Scientific, London, 1997.
15. Hawkins, P, et al: Localization of MN blood group antigens in kidney. Transplant Proc 17:1697, 1985.
16. Belzer, FO, Kountz, SL, and Perkins, HA: Red cell cold autoagglutinins as a cause of failure of renal transplantation. Transplantation 11:422, 1971.
17. Lutz, P, and Dzik, WH: Molecular biology of red cell blood group genes. Transfusion 32:467, 1992.
18. Darnborough, J, Dunsford, I, and Wallace, JA: The En^a antigen and antibody: A genetical modification of human RBCs affecting their blood grouping reactions. Vox Sang 17:241, 1969.
19. Furuhjelm, V, et al: The red cell phenotype En(a-) and anti-En^a: Serological and physiochemical aspects. Vox Sang 17:256, 1969.
20. Metaxas, MN, and Metaxas-Buhler, M: M^k: An apparently silent allele at the MN locus. Nature 202:1123, 1964.
21. Tokunaga, E, et al: Two apparently healthy Japanese individuals of type M^{k}M^k have erythrocytes which lack both the blood group MN and Ss-active sialoglycoproteins. J Immunogenet 6:383, 1979.
22. Tippett, P, et al: The Miltenberger subsystem: Is it obsolescent? Transfus Med Rev 6:170, 1992.
23. Lobo, C, et al: Glycophorin C is the receptor for the Plasmodium falciparum erythrocyte binding ligand PfEBP-2(baebl). Blood 101:4628, 2003.
24. Levine, P, et al: Isoimmunization by a new blood factor in tumor cells. Proc Soc Exp Biol 77:403, 1951.
25. Sanger, R: An association between the P and Jay systems of blood groups. Nature 176:1163, 1955.
26. Matson, GA, et al: A "new" antigen and antibody belonging to the P blood group system. Am J Hum Genet 11:26, 1959.
27. Ikin, EW, et al: P$_1$ antigen in the human foetus. Nature 192:883, 1961.
28. Arndt, PA, et al: An acute hemolytic transfusion reaction caused by an anti-P$_1$ that reacted at 37°C. Transfusion 38:373, 1998.
29. Hellberg, A, Poole, J, and Olsson, ML: Molecular basis of the globoside-deficient P^k blood group phenotype. J Biol Chem 277:29455, 2002.
30. Furukawa, K, et al: Molecular basis for the p phenotype. J Biol Chem 275:37752, 2000.
31. Koda, Y, et al: Three-base deletion and one-base insertion of the (1,4)galactosyltransferase gene responsible for the p phenoype. Transfusion 42:48, 2002.
32. Cameron, GL, and Staveley, JM: Blood group P substance in hydatid cyst fluids. Nature 179:147, 1957.
33. Roland, FP: P$_1$ blood group and urinary tract infection. Lancet 1:946, 1981.
34. Cantin, G, and Lyonnais, J: Anti-PP$_1$P^k and early abortion. Transfusion 23:350, 1983.
35. Shirey, RS, et al: Plasmapheresis and successful pregnancy after fourteen miscarriages in a P$_1^k$ with anti-P [abstract]. Transfusion 24:427, 1984.
36. Shechter, Y, et al: Early treatment by plasmapheresis in a woman with multiple abortions and the rare blood group p. Vox Sang 53:135, 1987.
37. Tippett, P, et al: An agglutinin associated with the P and the ABO blood group systems. Vox Sang 10:269, 1965.
38. Wiener, AS, et al: Type-specific cold autoantibodies as a cause of acquired hemolytic anemia and hemolytic transfusion reactions: Biologic test with bovine red cells. Ann Intern Med 44:221, 1956.
39. Marsh, WL, and Jenkins, WJ: Anti-i: A new cold antibody. Nature 188:753, 1960.
40. Yu, L, et al: Molecular basis of the adult i phenotype and the gene responsible for the expression of the human blood group I antigen. Blood 98:3840, 2001.
41. Taney, FA, Lee, LT, and Howe, C: Cold hemagglutinin crossreactivity with Mycoplasma pneumoniae. Infect Immun 22:29, 1978.
42. Moores, PP, et al: Some observations on "Bombay" bloods with comments on evidence for the existence of two different O$_h$ phenotypes. Transfusion 15:237, 1975.
43. Yu, L, et al: The molecular genetics of the human I locus and molecular background explain the partial association of the adult i phenotype with congenital cataracts. Blood 101:2081, 2003.
44. Curtain, CC, et al: Cold haemagglutinins: Unusual incidence in Melanesian populations. Br J Haematol 11:471, 1965.
45. Booth, PB, Jenkins, WL, and Marsh WL: Anti-I^T: A new antibody of the I blood group system occurring in certain Melanesian sera. Br J Haematol 12:341, 1966.
46. Garratty, G, et al: Autoimmune hemolytic anemia in Hodgkin's disease associated with anti-I^T. Transfusion 14:226, 1974.
47. Garratty, G, et al: An IgG anti-I^T detected in a Caucasian American. Transfusion 12:325, 1972.
48. Levine, P, et al: A new human hereditary blood property (Cellano) present in 99.8 percent of all bloods. Science 109:464, 1949.
49. Allen, FH, and Lewis, SJ: Kp^a (Penney), a new antigen in the Kell blood group system. Vox Sang 2:81, 1957.
50. Allen, FH, Lewis, SJ, and Fudenberg, HH: Studies of anti-Kp^b, a new alloantibody in the Kell blood group system. Vox Sang 3:1, 1958.
51. Giblett, ER: Js, a "new" blood group antigen found in negroes. Nature 181:1221, 1958.
52. Walker, RH, et al: Anti-Js^b, the expected antithetical antibody of the Sutter blood group system. Nature 197:295, 1963.
53. Chown, F, Lewis, M, and Kaita, H: A "new" Kell blood group phenotype. Nature 180:711, 1957.
54. Allen, FH, Krabbe, SM, and Corcoran, PA: A new phenotype (McLeod) in the Kell blood group system. Vox Sang 6:555, 1961.
55. Hughes-Jones, NC, and Gardner, B: The Kell system: Studies with radioactively labelled anti-K. Vox Sang 21:154, 1971.
56. Yamaguchi, H, et al: A "new" allele, Kp^c, at the Kell complex locus. Vox Sang 36:29, 1979.
57. Gavin, J, et al: The red cell antigen once called Levay is the antigen Kp^c of the Kell system. Vox Sang 36:31, 1979.
58. Marsh, WL, et al: Naturally occurring anti-Kell stimulated by E. coli enterocolitis in a 20-day-old child. Transfusion 18:149, 1978.
59. Lee, S, Russo, D, and Redman, CM: The Kell blood group system: Kell and XK membrane proteins. Semin Hematol 37:113, 2000.
60. Guévin, RM, Taliano, V, and Waldmann, O: The Côté serum, an antibody defining a new variant in the Kell system [abstract]. 24th Annual Meeting Abstract Booklet. American Association of Blood Banks, Washington, DC, 1971.
61. Strange, JJ, et al: Wk^a (Weeks), a new antigen in the Kell blood group system. Vox Sang 27:81, 1974.
62. Sabo, B, et al: Confirmation of K^{11} and K^{17} as alleles in the Kell blood group system. Vox Sang 29:450, 1975.
63. Eicher, C, et al: A new low incidence antigen in the Kell system: K24 (Cls) [abstract]. Transfusion 25:448, 1985.
64. Van der Hart, M, Szaloky, A, and Van Loghem, JJ: A "new" antibody associated with the Kell blood group system. Vox Sang 15:456, 1968.
65. Lee, S, Russo, D, and Redman, C: Functional and structural aspects of the Kell blood group system. Trans Med Rev 14:93, 2000.
66. Giblett, ER, et al: Kell phenotypes in chronic granulomatous disease: A potential transfusion hazard. Lancet 1:1235, 1971.
67. Marsh, WL, Uretsky, SC, and Douglas, SD: Antigens of the Kell blood group system on neutrophils and monocytes: Their relation to chronic granulomatous disease. J Pediatr 87:1117, 1975.
68. Marsh, WL, and Redman, CM: Recent developments in the Kell blood group system. Transfus Med Rev 1:4, 1987.
69. McGinnis, MH, Maclowry, JD, and Holland, PV: Acquisition of K:1-like antigen during terminal sepsis. Transfusion 24:28, 1984.
70. Marsh, WL, Dinapoli, J, and Øyen, R: Autoimmune hemolytic anemia caused by anti-K13. Vox Sang 36:174, 1979.
71. Cutbush, M, Mollison, PL, and Parkin, DM: A new human blood group. Nature 165:188, 1950.
72. Ikin, EW, et al: Discovery of the expected hemagglutinin, anti-Fy^b. Nature 168:1077, 1951.
73. Sanger, R, Race, RR, and Jack, J: The Duffy blood groups of New York Negroes: The phenotype Fy(a−b−). Br J Haematol 1:370, 1955.
74. Miller, LH, et al: Erythrocyte receptors for (Plasmodium knowlesi) malaria: Duffy blood group determinants. Science 189:561, 1975.
75. Pogo, AO, and Chaudhuri, A: The Duffy protein: A malarial and chemokine receptor. Semin Hematol 37:122, 2000.
76. Beattie, KM: The Duffy blood group system: Distribution, serology and genetics. In Pierce, SR, and Macpherson, CR (eds): Blood Group Systems: Duffy, Kidd and Lutheran. American Association of Blood Banks, Arlington, VA, 1988.
77. Donahue, RP, et al: Probable assignment of the Duffy blood group locus to chromosome 1 in man. Proc Natl Acad Sci USA 61:949, 1968.
78. Chown, B, Lewis, M, and Kaita, H: The Duffy blood group system in Caucasians: Evidence for a new allele. Am J Hum Genet 17:384, 1965.
79. Yazdanbakhsh, K, et al: Molecular mechanisms that lead to reduced expression of Duffy antigens. Transfusion 40:310, 2000.

80. Albrey, JA, et al: A new antibody, anti-Fy3, in the Duffy blood group system. Vox Sang 20:29, 1971.
81. Behzad, O, et al: A new anti-erythrocyte antibody in the Duffy system: Anti-FY4. Vox Sang 24:337, 1973.
82. Colledge, KI, Pezzulich, M, and Marsh, WL: Anti-Fy5: An antibody disclosing a probable association between the Rhesus and Duffy blood group genes. Vox Sang 24:193, 1973.
83. Nichols, ME, et al: A new Duffy blood group specificity defined by a murine monoclonal antibody. J Exp Med 166:776, 1987.
84. Mason, SJ, et al: The Duffy blood group determinants: Their role in susceptibility of human and animal erythrocytes to *Plasmodium knowlesi* malaria. Br J Haematol 36:327, 1977.
85. Miller, LH, et al: The Duffy blood group phenotype in American blacks infected with *Plasmodium vivax* in Vietnam. Am J Trop Med 27:1069, 1978.
86. Spencer, HC, et al: The Duffy blood group and resistance to *Plasmodium vivax* in Honduras. Am J Trop Med 27:664, 1978.
87. Hadley, TJ, and Peiper, SC: From malaria to chemokine receptor: The emerging physiologic role of the Duffy blood group antigen. Blood 89:3077, 1997.
88. Allen, FH, Diamond, LK, and Niedziela, B: A new blood group antigen. Nature 167:482, 1951.
89. Plaut, G, et al: A new blood group antibody, anti-Jk^b. Nature 171:431, 1953.
90. Pinkerton, FJ, et al: The phenotype Jk(a−b−) in the Kidd blood group system. Vox Sang 4:155, 1959.
91. Heaton, DC, and McLoughlin, K: Jk(a−b−) red blood cells resist urea lysis. Transfusion 22:70, 1982.
92. Sinor, LT, et al: Dot-blot purification of the Kidd blood group antigen [abstract]. Transfusion 26:561, 1986.
93. Okubo, Y, et al: Heterogeneity of the phenotype Jk(a−b−) found in Japanese. Transfusion 26:237, 1986.
94. Patten, E, et al: Autoimmune hemolytic anemia with anti-Jk^a specificity in a patient taking Aldomet. Transfusion 17:517, 1977.
95. Sosler, SD, et al: Acute hemolytic anemia due to a chloropropamide-dependent autoanti-Jk^a [abstract]. Transfusion 19:641, 1979.
96. Judd, WJ, Steiner, EA, and Cochrane, RK: Paraben-associated autoanti-Jk^a antibodies. Transfusion 22:31, 1982.
97. Ellisor, SS, et al: Autoantibodies mimicking anti-Jk^b plus anti-Jk3 associated with autoimmune hemolytic anemia in a primipara who delivered an unaffected infant. Vox Sang 45:53, 1983.
98. Obarski, G, et al: The Jk(a−b−) phenotype, probably occurring as a transient phenomenon [abstract]. Transfusion 27:548, 1987.
99. McGinnis, MH: The ubiquitous nature of human blood group antigens as evidenced by bacterial, viral and parasitic infections. In Garraty, G (ed): Blood Group Antigens and Disease. American Association of Blood Banks, Arlington, VA, 1983.
100. Callender, ST, Race, RR, and Paykos, ZV. Hypersensitivity to transfused blood. Br Med J 2:83, 1945.
101. Cutbush, M, and Chanarin, I: The expected blood group antibody, anti-Lu^b. Nature 178:855, 1956.
102. Crawford, MN, et al: The phenotype Lu(a−b−) together with unconventional Kidd groups in one family. Transfusion 1:228, 1967.
103. Darnborough, J, et al: A "new" antibody anti-Lu^{a}Lu^b and two further examples of the genotype Lu(a−b−). Nature 198:796, 1963.
104. Francis, BJ, and Hatcher, DE: Hemolytic disease of the newborn apparently caused by anti-Lu^a. Transfusion 1:248, 1961.
105. Parsons, SF, et al: Evidence that the Lu^b blood group antigen is located on red cell membrane glycoproteins of 85 and 78 kD. Transfusion 27:61, 1987.
106. Daniels, G, and Khalid, G: Identification, by immunoblotting, of the structures carrying Lutheran and para-Lutheran blood group antigens. Vox Sang 57:137, 1989.
107. Daniels, GL, et al: The red cell antigens Au^a and Au^b belong to the Lutheran system. Vox Sang 60:191, 1991.
108. Parsons, SF, Mawby, WJ, and Anstee, DJ: Lutheran blood group glycoprotein is a new member of the immunoglobulin superfamily of proteins [abstract]. Vox Sang (suppl 2):67:1, 1994.
109. Poole, J: Review: The Lutheran blood group system—1991. Immunohematology 8:1, 1992.
110. Udden, MM, et al: New abnormalities in the morphology, cell surface receptors, and electrolyte metabolism in In(Lu) erythrocytes. Blood 69:52, 1987.
111. Norman, PC, Tippett, P, and Beal, RW: A Lu(a−b−) phenotype caused by an X-linked recessive gene. Vox Sang 51:49, 1986.
112. Marsh, WL: Anti-Lu5, anti-Lu6 and anti-Lu7: Three antibodies defining high incidence antigens related to the Lutheran blood group system. Transfusion 12:27, 1972.
113. MacIlroy, M, McCreary, J, and Stroup, M: Anti-Lu8, an antibody recognizing another Lutheran-related antigen. Vox Sang 23:455, 1972.
114. Molthan, L, et al: Lu9, another new antigen of the Lutheran blood group system. Vox Sang 24:468, 1973.
115. Judd, WJ, et al: Anti-Lu14: A Lutheran antibody defining the product of an allele at the Lu8 blood group locus. Vox Sang 32:214, 1977.
116. Salmon, C, et al: Un nouvel antigene de groupe sanguin erythrocytaire present chez 80% des sujets du race blanche. Nouv Rev Fr Hematol 1:649, 1961.
117. Frandson, S, et al: Anti-Au^b: The antithetical antibody to anti-Au^a. Vox Sang 56:54, 1989.
118. Zelinski, T, et al: Assignment of the Auberger red cell antigen polymorphism to the Lutheran blood group system: Genetic justification. Vox Sang 61:275, 1991.

ten

The Red Cell Surface Antigen Terminology and Miscellaneous Blood Groups

Deirdre DeSantis Parsons, MS, MT(ASCP)SBB, CLS(NCA)

O B J E C T I V E S

On completion of this chapter, the learner should be able to:

1. Describe the terminology for RBC surface antigens and the four groups into which "authenticated" antigens may be classified.
2. Define the following terms and provide three examples of each: high-incidence antigen, low-incidence antigen.
3. Discuss the notable characteristics of antigens (and corresponding antibodies) in the following blood group systems:
   Diego (DI) blood group system
   Cartwright (YT) blood group system
   XG blood group system
   Scianna (SC) blood group system
   Dombrock (DO) blood group system
   Colton (CO) blood group system
   Chido/Rodgers (CH/RG) blood group system
   Gerbich (GE) blood group system
   Knops (KN) blood group system
4. Discuss the notable characteristics of the following antigens (and corresponding antibodies) that are classified into a system, collection, series, or the miscellaneous white blood cell (WBC) antigen heading.
   Cromer (CROM) antigens
   Indian (IN) antigens
   Cost (Cs^a) antigen
   JMH antigen
   Vel antigen
   Sid (Sd^a) antigen
   Bg antigens

Terminology for RBC Surface Antigens

More than 350 RBC surface antigens have been described since the discovery of the ABO system by Landsteiner in 1900. Over this time, numerous nomenclatures, systems of classification, and antigenic representations have been introduced, which has led to inconsistency in terminology. Historically, approaches to naming antigens included using all, part, or some derivation of the name of the first antibody maker or reactive donor, using the name of the scientist discovering the antigen, adopting the name of the country of the antibody producer, or deriving letters from related descriptive terminology such as "I" for indivduality and "U" for universal.[1] The Diego, Dombrock, Colton, Cromer, Gerbich, Knops, and Scianna blood group systems presented in this chapter were all named after their respective antibody makers.

The terminology for RBC surface antigens was initiated to develop a standard numeric system for describing and reporting RBC antigens in a format that is both eye- and computer-readable. The first monograph of this numeric system was released in 1990, and numerous amendments have been made.

Through ongoing advances in gene mapping, many blood group antigens have been reclassified, new blood group systems have been created, new antigens have been discovered,

and a few antigens have been determined to be obsolete.[2] In keeping with the genetic basis for RBC antigens, the International Society of Blood Transfusion (ISBT) organized a working party to develop a world standard for terminology that would provide a uniform numeric system suitable for electronic data processing equipment.[3] This terminology for RBC surface antigens assigns a six-digit identification number to each authenticated blood group antigen. The first three numbers represent the blood group system, collection, or series (e.g., 004 for the RH system), and the last three numbers represent antigen specificity (e.g., 001 for the D antigen). Accordingly, the ISBT number for the D antigen would be 004001. The original (alphabetical) names for the systems and most antigens have not been changed; however, the symbols for each system have been converted to capital letters (e.g., from Rh to RH). An alternative method for identifying antigens in a blood group system according to ISBT would be the system symbol followed by the antigen number (e.g., RH1 for the D antigen). See Table 10–1 for an abbreviated listing of the blood group systems and the related ISBT terminology and numbers. Phenotypes are designated by the system symbol with a colon followed by the specificity numbers separated by commas. Any negative result (or absent antigen) would be preceded by a minus sign. The phenotype DcEe would be represented in the ISBT system as RH:1, –2, 3, 4, 5. This

TABLE 10–1   Abridged ISBT Terminology for RBC Surface Antigens in Blood Group Systems*

ISBT System Number	System	Symbol	Antigen	Chromosomal† Number	Total No. of AGs
001	ABO	ABO	A	9q	4
	ABO	ABO	B		
	ABO	ABO	A, B		
	ABO	ABO	A1		
002	MNS	MNS	M	4q	43
	MNS	MNS	N		
	MNS	MNS	S		
	MNS	MNS	s		
	MNS	MNS	U		
003	P	P	P1	22q	1
004	Rh	RH	D	1p	55
	Rh	RH	C		
	Rh	RH	E		
	Rh	RH	c		
	Rh	RH	e		
	Rh	RH	Cʷ		
005	Lutheran	LU	Luᵃ	19q	21
	Lutheran	LU	Luᵇ		
	Lutheran	LU	Lu3		
	Lutheran	LU	Lu4		
	Lutheran	LU	Lu5		
	Lutheran	LU	Lu6		
	Lutheran	LU	Lu7		
006	Kell	KEL	K	7q	27
	Kell	KEL	k		
	Kell	KEL	Kpᵃ		
	Kell	KEL	Kpᵇ		
	Kell	KEL	Ku		
	Kell	KEL	Jsᵃ		
007	Lewis	LE	Leᵃ	19p	6
	Lewis	LE	Leᵇ		
008	Duffy	FY	Fyᵃ	1q	6
	Duffy	FY	Fyᵇ		
	Duffy	FY	Fy3		
	Duffy	FY	Fy4		
	Duffy	FY	Fy5		
	Duffy	FY	Fy6		

ISBT System Number	System	Symbol	Antigen	Chromosomal† Number	Total No. of AGs
009	Kidd	JK	Jk^a	18q	3
	Kidd	JK	Jk^b		
	Kidd	JK	Jk3		
010	Diego	DI	Di^a	17q	21
	Diego	DI	Di^b		
	Diego	DI	Wr^a		
	Diego	DI	Wr^b		
011	Cartwright	YT	Yt^a	7q	2
	Cartwright	YT	Yt^b		
012	Xg	XG	Xg^a	Xp	2
013	Scianna	SC	Sc^a	1p	4
	Scianna	SC	Sc^b		
	Scianna	SC	Sc3		
	Scianna	SC	Rd		
014	Dombrock	DO	Do^a	12p	5
	Dombrock	DO	Do^b		
	Dombrock		Gy^a		
	Dombrock		Hy		
	Dombrock		Jo^a		
015	Colton	CO	Co^a	7p	3
	Colton	CO	Co^b		
	Colton	CO	Co3		
016	Landsteiner-Wiener	LW	Lw^a	19p	3
	Landsteiner-Wiener	LW	Lw^{ab}		
	Landsteiner-Wiener	LW	LW^b		
017	Chido/Rodgers	CH	Ch1	6p	9
	Chido/Rodgers	CH	Ch2		
	Chido/Rodgers	CH	Ch3		
	Chido/Rodgers	CH	Rg1		
	Chido/Rodgers	CH	Rg2		
018	H	H	H	19q	1
019	Kx	XK	Kx	Xp	1
020	Gerbich	GE	Ge2	2q	8
	Gerbich	GE	Ge3		
	Gerbich	GE	Ge4		
021	CROMER	CROM	Cr^a	1q	11
	CROMER	CROM	Tc^a		
	CROMER	CROM	Tc^b		
	CROMER	CROM	Tc^c		
022	Knops	KN	Kn^a	1q	8
	Knops	KN	Kn^b		
	Knops	KN	McC^a		
	Knops	KN	Sl1		
	Knops	KN	Yk^a		
023	Indian	IN	In^a	11p	2
	Indian	IN	In^b		
024	Ok	OK	OK^a	19p	1
025	Raph	RAPH	MER2	11p	1
026	John Milton Hagen	JMH	JMH	15q	1
027	I	I	I	6p	1
028	Globoside	GLOB	P	3q	1
029	GIL	GIL	GIL	9p	1

*Only the more commonly known antigens are presented. The antigen listing for the following blood group system is incomplete: MNS, RH, LU, KEL, DI, GE, CROM, and KN.

†The gene location is designated by the chromosomal number, and the p (short)or q(long) arm.

AG = antigens

numeric system is designed as an alternative terminology for computer use and is not practical for verbal and publication purposes.

All authenticated antigens are assigned to a system, a collection, a low-incidence series, or a high-incidence series. To meet the criteria for a blood group system, an antigen must be an inherited character that is controlled by a single gene or by two genes so closely linked that recombination is seldom observed. In addition, "the names must be assigned to a unique chromosomal locus or be inherited discretely from any other gene."[3] The last requirement is the serologic defi-

nition of each antigen through testing with the corresponding antibody.

So far, 29 blood group systems have been established, and more than 350 antigens have been catalogued into these systems with an ISBT number.[4] The Blood Group Terminology website (www.iccbba.com/page25.htm), hosted by the International Council for Commonality in Blood Banking Automation, Inc., presents the most current tables on blood group systems, collections, low-incidence series, and high-incidence series, with information updated as new discoveries are made.

Collections include antigens that demonstrate a biochemical, serologic, or genetic relationship but do not meet the criteria for independent inheritance. Antigens classified as a collection are assigned a 200 number. For instance, the COST collection has been designated as ISBT 205. See **Table 10–2** for a listing of the ISBT collections. All remaining RBC antigens that are not associated with a system or a collection are catalogued into the 700 series of low-incidence antigens or the 901 series of high-incidence antigens. Refer to **Table 10–3** for an abbreviated listing of high-incidence antigens according to ISBT. High-incidence and low-incidence antigens represent antigens observed in more than 90 percent or less than 1 percent of most random populations, respectively.

More than 350 RBC surface antigens have been described that may or may not represent independent blood group systems. Accordingly, it would be difficult to try to present all of the known RBC surface antigens. Only the more commonly studied blood group systems are briefly addressed here, depending on the information currently available. Antigens are grouped into a blood group system, collection, series, or the miscellaneous WBC heading.

The Diego Blood Group System: DI (ISBT 010)

The Diego system is composed of two sets of independent pairs of antithetical antigens: Di^a/Di^b and Wr^a/Wr^b as well as 17 low-incidence antigens for a total of 21 antigens. Represented in each antithetical pair are high-incidence Di^b and Wr^b and low-incidence Di^a and Wr^a. In 1953 the discovery of anti-Di^a antibody defined the Di^a specificity,[5] and in 1967 the antithetical Di^b antigen was characterized with the newly identified anti-Di^b antibody. The DI antigens are inherited as codominant alleles on chromosome 17. **Table 10–1** provides a complete listing of the chromosomal assignments for all ISBT blood group systems. Di^a antigen is described as a low-incidence antigen (0.01 percent) rarely noted in white populations and more commonly noted in individuals of Asian origin. The Di^a antigen has served as a useful tool in anthropologic studies of Mongolian ancestry.

South American Indians have been shown to have an incidence of Di^a as high as 54 percent in some areas, Chippewa Indians an incidence of 11 percent, Chinese an incidence of 5 percent, and Japanese an incidence of 12 percent.[6–8] Di^b is a high-incidence antigen found in all other ethnic groups. The $Di(a-b-)$ phenotype has not been reported. Di^a and Di^b antigens are located on the anion exchange protein, AE-1 (also known as erythrocyte band 3),[7] which is an integral transport protein involved in the anion exchange of bicarbonate for chloride in the RBC membrane.[9] **Figure 10–1** provides a possible molecular representation of the location of the DI antigens on the AE-1 transporter protein. AE-1 also serves as a major instrinsic structural protein that interacts with the RBC membrane cytoskeleton; interestingly, mutations in AE-1 can result in hereditary spherocytosis,[10] congenital acanthocytosis,[11] and Southeast Asian ovalocytosis.[12]

The Di^a and Di^b antigens are well developed at birth and are described as resistant to all standard enzymes and reducing agents **(Table 10–4)** such as dithiothreitol (DTT). Both anti-Di^a and anti-Di^b are characterized as RBC-stimulated IgG antibodies that do not bind complement and are reactive in indirect antiglobulin testing (IAT). Anti-Di^b is reported to show dosage. Although both antibodies have been associated with causing moderate-to-severe transfusion reactions and hemolytic disease of the newborn (HDN), milder forms of HDN are noted with anti-Di^b. When the need arises, locating Di^b-negative donors is challenging due to the scarcity of reagent. Recently, a DNA-based polymerase chain reaction method has been developed to identify Di^b negative donors.[13]

The Wright antigens, discovered in 1953,[14] include two allelic antigens: Wr^a, a low-incidence antigen occurring in less than 0.01 percent of the random population, and Wr^b, a high-incidence antigen occurring in 99.9 percent of the random population. Historically, most RBC surface antigens have been identified and catalogued according to classical family studies and population statistics. The Wright antigens were first classified as an independent blood group system and later as a collection. The work of Bruce and coworkers[15] revealed that the Wr^a antigen represents amino acid Lys-658 and the Wr^b antigen Glu-658, which are housed on the

TABLE 10–2   Antigen Collections According to ISBT

Collection			Antigen		
Number	Name	Symbol	Number	Symbol	Comments
205	Cost	COST	205001	Cs^a	Cs^a: high-frequency antigen with variable expression.
			205002	Cs^b	Antibodies: IgG, IAT, high-titer
					Significance: HTR: no; HDN: no
					Anti-Cs^b extremely rare
207	Ii	I	207002	i	Refer to Chapter 9
208	Er	ER	208001	Er^a	Er^a antigen: high frequency. Er^b antigen: low frequency.
			208002	Er^b	Antibodies: Er^a, IgG, IAT
					Significance: HTR: no; HDN: no
					Anti-Er^b extremely rare
209		GLOB	209002	p^k	Formerly in P_1 system
			209003	LKE	Refer to Chapter 9
210			210001	Le^c	Formerly in Lewis system
			210002	Le^d	Refer to Chapter 8

TABLE 10–3   Notable Antigens in the High-Incidence Series (901)

Antigen	Name		Ig Class	HDN	HTR	ISBT Number
Vel			IgM and few IgG	No	Rare Severe Hemolytic	901.001
Comments		• Binds complement—few hemolytic • IAT reactively optimally with enzyme-treated cells • Red cell-stimulated • Vel(−) incidence: 1 in 4000 with higher frequency in Swedish populations • Weak expression on cord cells				
Lan	Langereis		IgG1 and IgG3	Mild	Rare Severe	901.002
Comments		• Few bind complement • IAT reactivity • Red cell-stimulated				
At^a	August		IgG	No	Few Moderate	901.003
Comments		• IAT reactivity • Red cell-stimulated • At(^{a}−) noted in blacks only				
Sd^a	Sid		IgM and few IgG	No	Very rare	901.012
Comments		• RT and IAT reactivity—enhanced by enzymes • Red cell-stimulated • Variable expression in adults with the most on polyagglutinable Cad cells: super-Sid (Chapter 22) • Mixed-field agglutinates, shiny and refractile hemagglutination inhibition with Sd(^{a}+) urine which is carried by Tamm Horsfall glycoprotein • Depressed antigen expression during pregnancy • Weak expression on cord cells				

anion transporter AE-1. The Wr antigens, like the Diego antigens, are then linked with anion exchange in the RBC membrane.[9] As a result, the Wright antigens were reclassified to the Diego blood group system. Worthy of mention, cells lacking glycophorin A are also negative for Wr^a and Wr^b, suggesting an important association between AE-1 and glycophorin A.[16]

Although the antigen Wr^a is extremely rare, the antibody anti-Wr^a has been reported quite frequently. Two types of anti-Wr^a have been observed, a non-RBC stimulated IgM and an immune-stimulated IgG. Non-RBC stimulated anti-Wr^a is frequently found in the serum of individuals who have never been pregnant or received transfusions. RBC-stimulated anti-Wr^a is typically an IgG$_1$ antibody that is reactive only in IAT testing. The IgG anti-Wr^a is reported to cause mild-to-severe HDN and transfusion reactions.

Only a few examples anti-Wr^b alloantibody have been described, so little is known about its clinical significance.[8] Anti-Wr^b may commonly be found as a warm autoantibody in patients with autoimmune hemolytic anemia.

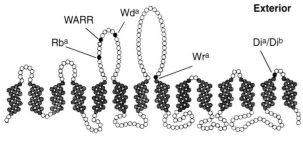

■ **FIGURE 10–1**   A molecular illustration of the Diego antigens on the AE-1 transporter molecule.

The Cartwright Blood Group System: YT (ISBT 011)

The Cartwright blood group system was discovered in 1956 with the observation of Yt^a.[17] The YT system is composed of two antigens: Yt^a, a high-incidence antigen presenting in 99.8 percent of the general population, and the antithetical partner, Yt^b, a low-incidence antigen presenting in 8 percent of the general population. Three phenotypes have been described, virtually with the same frequencies in both white and black populations: Yt(a+b−) occurs in 91.9 percent, Yt(a+b+) in 7.8 percent, and Yt(a−b+) in 0.3 percent.[18] The null phenotype Yt(a−b−) has not been observed. The YT antigens are located on acetylcholinesterase (AchE), which is an enzyme involved in neurotransmission.[19] AchE has been shown to be present in erythroid and nerve cells; distribution on other tissues remains undefined.[8]

The Yt^a and Yt^b antigens are inherited as codominant alleles on chromosome 7. Whereas Yt^a and Yt^b are sensitive to reducing agents, Yt^a has been shown to be variably sensitive to certain enzymes (see **Table 10–4**). The Yt^a antigen is not well developed at birth; therefore, cord blood is usually Yt^a-negative. Conversely, in adults, the Yt^a antigen is described as strongly immunogenic, which accounts for the relative frequency of the anti-Yt^a antibody. One noteworthy case has been reported of a Yt^a antigen–positive individual presenting with an alloanti-Yt^a, suggesting heterogeneity in antigen expression.[18]

The Yt^b antigen is well developed at birth but appears to be a poor immunogen. In fact, only a few examples of anti-Yt^b have been observed in patients who have been frequently transfused and who have produced multiple antibodies.[6]

Both anti-Yt^a and anti-Yt^b are IgG antibodies, mostly of the IgG1 and IgG4 subclasses. YT antibodies are reactive in IAT and are considered to be clinically important because they are

TABLE 10–4   Effect of Enzyme and Chemical Treatment*

System	Ficin/Papain	α-Chymotrypsin	Trypsin	Pronase	DTT 0.2M	Chloroquine
Diego	R	R	R	R	R	R
YT	V	S	R	S	S	R
XG	S	S	S	S	R	NR
Scianna	R	R	R	W	V	R
Dombrock	R	W	S	S	S	R
Colton	R	R	R	R	R	R
Chido/Rodgers	S	S	S	S	R	R
Gerbich	V**	R	S	V	R	R
Cromer	R	S	R	S	W/R	R
Knops	R	S	S	V	W/S	R
Indian	S	S	S	S	S	R
JMH	S	S	S	S	S	R

R = resistant; S = sensitive; V = variable; W = weakened; NR = not reported
* Note these are generalizations regarding antigen reactivity, and exceptions may be reported.
** Ge2 and Ge4 antigens are sensitive, and Ge3 antigens are resistant.

predominantly RBC-stimulated. Anti-Yt[a] has been associated with transfusion reaction; however, cases are documented of Yt[a] antigen–negative patients receiving Yt[a] antigen–positive RBCs without adverse consequences.[20] A number of RBC survival studies as well as cellular assay studies have been conducted with inconclusive results regarding the clinical potential of YT antibodies.[21,22] No reports have related YT antibodies to HDN.

The XG Blood Group System: XG (ISBT 012)

The XG blood group was discovered in 1962,[23] and other examples soon followed.[24,25] At present only the Xg[a] antigen has been identified with no known antithetical partner. For that reason, the XG phenotype is expressed as either Xg(a+) or Xg(a−), with Xg representing allele absence. Xg[a] is represented as XG1 in ISBT terminology. The blood group is unique in that the gene that encodes for the Xg allele is located on the petite (short) arm of the X chromosome. Family studies have confirmed the inheritance of the Xg[a] antigen on an X-linked basis; thus, a difference in the frequency of the Xg[a] antigen is noted between the sexes. Approximately 89 percent of the female population expresses Xg[a], whereas 66 percent of the male population expresses Xg[a]. The incidence of Xg[a] differs little across most populations.[8]

Males are hemizygotes for the XG gene, inasmuch as they carry only one X chromosome. Men, then, may be of genotype Xg^a or Xg, whereas women may be Xg^aXg^a, Xg^aXg, or $XgXg$. Thus, the mating of an Xg(a+) man with an Xg(a−) woman would produce all Xg(a+) daughters and Xg(a−) sons.

The infrequently encountered anti-Xg[a] antibodies are predominantly IgG immunoglobulins reactive in the IAT testing. The antigen is sensitive to most enzymes (see **Table 10–4**) but not reducing agents such as DTT. These antibodies are described variably to bind complement and react in IAT testing. Most Xg[a] antibodies are the result of RBC stimulation but have not been attributed to causing transfusion reactions or HDN. Consequently, Xg[a] antigen does not appear to be an effective immunogen. A single example of autoanti-Xg[a] has been reported.[26]

A modern addition to the XG system is the CD99 antigen, which is produced by the *MIC2* gene. The *XG* and *MIC2* genes are located in close proximity on the short arm of the X chromosome.[27] Given that Xg[a] and CD99 are encoded by these closely linked genes, CD99 has been assigned to the XG system as XG2. The CD99 antigen is described to have receptor and cell adhesion functions and to be found on most human cells.[28] It is not surprising, then, that XG transcripts have been detected on erythroid as well as numerous nonerythroid tissues such as the heart, placenta, skeletal muscle, trachea, prostate, thyroid, and spinal cord.[29]

The Scianna Blood Group System: SC (ISBT 013)

The SC system is composed of the Sc1 and Sc2 antithetical alleles, the high-incidence Sc3, and the low-incidence Radin (Rd) antigen. Sc1 and Sc2 are inherited as codominant characters on chromosome 1. Although the antithetical relationship of the Sc1 and Sc2 antigens was not realized until 1967,[30] the Sc1 antigen was first identified as the Sm antigen in 1962[31] and the Sc2 antigen as the rare Bu[a] antigen a year later.[32] Sc1 is a high-incidence antigen, occurring in approximately 100 percent of the random population. Sc2 is a low-incidence antigen, occurring in less than 1 percent of Northern Europeans.[6]

The newest antigen in the SC system is Radin. Until its genomic position was recently proved to reside on the Scianna locus, Rd was catalogued in the series of low-incidence antigens.[33]

The Sc1 and Sc2 antigens are resistant to most standard enzymes while sensitive to reducing agents (see **Table 10–4**). At present the function of these antigens remains unknown; however, their molecular basis has only just been defined, marking Scianna as the last blood group to have its molecular basis characterized. The Scianna antigens are shown to be expressed by the RBC adhesion protein ERMAP in humans.[33] The function of ERMAP is not completely clear, but it is understood to be expressed throughout erythropoiesis.[34]

The anti-Sc1 and anti-Sc2 antibodies are rarely observed. Most anti-Sc1 and anti-Sc2 antibodies are IgG, RBC-stimulat-

ed, and react in IAT testing. Anti-Sc1 has been described to bind complement, whereas anti-Sc2 has not. Neither anti-Sc1 nor anti-Sc2 has been implicated in transfusion reactions; however, anti-Sc2 has been described in causing mild HDN.[6] Anti-Rd is also viewed to be clinically important due to its association with HDN. A few cases of autoanti-Sc1 have been noted.

The Sc3 antigen has high frequency and is expressed on RBCs carrying the Sc1 and/or the Sc2 antigens, but it does not appear in the null phenotype Sc:−1−2. Sc3 was identified after anti-Sc3 was observed in two Sc:−1−2 individuals from the Marshall Islands and Papua New Guinea, respectively.[35] Later, six other individuals with the Sc null phenotype were found in the same New Guinea village. Anti-Sc3 reacts with all RBCs except Sc:−1−2 cells. The antibody does not reveal a discrete specificity in adsorption studies. Anti-Sc3 is characterized as IgG, RBC–stimulated, and reacting in the IAT phase of testing. With regard to clinical importance, the antibody has been linked to causing mild transfusion reactions. No cases of HDN have been reported.

The Dombrock Blood Group System: DO (ISBT 014)

Since the initial discovery of the Dombrock blood group in 1965 with the Do[a] antigen,[36] four more antigens have been added to the system. The antithetical partner, Do[b], was reported in 1973 when the antibody anti-Do[b] was observed.[37] Immunochemical and serologic findings linked the high-incidence Gregory (Gy[a]) antigen with Dombrock, but it was not catalogued in the DO blood group system until a sample negative for the Gy[a] antigen was also shown to lack both the Do[a] and Do[b] antigens.[38] Moreover, the sample was negative for the high-incidence antigens Holley (Hy) and Joseph (Jo[a]), which were subsequently assigned to the DO system. The DO gene is assigned to the short arm of chromosome 12.

The null phenotype in the Dombrock system demonstrates an absence of Do[a], Do[b], Gy[a], Hy, and Jo[a] antigens due to all residing on a glycosylphosphatidylinositol (GPI)-linked glycoprotein that anchors them to the RBC membrane.[38] This DO glycoprotein is part of the mono-ADP-ribosyltransferase family and may be involved in the regulation of cellular protein function.[39] In addition, a total absence of DO expression is observed in paroxysmal nocturnal hemoglobinuria III RBCs, which are deficient in all GPI-anchored glycoproteins.[40]

Do[a] and Do[b] are inherited as codominant alleles and are described as resistant to ficin/papain treatment and sensitive to trypsin, pronase, and reducing agents (see **Table 10–4**). The incidence of the Do[a] antigen is variable, with 67 percent of whites, 56 percent of blacks and Native Americans, and 24 percent of Japanese carrying the antigen. The Do[b] antigen may be observed in nearly 82 percent of whites and 89 percent of blacks. Four phenotypes have been described in the Dombrock system with the following frequencies in whites: Do(a+b−) at 18 percent, Do(a+b+) at 49 percent, and Do(a−b+) at 33 percent. The Do[null] phenotype has been noted infrequently in white and Japanese populations and, as previously noted, the Gy[a], Hy, and Jo[a] antigens are also lacking.

The infrequently encountered Dombrock system antibodies are characterized as weakly reacting IgG, RBC-stimulated, and unable to bind complement. The DO antibodies react optimally in IAT with polyethylene glycol or enzyme enhancement. These antibodies are more often observed in combination with other antibodies, with the exception of anti-Gy[a], which often occurs alone. Interestingly, all known cases of Gy(a−) pregnant woman show the presence of anti-Gy[a] in their serum, suggesting that the Gy[a] antigen is highly immunogenic.[40]

None of the Dombrock antibodies are associated with clinical HDN, although positive direct antiglobulin testing has been recorded. The DO antibodies are reported to cause acute to delayed transfusion reactions.[41]

The Colton Blood Group System: CO (ISBT 015)

The Colton system is composed of three antigens: Co[a], Co[b], and Co3 (formerly Co[ab]). Co[a] and Co[b] are antithetical partners inherited as codominant antigens on chromosome 7. The Colton blood group system was discovered in 1967 when the antibody to the Co[a] antigen was described.[42] Co[b] was defined in 1970 when the antibody anti-Co[b] was observed.[43] Co[a], a high-frequency antigen, is present in 99.9 percent of most random populations. Co[b] is noted in 10 percent of most random populations. Three phenotypes have been described in the Colton system with the following approximate frequencies: Co(a+b−), 90 percent; Co(a+b+), 9.5 percent; Co(a−b+), 0.5 percent; and Co(a−b−), less than 0.01 percent. All three CO antigens are described to be resistant to all enzymes and reducing agents (see **Table 10–4**). So far, only seven cases of the Colton null phenotype have been documented.[44] Disease associations have linked the Co(a−b−) phenotype with monosomy-7 of the bone marrow, which can result in myeloid leukemia and preleukemic dysmyelopoietic syndromes.[45,46]

The CO antigens are located on the integral transmembrane protein known as Aquaporin-1 (AQP1), which forms primary plasma membrane water channels for the regulation of osmotic water transport. In addition to being present on the RBC membrane, AQP1 and the CO antigens are expressed in the tissues of the proximal and descending tubules and the collecting ducts of the kidney and are believed to account for 80 percent of the reabsorption of water. A lack of AQP1 expression corresponds to the Colton null phenotype.[47]

Although encountered rarely, both anti-Co[a] and anti-Co[b] are IgG, RBC-stimulated, and reactive in IAT. Anti-Co[b] has been shown to bind complement weakly. Both anti-Co[a] and anti-Co[b] have been associated with acute to delayed transfusion reactions. Unlike the anti-Co[a], reports have implicated anti-Co[b] as causing subclinical to mild HDN only. Of the known examples of anti-Co[b], most were noted in individuals with multiple antibodies, suggesting that the Co[b] antigen may be a poor immunogen.[48]

The Co3 antigen has a high incidence and is present on RBCs carrying the Co[a] and/or the Co[b] antigens, but it is not expressed in the null phenotype Co(a−b−). Anti-Co3 reacts with all RBCs except Co(a−b−) cells. The antibody does not demonstrate a discrete specificity in adsorption studies. Anti-Co3 is characterized as potent IgG, RBC-stimulated, complement binding, and reacting in the IAT phase of testing. With regard to clinical importance, the antibody has been associated with causing severe HDN and one mild hemolytic transfusion reaction (HTR).

The Chido/Rodgers Blood Group System: CH/RG (ISBT 017)

The Chido/Rodgers blood group system includes nine antigens, which are subdivided into six Chido antigens, two Rodgers antigens, and the WH antigen. CH1, CH2, CH3, RG1, and RG2 are described as high-incidence antigens, with CH1 being noted in approximately 100 percent and RG1 in 98 percent of all random populations. None of the antigens have been shown to be antithetical. The antigens are located on the C4 complement component and adsorbed from plasma onto the RBC membrane. All of the CH/RG antigens are poorly expressed on cord cells, sensitive to treatment with most enzymes such as ficin/papain and pronase, and resistant to reducing agents such as DTT (see Table 10–4). Historically, the Chido/Rodgers system antibodies were collectively grouped as high-titer, low-avidity (HTLA) along with other antibodies sharing common serologic properties (Table 10–5). HTLA antibodies are characterized as weak and variably reacting IgG antibodies, reacting in the IAT phase of testing. Agglutination strength seldom exceeds 1+ because of low avidity (poor binding), and reaction patterns are not always reproducible. These antibodies demonstrate similar weak reactivity at dilutions of 1:64 and higher. Generally, they are of the IgG2 and IgG4 subclasses and are considered clinically insignificant. With advances in gene mapping and immunochemical studies, most of the HTLA antigens have been assigned to independent blood group systems or the high-incidence series (901). Subsequently, the term HTLA is regarded to be out of favor.[49] The Chido antigens were first described in 1967 by Harris when three antibody producers presented with "nebulous" reacting antibodies directed toward a common high-frequency antigen that created problems in compatibility testing.[50] Soon after, Chido-specific substance was identified in plasma and serum by the ability to neutralize anti-Ch antibodies.[51] Anti-Rg was not described until 1976 when a similar but separate antibody demonstrated weak and variable reactivity.[52]

Because of the observation that many serum samples containing antibodies to Chido/Rodgers system antigens also contained WBC-associated antibodies such as anti-Bg[a], it was postulated that the CH/RG antigens were associated with the human leukocyte antigen (HLA) system. The alleles for RG and CH have been located on two closely linked genes known as *C4A* and *C4B* on chromosome 6, substantiating the link with the HLA system.[53] The CH and RG antigens are not integral to the RBC membrane inasmuch as they are adsorbed onto the cell surface from plasma. The null CH and RG phenotypes, because of C4 deletion, have been associated with a number of autoimmune diseases such as systemic lupus erythematosus,[54] Graves' disease, and rheumatoid arthritis.

Antibodies to Chido or Rodgers are usually stimulated in multitransfused individuals lacking one or more of the corresponding antigens. As noted, these antibodies are IgG, weakly reactive in the IAT phase of testing, and are destroyed by enzyme treatment (see Table 10–4). Antibody producers are routinely given transfusions of antigen-positive RBCs without evidence of increased RBC destruction. However, severe anaphylactic reactions have been reported in a few of the CH/RG system antibody-producing patients transfused with large amounts of plasma products such as fresh frozen plasma and platelets.[55] Anti-Ch/Rg system antibodies have not been implicated in causing HDN.

The presence of antibodies to Chido or Rodgers antigens often complicates pretransfusion testing and antibody identification because the antibodies present with weak and variable serologic patterns that are not reproducible. It is important to identify their presence, inasmuch as they may obscure the detection of more important underlying alloantibodies, such as anti-K, Jk[a], Fy[a], C, or Vel. Two procedures, antibody screening with C4-coated RBCs[56] and plasma inhibition, are routinely used to confirm the identity of suspected anti-Ch or anti-Rg antibodies. Antibody screening with C4-coated RBCs is particularly useful for the rapid identification and differentiation of antibodies to Chido or Rodgers antigens from other antibodies with similar serologic reactivity (see Table 10–4). Plasma inhibition is a valuable tool in compatibility testing and antibody identification procedures in that the anti-Ch/Rg antibodies are removed from the test system, thereby allowing for the detection of possible underlying alloantibodies (see the Procedural Appendix at end of this chapter). Underlying alloantibodies have been reported in approximately 25 percent of samples being investigated for presenting with "nebulous" reactivity. In addition, anti-Ch and anti-Rg are the only antibodies formerly classified as HTLAs that may be neutralized or inhibited by plasma that is positive for these antigens. Caution must be exercised when using plasma inhibition because other antibodies—anti-Le[a] and anti-Le[b]—may also be neutralized by plasma or serum containing the corresponding Lewis substance. Plasma inhibition, then, should not be the only method used to identify Ch or Rg antibodies.

The Gerbich Blood Group System: GE (ISBT 020)

The Gerbich blood group is a complex system that is composed of three high-incidence antigens (Ge2, Ge3, and Ge4)

TABLE 10–5	Antibodies Formerly Classified as HTLAs Due to Similar Serologic Reactivity	
Antibody	**Name**	**ISBT Class**
Anti-Ch	Chido	Blood group system: CH/RG
Anti-Rg	Rodgers	Blood group system: CH/RG
Anti-Kn	Knops	Blood group system: KN
Anti-McC	McCoy	Blood group system: KN
Anti-Yk[a]	York	Blood group system: KN
Anti-Sl	Swain-Langley	Blood group system: KN
Anti-Cs[a]	Cost	Collection 205: COST
Anti-JMH	John Milton Hagen	Blood group system: JMH

and four low-incidence antigens (Wb, Ls^a, An^a, and Dh^a). The GE antigens were first reported in 1960 when three antibodies were described as reacting with the RBCs of all individuals but not with the original three propositi.[57] Soon after, a fourth antibody with similar, but not identical, serologic reactivity was characterized.[58] Accordingly, it was proposed that more than one antibody specificity was represented by these samples. The development of monoclonal GE antibody led to the revision of the GE system in that the Ge2, Ge3, and Ge4 antigens were authenticated, and the Ge1 antigen was declared obsolete. Examples of anti-Ge2, anti-Ge3, and anti-Ge4 have been used to define the three GE negative phenotypes presented in **Table 10–6**. Two forms of the GE null phenotype have been identified as the Leach types PL and LN, as a result of deletions in exons 3 and 4 and a deletion of nucleotide 134, respectively.[59]

The seven GE antigens are inherited on chromosome 2 and are expressed on RBC membrane sialoglycoproteins glycophorins C (GPC) and/or glycophorin D (GPD). GPC and GPD are associated with the RBC membrane band 4.1, which is integral for maintaining normal erythrocyte skeleton and shape. Individuals of the Leach phenotype (GE: −2, −3, −4) present with a change in erythrocyte morphology in the form of elliptocytosis.[60] The incidence of Ge2, Ge3, and Ge4 is cited to be 100 percent in all populations except Melanesians, in whom the incidence of Ge3 is reported to be 50 percent.[6] The Ge2, Ge3, and Ge4 antigens are resistant to standard reducing agents, with Ge2 and Ge4 being sensitive to ficin, papain, and trypsin (see **Table 10–4**). Ge3 is resistant to ficin and papain but sensitive to trypsin. Antibodies to high-incidence GE antigens are described to be predominantly IgG, RBC-stimulated, variably binding complement, and reacting in the IAT phase of testing. Anti-Ge2 and anti-Ge3 have also been noted as non-RBC stimulated IgM immunoglobulins and as autoantibodies. Anti-Ge2 and anti-Ge3 are implicated in causing acute to delayed transfusion reactions but not in cases of clinical HDN. Not much information is available on the clinical significance of anti-Ge4 as only one example has been reported. Likewise, little is known about the pathogenicity of the antibodies to the low-incidence GE antigens: anti-Wb, anti-Ls^a, anti-An^a, and anti-Dh^a.[4] All four are described as predominantly IgG with an IgM component and as not binding complement. Anti-Wb and anti-Ls^a are generally non-RBC stimulated.

The Cromer Blood Group System: CROM (ISBT 021)

The Cromer system is composed of eight high-incidence antigens (Cr^a, Tc^a, Dr^a, Es^a, IFC, UMC, WES^b, and GUTI)[61] and three low-incidence antigens (Tc^b, Tc^c, and WES^a). In 1965 the Cr^a antigen was reported by Stroup and McCreay in a black woman after delivery.[62]The CROM antigens are distributed on the membranes of RBCs, platelets, granulocytes, lymphocytes and placental tissue as well as in lower soluble quantities in plasma and urine. Most Cromer antigens are characterized as sensitive to chymotrypsin and pronase treatment and resistant to all other enzymes (see **Table 10–4**). Reducing agents such as DTT have little effect, causing only slightly weakened antigen expression. All are carried by decay accelerating factor (DAF or CD55), which is involved with the regulation of complement activation by accelerating the decay of the C3 and C5 convertases. DAF served as an integral intrinsic membrane glycoprotein that is anchored by GPI. The locus for the CROM antigens is encoded on chromosome 1.

The null phenotype, Inab, lacks all CROM antigens as well as DAF and is possibly linked with chronic intestinal conditions, given that DAF is thought to be an attachment site for *Escherichia coli* on epithelial cells.[63] Inab(−) individuals often produce anti-IFC, which is reactive with all samples except Inab RBCs. To date, Inab phenotype has been identified in six propositi, with the last described as being transient and acquired rather than inherited.[64] A total absence of Cromer expression is also observed in paroxysmal nocturnal hemoglobinuria III RBCs, which are deficient in all GPI anchored glycoproteins including DAF. Additionally, a weakened expression of all high-incidence Cromer antigens is observed in all Dr(a−) individuals.

Antibodies to Cromer system antigens are described as predominantly IgG1, RBC-stimulated, and reactive in IAT testing. Neutralization can be accomplished with concentrated serum, plasma, or urine. The Cromer system antibodies are rarely observed, with the majority of examples presenting in black individuals. Anti-Cr^a has been associated with mild transfusion reactions; however, cases are documented of Cr(a−) negative patients receiving Cr(a+) positive RBCs without adverse consequences.[65] A number of RBC survival studies as well as cellular assay studies have been conducted with inconclusive results regarding the clinical potential of Cromer system antibodies.

Because the placenta carries high levels of DAF, maternal antibodies to Cromer antigens are thought to be absorbed onto the tissue. This absorption is believed to prevent the passage of maternal antibody into fetal circulation, thereby limiting the occurrence of HDN. To date, no cases of Cromer related HDN have been reported.

The Knops Blood Group System: KN (ISBT 022)

The Knops blood group system is composed of eight antigens: Kn^a (Knops), Kn^b, McC^a (McCoy), Sl1 (Swain-Langley), Yk^a (York), McC^b, Sl2 (Vil), and Sl3.[4,66,67] Three pairs of antithetical alleles, Kn^a and Kn^b, McC^a and McC^b, and Sl1 and Sl2, are described. No antithetical partner has been identified for Yk^a. Although variations across ethnic groups are evident, Kn^a, McC^a, Sl1, and Yk^a are high-incidence antigens in most populations. Whereas Kn^b is a low-incidence antigen, noted in 4.5 percent of whites, the McC^b antigen is present in 45 percent of African Americans and has not been observed in white populations.

The first antigen to be reported was Kn^a in 1970,[68] with the most recent being the SL3 antigen that, due to molecular complexities, was provisionally assigned to the KN system in 2003.[4] Knops system antigens are notably resistant to ficin/papain treatment but destroyed or weakened by trypsin,

TABLE 10–6	Gerbich Negative Phenotypes	
Phenotype	**Type**	**Antibody**
GE: −2, 3, 4	Yus	Anti-Ge2
GE: −2, −3, 4	Gerbich	Anti-Ge2 or anti-Ge3
GE: −2, −3, −4	Leach types: PL LN	Anti-Ge2 or anti-Ge3

α-chymotrypsin, and reducing agents such as DTT (see **Table 10–4**). All are expressed poorly on cord cells and depressed in patients presenting with autoimmune disease and the Lu(a−b−) phenotype because of the influence of the *In(Lu)* gene.[69]

The alleles for the KN blood group have been located on chromosome 1, with the antigens residing on complement receptor 1 (CR1 or CD35). On erythrocytes, CR1 participates in an immune adherence mechanism whereby the receptor attaches to C3b-marked complexes and delivers them to the liver for removal.[70] Certain autoimmune diseases, such as systemic lupus erythematosus and chronic cold agglutinin disease, have been implicated in depressing the expression of the KN antigens caused by loss of erythrocyte CR1.[71]

The antibodies directed toward the KN blood group antigens were formerly described as having the serologic properties of HTLA antibodies. For more information on HTLA antibodies, refer to the Chido/ Rodgers blood group system in this chapter. Advances in gene mapping and immunochemical studies led to the assignment of the Knops, McCoy, York, and Swain-Langley antigens (formerly in the HTLA category) to the KN blood group system. The antibodies to KN antigens are characterized as IgG, RBC-stimulated, and reacting weakly and variably at the IAT phase of testing. The Knops system antibodies are considered of little clinical importance inasmuch as none have been attributed to causing clinical HDN or HTR. Nevertheless, their reactivity in serologic testing could mask the presence of an underlying antibody of clinical significance.

The Indian Blood Group System: IN (ISBT 023)

The Indian (IN) blood group system was discovered in 1973 by Badakere and associates.[72] The IN system is composed of two antithetical antigens, In[a] and In[b], which are of relatively low and high incidence, respectively. The frequency of In[a] is higher in Iranians and Arabs (11 percent) and much lower in whites, blacks, and Asians (0.1 percent). In[b] is noted in 96 percent of whites and 96 percent of Indians.[6] The antigens are inherited as codominant alleles on chromosome 11. Most enzymes and reducing agents (see **Table 10–4**) denature the IN antigens, which are poorly expressed on cord cells and probably depressed during pregnancy. Furthermore, In[b] expression may also be depressed in individuals presenting with the Lu(a−b−) phenotype, owing to the *In(Lu)* gene. The IN antigens are carried on the the the CD44 glycoprotein, which is present on most tissues. CD44 is a major component of the RBC membrane known for its involvement in T- and B-cell activation, WBC adhesion activities, as well as a host of other immune-mediated interactions.[8] The high incidence AnWJ antigen is found on an isoform of CD44, but so far has not been catalogued in the Indian blood group system.

Antibodies to IN antigens are characterized as IgG, RBC-stimulated, and reactive in IAT testing. The IN antigens are described as effective immunogens inasmuch as the corresponding Indian system antibodies are not exceedingly uncommon. Even so, only a few reports have linked anti-In[b] with causing HTR, and anti-In[a] has not yet been implicated. Neither In[a] nor In[b] antibodies have been associated with clinical HDN.

The John Milton Hagen Blood Group System: JMH (ISBT 026)

The high-frequency antigen JMH is the lone antigen in the John Milton Hagen blood group system. Originally listed in the high-incidence antigen series (#901007), JMH was reassigned to its own blood group system once the encoding gene was located on chromosome 15. The JMH antigen resides on the semaphorin CDw108, which is another GPI-linked protein in the RBC membrane. The function of CDw108 is unclear. Most cases of JMH antigen–negative RBCs are observed in the elderly and are attributed to an unexplained acquired mechanism of aging. A total absence of JMH expression is also observed in paroxysmal nocturnal hemoglobinuria III RBCs, which are deficient in all GPI anchored glycoproteins, including CDw108. The JMH antigens are detroyed by most standard enzymes and reducing agents (see **Table 10–4**) but not by sialidase.

Anti-JMH is usually IgG, predominantly of the IgG4 subclass. Individuals presenting with anti-JMH in their serum frequently have no history of pregnancy or transfusion. Auto anti-JMH is routinely found in the elderly who weakly express JMH on RBCs. Early records describe anti-JMH as having the serologic properties of HTLA antibodies, reacting weakly, and often being of high titer (even though undiluted samples of anti-JMH react weakly). JMH antibodies are viewed to be of little clinical importance, inasmuch as none have been associated with causing clinical HDN or HTR. In fact, several cases document the transfusion of JMH antigen–positive blood into patients with anti-JMH without adverse consequence.[73]

Collections and Notable Antigens of the High-Incidence Series

The RBC antigen collections and a few notable antigens in the high-incidence series are presented in **Tables 10–2** and **10–3**. Other texts, such as *Human Blood Groups* by Daniels,[8] *Applied Blood Group Serology* by Issitt and Anstee,[74] and *The Blood Group Antigen Facts Book* by Reid and Francis-Lomas,[6] provide additional information on these and other antigens.

The Miscellaneous WBC Antigens: Bg

The three specificities of Bennett-Goodspeed (Bg) antigens are Bg[a], Bg[b], and Bg[c]. The corresponding Bg antibodies are directed toward human leukocyte antigens (HLA). Bg antigens are gene products of the major histocompatibility complex (MHC) that are categorized into class I and class II antigens. For the purposes of transfusion practice, only class I antigens are addressed here. Class I antigens are assigned into three groups, HLA-A, HLA-B, and HLA-C, which are distributed on all nucleated cells as well as on a number of nonnucleated cells. RBCs and platelets are nonnucleated cells that contain nuclei during their developmental stages and sometimes carry residual amounts of HLA (Bg) antigen at maturity. Accordingly, weak and obscure Bg reactivity may be observed in serologic testing. Given that the Bg antigens are located primarily on leukocytes, they are not eligible for assignment to the ISBT terminology for RBC surface antigens.

The Bg[a] antigen corresponds with HLA-B7, Bg[b] with HLA-

TABLE 10–7	Bg Antigens and HLA	
Bg Antigen	**Related HLA Antigen**	**Comments**
Bg^a	B-7	• Formerly known as Bennett-Goodspeed
Bg^b	B-17	• WBC antigens
		• Weak and variable IAT reactively
Bg^c	A-28	• Clinically benign

B17, and Bg^c with HLA-A28 **(Table 10–7)**. Cross-reactivity with antigens in cross-reactive groups can be observed. Bg antigens are resistant to treatment with enzymes (e.g., ficin/papain) and reducing agents such as DTT. RBC expression of Bg or HLA antigens varies with the specificity of the HLA antigen, from individual to individual and within the same individual over a lifetime.[8] Transient increases in some Bg antigens have been observed in various disease states, such as infectious mononucleosis, leukemia, polycythemia, and hemolytic anemia.[75]

The Bg antibodies are characterized as IgG and reacting weakly and variably in IAT, with only one or two panel cells that happen to carry higher amounts of Bg antigen. They are more commonly detected in multiply transfused or multiparous individuals. Reactivity is seldom reproducible. Serologically, Bg antibodies are described as "nuisance" antibodies whose reactivity can be destroyed by treating RBC antigens with chloroquine or EDTA glycine-HCL. Because platelets express variable amounts of HLA-A, HLA-B, and HLA-C (weak or absent), commercial human platelet concentrate is routinely used to adsorb anti-Bg from serum.[76] The absorbed serum is then tested for significant underlying alloantibody without interference.

Serum samples from individuals with multiple transfusions presenting with anti-Bg antibodies also often contain anti-Ch, anti-Rg, or anti-Kn. Bg antibodies have historically been reported as contaminants in commercial reagents, especially polyclonal antisera however, chloroquine is used for inactivation.[61] The Bg antibodies are widely considered to be clinically benign because they are not associated with causing HDN and, except in rare instances, HTR. Three cases of HTR have been attributed to Bg antibodies, leading serologists to consider HLA antibodies as a cause when no RBC antibody is detected.[77]

SUMMARY CHART:
Important Points to Remember (SBB)

➤ The terminology for RBC surface antigens according to ISBT provides a standard numeric system for naming authenticated RBC antigens that is suitable for electronic data processing equipment.

➤ In the ISBT system, RBC antigens are assigned a six-digit identification number, and the symbols are converted to capital letters. All antigens are catalogued into one of the following four groups:

　➤ A blood group system if controlled by one discrete gene or by two closely linked genes

　➤ A collection if shown to share a biochemical, serologic, or genetic relationship

➤ The high-incidence series (901) if independently noted in more than 90 percent of most populations

➤ The low-incidence series (700) if independently noted in less than 1 percent of most populations

➤ The discovery that the Wright antigens are located on the same transport protein (AE-1) as the Diego antigens led to their assignment to the Diego system (DI).

➤ The low-incidence antigen, Di^a, is a useful anthropologic marker for Mongolian ancestry.

➤ Anti-Di^a, anti-Di^b, and anti-Wr^a are generally considered to be clinically significant, inasmuch as all have been described to cause severe HTR and HDN.

➤ Anti-Yt^a is a fairly common antibody that is associated with mild HTR.

➤ The Xg^a antigen is found on the short arm of the X chromosome and is seen in higher frequency in females (89%) than in males (66%).

➤ The Scianna system (SC) is composed of the antithetical Sc1 and Sc2 antigens as well as the high-incidence Sc3 antigen, which is present on all Sc1- and/or Sc2-positive cells.

➤ The rare null phenotype in the SC system has been observed only in the Marshall Islands and New Guinea.

➤ In addition to the Do^a and Do^b antigens, the Gy^a, Hy, and Jo^a antigens are assigned to the Dombrock system (DO).

➤ Antibodies to the DO antigens have been reported to occasionally cause moderate HTR.

➤ The Colton system (CO) is composed of the antithetical Co^a and Co^b antigens as well as the high-frequency CO3 antigen, which is present on all Co^a-positive and/or Co^b-positive cells.

➤ The rare antibodies in the CO system have been associated with causing mild HTR and HDN.

➤ The nine antigens in the Chido/Rodgers system are located on the complement fragments C4B and C4A, respectively.

➤ The clinically insignificant CH and RG antibodies present with weak and nebulous reactivity at IAT and may be identified by plasma inhibition methods and adsorption with C4-coated cells.

➤ The 11 Cromer antigens are carried on the decay accelerating factor and are distributed in body fluids and on RBCs, WBCs, platelets, and placental tissue.

➤ The rare anti-CROM antibodies have been noted only in black individuals and associated with mild HTR.

➤ In addition to the Kn^a and Kn^b antigens, the McC, Yk, and Sl antigens are assigned to the Knops system (KN).

➤ The KN antigens are located on complement receptor 1 (CR1) with expression being depressed by the *In(Lu)* gene and autoimmune disease.

➤ The clinically insignificant KN antibodies present with weak and "nebulous" reactivity at IAT.

➤ The In^a antigen is more prevalent in Arab and Iranian populations, with In^a and In^b antigen expression being depressed by the *In(Lu)* gene.

➤ Antibodies directed against the Vel antigen have occasionally been described to cause hemolysis in the test tube and severe hemolytic reactions.

➤ Anti-Sd^a antibodies present with weak reactivity at IAT, which appears shiny and refractile under the microscope and may be inhibited with Sd-positive urine.

➤ Bg^a, Bg^b, and Bg^c WBC antigens correspond with the class I HLA antigens B-7, B-17, and A-28, respectively.

➤ The clinically insignificant anti-Bg antibodies present with weak and variable reactivity at IAT, which may be destroyed by chloroquine or EDTA glycine-HCL treatment.

REVIEW QUESTIONS

1. Which blood group system is under control of a gene located on the short arm of the X chromosome?
   a. GE
   b. DI
   c. YT
   d. XG

2. Which of the following presents with depressed or absent antigen expression due to the *In(Lu)* regulator gene?
   a. GE and DI
   b. KN and IN
   c. CROM and CH/RG
   d. IN and GE

3. Mutations in the carrier molecule for this blood group system may result in changes of RBC shape in the forms of elliptocytosis, acanthocytosis, or ovalocytosis.
   a. DI
   b. DO
   c. CO
   d. SC

4. According to the RBC surface antigen terminology by ISBT, all authenticated antigens may be assigned to a blood group system, provided they are:
   a. Controlled by a single gene or by two closely linked genes
   b. Inherited from multiple regulator genes
   c. Shown not to follow mendelian principles
   d. Shown to share serologic characteristics with other members of the blood group system

5. The antibody to this RBC antigen in the 901 series demonstrates mixed-field agglutination that appears shiny and refractile under the microscope.
   a. Vel
   b. JMH
   c. Lan
   d. Sd^a

6. The antibody to this RBC antigen in the 901 series has been associated with causing severe immediate HTR.
   a. Anti-JMH
   b. Anti-Bg^a
   c. Anti-Vel
   d. Anti-Sd^a

7. Which of the following antibodies is directed toward HLA antigens and may be inactivated by chloroquine or EDTA glycine-HCL treatment?
   a. Anti-Ch2
   b. Anti-Yk^a
   c. Anti-Bg^a
   d. Anti-Kn^b

8. The most useful methods for rapidly identifying antibodies in the CH/RG blood group system are:
   a. Prewarmed technique and titration studies
   b. Plasma inhibition and adsorption with C4-coated cells
   c. DTT and chloroquine treatment
   d. Trypsin and chymotrypsin treatment

9. The following antibodies are generally considered clinically insignificant because they have not been associated with causing increased destruction of RBCs, HDN, or HTR.
   a. Anti-Do^a and anti-Co^a
   b. Anti-Ge3 and anti-Wr^a
   c. Anti-Ch2 and anti-Kn^a
   d. Anti-Di^b and anti-Yt^a

10. Match the system name in Column II with the correct antibody in Column I.

Column I	Column II
1. Anti-Ch3	a. Chido/Rodgers
2. Anti-Yt^b	b. Knops
3. Anti-Di^a	c. XG
4. Anti-Xg^a	d. Scianna
5. Anti-McC^a	e. Cartwright
6. Anti-Sc2	f. Diego
7. Anti-Co^b	g. Colton
8. Anti-Ge3	h. Dombrock
9. Anti-Yk^a	i. Gerbich
10. Anti-Wr^b	

REFERENCES

1. Garrity, G, et al: Terminology for blood group antigens and genes: Historical origins and guidelines for the new millennium. Transfusion 40:477, 2000.
2. Daniels, J, et al: Blood group terminology 1995, from the ISBT working party on terminology for red cell surface antigens. Vox Sang 69:265, 1995.
3. Issit, PD, and Moulds, JJ: Blood group terminology suitable for use in electronic data processing equipment. Transfusion 32:7, 1992.
4. Daniels, G, et al: International Society for Blood Transfusion Committee on terminology for red cell surface antigens: Vancouver Report. Vox Sang 84:244, 2003.

5. Levine, P, et al: The Diego blood factor. Nature 77, 1956.
6. Reid, M, and Francis-Lomas, C: The Blood Group Antigen Facts Book. Academic Press, New York, 1997.
7. Bruce, LJ, et al: Band 3 Memphis variant II: Altered stilbene disulfonate binding and the Diego (Di^a) blood group antigen are associated with the human erythrocyte band 3 mutation Pro → Leu. J Biol Chem 269, 1994.
8. Daniels, G: Human Blood Groups, ed 2. Blackwell Science, Oxford, 2002.
9. Silberstein, LS (ed): Molecular and Functional Aspects of Blood Group Antigens. American Association of Blood Banks. Bethesda, MD, 1995.
10. Jarolim, P, et al: Mutations conserved arginines in the membrane domain of erythroid band 3 lead to a decrease in membrane-associated band 3 and to the phenotype of hereditary spherocytosis. Blood 85, 1995.
11. Bruce, LJ: Band 3HT, a human red-cell variant associated with acanthocytosis and increased anion transport carries the mutation Pro → Leu in the membrane domain of band 3. Biochem J 293, 1993.
12. Schofield, AE, et al: Basis of unique red cell membrane properties in hereditary spherocytosis. J Mol Biol 223, 1992.
13. Wu, G, et al: Development of a DNA-based genotyping method for the Diego blood group system. Transfusion, 42,1553, 2002.
14. Holman, CA: A rare new blood group antigen (Wr^a). Lancet 2:119, 1953.
15. Bruce, LJ, et al: Changes in the blood group Wright antigens are associated with a mutation at amino acid 658 in human erythrocyte band 3: A site of interaction between band 3 and glycophorin A under certain conditions. Blood 85, 1995.
16. Auffrye, I, et al: Glycophorin A dimerization and band 3 interaction during membrane biogenesis; in vivo studies in human glycophorin A transgenic mice. Blood 97:2872, 2001.
17. Eaton, BR, et al: A new antibody, anti-Yt^a, characterizing a blood group antigen of high incidence. Br J Haematol 2:333, 1956.
18. Mazzi, G, et al: Presence of anti-Yt^a antibody in a Yt(a+) patient. Vox Sang 66, 1994.
19. Spring, FA, Gardner, B, and Anstee, DJ: Evidence that the antigens of the Yt blood group system are located on human erythrocyte acetylcholinesterase. Blood 80:21, 1992.
20. Mohandas, K, Spivak, M, and Dehanhanty, C: Management of patients with anti-Cartwright (Yta). Transfusion 25:381, 1985.
21. Davey, R, and Simpkins, S: Chromium survival of Yt (a+) red cells as a determinant of in vivo significance of anti-Yt^a. Transfusion 21:702, 1981.
22. Eckrich, R, Mallory, D, and Sandler, S: Correlation of monocyte monolayer assays and post-transfusion survival of Yt(a+) red cells in patients with anti-Yta. Immunohematology 11:81, 1995.
23. Mann, J, et al: A sex-linked blood group. Lancet 1:8, 1962.
24. Cook IA, et al: A second example of anti-Xg^a. Lancet 10:857, 1963.
25. Sausais, L, et al: Characteristic of a third example of Anti-Xg^a [abstract]. Transfusion 4:312, 1964.
26. Yokoyama, M, et al: The first example of autoanti-Xg^a. Vox Sang 12:198, 1967.
27. Smith, M, and Goodfellow, P: The genomic organization of the human psuedoautosomal gene MIC2 and the detection of related locus. Hum Mol Genet 2:417, 1993.
28. Schlossman, SF, et al: CD antigens. Blood 83, 1994.
29. Fouchet, C, et al: A study of the co-regulation and tissue specificity of XG and MIC2 gene expression in eukaryotic cells. Blood 95:5,1819–1826, 2000.
30. Lewis, M, Chown, B, and Kaita, H: On blood group antigens Bu(a) and Sm. Transfusion 7:92, 1967.
31. Schmidt, PR, Griffitts, JJ, and Northam, FF: A new antibody anti-Sm, reacting with a high-incidence antigen. Cited by Race, RR, and Sanger, R, 1962.
32. Anderson, C, et al: An antibody defining a new blood group antigen, Bu^a. Transfusion 3:30, 1963.
33. Franz, F, Wagner, J, and Flegel, W: Scianna antigens including Rd are expressed by ERMAP. Blood, 101:752, 2003.
34. Xu, H, et al: Cloning and characterization of human erythroid membrane-associated protein, human ERMAP. Genomics 76:2, 2001.
35. Nason, SG, et al: A high incidence antibody (anti-Sc3) in the serum of a SC:−1, −2 patient. Transfusion 20:531, 1980.
36. Swanson, JL, et al: A "new" blood group antigen, Do^a. Nature 206:313, 1965.
37. Molthan, L, et al: Enlargement of the Dombrock blood group system: The finding of anti-Do^b. Vox Sang 24:382, 1973.
38. Banks, JA, Hemming, M, and Poole, J: Evidence that the Gy^a, Hy, and Jo^a antigens belong to the Dombrock blood group system. Vox Sang 68, 1995.
39. Gubin A, et al: Identification of Dombrock blood group glycoprotein as a polymorphic member of the ADP-ribosyltransferase gene family. Blood 96:2621, 2000.
40. Reid, M: Dombrock blood group system: A review. Transfusion 43:107, 2003.
41. Halverson, G, et al: The first reported case of anti-Do^b causing an acute hemolytic transfusion reaction. Vox Sang 66, 1994.
42. Heisto, H, et al: Three examples of a red cell antibody, anti-Co^a. Vox Sang 12:18, 1967.
43. Giles, CM, et al: Identification of the first example of anti-Co^b. Br J Haematol 19:267, 1970.
44. Joshi, S, et al: An AQP1 null allele in an Indian woman with Co(a−b−) phenotype and high-titer anti-Co3 associated with mild HDN. Transfusion 41:1273, 2001.
45. De la Chapelle, A, et al: Monosomy-7 and the Colton blood groups. Lancet 2:817, 1975.
46. Parsons, SF, et al: A novel form of congenital dyserythropoietic anemia associated with deficiency of erythroid CD44 and a unique blood group phenotype [In(a−b−), Co(a−b−)]. Blood 83, 1994.
47. Chretien, S, and Cartron, J: A single mutation inside the NPA motif of Aquaporin-1 found in a Colton-null phenotype. Blood 93:4021, 1999.
48. Hoffman, JJML, and Overbeeke, MAM: Characteristics of anti-Co^b in vitro and in vivo: A case study. Immunohematology 1:12, 1996.
49. Moulds, JM, and Laird-Fryer, B (eds): Blood Groups: Chido/Rodgers, Knops/McCoy/York and Cromer. American Association of Blood Banks, Bethesda, MD, 1992.
50. Harris, JP, et al: A nebulous antibody responsible for crossmatching difficulties (Chido). Vox Sang 30, 1967.
51. Middleton, J, and Crookston, MC: Chido substance in plasma. Vox Sang 12, 1972.
52. Longster, G, and Giles, CM: A new antibody specificity: Anti-Rg^a reacting with a red cell and serum antigen. Vox Sang 30, 1976.
53. Tilley, CA, et al: Localization of Chido and Rodgers determinants to the C4d fragment of human C4. Nature 273, 1978.
54. Moulds, JM: Incidence of Rodgers-negative individuals in systemic lupus erythematosus patients. Immunohematology 4:6, 1990.
55. Westhoff, CM, et al: Severe anaphylactic reactions following transfusions of platelets to a patient with anti-Ch. Transfusion 6:32, 1992.
56. Judd, JW, et al: The rapid identification of Chido and Rodgers antibodies using C4d-coated red blood cells. Transfusion 21, 1981.
57. Rosenfield, RE, et al: Ge, a very common red cell antigen. Br J Haemat 6, 1960.
58. Barnes, R, and Lewis, TLT: A fourth example of anti-Ge. Lancet 2, 1961.
59. Reid, ME, and Spring, FA: Molecular basis of glycophorin C variants and their associated blood group antigens. Transfus Med 4, 1994.
60. Telen, MJ, et al: Molecular basis for elliptocytosis associated with glycophorin C and D deficiency in the Leach phenotype. Blood 78, 1991.
61. Storry, J, et al: GUTI: a new antigen in the Cromer blood group system. Transfusion 43:340, 2003.
62. Stroup, M, and McCreary, J: Cr^a, another high frequency blood group factor [abstract]. Transfusion 15, 1975.
63. Moulds, J, et al: Human blood groups: Incidental receptors for viruses and bacteria. Transfusion 36: 362, 1996.
64. Matthes, T, et al: Acquired and transient RBC CD55 deficiency (Inab phenotype) and anti-IFC. Transfusion 42:1448, 2002.
65. Storry, J, and Reid, M: The Cromer blood group system: A review. Immunohematology 18:95, 2002.
66. Daniels, G, et al: ISBT working party on terminology for red cell surface antigens: Report and Guidelines. Vox Sang 8067:193, 2001.
67. Moulds, J, Zimmerman, P, and Doumbo, O: Expansion of the Knops blood group system and the subdivision of Sl^a. Transfusion 42:215, 2002.
68. Helgeson, M, et al: Knops-Helgeson (Kn^a): A high-frequency erythrocyte antigen. Transfusion 10, 1970.
69. Daniels, GL: The effect of *In(Lu)* on some high-frequency antigens. Transfusion 26, 1986.
70. Ahearn, JM, and Fearon, DT: Structure and function of the complement receptor, CR1 (CD35) and CR2 (CD21). Adv Immunol 46, 1989.
71. Ross, GD: Disease-associated loss of erythrocyte complement receptors (CR1, C3b receptors) in patients with systemic lupus erythematosus and other diseases involving autoantibodies and/or complement activation. J Immunol 135, 1985.
72. Badakere, SS, et al: Evidence of a new blood group antigen in the Indian population (a preliminary report). Ind J Med Res 62, 1973.
73. Baldwin, M, et al: In vivo studies of the long term ^{51}Cr red cell survival of serologically incompatible red cell units. Transfusion 25:34, 1985.
74. Issitt, P, and Anstee, D: Applied Blood Group Serology, ed 4. Montgomery Scientific, Durham, NC, 1998.
75. Morton, JA, et al: Changes in red cell Bg antigens in haematological disease. Immunol Commun 9:173, 1980.
76. Organon Teknika package insert for human platelet concentrate. Durham, NC, 1992.
77. Benson, K, et al: Acute and delayed transfusion reactions secondary to HLA alloimmunization. Transfusion 43:753, 2003.

Plasma Inhibition Studies*

Materials and Methods

Serum (plasma) and cells: unknown patient serum, indicator cells (screening cells), Chido-Rodgers–positive plasma: Ch(a+) Rg(a+) plasma, Ch(a+) Rg(a−) plasma

1. Set up two sets of each of the following mixtures, and incubate at room temperature for 15 minutes:
   a. 2 drops unknown serum, 1 drop Ch(a+) Rg(a−) plasma
   b. 2 drops unknown serum, 1 drop Ch(a−) Rg(a+) plasma
   c. 2 drops unknown serum, 1 drop Ch(a+) Rg(a+) plasma
2. Incubate a set of selected screening cells with the foregoing three mixtures for 60 minutes at 37°C. Wash three times with saline, and convert to the antihuman globulin test.
3. If multiple alloantibodies are suspected after the previous results are obtained, test a complete genotyped panel of donors with the appropriate mixture.

Interpretation of Results

1. If mixture A is reactive with both screening cells and mixtures B and C are nonreactive, the antibody is anti-Rg^a and no other alloantibodies are detected in the unknown serum.
2. If mixture B is reactive and mixtures A and C are nonreactive with the screening cells, the antibody is anti-Ch^a and no other alloantibodies are detected in the unknown serum.
3. If mixture C is reactive and either mixture A or mixture B is nonreactive, it could mean that there is not sufficient quantity of Ch^a or Rg^a substance in the Ch^a- or Rg^a-positive plasma to inhibit the antibody but that there is enough in mixture A or mixture B plasma to inhibit the antibody.
4. If all three mixtures are nonreactive, the serum antibody is too weak to allow dilution studies.
5. If one screening cell is negative and the other positive with any of the mixtures, then anti-Ch^a and anti-Rg^a and a second or third antibody may be present in the serum. The appropriate mixtures should then be incubated with a panel of selected genotyped cells.

---

*From Moulds, MK: Serological investigation and clinical significance of high-titered, low-avidity (HTLA) antibodies. Am J Med Tech 10:794, 1981, with permission.

CHAPTER eleven

Donor Screening and Component Preparation

Virginia C. Hughes, MS, MT(ASCP)SBB, CLS(NCA)I, **and**
Patricia A. Wright, BA, MT(ASCP)SBB

OBJECTIVES

On completion of this chapter, the learner should be able to:

1. State the governing agencies that regulate the immunohematology laboratory.
2. State the minimum acceptable levels for the following tests in allogeneic and autologous donation:
   - Weight
   - Temperature
   - Pulse
   - Blood pressure
   - Hemoglobin
   - Hematocrit
3. Differentiate between acceptable donation and permanent deferral given various medical conditions.
4. Differentiate among the four different types of autologous donations.
5. Describe the procedure for a whole blood donation including arm preparation, blood collection, and postphlebotomy care instructions for the donor.
6. Differentiate among mild, moderate, and severe donor reactions and list recommended treatments for each.

7. List the tests required for allogeneic, autologous, and pheresis donation.
8. State the acceptable interval of donation for allogeneic donors.
9. State the acceptable interval of donation for pheresis donors.
10. List the labeling criteria for a unit of allogeneic and autologous blood.
11. Identify the storage conditions, shelf life, quality control requirements, and indications for use for the following:
    - Red blood cells (RBCs)
    - RBCs irradiated
    - RBCs leukoreduced
    - Random platelets
    - Apheresis platelets
    - Random platelets irradiated
    - Apheresis platelets irradiated
    - Random platelets leukoreduced
    - Apheresis platelets leukoreduced
    - Washed RBCs
    - Washed random platelets
    - Washed apheresis platelets
    - Pooled random platelets
    - Frozen, deglycerolized RBCs
    - Fresh frozen plasma
    - Liquid plasma
    - Whole blood modified
    - Cryoprecipitate
    - Granulocyte concentrates
    - Factor VIII concentrates
    - Factor IX concentrates
    - Factor XIII concentrates
    - $Rh_o(D)$ immunoglobulin
    - Normal serum albumin
    - Immune serum globulin
    - Plasma protein fraction
    - Antithrombin III concentrates

Governing Agencies

The agencies charged with regulating processes and procedures in the immunohematology laboratory include the AABB (American Association of Blood Banks), FDA (U.S. Food and Drug Administration), CAP (College of American Pathologists), and JCAHO (Joint Commission on Accreditation of Healthcare Organizations). The first two are more specifically involved in donor screening regulations and are described in the following paragraphs. All organizations conduct inspections of hospital blood banks by reviewing policies and procedures for accreditation purposes.

AABB

The AABB was established in 1947. It is an international association of blood banks that includes hospital and community blood centers, transfusion and transplantation centers, and individuals involved in transfusion medicine. Its members consist of medical laboratory technicians, medical technologists, registered nurses, laboratory managers, physicians, transfusion medicine fellows, and researchers involved in transfusion medicine.[1] The mission of the AABB is to establish and provide the highest standard of care for patients and donors in all aspects of transfusion medicine. The AABB has published books on transfusion medicine throughout its existence; two resources that are vital to donor screening procedures are *AABB Standards* and *AABB Technical Manual*. The specific regulations for donor screening and component preparation are discussed in these publications and will be referred to throughout this chapter.

FDA

The FDA inspects blood banks on an annual basis; its regulations for donor screening are outlined in the *Code of Federal Regulations (CFR)*, parts 211, 600–799. Under the auspices of the FDA, blood is regarded both as a biologic and a drug. In 1988 the Center for Biologics Evaluation and Research (CBER) was formed. CBER is responsible for regulating the collection of blood and blood components used for transfusion and for the manufacture of pharmaceuticals derived from blood and blood components. CBER develops and enforces quality standards, inspects blood establishments, and monitors reports of errors, accidents, and adverse clinical events.[2] In the early 1990s the FDA began to treat blood establishments such as manufacturers, requiring strict compliance toward all aspects of transfusion medicine including donor selection and screening. The FDA differs from the AABB in that the former is responsible for licensing of reagents and blood products as well as blood center inspections.

Donor Screening

Donor screening encompasses the medical history requirements for the donor, the (mini) physical examination, and serologic testing of the donor blood. Any one of these areas may preclude a potential donor from the donation process. The medical history information and physical examination are designed to answer two questions: (1) Will a donation of approximately 450 mL of whole blood at this time be harmful to the donor? (2) Could blood drawn from this donor at this time potentially transmit a disease to the recipient?

Registration

As outlined in *Standards*, blood collection facilities must confirm donor identity and link the donor to existing donor records.[3] Most facilities require a photographic identification such as a driver's license or school identification card. The following is a list of information used by the collection facility in the registration process and is kept on record by use of a single donation record form (Fig. 11–1):

- **Name (first, last, MI)**
- **Date and time of donation**
- **Address**
- **Telephone**
- **Gender**
- **Age or date of birth.** The minimum age for an allogeneic

JAN 2003

SINGLE DONATION RECORD

LIFESouth
Community Blood Centers

Location:

4039 West Newberry Road • Gainesville, Florida 32607 • (352) 334-1000

SEX:	ETHNIC:	STUDENT:	NEW CARD:	DATE DRAWN:	
CALL OK?		BIRTH DATE:		# PREV. DONATIONS:	PREVIOUS REACTION:
CALL STATUS:		HLA TYPING:			
CALL OK?		HLA TYPING DATE:		LAST DONATION DATE:	

CREDIT FOR:

COMMENTS:

REMARKS:

DEFERRAL INFO:	NUMBER	NEXT DONATION DATE:	INITIALS:
DEFERRAL ○ PD ○			

LAB ONLY

POSITIVE ANTIBODIES:

POSITIVE ANTIGENS:

NEGATIVE ANTIGENS:

ABO Prescreening (First Time Donor)

ABO SLIDE TYPE:		PER DONOR TYPE:		INITIALS:
○ 0 ○ 1		○ A ○ B		
○ 2 ○ 1,2		○ O ○ AB		

Collection Information

Donor Reaction: ○ Type 1   ○ Type 2   ○ Type 3

○ Apheresis RBC Loss (if > 50ml):   mL

○ Enter/Remove Donor Comment:

DRAWN UNIT INFORMATION

○ QNS <= 50 mL   ○ QNS > 50 mL   ○ Long Draw Discard

○ Low Volume   ○ Overdraw   ○ Air Contaminated

First Stick Information

BAG INFO: ○ ASA	BAG LOT NUMBER:	BAG EXPIRATION:

BAG TYPE:

			SCALE NUMBER:
CPDA-1:	○	1 ○	○ Fenwal ○ Donormatic
Additive:	○	2 ○	
ACD-A:	○	3 ○	VENIPUNCTURE: START TIME:
___	○	4 ○	
		5 ○	DISCONNECT: END TIME:

FRONT DESK	COMMENTS:	AMOUNT DRAWN:
		mL

CRBCIS Lab Information

CMV:	CMV DATE:	BLOOD TYPE:	FIRST UNIT NUMBER
LAB CMV:	INITIALS	LAB TYPE INITIALS	

Second Stick Information

BAG INFO: ○ ASA	BAG LOT NUMBER:	BAG EXPIRATION:

BAG TYPE:

			SCALE NUMBER:
CPDA-1:	○	1 ○	○ Fenwal ○ Donormatic
Additive:	○	2 ○	
ACD-A:	○	3 ○	VENIPUNCTURE: START TIME:
___	○	4 ○	
		5 ○	DISCONNECT: END TIME:

COMMENTS:	AMOUNT DRAWN:
	mL

SECOND UNIT NUMBER

■ FIGURE 11–1   Single donation record form. (LifeSouth Blood Center, Montgomery, AL, with permission.)

donation is 17 years; there is no upper age limit. For autologous donation (donating blood to be used for oneself [donor-patient]), there is no age restriction; however, each donor-patient must be evaluated by the blood bank medical director.

- **Consent to Donate.** Donors should be given educational materials informing them of the risks of the procedure, signs and symptoms associated with the human immunodeficiency virus infection and AIDS, and the opportunity to decline from the donation process if they believe their blood is not safe or they are uncomfortable with the procedure **(Fig. 11–2)**.

Additional information that may be helpful includes the donor's social security number, the name of the patient for whom the blood is intended (directed donation), race of the donor for unique phenotypes, and cytomegalovirus (CMV) status. The latter may be helpful because some patient groups

(e.g., neonates) require CMV-negative blood in certain circumstances.

Medical History Questionnaire

Obtaining an accurate medical history of the donor is essential to ensure benefit to the recipient. The medical history questions have been developed and revised as necessary by the AABB and FDA. The interviewer should be familiar with the questions, and the interview should be conducted in a secluded area of the blood center. The questions are designed so that a simple "yes" or "no" can be answered but elaborated if indicated **(Fig. 11–3).** The medical history is conducted on the same day as the donation.

1. **Have you donated blood in the past 8 weeks or plasma or platelets in the past 48 hours?** The time interval between

---

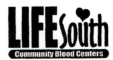

Responsibilities of a Blood Donor & Important Information about Donating Blood

Please read the following information before you decide that you want to donate blood today.

Interview Process

Donating blood is typically a pleasant experience, and it benefits the entire community. LifeSouth has a number of procedures that we apply routinely to every donor. These procedures help ensure your safety, as the blood donor, as well as the safety of the patient receiving your blood.

During a private interview, our staff member will ask you medical questions about your health and lifestyle. Note the following:

- Some questions will be about sexual activity, illegal drug use, your travel history, and some infectious diseases.
- It is extremely important that you answer all questions truthfully.
- All information you give us is strictly confidential.
- If you feel uncomfortable about disclosing such information, you should not donate.
- If you do not want to answer a question, during the interview, you can simply walk away with no questions asked.

Post-donation Activities

If you donate blood, we ask that, for the remainder of the day, you not participate in strenuous activity or in critical work where safety requires your maximum abilities. We ask you to avoid strenuous activity because performing strenuous activities after blood donation can cause you to feel lightheaded and possibly faint.

A Window Period

There is a period of time early in HIV infection when a person can be infectious and transmit

the disease to a patient even though blood tests are negative. This is why LifeSouth cannot rely completely on lab tests to ensure the safety of patients who may receive your blood. We need your cooperation by having you truthfully answer all questions during the interview. This is your responsibility as a blood donor.

If you want to find out your HIV status, do not donate blood, but rather contact the local Health Department where you can get a quick, anonymous, and free HIV test.

Testing

Your blood will be tested for various infectious agents. Two of the tests, for HIV and hepatitis C, are unlicensed and part of a federally recommended research program. Blood that tests positive will not be used for transfusion. If any of your tests are positive, you may not be able to donate blood in the future. You can choose not to be tested, however, if you so choose, we can't accept your blood donation. Sometimes tests are falsely positive which means that, although your blood tests positive, you don't have the disease.

Notification

You will be notified by letter of any positive test that affects your status as a blood donor. Notification may be delayed up to 50 days. It may be necessary to draw additional samples to better understand and interpret the results and provide you with a thorough explanation.

A.   **Thank you for considering donating blood today.**

Revised January 2001

■ **FIGURE 11–2** A, Responsibilities of a blood donor. (LifeSouth Blood Center, Montgomery, AL, with permission.) B, Informed consent. (LifeSouth Blood Center, Montgomery, AL, with permission.)

Donor Release:

I have read and I understand the information contained in the *Responsibilities of a Blood Donor and Important Information About Donating Blood* Information sheet. I understand that if my behavior or physical condition puts me at risk to transmit AIDS or any other disease, I should not donate blood. The medical history I have given is truthful and accurate to the best of my knowledge. I have not participated in activities considered high risk for acquiring and transmitting AIDS.

I give my permission for all laboratory testing necessary to provide safe blood to the recipient including tests to detect exposure to hepatitis, AIDS, and other transfusion-transmitted diseases. Some of these tests may be unlicensed and for research only. Some positive test results are routinely reported to the State Health Department as required by law for notification of sexual partners. I realize that LifeSouth is not a testing center and that by giving blood I am not guaranteed that disease testing will be performed.

Although donating blood is normally a pleasant experience, I realize that short-term side effects can occur, such as bruising, dizziness, or fainting, and that, in rare cases, a donor may experience infection or nerve damage.

I voluntarily donate my blood to the LifeSouth Community Blood Centers to be used as the blood center deems advisable.

Donor: _____   Date: _____

B.

■ **FIGURE 11–2**   *(continued)*

allogeneic whole blood donations is 8 weeks or 56 days. If the prospective donor has participated in a pheresis donation (platelets, plasma, granulocytes), at least 48 hours must pass before donating whole blood.[4]

2. **In the past 12 months have you been under a doctor's care, been pregnant, or had a major illness or surgery? If yes, what and when?** If the donor's response is a "yes," the interviewer must investigate further. Prospective donors who have recently undergone surgery need to be evaluated by the medical director; if blood or its components were transfused during surgery, the donor must be deferred for 12 months from the time the product was transfused. If the surgery involved a biopsy, the site and reason for the biopsy should be determined; patients with lymphoma and AIDS have had lymph node biopsies, and these diagnoses are cause for deferral. A donor who has been hospitalized for AIDS must be permanently deferred.[5]

3. **Do you currently have an infection or are you taking antibiotics for an infection?** Donors currently taking antibiotics for an infection or for prophylaxis after dental surgery may be deferred temporarily until the infection has cleared up. Donors who have taken tetracyclines or other antibiotics used to treat acne are acceptable for donation. All drugs and medications must be cleared by the blood collection facility and/or blood bank medical director.

4. **Have you ever had heart problems, lung problems (other than asthma), or a bleeding problem?** A history of cardiovascular, coronary, or rheumatic heart disease is usually cause for deferral; however, in the absence of disability or restrictions by the patient's physician, the donor may be accepted on a case-by-case basis by the blood bank director. Active pulmonary tuberculosis or other active pulmonary disease is cause for deferral. A history of cancer, leukemia, or lymphoma is generally a cause for indefinite deferral. Any donor presenting with a history of cancer should be reviewed by the blood bank medical director. The exceptions include basal or squamous cell cancer, carcinoma in situ of the cervix, and papillary thyroid carcinoma that has been surgically

removed. Donors indicating a history of a bleeding problem following surgery, invasive dental procedures, cuts, or abrasions must be further evaluated by the blood bank director. Diseases of the blood such as hemophilia, von Willebrand's disease, sickle cell anemia, thalassemia, Kaposi's sarcoma, polycythemia, or a history of receiving clotting factor concentrates are causes for indefinite deferral.

5. **Have you ever had hepatitis? If yes, when?** Donors with a history of hepatitis after their 11th birthday or a confirmed positive test for hepatitis B surface antigen (HBsAg) or a repeatedly reactive test for anti-HBc should be indefinitely deferred.[6] Donor suitability with regard to the age restriction for hepatitis can be assessed by the medical director; recollections of symptoms, diagnoses, and laboratory data can be helpful in making the decision if the donor is suitable for whole blood donation. The FDA stipulates that a history of an elevated alanine aminotransferase or a reactive test for antibodies to hepatitis A virus or antibodies to hepatitis B surface antigen should not exclude a potential donor without additional clinical evidence of viral hepatitis. If viral hepatitis before the age of 11 years is suspected, the donor should be deferred temporarily until the circumstances are investigated and medical opinion concludes there is no history or diagnosis of viral hepatitis after age 11.

6. **Have you ever had a positive test for HIV?** Persons with clinical or laboratory evidence of HIV infection should be permanently deferred.

7. **Have you ever had babesiosis or Chagas' disease? If malaria, when?** A history of babesiosis or Chagas' disease is cause for indefinite deferral. There are 70 known species of *Babesia* and at least five are identified as infecting humans. *Babesia microti* utilizes the vector *Ixodes scapularis* to infect the human and transmit the parasite. The *Babesia* organism penetrates the erythrocyte where the trophozoite multiplies; upon lysis of the RBC merozoites are released into the blood where they are free to infect other RBCs. Transfusion-associated infection with *Babesia* carries an incubation period of 2 to 8 weeks;

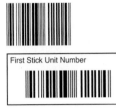

First Stick Unit Number

Donor Physical

			Acceptable	Pass	Fail
Examiner:		42Hgb:	≥ 2.5	○	○
Interviewer:		45Temp:	95.0 to 99.5 F	○	○
45Arm Insp:	Pass○ Fail○	44Pulse:	50 to 100 bpm	○	○
42CuSO4:	Pass○ Fail○	43B/P:	90-180 / 50-100	○	○

Thermometer ID:		HemoCue ID:	

Medical History Questions

		Yes	No
1.	Is the information on the front of this form correct?	○	○
2.	Are you feeling well today?	○	○
3.	Do you weigh less than 110 pounds? If yes, list weight:	○	○
4.	Have you donated blood in the last 8 weeks or a double unit of red cells in the last 16 weeks, or plasma or platelets in the last 48 hours?	○	○
5.	In the past 12 months have you been under a doctor's care, been pregnant, or had a major illness or surgery? If yes, what & when?	○	○
6.	Do you currently have an infection or are you taking antibiotics for an infection?	○	○
7.	Have you ever had heart problems, lung problems (other than asthma), or a bleeding problem?	○	○
8.	Have you ever had hepatitis? If yes, when?	○	○
9.	Have you ever had a positive test for the HIV or AIDS virus?	○	○
10.	Have you ever had malaria, babesiosis, or Chagas' disease? If malaria, when?	○	○
11.	Have you ever had cancer including leukemia or lymphoma? If yes, what & when? Chemotherapy? ○ YES ○ NO	○	○
12.	Have you ever taken any of these drugs: Tegison, Soriatane, Accutane, Proscar, Propecia, or Avodart? If yes, what & when.	○	○
13.	In the past 36 hours have you taken aspirin or anything with aspirin in it?	○	○
14.	In the past 4 weeks have you had any vaccinations, shots or immunizations?	○	○
15.	In the past 8 weeks have you received the smallpox vaccine or had close contact with the vaccination site of anyone who has?	○	○
16.	In the past 3 years have you been out of the US or Canada? If yes, record where and check one. ○ Non-malarial ○ Malarial, Date:	○	○
17.	Have you ever taken money or drugs in exchange for sex?	○	○
18.	Have you ever taken street drugs by needle?	○	○
19.	Have you ever taken clotting factor concentrates for a bleeding problem, such as hemophilia, or had sex with someone who has?	○	○
20.	*For men*: Have you ever had sex with another man? *For women*: In the past 12 months have you had sex with a man who had sex with another man?	○	○
21.	Since 1977, have you been in Africa?	○	○
	21a) Were you born in or have you lived in Cameroon, Central African Republic, Chad, Congo, Equatorial Guinea, Gabon, Niger, or Nigeria?	○	○
	21b) Have you received a blood transfusion or any other medical treatment with a product made from blood in any of these countries?	○	○
22.	Have you had sex with anyone who, since 1977, was born in or lived in Cameroon, Central African Republic, Chad, Congo, Equatorial Guinea, Gabon, Niger, or Nigeria?	○	○
23.	Have any of your blood relatives had Creutzfeldt-Jakob Disease (CJD)?	○	○
24.	Since 1980, have you injected bovine (beef) insulin?	○	○
25.	Have you ever received growth hormone or had a dura mater (or brain covering) graft?	○	○
26.	Between 1980 and 1996, did you spend a total time of 6 months or more associated with a U.S. military base in Europe or Turkey*?	○	○

■ **FIGURE 11–3** Medical history questionnaire. (LifeSouth Blood Center, Montgomery, AL, with permission.)

Medical History Questions

		Yes	No
27.	Since 1980 have you lived in or traveled to Europe, including the United Kingdom?	○	○
	27a) From 1980 through 1996, did you spend a total of 3 months or more in the United Kingdom (England, Northern Ireland, Scotland, Wales, the Isle of Man, the Channel Islands, Gibraltar, or the Falkland Islands)?	○	○
	27b) Since 1980, have you received a blood transfusion in the United Kingdom?	○	○
	27c) Since 1980, have you spent time that adds up to 5 years or more in Europe (including time spent in the U.K. from 1980 through 1996)?	○	○
In the past 12 months have you:			
28.	Had close contact with someone with symptomatic viral hepatitis or been given Hepatitis B Immune Globulin (after hepatitis exposure)?	○	○
29.	Had a tattoo applied, ear or skin piercing or acupuncture?	○	○
30.	Had contact with someone else's blood through an accidental needle stick or mucosal exposure?	○	○
31.	Received a blood transfusion or had an organ or tissue transplant or a skin or bone graft? If yes, when?	○	○
32.	Been a victim of rape? If yes, when?	○	○
33.	Been treated for a sexually transmitted disease including syphilis?	○	○
34.	Been in prison or jail? If yes, when?	○	○
35.	Had sex with a prostitute or anyone else who takes money or drugs or other payment for sex? If yes, when?	○	○
36.	Had sex with someone who has ever taken street drugs by needle? If yes, when?	○	○
37.	Had sex with anyone who has HIV or AIDS or a positive test for HIV or AIDS? If yes, when?	○	○

Comments:

○ THERAPEUTIC   ○ AUTOLOGOUS

* 1980 to 1990: Belgium, The Netherlands, or Germany; 1980 to 1996: Spain, Portugal, Turkey, Italy or Greece.

JAN 2003

■ **FIGURE 11-3** *(continued)*

symptoms may include malaise, fatigue, anorexia, arthralgias, nausea, vomiting, abdominal pain, and fever reaching temperatures of 40°C.

Chagas' disease, also known as American trypanosomiasis, is caused by the protozoan parasite *Trypanosoma cruzi*. The vector responsible for transmission of the parasite is the hematophagous bug belonging to the family *Reduviidae*. Transmission occurs when mucous membranes or breaks in the skin are contaminated with the feces of infected hematophagous bugs.[7] Chagas' disease is endemic in parts of Central and South America and Mexico, where an estimated 16 to 18 million persons are infected with *T. cruzi*. An estimated 25,000 to 100,000 Latin American immigrants living in the United States are infected with *T. cruzi*. Chagas' disease may be transmitted congenitally by breast feeding, organ transplants, or blood transfusion.[7]

8. **Have you ever taken the following drugs: Tegison, Soriatane, Accutane, Dutasteride, Proscar, or Propecia? If yes, what and when?** Tegison or etretinate is characterized as being potentially teratogenic; any donor who has taken this drug should be permanently deferred. Donors who have ingested Accutane or Proscar should be deferred from donating blood for at least 1 month after taking the last dose.[8] Dutasteride or AVODART is used in the treatment of symptomatic benign prostatic hyperplasia. The FDA has advised blood centers that males using this drug should not donate blood until at least 6 months after the last dose for fear of transfusion to a pregnant female.[9] Dutasteride is considered teratogenic and may cause birth defects. Soriatane carries a deferral of 3 years.

9. **In the past 36 hours, have you taken aspirin or anything with aspirin in it?** Donors who have taken piroxicam, aspirin, or anything with aspirin in it within 3 days of donation may not be a suitable donor for platelet concentrates or platelet pheresis; these medications inhibit platelet function.

10. **In the past 4 weeks, have you had any vaccinations, shots, or immunizations?** If a potential donor has received a live attenuated or bacterial vaccine such as measles (rubeola), mumps, polio, typhoid, or yellow fever, there is a 2-week deferral; if the donor has received a live attenuated vaccine for German measles (rubella) or chickenpox, there is a 4-week deferral.[10] There is however, no deferral for toxoids or killed or synthetic viral, bacterial, or rickettsial vaccines if the donor is symptom-free and afebrile.

11. **In the past 3 years, have you been out of the United States or Canada? If yes, where?** Persons who have traveled to areas or countries considered endemic for malaria may be accepted as blood donors 1 year after returning from the endemic area, provided they are symptom-free of any malaria-related illness.

    Immigrants, refugees, or citizens coming from a country in which malaria is considered endemic may be accepted as blood donors 3 years after departure. After 3 years, donors free of any symptoms related to malaria may be accepted as blood donors.[11]

12. **At any time since 1977, have you taken money or drugs for sex? In the past 12 months, have you had sex, even once, with anyone who has done so? In the past 12 months, have you given money or drugs to anyone to have sex with you?** Men or women who have engaged in sex for money or drugs since 1977 and persons who have engaged in sex with such people during the preceding 12 months should not donate blood or its components.

13. **In the past 12 months, have you had sex with anyone who has ever used a needle, even once, to take any drug (including steroids)? In the past 12 months, have you ever had sex, even once, with anyone who has ever taken clotting factor concentrates for a bleeding problem such as hemophilia?** The FDA mandates persons who have had sex with any person who is a past or present IV drug user should be deferred for 12 months; additionally, persons who have had sex with any person with hemophilia or related blood disorder who has received factor concentrates should be deferred for 12 months.

14. *Male donors:* **Have you had sex with another male, even once, since 1977?** *Female donors:* **In the past 12 months, have you had sex with a male who has had sex, even once since 1977, with another male?** Men who have engaged in sex with another man since 1977 should be permanently deferred; women who have had sex with men who have had sex with another man even once since 1977 should be deferred for 12 months.[12] There is no tangible evidence of HIV being transmitted by close contact; therefore, potential donors who meet the definition of being in close contact with someone with AIDS or an HIV-positive individual should not be deferred.[13]

15. **Are you giving blood today in order to be tested for the AIDS virus?** Although there are no specific requirements by either the FDA or AABB, this question is asked to ascertain the possible motive for donating blood for the sole purpose of testing blood for the HIV virus.

16. **Do you understand that if you have the AIDS virus, you can give it to someone else, even though you may feel well and test negative for HIV?** The FDA stipulates prospective donors should be informed about the "window period" of the HIV virus. The window period occurs when the donor is infected with the virus but the antibodies are not yet detectable by current screening methods.

17. **Have you read and understood all the donor information presented to you, and have all your questions been answered?** Prospective donors must be provided information about the collection procedure and any risks involved; they should also be informed about high-risk behavior related to the AIDS virus and confidential unit exclusion (CUE) in a language they can understand. They should be given the opportunity to ask questions regarding any aspect of the collection procedure.

18. **Have you had sex with anyone since 1977 who was born in or lived in Cameroon, Central African Republic, Chad, Congo, Equatorial Guinea, Gabon, Niger, or Nigeria?** Donors who answer yes to this question should be indefinitely deferred. The basis for this deferral is the risk of exposure via sexual contact and the widespread use of nonsterile needles in these countries.

19. **Have any of your blood relatives had Creutzfeldt-Jakob Disease (CJD)?**

20. **Since 1980, have you injected bovine (beef) insulin?**

21. **Have you ever received growth hormone or had a dura mater graft?**

22. **Between 1980 and 1996, did you spend a total time of 6 months or more associated with U.S. military bases in Europe or Turkey?**

23. **Since 1980, have you lived in or traveled to Europe?**

Questions 19 through 23 are related to CJD and vCJD (variant Creutzfeldt-Jakob Disease). CJD was first described in the 1920s and is a fatal disease with a mean survival of about 5 months. CJD is a member of a group of neurologic disorders known as the transmissible spongiform encephalopathies or prion diseases, which affect sheep, cows, and humans. The prion hypothesis states the agent is composed of an abnormally folded form of a host protein or prion protein. The abnormal protein accumulates in the central nervous system in prion diseases, and the infectious agent is resistant to most forms of degradation.[14] The disease results in progressive dementia and spongiform alterations in the brain. CJD may be transmitted by corneal transplants, human dura mater grafts, pituitary-derived human growth hormone, and neurosurgical instruments.[15]

vCJD is also a fatal disease with degenerative neurologic manifestations discovered in the United Kingdom (UK) in 1996. To date, there are 73 confirmed cases of vCJD in the UK,[16] 2 cases in France, and 1 case in the Republic of Ireland. Persons with the variant type comprise a younger age group than those with classic CJD, with a median age at death of 28 years.[17] vCJD is thought to be transmitted by persons who have consumed meat from cattle with bovine spongiform encephalopathy or "mad cow disease." With regard to donor deferral, the FDA took a proactive role mandating the following:

- Donors who spent 6 months or more cumulatively in the UK from 1980 to 1996 were indefinitely deferred.
- Donors who injected bovine insulin manufactured since 1980 from cattle in the UK were indefinitely deferred.[18]

24. **In the past 12 months, have you had close contact with someone with symptomatic viral hepatitis or have you been given hepatitis B immune globulin (after hepatitis exposure)?** "Close contact" can be defined as cohabitation or being in close quarters with someone for an extended time. Close contact with a person with viral hepatitis carries a 12-month deferral.

25. **In the past 12 months, have you had a tattoo applied, ear**

or skin piercing, or acupuncture? Prospective donors who have been exposed to blood or body fluids via an accidental needlestick or other injury should be deferred for 12 months; persons who have received a tattoo also should be deferred for 12 months.[19]

26. **In the past 12 months, have you received a blood transfusion or had an organ or tissue transplant or a skin or bone graft? If yes, when?** Donors who during the preceding 12 months have received a blood transfusion (blood or its components) or other human tissues known to be possible sources of blood-borne pathogens should be deferred for 12 months from the time of receiving the blood product or graft.

27. **In the past 12 months, have you been treated for a sexually transmitted disease, including syphilis?** Prospective donors with a history of syphilis or gonorrhea or treatment for either or a reactive screening test for syphilis should be deferred for 12 months after completion of therapy. The agent that causes syphilis, *Treponema pallidum*, may live for 1 to 5 days in cold storage so that a fresh unit of RBCs may transmit infection; at room temperature, however, this agent thrives very well, placing platelet concentrates above RBCs as potentially supporting transfusion-transmitted syphilis. To date, however, only three cases of transfusion-transmitted syphilis have been documented.[20,21–23]

28. **In the past 12 months, have you been in prison?** Donors should be deferred for 12 months if they have been incarcerated in a correctional institution in the past 12 months. In 1995, the FDA recommended that individuals who were inmates of correctional institutions and individuals who have been incarcerated for more than 72 consecutive hours during the previous 12 months be deferred for 12 months from their last date of incarceration.[24]

29. **Female Donors: In the past 6 weeks, have you been pregnant or are you pregnant now?** The AABB mandates existing pregnancy or pregnancy in the past 6 weeks as cause for deferral. Exceptions can be made by the blood bank medical director for an autologous donation if complications are anticipated at delivery. A first trimester or second trimester abortion or miscarriage is not cause for deferral. A 12-month deferral would apply if the woman received a transfusion during her pregnancy.

West Nile Virus Donor Deferral

Since its appearance in the United States about 4 years ago, West Nile virus (WNV) has spread at an alarming rate across the country. WNV is spread via the female mosquito of the *Culex* family and is categorized as a flavivirus. It was first isolated in 1937 from the blood of a febrile woman in the West Nile district of Uganda in Eastern Africa. To date there have been reports of infection from 44 states and the District of Columbia.[25] Transmission has been reported via person-to-person by blood transfusion, organ transplantation, intrauterine transmission, and breast-feeding. As a result the FDA offered recommendations on donor deferral of patients suspected of being exposed to WNV. A potential donor diagnosed with WNV infection should be deferred until 14 days after the condition is resolved and at least 28 days from the onset of febrile illness or diagnosis of WNV, whichever date is later. Donors with an otherwise unexplained predonation febrile illness suggesting WNV infection (in a community of active viral transmission) should be deferred for 28 days after the onset of illness or 14 days after resolution of the condition, whichever date is later.[26] Additionally, a new recommendation includes asking donors if they have had a history of fever with headache 1 week prior to donation; if donors answers "yes," they should be deferred for 28 days from the date of interview.

Donor samples can be screened for WNV using the FDA-approved WNV IgM capture ELISA (PanBio Limited of Australia) and the Procleix WNV Assay (Gen-Probe Inc.). The Procleix WNV Assay is a nucleic acid amplification test (NAT) available in the United States under an investigational new drug. A nationwide testing of WNV using NAT technology began in 2003.[25]

Severe Acute Respiratory Syndrome (SARS)

SARS is a respiratory illness that has been reported in Asia, North America, Europe, and Canada. Approximately 38 cases have been documented in the United States.[27] SARS is spread by person-to-person contact such as touching the skin of other people or objects contaminated with infectious droplets; other routes of transmission have yet to be elucidated. Symptoms include a fever higher than 100.4°F, headaches, and malaise. After 7 days, infected persons may present with a dry cough and dyspnea. The FDA recommends travelers to areas of the world affected by SARS be deferred from donating blood for 14 days after their return to the United States. The regions affected include the People's Republic of China, Hanoi, Vietnam, Singapore, and Toronto, Canada. Individuals who have had an acute case of SARS will be deferred from donating until 28 days after becoming asymptomatic and after any prescribed treatment is complete.[28] Additionally, the FDA recommends the following questions be asked the potential donor in the interview process:

- In the past 28 days, have you been ill with SARS or suspected SARS?
- In the past 14 days, have you cared for, lived with, or had direct contact with body fluids of a person with SARS or suspected SARS?
- In the past 14 days, have you traveled to, traveled through, or resided in areas affected by SARS?[28]

Confidential Unit Exclusion (CUE)

Although CUE is not mandated by the AABB *Standards* or the FDA, most blood centers include the CUE as part of the donation process. The rationale for the CUE is to provide an opportunity for those donors who felt pressure to donate in the workplace or at a community blood drive to indicate their blood should not be transfused.[29] There are many ways this can be carried out; most procedures avoid face-to-face contact with the donor representative for answering the question "should my blood be used for donation?" One method used by LifeSouth Blood Center (Montgomery, AL) asks the donor to select a barcode (use or do not use), and the donor simply peels the sticker and places it on his or

Confidential Self-Exclusion

The truthful answering of the donor history questions is vital in providing disease free blood to patients. Sometimes this is difficult. If you have any reason to think your blood should not be given to another person and were unable to indicate this, please use this confidential procedure to let us know.

Thank you.

A.

Instructions

1. Select the appropriate label

   USE   Your blood may be given to another.

   DON'T USE   Your blood *will not* be given to another. (It will be destroyed.)

2. Attach the bar code label to the bag your blood will be collected into. If you do not select a label, you *cannot* donate.

3. Discard the remaining portion of this form.

   Only a computer scanner in the lab will be able to read your reply. Nobody in the donor room or the mobile will know your answer.

   All units will be tested and the donor notified of any positive results.

   Some positive test results are routinely reported to the state health department as required by law for notification of sexual partners.

   Thank you for your generous blood donation and helping save a life.

USE	DON'T USE

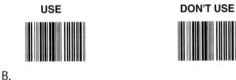

B.

■ **FIGURE 11–4** A, Confidential unit exclusion. (LifeSouth Blood Center, Montgomery, AL, with permission.) B, Confidential unit exclusion. (LifeSouth Blood Center, Montgomery, AL, with permission.)

her paperwork. The donor center representative then scans the barcode when processing the donor paperwork to determine the result of the CUE (**Fig. 11–4**). Other facilities simply have the donor check a box (use or do not use) in private.

Whichever method is used, *Standards* does mandate that the donor will be informed that the blood will be subjected to testing and that there will be notification to the donor of any positive infectious disease test results.

The Physical Examination

The donor center representative evaluates the prospective donor with regard to general appearance, weight, temperature, pulse, blood pressure, hemoglobin, and presence of skin lesions. A blood bank physician should be available on site to evaluate any special considerations.

- *General Appearance.* The donor center representative should observe the prospective donor for presence of excessive anxiety, drug or alcohol influence, or nervousness. If

possible, this should be done in a gentle manner so as to not deter the donor from donations in the future.

- *Weight. Standards* mandates a maximum of 10.5 mL/kg of donor weight for whole blood collection inclusive of pilot tubes for testing. If the donor weighs less than 110 pounds, the amount of blood collected must be proportionately reduced as well as that of the anticoagulant. The following formula can be utilized for this purpose:

- **Amount of blood to be drawn:**

$$\frac{\text{Donor's weight (lb)} \times 450 \text{ mL}}{110 \text{ lb}} = \text{Allowable amount (mL)}$$

- **Amount of anticoagulant needed:**

$$\frac{\text{Allowable amount}}{100} \times 14 = \text{Anticoagulant needed (mL)}$$

- **Amount of anticoagulant to remove:**

$$63 \text{ mL} - \text{anticoagulant (mL)} = \text{Anticoagulant to remove (mL)}$$

- *Temperature. Standards* mandates the donor temperature must be less than or equal to 37.5°C or 99.5°F.[30] Donors are asked not to drink coffee or hot beverages while waiting to donate as this may affect the temperature on occasion. Oral temperatures that are lower than normal are not cause for deferral.

- *Pulse.* The pulse of the donor should be between 50 and 100 bpm. Often, a donor who is athletic will have a pulse less than 50 bpm, which is not cause for deferral. The pulse should be counted for at least 15 seconds; any irregularities should be evaluated by a blood bank physician.

- *Blood Pressure.* The systolic blood pressure of a potential donor should be less than or equal to 180 mm Hg and the diastolic less than or equal to 100 mm Hg. Blood pressure readings above these levels should be evaluated by a blood bank physician.

- *Hemoglobin.* The hemoglobin level of the donor should be greater than or equal to 12.5 g/dL, and the hematocrit level greater than or equal to 38 percent for allogeneic donation. For autologous donation, the hemoglobin/hematocrit level should be greater than or equal to 11 g/dL and 33%, respectively.[31] The methods used for measuring hemoglobin include the copper sulfate method[32] or point-of-care instruments using spectrophotometric methodology.[33] A hematocrit or packed cell volume can be determined manually by centrifugation[34] or calculated using the RBC count and mean corpuscular volume; blood is usually acquired via a finger stick.

- *Skin Lesions.* Prior to donation, the donor's arms should be inspected for skin lesions. Evidence of skin lesions (e.g., multiple puncture marks) is cause for indefinite deferral. Skin disorders that are not cause for deferral include poison ivy and other rashes; these, however, should be evaluated by a blood bank physician.

Informed Consent

AABB Standards mandates that informed consent of allogeneic, autologous, and apheresis donors be obtained before donation. The donor must be informed of the risks of the procedure and also of the tests that are performed to reduce the risk of infectious disease transmission to the recipient. The donor must be able to ask questions concerning any element of the collection or testing process. If the donor is a minor or is unable to comprehend the informed consent protocol, applicable state law provisions will intercede. An example of an informed consent is shown in **Figure 11–2.**

Autologous Donors

An autologous donor is one who donates blood for his or her own use; thus, such a donor is referred to as the donor-patient. Autologous blood is safer than allogeneic blood. There is no risk of disease transmission, transfusion reactions, or alloimmunization to white blood cells, RBCs, platelets, or plasma proteins. Autologous blood transfusion is a viable and common alternative therapy for many patients undergoing transfusion. There are four different types of autologous donation:

1. Preoperative collection
2. Acute normovolemic hemodilution
3. Intraoperative collection
4. Postoperative collection

Each type of autologous donation and its requirements will be described briefly.

Preoperative Collection

Indications for preoperative collection include patients undergoing orthopedic procedures, vascular surgery, cardiac or thoracic surgery, and radical prostatectomy. Although some women do participate in an autologous collection program during pregnancy for unforeseen complications, blood is seldom needed except in cases in which the mother has multiple antibodies to high-frequency antigens or risk for placenta previa or intrapartum hemorrhage.[35] A schedule for collection should be established with the donor-patient. The maximal surgical blood order schedule can provide guidance for surgical procedures to estimate the number of units needed for transfusion. The last blood collection should occur no sooner than 72 hours before the scheduled surgery to allow for volume repletion.

Requirements for autologous donation are considerably less stringent than those for allogeneic donations. Autologous donations, however, do require the order of the donor-patient physician **(Fig. 11–5)**; a minimum hemoglobin/hematocrit level of 11 g/dL and 33 percent, respectively; and deferral of the donor-patient when there is a risk of bacteremia.[36] In the past, the autologous units that were not used by the donor-patient could be crossed-over into the homologous inventory; this is no longer allowed. *Standards* states that only in exceptional circumstances could a unit labeled as autologous be used for another recipient and that this decision must be approved by the medical director on a case-by-case basis.[36]

A low-volume unit is defined as containing between 300 to 405 mL of blood. If a low-volume unit is collected, it is important the unit be labeled as "low-volume unit" and that plasma is not transfused. For autologous donors weighing less than 50 kg, a 450-mL bag is usually used, and there should be a reduction in the volume of blood collected. Units collected with a volume of less than 300 mL require approval by the medical director.

Units collected for autologous use must be labeled appropriately. The label should include the patient's full name, medical record number or ID number, expiration date of the unit, and the name of the facility where the donor-patient will be transfused. The label must also clearly state "For Autologous Use Only" **(Fig. 11–6)**.

The ABO group is determined for each autologous collection via testing with anti-A and anti-B for RBC antigens and testing with A_1 cells and B cells for expected antibodies. The collecting facility must determine ABO and Rh types on all units. The transfusing facility, if different from the collecting facility, must retest ABO and Rh types. The exceptions to this rule are if the collecting facility tests segments from the units or confirms donor ABO and Rh using a computer-validated system. Additionally, all units are tested for the D antigen by using the anti-D reagent. In the event the initial test for D antigen is negative, a test for weak D is performed. When either test is positive, the unit is labeled as Rh-positive; if both tests yield negative reactions, the unit is labeled as Rh-negative.

If the autologous unit is to be transfused outside the collecting facility, the following infectious disease markers must be tested: HBsAg, anti-HBc, anti-HCV, anti-HIV-1/2, HIV-1 Ag, anti-HTLV I/II, and a serologic test for syphilis.[37] According to AABB *Standards*, the testing must be done before the unit is shipped at 30-day intervals. If any of the markers yield a positive or reactive result, the patient's physician and transfusing facility must be notified of the result.[38]

Autologous units are labeled differently than allogeneic units and directed units. The former generally have a distinct green label and tag **(Fig. 11–7)**. This is done both to ensure the unit is linked correctly with the donor-patient and to make the blood bank technologists aware that certain patients do have autologous units on the shelf and must be transfused before allogeneic units; more specifically, the oldest units should be transfused first. Blood banks should have a system in place to ensure autologous units are selected first.

Acute Normovolemic Hemodilution

This type of autologous collection involves removal of whole blood from a patient with infusions of crystalloid or colloid before surgical blood loss. The blood is collected in standard blood bags containing anticoagulant/preservative and stored at room temperature. The "shed" blood is normally reinfused to the patient within 8 hours of collection; this short interval conserves viability of platelets and coagulation factors. Blood should be properly labeled and must contain the patient's full name, medical record number, date and time of collection, and the label For Autologous Use Only. If blood is collected from an open system such as a central venous line, it may be stored for up to 8 hours at room temperature or 24 hours in a monitored refrigerator. Blood units for acute normovolemic hemodilution (ANH) are reinfused in the reverse order of collection so that the last unit reinfused carries the highest hematocrit level. This procedure has been well documented in the literature.[39,40] In one case, a 65-year-old patient scheduled for a radical prostatectomy underwent an ANH. Approximately 2360 g of blood was removed and replaced with

LIFESouth
Community Blood Centers
1221 Northwest 13th Street
Galnesville, Florida 32601
(352) 334-1000

Branch Location: _____

*An appointment is recommended for this service. Please contact your local blood bank for information.

[Reset Form]

Request For Autologous Collections

Patient's Name _____ SS# _____ Birth Date _____

Patient's Phone Number _____ Patient's Address _____

Date of Surgery/Transfusion _____ Diagnosis _____ Hospital _____

If patient is also under treatment for, or has any, preexisting medical condition(s), please indicate below.

_____, MD   Condition _____

_____, MD   Condition _____

_____, MD   Condition _____

Please list all medications prescribed for this patient: _____

_____

LifeSouth Community Blood Centers will process and store this blood for subsequent replacement transfusion. The number of units drawn and the interval between donations will be determined by the patient's hemoglobin and anticipated blood requirements, and will be at the discretion of the blood center's Medical Director. Units will be held only until outdate (42 days from the date drawn) unless specific arrangements are made with the blood center prior to that date. Blood should not be drawn from the donor-patient within 72 hours of the time of anticipated surgery or transfusion. A cardiac release is required for all patients with a history of cardiac problems; units will not be collected until the blood center has received written release from the patient's cardiologist.

Physicians will be notified in writing of abnormal test results as soon as possible. It is the responsibility of the ordering physician to notify the patient.

Physicians, please complete:
I have explained the reasons for and risks involved in autologous collection to this patient and have considered the need for iron supplementation:

#Units _____

• Packed Cells   Signature, MD _____ Date _____

• Whole Blood   Physician (printed name) _____

• Fresh Frozen Plasma   Phone _____

• Cryoprecipitated AHF

.... **Blood Center Use Only** ....

Verbal Order _____ Taken by _____ Date _____

Donation Date _____ Unit Number _____   Donation Date _____ Unit Number _____

Donation Date _____ Unit Number _____   Donation Date _____ Unit Number _____

Apr 99   ver 1.0

■ **FIGURE 11–5**   Autologous donation permission form. (LifeSouth Blood Center, Montgomery, AL, with permission.)

1500 mL of colloids and 2000 mL of crystalloid solution. Retransfusion was started after a blood loss of 1800 mL, or a transfusion trigger of 20 percent. The patient remained hemodynamically stable throughout the operation.[41] Hospitals should devise their own guidelines and policies for this type of collection.

Intraoperative Collection

This type of autologous collection involves collecting and reinfusing blood lost by a patient during surgery. Most programs use devices that are capable of collecting the shed blood, washing it with saline, and then concentrating the

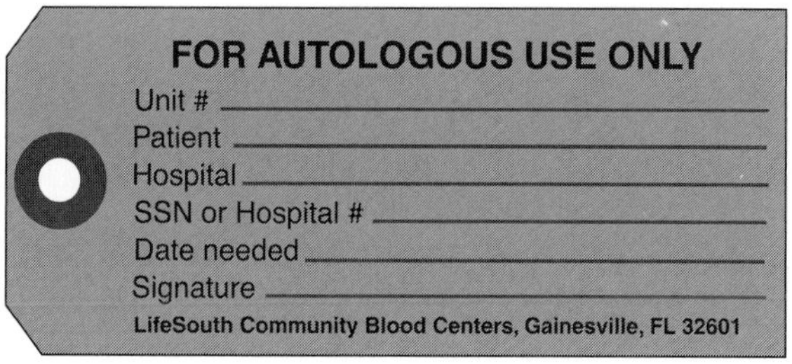
FOR AUTOLOGOUS USE ONLY
Unit # ______
Patient ______
Hospital ______
SSN or Hospital # ______
Date needed ______
Signature ______
LifeSouth Community Blood Centers, Gainesville, FL 32601

■ **FIGURE 11–6** Autologous donation label. (LifeSouth Blood Center, Montgomery, AL, with permission.)

RBCs with hematocrits in the range of 50 to 60 percent. The vacuum setting on the device should be less than 100 torr to guard against possible hemolysis of recovered blood.[42] Several studies have associated disseminated intravascular coagulation with shed blood that has undergone coagulation/fibrinolysis and hemolysis.[43–45] For this reason, intraoperative blood collection is contraindicated when procoagulants are applied to the surgical field; special attention should be paid to contact surfaces in the collection process that may precipitate coagulation. This type of collection has been used in cardiothoracic, major orthopedic, and cardiac surgery and vascular surgeries such as liver transplantation.

As with ANH, blood must be labeled with patient's full name, medical record number, date and time of collection, and For Autologous Use Only. Blood may be stored at room temperature for up to 6 hours or at 1° to 6°C for up to 24 hours as long as the latter temperature is begun within 4 hours from the end of collection. Hospitals should establish their own policies and procedures for this type of collection.

Postoperative Blood Collection

In this type of autologous collection, blood is collected from a drainage tube placed at the surgical site. It is reinfused with or without processing via a microaggregate filter to screen out any debris. This blood is characterized as being dilute, partially hemolyzed, and defibrinated. It is recommended that no more than 1400 mL be reinfused.[46] Surgeries that have used postoperative blood collection include orthopedic (e.g., arthoplasty) and cardiac. The volume of reinfused drainage blood has been reported to be as much as 3000 mL, with a corresponding RBC volume of 174 to 704 mL or 0.75 to 3.5 units of blood.[47]

Blood must be reinfused within 6 hours of collection or it is to be discarded. Hospitals should establish their own policies and procedures for this type of collection.

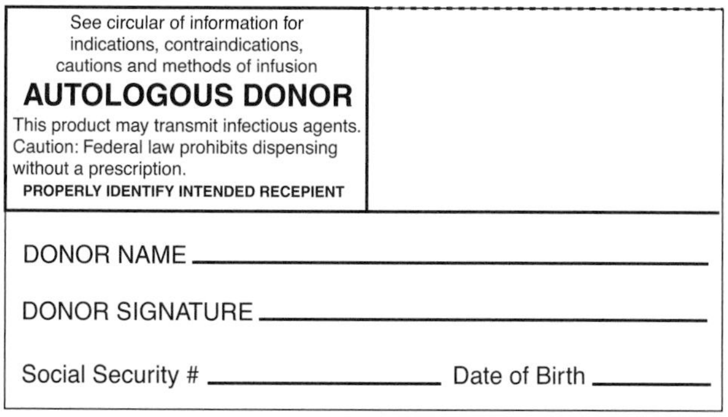
See circular of information for indications, contraindications, cautions and methods of infusion
AUTOLOGOUS DONOR
This product may transmit infectious agents.
Caution: Federal law prohibits dispensing without a prescription.
PROPERLY IDENTIFY INTENDED RECEPIENT
DONOR NAME ______
DONOR SIGNATURE ______
Social Security # ______ Date of Birth ______

■ **FIGURE 11–7** Autologous donation label. (LifeSouth Blood Center, Montgomery, AL, with permission.)

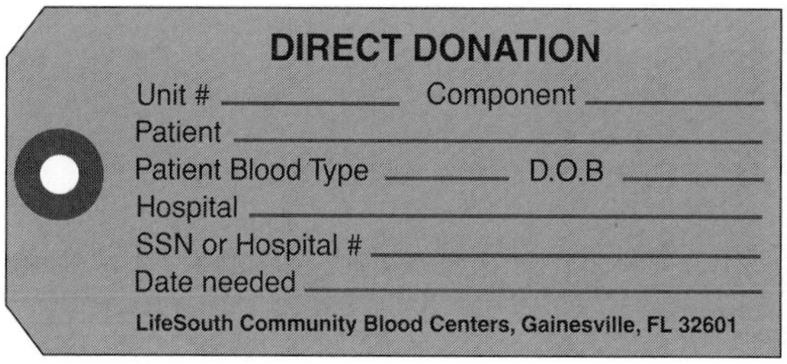
DIRECT DONATION
Unit # ______ Component ______
Patient ______
Patient Blood Type ______ D.O.B ______
Hospital ______
SSN or Hospital # ______
Date needed ______
LifeSouth Community Blood Centers, Gainesville, FL 32601

■ **FIGURE 11–8** Directed donation tag. (LifeSouth Blood Center, Montgomery, AL, with permission.)

Directed Donors

A directed donation is a unit collected under the same requirements as those for allogeneic donors, except that the unit collected is *directed* toward a specific patient. Often, when a friend or family member needs blood the donor center will accommodate these directed donations so that the required testing may be done as soon as possible and, if the blood is compatible, it can be used by the patient. The tag for the directed unit is a distinct color (e.g., yellow, salmon) to differentiate it from autologous tags **(Fig. 11–8).** If the donor is a blood relative, the unit must be irradiated to prevent graft versus host disease where viable T cells from the donor enter the patient's circulation and mount an attack against patient cells and tissue.[48]

A system should be in place to ensure directed units from blood relatives are irradiated; the method used by LifeSouth Community Blood Centers is a red stamp on the back of the directed donation tag, with respective boxes to indicate "yes" or "no" for irradiation. When processing the directed unit, the donor center technician would check this box before placing it on the respective blood shelf.

Pheresis Donation

A pheresis donor may be characterized into one or all of the following:

1. Plateletpheresis
2. Plasmapheresis
3. Leukopheresis
4. Double RBC pheresis
5. Stem cell pheresis.

Each of these procedures carries with it its own requirements for the donor as regulated by the AABB and FDA and by guidelines offered by the American Society for Apheresis (ASFA). We begin with a basic definition of apheresis.

Most apheresis centers use an automated cell separator device whose centrifugal force separates blood into components based on differences in density. Blood collected from the donor is anticoagulated and pumped into a rotating bowl or chamber. Components of blood are separated out based on cellular density. The desired fraction (e.g., platelets) is collected, and the remaining elements are returned to the donor.

Plateletpheresis

The donor criteria for plateletpheresis donors are similar to those for whole blood, with a few differences. Plateletpheresis donors may donate more often. The interval between donations is at least 2 days, not to exceed more than twice a week or more than 24 times a year.[49] Donors who have ingested aspirin or aspirin-containing medications are deferred. Although a platelet count is not required on the first donation, it is required if the interval between donations is less than 4 weeks; in that case the platelet count must be above $150,000/\mu L$. Any abnormal results must be cleared by the blood bank medical director or physician in the case of special circumstances.

Plasmapheresis

A plasmapheresis donor may be characterized as either "occasional" or "serial."[49] In the former, the donor undergoes pheresis not more often than once every 4 weeks, and donor selection mimics that of whole blood collection; in the latter, donation is more frequent than once every 4 weeks, and additional requirements apply.

At least 48 hours should elapse before the subsequent donation, with a maximum of 2 donations in a 7-day period; and serum or plasma must be tested for total protein and serum protein electrophoresis or quantitative immunoglobulins. Results must be within normal limits.

Leukopheresis

Special agents are required in the procedure for collection of granulocytes from the leukopheresis donor. These may include hydroxyethyl starch, corticosteroids, or growth factors such as granulocyte-colony stimulating factor.[50] The informed consent must include specific permission for any of these agents used in the procedure. AABB *Standards* states that any of these drugs or agents used to facilitate leukopheresis will not be used on donors whose medical history suggests that such a drug will exacerbate previous disease.[51]

Double RBC Pheresis

Both the AABB and FDA have approved procedures for removal of two allogeneic or autologous RBC units every 16 weeks by an automated method. The specifications for these donors are based primarily on weight, height, and hematocrit level. For male donors, weight must be at least 130 pounds, and height 5'1"; for females, weight of at least 150 pounds, and height 5'5". The hematocrit level for both sexes must be a minimum of 40 percent.[52]

Whole Blood Collection

Once the donor has satisfied requirements of the screening process and has been registered, whole blood collection can

proceed. This procedure is to be done only by trained personnel working under the direction of a qualified licensed physician. This section describes the identification of the donor, aseptic technique, venipuncture, collection of pilot tubes and whole blood unit, postdonation instructions, and adverse donor reactions.

Donor Identification

A numeric or alphanumeric system is used to link the donor to the donor record, pilot tubes, blood container, and all components made from the original collection. Care must be taken to avoid duplicate numbers, voided numbers, or other mistakes in the labeling system. These must be investigated and kept on record.

AABB *Standards*[53] states that the trained phlebotomist must identify the donor record and ensure that the donor name and identification numbers match. The phlebotomist should ask the donor to state and/or spell his or her name. At this time, the phlebotomist can attach all labels to blood bags, donor record, and pilot tubes.

Aseptic Technique

For blood collection, most blood centers use an iodine compound such as PVP-iodine or polymeriodine complex. Using a tourniquet or blood pressure cuff, the venipuncture site is identified, and the area is scrubbed at least 4 cm in all directions from the site for a minimum of 30 seconds. The area is then covered with a dry sterile gauze pad until the venipuncture is performed. Donors who are allergic or sensitive to iodine compounds may use chlorhexidrine gluconate and isopropyl alcohol. All methods must be approved by the FDA[54] (Box 11–1).

Collection Procedure

1. Confirm donor identity, and make the donor as comfortable as possible.
2. Select a firm large vein in the antecubital space that is free of any skin lesions or scarring. Both arms should be inspected.
3. Prepare the site using an FDA-approved cleansing method.
4. Inspect the blood bags for any defects or discoloration.
5. Ensure the balance system is adjusted to the volume being drawn; ensure counterbalance is level. Place hemostats on the tubing to prevent air from entering the line.
6. Reapply tourniquet or blood pressure cuff (40 to 60 mm Hg) to increase distention of the vein.
7. Uncover the sterile gauze, and perform the venipuncture immediately. Check the position of the needle, and tape the tubing to the donor's arm to hold needle in place. Cover with a sterile gauze.
8. Release the hemostat, and ask the donor to open and close hand every 10 to 12 seconds during collection procedure.
9. Reduce the pressure on the cuff to approximately 40 mm Hg.
10. Continue to monitor the patient throughout the entire collection process. The donor should never be left unat-

BOX 11–1
Arm Preparation Methods

Method I

1. Scrub the site (2 × 2 inches) for 30 sec using an aqueous Iodophor scrub solution (0.7%). Iodophor is a polyvinyl pyrrolidone-iodine or poloxamer iodine complex.
2. Apply iodophor complex and let stand for 30 sec. Use a concentric spiral motion, starting in the center and moving outward. Do not go back to the center. Removal of the iodophor solution is not necessary.
3. Site is now ready for venipuncture. Cover with sterile gauze until ready for needle insertion.
4. If the donor bends the arm, or the prepared site is touched with the fingers or other nonsterile object, the arm preparation must be repeated.

Method II

1. Apply a minimum of 1 mL of One Step Gel directly to the venipuncture site by squeezing the gel bottle directly over the intended area.
2. Using a sterile applicator and while holding it at an approximate 30° angle, begin scrubbing in a circular motion about a 1 inch area directly over the venipuncture site. Continue this for a minimum of 30 sec.
3. After scrubbing for 30 sec, use the same applicator to begin at intended site of venipunctures, and move gradually outward in concentric circles to form a total prepared area measuring at least 3 inches in diameter.
4. Using a second sterile applicator and starting from the center of the 3-inch prepared area, remove excess gel by moving gradually outward in concentric circles.
5. Allow site to air dry according to manufacturer's instructions.
6. If the donor bends the arm or the prepared site is touched with the fingers or with any other nonsterile object, the arm preparation must be repeated.

tended. Mix blood and anticoagulant periodically during the procedure. (e.g. every 45 seconds)

11. When the primary bag has tripped the scale, the donor can stop squeezing, and tubing can be clamped. A unit containing a volume of 405 to 550 mL should weigh between 429 to 583 g + the weight of the container and anticoagulant.[55] The conversion 1.06 g/mL is used to convert grams to mL. If the volume collected is in the low volume range (300 to 404 mL), the unit must be labeled as a Low Volume Unit,[56] and fresh frozen plasma (FFP) cannot be made from this unit as it would not contain adequate levels of coagulation factors.

12. Before the needle is removed from the donor's arm, pilot tubes are filled. The pressure is reduced to 20 mm Hg or less and, depending on the tubing of the bag, the tubes are filled:

➤ In-line needle. A hemostat or metal clip is used to seal tubing distal to the needle. The connector is opened, the needle is inserted into the pilot tube, the hemostat is removed, and tubes are filled. The donor needle can now be removed.[55]

➤ Straight-tubing assembly. Place hemostats approximately four segments from the needle. Tighten the loose knot made previously in the tubing; release the hemostats, and strip a segment of tubing between knot and needle. Secure hemostat and cut tubing in stripped area of segment. Fill required tubes by releasing hemostats. This is an open system, and appropriate biohazard precautions should be followed. Reapply hemostats and remove needle from donor's arm.[55]

13. Once the needle has been removed from the donor's arm, apply pressure over gauze, and ask the donor to raise his or her arm, continuing to exert pressure over the site. When the bleeding has stopped, the donor can lower his or her arm, and an appropriate bandage can be applied.

14. The needle assembly should be discarded into an appropriate biohazard receptacle. The tubing should be stripped to allow proper mixing of anticoagulant/preservative with blood.

15. Make a hermetic seal to the segments, and apply an appropriate identification label to one segment for storage. A dielectric sealer is generally used for heat sealing. Place blood at the appropriate temperature. Units in which platelets will be made must be stored at room temperature (20° to 24°C); all others can be stored at 1° to 6°C.

Postdonation Instructions

Most blood centers have a designated postdonation area where donors can sit and replenish their fluids. An example of postdonation instructions is shown in **Figure 11–9.**

Donor Reactions

Most donors tolerate the withdrawal of a unit of blood without incident; however, in the event an adverse reaction does occur, the donor room staff must be well trained and able to react immediately to the donor's need. Donor reactions cover a wide spectrum from nervousness and fainting to loss of consciousness. The donor staff should be trained in CPR. Reactions can generally be divided into three categories: mild, moderate, and severe.

Mild Reactions

Reactions in this category encompass one or more of the following: syncope or fainting, nausea or vomiting, hyperventilation, twitching, and muscle spasm. Syncope may be idiopathic with no known cause or be brought about by the sight of blood or by watching someone else give blood. The donor may show signs of sweating, dizziness, pallor, or convulsions. The following instructions apply for a donor who has fainted:

1. Remove the tourniquet and withdraw needle
2. Place cold compresses on the donor's forehead
3. Raise the donor's legs above the level of the head
4. Loosen tight clothing and secure airway
5. Monitor vital signs

Donors who are extremely nervous may exhibit sudden twitching or muscle spasms. If this happens, try to disengage

LifeSouth Community Blood Centers
1221 NW 13th Street
Gainesville, FL 32601

Post Donation Recommendations

Date:	Location:	Branch:

Donor Recommendations

Please read the following instructions and sign at the bottom.

1. Contact the blood center:

   - If any illness arises after your donation.

   - If you develop a headache and fever of 101°F or higher within 14 days following your donation or if you become diagnosed with West Nile Virus infection.

   - If you have any questions about your donation or if you remember something about your medical or personal history that may affect your blood donation.

2. Do not smoke for one-half hour.

3. Eat and drink something before leaving.

4. Do not leave until released by the donor technician.

5. Drink more fluids (nonalcoholic) than usual in the next four hours, especially fruit juices.

6. Leave the bandage on for a few hours, and then you may remove it. If there is any bleeding from the puncture site, raise arm, and apply direct pressure.

7. If you feel faint or dizzy, either lie down or sit down with head between the knees.

8. Do not perform strenuous activities or engage in critical work where safety requires your maximum abilities.

9. If any symptoms persist, either return to blood center or see your doctor.

Signatures

_____   _____

_____   _____

_____   _____

_____   _____

_____   _____

_____   _____

_____   _____

_____   _____

Thank you for your blood donation.

■ **FIGURE 11–9**   Postdonation instructions. (LifeSouth Blood Center, Montgomery, AL, with permission.)

the hyperventilation sequence by engaging in conversation with the donor and having the donor breathe into a paper bag, if necessary. It is not advised to give oxygen to these donors.

If the donor starts to feel nauseated or starts to vomit, the following instructions apply:

1. Instruct the donor to breathe slowly
2. Apply cold compresses to the forehead
3. Turn the donor's head to one side and provide an appropriate receptacle
4. The donor may be given water after vomiting has ceased

Moderate Reactions

A moderate reaction can include any of the reactions listed above in addition to loss of consciousness. The donor may have a decreased pulse rate, may hyperventilate, and exhibit a fall in systolic pressure to 60 mm Hg. The following instructions apply:

1. Check vital signs frequently
2. Administer 95 percent oxygen and 5 percent carbon dioxide

Severe Reactions

The presence of convulsions exhibited by the donor defines severe reactions. Convulsions can be caused by cerebral ischemia, marked hyperventilation, or epilepsy. The former is associated with vasovagal syncope or reduced blood flow to the brain owing to the shock symptoms, and hyperventilation is caused by marked depletion of carbon dioxide. The following should be followed by the donor room personnel:

1. Call for help immediately; notify blood bank physician
2. Try and restrain the donor to prevent injury to self or others
3. Ensure an adequate airway

In the event of cardiac or respiratory difficulties, the donor room staff should perform CPR until medical help arrives.

Hematomas

A hematoma is a localized collection of extravasated blood under the skin, resulting in a bluish discoloration. It is caused by the needle going through the vein, with subsequent leakage of blood. If a hematoma develops, the following instructions apply:

1. Remove the tourniquet and needle from donor's arm
2. Apply pressure with sterile gauze pads for 7 to 10 minutes, with the donor raising his or her arm above the heart
3. Apply ice to the area for 5 minutes

Donor Records

Donor records must be retained by the blood collection facility as mandated by the FDA and AABB. There must be a system to ensure the confidentiality of the donor is not compromised and that donor records are not altered. There must be policies on record-keeping and storage, and the blood bank staff should be well trained on these policies and procedures.

The minimum retention time for donor records varies from 5 to 10 years to indefinite retention.[56] Table 11–1 lists minimum retention times for various donor records.

Donor Processing

The donor unit collected must be tested and *processed* by blood bank technologists before it can be made available for transfusion. The tests performed on donor blood include the following:

- ABO/Rh
- Antibody screen
- HBsAg
- Anti-HBc
- Anti-HCV and NAT
- Anti-HIV 1/2 and NAT
- WNV RNA
- Anti-HTLV I/II
- Serologic test for syphilis
- WNV RNA

TABLE 11–1 Retention of Donor Records	
Donor Record	**Retention Time (years)**
Donor ABO/Rh	10
Donor antibody screen	10
Informed consent for donation	10
Medical director approval for donation interval	5
Physical examination	10
Medical history information	10
Identification number of donor unit	10
Viral marker testing results	10
Quarantine of donor unit	10
Repeat testing of donor blood	5
ID of donor processing tech	10
Plt count for frequent platelet pheresis	5
Sedimenting agent of leukopheresis	5
Notification of abnormal results	10/indefinite

Modified from *AABB Standards*, American Association of Blood Banks, Bethesda, MO 2002, p. 32.

ABO/Rh

Testing for the donor's ABO group must include both forward and reverse grouping. The ABO group must be determined by testing the donor RBCs with anti-A and anti-B reagents and by testing the donor serum or plasma with reagent A_1 cells and B cells.

The Rh type of the donor should be determined by testing with anti-D reagent at the immediate spin phase. In the event the initial testing is negative, a test for weak D should be performed. This involves a 37°C incubation and an antihuman globulin (AHG) phase. If both the immediate spin and test for weak D are negative, label the donor as Rh-negative; if, however, any part of the testing yields a positive test for D, the donor unit should be labeled as Rh-positive.

Antibody Screen

AABB *Standards* requires that donors with a history of pregnancy or transfusion be tested for unexpected antibodies to RBC antigens.[57] In the case of donors, a pooled screening cell is usually tested against donor serum or plasma. The pooled screening cell contains antigens directed toward significant alloantibodies. A control system must be in place for the method used. For example, in the tube system, cells sensitized with IgG are added to all negative tubes after the AHG phase; if the Gel system is used, the blood center must follow the manufacturer's guidelines. Most blood centers choose to perform a test for unexpected antibodies on all donors, not just those with a history of pregnancy or transfusion. The introduction of automated instruments for donor processing has helped to lessen the tedious workload of ABO/Rh and antibody screens on donors. See the later section on automation.

HBsAg

The test procedure used must be one approved by the FDA[58] or a documented equivalent method. The methods currently approved are the radioimmunoassay (RIA), enzyme-linked immunosorbent assay (ELISA), and reverse passive hemagglutination (RPHA). Of the three, the ELISA is the most common procedure used. In this method, serum or plasma is incubated with antigen to HBsAg. An enzyme-conjugate mixture is added, and if the antibody is specific to the antigen, a color change develops and can be quantified spectrophotometrically.

If the ELISA yields negative results, no further testing is warranted; however, in the case of reactive results, the screening test must be repeated in duplicate, and a positive result is one in which one or both of the repeated tests are positive. All components must be discarded when results are positive.

A supplemental test for HBsAg is neutralization.[59] In this method, the donor specimen is reacted with serum known to contain antibody to HBsAg. If the positive reaction dissipates upon incubation by at least 50 percent, the original screening result is confirmed as a true positive as long as controls work as expected.

In the event the donor unit is needed in an emergency that precludes completion of viral marker testing, a notation indicating testing is not yet completed must be conspicuously attached to the unit. If positive tests are found, the transfusion service must be notified as soon as possible.

Anti-HBc

Antibody to the core or interior protein on the hepatitis B virus has been implicated in hepatitis C disease. This test was once part of surrogate testing, along with its counterpart alanine transferase (ALT). In 1995 a National Institutes of Health consensus panel voted to discontinue the ALT test for blood donors because of the increased sophistication and sensitivity for anti-HCV testing[60]; however, testing for anti-HBc has remained a requirement of blood donors in the prevention of post-transfusion hepatitis B. The methods employed are similar to those for HBsAg.

Anti-HCV and NAT

The hepatitis C virus was identified in 1988[61] and was initially referred to as non-A, non-B hepatitis. Screening tests for anti-HCV involve enzyme immunoassay (EIA) methods whose sensitivity has increased through three generations of screening kits. Current assays detect antibodies to c200, c22–3, and NS-5 proteins of the HCV genome. In 1999 NAT for HCV RNA was implemented as a donor screening assay under FDA-sanctioned Investigational New Drug applications.[62] NAT is able to detect small amounts of viral nucleic acid in blood before antibodies or viral proteins such as HCV core antigen are detectable by current methods. The window period for detection of HCV is reduced by approximately 70 percent, from a mean of 82 days to 25 days.[63]

Confirmatory methods include the RIBA (recombinant immunoblot assay). In this assay, fusion of HCV antigens to human superoxide dismutase and a recombinant superoxide dismutase is incorporated to detect nonspecific reactions. The test is reported as positive, negative, or indeterminate. An individual who is positive by RIBA is considered to have the HCV antibody.

Anti-HIV-1/2 and NAT

All donor units must be screened for the presence of the HIV-1/2 antibody using an FDA-approved EIA method.[58] If the initial screening test is negative, the unit is suitable for transfusion; if it is positive, the test must be repeated in duplicate. If any one of the duplicate tests is reactive, the unit must be discarded as well as any in-date components from prior donations.

Confirmation tests for HIV include the Western blot (Wb) and the immunofluorescence assay (IFA).

The Wb is performed using donor serum. HIV virus material is separated into bands according to their molecular weight. Material is transferred to a nitrocellulose membrane, and donor serum is added. If antibodies to HIV are present, they will bind to specific bands. Results are expressed as positive, negative, or indeterminate.

In the IFA technique, cells infected with HIV are fixed onto a slide. Donor serum is added and incubated with the fixed cells. If the donor serum contains antibody to HIV, the antibody will bind to corresponding antigen on the cells. A fluorescent labeled anti-IgG is added, and reactivity is determined using a fluorescent microscope.

HIV-1 testing for blood donations began in 1999 and has effectively reduced the window period from 16 to 10 days. This test has replaced the HIV-1 Ag test once required by the AABB and FDA. Testing is done in pools of 16 or on an individual basis. Chapter 19 provides additional information on NAT testing for HIV.

WNV RNA

As previously discussed, outbreaks of WNV in the United States prompted donor testing for antibodies to WNV and, in 2003, NAT testing to detect RNA to the virus. Donor units are screened in pools of 6 or 16, and if the pool is reactive individual units are tested.[64] The Procleix WNV assay (Gen-Probe Inc) is a NAT test currently available in the United States under the FDA investigational New Drug Guidelines.

Anti-HTLV-I/II

The HTLV-I virus or human T-cell lymphotrophic virus type I is the causative agent of adult T-cell leukemia and has been associated with a neurologic disorder called HTLV-associated myelopathy. HTLV-II has been shown to have about 60 percent homology with type I and is prevalent among intravenous drug users in the United States.[65] Persons can contract both viruses from transfusion via infected lymphocytes. Screening for HTLV-I began in 1988; a combined HTLV-I/II was approved 10 years later in 1998. This is an EIA screening test that utilizes viral lysates from both viruses.

As with the other viral markers, a donation that is repeatedly reactive with EIA may not be used for transfusion. It is recommended that if another EIA kit is used by another manufacturer and that test is also positive, the donor should be indefinitely deferred.[66] Confirmatory tests include Western blot, RIPA, and NAT testing.

Syphilis

A serologic test for syphilis is required by both the AABB and FDA. Screening tests include the rapid plasma reagin and the Venereal Disease Research Laboratory. Both tests are based on reagin, or antibody directed toward cardiolipin particles. Cardiolipin-like antibodies have been documented in persons with untreated infections from syphilis. Antibody will agglutinate cardiolipin carbon particles in the form of visible flocculation.

The confirmatory test for syphilis is the FTA-ABS or fluorescent treponemal antibody absorption test. In this test, indirect immunofluorescence is used to detect antibodies to the spirochete *T. pallidum*, the agent that causes syphilis.

There have never been any documented cases of transfusion-transmitted syphilis. The spirochete that causes syphilis, *T. pallidum*, cannot survive more than 72 hours in citrated blood stored at 1° to 6°C, which would make platelets the only component capable of transmitting infection.

A serologic test for syphilis is also done because the disease is characterized as being sexually transmitted and places the donor at higher risk for possible exposure to hepatitis and HIV.

Automation

The blood banking industry has capitalized on the Gel Technology and Solid Phase automated test systems. The automated instruments on the market today use these methodologies to increase the efficiency and productivity of donor testing. They include the ABS2000, ROSYS Plato, ABS$_{HV}$, and Dynex dias Plus by Immucor (Norcross, GA), and the Tecan Megaflex and ProVue by Ortho-Clinical Diagnostics (Raritan, NJ). These systems are capable of performing ABO/Rh and antibody screens in the processing of donor blood in addition to donor crossmatching on the transfusion side. The Ortho Summit is a fully automated system capable of performing infectious disease assays to satisfy viral marker testing on donor units **(Fig. 11–10)**.

Solid Phase Technology

The ABS2000[67] **(Fig. 11–11)** is credited as being the first fully automated walk-away system designed to automate routine, labor-intensive processing, thus allowing technologists to complete other tasks. It performs ABO/Rh using hemagglutination and antibody screens/crossmatches using solid phase technology. The ABS2000 uses a barcode scanner to log reagents and samples, transfer specimens by automated pipetting, prepare RBC suspensions, incubate, wash, centrifuge, and read and interpret results. The on-line microprocessor can be interfaced with the data management system of the blood bank or blood center. Whereas the ABS2000 can perform low- to medium-volume workloads, the ROSYS

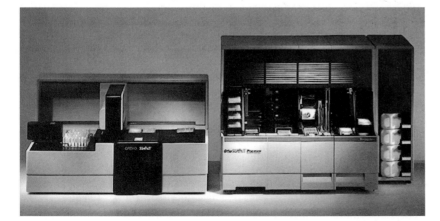

■ **FIGURE 11–10** Ortho Summit Instrument for Infectious Disease Testing. (Ortho Clinical Diagnostics, Raritan, NJ, with permission.)

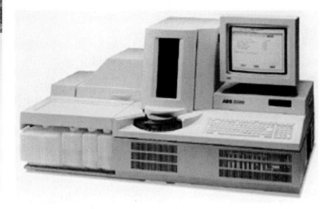

■ FIGURE 11–11 ABS2000 Instrument. (Immucor Inc, Norcross, GA, with permission.)

Plato[68] **(Fig. 11–12)** and ABS_{HV}[69] can perform medium-to high-volume testing. These instruments also use a barcode scanner to positively identify samples, pipet reagent and samples, incubate, wash, and interpret results at volumes of 1800 tests per shift. The Dias Plus System[70] performs high-volume testing (more than 300 tests per hour) and uses a robotic system and a closed washing system, thus minimizing biohazard exposure. This instrument is designed for 24-hour operation and high throughput. The newest addition to the Immucor line of automated instruments is the Galileo **(Fig. 11–13).** The Galileo is available in Europe and has acquired FDA clearance to be marketed in the United States. It is fully automated, bidirectional interface, and capable of medium- to high-volume testing for ABO, Rh, antibody screen donor testing, and compatibility testing.

The Gel System

Gel Technology was approved by the FDA in 1994 for blood banking procedures in the United States.[69] Ortho Clinical Diagnostics and Micro Typing Systems Inc (Pompano Beach, FL) nicely packaged this technology into a "gel card" containing six microtubes or gel chambers. Each chamber contains dextran acrylamide gel particles that facilitate trapping agglu-

tinates if agglutination of antibody and RBCs has occurred. The tests performed by this technology include ABO/Rh, direct antiglobulin testing, antibody screens and identification, and crossmatches. The semiautomated Tecan Megaflex[69] uses a barcode scanner to positively identify donor samples, pipets to transfer reagents and prepare RBC suspensions, a photo-optical centrifuge to read agglutination, and a microprocessor to process reports and interpret data (see **Fig. 15–13).** Gel technology does not require washing. The new ProVue is credited as the first fully automated blood banking system for use with the ID-Micro Typing System (ID-MTS) Gel Test. Micro Typing Systems has recently received clearance from the FDA to begin marketing the Ortho ProVue. It offers high volume testing and STAT capabilities to the blood bank laboratory (see **Fig. 15–12).**

Component Preparation

A single blood donation can provide transfusion therapy to multiple patients in the form of RBCs, platelets, fresh frozen plasma, and cryoprecipitate. Other products such as derivatives of plasma (e.g., immune serum globulin) also benefit patients in various disease states. This section describes the manufacturing process of all components used in transfusion therapy.

Whole Blood Modified

Whole blood contains RBCs and plasma, with a hematocrit level of approximately 38 percent. When the cryoprecipitate antihemophilic factor has been removed from the unit of whole blood, whole blood is referred to as whole blood modified.[71] The appropriate storage temperature is 1° to 6°C, and the shelf-life is dependent on the preservative used: that of ACD and CPD is 21 days, and that of CPDA-1 is 35 days.

Whole Blood Irradiated

Whole blood that has been irradiated to inhibit T-cell proliferation in the recipient has an expiration date of 28 days from the date of irradiation or the original outdate of the unit, whichever is sooner.

RBCs

RBCs are prepared by separating the RBCs from the plasma using a method that results in a final hematocrit level of less than or equal to 80 percent, depending on the anticoagulant/preservative used in collection.[72] RBCs are useful in patients who require the increased RBC mass but may be at risk of circulatory overload; for example, patients with anemia in addition to cardiac failure. RBCs can be prepared any time during the normal dating period by centrifugation or sedimentation. There is variation in the amount of plasma removed from the unit, depending on the anticoagulant-perservative solution used. When CPDA-1 is used, 200 to 250 mL of plasma can be removed. If additive solutions are employed, an additional 50 mL of plasma can be removed because 150 mL of adenine-saline is added back to the cells, achieving the desired hematocrit level of less than 80 percent.

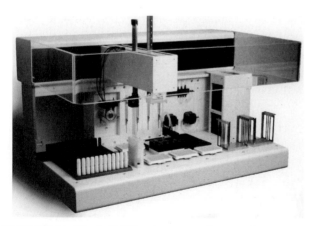

■ FIGURE 11–12 ROSYS Plato Instrument. (Immucor Inc, Norcross, GA, with permission.)

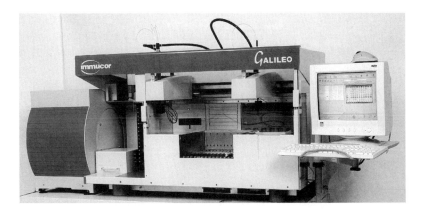

■ **FIGURE 11–13** Galileo Instrument.
(Immucor Inc, Norcross, GA, with permission.)

The following serves as a general procedure for RBC production using centrifugation:

1. Weigh and balance each unit.
2. Load units into a swinging bucket apparatus, making sure each unit is balanced. An assortment of rubber weights is generally used.
3. Centrifuge whole blood using a heavy spin. ($5000 \times g$ for 5 minutes in a refrigerated centrifuge). Temperature setting should be 4°C.
4. When the centrifuge has stopped completely, place the unit carefully onto an expressor and release the spring.
5. Express the plasma into the attached satellite bag. If more than one satellite bag is attached, apply hemostats to one of the bags so that the plasma will flow into only one bag. Remove the appropriate amount of plasma by using a scale. Approximately 230 to 256 g of plasma will yield a hematocrit level between 70 and 80 percent.[73]
6. When the appropriate amount of plasma has been removed, hemostats can again be applied to the satellite bag until such time as a dielectric heat sealer can separate the tubing. Always ensure the satellite bags have the same donor number as the primary bag.
7. Store the RBCs at 4°C. The plasma is stored depending on the product desired (FFP, liquid plasma, etc.).
8. Quality control on the hematocrit level of the RBCs is performed monthly; 75 percent of samples tested must yield a hematocrit level of 80 percent or less.

RBC Aliquots

Aliquotted RBCs is the product most often transfused during the neonatal period or infants younger than 4 months of age. Indications for transfusion include anemia caused by spontaneous fetomaternal or fetoplacental hemorrhage, twin-twin transfusion, obstetric accidents, and internal hemorrhage. Blood drawn from infants for laboratory testing (iatrogenic anemia) also may warrant a neonatal transfusion if more than 10 percent of the blood volume has been removed. Transfusions for neonates require only small volumes of RBCs (10 to 25 mL); several aliquots may be prepared from a single-donor unit. A multiple pack system or a quad pack is available for use when a single unit of whole blood is collected in a bag with four integrally attached containers; such a system can increase the number of transfusions an infant can receive

from one donor. Each pack retains the original outdate of the primary bag within a closed system. Sterile connecting devices can be used to maintain a closed system in attaching Pedipaks to a unit of RBCs.

The precise volume of blood desired can be aspirated into a syringe through a large-bore needle inserted through an injection site coupler. The filled syringe should be closed securely with a sterile cap and labeled with expiration date, patient identification, volume transfused, preservative, and ABO type. The aliquotted blood has an expiration time of 24 hours and should be stored at 1–6°C until issued.

Initial testing for neonates includes ABO, Rh, and antibody screen for unexpected antibodies, which can be performed on serum or plasma from the infant or mother. *AABB Standards*[74] states repeat ABO and Rh typing may be omitted for the remainder of the neonate's hospital admission; in the event the initial screen for RBC antibodies is negative, it is not necessary to crossmatch donor RBCs for the initial or subsequent transfusions. If the antibody screen is positive for clinically significant RBC antibodies, the neonate must receive blood that does not contain the corresponding antigen or is compatible by the antiglobulin crossmatch.

The anticoagulant most often used for neonate transfusions is CPDA-1. A transfusion of 10 mL/kg in a unit with a hematocrit level of 80 percent should raise the hemoglobin by 3 g/dL.[75] Some institutions, however, have begun using additive solutions for neonatal transfusions when the volume transfused is minimal. Concerns with additive solutions involve the constituents adenine and mannitol and their toxic effects on the renal system. Most physicians advocating the use of additive solutions do so in the limited setting of small-volume transfusions.

RBCs Irradiated

Patients who are immunocompromised or who are receiving a bone marrow or stem cell transplant, fetuses undergoing a intrauterine transfusion, and recipients of units from blood relatives or of HLA selected platelets must receive irradiated blood and/or platelets to inhibit the proliferation of T cells and subsequent transfusion-associated graft-versus-host disease. RBCs, platelets, and granulocyte concentrates contain viable T lymphocytes.

Both the FDA and AABB recommend a minimum dose of

gamma irradiation of 25 Gy to the central portion of the blood unit, with no less than 15 Gy delivered to any part of the blood unit.[76] Irradiation is generally performed using cesium-137 or cobalt-60. To confirm a product was irradiated, a radiochromic film label is affixed to the component before it is placed into the metal canister of the irradiator. Darkening of the film confirms irradiation requirements. Each facility should have a protocol and procedure for irradiation of blood components, training of personnel using the irradiator, and issuing of irradiated components. The expiration date of platelets that have been irradiated does not change from the original outdate; however, the expiration of RBCs irradiated is 28 days from the time of irradiation or the original outdate, whichever is sooner.

RBCs Leukoreduced

RBCs leukoreduced are products in which the absolute WBC count in the unit is less than 5×10^6 and must contain at least 85 percent of the original RBC mass per *AABB Standards*.[77] There are two major categories of leukoreduced RBCs: prestorage and poststorage.

In prestorage leukoreduction, special filters procure at least a 99.9 percent removal of leukocytes by employing multiple layers of synthetic nonwoven fibers that trap leukocytes and platelets but that allow RBCs to flow through. The impetus for prestorage leukoreduction involved biologic response modifiers (BRMs) released from leukocytes during storage of the component that were found to promote febrile transfusion reactions. Examples of BRMs include proinflammatory cytokines (interleukin-1, interleukin-6, and tumor necrosis factor) and complement fragments (C5a and C3a).[78] There are three methods available in prestorage leukoreduction. In the first method, an in-line filter can be attached to the whole blood unit and filtered via gravity; RBCs and plasma can then be prepared. In the second method, plasma is initially removed from the whole blood unit, and then the blood is passed through an in-line reduction filter for the production of RBCs. In both these methods, random-donor platelets cannot be prepared as they would have been trapped in the filter. In the third method, a sterile docking device can be used to attach a leukocyte reduction filter to a unit of RBCs, which is allowed to flow via gravity.

In poststorage leukoreduction, leukocytes are removed in the blood bank prior to issuing blood or at the bedside before transfusion. Whereas centrifugation can procure counts less than 5×10^8, which can prevent most febrile hemolytic reactions to RBC concentrates, third-generation filters reduce leukocytes to levels of 5×10^6 or lower. Removal of leukocytes by centrifugation or filtration just before transfusion of blood should prevent reactions that are caused by leukocyte antibody in patient's plasma and leukocytes present in the transfused blood but will not prevent reactions caused by BRMs that originate from the leukocytes present in the component during storage. Studies suggest that the age of the RBC unit is a predictor of a febrile reaction and that the cytokine involvement may be cumulative.[79]

Leukocytes in transfusion have been associated with febrile nonhemolytic transfusion reactions and transfusion related acute lung injury as well as transmission of Epstein-Barr virus, CMV, and human T-cell lymphotrophic virus.

Filtration

Many types of filters are available that can produce an acceptable leukocyte-reduced product, depending on the purpose for the WBC reduction and the intended recipient.

Third-generation filters use selective adsorption of leukocytes or leukocytes and platelets. They are made of polyester or cellulose acetate and will produce a 2- to 4-log (more than 99.9 percent) reduction of the WBCs ($<5 \times 10^6$) or platelets, or both. These filters provide a leukocyte-reduced product with normal shelf-life and meet the 85 percent retention of original RBCs.

Freezing, Deglycerolizing, and Saline Washing

RBCs that have been frozen, thawed, deglycerolized, and washed produce a leukoreduced product. Arnaud and Meryman[80] recently discovered removal of the buffy coat at time of collection lowered the level of leukocytes to acceptable limits (1.9×10^6) after freezing and deglycerolization; instituting such a protocol may provide a possible economic alternative to leukocyte filtration after freezing. Saline washing during deglycerolization ensures all donor plasma is removed and can be used for patients with paroxysmal nocturnal hemoglobinuria and IgA deficiency with circulating anti-IgA. This product has a shelf-life of 24 hours because it is an open system and requires special equipment to carry out the procedure.

Frozen, Deglycerolized RBCs

Freezing RBCs with glycerol dates back to the 1950s.[81] Frozen RBCs can be stored for up to 10 years for those patients with rare phenotypes, for autologous use, and in the case of national emergencies in which blood cannot be dispositioned out to hospitals quickly enough to prevent expiration. The resulting deglycerolized product is free of leukocytes, platelets, and plasma due to the washing process. Cryoprotective agents can be categorized as penetrating and nonpenetrating. A penetrating agent involves small molecules that cross the cell membrane into the cytoplasm. The osmotic force of the agent prevents water from migrating outward as extracellular ice is formed, preventing intracellular dehydration. An example of a penetrating agent is glycerol. An example of a nonpenetrating agent is hydroxyethyl starch (HES). This comprises large molecules that do not enter the cell but instead form a shell around the cell, preventing loss of water and subsequent dehydration. HES as well as dimethylsulfoxide is used to freeze hematopoietic progenitor cells.

Two procedures used for deglycerolizing RBCs are the high glycerol and low glycerol methods. The methods differ in the equipment used, the temperature of storage, and the rate of freezing. Most blood centers practice the high glycerol method, which is outlined in Table 11–2.

High Glycerol (40 Percent Weight per Volume)

This method increases the cryoprotective power of the glycerol, thus allowing a slow, uncontrolled freezing process. The freezer is generally a mechanical freezer that provides storage at $-80°C$. This particular procedure is probably the one

TABLE 11-2   Key Steps in Freezing Red Cells Using High Glycerol Concentration

Preparation	Glycerolization	Deglycerolization
Weigh RBCs Adjust to 260–400 g 0.9% NaCl Prewarm RBCs and glycerol to 25°C	Place cells on a shaker and add 100 mL glycerol Stop agitation and allow cells to equilibrate 5–30 min	Thaw frozen cells at 37°C in water bath Deglycerolize cells using a continuous flow washer
Set glycerol bottles in a water bath for 15 min at 25–37°C	Let partially glycerolized cells flow into freezing bag; slowly add glycerol	Apply a deglycerolize label to transfer pack; ABO, Rh, WB unit #s and expiration date
Label the freezing bag with name of facility, whole blood unit #s, ABO, Rh, date collected, date frozen, cryoprotective agent, expiration, and "red blood cells frozen"	Maintain glycerolized cells at 24–32°C until ready to freeze (not to exceed 4 hours)	Dilute unit with hypertonic 12% NaCl and let equilibrate for 5 min
	Freeze at ≤ 65°C	Wash with 1.6% NaCl until residual glycerol is less than 1%; wash with 0.9% NaCl plus 0.2% dextrose; Store at 1–6°C

most widely used because the equipment is fairly simple and the products require less delicate handling. It does, however, require a larger volume of wash solution for deglycerolization. RBCs are frozen within 6 days of collection when the preservative is CPD or CPDA-1 and up to 42 days when preserved in AS-1, AS-3, and AS-5. *AABB Standards*[82] states RBCs must be placed in the freezer within 4 hours of opening the system. It is advisable to freeze a sample of donor serum in the event additional testing is required for donor screening.

The thawing process takes approximately 30 minutes and involves immersion of units into a 37°C waterbath and washing the RBCs with solutions of decreasing osmolarity (e.g., 12% NaCl, 1.6% NaCl, 0.9% NaCl, + 0.2% dextrose). An exception to this rule is a donor with sickle trait in which RBCs would hemolyze upon suspension in hypertonic solutions; in this case the cells would be washed in 12% NaCl and then 0.9% NaCl with 0.2% dextrose, omitting the 1.6% solution. Automated continuous-flow instruments can be utilized for washing. Once the RBCs have been deglycerolized, the unit is considered an open system with an expiration date of 24 hours and is stored at 1° to 6°C.

Low Glycerol (20 Percent Weight per Volume)

In this method, the cryoprotection of the glycerol is minimal, and a very rapid, more controlled freezing procedure is required. Liquid nitrogen (N_2) is routinely used for this method. The frozen units must be stored at about −120°C, which is the temperature of liquid N_2 vapor. Because of the minimal amount of protection by the glycerol, temperature fluctuations during storage can cause RBC destruction.

The quality control procedures necessary for RBC freezing include all of the standard procedures for monitoring refrigerators, freezers, water baths, dry thaw baths, and centrifuges. They also include procedures to ensure good RBC recovery (80 percent), good viability (70 percent survival at 24 hours post-transfusion), and adequate glycerol removal (less than 1

percent residual intracellular glycerol). Valeri et al[83] froze RBCs for up to 37 years by using the high glycerol method (40 w/v) and yielded an average RBC recovery of 75 percent, with 1 percent hemolysis. Although researchers are attempting to freeze cells for more than 10 years, the FDA has not yet been swayed to change the maximum storage time. Studies have also shown that frozen, deglycerolized RBCs that have been irradiated (25 Gy) yield results similar to those of RBC recovery and post-transfusion survival rather than to those units not irradiated.[84] Cells should be frozen within 6 hours of collection unless they have been rejuvenated. Rejuvenation serves to increase the levels of 2,3-DPG and ATP in RBCs stored in citrate/phosphate/dextrose (CPD) or CPDA-1 using an FDA approved solution. RBCs can be rejuvenated up to 3 days after expiration and then glycerolized and frozen. The following comprise quality control procedures for deglycerolization:

1. RBC recovery can be determined by estimating the recovered RBC mass:

$$\% \text{ Recovery} = \frac{\text{wt. of DRBC (g)} \times \text{Hct of DRBC} \times 100}{\text{wt. of liquid RBC (g)} \times \text{Hct of liquid RBC}}$$

DRBC = deglycerolized RBCs

2. A post-transfusion survival study should be done when the program is first being set up to ensure the proper use of the equipment and procedure. If the procedure being used is standard, with data already published in the literature, these survival studies are not required.

3. Glycerol must be removed to a level of less than 1 percent residual. The published procedures should accomplish this. It is important, however, to perform this check on each unit before releasing it for transfusion.
   - Measure the osmolarity of the unit using an osmometer. The osmolarity should be about 420 mOsm (maximum 500 mOsm).
   - Perform a simulated transfusion. Place one segment (approximately 3 inches) of deglycerolized

cells into 7 mL of 0.7 percent NaCl. Mix, centrifuge, and check for hemolysis. Compare with a standard hemoglobin color comparator. If the hue exceeds the 500 mOsm level, hemolysis is too great, and the unit is not suitable for transfusion. Postdeglycerolized tests include confirmation of ABO, Rh, and a direct antiglobulin test.

Platelet Concentrates

Platelet concentrates can be produced during the routine conversion of whole blood into concentrated RBCs or by apheresis; more and more blood centers are producing apheresis platelets because of the high yield and minimal RBC contamination. Platelets have widespread use for a variety of patients: actively bleeding patients who are thrombocytopenic (less than 50,000/μL) due to decreased production or decreased function, cancer patients during radiation and chemotherapy because of induced thrombocytopenia (less than 20,000/μL), and thrombocytopenic preoperative patients (less than 50,000/μL). Prophylactic platelet transfusion is not usually indicated or recommended in disseminated intravascular coagulation (DIC) or idiopathic thrombocytopenic purpura (ITP). In both cases, there is an induced thrombocytopenia owing to increased destruction in ITP and consumption in DIC.

Platelet concentrates prepared from whole blood are generally referred to as random-donor platelets to distinguish them from single-donor platelets produced by apheresis. Random-donor platelet concentrates should contain at least 5.5×10^{10} platelets, are stored at 20° to 24°C with continuous agitation, contain sufficient plasma to yield a pH of greater than or equal to 6.2, and have a shelf-life of 5 days.[85] Apheresis or single-donor platelets contain at least 3.0×10^{11} platelets, are stored at 22° to 24°C with agitation, contain approximately 300 mL of plasma, and also have a shelf-life of 5 days.[85] Single-donor platelets are generally indicated for patients who are unresponsive to random platelets due to HLA alloimmunization or to limit the platelet exposure from multiple donors. However, as more blood suppliers are instituting apheresis platelets as their platelet product of choice, patients without the aforementioned restrictions are receiving single-donor platelets.

Whole blood used for the preparation of platelet concentrates must be drawn by a single nontraumatic venipuncture, and the concentrate must be prepared within 6 hours of collection. The following is a general procedure for preparing random-donor platelets:

1. Maintain the whole blood at 20° to 24°C before and during platelet preparation.
2. Set the centrifuge temperature at 22°C. The rpm and time must be specifically calculated for each centrifuge. It will generally be a short (2 to 3 minute), light (3200 rpm) spin. This spin should separate most of the RBCs but leave most of the platelets suspended in the plasma.
3. Platelet preparation should be done in a closed, multibag system.
4. Express off the platelet-rich plasma into one of the satellite bags. Enough plasma must remain on the RBCs to maintain a 70 to 80 percent hematocrit level.

5. Seal the tubing between the RBC and the plasma. Disconnect the RBC and store it at 4°C.
6. Recentrifuge the platelet-rich plasma at 22°C using a heavy spin (approximately 3600 rpm for 5 minutes). This will separate the platelets from the plasma.
7. Express the majority of the plasma into the second satellite bag, leaving approximately 50 to 70 mL on the platelets. The volume is important to maintain the pH above 6.2 during storage.
8. Seal the tubing between the bags and separate. Make segments for both the platelets and the plasma for testing purposes.
9. The plasma can be stored as FFP, single-donor plasma frozen within 24 hours (PF24), or liquid recovered plasma. Be sure to record the plasma volume on the bag.
10. Allow the platelet concentrate to lie undisturbed for 1 to 2 hours at 20° to 24°C. Be sure the platelet button is covered with the plasma. Platelets should be resuspended. Gentle manipulation can be used if needed.
11. Shelf-life is 5 days from the date of collection. If the system is opened, transfusion must occur within 6 hours. The volume, expiration date, and time (if indicated) must be on the label.
12. All of the units for a single dose (typically 6 to 8 units for an adult) can be pooled into a single bag before transfusion. Once pooled, the product must be transfused within 4 hours of pooling.[86] The pooled unit must be given a unique pool number, which must be placed on the label.

The quality control procedures must include a platelet count (5.5×10^{10} for random donor, 3.0×10^{11} for single donor), pH (6.2 or greater), and volume (must be sufficient to maintain an acceptable pH until the end of the dating period). A new standard, included in the 22nd edition of *Standards,* requires transfusion services to have methods in place to limit and detect bacterial contamination in platelet components. This will include improved phlebotomy techniques, culture and staining methods to detect bacterial organisms, dipsticks to detect bacterial levels, and a swirling technique to detect metabolic changes in platelets. These procedures are performed monthly, depending on the production volume at the end of the product's dating period. Generally one to four units are tested per month. Ninety percent of all units tested must meet or exceed the minimum standards. Temperature monitoring must be performed during each major stage of production, and records must be maintained of all procedures performed.

Platelets, either random-donor or single-donor, can be irradiated if the patient's diagnosis indicates that it is appropriate. The irradiation requirements are the same for RBCs and does not affect the shelf-life of the platelet product.

Platelet Aliquots

Transfusion of platelet concentrates is indicated for neonates whose counts fall below 50,000/μL and who are experiencing bleeding. Factors that may be associated with thrombocytopenia include immaturity of the coagulation system, platelet dysfunction, increased destruction of platelets, dilu-

70. http://www.immucor.com/DiasPlus.htm
71. Menitove, JE (ed): Standards for Blood Banks and Transfusion Services, ed 19. American Association of Blood Banks, Bethesda, MD, 1999, p 26.
72. Menitove, JE (ed): Standards for Blood Banks and Transfusion Services, ed 21. American Association of Blood Banks, Bethesda, MD, 2002, p 31.
73. Brecher, ME (ed): Technical Manual, ed 14. American Association of Blood Banks, Bethesda, MD, 2002, p 738.
74. Menitove, JE (ed): Standards for Blood Banks and Transfusion Services, ed 21. American Association of Blood Banks, Bethesda, MD, 2002, p 46.
75. Triulzi, DJ (ed): Blood Transfusion Therapy: A Physician's Handbook, ed 7. American Association of Blood Banks, Bethesda, MD, 2002, p 73.
76. Butch, SH, and Tiehen, A: Blood Irradiation: A User's Guide. American Association of Blood Banks, Bethesda, MD, 1996, p 4.
77. Menitove, JE (ed): Standards for Blood Banks and Transfusion Services, ed 21. American Association of Blood Banks, Bethesda, MD, 2002, p 32.
78. Heddle, NM, and Kelton, JG: Febrile nonhemolytic transfusion reactions. In Popovsky, MA: Transfusion Reactions. American Association of Blood Banks, Bethesda, MD, 1996, p 56.
79. Heddle, NM, et al: A prospective study to identify the risk factors associated with acute reactions to platelet and red cell transfusions. Transfusion 33:794, 1993.
80. Arnaud, FG, and Meryman, HT: WBC reduction in cryopreserved RBC units. Transfusion 43:517, 2003.
81. Smith, AU: Prevention of haemolysis during freezing and thawing of red blood cells. Lancet 2:910, 1950.
82. Menitove, JE (ed): Standards for Blood Banks and Transfusion Services, ed 21. American Association of Blood Banks, Bethesda, MD, 2002, p 31.
83. Valeri, CR, et al: An experiment with glycerol-frozen red blood cells stored at −80 degrees C for up to 37 years. Vox Sang 79:168, 2000.
84. Suda, BA, et al: Characteristics of red cells irradiated and subsequently frozen for long-term storage. Transfusion 33:389, 1993.
85. Menitove, JE (ed): Standards for Blood Banks and Transfusion Services, ed 21. American Association of Blood Banks, Bethesda, MD, 2002, p 35.
86. Ibid, p 61.
87. Brecher, ME (ed): Technical Manual, ed 14. American Association of Blood Banks, Bethesda, MD, 2002, p 528.
88. Menitove, JE (ed): Standards for Blood Banks and Transfusion Services, American Association of Blood Banks, Bethesda, MD, 2002, p 62.
89. Brecher, ME (ed): Technical Manual, ed 14. American Association of Blood Banks, Bethesda, MD, 2002, p 166.
90. Triulzi, DJ: Blood Transfusion Therapy: A Physician's Handbook, ed 7. American Association of Blood Banks, Bethesda, MD, 2002, p 28.
91. Brecher, ME (ed): Technical Manual, ed 14. American Association of Blood Banks, Bethesda, MD, 2002, p 469.
92. Erhardtsen, E: Ongoing NovoSeven® trials. Intensive Care Med 28:2, 2002.
93. Hedner, U: Recombinant factor VIIa (NovoSeven) as a hemostatic agent. Semin Hematol 38:43, 2001.
94. Hedner, U. Recombinant factor VIIa (NovoSeven) as a hemostatic agent. Dis Mon 49:39, 2003.
95. Astermark, J, et al: Antibodies to factor VIIa in patients with haemophilia and high-responding inhibitors. Br J Haematol 119:342, 2002.
96. Hoffman, M, and Monroe, DM: The action of high-dose factor VIIa in a cell-based model of hemostasis. Dis Mon 49:14, 2003.
97. Saba, HI, et al: Efficacy of NovoSeven® during surgery on a haemophiliac with previous history of inhibitors. Haemophilia 9:131, 2003.
98. Lee, CA: The evidence behind inhibitor treatment with porcine factor VIII. Pathophysiol Haemost Thromb 32 (suppl 1): 5, 2002.
99. Freedman, J et al: Platelet activation and hypercoagulability following treatment with porcine factor VIII (HYATE:C). Am J Hematol 69:192, 2002.
100. Suiter, TM: First and next generation native rFVIII in the treatment of hemophilia A. What has been achieved? Can patients be switched safely? Semin Thromb Hemost 28:277, 2002.
101. Triulzi, DJ (ed): Blood Transfusion Therapy: A Physician's Handbook. American Association of Blood Banks, Bethesda, MD, 2002, p 43.
102. Roth, DA, et al: Human recombinant factor IX: Safety and efficacy studies in hemophilia B patients previously treated with plasma-derived factor IX concentrates. Blood 98:3600, 2001.
103. The European Agency for the Evaluation of Medicinal Products: Note for guidance on the clinical investigation of recombinant factor VIII and IX products http://www.emea.eu.int/pdfs/human/ich/013595en.pdf Accessed Jan. 1997.
104. Gootenber, JE: Factor concentrates for the treatment of factor XIII deficiency. Curr Opin Hematol 5:372, 1998.
105. Dardik, R et al: Factor XIII mediates adhesion of platelets to endothelial cells through alpha(v)beta(3) and glycoprotein IIb/IIIa integrins. Thromb Res 105:317, 2002.
106. George, JN: Initial management of adults with idiopathic (immune) thrombocytopenic purpura. Blood Rev 16:37, 2002.
107. Triulzi, DJ (ed): Blood Transfusion Therapy: A Physician's Handbook. American Association of Blood Banks, Bethesda, MD, 2002, p 53.
108. Konkle, BA, et al: Use of recombinant human antithrombin in patients with congenital antithrombin deficiency undergoing surgical procedures. Transfusion 43:390, 2003.
109. http://www.show.scot.nhs.uk/snbts/isbt128.htm

twelve

Detection and Identification of Antibodies

Kathleen S. Trudell, MT (ASCP), SBB

OBJECTIVES

On completion of this chapter, the learner should be able to:

1. Differentiate between the following antibodies: expected and unexpected, immune, naturally occurring, passive, autoantibody and alloantibody, warm and cold.
2. Define what makes an antibody clinically significant.
3. Discuss which patient populations require an antibody screen.
4. Discuss the composition of screening cell sets.
5. Describe the impact of various enhancement media on antibody detection.
6. Compare and contrast antibody detection methods.
7. List the limitations of the antibody screen.
8. Interpret the results of an antibody identification panel.
9. Summarize the exclusion and inclusion methods.
10. Correlate knowledge of the serologic characteristics of commonly encountered antibodies with antibody identification panel findings.
11. Select cells to increase the probability of correct antibody identification.
12. Discuss antigen-typing techniques.
13. Calculate the number of red blood cell (RBC) units that must be antigen-tested to fulfill a physician's request for crossmatch.
14. Recognize when additional panel cells should be tested and select appropriate cells.
15. Explain the principles behind enzyme and neutralization techniques.
16. Given a patient's history and initial results, choose the correct method for performing an adsorption.
17. Describe three techniques for elution and give an example of when each would be used.
18. Discuss three chemicals used in preparing a partial elution and the advantages of use.
19. Outline the antibody titer level procedure.
20. Calculate the antibody titer level and score.
21. Given a patient scenario, recommend additional steps to be taken in resolving complex antibody identification.
22. Outline the steps used to investigate a warm autoantibody.

Introduction

Antibody detection plays a critical role in transfusion medicine. It is a key process in pretransfusion compatibility testing. It aids in the detection and monitoring of patients who are at risk of delivering infants with hemolytic disease of the newborn (HDN). It is one of the principle tools for investigating potential hemolytic transfusion reactions and immune hemolytic anemias. The focus of antibody detection methods is on "irregular" or "unexpected" antibodies, as opposed to the "expected" antibodies of the ABO system. These unexpected antibodies may be immune alloantibodies, produced in response to RBC stimulation through transfusion, transplantation, or pregnancy. Other unexpected antibodies may be "naturally occurring," produced without RBC stimulation. Naturally occurring antibodies may form as a result of exposure to environmental sources, such as pollen, fungus, and bacteria, which may have structures similar to some RBC antigens. Another category of antibody is the passively acquired antibody. Passively acquired antibodies are produced in another individual and then transmitted to the patient through plasma-containing blood products or derivatives such as intravenous immunoglobulin (IVIG).

Of greatest concern are the unexpected antibodies that cause decreased survival of RBCs that possess the target antigen. These antibodies are deemed "clinically significant." Clinically significant antibodies are usually IgG antibodies that react at 37°C or in the antihuman globulin (AHG) phase of the indirect antiglobulin test. (I AT)

Autoantibodies complicate the detection of clinically significant antibodies. Autoantibodies are directed at antigens expressed on one's own RBCs. Because they react with all cells tested, autoantibodies may mask the presence of clinically significant alloantibodies.

After detection, an antibody identification panel is performed to determine the specificity of the antibody. Once the antibody is identified, the clinical significance can be ascertained, and the appropriate transfusion considerations are put into place.

This chapter will discuss antibody detection and identification methods as well as resolution of complex antibody cases.

Antibody Screen

Only a small percentage of the population (between 0.2 and 2 percent) has detectable RBC antibodies.[1-3] However, certain populations require careful screening. The American Association of Blood Banks (AABB) *Standards* requires the use of an antibody screen to detect clinically significant antibodies as part of pretransfusion testing on the recipient.[4] The method must include incubation at 37°C and the use of an antiglobulin test. An antibody screen is included in standard prenatal testing for obstetric patients in order to evaluate the risk of HDN in the fetus and to evaluate the mother's candidacy for Rh-immune globulin prophylaxis (RhIG). [5] The third group in which an antibody screen is required is donors of allogeneic blood and blood products and stem/progenitor cells.[6-8] When antibodies are detected in a blood donor, the resulting components will be labeled with the identity of the antibody (with the exception of cryoprecipitate and washed or frozen/deglycerolized RBCs). These donors may be used as a source of antigen-typing sera as well as antigen-negative RBC units. Antibodies detected in stem cell donors indicate that additional processing steps may be required to reduce the plasma in the product.

Tube Technique

Method

The traditional method of detecting antibodies is an indirect antiglobulin test performed in a test tube (**Fig. 12–1**). In this method, the patient's serum or plasma is tested against RBCs with known antigens. The test may include an immediate spin phase to detect antibodies reacting at room temperature. This phase is not required and may lead to the detection of clinically insignificant cold antibodies. The test must include a 37°C incubation phase. During this phase, immunoglobulin G (IgG) molecules sensitize antigen-carrying RBCs. Enhancement media may be added to increase the degree of sensitization. Depending on the enhancement added, the tubes might be centrifuged and observed for hemolysis or agglutination following the incubation. To observe for hemolysis, the tube is carefully removed from the centrifuge so as not to dislodge the RBC button. The supernatant is observed

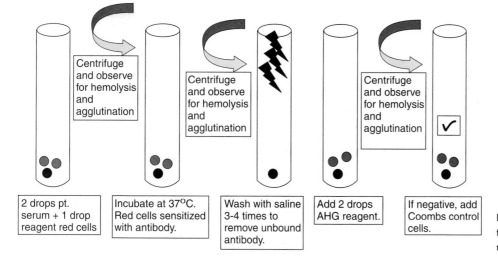

| 2 drops pt. serum + 1 drop reagent red cells | Incubate at 37°C. Red cells sensitized with antibody. | Wash with saline 3-4 times to remove unbound antibody. | Add 2 drops AHG reagent. | If negative, add Coombs control cells. |

■ FIGURE 12–1 Steps for performing the tube antibody screen test.

CELL	Rh								MNS				Lutheran		P	Lewis		Kell		Duffy		Kidd					
	D	C	E	c	e	f	V	Cʷ	M	N	S	s	Luᵃ	Luᵇ	P₁	Leᵃ	Leᵇ	K	k	Fyᵃ	Fyᵇ	Jkᵃ	Jkᵇ				
R1R1-29	+	+	0	0	+	0	0	0	+	0	+	0	0	+	+	+	0	0	+	+	0	+	0				
R2R2-45	+	0	+	+	0	0	0	0	+	+	0	+	0	+	+	0	+	+	+	+	0	0	+				
rr-86	0	0	0	+	+	+	0	0	0	+	0	+	0	+	+	+	0	0	+	0	+	+	+				

■ **FIGURE 12–2**   Antigen profile of 3-cell structure set.

for pink or red discoloration. To observe for agglutination, the tube is gently tilted or rolled to dislodge the cell button. The degree of reactivity is graded as 0 (negative, no agglutination present) to w+ (barely visible to the naked eye) to 4+ (one solid agglutinate) (see **Color Plate 2**). The degree of agglutination should be judged only after all of the cells have been dislodged from the bottom of the test tube. The tubes are then washed with saline a minimum of three times to remove all unbound antibody. AHG or Coombs' serum is added to each tube. The antibody in this reagent will create a bridge between sensitized RBCs, resulting in observable agglutination. If no antibodies are present, no sensitized RBCs will be present, and there will not be agglutination. With the addition of the AHG reagent, the tubes are centrifuged and examined for hemolysis and agglutination. In this phase, hemolysis may appear as a loss of cell button mass. Again depending on the enhancement media, the agglutination reactions may be observed macroscopically only, or macro- and microscopically. All negative tests will have Coombs' control cells (check cells) added to confirm the negative test.

RBC Reagents

The RBC reagents used in the antibody screen come from group O individuals who have been typed for the most common, and the most significant, RBC antigens. Group O cells are used so that anti-A and anti-B will not interfere in the detection of antibodies to other blood group systems. The cells are suspended at a concentration between 2 and 5 percent in a preservative diluent, which maintains the antigens and prevents hemolysis. The screening cells are packaged in sets of two or three cells with varied antigen expression. Within the set, there should be one cell that is positive for each of the following antigens: D, C, c, E, e, K, k, Fyᵃ, Fyᵇ, Jkᵃ, Jkᵇ, Leᵃ, Leᵇ, P₁, M, N, S, and s. Other antigens may be expressed as well. Each set of screening cells will be accompanied by an antigen profile sheet, detailing which antigens are present on each cell. These profiles are lot-specific and should not be interchanged. **Figure 12–2** shows an example of a three-cell profile.

Ideally, there will be homozygous expression of many of the antigens within the screening cell set, allowing for detection of antibodies that show dosage. A cell with homozygous expression is from an individual who inherited only one allele at a given locus. Therefore, the cell surface has a "double dose" of that antigen. A cell with heterozygous antigen expression is from a person who inherited two different alleles at a locus. The alleles "share" the available antigen sites on the cell surface. In **Figure 12–3**, the pair of chromosomes on the left both possess the same allele, giving rise to the "homozygous" RBC. The pair of chromosomes on the right each possess a different allele, resulting in the "heterozygous"

cell. Certain antibodies, such as those of the Kidd system, may be detected only when tested against a cell expressing one allele (homozygous). Antibodies that react more strongly with a "homozygous" cell are said to show dosage. Refer to **Table 12–1** for a list of antibodies that may show dosage. **Table 12–2** gives an example of RBC phenotypes, comparing homozygous and heterozygous expression.

When testing blood donors, it is acceptable to use a pooled screening reagent that contains cells from at least two different individuals. These reactions should be carefully observed for mixed field agglutination, as the target antigen may only be expressed on one cell in the pool.

Using commercially prepared screen cells to detect antibodies is superior to relying on the crossmatch alone to ensure compatibility with a donor RBC unit. The screen cell sets will test for most clinically significant antigens, whereas the crossmatched unit of blood will possess only some of those antigens. The screen cell sets will have cells with homozygous expression of many antigens, making it more reliable in the detection of weakly reacting antibodies. Donor units may or may not have homozygous antigen expression, so it is possible that weak antibodies may not be detected by crossmatch alone. As RBCs age, antigen expression begins to weaken. Commercially prepared screen cell sets are diluted in a preservative to maintain antigen integrity.

Enhancement Reagents

Various enhancement reagents, or potentiators, may be added to the cell/serum mixture before the 37°C incubation phase to increase the sensitivity of the test system. These reagents may also allow for a shortened incubation time.

22% Albumin: In an electrolyte solution, negatively charged RBCs are surrounded by cations, which in turn are surrounded by anions. The effect is to produce an ionic cloud around each RBC, forcing the cells apart. The difference in electrical potential between the surface of the RBC and the outer layer of the ionic cloud is called the zeta potential. Albumin works by reducing the zeta potential, dispersing the

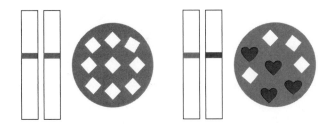

■ **FIGURE 12–3**   Homozygous inheritance versus heterozygous inheritance.

TABLE 12–1   Some Blood Group Systems that Exhibit Dosage

Rh (except D)
Kidd
Duffy
MNSs
Lutheran

charges, thus allowing the RBCs to approach each other, increasing the chances of agglutination. In **Figure 12–4**, the top illustration demonstrates the repulsion of RBCs due to the surrounding electrical charges. The lower figure illustrates that once those charges are dispersed by albumin (or some other enhancement reagent), the RBCs may approach each other more closely.

2. **Low Ionic Strength Solution (LISS):** LISS contains glycine in an albumin solution. In addition to lowering the zeta potential, LISS increases the uptake of antibody onto the RBC during the sensitization phase. This increases the possibility of agglutination.

3. **Polyethylene Glycol (PeG):** PeG in a LISS solution removes water from the test system, thereby concentrating any antibodies present. This increases the degree of RBC sensitization. PeG can cause nonspecific aggregation of cells, so centrifugation after the 37°C incubation is not performed. Generally, PeG test systems are more sensitive than LISS, albumin, or saline systems. However, in patients with elevated levels of plasma protein, such as in multiple myeloma, PeG is not appropriate for use due to increased precipitation of proteins.[9]

AHG Reagents

The addition of AHG reagent allows for the agglutination of incomplete antibodies. AABB *Standards* requires that the reagent contain anti-IgG when used for antibody detection and pretransfusion compatibility testing.[10] Polyspecific AHG reagent (also called polyvalent or broad spectrum Coombs' serum) contains antibodies to both IgG and complement components, either C3 and C4 or C3b and C3d. It has been suggested that antibodies to the C3 components, especially C3d, are more desirable in the reagent, as these are more abundant on the RBC surface during complement activation and lead to fewer cases of false-positive reactions.[11] The presence of complement in the Coombs' serum may lead to the detection of clinically insignificant antibodies. Relatively few examples of clinically significant antibodies, most notably Jk[a], react with complement alone.[12] To avoid time-consuming investigations of insignificant antibodies, many technologists choose to use monospecific AHG reagent containing anti-IgG only.

TABLE 12–2   Examples of Some RBC Phenotypes and Whether They Come from Homozygous or Heterozygous Individuals

Jk(a–b+)	Homozygous
Jk(a+b+)	Heterozygous
Fy(a+b–)	Homozygous
Fy(a+b+)	Heterozygous

Any test that is negative following the addition of the reagent should be controlled by the addition of Coombs' trol cells. These are Rh-positive cells that have been c with anti-D. These antibody-coated cells should agglutinate when added to the negative test due to the anti-IgG present in the AHG reagent. The addition of the Coombs' control cells proves that there was adequate washing performed before the addition of the AHG reagent, that the AHG reagent was added, and that the reagent was working properly. If the Coombs' control cells fail to agglutinate, the antibody screen must be repeated.

Use of the tube test remains popular, due to the flexibility of the test system, use of commonly available laboratory equipment, and relative inexpensiveness. The disadvantages include the instability of the reactions and subjective nature of grading by the technologist, the amount of hands-on time for the technologist, and problems related to the failure of the washing phase to remove all unbound antibody.

Gel Technique

The antibody screen may also be performed using a microtubule filled with a dextran acrylamide gel. The screening cells used for this technique meet the same criteria as for the tube test but are suspended in LISS to a concentration of 0.8 percent. With this technique, the patient's serum or plasma specimen and screen cells are added to a reaction chamber that sits above the gel. There are up to six chamber/gel microtubules contained in a plastic card, about the size of a credit card. The card is incubated at 37°C for 15 minutes to 1 hour,[13] thus allowing sensitization to occur. The card is then centrifuged for 10 minutes. During this time, the RBCs are forced out of the reaction chamber down into the gel. The gel contains anti-IgG. If sensitization occurred, the anti-IgG will react with the antibody-coated cells, resulting in agglutination. The agglutinated cells will be trapped within the gel (because of the action of the anti-IgG and because the agglutinates are too large to pass through the spaces between gel particles.). If no agglutination occurred, the cells will form a pellet at the bottom of the microtubule **Fig. 12–5**.

There are numerous advantages to the gel technique. It is reported to be as sensitive as the PeG tube test method.[14] The omission of the washing and Coombs' control steps results in fewer hands-on steps for the technologist to perform. Reactions are stable for up to 24 hours and may be captured electronically, leading to standardized grading of reactions, and easier review by a supervisor. Mixed field reactions may be more readily detected with the gel technique. One of the greatest advantages is the ability to automate many of the pipetting and reading steps, thereby allowing increased productivity. Disadvantages include the need for incubators and centrifuges that can accommodate the gel cards.

Solid Phase Technique

A third method that is commonly used to perform the antibody screen is solid phase testing. With this method, RBC antigens coat microtiter wells instead of being present on intact RBCs **(Fig. 12–6A)**. The patient's serum or plasma is added to each well in the screen cell set along with LISS. Incubation at 37°C allows for sensitization **(Fig. 12–6B)**. The wells are then washed to remove unbound antibody. Rather

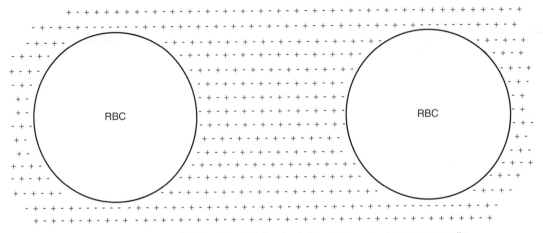

Electrical charges surrounding Red Blood Cells prior to the addition of enhancement media.

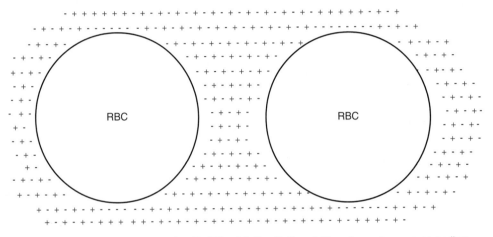

Electrical charges surrounding Red Blood Cells with the addition of an enhancement medium.

■ **FIGURE 12–4**   Use of enhancement reagents can lower the zeta potential, allowing for better interaction between RBCs and increasing the possibility of agglutination.

than AHG reagent, indicator cells are added. These cells are coated with anti-IgG. The wells are then centrifuged for several minutes. If sensitization occurred, the indicator cells react with the antibody bound to the antigens coating the microtiter well, forming a diffuse pattern in the well **(Fig. 12–6C)**. If no sensitization occurred (a negative reaction), the indicator cells form a pellet in the bottom of the well **(Fig. 12–6D)**.

The solid phase test has been successfully automated. Such instruments may perform pipetting steps and make determinations of the degree of reactivity by taking multiple readings of each well. Other advantages include a smaller sample size (when compared with the tube test), making it ideal in a pediatric setting, and a LISS reagent that changes color when added to serum or plasma. This ensures that an adequate sample is present in the test system. Among the disadvantages is that with such a small sample and reagent volume, careful pipetting is necessary when performing the test manually. An inadequate volume of indicator cells may result in a pattern similar to that of a weak positive reaction. Staff should be carefully trained to visually interpret results if automation is

not used. Staff members who have primarily used the tube test previously may interpret the diffuse positive pattern as a negative reaction and the dense pellet of the negative reaction as a positive (4+) reaction. Incubators, washers, and centrifuges that can hold the wells are among the special equipment needed for this method. A final disadvantage is the need to run a positive and negative control with each batch of tests, which adds to the expense of this method.

Interpretation

Agglutination or hemolysis at any stage of testing is a positive test result, indicating the need for antibody identification studies. However, evaluation of the antibody screen results (and autologous control, if run at this time) can provide clues and give direction for the identification and resolution of the antibody or antibodies. The investigator should consider the following questions:

1. **In what phase(s) did the reaction(s) occur?**
   Antibodies of the immunoglobulin M (IgM) class react best at low temperatures and are capable of causing agglu-

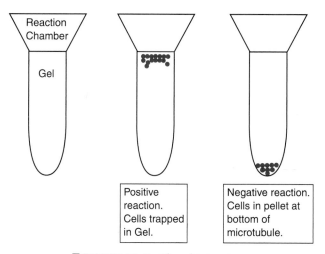

Reaction
Chamber

Gel

Positive reaction. Cells trapped in Gel.

Negative reaction. Cells in pellet at bottom of microtubule.

■ FIGURE 12–5   The gel test system.

tination of saline-suspended RBCs (immediate spin reading). Antibodies of the IgG class react best at the AHG phase. Of the commonly encountered antibodies, anti-N, anti-I, and anti-P$_1$ are frequently IgM, whereas those directed against Rh, Kell, Kidd, and Duffy antigens are usually IgG. Lewis and M antibodies may be IgG, IgM, or a mixture of both.

2. **Is the autologous control negative or positive?**
   The autologous control is the patient's cells tested against the patient's serum in the same manner as the antibody screen. A positive antibody screen and a negative autologous control indicate that an alloantibody has been detected. A positive autologous control may indicate the presence of autoantibodies or antibodies to medications. If the patient has been recently transfused, the positive autologous control may be caused by alloantibody coating circulating donor RBCs. Evaluation of samples with positive autologous control or direct antiglobulin test (DAT) results is often complex and may require a great deal of time and experience on the part of the investigator. Some technologists choose to omit the autologous control when performing the antibody screen and include it only when performing antibody identification studies.

3. **Did more than one screening cell sample react; if so, did they react at the same strength and phase?**
   More than one screening cell sample may be positive when the patient has multiple antibodies, when a single antibody's target antigen is found on more than one screening cell, or when the patient's serum contains an autoantibody. A single antibody specificity should be suspected when all cells react at the same phase and strength. Multiple antibodies are most likely when cells react at different phases and strengths, and autoantibodies are suspected when the autologous control is positive. **Figure 12–7** provides several examples of antibody screen results with possible causes.

4. **Is hemolysis or mixed-field agglutination present?**
   Certain antibodies, such as anti-Le^a, anti-Le^b, anti-PP^{1}P^k, and anti-Vel, are known to cause in-vitro hemolysis. Mixed-field agglutination is associated with anti-Sd^a and Lutheran antibodies.

5. **Are the cells truly agglutinated, or is rouleaux present?**
   Serum from patients with altered albumin-to-globulin ratios (e.g., patients with multiple myeloma) or who

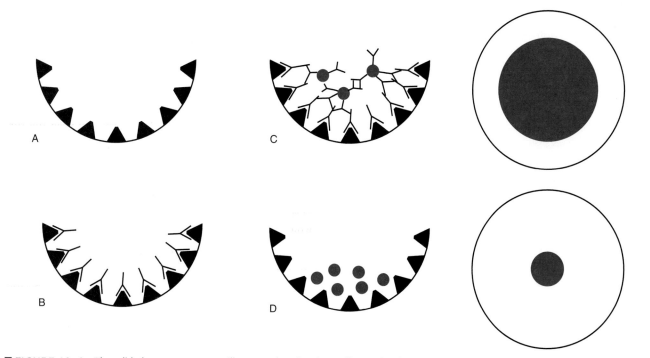

■ FIGURE 12–6   The solid phase test system. *A* illustrates the microtiter well coated with RBC antigens. In *B*, the patient's antibody has attached to the RBC antigens in the microtiter well. For *C* and *D*, the figure on the left is a detailed side view of what is taking place in the well, on a cellular level, and the figure on the right is the view looking down into the well, as the technologist would view it for grading purposes. *C* illustrates the reaction between the patient's antibodies and the indicator cells. In *D*, when no patient antibody is present, the indicator cells form a pellet at the bottom of the well.

			Results	**Possible Interpretation**
cell	IS	37°	AGT (poly)	1. Single alloantibody
SC I	neg	neg	neg	2. Two alloantibodies, antigens only present on cell II
SC II	neg	neg	2+	
auto	neg	neg	neg	3. Probably IgG antibody
cell	IS	37°	AGT	1. Multiple antibodies
SC I	neg	1+	3+	2. Single antibody (dosage)
SC II	neg	neg	1+	3. Probable IgG
auto	neg	neg	neg	
cell	IS	37°	AGT	1. Single or multiple antibodies
SC I	1+	neg	neg	2. Probably IgM antibodies
SC II	2+	neg	neg	
auto	neg	neg	neg	
cell	IS	37°	AGT	1. Multiple antibodies, warm and cold
SC I	2+	neg	1+	
SC II	3+	1+	2+	2. Potent cold antibody binding complement in AGT
auto	neg	neg	neg	
cell	IS	37°	AGT	1. Single warm antibody, antigen present on both cells
SC I	neg	neg	1+	
SC II	neg	neg	1+	2. Antibody to high-frequency antigen
auto	neg	neg	neg	3. Complement binding by a cold antibody not detected at IS
cell	IS	37°	AGT	1. Warm antibodies
SC I	neg	neg	3+	2. Transfusion reaction
SC II	neg	neg	3+	3. Probable IgG antibody
auto	neg	neg	3+	4. Warm autoantibody

■ **FIGURE 12–7**   Examples of reactions that may be obtained in antibody screening tests.

have received high-molecular-weight plasma expanders (e.g., dextran) may cause nonspecific aggregation of RBCs, known as rouleaux. Rouleaux is not a significant finding in antibody screening tests, but is easily confused with antibody-mediated agglutination. Knowledge of the following characteristics of rouleaux helps in differentiation between rouleaux and agglutination:

- Cells have a "stacked coin" appearance when viewed microscopically (see **Color Plate 2**).
- Rouleaux is observed in all tests containing the patient's serum, including the autologous control and the reverse ABO typing.
- Rouleaux does not interfere with the AHG phase of test-

ing because the patient's serum is washed away prior to the addition of the AHG reagent.
- Unlike agglutination, rouleaux is dispersed by the addition of one to three drops of saline to the test tube.

Limitations

Screening reagents and methods is designed to detect as many clinically significant antibodies as possible but not to detect those antibodies that are insignificant. When using a three-cell screen, a negative result with all three cells gives the technologist 95 percent confidence that no clinically significant antibodies are present.

Despite this, there are limitations to the antibody screen. The screen will not detect antibodies when the antibody titer level has dropped below the level of sensitivity for the screening method employed. One study, which reviewed antibodies detected over a 20-year period, showed that 26 percent of antibodies became undetectable over time, with a median time of 7 months.[15] The screen will also not detect antibodies to low-frequency antigens that are not present on any of the cells in the screen cell set.

Several factors may influence the sensitivity of the antibody screen. These include:

- **Cell-to-serum ratio.** When antibody is present in the test system in excess (when related to antigen), false-negative reactions occur as a result of prozone. When the antigen is in excess, false-negative reactions occur due to postzone. A ratio of two drops of serum to one drop of cells usually gives the proper balance between antigen and antibody to allow sensitization and agglutination to occur. Occasionally, when an antibody is weak, the amount of serum in the test system may be increased to four drops, providing more antibodies to react with the available antigens. This should be done only when potentiators have not been included in the test system.
- **Temperature.** The optimal temperature at which an antibody reacts can be a tool used in detection and identification. When performing pretransfusion compatibility testing, the focus is on clinically significant antibodies, which generally react at 37°C or with AHG. Technologists may omit the immediate spin and room temperature phases to limit the detection of insignificant cold antibodies. **Table 12–3** summarizes the optimal temperature of reactivity for some of the most common antibodies.
- **Length of incubation.** Antigen/antibody reactions are in dynamic equilibrium. If too little contact time is allowed, there will not be enough cells sensitized to detect with routine methods. If the incubation time is allowed to continue for too long, bound antibody may begin to dissociate from the cell. Incubation time is dependent on the medium in which the reaction takes place. A saline environment may require an incubation of 45 minutes to 1 hour, whereas potentiators may shorten the incubation time to as little as 10 minutes.
- **pH.** Most antibodies react best at a neutral pH between 6.8 and 7.2[16]; however, some examples of anti-M demonstrate enhanced reactivity at a pH of 6.5.[17] Acidifying the test system may aid in distinguishing anti-M from other antibodies.

Antibody Identification

Once an antibody has been detected, additional testing is necessary to identify the antibody and determine its clinical significance. The method used should be as sensitive as that used for detection.

Patient History

Information concerning the patient's age, sex, race, diagnosis, transfusion and pregnancy history, medications, and intravenous solutions may provide valuable clues in antibody identification studies, especially with complex cases. The patient's race may be valuable as some antibodies are associated with a particular race. For example, anti-U is associated with persons of African descent because most U-negative individuals are found in this race.

Transfusion and pregnancy history are helpful because patients who have been exposed to "non-self" RBCs via transfusion or pregnancy are more likely to have produced immune antibodies. Naturally occurring antibodies (e.g., anti-M, Le[b]) should be suspected in patients with no transfusion or pregnancy history. Medications such as IVIG, RhIG, and antilymphocyte globulin may passively transfer antibodies such as anti-A or anti-B, anti-D, and antispecies antibodies, respectively. This will result in the presence of an unexpected serum antibody that is likely to confound the interpretation of antibody identification.

The patient's history is especially important when the autologous control or DAT is positive. Certain infectious and autoimmune disorders are associated with production of RBC autoantibodies, and some medications are known to cause positive DATs. Furthermore, in a patient transfused within the past 3 months, a positive DAT result may indicate a delayed hemolytic transfusion reaction.

Information regarding recent transfusions is also important when antigen-typing the patient's RBCs. Antigen-typing results must be interpreted carefully when the patient has recently received a transfusion because positive reactions may be caused by the presence of donor RBCs in the patient's circulation. Positive reactions caused by donor RBCs usually

Phase	Room Temperature (immediate Spin)	37°C Incubation	Antiglobulin Phase
TABLE 12–3 Optimal Temperature of Reactivity for Some Common Antibodies			
Antibodies	Cold autoantibodies (I, H, IH) M, N P$_1$ Le^a, Le^b Lu^a	Potent cold antibodies (especially if causing hemolysis) D, E K	Rh antibodies K Duffy Kidd S,s Lu^b Xg^a
Immunoglobulin Class	IgM	IgG	IgG
Clinically Significant	No	Yes	Yes

show mixed-field agglutination, but this depends on how recently the transfusion was given and how much blood was transfused.

Reagents

An antibody identification panel is a collection of 11 to 20 group O cells with various antigen expression. The pattern of antigen expression should be diverse enough that it will be possible to distinguish one antibody from another and should include cells with homozygous expression of Rh, Duffy, Kidd, and MNSs antigens. A profile sheet specifying the antigens on each cell and providing a place to record reactions accompanies each panel **(Fig. 12–8)**. As with the screen cells, the profile sheet is lot-specific and should not be interchanged with that of another panel. The profile sheet will often indicate the presence of rare cells, which are positive for low-frequency antigens or negative for high-frequency antigens.

Exclusion

When interpreting panel results, the first step is to exclude antibodies that could not be responsible for the reactivity seen. To do this, the cells that gave a negative reaction in all phases of testing are examined. The antigens on these negatively reacting cells will probably not be the target of the antibody. Generally, it is advisable to perform this "rule-out" technique only if the antigen is homozygously expressed on the cell. This avoids excluding a weak antibody that is showing dosage. Exceptions are made for low-frequency antigens that are rarely expressed homozygously. These include K, Kp^a, Js^a, and Lu^a. In **Figure 12–9**, cell numbers 1, 3, 4, 6, 7, 10, and 11 reacted positively and cannot be used for exclusions. Cell number 2 reacted negatively and can be used to exclude D, C, e, C^w, K, Kp^b, Js^b, Fy^b, Jk^a, P$_1$, M, S, Lu^b, and Xg^a. Cell number 5 can be used to exclude k, Jk^b, and Le^b. Cell number 8 is used to rule out c, Le^a, and Lu^a, and cell number 9 eliminates N and s. This leaves anti-E, -Kp^a, -Js^a, and -Fy^a as possible antibodies present.

Evaluation of Panel Results

After each negatively reacting cell has been evaluated, the remaining antigens should be examined to see if the pattern of reactivity matches a pattern of antigen-positive cells (inclusion technique). Evaluation of panel results should be carried out in a logical step-by-step method to ensure proper identification and to avoid missing antibody specificities that may be masked by other antibodies. A logical approach to antibody identification is outlined here, using a series of questions and the example illustrated in **Figure 12–9**.

In what phase(s) and at what strength(s) did the positive reactions occur? Do all of the positive cells react to the same degree? Carefully grading the observed reactions may aid in antibody identification. The strength of the reaction does not indicate the significance of the antibody, only the amount of antibody available to participate in the reaction. A stronger reaction may be due to dosage ("homozygous" cells reacting more strongly than "heterozygous" cells). Different reaction strengths could also indicate the presence of more than one antibody. A cell that possesses more than one of the target antigens may react more strongly than a cell possessing only one of the target antigens. A third possibility is an antigen with variable expression. I, P$_1$, Le^a, Le^b, Vel, Ch/Rg, and Sd^a antigens are expressed more strongly on some cells than on others; antibodies to these antigens may react more strongly with one cell than another.

Do all of the positive cells react at the same phase, or do any react at different or multiple phases? Reactions of certain cells at one phase and different cells at another phase may indicate the presence of multiple antibodies. Cells that react at multiple phases may also be a sign of an antibody showing dosage, with the homozygous cells reacting at an earlier phase than the heterozygous cells. Phase of reactivity may be helpful in establishing the clinical significance of an antibody. IgM antibodies, which are usually not significant, most often react at the immediate spin phase, room temperature or colder. Clinically significant IgG antibodies are most often detected during the AHG phase. Some potent IgG anti-

Donor	Cell number	D	C	c	E	e	C^w	K	k	Kp^a	Kp^b	Js^a	Js^b	Fy^a	Fy^b	Jk^a	Jk^b	Le^a	Le^b	P$_1$	M	N	S	s	Lu^a	Lu^b	Xg^a			
R$_1$R$_1$	1	+	+	0	0	+	0	0	+	0	+	0	+	+	+	+	0	0	+	+	+	+	+	+	0	+	+			
R$_1$r	2	+	+	+	0	+	+	+	+	0	+	0	+	+	0	0	+	0	+	0	+	0	+	+	0	+	+			
R$_1$R$_1$	3	+	+	0	0	+	0	0	+	0	+	0	+	0	+	+	+	0	+	+	0	+	0	+	+	+	+			
R$_2$R$_2$	4	+	0	+	+	0	0	0	+	0	+	0	+	+	0	+	0	+	0	+	+	0	+	0	0	+	+			
r'r	5	0	+	+	0	+	0	0	+	0	+	0	+	0	0	0	0	+	0	+	+	0	+	+	0	+	0			
r"r"	6	0	0	+	+	0	0	0	+	0	+	0	+	+	0	+	0	0	0	+	0	+	0	+	0	+	+			
rr K	7	0	0	+	0	+	0	+	+	0	+	0	+	+	0	0	+	0	+	+	0	+	0	+	0	+	+			
rr	8	0	0	+	0	+	0	0	+	0	+	0	+	0	+	0	+	0	0	+	0	+	0	+	0	0	+			
rr	9	0	0	+	0	+	0	0	+	0	+	0	+	+	0	+	0	0	+	+	+	+	0	+	0	+	0			
R$_1$r	10	+	+	+	0	+	0	0	+	0	+	0	+	+	0	+	+	0	+	+	0	0	+	0	+	+			
R$_0$	11	+	0	+	0	+	0	0	+	0	+	0	+	+	+	0	+	0	+	+	0	0	+	+	0	+	+			
	Patient Cells																													

■ FIGURE 12–8   Antibody identification profile sheet: + indicates the antigen is present on the cell; 0 indicates the antigen is not present.

Donor	Cell number	D	C	c	E	e	Cw	K	k	Kpa	Kpb	Jsa	Jsb	Fya	Fyb	Jka	Jkb	Lea	Leb	P1	M	N	S	s	Lua	Lub	Xga	IS	37	AHG	CC
R1r	1	+	+	+	0	+	0	0	0	+	0	+	0	+	+	+	+	0	+	+	+	+	+	+	0	+	+	0	0	2+	
R1R1	2	+	+	0	0	+	+	+	+	+	0	+	0	0	+	+	0	0	0	+	+	0	+	0	0	+	+	0	0	0	3+
R2R2	3	+	0	+	+	0	0	0	+	0	+	0	+	+	0	0	+	0	+	+	0	+	0	+	0	+	+	0	0	3+	
R0r	4	+	0	+	0	+	0	0	+	0	+	0	+	+	0	+	+	+	0	0	+	0	+	+	0	+	0	0	0	3+	
r'r	5	0	+	+	0	+	0	0	+	0	+	0	+	0	0	0	+	0	+	+	+	0	+	0	+	+	0	0	0	0	3+
r"r	6	0	0	+	+	+	0	0	+	0	+	0	+	+	+	+	0	+	0	+	+	0	+	0	+	+	0	0	0	2+	
rr K	7	0	0	+	0	+	0	+	+	0	+	0	+	+	+	+	+	+	0	+	0	+	+	0	+	+	0	0	0	2+	
rr	8	0	0	+	0	+	0	0	+	0	+	0	+	0	+	+	0	+	0	+	+	+	0	+	+	0	+	0	0	0	3+
r'r"	9	0	+	+	+	+	0	0	+	0	+	0	+	0	0	+	+	0	0	+	+	0	+	0	+	+	0	0	0	0	3+
rr	10	0	0	+	0	+	0	0	+	0	+	0	+	+	0	+	0	+	0	+	+	0	+	0	0	+	+	0	0	3+	
R1r	11	+	+	+	0	+	0	0	+	0	+	0	+	+	0	+	0	+	0	+	+	+	+	+	0	+	+	0	0	2+	
	Patient Cells																											0	0	0	3+

■ **FIGURE 12–9**   Sample panel demonstrating anti-Fy^a.

bodies, such as D, E, and K, may become evident following the 37°C incubation phase. In the case presented in **Figure 12–9**, all reactions occurred in the AHG phase with strengths of both 2+ and 3+. Multiple antibodies or a single antibody showing dosage should be considered.

Does the serum reactivity match any of the remaining specificities? When a single alloantibody is present, the pattern of reactivity usually matches a pattern exactly. In our example, the serum reactivity perfectly matches the Fy^a pattern. The serum gave uniform positive results with all Fy^a-positive cells (1, 3, 4, 6, 7, 10, and 11) and negative results with all of the Fy^a-negative cells (2, 5, 8, and 9). The reason for the variation in strength in the AHG phase is due to dosage; all cells yielding 2+ reactions were heterozygous for Fy^a, and all cells yielding 3+ reactions were homozygous for Fy^a.

Are all commonly encountered RBC antibodies ruled out? As mentioned above, in this case anti-E, -Kp^a, and -Js^a were not ruled out. None of the cells on this panel were positive for Kp^a or Js^a, so they cannot be the cause of the observed reactions. These two antigens are characterized as low-frequency antigens occurring in less than 5 percent of the population. Antibodies to low-frequency antigens are uncommon because of the small chance of being exposed to the antigen; therefore, it may not be necessary to rule them out. In contrast, if a commonly encountered antibody is not ruled out, it is important to test selected cells that will rule out the presence of the antibody. In this example, anti-E still needs to be ruled out. A negative result when testing an E+ e− Fy^a-RBC sample would exclude anti-E (see section on selected cell panels below).

Is the autologous control (last row in panel antigen profile) positive or negative? In the example shown, the autocontrol is negative, indicating that the positive reactions are caused by alloantibody, not by autoantibody. The presence of autoantibodies complicates the process of antibody identification and is discussed briefly in Special Problems in Antibody Identification.

Is there sufficient evidence to prove the suspected anti-body? Conclusive antibody identification requires testing the patient's serum with enough antigen-positive and antigen-negative RBC samples to ensure that the pattern of reactivity is not the result of chance alone. Testing the patient's serum with at least three antigen-positive and three antigen-negative cells (also known as the "3 and 3 rule") will result in a probability (*P*) value of 0.05.[18] A *P* value is a statistical measure of the probability that a certain set of events will happen by random chance. A *P* value of 0.05 or less is required for identification results to be considered valid, and it means that there is a 5 percent (1 in 20) chance that the observed pattern occurred for reasons other than a specific antibody reacting with its corresponding antigen. Stated another way, it means that the interpretation of the data will be correct 95 percent of the time. When multiple antibodies are present, the 3 and 3 rule must be applied to each specificity. For example, if anti-K and anti-E are both suspected, the 3 and 3 rule would be fulfilled if three K−E− cells reacted negatively, three K+E− cells reacted positively, and three K−E+ cells reacted positively. Other researchers have derived formulas where *P* 0.05 is fulfilled with two positive cells and three negative cells[19] or two positive cells and two negative cells.[20]

Testing of RBCs selected from other panels is necessary when inadequate numbers of antigen-positive or antigen-negative cells are tested. In our example, the patient's serum reacted with seven Fy^a-positive cells (1, 3, 4, 6, 7, 10, and 11) but did not react with four Fy^a-negative cells (2, 5, 8, and 9). As a result, selected cells are not required in this case, and the identification of anti-Fy^a is conclusive.

Is the patient lacking the antigen corresponding to the antibody? Individuals cannot make alloantibodies to antigens that they possess; therefore, the last step in identification studies is to test the patient's RBCs for the corresponding antigen. A negative result is expected and indicates that identification results are correct. If the patient's RBCs are positive for the corresponding antigen, misidentification of the antibody or a false-positive typing are the most likely explanations. Antigen typing is also useful in the resolution of complex cases because it eliminates many possibilities.

[handwritten margin note: 95% probability]

For example, an R_1R_1, K-negative, Fy(a−b+), Jk(a+b+), M+N+S+s+ patient could form only anti-c, anti-E, anti-K, or anti-Fy[a]. It is not practical to do extended typing on all patients with antibodies; however, judicious use of this procedure can be helpful, especially in patients who chronically receive transfusions and are at risk for alloimmunization, such as patients with sickle cell disease or thalassemia.

Phenotyping may be complicated when a patient has a positive DAT or when the patient has been transfused in the last 3 months. When the DAT is positive due to IgG coating the cells, typing reagents employing the indirect antiglobulin test (IAT) may give invalid results. The coating antibody blocks the antigens sites, preventing the typing serum from reacting. The AHG reagent will react with the coating antibody, yielding a false-positive reaction. Removal of the antibody coating (elution) will be necessary in order to get an accurate phenotype. Two reagents useful in stripping antibody from the RBC surface, while leaving the membrane intact to allow phenotyping, are chloroquine diphosphate and acid glycine/EDTA.[21] In the chloroquine diphosphate method, washed RBCs are incubated with the reagent at room temperature for 30 minutes to 2 hours. The cells are washed to remove the chloroquine diphosphate. When the treated cells yield a negative DAT, they may then be phenotyped. Rh antigens may show diminished reactivity with this method. Acid glycine/EDTA (EGA) is a rapid method for antibody removal. Kell antigens are denatured when using this method; so patient cells cannot be reliably typed for these antigens.

In cases where the coating antibody resists elution, an absorption method has been described.[22] RBCs to be phenotyped are incubated with diluted antiserum. Following incubation, the cell/antiserum mixture is centrifuged. The supernatant is harvested and tested against a cell with heterozygous antigen expression. If the patient's cell is positive for the target antigen, the antibody will have been absorbed from the diluted antiserum, and the supernatant will react negatively. If the patient's cells are negative for the target antigen, the antibody will remain in the antiserum, and the supernatant will be positive when tested against the heterozygous cell.

Recently transfused patients present a different challenge. Mixed field reactions are common when phenotyping these patients; the donor cells that stimulated antibody formation react with the typing serum, whereas the patient's autologous cells do not react. To get an accurate phenotype of the patient's autologous cells, reticulocyte typing can be performed. For this technique, the patient's cells are drawn into microhematocrit tubes and centrifuged. Because reticulocytes are less dense than mature RBCs, the patient's reticulocytes should be at the top of the RBC layer. These cells can be harvested and used for antigen typing.[23]

Antigen typing is routinely performed using the tube technique, solid phase technique,[24] or gel technique.[25] Positive and negative controls should be performed on each antisera used for antigen typing. The positive control should have heterozygous expression of the antigen to ensure that the antiserum can detect weak forms of the antigen. The negative control should lack the target antigen. Flow cytometry has been used to detect small quantities of antigens, and fetal antigen typing may be accomplished through polymerase chain reaction techniques.[26]

Additional Techniques for Resolving Antibody Identification

There may be times when the first antibody identification panel performed does not produce a clear specificity. When multiple specificities remain following exclusion/inclusion techniques, additional testing is necessary.

Selected Cell Panels

Perhaps the easiest technique is to test additional cells. The cells selected for testing should have minimal overlap in the antigens they possess. **Figure 12–10** shows the results of an initial panel in which anti-E, -Kp[a], -Js[a], -Fy[a] and -Jk[b] are not excluded. The lower section of **Figure 12–10** shows a selected cell panel that could be used to differentiate between those antibodies. Anti-Jk[b] appears to be present in the sample. Anti-Fy[a] is eliminated by selected cell number 1, and anti-E is eliminated by selected cell number 3. Finding cells that are positive for low-frequency antigens such as C[w], Kp[a], Js[a], and Lu[a] may not be possible in many cases.

Selected cell panels are also used when a patient has a known antibody and the technologist is attempting to determine if additional antibodies are present. **Figure 12–11** is an example of a selected cell panel for a patient with a known anti-Fy[a]. The panel cells selected are each negative for Fy[a] but possess examples of other common, significant antigens.

Enzymes

When it appears that multiple antibodies may be present in a sample, treatment of the panel cells with enzymes may help separate the specificities and allow for identification. Ficin, papain, trypsin, and bromelin are all commonly used to treat RBCs. Enzymes modify the RBC surface by removing sialic acid residues and by denaturing or removing glycoproteins. The effect is to destroy certain antigens and enhance expression of others. **Table 12–4** reviews how enzymes affect various antigens.

Enzymes may be utilized in place of enhancement media, such as LISS or PeG, in a one-step enzyme test method. A second, more sensitive method uses enzymes to treat the panel RBCs first, and then the antibody identification panel is performed using the treated cells. Because enzymes destroy some antigens, the exclusion technique cannot be used on the enzyme panel alone. The enzyme panel should be compared with a panel using the same cells untreated. Observing which cells reacted positively in the untreated panel but did not react (or gave weaker reactions) with the treated panel will aid the technologist in identification. Similarly, observation of

TABLE 12–4   The Effect of Proteolytic Enzymes on Select Antigen-Antibody Reactions

Enhanced	Inactivated
Rh	Duffy
Kidd	MNS
Lewis	Xg[a]
P_1	
I	
ABO	

Donor	Cell number	D	C	c	E	e	Cw	K	k	Kpa	Kpb	Jsa	Jsb	Fya	Fyb	Jka	Jkb	Lea	Leb	P1	M	N	S	s	Lua	Lub	Xga	IS	37	AHG	CC
R₁r	1	+	+	+	0	+	0	0	0	+	0	+	0	+	+	+	+	+	0	+	+	+	+	+	0	+	+	0	0	1+	
R₁R₁	2	+	+	0	0	+	+	+	+	0	+	0	+	0	+	0	0	0	+	+	0	+	0	0	+	+	+	0	0	0	3+
R₂R₂	3	+	0	+	+	0	0	0	+	0	+	0	+	+	0	+	+	0	+	+	0	+	0	+	0	+	+	0	0	1+	
R₀r	4	+	0	+	0	+	0	0	+	0	+	0	+	+	0	+	+	+	0	0	+	0	+	+	0	+	0	0	0	1+	
r'r	5	0	+	+	0	+	0	0	+	0	+	0	+	0	0	+	0	0	+	+	+	0	+	+	0	+	0	0	0	0	3+
r"r	6	0	0	+	+	+	0	0	+	0	+	0	+	+	+	0	+	0	+	+	0	+	0	+	0	+	+	0	0	2+	
rr K	7	0	0	+	0	+	0	+	+	0	+	0	+	+	+	+	+	0	+	0	+	+	0	+	0	+	+	0	0	1+	
rr	8	0	0	+	0	+	0	0	+	0	+	0	+	0	+	0	+	0	+	+	+	+	0	+	0	+	+	0	0	0	3+
r'r"	9	0	+	+	+	+	0	0	+	0	+	0	+	0	0	+	0	0	+	+	0	+	0	+	0	+	+	0	0	0	3+
rr	10	0	0	+	0	+	0	0	+	0	+	0	+	+	+	0	+	0	+	+	+	0	+	0	0	+	+	0	0	1+	
R₁r	11	+	+	+	0	+	0	0	+	0	+	0	+	+	+	+	0	+	0	+	+	+	+	+	0	+	+	0	0	2+	
	Patient Cells																												0	0	0	3+
Selected Cell Panel																																
R₁R₁	SS1	+	+	0	0	+	0	+	+	0	+	0	+	+	0	+	0	0	+	+	0	+	+	+	0	+	0	0	0	0	3+
rr	SS2	0	0	+	0	+	0	0	+	0	+	0	+	+	+	0	+	+	0	+	0	+	+	0	0	+	+	0	0		3+
R₂R₂	SS3	+	0	+	+	0	0	0	+	0	+	0	+	0	+	+	0	0	+	0	+	0	+	0	0	+	0	0	0	0	3+

■ **FIGURE 12-10**   Selected cell panel.

cells that reacted more strongly or at an earlier phase in the enzyme panel than in the untreated panel may lead to identification.

Neutralization

Other substances in the body and in nature have antigenic structures similar to RBC antigens. These substances can be used to neutralize antibodies in serum, allowing for separation of antibodies or confirmation that a particular antibody is present. The patient's serum is first incubated with the neutralizing substance, allowing the soluble antigens in the substance to bind with the antibody. An antibody identification panel is performed using the treated serum. The neutralizing substance inhibits reactions between the antibody and panel RBCs. Use of a control (saline and serum) is necessary to prove that the loss of reactivity is due to neutralization and not to dilution of antibody strength by the added substance. In **Figure 12-12**, positive reactions are seen in cells 1 to 4, 7, and 8. When the serum is incubated with Lewis' substance, positive reactions are seen in only cells 3, 4, and 7, which matches the pattern of anti-Kell. Anti-Le^b activity has been inhibited by Lewis' substance. This technique is helpful when multiple antibodies are suspected. **Table 12-5** lists some of the antibodies that can be neutralized and the source of corresponding neutralizing substance. Lewis and P₁ substances may be prepared commercially.

Adsorption

Antibodies may be removed from serum by adding the target antigen and allowing the antibody to bind to the antigen (similar to the neutralization technique). In the adsorption method, the antigen/antibody complex is composed of solid precipitates and is removed from the test system by centrifugation. The absorbed serum is tested against an RBC panel. The adsorbent is typically composed of RBCs but may be another antigen-bearing substance.

Donor	Cell number	D	C	c	E	e	Cw	K	k	Kpa	Kpb	Jsa	Jsb	Fya	Fyb	Jka	Jkb	Lea	Leb	P1	M	N	S	s	Lua	Lub	Xga	Peg/IgG	CC		
	1	+	+	0	0	+	0	0	+	0	+	0	+	0	+	+	0	0	+	+	+	+	0	0	+	+	0	2+		
	2	+	+	0	0	+	+	0	+	+	+	0	+	0	+	+	+	0	+	+	+	0	+	0	0	+	0	2+		
	3	+	0	+	+	0	0	+	+	0	+	0	+	0	+	0	+	0	0	0	0	+	0	+	0	+	+	0	2+		
	4	0	+	+	0	+	0	0	+	0	+	0	+	0	0	+	+	+	0	+	+	0	+	+	0	+	+	0	2+		
	Patient Cells																											0	2+		

■ **FIGURE 12-11**   Selected cell panel for a patient with known antibody.

CELL	D	C	E	c	e	f	V	Cw	M	N	S	s	Lua	Lub	P1	Lea	Leb	K	k	Fya	Fyb	Jka	Jkb	Albumin 37C	AHG	Control: Serum + Saline AHG	Serum + Lewis Substance AHG
1. r'r-2	0	+	0	+	+	+	0	0	+	+	0	+	0	+	0	0	+	0	+	+	0	+	+	0	2+	2+	0
2. R1wR1 -1	+	+	0	0	+	0	0	+	+	+	+	0	+	+	+	0	+	0	+	0	+	+	0	0	2+	2+	0
3. R1R1-6	+	+	0	0	+	0	0	0	0	+	0	+	0	+	+	+	0	+	+	0	+	+	0	0	2+	2+	2+
4. R2R2-8	+	0	+	+	0	0	0	0	+	+	+	+	0	+	+	0	+	+	0	0	+	0	+	0	2+	2+	2+
5. r"r-3	0	0	+	+	+	+	0	0	+	+	+	0	0	+	+	+	0	0	+	0	+	0	+	0	0	0	0
6. rr-32	0	0	0	+	+	+	+	0	+	0	+	0	0	+	+	0	0	0	+	+	+	+	0	0	0	0	0
7. rr-10	0	0	0	+	+	+	0	0	+	+	+	+	0	+	0	0	+	+	+	0	+	+	0	0	2+	2+	2+
8. rr-12	0	0	0	+	+	+	0	0	0	+	0	+	0	+	+	0	+	0	+	0	+	0	+	0	2+	2+	0
9. Ro-4	+	0	0	+	+	+	0	0	+	0	0	+	0	+	0	+	0	0	+	0	0	0	+	0	0	0	0
Cord cell	/	/	/	/	/	/	/	/	/	/	/	/	/	/	/	0	0	/	/	/	/	/	/				
Patient																								0	0	0	0

DIRECT ANTIHUMAN GLOBULIN TEST

Poly	*negative*
IgG	
C3	

■ FIGURE 12–12   Neutralization using Lewis' substance in a serum containing anti-Le^b and anti-Kell.

Commercial Reagents for Adsorption

Human platelet concentrate is used to adsorb Bg-like antibodies from serum. The HLA antigens present on platelets bind the HLA-related Bg antibodies,[27] leaving other specificities in the serum. Antibody identification can be performed on the adsorbed serum.

Rabbit erythrocyte stroma (RESt) performs a similar function with some cold-reacting autoantibodies. RESt possesses I, H, and IH-like structures. Incubating the patient's serum at 4°C with RESt will remove these insignificant antibodies, which may interfere with the detection of clinically significant warm-reacting antibodies. Most other antibody specificities remain unaffected by RESt adsorption.[28] However; RESt also possesses structures similar to B and P$_1$ antigens. Because RESt may absorb anti-B, reverse grouping and crossmatching with RESt-adsorbed serum is not recommended.

Autoadsorption

Autoantibodies are commonly removed through adsorption techniques. Perhaps the simplest is adsorption using the

TABLE 12–5   Sources of Substances for Neutralization for Certain Antibodies

Anti-P$_1$	Hydatid cyst fluid, pigeon droppings, turtledoves' egg whites
Anti-Lewis	Plasma or serum
Anti-Chido, Anti-Rodgers	Plasma or serum
Anti-Sd^a	Urine
Anti-I	Human breast milk

patient's own cells. The autologous cells are first washed thoroughly to remove unbound antibody. They may then be treated to remove any autoantibody coating the cells. The cells are then incubated with the patient's serum for up to 1 hour. Temperature of incubation will depend on the thermal range of the autoantibody being removed, generally 4°C for cold-reacting autoantibodies and 37°C for warm-reacting autoantibodies. The sample is inspected for signs of agglutination throughout the incubation period. If agglutination appears, all the RBC binding sites are saturated with autoantibody. The serum is harvested and incubated with a new batch of autologous cells. When no agglutination is apparent during incubation, the harvested serum is tested against the patient's RBCs. If no reactivity is observed, the absorption is complete. However, if a reaction is observed, autoantibody remains in the serum, and further absorption is necessary. It is not unusual for three to six sets of cells to be used for autoadsorption. With some powerful warm autoantibodies, the technologist may be unable to remove the autoantibody completely and must settle for diminished reactivity. **Figure 12–13** illustrates the steps in performing an autoadsorption. In the first set of figures, the patient's cell is coated with autoantibody. Autoantibody can be seen free in the serum, along with an alloantibody. The cells are washed and then treated to remove the autoantibody. They are incubated with the patient's serum (middle figure). The autoantibody begins to adsorb onto the patient's cells and is removed from the serum. In the last set of figures, the autoantibody has once again coated the patient's cells, leaving only the alloantibody in the serum. The serum is separated from the autologous cells, and an antibody identification panel is performed to reveal any alloantibodies that had previously been masked by the autoantibody. **Figure 12–14** shows an example of an anti-

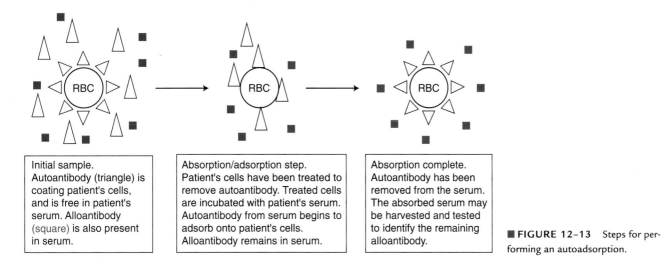

| Initial sample. Autoantibody (triangle) is coating patient's cells, and is free in patient's serum. Alloantibody (square) is also present in serum. | Absorption/adsorption step. Patient's cells have been treated to remove autoantibody. Treated cells are incubated with patient's serum. Autoantibody from serum begins to adsorb onto patient's cells. Alloantibody remains in serum. | Absorption complete. Autoantibody has been removed from the serum. The absorbed serum may be harvested and tested to identify the remaining alloantibody. |

■ FIGURE 12–13   Steps for performing an autoadsorption.

body identification panel before and after warm autoadsorption. Anti-K is apparent in the postadsorption panel.

Homologous Adsorption

When a patient is so anemic that there are not enough RBCs available to perform an adequate number of adsorptions or if the patient has been recently transfused (donor cells in the specimen may adsorb alloantibodies), homologous or differential adsorptions may be employed in place of autoadsorption. For homologous adsorption, the patient is phenotyped, and then phenotypically matched cells are used for the adsorption in place of autologous cells. If an exact match cannot be made, the focus is on finding cells that lack the antigens to which the patient may form antibodies. For example, if the patient types as R_1R_1, K–, Fy^a+, Fy^b+, Jk^a–, Jk^b+, S+, s–; then anti-E, anti-c, anti-K, anti-Jk^a, and anti-s may be formed by the patient. The homologous donor cells must be negative for E, c, K, Jk^a, and s antigens in order for those antibodies to remain in the adsorbed serum.

Differential Adsorption

When phenotyping the patient is difficult because of a positive DAT or recent transfusion, differential absorption is performed. For this method, the patient's serum sample is divided into a minimum of three aliquots. Each aliquot is adsorbed using a different cell. One cell is usually R_1R_1, one is usually R_2R_2, and the third is usually rr. Among the three, one must be negative for K, another negative for Jk^a, and the third negative for Jk^b. The cells are treated with an enzyme to render them negative for antigens of the Duffy and MNSs systems. Following adsorption, antibody identification panels are performed separately on each aliquot, and the reactivities are compared to reveal underlying alloantibodies. See Chapter 21 for a more complete discussion.

Adsorption may also be performed when multiple alloantibodies are present in order to separate the specificities. The adsorbing cell must be antigen-positive for one suspected specificity but negative for others. Following adsorption, the serum is tested to see which, if any, additional alloantibodies have been unmasked.

Donor	Cell number	D	C	c	E	e	Cw	K	k	Kpa	Kpb	Jsa	Jsb	Fya	Fyb	Jka	Jkb	Lea	Leb	P1	M	N	S	s	Lua	Lub	Xga	Peg/IgG	CC	Absorbed serum	CC
R1R1	1	+	+	0	0	+	0	0	+	0	+	0	+	+	0	+	+	0	+	+	+	+	+	0	+	+	+	2+		0	3+
R1R1	2	+	+	0	0	+	+	+	+	0	+	0	+	+	+	0	+	0	+	+	+	0	+	+	0	+	+	3+		2+	
R2R2	3	+	0	+	+	0	0	0	+	0	+	0	+	0	+	0	+	0	+	+	+	+	+	0	0	+	+	2+		0	3+
R0r	4	+	0	+	0	+	0	0	+	0	+	0	+	0	0	+	+	0	+	+	+	0	+	0	0	+	0	2+		0	3+
r'r	5	0	+	+	0	+	0	0	+	0	+	0	+	0	+	+	0	+	0	0	0	0	+	0	+	0	+	2+		0	3+
r"r	6	0	0	+	+	+	0	0	+	0	+	0	+	0	+	+	+	0	+	+	+	+	+	0	+	+	+	3+		2+	
rr	7	0	0	+	0	+	0	0	+	0	+	0	+	0	+	+	+	+	0	0	+	0	+	0	+	0	+	2+		0	3+
rr	8	0	0	+	0	+	0	0	+	0	+	0	+	0	+	0	+	0	+	+	+	0	+	+	0	+	+	2+		0	3+
rr	9	0	0	+	0	+	0	0	+	0	+	0	+	0	+	+	0	0	+	0	+	+	+	0	+	0	0	2+		0	3+
rr	10	0	0	+	0	+	0	+	+	0	+	0	+	0	+	0	+	+	0	+	0	+	0	+	0	+	+	3+		2+	
R0r	11	+	0	+	0	+	0	0	+	0	+	0	+	+	+	0	+	0	+	+	0	+	0	+	0	+	+	2+		0	3+
Patient Cells																												2+		0	3+

■ FIGURE 12–14   Panel using warm autoadsorption technique.

DAT and Elution Techniques

Detection of antibodies coating RBCs is valuable when investigating suspected hemolytic transfusion reactions, HDN, and autoimmune and drug-induced hemolytic anemias. DAT is used to detect in-vivo sensitization of RBCs. The patient's cells are washed thoroughly to remove any unbound antibody, and then AHG reagent is added. If IgG antibody or complement is fixed to the cell, agglutination will be observed. If neither is present, no agglutination will be observed. Coombs' control cells are added to validate the negative test.

When IgG antibodies are detected, the next step is to dissociate the antibodies from the cell surface to allow for identification. Elution techniques are used to release, concentrate, and purify antibodies. The methods used to remove the antibody change the thermodynamics of the environment, change the attractive forces between antigen and antibody, or change the structure of the RBC surface. The antibody is then freed into a solution known as an eluate. The eluate may be tested against an RBC panel to identify the antibody. A total elution, in which antibody is released and the RBC antigens are rendered useless, is necessary when performing antibody identification. Partial elution, in which antibody is removed but RBC antigens remain intact, is useful when stripping antibody from RBCs to allow for phenotyping or preparing RBCs for autoadsorption. Chloroquine diphosphate and EGA are examples of chemicals used for this purpose.

Temperature

The simplest elution methods involve changing the temperature of the antigen/antibody environment. Heat may be used to remove antibody when washed, coated RBCs are suspended in an equal volume of saline or albumin. The gentle heat method, performed at 45°C, allows for antibody removal while leaving the RBC intact.[29] Elution performed at 56°C is a total elution method, allowing for antibody identification.[30] The Lui freeze method[31] also produces a total elution. With this method, washed, coated RBCs suspended in saline or albumin are frozen at −18°C or colder until solid. The mixture is then thawed rapidly, causing the RBCs to burst, freeing the bound antibody. Temperature-dependent elutions are best at detecting IgG antibodies directed against antigens of the ABO system.

pH

A common and relatively quick and easy method for total elution in order to detect non-ABO antibodies is acid elution.[32,33] In this method, the washed antibody-coated cells are mixed with a glycine acid solution at a pH of 3.0. The antigen/antibody bond is disrupted, and the antibody is released into the acidic supernatant. The supernatant is harvested, and the pH is neutralized so that antibody identification testing can take place. Citric acid and digitonin acid are also used in similar methods.

Organic Solvents

Several organic solvents have been used in total elution methods, among them dichloromethane, xylene, and ether. These solvents act on the lipids in the RBC membrane to reduce surface tension and lead to the reversal of the van der Waal forces that hold antigens and antibodies together.[34,35] Organic eluates are very potent as compared with the temperature-dependent eluates and are best for detecting non-ABO antibodies. However, these procedures are time-consuming, and the chemicals pose several health and safety hazards as they are carcinogenic and flammable.

The most critical step in preparing any eluate is the original washing, which is used to remove unbound immunoglobulins. If allowed to remain in the test system, these antibodies will contaminate the final eluate and yield false-positive results. As a control, the last wash supernatant should be run in parallel with the eluate to detect the presence of unbound antibody. The last wash should be nonreactive, or the eluate results are invalid.

Antibody Titration

Once identified, it is sometimes useful to quantify the amount of antibody present. While techniques employing flow cytometry, radioimmunoassay, or enzyme-linked immunoassay may give more precise results, these methods are not readily available in every laboratory. Performing an antibody titration can help determine antibody concentration levels. Twofold serial dilutions of serum containing an antibody are prepared and tested against a suspension of RBCs that possesses the target antigen. The titer level is the reciprocal of the greatest dilution in which agglutination is observed. A score may also be assigned, based on the strength of reactivity. Each reaction is given a value, and the score is determined by adding up the individual values. After the initial titer, the specimen should be frozen. When new specimens are submitted for titer, the initial titer specimen should be tested in parallel to control variability among technologists and the relative strength of the target antigen on the cells being used. A comparison of the current specimen's results and the initial specimen's current results should be made. A change in titer level of 2 or more tubes (fourfold increase) or a change in score of 10 or more is considered to be significant. **Table 12–6** shows an example of titer level results that indicate a significant increase in antibody levels.

When performing the antibody titer, careful preparation of dilutions is necessary. Contamination from a tube with a higher antibody concentration can lead to falsely elevated titer level results. Changing pipette tips between each tube when preparing the dilutions and working/reading from the most diluted tube to the least diluted can help avoid this problem.

Selection of the cell containing the target antigen should be consistent throughout the series of titer level studies. If a cell with homozygous antigen expression was used for the initial titer, then all subsequent titer specimens should be tested against a homozygous cell. The method used must also be consistent. It has been reported that titers using the gel method are more sensitive than those using the tube method and therefore result in a higher titer level.[36] The technologist must make the test systems as identical as possible in order to make valid comparisons between samples.

Titer level studies are useful in monitoring the obstetric patient who has an IgG antibody that may cause HDN. An increase in antibody titer level during pregnancy suggests that the fetus is antigen-positive and therefore at risk of devel-

TABLE 12–6 Titer and Score of Anti-D*

	1:2	1:4	1:8	1:16	1:32	1:64	1:128	
Previous sample	2+	2+	1+	w+	0	0	0	Titer 16
Score	8	8	5	2	0	0	0	Score 23
Current sample	3+	3+	2+	2+	1+	w+	0	Titer 64
Score	10	10	8	8	5	2	0	Score 43

*Score values: 4+ = 12, 3+ = 10, 2+ = 8, 1+ = 5, w+ = 2

oping HDN. An increasing titer level may indicate the need for intrauterine exchange transfusion. An antibody titer may also be used to help differentiate immune anti-D from passively acquired anti-D from RhIG. The titer level in RhIG is rarely above 4.[37]

Performing a titer is one way to confirm the presence of antibodies belonging to the group collectively known as HTLA (high titer, low avidity). These high-frequency antibodies are observed at the AHG phase of testing with weakly positive reactions. These weak reactions persist through extensive dilutions (as high as 2048).[38] Examples of these antibodies include anti-Ch, -Rg, -Cs[a], -Yk[a], -Kn[a], -McC[a], and -JMH. These antibodies are usually not clinically significant but may mask significant antibodies.

Providing Compatible Blood Products

The relative difficulty in providing compatible blood products is determined by the frequency of the antigen in the population and by the clinical significance of the antibody. If the antibody does not cause decreased survival of antigen-positive RBCs, then use of random blood products that are crossmatch-compatible is acceptable. Examples of such antibodies include anti-M, -N, -P$_1$, -Le[a], and -Le[b].[39]

When the patient sample contains a clinically significant antibody or the patient has a past history of a clinically significant antibody, units for transfusion must be antigen-negative. The crossmatch technique must demonstrate compatibility at the AHG phase.[40] If the patient sample is plentiful, the technologist may choose to crossmatch units, then antigen-type those that are crossmatch-compatible. If the sample is limited or if the antibody is no longer detectable in the serum, units should be antigen-typed first, then crossmatched.

Knowing the incidence of the antigen in the population is helpful when determining the number of units that must be antigen-typed to find a sufficient number to fill the crossmatch request. The number of units requested is divided by the frequency of antigen-negative individuals. For example, if a crossmatch for 2 units is received for a patient with anti-E, the calculation would be 2 (units requested)/0.70 (the frequency of E-negative individuals). The result is 2.8, meaning that 3 units would need to be typed for E in order to find 2 E-negative units. When multiple specificities are present, the frequencies of antigen negative are multiplied together. If E-negative, c-negative units were required in the above example, the calculation would be 2/(0.70 × 0.20) = 14.3. Fourteen or fifteen units would have to be antigen-typed for E and c in order to find two units that are negative for both antigens.

In certain cases, knowing the ethnicity of the donor is helpful when selecting units for antigen testing because the frequency of some antigens varies between the races. For example, when searching for units that are Fy[a]-negative, it may be prudent to screen black donors as 90 percent will be negative for Fy[a] compared with only 34 percent of whites.

It has been proposed by some transfusion medicine experts that certain populations, particularly sickle cell and beta-thalassemia patients, receive units that are phenotypically matched.[41,42] These multiply transfused patients seem more likely to make alloantibody than the general population; if they are immunized, it may be difficult to find compatible blood. When the number of antigens that must be negative makes it difficult to find suitable units, rare-donor registries may be consulted. These registries maintain lists of donors and may provide frozen units of rare phenotypes. Another approach is to transfuse units that are phenotypically matched for Rh antigens and K, as these antigens are the most immunogenic.[43]

Resolving Difficult Antibody Identification Problems

Case One: Multiple Antibodies

Suspect multiple antibodies when all or most of the screen and panel cells are positive but reactions are at different strengths or in different phases and the autocontrol is negative. When using inclusion techniques, no single antibody accounts for all of the reactions seen.

Resolution may include performing a selected cell panel to exclude certain specificities. Several sets of cells may need to be tested in order to narrow the list of possible antibodies (see **Fig. 12–10**). Enzyme techniques may allow for separation of antibodies. In **Figure 12–15**, the specificity of the antibodies was unclear after the initial panel. After repeating the panel using ficin-treated cells, it appears that the antibodies present are anti-K and anti-Fy[b]. The enzyme treatment removed the Fy[b] antigens, allowing the anti-K to present clearly. Anti-C and anti-Jk[a] were also not eliminated by the initial panel. However, one would expect these antibodies to demonstrate enhanced reactivity with the ficin-treated cells. Anti-Jk[a] may be excluded using cell 8 of the ficin panel. Whereas anti-C cannot be excluded using a homozygous cell, the pattern of reactivity and lack of response to enzyme treatment suggest it is not present in this sample. Testing a C+, c−, K−, Fy[b]− cell would be necessary for exclusion. In other cases, neutralization and absorption techniques may also be useful in separating multiple antibodies.

Donor	Cell number	D	C	c	E	e	Cw	K	k	Kpa	Kpb	Jsa	Jsb	Fya	Fyb	Jka	Jkb	Lea	Leb	P1	M	N	S	s	Lua	Lub	Xga	Peg/IgG	CC	Ficin/IgG	CC
R1r	1	+	+	+	0	+	0	0	+	0	+	0	+	+	+	+	+	0	+	+	+	+	+	+	0	+	+	1+		0	3+
R1R1	2	+	+	0	0	+	+	+	+	0	+	0	+	0	+	+	0	0	0	+	+	0	+	0	0	+	+	3+		2+	
R2R2	3	+	0	+	+	0	0	0	+	0	+	0	+	+	0	0	+	0	+	+	0	+	0	+	0	+	+	0	3+	0	3+
R0r	4	+	0	+	0	+	0	0	+	0	+	0	+	+	+	0	+	+	+	0	0	+	0	+	0	+	0	0	3+	0	3+
r'r	5	0	+	+	0	+	0	0	+	0	+	0	+	0	+	0	0	0	+	0	+	+	+	0	+	+	0	0	3+	0	3+
r"r	6	0	0	+	+	+	0	0	+	0	+	0	+	+	+	+	0	+	0	+	+	0	+	0	+	0	+	1+		0	3+
rr K	7	0	0	+	0	+	0	+	+	0	+	0	+	+	+	+	+	0	+	0	+	+	0	+	0	+	+	2+		2+	
rr	8	0	0	+	0	+	0	0	+	0	+	0	+	0	+	+	0	+	0	+	+	+	+	0	+	+	0	2+		0	3+
r'r"	9	0	+	+	+	+	0	0	+	0	+	0	+	0	+	+	0	0	+	+	0	+	0	+	0	+	+	2+		0	3+
rr	10	0	0	+	0	+	0	0	+	0	+	0	+	+	0	+	+	0	+	+	+	0	+	0	0	+	+	0	3+	0	3+
R1r	11	+	+	+	0	+	0	0	+	0	+	0	+	+	+	0	+	0	+	+	+	+	+	+	0	+	+	1+		0	3+
Patient Cells																												0	3+	0	3+

■ FIGURE 12–15   Enzyme panel.

Case Two: Antibody to a High-Frequency Antigen

High-frequency antigens are those that are present in almost all individuals (98 percent or more). Suspect an antibody to a high-frequency antigen when all or most screen and panel cells are positive, with reactions in the same phase and same strength, and a negative autocontrol (Fig. 12–16). The testing of additional cells that lack the antigen would be most useful. Panel cells that are negative for these high-frequency antigens are usually indicated on the antigen profile sheet (see cell 10), or you may refer to the manufacturer's extended typing list, which usually accompanies the panel set. If antigen-negative cells are not readily available, it may be necessary to consult a reference laboratory that maintains a stock of rare cells. For this case, the ideal solution is to test two additional Yt^a-negative cells, which would provide 95 percent confidence of correct antibody identification. Any other antibodies not excluded at that point may require patient phenotyping or absorption studies to confirm their presence or absence.

Knowing the ethnicity of the patient may give clues as to the identity of the antibody, as antigen frequencies vary among races. An example is the U antigen, which is present in virtually all whites and all but about 1 percent of blacks. Anti-U is produced mainly in multiparous black females or those who have been repeatedly transfused.

Donor	Cell number	D	C	c	E	e	Cw	K	k	Kpa	Kpb	Jsa	Jsb	Fya	Fyb	Jka	Jkb	Lea	Leb	P1	M	N	S	s	Lua	Lub	Xga	Peg/IgG	CC
R1R1	1	+	+	0	0	+	0	0	+	0	+	0	+	+	0	+	+	+	0	+	+	+	+	+	0	+	+	2+	
R1R1	2	+	+	0	0	+	+	+	+	0	+	0	+	+	+	0	+	0	+	+	+	0	+	+	0	+	+	2+	
R2R2	3	+	0	+	+	0	0	0	+	0	+	0	+	0	+	0	+	0	+	+	+	+	+	0	0	+	+	2+	
R0r	4	+	0	+	0	+	0	0	+	0	+	0	+	0	0	+	+	+	0	+	+	+	0	+	0	+	0	2+	
r'r	5	0	+	+	0	+	0	0	+	0	+	0	+	+	0	+	0	0	0	0	0	+	0	+	0	+	0	2+	
r"r	6	0	0	+	+	+	0	+	+	0	+	0	+	+	+	+	0	+	+	+	+	+	+	0	+	+		2+	
rr Co^b +	7	0	0	+	0	+	0	0	+	0	+	0	+	+	+	+	+	+	0	0	+	+	0	+	0	+	+	2+	
rr	8	0	0	+	0	+	0	0	+	0	+	0	+	0	+	0	+	0	+	+	+	0	0	+	0	+	+	2+	
rr	9	0	0	+	0	+	0	0	+	0	+	0	+	0	+	+	0	+	0	+	+	+	+	0	+	0		2+	
rr Yt(a)$^-$	10	0	0	+	0	+	0	+	+	0	+	0	+	0	+	+	+	0	+	+	0	+	0	+	0	+	+	0	3+
R0r	11	+	0	+	0	+	0	0	+	0	+	0	+	+	+	0	+	0	+	+	0	+	0	+	+	0	+	+	2+	
Patient Cells																												0	3+

■ FIGURE 12–16   Panel performed on a patient with an antibody to a high-frequency antigen.

Finding compatible blood for patients with an antibody to a high-frequency antigen may be a challenge. Autologous donations should be encouraged. Other sources of antigen-negative blood may include family members and the rare donor registry. Fortunately, because these antigens do occur so frequently, it is rare to find a patient with an antibody to one of them.

Antibodies to the so-called HTLA antigens also fall under this category. Although these antibodies are usually not clinically significant themselves, up to 25 percent of patients with an HTLA antibody also make clinically significant antibodies.[44] It is not necessary to determine the specificity of the HTLA antibody, but removal of these antibodies is usually necessary to identify any underlying alloantibodies. Some HTLA antibodies, notably anti-Ch and anti-Rg, may be neutralized by normal serum, which contains complement. Routine blood bank enzymes will destroy anti-Ch, -Rg, and -JMH, whereas anti-Kn^a and -McC^a are destroyed by dithiothreitol (DTT).

Case Three: Antibody to a Low-Frequency Antigen

Low-frequency antigens are present in less than 10 percent of the population. Antibodies to these antigens are uncommon because exposure to the antigen is rare. The antibody screen will most likely be negative, therefore no panel will have been performed. Antibodies to these antigens should be suspected when an antiglobulin crossmatch is incompatible and other sources of explanation, such as ABO incompatibility or positive donor DAT, have been eliminated. These antibodies may also be suspected when an infant has a positive DAT and there is no known blood group discrepancy between mother and infant.

Testing with additional antigen-positive cells will be required to confirm the specificity. Panel cells that are positive for these rare antigens are normally indicated on the panel profile sheet or listed on the extended typing form. In Figure 12–17, positive reactions were seen only with cell 4 that matched the pattern of anti-Js^a. All other antibodies could be ruled out except for the other low-frequency, anti-Lu^a. Testing two other cells positive for the Js^a antigen to satisfy the 3 and 3 rule and phenotyping the patient for the Js^a antigen should be done to complete the antibody identification workup. If additional cells are not readily available, consult a reference laboratory. Because these antigens are infrequent, finding antigen-negative units for crossmatch is usually not difficult

Case Four: Cold-Reacting Autoantibodies

Most adult sera contain low titers of cold-reacting autoantibodies, most notably autoanti-I, -H, and -IH. These antibodies are usually IgM and of no clinical significance. They are troublesome in that they may interfere with the detection of significant antibodies, resulting in prolonged workups and delayed transfusions.

Cold-reacting autoantibodies may be suspected when the screening cells, panel cells, and the autocontrol are all positive at the immediate spin phase and get weaker or disappear with incubation at 37°C (Fig. 12–18). In this case, reactions were reduced at 37°C and were no longer apparent at the AHG phase. The use of cord blood cells, which lack the I antigen, confirms the presence of anti-I in this sample.

Certain autoantibodies may fix complement and are only detected at the AHG phase when using complement containing AHG reagent. These autoantibodies may be mistaken for weakly reacting IgG antibodies. Many laboratories avoid detection of cold autoantibodies by omitting the immediate spin phase of the antibody screen and by using monospecific anti-IgG Coombs' serum.

One of the least complex methods used to prevent these autoantibodies from interfering is the prewarm technique. In this procedure, the serum being tested and the screening or panel cells are heated to 37°C in separate test tubes. Once at 37°C, a drop of cells is added to the tube containing the

Donor	D	C	c	E	e	K	k	Js^a	Js^b	Fy^a	Fy^b	Jk^a	Jk^b	Le^a	Le^b	P1	M	N	S	s	Lu^a	Lu^b	IS	37	IgG	CC
1	+	+	+	0	+	0	+	0	+	0	+	0	+	+	0	+	+	+	0	+	0	+	0	0	0	3+
2	+	+	0	0	+	0	+	0	+	0	+	0	+	+	0	+	+	+	+	+	0	+	0	0	0	3+
3	+	0	0	+	+	0	+	0	+	+	+	0	+	+	+	0	+	+	+	+	0	+	0	0	0	3+
4	+	+	+	0	+	0	+	+	+	+	+	+	+	+	+	0	+	+	+	0	0	+	0	1+	2+	NT
5	+	+	+	0	+	0	+	0	+	+	0	+	+	0	0	+	0	+	0	+	0	+	0	0	0	3+
6	0	0	+	0	+	0	+	0	+	+	0	+	0	+	+	+	0	+	+	0	+	+	0	0	0	3+
7	0	0	+	0	+	+	+	0	+	+	0	+	0	+	0	+	+	0	+	0	0	+	0	0	0	3+
8	0	0	+	+	0	0	+	0	+	+	+	0	+	0	+	0	+	0	+	0	0	+	0	0	0	3+
9	0	0	+	0	+	0	+	0	+	0	0	0	+	0	+	+	+	+	+	0	0	+	0	0	0	3+
10	+	0	+	0	+	0	+	0	+	0	+	+	+	0	+	+	+	+	0	+	0	+	0	0	0	3+
11	+	+	0	+	0	0	+	0	+	0	+	+	0	+	0	+	+	0	+	+	0	+	0	0	0	3+
12	+	+	0	0	+	0	+	0	+	+	+	+	0	+	0	+	+	0	0	+	0	+	0	0	0	3+
PC																							0	0	0	3+

■ FIGURE 12–17 Panel performed on a patient with an antibody to a low-frequency antigen.

Donor	Cell number	D	C	c	E	e	Cw	K	k	Kpa	Kpb	Jsa	Jsb	Fya	Fyb	Jka	Jkb	Lea	Leb	P1	M	N	S	s	Lua	Lub	Xga	IS	37	AHG	CC
R1R1	1	+	+	0	0	+	0	0	+	0	+	0	+	+	0	+	+	0	+	+	+	+	+	+	0	+	+	2+	W+	0	3+
R1R1	2	+	+	0	0	+	+	+	+	0	+	0	+	+	+	0	+	0	+	+	+	0	+	+	0	+	+	2+	W+	0	3+
R2R2	3	+	0	+	+	0	0	0	+	0	+	0	+	0	+	0	+	0	+	+	+	+	+	0	0	+	+	2+	W+	0	3+
R0r	4	+	0	+	0	+	0	0	+	0	+	0	+	0	0	+	+	0	+	+	+	0	+	0	0	+	0	2+	W+	0	3+
r'r	5	0	+	+	0	+	0	0	+	0	+	0	+	+	0	+	0	0	0	0	0	+	0	+	0	+	0	2+	W+	0	3+
r"r	6	0	0	+	+	+	0	+	+	0	+	0	+	0	+	+	+	0	+	+	+	+	+	+	0	+	+	2+	W+	0	3+
rr	7	0	0	+	0	+	0	0	+	0	+	0	+	+	+	+	+	+	0	0	+	+	0	+	0	+	+	2+	W+	0	3+
rr	8	0	0	+	0	+	0	0	+	0	+	0	+	+	0	+	0	+	0	+	+	0	0	+	0	+	+	2+	W+	0	3+
rr	9	0	0	+	0	+	0	0	+	0	+	0	+	0	+	+	0	0	+	0	+	0	+	+	+	0	+	2+	1+	0	3+
rr	10	0	0	+	0	+	0	+	+	0	+	0	+	0	+	+	+	0	+	0	+	0	+	0	+	0	+	2+	1+	0	3+
R0r	11	+	0	+	0	+	0	0	+	0	+	0	+	+	+	0	+	0	+	+	0	+	0	+	0	+	+	2+	1+	0	3
I neg	Cord Cell																											0	0	0	3+
	Patient Cells																											2+	1+	0	3+

■ FIGURE 12-18   Panel performed on a patient with a cold autoantibody.

serum, and the test proceeds with incubation, washing, and AHG steps. The wash step uses saline that has also been maintained at 37°C so that at no time is the test system allowed to drop below that temperature, thus avoiding the optimal temperature range of the autoantibody. Because this method does not usually have enhancement media in the system, it is possible to fail to detect some weak significant antibodies. Also, the warm saline may result in the dissociation of some significant antibodies from the cells.

A more complex method, discussed previously, is adsorption. The patient's autologous cells may be incubated with the patient's serum at 4°C to remove the autoantibody before antibody detection steps are performed. This method provides autoantibody-free serum for antibody detection and identification procedures and for compatibility testing. If the autoantibody is particularly strong or if the patient has been recently transfused, RESt may be used to perform the adsorption instead of the patient's cells. RESt-adsorbed serum is not suitable for crossmatch as anti-B may be removed.

Sulfhydryl compounds, such as DTT and 2-mercaptoethanol, are known to break the disulfide bonds in IgM. Treating the patient's serum with such a reagent before the antibody detection test will denature the cold autoantibody. IgG antibodies are not affected by these reagents and will remain detectable. A control of saline and serum is tested in parallel with the treated serum to ensure that the autoantibody was truly denatured, not merely diluted.

Although it is not necessary to determine the specificity of the cold autoantibody, testing against additional cells may confirm its presence. Cord blood cells that lack the I antigen are of particular value for this purpose. A cold panel, consisting of group O adult cells (H and I antigens), group O cord cells (H and i antigens), group A₁ adult cells (I antigen), and an autocontrol, may be tested at 4°C to determine the specificity of the cold autoantibody, if desired (Fig. 12–19).

Case Five: Warm-Reacting Autoantibodies

Warm-reacting autoantibodies are some of the most challenging to work up. Warm autoantibodies are uncommon, but they may occur secondary to chronic lymphocytic leukemia, lymphoma, systemic lupus erythematosus, and other autoimmune diseases or as a result of drug therapy. Suspect a warm autoantibody when all cells, including the autocontrol, are reactive at the AHG phase and react at the same strength. If an underlying alloantibody is present, cells that possess that antigen may react stronger than those that are antigen-negative. Removal of the warm autoantibody to allow for detection of alloantibody is of primary importance. It is not necessary to determine the specificity of the autoantibody, although many seem to have Rh-specificity.

Warm autoantibodies are IgG antibodies that are found coating the patient's cells and free in the patient's serum. Adsorption techniques are used to remove the antibody from the serum. Autoadsorption is the method of choice when possible. The patient's cells must first be stripped of autoantibody before they can be used to adsorb autoantibody from the

CELL	IS	RT	18°C	4°C
A₁	0	0	1+	2+
A₂	1+	2+	4+	4+
B	0	0	2+	3+
O adult	2+	3+	4+	4+
O cord	0	0	1+	2+
Auto	0	0	1+	2+

■ FIGURE 12-19   Cold antibody screen performed on an AB patient with autoanti-IH.

serum. Partial elution using gentle heat or chemical methods is used to produce an antibody-free cell. ZZAP is one chemical that works particularly well for this. It is composed of DTT and papain, resulting in the destruction of enzyme-sensitive antigens and denaturing Kell, LW, Dombrock, Knops, and Cromer antigens. Once the autoantibody has been removed from the cells, the treated cells can be mixed with the patient's serum to absorb autoantibody from the serum. Multiple steps are necessary to treat the cells and adsorb the autoantibody, which is very time-consuming. The adsorbed serum is then tested for alloantibody. See **Figure 12–14** for an example of warm autoantibody autologous adsorption. The pattern of reactivity matches that of anti-Kell. Positive reactions in the autoabsorbed serum were found in cells 2, 6, and 10, which were positive for the Kell antigen. All other antibodies could be ruled out except for C_w, Kp^a, Lu^a, and Js^a. These are low-frequency antigens and generally do not need to be ruled out. Additional phenotyping strategies should be employed to determine if the patient is negative for the Kell antigen. Transfusion requirements include units negative for the Kell antigen that appear to be less incompatible with the warm autoantibody than the patient's own cells (least incompatible).

When patient cells are limited or when the patient has been recently transfused, allogeneic cells are used for adsorption. The cells used for homologous or differential adsorption are usually treated with enzymes or with ZZAP to enhance certain antigens and facilitate autoantibody removal. These treatment and adsorbing steps are time-consuming. There is an alternative method, in which PEG is used to enhance antibody removal, cutting the processing time approximately in half while still providing for adequate autoantibody removal.[45,46]

Finding RBC units that are compatible with a patient who has a warm autoantibody may be difficult. If after the absorption no clinically significant antibodies are detected, an immediate spin crossmatch to detect ABO incompatibility is all that is necessary. If clinically significant antibodies are present, then antigen-negative units should be crossmatched using an antiglobulin technique. The warm autoantibody frequently interferes with this testing, making interpretation of results difficult.

Some transfusion medicine experts believe that repeating the full warm autoantibody workup is unnecessary if the patient's serologic picture has remained unchanged when compared with previous results.[47,48] They advocate transfusing with units that are phenotypically matched for Rh and K antigens in order to reduce the risk of alloimmunization.

SUMMARY CHART:
Important Points to Remember (MT/MLT)

► The purpose of the antibody screen is to detect *unexpected* antibodies, which make up approximately 0.2–2% of the general population. The antibodies may be classified as immune (the result of RBC stimulation in the patient), passive (transferred to the patient through blood products or derivatives), or naturally occurring (the result of environmental factors).

Antibodies may also be classified as alloantibodies, directed at foreign antigens, or autoantibodies, directed at one's own antigens.

► A clinically significant antibody is one that results in the shortened survival of RBCs possessing the target antigen. Clinically significant antibodies are IgG antibodies that react best at 37°C and/or in the AHG phase. They are known to cause hemolytic transfusion reactions and HDN.

► Screening cells are commercially prepared group O cell suspensions obtained from individual donors who are phenotyped for the most commonly encountered and clinically important RBC antigens.

► RBCs from a homozygous individual have a double dose of a single antigen, which results from the inheritance of two genes that code for the same antigen, whereas heterozygous individuals carry only a single dose each of two different antigens. (Each gene codes for a different antigen.)

► Antibodies in the Kidd, Duffy, Lutheran, Rh, and MNSs blood group systems show *dosage* and yield stronger reactions against RBCs with homozygous expression of their corresponding antigen.

► Enhancement reagents, such as LISS and PEG, are solutions added to serum and cell mixtures in the IAT to promote antigen-antibody binding or agglutination.

► Coombs' control cells are RBCs coated with human IgG antibody, which are added to all AHG-negative tube tests to ensure that there was an adequate washing step performed and that the AHG reagent is present and functional in the test system.

► Gel and solid phase testing are alternatives to tube testing. These methods may be automated to increase efficiency.

► The antibody exclusion method rules out possible antibodies based on antigens that are present on negatively reacting cells.

► Conclusive antibody identification is achieved when the serum containing the antibody is reactive with at least three antigen-positive cells (i.e., reagent cells that express the corresponding antigen), negative with at least three antigen-negative cells (i.e., reagent cells that do not express the corresponding antigen), and the patient's RBCs phenotype negative for the corresponding antigen.

► The DAT detects cells that were sensitized with antibody in vivo. Elution methods are used to free antibody from the cell surface to allow for identification.

► The calculation for determining the number of random donor units screened for patients with an antibody is described as dividing the number of antigen-negative units desired for transfusion by the incidence of antigen-negative individuals in the donor population.

► The relative quantity of an RBC antibody can be determined by testing serial twofold dilutions of serum against antigen-positive RBCs; the reciprocal of the highest serum dilution showing agglutination is the antibody titer.

REVIEW QUESTIONS

1. Based on the following phenotypes, which pairs of cells would make the best screening cells?
   a. Cell 1: Group A, D+C+c−E−e+, K+, Fy(a+b−), Jk(a+b−), M+N−S+s−
      Cell 2: Group O, D+C−c+E+e−, K−, Fy(a−b+), Jk(a−b+), M−N+S+s+
   b. Cell 1: Group O, D−C−c+E+e+, K−, Fy(a−b+), Jk(a+b+), M+N−S+s+
      Cell 2: Group O, D+C+c−E−e+, K−, Fy(a+b−), Jk(a+b−), M−N+S−s+
   c. Cell 1: Group O, D+C+c+E+e+, K+, Fy(a+b+), Jk(a+b+), M+N−S+s+
      Cell 2: Group O, D−C−c+E−e+, K−, Fy(a+b−), Jk(a+b+), M+N+S−s+
   d. Cell 1: Group O, D+C+c−E−e+, K+, Fy(a−b+), Jk(a−b+), M−N+S−s+
      Cell 2: Group O, D+C−c+E+e−, K−, Fy(a+b−), Jk(a+b−), M+N−S+s−

2. Antibodies are ruled out using cells that are homozygous for the corresponding antigen because:
   a. Antibodies show dosage
   b. Multiple antibodies may be present
   c. It results in a *P* value of .05 for proper identification of the antibody
   d. All of the above

3. A request for 8 units of packed RBCs was received for patient LF. The patient has a negative antibody screen, but one of the 8 units was 3+ incompatible at the AHG phase. Which of the following antibodies may be the cause?
   a. Anti-K
   b. Anti-Le^a
   c. Anti-Kp^a
   d. Anti-Fy^b

4. The physician has requested two units of blood for patient DB, who has both anti-L and anti-Q. The frequency of antigen L is 45%, and the frequency of antigen Q is 70% in the donor population. Approximately how many units will need to be antigen-typed for L and Q to fill the request?
   a. 8
   b. 12
   c. 2
   d. 7

5. Anti-Sd^a has been identified in patient ALF. What substance would neutralize this antibody and allow detection of other alloantibodies?
   a. Saliva
   b. Hydatid cyst fluid
   c. Urine
   d. Human breast milk

6. Patient JM appears to have a warm autoantibody. She was transfused 2 weeks ago. What would be the next step performed in order to identify any alloantibodies that might be in her serum?
   a. Acid elution
   b. Warm autoadsorption using autologous cells
   c. Warm differential adsorption
   d. RESt adsorption
   For Question 7, refer to **Figure 12–20.**

7. What is the titer and score for this prenatal anti-D titer?
   a. Titer = 64 , score = 52
   b. Titer = 32, score = 52
   c. Titer = 32, score = 21
   d. Titer = 32, score = 52
   For Questions 8–10, refer to **Figure 12–21.**

8. Select the antibody/ies most likely responsible for the reactions observed:
   a. Anti-E and anti-K
   b. Anti-Fy^a
   c. Anti-e
   d. Anti-Jk^b

9. What additional cells need to be tested to be 95% confident that the identification is correct?
   a. Three e-negative cells that react negatively and one additional e-positive cell that reacts positively
   b. One additional E-positive cell to react positively and one additional K-positive cell to react positively
   c. Two Jk^b homozygous positive cells to react positivel and one Jk^b heterozygous positive cell to react negatively
   d. No additional cells are needed

10. Using the panel in **Figure 12–21**, select cells that would make appropriate antigen typing controls when typing for the C antigen.
    a. Cell number 1 for the positive control and cell number 2 for the negative control
    b. Cell number 1 for the positive control and cell number 6 for the negative control
    c. Cell number 2 for the positive control and cell number 4 for the negative control
    d. Cell number 4 for the positive control and cell number 5 for the negative control

Dilution	1:1	1:2	1:4	1:8	1:16	1:32	1:64	1:128	1:256	1:512	1:1024	Saline control
Results	4+	4+	3+	2+	1+	1+	0	0	0	0	0	0

■ **FIGURE 12–20** Anti-D titer results for Question 7.

Donor	Cell number	D	C	c	E	e	Cw	K	k	Kpa	Kpb	Jsa	Jsb	Fya	Fyb	Jka	Jkb	Lea	Leb	P1	M	N	S	s	Lua	Lub	Xga	IS	37	AHG	CC
R1R1	1	+	+	0	0	+	0	0	+	0	+	0	+	+	+	+	+	0	0	+	+	+	+	+	0	+	+	0	0	0	3+
R1r	2	+	+	+	0	+	+	+	+	0	+	0	+	+	0	0	+	0	+	0	+	0	+	+	0	+	+	0	0	3+	
R1R1	3	+	+	0	0	+	0	0	+	0	+	0	+	+	0	+	+	+	0	+	+	0	+	0	+	+	+	0	0	0	3+
R2R2	4	+	0	+	+	0	0	0	+	0	+	0	+	+	0	+	0	+	0	+	+	0	+	0	0	+	+	0	2+	3+	
r'r	5	0	+	+	0	+	0	0	+	0	+	0	+	+	0	+	0	+	0	+	0	+	0	+	0	+	+	0	0	0	3+
r"r"	6	0	0	+	+	0	0	0	+	0	+	0	+	0	+	0	+	0	+	+	0	+	0	+	0	+	+	0	2+	3+	
rr K	7	0	0	+	0	+	0	+	+	0	+	0	+	+	0	+	0	0	+	+	+	0	+	0	0	+	+	0	0	3+	
rr	8	0	0	+	0	+	0	0	+	0	+	0	+	0	+	+	0	0	+	0	+	0	0	+	0	+	+	0	0	0	3+
rr	9	0	0	+	0	+	0	0	+	0	+	0	+	+	0	+	+	0	+	0	+	+	0	0	0	+	+	0	0	0	3+
R1r	10	+	+	+	0	+	0	0	+	0	+	0	+	+	0	+	0	+	0	+	+	+	0	0	0	+	0	+	0	0	3+
R0	11	+	0	+	0	+	0	0	+	0	+	0	+	+	+	+	0	+	0	+	+	+	0	0	0	+	0	+	0	0	3+
Patient Cells																													0	0	0	3+

■ FIGURE 12–21   Panel study for Questions 8–10.

REFERENCES

1. Giblett, ER: Blood group alloantibodies: An assessment of some laboratory practices. Transfusion 1977; 17:299.
2. Boral, L, and Henry, IB: The type and screen: A safe alternative and supplement in selected surgical procedures. Transfusion 1977; 17:163.
3. Mollison, PL, Engelfreit, CP, and Contreras, M: Blood Transfusion in Clinical Medicine, ed 9. Blackwell Scientific Publications, Oxford, England, 1993, p 111.
4. Standards for Blood Banks and Transfusion Services, ed 21. American Association of Blood Banks, Bethesda, MD, 2002.
5. Judd, WJ, Luban, NLC, Ness, PM, et al. Prenatal and perinatal immunohematology: Recommendations for serologic management of the fetus, newborn infant, and obstetric patient. Transfusion 1990; 30:175.
6. Standards for Blood Banks and Transfusion Services, ed 21. American Association of Blood Banks, Bethesda, MD, 2002.
7. Standards for Hematopoietic Progenitor Cell Services, ed 2. American Association of Blood Banks, Bethesda, MD, 2002.
8. Standards for Hematopoietic Progenitor Cell Collection, Processing, and Transplantation, ed 2. Foundation for the Accreditation of Cellular Therapy, 2002.
9. Issitt, PD, and Anstee, DJ: Applied Blood Group Serology, ed 4. Montgomery Scientific Publications, Durham, NC, 1998, p 47.
10. Standards for Blood Banks and Transfusion Services, ed 21. American Association of Blood Banks, Bethesda, MD, 2002.
11. Mollison, PL, Engelfreit, CP, and Contreras, M: Blood Transfusion in Clinical Medicine, ed 9. Blackwell Scientific Publications, Oxford, England, 1993, p 337.
12. Issitt, PD, and Anstee, DJ: Applied Blood Group Serology, ed 4. Montgomery Scientific Publications, Durham, NC, 1998, pg 132.
13. Kosanke, J, Dickstein, B, and Davis, K: Evaluation of incubation times using the ID-Micro Typing system (abstract). Transfusion 2000; 42:108S.
14. Ciavarella, D, Pate, L, and Sorenson, E: Serologic comparisons of antibody detection and titration methods: LISS, PeG, gel (abstract). Transfusion 2002; 42:108S.
15. Schonewille, H, Haack, HL, and van Zijl, AM: RBC antibody persistence. Transfusion 2000; 40:1127.
16. South, SF: Use of the direct antiglobulin test in routine testing. In Wallace, ME, and Levitt, JS (eds): Current Application and Interpretation of the Direct Antiglobulin Test. American Association of Blood Banks, Arlington, VA, 1988, p 25.
17. Issitt, PD, and Anstee, DJ: Applied Blood Group Serology, ed 4. Montgomery Scientific Publications, Durham, NC, 1998, p 470.
18. Fisher, RA: Statistical methods and scientific inference, ed 2. Oliver and Boyd, Edinburgh, Scotland, 1959.
19. Harris RE, and Hochman, HG. Revised p values in testing blood group antibodies. Transfusion 1986; 26:494.
20. Kanter, MH, Poole, G, and Garretty, G: Misinterpretation and misapplication of p values in antibody identification: The lack of value of a p value. Transfusion 1997; 37:816.
21. Brecher, M (ed): Technical Manual, ed 14. American Association of Blood Banks, Bethesda, MD, 2002, p 683.
22. Kosanke, J, and Arrighi, S. Antigen typing red cells that are resistant to IgG reduction (abstract). Transfusion 2000; 40:119S.
23. Brecher, M (ed): Technical Manual, ed 14. American Association of Blood Banks, Bethesda, MD, 2002, p 685.
24. Morelati, F, Revelli, N, Musella, A, et al: Automated red cell phenotyping (abstract). Transfusion 2001; 41:110S.
25. Lowe, L. Use of MTS IgG gel cards for red blood cell antigen typing (abstract). Transfusion 2002; 42:109S.
26. Bennett, PR, Le Van Kim, C, Dolon, Y, et al: Prenatal determination of fetal RhD type by DNA amplification. N Engl J Med 1993; 329:607–610.
27. Aster, RH, Miskovich BH, and Rodey GE: Histocompatibility antigens of human plasma; localization to HLD-3 lipoprotein fraction. Transplantation 1973; 16:205.
28. Marks, MR, Reid, ME, and Ellisor, SS: Adsorption of unwanted cold autoagglutinins by formaldehyde-treated rabbit red blood cells (abstract). Transfusion 1980; 20:629.
29. Brecher, M (ed): Technical Manual, ed 14. American Association of Blood Banks, Bethesda, MD, 2002, p 682.
30. Landsteiner, K, and Miller, CP: Serologic studies on the blood of primates: II. The blood group of anthropoid apes. J Exp Med 1925; 42:853.
31. Feng, CS, Kirkley, KC, and Eicher, CA, et al: The Lui elution technique: A simple and efficient method for eluting ABO antibodies. Transfusion 1985; 25:433.
32. Rekkvig, OP, and Hannestad, K: Acid elution of blood group antibodies from intact erythrocytes. Vox Sang 1977; 33:280.
33. Judd, WJ: Methods in immunohematology, ed 2. Montgomery Scientific Publications, Durham, NC, 1994.
34. van Oss, CJ, Absolom, DR, and Neumann, AW: The "hydrophobic effect": Essentially a van der Waals interaction. Colloid Polymer Sci 1980; 1:424.
35. van Oss, CJ, Absolom, DR, and Neumann, AW: Applications of net repulsive van der Waals forces between different particles, macromolecules, or biological cells in liquids. Colloid Polymer Sci 1980; 1:45.
36. Ciavarella, D, Pate, L, and Sorenson, E: Serologic comparisons of antibody detection and titration methods: LISS, PeG, gel (abstract) Transfusion 2002; 42:108S.
37. Brecher, M (ed): Technical Manual, ed 14. American Association of Blood Banks, Bethesda, MD, 2002, p 417.
38. Schulman, IA, and Petz, LD. Red cell compatibility testing: Clinical significance and laboratory methods. In Petz, LD, Swisher, SN, and Kleinman, S (eds): Clinical Practice of Transfusion Medicine, ed 3. Churchill Livingstone, New York, 1996, p 199.
39. Brecher, M (ed): Technical Manual, ed 14. American Association of Blood Banks, Bethesda, MD, 2002, p 508
40. Standards for Blood Banks and Transfusion Services, ed 21. American Association of Blood Banks, Bethesda, MD, 2002, p 46.
41. Tahhan, HR, Holbrook, CT, Braddy, LR, et al: Antigen-matched donor blood in the transfusion management of patients with sickle cell disease. Transfusion 1994; 34:562.
42. Matteocci, A, Palange, M, Dionisi, M, et al. Retrospective study on the red cell alloimmunization after multiple blood transfusions (abstract). Transfusion 2001; 41:112S.
43. Vichinsky, EP, Luban, NLC, Wright, E, et al: Prospective RBC phenotype matching in a stroke-prevention trial in sickle cell anemia: A mulitcenter transfusion trial. Transfusion 2001; 41:1086.
44. Moulds, MK: Special serologic technics useful in resolving high-titer, low-avidity antibodies. In Recognition and Resolution of High-Titer, Low-Avidity Antibodies: A Technical Workshop. American Association of Blood Banks, Washington, DC, 1979.
45. Cheng, CK, Wong, ML, and Lee, AW: PEG adsorption of autoantibodies and detection of alloantibodies in warm autoimmune hemolytic anemia. Transfusion 2001; 41:13.
46. Leger, RM, and Garratty, G: Evaluation of methods for detecting alloantibodies underlying warm autoantibodies. Transfusion 1999; 39:11.
47. Sanguin, J, Angus, N, and Sutton, DM: Repeated serological testing of patients with warm autoimmune hemolytic anemia may not be necessary (abstract). Transfusion 2001; 41:106S.
48. Judd, WJ: Investigation and management of immune hemolysis: Autoantibodies and drugs. In Wallace, ME, and Levitt, JS (eds): Current Applications and Interpretations of the Direct Antiglobulin Test. American Association of Blood Banks, Arlington, VA, 1988, p 47.

thirteen

Pretransfusion Compatibility Testing

Mary P. Nix, MS, MT(ASCP)SBB, and
William B. Zundel, MS, MT(ASCP)SBB

OBJECTIVES

Upon completion of this chapter, the learner will have the opportunity to:

1. Recognize appropriate methods for proper patient identification in sample collection.
2. Outline the procedure for testing of donor and patient specimens.
3. Select appropriate donor units based on availability, presence, or absence of unexpected alloantibody in the patient.
4. Compare and contrast crossmatch procedures.
5. Resolve incompatibilities in the crossmatch.
6. Explain compatibility testing procedures and protocols in special circumstances.
7. State the limitations of compatibility testing procedures.
8. Describe a scheme for effective blood utilization.
9. List the steps necessary to reidentify the patient before transfusion.
10. Discuss future issues of compatibility testing.

Pretransfusion compatibility testing is a series of testing procedures and processes with the ultimate objective of ensuring the best possible results of a blood transfusion. Much of this textbook thus far has dealt with how to perform testing procedures (i.e., ABO, Rh, antibody detection, etc.) and processes of pretransfusion compatibility testing. This chapter is a comprehensive examination of their application in enhancing the safety of blood transfusion. That is, transfused red blood cells (RBCs) should have an acceptable survival rate, and there should not be significant destruction of the recipient's own RBCs. **Box 13–1** represents the results of a study of consensus pretransfusion compatibility testing procedures and

processes.[1] Strict adherence to and application of each parameter of pretransfusion compatibility testing is imperative to the management of safe blood transfusion therapy. Each parameter must also be considered in any comprehensive review of the process used to select blood for a recipient.

Pretransfusion compatibility testing cannot guarantee normal survival of transfused RBCs in the recipient's circulation. The potential benefits of RBC transfusion should always be weighed against the potential risks any time this form of therapy is considered. Although adverse responses to transfusion cannot always be avoided, results are much more likely to be favorable if pretransfusion compatibility testing is care-

BOX 13–1
Consensus PRE-TXN Practices, 2001

- ABO Testing
  Tube method using monoclonal reagents
  Patient sample ≤3 days old if, within past 3 months, patient has been
    Pregnant
    Transfused
- Rh testing
  Tube method using monoclonal/polyclonal blend reagent
  Patient sample ≤3 days old if, within past 3 months, patient has been
    Pregnant
    Transfused
- Historical record check
  Every patient, every time
- Screening for unexpected alloantibodies
  Tube method using three vial sets (not pooled) of reagent RBCs and LISS enhancement media; PEG enhancement media on the increase
  Gel method on the increase
  Detect clinically significant alloantibodies reactive at 37°C
  Although not required, most labs still read for hemolysis and agglutination before and after addition of AHG; only a reading after addition of AHG is required
  DAT and autocontrol are not required
- Alloantibody identification
  Tube method with LISS enhancement media
  Gel method on the increase
  Additional methods may be useful:
    Prewarm serum
    Increase serum-to-cell ratio
    Enzyme-treated reagent RBCs
    PEG
- Management of previously identified alloantibodies
  Honor all clinically significant alloantibodies, even if currently undetectable
  It is not necessary to reidentify previously identified alloantibodies
- Crossmatch
  Serologic
    Use immediate spin only if
      No alloantibody has been currently or historically identified
    Use AHG crossmatch if
      An alloantibody has been currently or historically identified
  Electronic
    Use only when immediate spin crossmatch would have been used

Reprinted with permission from Shulman, IA, et al: Pretransfusion compatibility testing for red blood cell administration. Current Opinion in Hematology 8: 397–404, 2001. Table 2, page 402.

fully performed and results of laboratory testing show no incompatibility between donor and patient.

Identification, Collection, and Preparation of Samples

Positive Recipient Identification

The major cause of transfusion-associated fatalities is clerical error resulting in incorrect ABO groupings. In a study of

transfusion errors in New York state over a 10 year period, 47 percent of errors involved the identification of the patient or the blood at bedside.[2] Clerical error is the greatest threat to safe transfusion therapy. The most common cause of error is misidentification of the recipient. Examples include misidentification of the recipient when the blood sample is drawn, mix-up of samples during handling in the laboratory, and misidentification of the recipient when the transfusion is given. Exact procedures for proper identification of the recipient, recipient sample, and donor unit must be established and utilized by all staff responsible for each aspect of transfusion therapy.

To prevent collection of samples from the wrong patient, the recipient's wristband identification must always be compared with the requisition form (blood request form). The request form must state the intended recipient's full name and unique hospital identification number.[3] Other information such as age, date of birth, address, sex, and name of requesting physician can be used to further verify patient identity but is not required on the form. Printing must be legible, and indelible nameplate impressions or computer printouts are preferable to handwritten forms. Any discrepancies must be completely resolved before the sample is taken. Nameplates on the wall or bed labels must never be used to verify identity; the patient specified may no longer occupy that bed. If the patient does not have a wristband or if the patient's identity is unknown, some form of positive identification must be attached to the patient before collection of samples. This may be a temporary tie tag or a wristband or ankle band; it should not be removed until proper identification has been attached to the patient and the person collecting the recipient sample confirms verification of identity.

In some transfusing facilities, if the patient does not have a wristband and is coherent, it is permissible to ask the patient to state his or her full name and to spell it out. If the date of birth or home address is printed on the requisition form, the patient might be asked to state this information. Occasional errors can result from two patients with the same name being mistaken for each other. The phlebotomist should never offer a name and ask the patient to confirm that it is correct (e.g., "Are you Mr. Jones?"). Some disoriented patients may answer yes to any question. If the patient is very young or is incoherent, some other reliable professional individual who knows the patient must confirm the identity and document this on the requisition form. Commercially manufactured identification systems using preprinted tags and numbers (**Figs. 13–1, 13–2,** and **13–3**) are especially useful in patient and donor verification. Whatever procedure is adopted, it must be an integral part of the blood bank's standard operating procedure (SOP) manual, thus resulting in the requirement of all blood bank personnel demonstrating competency in the process.[4]

Collecting Patient Samples

After positive identification has been accomplished, blood samples should be drawn, using careful technique to avoid hemolyzing the sample. In-vitro hemolysis of recipient samples for pretransfusion testing cannot be used because it can mask hemolysis caused by antigen-antibody complexes that activate complement to completion. There are patients experiencing in-vivo hemolytic processes (such as hemolytic ane-

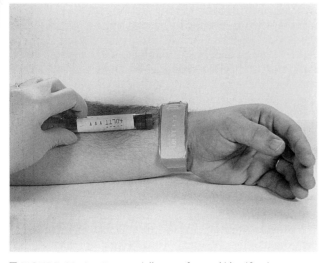

■ FIGURE 13–1   Commercially manufactured identification systems. Compare preprinted label with the patient armband.

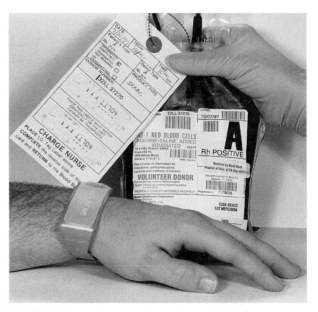

■ FIGURE 13–3   Commercially manufactured identification systems. Pretransfusion comparison of recipient armband and donor *unit* bag.

mia) who will do so no matter how well the collection procedure is performed. The hemolysis occurs in the patient prior to collection and cannot be avoided. In these circumstances, care must be taken to note the extent of hemolysis present in the patient serum/plasma and observe for any increases during each stage of testing.

Serum or plasma may be used for pretransfusion testing. Most blood bank technologists prefer serum because plasma may cause small fibrin clots to form, and these may be difficult to distinguish from true agglutination. Also, plasma may inactivate complement so that some antibodies may not be detected. About 10 mL of blood is usually sufficient for all testing procedures if there are no known serologic problems.

Tubes must be labeled before they leave the recipient's bedside. If imprinted labels are used, they must be compared with the recipient's wristband and requisition form before the tubes are used. Labels must be attached to the tubes at the

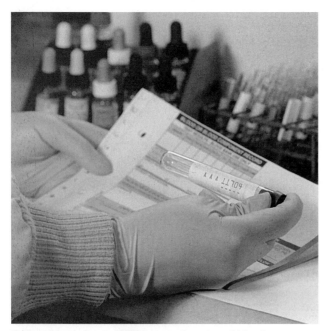

■ FIGURE 13–2   Confirm that sample and requisition form agree.

bedside in a tamper-proof manner that will make removal and reattachment impossible. All writing must be legible and indelible, and each tube must be labeled with the patient's full name, unique identification number, and date of sample collection.[5] The phlebotomist must initial or sign the label and add additional pertinent information as required by the facility's SOP.

To avoid contamination with materials that may cause confusing serologic results, blood samples should not be taken from intravenous (IV) tubing lines. Venous samples are not to be drawn from above an infusion site but are to be drawn from below the site. For example, if a patient has an IV line in the antecubital area of the arm, below the site would include any vein below the angle of the arm to the hand. If a sample must be taken from an IV line, the line should be disconnected for 5 to 10 minutes, the first 10 mL of blood drawn should be discarded, and then the sample for testing should be obtained.

When a specimen is received in the laboratory, blood bank personnel must confirm that the information on the sample and requisition form agree. All discrepancies must be resolved before the sample is accepted, and if any doubt exists, a new sample must be drawn. Receipt of an unlabeled specimen requires that a new sample be obtained.[6]

Recipient samples should be tested as soon as possible after collection. Recipient serum should also be separated from the patient's RBCs as soon as possible after the sample has clotted. If testing cannot be performed immediately, samples should be kept at 1° to 6°C.

As noted in Chapter 3, recent pregnancy or transfusion indicates an opportunity for a humoral immune response. Antibody production occurs over a predictable range of time, but the exact time varies from patient to patient. Specimens used in compatibility testing should ideally be collected during the critical phases of the immune response. In an attempt to capture this important time for each patient, serum obtained from samples fewer than 72 hours after collection must be used for antibody screening and crossmatch testing if the patient was pregnant, received RBC products by transfusion within the last 3 months, or if these histories are unknown.[7]

Patient RBCs can be obtained from either clotted or anticoagulated samples. They can be washed before use to remove plasma or serum, which may interfere with some testing procedures. A 2 to 5 percent saline suspension of RBCs is used for most serologic testing procedures; however, the manufacturer's directions should be consulted for the proper cell concentration to use for typing tests performed with licensed reagents. A method for preparing a button of washed RBCs suitable for performing one test is given in Procedural Appendix 1.

Donor Samples

Samples for donor testing must be collected at the same time as the full donor unit. Depending on the method used for testing, clotted and/or anticoagulated pilot samples are obtained. The donor information and medical history card, the pilot samples for processing, and the collection bag must be labeled with the same unique number before starting the phlebotomy, and the numbers must be verified again immediately after collection.[8] The donor number is used to identify all records of testing and eventual disposition of all component parts of the unit of blood. More detailed information on donor samples can be found in Chapter 11.

RBCs for donor pretransfusion compatibility testing can be prepared from the segmented tubing through which the donor blood was collected. The tubing or segment is attached to the collection bag, and each segment is imprinted with the same number. These numbers are different from the donor unit number but nonetheless are a positive means of sampling a given unit of blood.

Donor RBCs can be obtained from the segments in a number of ways that permit several procedures to be performed from the same segment. One technique that works well for sampling is using a lancet to make a tiny hole in the segment through which a single drop of blood can be expressed easily and then disposing the lancet in a biohazard sharps container. The hole is essentially self-sealing, so the rest of the blood in the segment remains uncontaminated. Another technique is to cut the RBC end of the segment tubing with scissors and use an applicator stick to remove cells or express a drop by squeezing the tubing. Commercially manufactured segment cutters eliminate the need for scissors, thus enabling dispensing the RBCs into a test tube in one motion. The segment may be stored with the cut end down in a properly labeled test tube and covered or stoppered to minimize contamination and maintain RBC integrity. The contents of the segment should preferably not be emptied into a test tube for storage because of the increased risk of contamination. Regardless of the method used to harvest cells from a segment, it is important that engineering and/or work practice controls be used to eliminate or minimize aerosol production when the segment is cut or opened. Refer to Chapter 25 for additional information on safety procedures.

Both donor and recipient samples must be stored for a minimum of 7 days following transfusion.[9] The samples should be stoppered, carefully labeled, and refrigerated at 1° to 6°C. They should be adequate in volume so they can be

reevaluated if the patient experiences any adverse reaction to the transfusion.

Compatibility Testing Protocols

Testing of the Donor Sample

According to the *Code of Federal Regulations*[10] and the American Association of Blood Banks (AABB) *Standards*,[11] ABO and Rh grouping (including a test for weak D) and tests intended to prevent disease transmission must be performed on a sample of blood taken at the time of collection from the donor. A screening test for unexpected antibodies to RBC antigens is required by AABB *Standards* on samples from donors who reveal a history of prior transfusion or pregnancy.[12] Testing is performed by the facility collecting the donor unit, and results must be clearly indicated on all product labels appearing on the unit.

The transfusing facility is required by AABB *Standards*[13] to confirm the ABO cell grouping on all units and Rh typing on units labeled Rh-negative. Repeat weak-D testing is not required. The transfusing facility is not required to repeat any other testing procedure. The sample used for this testing must be obtained from an attached segment on the donor unit.

All testing must be performed using in-date licensed reagents according to manufacturers' directions and protocol established in the written SOP of the facility. A detailed explanation of the processing of donor blood can be found in Chapter 11.

Testing of the Patient Sample

A record must be maintained of all results obtained in testing patient samples. Some large transfusion services keep this information on a computerized retrieval system for ready access. However, when computer records are not available, these transfusion services must have another system that permits retrieval of patient testing results.[14]

Ideally, the same unique identification number should be assigned each time a patient is admitted to a health-care facility for treatment. The number can then be used as a method for positive identification by comparing results of previous and current testing. Verification of previous results helps establish that the current samples were collected from the correct individual. Any discrepancies between previous and current results must be resolved before transfusion is initiated. A new sample should be collected from the patient, if necessary, to resolve the problem.

ABO, Rh, and unexpected antibody screening test results should be included in the record. Notations concerning unusual serologic reactions and the identity of unexpected antibodies in the patient's serum should also be included in the record. This may be the most important information. Sometimes an unexpected antibody can drop below detectable levels in a patient's serum, and previous records are the only source of information regarding its presence, identity, and clinical significance.

ABO, Rh grouping, and antibody screening of the patient's serum can be performed in advance of or at the same time as the crossmatch. If the patient has had a transfusion or has been pregnant within the last 3 months or if the history is unavailable or uncertain, the sample must be obtained from the patient within 3 days of the scheduled transfusion.[15] An accurate medical history, including information on medications, recent blood transfusions, and previous pregnancies, may help to explain unusual results.

ABO Grouping

Determination of the patient's correct ABO group is the most critical pretransfusion serologic test. ABO grouping can be performed on slides or in tubes, using solid-phase RBC adherence or column gel technology. Testing is performed in a manner similar to that described in Chapter 6, using potent licensed reagents according to the manufacturer's directions. If the ABO forward and reverse grouping results do not agree, additional testing must be conducted to resolve the discrepancy. Useful information on resolving ABO grouping discrepancies has also been presented in Chapter 6. If the patient's ABO group cannot be satisfactorily determined and immediate transfusion is required, group O–packed RBCs should be used.

Rh Typing

Rh typing is performed using anti-D blood typing reagents. Tube or slide tests should be performed according to the manufacturer's directions for the reagent, which may or may not include the use of a suitable diluent control. When indicated, these controls must be run in parallel when Rh typing tests are performed on patient samples to avoid incorrect designation of Rh-negative patients as Rh-positive. If the diluent control is positive, the result of the Rh typing test is invalid. In such a case, a direct antiglobulin test (DAT) should be performed on the patient's RBCs to determine whether uptake of autoantibodies or alloantibodies (if the recipient has been recently transfused) is responsible for the positive control. If the DAT is positive, accurate Rh typing can sometimes be performed using saline-active or chemically modified Rh blood typing serum with an appropriate diluent or 8 percent albumin control. If the Rh type of the recipient cannot be determined and transfusion is essential, Rh-negative blood should be given. Currently, most monoclonal or monoclonal blend anti-D reagents are room temperature–reactive and do not require the use of a control. See Chapter 7 for more in-depth discussion.

The test for weak D is unnecessary when testing transfusion recipients.[16] Individuals typing as Rh-negative in direct testing should receive Rh-negative blood, and those typing as Rh-positive in direct testing should receive Rh-positive blood. There are those in the blood bank community who prefer complete Rh typing of all recipients to conserve Rh-negative blood for Rh-negative patients. Female patients whose RBCs type as weak D are considered Rh-positive (see Chapter 7) and may receive Rh-positive blood during transfusion.

Some patients who type as Rh-positive, whether by direct or indirect testing, may produce anti-D following transfusion of Rh-positive RBC components (see Chapter 7). This occurs rarely and does not justify the routine transfusion of Rh-negative blood to these Rh-positive patients until the antibody is detected.

Antibody Screening

The recipient's serum or plasma must be tested for clinically significant unexpected antibodies. The object of the antibody screening test is to detect as many clinically significant unexpected antibodies as possible. In general, "clinically significant unexpected antibody" refers to antibodies that are reactive at 37°C and/or in the antihuman globulin test and are known to have caused a transfusion reaction or unacceptably short survival of transfused RBCs. **Table 13–1** lists these antibodies.[17]

TABLE 13–1	Clinical Significance of 37° C-Reactive Antibodies	
Usually*	**Very Unusual (if ever)†**	**Sometimes**
ABO	Bg(HLA)	Cartwright (e.g.,Yt^a)‡
Rh	Ch/Rg (complement C4)	Lutheran (e.g., Lu^b+)‡
Kell	Le^b	Gerbich‡
Duffy	JMH	Dombrock‡
S, s, U	Xg^a	M, N‡
P		Le^a
		Vel
		LW
		Ii
		H
		At^a
		In^b
		Mi^a
		Cs^a

* These antibodies usually cause obvious clinical symptoms and decreased RBC survival. Sometimes no obvious clinical symptoms occur.

† These antibodies rarely (if ever) cause clinically obvious symptoms, but there are some data to suggest that some unusual examples of Bg [36, 39–41], anti-Kn/Mc/Yk [36, 42], and JMH [36, 43] cause shortened RBC survival.

‡ These antibodies rarely cause acute severe HTR, but when they are "clinically significant" they may cause obvious clinical symptoms (e.g., jaundice); they more often cause only shortened RBC survival.

Reprinted with permission from Garratty, G: Evaluating the clinical significance of blood group alloantibodies that are causing problems in pretransfusion testing. Vox Sanguinis 74: 285–290, 1998. Table 1, Page 289.

The incidence of unexpected alloantibodies depends on the fact that antibody formation is the result of exposure to a foreign RBC antigen and the patient's ability to respond to that exposure. This occurs by allogeneic transfusion of RBCs, pregnancy, or transplantation. The incidence of unexpected antibodies in the general patient population, therefore, is low: 1.64 percent in one large study[18] and 0.78 percent in another.[19] It follows, then, that the more frequently a patient is exposed to foreign RBC antigens, the more likely that patient will produce unexpected alloantibodies. This is evidenced by a study of multiply transfused sickle cell patients in which 29 percent of pediatric and 47 percent of adult multiply transfused sickle cell patients developed clinically significant alloantibodies.[20]

Detection of unexpected antibodies is important for the selection of donor RBCs that will have the best survival rate in the patient's circulation and reduce the risk of hemolytic transfusion reaction. Refer to Chapter 12 for a complete discussion of the detection and identification of unexpected clinically significant alloantibodies.

Antibody screening tests should demonstrate the presence of all potentially clinically significant alloantibodies in the recipient's serum/plasma and indicate the need for further studies. All antibodies encountered in the screening test must be identified to determine potential clinical significance and to allow a logical decision to be made whether there is a need to select antigen-negative units for transfusion.

Selection of Appropriate Donor Units

In almost all cases, the first choice for transfusion is blood and blood components of the patient's own ABO and Rh group. This is defined as ABO group–specific. When blood and blood components of the patient's ABO blood group are not available or some other reason precludes their use, units selected must lack any antigen against which the recipient has a clinically significant antibody. It is completely acceptable, however, to use blood and blood components that do not contain all of the antigens carried on the patient's own RBCs (e.g., group A– or B–packed RBCs can be safely given to a group AB recipient). When a recipient must be given blood of a different ABO group, only packed RBCs can be given. Whole blood cannot be administered in these situations because incompatible preformed ABO antibodies are present in the whole blood plasma. For example, group A whole blood cannot be transfused into a group AB recipient because the plasma of the group A whole blood has anti-B antibodies present. Group O packed RBCs can be safely used for all patients; however, conservation of a limited supply of group O blood should

dictate its use for recipients of other ABO types only in special circumstances. If ABO group–specific blood is not available or is in less than adequate supply, alternative blood groups are chosen as summarized in **Table 13–2.**

Rh-negative blood can be given to Rh-positive patients; however, good inventory management should conserve this limited resource for use in Rh-negative recipients. But if the Rh-negative unit is near expiration, the unit should be given rather than wasted. Rh-positive blood should not be given to Rh-negative female patients of childbearing age. Transfusion of Rh-negative male patients and female patients beyond menopause with Rh-positive blood is acceptable as long as no preformed anti-D is demonstrable in their sera. About 80 percent of Rh-negative patients who receive 200 mL or more of Rh-positive blood respond to such a transfusion by producing anti-D.[21] However, this outcome must sometimes be weighed against the alternatives of not transfusing at all if the supply of Rh-negative blood has been exhausted. If the formation of anti-D is unlikely to be of great significance (for example, in an Rh-negative elderly surgical patient), use of Rh-positive blood is judicious in the opinion of many technologists. In these situations, approval by or notification of the blood bank's medical director is necessary, according to the laboratory's SOP.

When an unexpected antibody is found in the patient's serum during an antibody screening test, donor units selected at random are crossmatched with the patient's serum. This should not be assumed to be the standard, although this may assist in the identification of the unexpected antibody. If a clinically significant antibody is identified, the serologically compatible units are then phenotyped with commercial antiserum to verify that they are antigen-negative for the corresponding antibody. For example, if a recipient has an anti-K1 antibody, the crossmatch-compatible donor RBC unit is tested with commercial anti-K1 antisera for the presence of the K1 antigen.

There is no need to provide antigen-negative RBCs for patients whose sera contain antibodies that are reactive only below 37°C because these antibodies are incapable of causing significant RBC destruction in vivo. Clinically significant or potent examples of anti-P1, anti-Le[a], anti-Le[b], and other typically cold reactive antibodies in patients' sera can be used to select appropriate donor units that are crossmatch-compatible in tests conducted at 37°C.[22]

Potent examples of IgG, warm reactive antibodies in patients' serum can also be used to select suitable donor units by direct crossmatch testing. Commercially prepared typing reagents must be used to select blood for patients whose serum contains weak examples of antibodies active at 37°C,

	Component ABO Group			
Recipient ABO Group	1st Choice	2nd Choice	3rd Choice	4th Choice
AB	AB	A	B	O
A	A	O		
B	B	O		
O	O			

TABLE 13–2 Suggested ABO Group Selection Order for Transfusion of RBCs

Reprinted with permission from: AABB Technical Manual 14th Edition, page 454, Table 21.1 Suggested ABO Group Selection Order for Transfusion of RBCs

antibodies that react well only with panel cells carrying homozygous expression of the corresponding antigens, and for patients whose serum no longer exhibit demonstrable in vitro reactivity but which previously was known to contain clinically significant IgG antibodies, such as anti-Jk^a, anti-K1, or anti-E.

Donor units should be selected so that the RBCs are of appropriate age for the patient's needs and will not expire before use. For efficient inventory management, units that will definitely be transfused should be selected from units close to their expiration date based on the needs of the recipient.

Donor units should be examined visually before compatibility testing for unusual appearance, correct labeling, and hermetic seal integrity. Donor units showing abnormal color change, turbidity, clots, incomplete or improper labeling information, or leakage of any sort should be returned to the collecting facility.

Crossmatch Testing

The crossmatch test has traditionally meant the testing of the patient's serum with the donor RBCs including an antiglobulin phase or simply an immediate spin phase to confirm ABO compatibility. The terms "compatibility test" and "crossmatch" are sometimes used interchangeably; they should be clearly differentiated. A crossmatch is only part of pretransfusion compatibility testing, as shown in **Box 13–1**.

The serologic crossmatch test has recently undergone much scrutiny, and there have been thoughts of eliminating it entirely. However, to many blood bankers, the serologic crossmatch still has a definite role.

Originally the serologic crossmatch preceded antibody screening as part of pretransfusion compatibility testing to check for unexpected alloantibodies. Considering that over 99 percent of clinically significant unexpected antibodies in patients' sera can be detected by adequate antibody screening procedures, many blood bankers abbreviate or altogether eliminate the serologic crossmatch. What, then, is the value of performing serologic crossmatching between patient and donor samples? Two main functions of the serologic crossmatch test can be cited:

1. It is a final check of ABO compatibility between donor and patient.
2. It may detect the presence of an antibody in the patient's serum that will react with antigens on the donor RBCs but that was not detected in antibody screening because the corresponding antigen was lacking from the screening cells.

The current AABB *Standards*[23] states that tests to detect ABO incompatibility are sufficient if:

1. No clinically significant antibodies were detected in the antibody screening process, and
2. No historical record exists of the detection of clinically significant unexpected antibodies

Elimination of advance crossmatch testing, for patients undergoing surgical procedures, in which blood is unlikely to be used, has been implemented successfully in many facilities. This is accomplished by using the "type and screen" in conjunction with the maximum surgical blood order schedule (MSBOS) approach or the abbreviated crossmatch. This leads to the next generation of crossmatch decisions: the computer crossmatch.

Serologic Crossmatch Tests

The serologic crossmatch test consists of mixing the recipient's serum with donor RBCs. Several procedures can be used for serologic crossmatch testing, including the immediate spin and antiglobulin crossmatch. The objective of testing is to select donor units that are able to provide maximal benefit to the patient, which should be kept in mind when developing the test protocol. A sample procedure for a one-tube crossmatch test is given in Procedural Appendix 2. Crossmatch methods can generally be categorized by the test phase in which the procedure ends.

Immediate Spin Crossmatch

When no clinically significant unexpected antibodies are detected and there are no previous records of such antibodies, a serologic test to detect ABO incompatibility is sufficient.[24] This is accomplished by mixing the recipient's serum with donor RBCs and centrifuging immediately (i.e., immediate spin). Absence of hemolysis or agglutination indicates compatibility.

The "type and screen" process involves testing the patient's blood sample for ABO, Rh, and unexpected antibodies. The patient sample is then stored in the blood bank refrigerator for future crossmatch if blood is needed for transfusion. This process has application for patients who may need blood but, because the process may not always require transfusion, the crossmatch is not performed until necessary. The type and screen, coupled with an immediate spin crossmatch, is referred to as an abbreviated crossmatch. Studies of the use of an abbreviated crossmatch show that it is a safe and effective method of pretransfusion testing. It has been calculated to be 99.9 percent effective in preventing occurrence of an incompatible transfusion.[25] Walker[26] was able to show that the frequency with which an incompatible antiglobulin crossmatch follows a negative screen is very low: 0.06 percent. Other studies confirm its safety with similar statistics.[27–30]

However, the immediate spin does not detect all ABO incompatibilities.[31] False reactions may be seen in the presence of other immediate spin-reactive antibodies (e.g., autoanti-I), in patients with hyperimmune ABO antibodies, when the procedure is not performed correctly (i.e., delay in centrifugation or reading), when rouleaux is observed, or when infants' specimens are tested. Adding ethylenediaminetetraacetic to the test system has been reported to eliminate some of the false-positive reactions, thus improving the sensitivity of the immediate spin crossmatch.[32]

Antiglobulin Crossmatch

The antiglobulin crossmatch procedure begins in the same manner as the immediate spin crossmatch, continues to a 37°C incubation, and finishes with an antiglobulin test. Several enhancement media may be applied to enhance antigen-antibody reactions. These may include albumin, low ionic strength solution (LISS), polyethylene glycol, and polybrene as discussed in Chapter 5. For greatest sensitivity, an antihuman globulin (AHG) reagent containing both anti-IgG and anticomplement may be selected for the final phase of this crossmatch method. However, many laboratories routinely use mono specific anti-IgG AHG reagents, as discussed in Chapter 5.

An auto-control, consisting of the patient's own cells and serum, may be tested in parallel with the crossmatch test. Although current AABB *Standards* no longer requires an auto-control, some technologists still find it useful. Perkins[33] calculated the predictive value of a positive auto-control (3.6 percent) when the antibody screen was negative and decided to continue using the auto-control in pretransfusion testing. Results of the auto-control help clarify possible explanations for positive results in the crossmatches and are discussed later in this chapter.

Interpretation of Results

Tubes (gel cards, etc.) should be carefully labeled so that the contents can be identified at any stage of the procedure. After centrifugation of tubes, the supernatant should be examined for hemolysis, which, if present, must be interpreted as a positive result. Results should be read against a white or lighted background, and a magnifying mirror or hand lens can be used to facilitate reading. The button of RBCs should be gently resuspended. A "tilt and wiggle" method of resuspension is ideal. The initial tilt, when the clear supernatant sweeps over the button of RBCs, immediately indicates a positive or negative reaction. A jagged or firm button edge is indicative of a positive reaction, whereas a smooth swirling of free cells off the RBC button indicates a negative reaction. Violent or excessive shaking or tapping of the tubes may yield false-negative results because weak reactions or fragile agglutinates may be shaken loose and misread as negative. After the button has been completely resuspended, the contents of the tube should be interpreted and positive results graded according to a scale used by all technologists in the facility according to the SOP. Uniform grading of reactions allows retrospective analysis of results by supervisory staff as well as comparison of serial results obtained on samples collected from the same patient. Results can be examined microscopically for verification, if desired. Review **Color Plate 2** for typical grading of agglutination reactions.

According to the *Code of Federal Regulations,*[34] all results must be recorded immediately in a permanent ledger by means of a logical system that allows them to be easily recalled; actual observations as well as interpretations must be recorded. All work should be signed or initialed by the technologist performing the test. If an incompatibility is found, the record should clearly show the location of results of the follow-up studies, and additional testing should be performed.

Resolving Incompatibilities in the Serologic Crossmatch

The primary objective of the crossmatch test is to detect the presence of antibodies in the recipient's serum, including anti-A and anti-B, that could destroy transfused RBCs. A positive result in the crossmatch test requires explanation, and the recipient should not receive a transfusion until the cause of the incompatibility has been determined. When the crossmatch test result is positive, the results of the autocontrol and antibody screening test should be reviewed to identify patterns that may help determine the cause of the problem.

Causes of Positive Results in the Serologic Crossmatch

A positive result in the serologic crossmatch test may be caused by any of the following:

1. **Incorrect ABO grouping of the patient or donor.** ABO grouping should be immediately repeated, especially if strong incompatibility is observed in a reading taken after immediate spin. Samples that bear undisputable identity with the original patient sample and the donor bag should be used for retesting.

2. **An alloantibody in the patient's serum reacting with the corresponding antigen on donor RBCs.** The autocontrol tube will be negative unless the patient has been recently transfused with incompatible RBCs. If the antibody screening test is positive, panel studies should allow identification of antibody specificity, which then permits selection of units lacking the offending antigens for compatibility testing. Chapter 12 provides further discussion of antibody detection and identification as well as examples for study.

   A. If RBCs of all donors tested are incompatible with the patient's serum and the antibody screening test is positive, suspect either an antibody directed against an antigen of high incidence or multiple antibodies in the patient's serum. Consult a reference laboratory if you are unable to identify the specificity. (Note: If the patient has ABO-compatible siblings, the siblings may lack the antigen(s) to which the patient has been sensitized and may be excellent potential donors in an emergency.)

   B. If the antibody screening test is negative and only one donor unit is incompatible, an antibody in the patient's serum may be directed against an antigen of relatively low incidence that is present on that donor's RBCs.

   C. If the antibody screening test is negative, the patient's serum may contain either naturally occurring (e.g., anti-A1) or passively acquired ABO agglutinins. Passive acquisition of anti-A, anti-B, or anti-A,B may occur after transfusion of non-ABO–specific blood products (e.g., platelets) or by organ (e.g., liver) or bone marrow transplantation. Checking the serum grouping result to confirm the presence of an unexpected reaction with A1 cells and/or checking the patient's transfusion and transplant histories is helpful in the investigation of these cases.

3. **An autoantibody in the patient's serum reacting with the corresponding antigen on donor RBCs.** The auto-control tube will be positive. The antibody screening test and tests of the patient's serum with donor cells will show positive results. Most autoantibodies have specificity for antigens of relatively high incidence. Panel adsorption and elution studies are important to assess whether underlying alloantibodies are also present. Techniques for management of patients with autoantibodies include, among other tests, auto-adsorption of the patient's serum to remove autoan-

tibody activity. Compatibility testing could then be performed using the autoabsorbed serum. Chapter 21 provides further discussion of autoantibodies and their serologic activity.

4. **Prior coating of the donor RBCs with protein, resulting in a positive antihuman globulin test.** If one isolated positive result is obtained, a DAT should be performed on the donor's RBCs. Donor cells that demonstrate a positive DAT will be incompatible with all recipients tested in the AHG phase, because the cells are already coated with immunoglobulin and/or complement.

5. **Abnormalities in the patient's serum.**

   A. Imbalance of the normal ratio of albumin and gamma globulin (A/G ratio), as in diseases such as multiple myeloma and macroglobulinemia, may cause RBCs to stick together on their flat sides, giving the appearance of stacks of coins when viewed microscopically. This is called rouleaux formation (see Color Plate 2). This property of the serum will affect all tests, including the auto-control. Strong rouleaux may mimic true agglutination; however, agglutination clumps are refractile when viewed under the microscope. Rouleaux are usually strongest after 37°C incubation but do not persist through washing before the AHG test. Problems with rouleaux can often be resolved using the saline replacement technique.[35] See Procedural Appendix 3 for a saline replacement procedure.

   B. The presence of high molecular weight dextrans or other plasma expanders may cause false-positive results in compatibility and other tests. However, Bartholomew[36] raised doubt that the use of dextran interferes with pretransfusion testing. In scenarios in which plasma expanders interfere, all tests, including the auto-control, are generally affected equally. Saline replacement may be useful to resolve the problem.

   C. An antibody against additives in the albumin reagents may cause false-positive results in compatibility tests. Rarely, a patient's serum reacts against the albumin in testing reagents. This occurs when the patient has antibodies to the stabilizing substances, such as caprylate, added to the albumin reagents.[37] Thus, caprylate-free albumin solutions should be used in testing.

6. **Contaminants in the test system.** Dirty glassware, bacterial contamination of samples, chemical or other contaminants in saline, and fibrin clots may produce false-positive compatibility test results. Refer to **Table 13–3** for suggestions for investigation of incompatible serologic crossmatches.

Computer Crossmatch

A report by Judd[38] indicated that an electronic (computer) crossmatch to detect ABO incompatibilities was as safe as the serologic immediate spin test. Many believe that the computer crossmatch is safer than the immediate spin because the of the integrity of the computer software to detect ABO incompatibility between the sample submitted for pretransfusion testing and the donor unit.[39] The computer crossmatch compares recent ABO serologic results and interpretations on file for both the donor and the recipient being matched and determines compatibility based on this comparison. An excellent model of the computer crossmatch SOP is Butch et al.[40] Annual savings, reduced sample requirements, reduced handling of biologic materials, and elimination of false reactions associated with the immediate spin crossmatch are additional benefits identified when using the computer crossmatch. Although the advantages outweigh the disadvantages, a pretransfusion testing survey indicated that only about 1 percent of facilities in the United States use nonserologic methods for crossmatching.[41]

Figure 13–4 is a flowchart that illustrates the necessary steps for a computer crossmatch to meet the AABB

TABLE 13-3	Investigation of Incompatible Major Crossmatches	
Observations	**Possible Interpretations**	**Comments**
Crossmatch:+ Auto-control:− Antibody screen:−	• Incorrect ABO grouping of patient or donor • Patient's serum may contain an ABO antibody • Alloantibody in patient's serum reacting with antigen donor's red cells but not present on screening cells	• Repeat ABO grouping: verify identity of sample. • Check patient's sample for subgroups; check patient's transfusion and transplantation histories. • Perform antibody identification tests on patient's serum and repeat crossmatch using units negative for the corresponding antigen. If studies are noninformative and patient is incompatible with only 1 unit, locate other compatible units.
Crossmatch:+ Auto-control:− Antibody screen:+	• Donor unit may have a positive DAT • Alloantibody in patient's serum reacting with antigens on donor's cells and screening cells	• Perform DAT on donor unit; if positive, do not use the unit. • Perform antibody identification studies on patient's serum and repeat crossmatch using units negative for the corresponding antigen. • If unable to identify antibody specificity, consult a reference laboratory.
Crossmatch:+ Auto-control:+ Antibody screen:+	• Both an autoantibody and alloantibody may be present in the patient's serum • Abnormalities in patient's serum owing to imbalance of A/G ratio • Plasma expanders • Caprylate antibodies • Contaminants	• Perform autoadsorption of patient serum to remove autoantibody (if not recently transfused), perform antibody identification tests, repeat compatibility tests using autoadsorbed serum. • If rouleaux are seen, use saline replacement technique. • Obtain new specimen. • Use caprylate-free reagents. • Repeat tests using fresh saline, new bottles of reagent, clean test tubes.

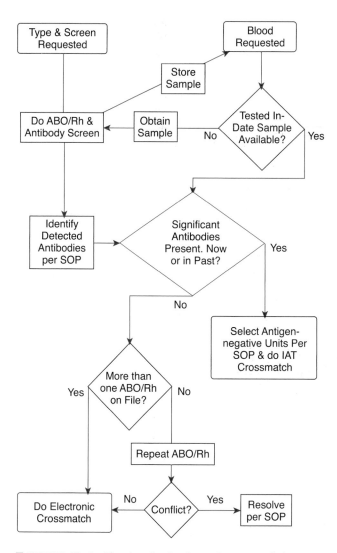

■ FIGURE 13–4 Flowchart for the electronic crossmatch that meets the requirements set forth by the AABB. Reprinted with permission from Judd, JW: Requirements for the Electronic Crossmatch. Vox Sanguinis 74: 409–417, 1998, Figure 1, page 410.

Standards.[42] The AABB *Standards* specifies that the computer crossmatch can be used only for the purpose of detecting an ABO incompatibility between the donor unit and the sample that was submitted for pretransfusion testing. Current testing for unexpected antibodies must be nonreactive, and there must not be any history of such antibodies. Also, at least two concordant patient ABO/Rh types must be on file or the computer crossmatch is not permissible.[43] One of the ABO determinations must be done on the current sample. Having a previous ABO result on file may serve as the second occasion. When there are no results on file, testing of the same sample by a second technologist, if possible, or testing of a second current sample is indicated. The computer system must have logic to notify the user of the following: discrepancies between the donor ABO group and Rh type on the unit label, and those determined by blood group confirmatory tests, and ABO incompatibility between the recipient and the donor unit. Additionally, the computer system must be validated to show that it can detect data entry discrepancies and ABO incompatibilities between patient and donor.[44]

Compatibility Testing in Special Circumstances

Emergencies

Blood component needs sometimes exceed pretransfusion testing requirements. In other words, the recipient may require the transfusion of RBC components prior to the completion of pretransfusion testing. Several approaches can be utilized in these circumstances. Some laboratories use an "emergency" compatibility testing procedure that employs a shortened incubation time, often with addition of LISS, to accelerate antigen-antibody reactions. Others maintain that regular procedures should be used in all circumstances and that blood should be issued before completion of the standard compatibility testing procedure, if necessary. They believe that there is greater danger in using an unfamiliar procedure under pressure than in releasing blood without completed testing. Although both lines of reasoning have merit, the ideal compromise may be to develop regular testing procedures that are most efficient so that they can be used in emergency and routine situations alike. Whatever the approach, the protocol for handling emergencies must be decided in advance of the situation and be familiar to all staff in the transfusion service. Adequate pretransfusion samples should be collected before transfusion of any donor blood, if possible, so that pretransfusion compatibility testing, if necessary, can subsequently be performed.

If blood must be issued in an emergency, the patient's ABO and Rh group should be determined so that group-compatible blood can be given. In extreme emergencies, when there is no time to obtain and to test a sample, group O Rh-negative packed cells can be used. If the patient is Rh-negative and large amounts of blood are likely to be needed, a decision should be made rapidly whether inventory allows and the situation demands transfusion of Rh-negative blood. Conversion to Rh-positive is best made immediately if the patient is a man or is a woman beyond childbearing age. Injections of Rh immunoglobulin to prevent formation of anti-D may sometimes be appropriate after the crisis has been resolved. This product is discussed in detail in Chapter 20.

Accurate records of all units issued in the emergency must be maintained. A conspicuous tie tag or label must be placed on each unit indicating that compatibility testing was not completed before release of the unit, and the physician must sign a release authorizing and accepting responsibility for using blood products prior to completion of pretransfusion testing, according to the *Code of Federal Regulations*.[45] Subsequent pretransfusion testing should be completed according to the chosen protocol, and any incompatible result should be reported immediately to the recipient's physician and the blood bank medical director.

Transfusion of Non–Group-Specific Blood

When donr units of an ABO group other than the recipient's own type have been transfused, such as giving a group A recipient large volumes of group O RBCs, testing the recipient's serum in a freshly drawn sample for the presence of unexpected anti-A and/or anti-B must be performed prior to giving any additional RBC transfusions. When serum from the freshly drawn sample is compatible with donor RBCs of the recipient's own ABO group, ABO group-specific blood may be given for the transfusion. If the serologic crossmatch reveals incompatibility, additional transfusions should be of the alternative blood group.

For example, if a group B patient has been given a large number of units of group O packed cells, anti-B may be present in adequate amounts to result in a positive reaction in an immediate spin crossmatch. Group O units should therefore be used for any additional transfusions.

Compatibility Testing for Transfusion of Plasma Products

Compatibility testing procedures are not required for transfusion of plasma products. However, for transfusion of large volumes of plasma and plasma products, a crossmatch test between the donor plasma and patient RBCs may be performed, although current *Standards* does not require a crossmatch test. The primary purpose for testing is to detect ABO incompatibility between donor and patient; therefore, an immediate spin crossmatch is sufficient.

Intrauterine Transfusions

Blood for intrauterine transfusion must be compatible with maternal antibodies capable of crossing the placenta. If the ABO and Rh groups of the fetus have been determined following amniocentesis, chorionic villus sampling, or percutaneous umbilical blood sampling, group-specific blood could be given provided that there is no fetomaternal ABO or Rh incompatibility. If the ABO and Rh groups of the fetus are not known, then group O Rh-negative RBCs should be selected for the intrauterine transfusion. The group O Rh-negative cells must lack any antigens against which the mother's serum contains unexpected antibodies (e.g., anti-K1, anti-Jk^a). Crossmatch testing is performed using the mother's serum sample.

Neonatal Transfusions

Blood for an exchange or regular transfusion of a neonate (younger than 4 months of age) should be compatible with any maternal antibodies that have entered the infant's circulation and are reactive at 37°C or AHG. Blood of the infant's ABO and Rh group can be used, as long as the ABO and Rh groups are not involved in the fetomaternal incompatibility. An initial pretransfusion specimen from the infant must be typed for ABO and Rh groups (only anti-A and anti-B reagents are required for ABO grouping, omitting the testing of the infant's serum with reagent RBCs).[46] Antibody detection testing can be performed using the maternal serum or, alternatively, using the infant's serum (e.g., cord serum) and/or an eluate prepared from the infant's RBCs. In addition, when cells selected for transfusion are not group O, the infant's serum or plasma must be tested to demonstrate the absence of anti-A (using A1 cells) and anti-B. This testing must include an antiglobulin phase.[47] It is unnecessary to repeat these pretransfusion tests during any one hospital admission, provided that the infant received only ABO-compatible and Rh-compatible transfusions and had no unexpected antibodies in the serum or plasma.[48] The presence of clinically significant antibodies, including anti-A and anti-B, indicates that cells lacking the corresponding antigen must be selected for transfusion until the antibody is no longer demonstrable in

the infant's serum.[49] A crossmatch does not have to be performed in these situations. **Box 13-2** summarizes the compatibility tests for infants (younger than 4 months old) and how frequently they must be performed.

For both intrauterine and infant (younger than 4 months) transfusions, blood should be as fresh as possible and no older than 7 days. Refer to Chapter 20 for additional information on neonatal transfusion.

Massive Transfusions

When the amount of whole blood or packed cell components infused within 24 hours approaches or exceeds the patient's total blood volume, the compatibility testing procedure may be shortened or eliminated at the discretion of the transfusion service physician following written policy guidelines.[50] If the patient is known to have a clinically significant unexpected antibody, all infused units should be tested for and lack the corresponding antigen, if time permits. The antibody in the patient's serum may not be demonstrable because of dilution with large volumes of plasma and other fluids. However, a rapid rise in antibody titer level and subsequent destruction of donor RBCs may occur if antigen-positive units are infused. The transfusion service physician may decide that it is better to give antigen-untested units than to hold up transfusion by waiting for the results of testing. The rationale is that it is important to give the patient a chance to survive and then to treat the immune-mediated anemia induced by massive transfusion of antigen-untested units. Again, the physician must sign a waiver of testing or a release form for all untested units for transfusion.

Specimens with Prolonged Clotting Time

Testing difficulties may be observed in blood samples from patients who have prolonged clotting times caused by coagulation abnormalities associated with disease or medications

---

BOX 13-2
Compatibility Tests for Infants Once per Admission

Routine:
ABO
Rh
Antibody screen
● Using maternal serum *or*
● Using infant's serum, especially when:
    ● No maternal specimen available
    ● Mother has clinically insignificant antibodies *or*
● Using infant's eluate
Additional:
IAT using infant serum and A₁ *and/or* B cells
● Cells can be reagent or donor (i.e., major crossmatch)
● Must be done if non-group O cells will be transfused
Antigen typing donor unit
● While infant antibody screen is positive
● Donor units must lack antigen corresponding to antibody
Every 3 Days:
Same tests as above when:
● ABO- or Rh-incompatible units are transfused *and/or*
● Unexpected antibodies are demonstrating via antibody screen

(such as heparin). A fibrin clot may form spontaneously when partially clotted serum is added to saline-suspended screening or donor RBCs. Complete coagulation of these samples can often be accelerated by addition of thrombin. One drop of thrombin, 50 U/mL, to 1 mL of plasma (or the amount of dry thrombin that will adhere to the end of an applicator stick) is usually sufficient to induce clotting.[51] A small amount of protamine sulfate can be added to counteract the effects of heparin in samples of blood collected from patients on this anticoagulant.[52]

Autologous Transfusion

Autologous transfusion refers to the removal and storage of blood or components from a donor for the donor's own possible personal use at a later time, usually during or after a surgical procedure. The ABO and Rh groups of the units must be determined by the facility collecting the blood. Tests for unexpected antibodies and tests designed to prevent disease transmission are not required when the blood will be used within the collecting facility.[53] These units must be labeled "For autologous use only."[54] According to AABB *Standards,* the pretransfusion testing and identification of the recipient and the blood sample are required and must conform to the protocols mentioned earlier in this chapter. However, tests for unexpected antibodies in the recipient's serum or plasma and a crossmatch test are optional.[55]

Limitations of Compatibility Testing Procedures

As mentioned in the introduction to this chapter, no current testing procedure can guarantee the fate of a unit of blood that is to be transfused. Even a compatible crossmatch cannot guarantee that the transfused RBCs will survive normally in the recipient. Despite careful and meticulous in-vitro testing, some compatible units will be hemolyzed in the patient. In some cases, even limited survival of donor cells may help to maintain a patient until the patient can begin to produce his or her own cells. Certainly no patient should be denied a transfusion if he or she needs one to survive, and donor cells that appear incompatible by in-vitro testing procedures may, in fact, survive quite well in vivo.

In-vivo compatibility can be determined using donor RBCs labeled with radioactive chromium (^{51}Cr) or technetium (^{99m}Tc) to measure the likelihood of successful transfusion when standard in-vitro testing procedures are inconclusive.[56,57] If a transfusion is needed to save a patient's life and all units are incompatible and if the ^{51}Cr studies indicate adequate survival of donor RBCs, then transfusion of an in-vitro incompatible unit may need to be considered. This decision should be made in consultation with the blood bank medical director and the patient's physician. The blood should be transfused slowly, and the patient should be monitored carefully.[58]

Effective Blood Utilization

Many blood bankers are acutely aware of the need to use blood efficiently due to limited blood supplies and increasing demands for blood. Technologists have observed that there have been many surgical procedures, such as dilatation and curettage and cholecystectomy, for which blood was routinely ordered but rarely used. Blood bankers also pointed out that for many other surgical procedures, more units were being ordered than were used.

The MSBOS was developed to promote more efficient utilization of blood. The goal of the MSBOS is to establish realistic blood ordering levels for certain procedures. Because variation exists in the surgical requirements of institutions, the standard blood orders should be based on the transfusion pattern of each institution and should be agreed on by the staff surgeons, anesthesiologists, and the blood bank medical director. See Chapter 16, **Box 16–8,** on page 314.

Utilization of a type and screen policy is another method to manage blood inventory levels efficiently and to reduce blood banking operating costs.[59–61] The type and screen method involves testing the recipient's blood sample completely for ABO, Rh groups, and unexpected antibodies. The specimen is refrigerated and kept available for immediate crossmatching if the need arises. The blood bank must ensure that the appropriate donor blood is available in case it is needed. The type and screen policy does not apply to patients with existing clinically significant unexpected alloantibodies because donor blood lacking the corresponding antigens must be available and should be fully crossmatched prior to surgery or transfusion.

A type and screen policy is most effective when a recipient does not have any clinically significant unexpected alloantibodies present or any abnormal serologic results in the ABO and/or Rh testing. If blood is needed quickly, the blood bank is then prepared to perform the immediate spin (or computer) crossmatch and release blood of the same ABO and Rh group as that of the recipient before release of the unit to the hospital floor. Once the blood is issued, both a 37°C incubation and AHG crossmatch can be performed using the same tube employed for the immediate spin crossmatch, if the antiglobulin crossmatch is the standard protocol used by the laboratory. If either the 37°C incubation or AHG phase of testing is positive, the patient's physician is notified immediately, and the transfusion of the unit of blood is stopped.

The application of the type and screen in combination with the MSBOS can greatly enhance the effectiveness of the blood utilization program in a health-care facility by minimizing the crossmatch-to-transfusion ratio, reducing blood bank personnel workload, and making efficient use of the blood on hand.

Reidentification of the Patient Before Transfusion

The reestablishment of the identity of the intended recipient and selected donor product is the final step leading to transfusion. The same careful approach used to properly identify the patient before sample collection must now be applied to verify that the recipient is indeed the same person who provided the initial blood sample for testing. In addition, the actual product and accompanying record of testing must be verified as relating to the same donor number.

After pretransfusion compatibility testing is completed, two records must be prepared. A statement of compatibility must be retained as part of the patient's permanent medical record if the blood is transfused, and a label or tie tag must be attached to the unit stating the identity of the intended recipient, the results of pretransfusion compatibility testing, and the donor number.[62] This identification must remain on the unit throughout the transfusion.

The original blood request form can be used conveniently to accomplish one or both of these record-keeping requirements. A multipart form is used in some facilities to record the history of pretransfusion testing and infusion of the unit. Useful information might include the initials or signature of the phlebotomist taking the sample, donor numbers, results of compatibility testing, initials or signature of the technologist performing the testing, and signatures of the persons who verify the identity of the recipient before infusion and who start the infusion. One copy of the form can be placed on the recipient's chart after the transfusion is completed, and the other is returned to the blood bank, if desired, for filing. The last copy of the form might be printed on heavier stock and perforated so that it can be torn off and attached to the unit in the laboratory. The most important feature of this system is that the patient's nameplate impression rather than a handwritten transcription identifies all forms used to identify the patient-donor combination. Many facilities now use computer-generated labels to attach to each form.

Other useful systems, mentioned earlier in this chapter, employ numbered strips or other unique coding systems that can be attached to the patient's wristband, to the compatibility form, and to the donor unit. Bar-coded identification symbols verified by portable laser scanner devices may be the system of choice in the near future for linking sample, patient, and donor products.

Whatever system is used, the information should be verified at least twice before the infusion of the product occurs. A copy of the original blood requisition form, placed on the recipient's chart after samples are collected, can be used as the request for release of the units from the blood bank. This allows another check of the nameplate impressions on all forms. Before blood is taken from the blood bank to the patient treatment area, the following records must be checked: ABO and Rh results, clinically significant unexpected antibodies, and adverse reactions to transfusion.[63] In addition, the person releasing and the person accepting the units should verify agreement between the donor numbers and ABO and Rh groups on the compatibility form and on the products themselves. The unit should also be inspected visually for any abnormalities in appearance, indicating contamination. If any abnormality is seen, the unit should not be issued unless specifically authorized by the medical director.[64]

Before transfusion is initiated, a reliable professional (and preferably two professionals) must once again verify identity of the patient and donor products. A system of positive patient identification by comparison of wristband identification and compatibility forms must be followed strictly. This is the most critical check and yet the most fallible, because the transfusion may take place in the operating suite or emergency room where the person responsible for identification may be involved with many other duties as well.

If a unit is returned to the blood bank for any reason, within the specified time for that laboratory, it should not be reissued if the container closure was opened or if the unit was allowed to warm above 10°C or to cool below 1°C.[65]

The Future of Compatibility Testing

Modern transfusion medicine is a rapidly progressing science. Technological advances will certainly affect the future prac-

tice of blood banking. Developments include the use of RBC substitutes such as modified hemoglobin solutions currently under investigation.[66,67] These substitutes can provide oxygen-carrying capacity and, because they are biologically inert and nonimmunogenic, can be administered with no requirements for crossmatching. They have been used in coronary artery bypass grafts[68] and could be used instantly at the scene of an accident or in the emergency room.[69] However, further research is needed to develop viable substitutes for blood products, and indications are that a range of products targeted at specific clinical indications, rather than one generic product, may emerge from this research.

Studies are ongoing in the biochemical modification of non–group O blood groups to phenotypically universal donor blood: the conversion of group B or A to resemble group O by the removal of A or B antigens from the RBC membrane.[70] This has great potential in helping to alleviate the problem of disproportions in certain blood group supplies. The concept of creating a universal blood donor supply is very compelling.

Automation with pretransfusion testing instruments, such as continuous-flow and batch analyzers, has streamlined compatibility testing, especially in large blood centers. Two of the most successful approaches have used microplates to perform either liquid agglutination tests or solid-phase RBC adherence tests. In addition to microplates is the column agglutination technology, whether using gel or glass beads in the column to capture agglutinates.[71,72] These methods provide efficient and economic compatibility tests for processing large numbers of donor specimens. Similar innovations are emerging to streamline blood banking testing in hospital transfusion services.

The use of gel technology is on the rise in hospital and transfusion services. The percentage of laboratories using a gel method increased from 7 percent in 1998 to 18 percent in 2001.[73] The gel test is sensitive for both antigen testing and antibody detection and identification and ABO and Rh typing.[74,75] Advantages of the gel system include standardized pipetting of reagents and specimens, reading of agglutination reactions, reviewing stable reaction endpoints up to 24 hours, and significantly reducing specimen volume. Disadvantages include longer turnaround time for ABO determinations and less sensitive detection of ABO antibodies in patient serum/plasma when compared with the tube method.[76]

The emergence of molecular biology techniques in blood bank testing is just now beginning. Nucleic acid amplification techniques, often based on polymerase chain reaction, have demonstrated application in blood typing[77] and in screening blood for hepatitis C. This testing process goes beyond the detection of antigenic determinants on the RBC membrane and goes directly into the genetic foundation of those antigens.

As a result of the French requirement to perform a final check of the ABO compatibility of the recipient and donor, several methods are available including:

1. A card with four columns containing reagent anti-A and anti-B (two for recipient and two for donor) and
2. A card with six wells, two for recipient and donor samples, and four with dried anti-A and anti-B for testing of the recipient and donor.[78]

The use of multiwavelength ultraviolet and visible light spectroscopy is currently under development and investigation as a potential quantitative blood grouping and typing procedure.

This process lends itself to automation as current blood bank automated instruments continue to experience difficulty determining and correctly interpreting weak reactions (i.e., A_2B or weak-D patients), whereas this method does not. [79,80]

Preparing for clinical care in space, National Aeronautics and Space Administration scientists showed that ABO and Coombs-sensitized standard blood grouping tests can be performed under microgravity. This was done using a closed self-operating system that automatically performed the tests and fixed the results onto filter paper for analysis on Earth. Agglutinates were smaller than usual; however, reaction endpoints were clear.[81] Although these researchers noted that additional experiments in space were needed to confirm and to quantify their results, these preliminary findings indicate yet another method for performing compatibility testing.

Finally, an automated flow cytometry system is currently being developed and investigated as to its application to pretransfusion compatibility testing. A study comparing flow cytometry with column agglutination and standard tube testing for ABO, Rh typing, and antibody detection revealed a system equivalent for each methodology. It is also quite comparable in many aspects, including sensitivity, accuracy, and specimen turnaround time.[82]

As information technology continues to grow, all aspects of patient care, including compatibility testing, may be computerized. In addition to performing an electronic crossmatch, computer systems now include electronic identification of the patient, automated testing, and electronic transfer of data. The success of these systems depends on interfacing automated testing instruments with bar-code readers and a laboratory computer.[83]

Our knowledge of compatibility testing is in a dynamic state, and we look forward to continuing developments in technical procedures to streamline and to safeguard transfusion practice. The challenge of modern blood banking will be to merge new technology with the assurance of beneficial results and positive outcomes for the patient.

SUMMARY CHART:

Important Points to Remember (MT/MLT)

I. **Collection and Preparation of Sample**
   - Most fatal transfusion reactions are caused by clerical errors.
   - Samples and forms must contain patient's full name and unique identity number.
   - Writing must be legible and indelible.
   - Date of collection must be written on sample.
   - Sample must be collected within 3 days of scheduled transfusion.
   - A blood bank specimen must have two unique patient identifiers, the date of collection, and initials or signature of the person who collected the sample

II. **Compatibility Testing**
   - Confirm blood type of donor.
   - Check patient records (history) for results of previous tests. Perform ABO grouping, Rh typing, and antibody screening on patient.
   - Select donor unit based on ABO group and Rh type of patient; further consider presence of antibodies in

patient by antigen-typing donor unit for the corresponding antigen.
   - Perform immediate spin or antiglobulin crossmatch based on current or historical serologic results.
   - Electronic crossmatch can replace immediate spin crossmatch when two blood types are on file for the patient and antibody screen is negative.
   - Positive results in the crossmatch may be caused by incorrect ABO grouping of patient or donor, alloantibody or autoantibody in patient reacting with the corresponding antigen on the donor RBCs, donor having a positive DAT, abnormalities in patient serum such as increased protein concentration (rouleaux) or contaminants in test system.

III. **Compatibility Testing in Special Circumstances**
   - Emergencies
     - May have to select uncrossmatched, group O, Rh-negative packed RBCs.
     - May want to give uncrossmatched, group O, Rh-positive packed RBCs if male patient or female patient beyond childbearing years.
     - May be able to provide type-specific, uncrossmatched RBCs.
   - Plasma products units
     - No compatibility testing required.
   - Transfusion to fetus
     - Compatibility testing performed using mother's sample.
     - Donor unit must lack antigen against maternal antibody.
     - Group O Rh-negative donor selected when fetal type is unknown or when type is known but is not compatible with mother's type.
   - Transfusion to infant
     - Maternal sample can be used for compatibility testing.
     - Initial sample from infant typed for ABO (front type) and Rh.
     - Donor unit selected should be compatible with both mother and baby.

REVIEW QUESTIONS

1. Compatibility testing:
   a. Proves that the donor's plasma is free of all irregular antibodies
   b. Detects most irregular antibodies on the donor's RBCs that are reactive with patient's serum
   c. Detects most errors in the ABO groupings
   d. Ensures complete safety of the transfusion

2. Which is true of rouleaux formation?
   a. It is a stacking of RBCs to form aggregates.
   b. It can usually be dispersed by adding saline.
   c. It can appear as an ABO incompatibility.
   d. It can cause a false-positive immediate spin crossmatch.

3. What type of blood should be given in an emergency transfusion when there is no time to type the recipient's sample?
   a. O Rh_0 (D)-negative, whole blood
   b. O Rh_0 (D)-positive, whole blood
   c. O Rh_0 (D)-positive, packed cells
   d. O Rh_0 (D)-negative, packed cells

4. A patient developed an anti-Jk^a antibody 5 years ago. The antibody screen is currently negative. To obtain suitable blood for transfusion, which procedures apply?
   a. Type the patient for the Jk^a antigen as an added part to the crossmatch procedure.
   b. Crossmatch random donors with the patient's serum, and release the compatible units for transfusion to the patient.
   c. Type the donor units for the Jk^a antigen, and then crossmatch the Jk^a negative units for the patient.
   d. Computer-crossmatch Jk^a negative donor units

5. A 26-year-old B Rh_0 (D)-negative female patient requires a transfusion. No B Rh_0 (D)-negative donor units are available. Which should be chosen for transfusion?
   a. B Rh_0 (D)-positive RBCs
   b. O Rh_0 (D)-negative RBCs
   c. AB Rh_0 (D)-negative RBCs
   d. A Rh_0 (D)-negative RBCs

6. Having checked the patient's prior history after having received the specimen and request, you:
   a. do not have to repeat the ABO and Rh if the name and hospital number agree
   b. do not have to repeat the indirect antiglobulin test (IAT) if the previous IAT was negative
   c. have to perform a crossmatch only if one has not been done within the last 2 weeks
   d. have to compare the results of your ABO, Rh, & IAT with the previous results.

7. The purpose of the immediate spin crossmatch is to:
   a. ensure survival of transfused RBCs
   b. determine ABO compatibility between donor and recipient
   c. detect cold-reacting unexpected antibodies
   d. meet computer crossmatch requirements

8. Which represents requirements set forth by the AABB for the performance of a computer crossmatch?
   a. Computer system must be validated on site
   b. Recipient antibody screen must be negative
   c. Two determinations of the recipient ABO and Rh must be performed
   d. Computer system must have logic

9. You have just received a request and sample for pretransfusion testing. Which is the *most* appropriate to do *first*?
   a. Perform the ABO grouping and Rh typing
   b. Complete the crossmatch
   c. Perform the IAT to see if the patient is going to be a problem

d. Check the records for prior type and screen results on the patient

10. Blood donor and recipient samples used in crossmatching must be stored for a minimum of how many days following transfusion?
    a. 2
    b. 5
    c. 7
    d. 10

11. Which is true regarding compatibility testing for the infant younger than 4 months old?
    a. A DAT is required.
    b. A crossmatch is not needed with the infant's blood when unexpected antibodies are present.
    c. Maternal serum cannot be used for antibody detection.
    d. To determine the infant's ABO group, RBCs must be tested with reagent anti-A, anti-B, and anti-A,B.

12. A nurse just called to request additional RBC units for a patient for whom you performed compatibility testing 4 days ago. They would like you to use the original specimen as you keep it for 7 days anyway. Your *most* appropriate course of action would be to:
    a. check to see if there is enough of the original specimen
    b. perform the compatibility testing on the original specimen
    c. request a new specimen in case the patient has developed a clinically significant unexpected antibody
    d. indicate that a new specimen is necessary because the patient has been recently transfused

13. A crossmatch is positive at AHG phase with polyspecific AHG reagent but is negative with monospecific anti-IgG AHG reagent. This may indicate the antibody:
    a. is a weak anti-D
    b. is a clinically insignificant Lewis antibody
    c. can cause decreased survival of transfused RBCs
    d. is a Kidd antibody

14. The emergency room requests six units of packed RBCs for a trauma patient prior to collection of the patient's specimen. The *most* appropriate course of action is to:
    a. release group O RBCs to ER with trauma patient identification on each unit sent
    b. refuse to release units until you get a patient sample
    c. indicate necessity for signed physician waiver for incomplete pretransfusion testing
    d. explain need of patient's ABO group prior to issuance of blood

15. Which is an example of the most common form of error associated with fatal transfusion reactions?
    a. Phlebotomist labels patient A tubes with patient B information
    b. Technologist enters results of patient A testing into patient B field
    c. Wrong RBC unit is tagged for transfusion
    d. Antibody below detectable levels during pretransfusion testing

REFERENCES

1. Shulman, I, et al, Pretransfusion compatibility testing for red cell administration. Cur Opin Hematol 8:397, 2001.
2. Linden, JV, et al: Transfusion error in New York State: An analysis of 10 years experience. Transfusion 40:1207, 2000
3. Standards for Blood Banks and Transfusion Services, ed 21. American Association of Blood Banks, Bethesda, MD, 2002, p 42, 5.11.2.
4. Ibid, p 3, 2.1.2
5. Ibid, p 42, 5.11.2–4.
6. Ibid, p 42, 5.11.1,5.
7. Ibid, p 44, 5.12.3.2.
8. Ibid, pp 10–13, 5.1.6.
9. Ibid, pp 42–43, 5.11.6, 5.11.6.1.
10. Code of Federal Regulations (CFR), Title 21, Food and Drugs. Office of the Federal Register, National Archives and Records Service, General Services Administration, Part 610, section 40, revised June 11, 2001, and Part 640, section 5 revised August 6, 2001.
11. Standards, op cit, pp 36–39, 5.8, and pp 43–45, 5.12.
12. Ibid, p 37, 5.8.3.1.
13. Ibid, p 43, 5.11.7.
14. Ibid, p 71, 6.2.5.2.
15. Ibid, p 44, 5.12.3.4.1.
16. Ibid, p 44, 5.12.2.
17. Garratty, G: Evaluating the clinical significance of blood group alloantibodies that are causing problems in pretransfusion testing. Vox Sang 74: 285, 1998.
18. Giblett, ER: Blood group alloantibodies: An assessment to some laboratory practices. Transfusion 17:299, 1977.
19. Spielmann, W, and Seidl, S: Prevalence of irregular red cell antibodies and their significance in blood transfusion and antenatal care. Vox Sang 26:551, 1974.
20. Aygun B, et al: Clinical significance of RBC alloantibodies and autoantibodies in sickle cell patients who received transfusion. Transfusion 42:37, 2002.
21. Mollison, PL: Blood Transfusion in Clinical Medicine, ed 9. Blackwell Scientific, Oxford, England, 1993, p 225.
22. Brecher, Mark E (ed): Technical Manual, ed 14. American Association of Blood Banks, Bethesda, MD, 2001, p 387.
23. Standards, op cit, p 46, 5.13.1.1.
24. Brecher, MD, (ed): Technical Manual, ed 14, American Association of Blood Banks, Bethesda, MD, 2002, p 385
25. Alexander D, and Henry JB: Immediate spin crossmatch in routine use: A growing trend in compatibility testing for red cell transfusion therapy. Vox Sang 70:48, 1996.
26. Walker, RH: On the safety of the abbreviated crossmatch. In Polesky, HF, and Walker, RH (eds): Safety in Transfusion Practices; CAP Conference, Aspen, 1980. College of American Pathologists, Skokie, IL, 1982, p 75.
27. Shulman, IA, et al: Experience with the routine use of an abbreviated crossmatch. Am J Clin Pathol 82:178, 1984.
28. Dodsworth, H, and Dudley, HAF: Increased efficiency of transfusion practice in routine surgery using pre-operative antibody screening and selective ordering with an abbreviated crossmatch. Br J Surg 72:102, 1985.
29. Garratty, G: Abbreviated pretransfusion testing. Transfusion 26:217, 1986.
30. Shulman, IA, et al: Experience with a cost-effective crossmatch protocol. JAMA 254:93, 1985.
31. Judd, WJ: Are there better ways than the crossmatch to demonstrate ABO incompatibility? Transfusion 31:192, 1991.
32. Shulman, IA, and Calderon, C: Effect of delayed centrifugation or reading on the detection of ABO incompatibility by the immediate-spin crossmatch. Transfusion 31:197, 1991.
33. Perkins, JT, et al: The relative utility of the autologous control and the antiglobulin test phase of the crossmatch. Transfusion 30:503, 1990.
34. CFR, op cit, part 606, section 160.
35. Green, TS: Rouleaux and autoantibodies (or things that go bump in the night). In Treacy, M (ed): Pre-Transfusion Testing for the 80s. American Association of Blood Banks, Washington, DC, 1980, p 93.
36. Bartholomew, JR, et al: A prospective study of the effects of dextran administration on compatibility testing. Transfusion 26: 431, 1986.
37. Golde, DW, et al: Serum agglutinins to commercially prepared albumin. In Weisz-Carrington, P: Principles of Clinical Immunohematology. Year Book Medical, Chicago, 1986, p 214.
38. Judd, JW: Requirements for the electronic crossmatch. Vox Sang 74: 409, 1998.
39. Ibid.
40. Butch, SH, et al: Electronic verification of donor-recipient compatibility: The computer crossmatch. Transfusion 34:105, 1994.
41. Maffei, LM, et al: Survey on pretransfusion testing. Transfusion 38:343, 1998.
42. Judd, JW: Requirements for the electronic crossmatch. Vox Sang 74: 409, 1998.
43. Ibid.
44. Standards, op cit pp 46–47, 5.13.2.
45. CFR, op cit, part 606, section 160.
46. Standards, op cit, pp 48–49, 5.15.
47. Ibid.
48. Ibid.
49. Ibid.
50. Ibid, p 50, 5.16.4.
51. Brecher, MD, (ed): Technical Manual, ed 14, American Association of Blood Banks, Bethesda, MD, 2002, p 381.
52. Ibid.
53. Standards, op cit, pp 38–39, 5.8.5.
54. Ibid, p 57, 5.6.1A.
55. Ibid, p 36, 5.8
56. Garratty, G: Evaluating the clinical significance of blood group alloantibodies that are causing problems in pretransfusion testing. Vox Sang 74:285, 1998.
57. Marcus CS, et al: Radiolabeled red cell viability II. ^{99m}Tc and ^{111}In for measuring the viability of heterologous red cells in vivo. Transfusion 7: 420, 1986.
58. Garratty, G: Evaluating the clinical significance of blood group alloantibodies that are causing problems in pretransfusion testing. Vox Sang 74:285, 1998.
59. Shulman, IA, et al: Experience with a cost-effective crossmatch protocol. JAMA 254:93, 1985.
60. Davis, SP, et al: Maximizing the benefits of type and screen by continued surveillance of transfusion practice. Am J Med Technol 49:579, 1983.
61. Issitt, PD: Applied Blood Group Serology, ed 4. Montgomery Scientific, Durham, NC, 1998, pp 892–893.
62. Standards, op cit, pp 11–12, 5.1.6.3.
63. Ibid, p 50–51, 5.17.
64. Ibid.
65. Ibid.
66. Chang, TMS: Future generations of red blood cell substitutes. J Intern Med 253:527, 2003.
67. Moore, EE: Blood substitutes: The future is now. J Am Coll Surg 196:1, 2003.
68. Moore, EE: op cit, p 7
69. Ibid.
70. Kruskall, MS, et al: Transfusion to blood group A and O patients of group B RBCs that have been enzymatically converted to group O. Transfusion 40:1290, 2000.
71. Sandler, SG: A fully automated blood typing system for hospital transfusion services. ABS2000 Study Group. Transfusion 40:201, 2000.
72. Morelati, R, et al: Evaluation of a new automated instrument for pretransfusion testing. Transfusion 38:959, 1998.
73. Shulman, I, et al: Pretransfusion compatibility testing for red cell administration. Curr Opin Hematol 8:397, 2001.
74. Weisbach, V, et al: Comparison of the performance of four microtube column agglutination systems in the detection of red cell alloantibodies. Transfusion 39:1045, 1999.
75. Dittmar, K, et al: Comparison of DATs using traditional tube agglutination to gel column and affinity column procedures. Transfusion 41:1258, 2001.
76. Langston, JL, et al: Evaluation of the gel system for ABO grouping and D typing. Transfusion 39:300, 1999.
77. St. Louis, M, et al: Extended blood grouping of blood donors with automatable PCR-ELISA genotyping. Transfusion 43:1126, 2003.
78. Migeot, V, et al: Reliability of bedside ABO testing before transfusion. Transfusion 42:1348, 2002.
79. Narayanan, S, et al: Ultraviolet and visible light spectrophotometric approach to blood typing: Objective analysis by agglutination. Transfusion 39:1051, 1999.
80. Narayanan, S, et al: UV-visible spectrophotometric approach to blood typing II: Phenotyping of subtype A_2 and weak D and whole blood analysis. Transfusion 42:619, 2002.
81. Morehead, RT, et al: Erythrocyte agglutination in microgravity. Aviat Space Environ Med 60:235, 1989.
82. Roback, JD, et al: An automatable format for accurate immunohemtology testing by flow cytometry. Transfusion 43:918, 2003.
83. Lau, FY, et al: Improvement in transfusion safety using a specially designed transfusion wristband. Transfusion Med 10:121, 2000.

PROCEDURAL APPENDIX 1

Preparation of Washed "Dry" Button of RBCs for Serologic Tests

1. Transfer one drop of 3%–5% suspension of RBCs into a 10 × 75 mm test tube filled 3/4 full with saline. Tube should be prelabeled to identify contents.
2. Centrifuge at time and speed calibrated for particular test to form tight button at the bottom of the tube.
3. Decant saline by quick inversion of the tube over a receptacle. Flick last drop of saline from cells by giving tube a quick shake while it is still in inverted position. (Reduce aerosol production by using engineering and/or work practice controls.) Tap inverted tube onto gauze or paper towel to remove residual saline.
4. Add serum directly to "dry" button of cells. Method can be used for antibody screening or identification procedures, compatibility testing, and cell typing using a tube technique.

Model One-Tube-Per-Donor-Unit Crossmatch Procedure

1. Into an appropriately labeled, 10×75 mm test tube, add 2 or 3 drops of recipient serum to achieve an approximate 2:1 ratio of serum to RBC. (Droppers used to dispense RBCs and serum should be of equivalent size.)

2. Dispense 1 drop of a washed, 2–5% suspension of donor RBCs. (Alternatively, prepare a washed "dry" button of donor RBCs, using the technique in Procedural Appendix 1.)

3. Centrifuge at time and speed that have been previously shown to give clear-cut differentiation between positive and negative results (15 sec in a Serofuge is usually adequate).

4. Observe supernatant for hemolysis that must be considered indicative of an antigen-antibody reaction. Resuspend cell button by gentle manipulation of the tube. Grade all positive results. Record observations. **Stop here for immediate spin crossmatch**.

5. Add 2 drops of LISS (or other enhancement medium, such as 22% albumin) to the tube (the enhancement medium may be omitted, if desired; incubating tubes for at least 30 min at 37°C). Mix and incubate for time indicated in enhancement media manufacturer's instructions at 37°C.

6. Centrifuge as above, observe supernatant for hemolysis, gently resuspend cell button, and record reaction results.

7. Wash 3 to 4 times using an automated instrument or manual washing technique. Decant saline completely from last wash and blot dry to achieve dry button.

8. Add 1 to 2 drops of AHG serum to tube. (Follow manufacturer's directions for use of reagent selected.) Centrifuge, gently resuspend cell button, and record reaction results.

9. Add 1 drop IgG-sensitized RBCs to each negative reaction test. Centrifuge and examine. Test must be positive, or results of procedure are invalid and test must be repeated.

Saline Replacement Procedure

This procedure has application for patients with abnormally high serum/plasma protein concentrations (such as a multiple myeloma patient whose RBCs demonstrate rouleaux formation in the test tube). The problem arises when attempting to distinguish between true agglutination and rouleaux. This applies to tests that use patient serum/plasma such as the ABO reverse (confirmatory) testing or antibody screen/panel testing. It also has application for facilities that use patient serum/plasma suspended RBCs for tests such as the ABO forward grouping and Rh typing.

Upon discovery that the observed agglutination may be caused by rouleaux:

1. Centrifuge the tube or tubes for time appropriate for test. Gently remove tube from centrifuge; with a pipette, carefully remove the patient's serum/plasma from the RBC button, noting volume removed.
2. Add volume of saline to tube equivalent to volume of serum/plasma removed. Resuspend RBCs in saline. Centrifuge for time appropriate for test.
3. Gently remove tube and observe for agglutination. Rouleaux will readily disperse in the saline, whereas true agglutination will persist.

fourteen

Orientation to the Modern Blood Bank Laboratory

Cara L. Calvo, MS, MT(ASCP)SH, CLS(NCA), and
Burlin Sherrick, MT(ASCP)SBB

OBJECTIVES

On completion of the chapter, the learner should be able to:

1. Describe a modern blood bank laboratory in terms of its operations, personnel, facilities, and equipment.
2. Explain the purpose of the following equipment used in a blood bank laboratory: apheresis machine, flatbed agitator, sterile docking device, and leukoreduction filter.
3. Summarize blood bank laboratory services in terms of policies, procedures, and tests performed.
4. Compare and contrast testing performed on donor units and recipient blood samples.
5. Apply knowledge of immunohematology theory and skills developed in classroom practice to actual work situations in the blood bank laboratory.

Introduction

Each year over 8 million volunteers donate 14 million units of whole blood in the United States,[1] collected primarily at blood centers like those operated by the American Red Cross and the American Blood Centers. In addition, in the United States approximately 27 million units of blood and blood products are transfused each year.[2] The blood bank laboratory is one of the most specialized and challenging workplaces in the field of laboratory medicine. Scientific discovery, technological innovation, and advances in medical informatics are played out on a daily basis against a backdrop of work routines unfamiliar to the newcomer. Underlying theories and principles of antigen-antibody reactions and their effects on blood are translated into clinical practice. The blood bank laboratory is a place of business where donated blood and blood products undergo extensive testing, and every task associated with the work performed is scrutinized to ensure the quality and safety of both the services and the products provided. The reg-ulating agency is the Food and Drug Administration (FDA), and the accrediting organization is usually the American Association of Blood Banks (AABB).

The purpose of this chapter is to serve as a tour through the typical blood bank and to describe the various sections within the department and the procedures that are performed. Although every blood bank may not contain all the sections described in this chapter, it is important for the student to understand and appreciate the complete scope of transfusion medicine.

Organization

For the purposes of this discussion, a blood bank laboratory is a facility involved in the collection, storage, processing, and distribution of human blood and blood products for transfusion.[3] Typically, it functions as a unit of a larger organization, such as a hospital department or community blood center, and follows the general operational guidelines of that organization. The larger organization stipulates the conditions under which the blood bank conducts business, such as hours of operations, and provides necessary facilities, equipment, and personnel. However, the blood bank laboratory also functions as a component of the heavily regulated health-care industry. This means that the blood bank laboratory also operates under constraint of laws administered by various governmental agencies (Table 14–1) and in accordance with standards established by nonregulatory accrediting organizations such as the AABB.[4,5]

Blood bank laboratories are located in a variety of settings, and the extent of services that a blood bank offers varies accordingly. For example, hospital blood banks may choose to collect and process blood components for their own use, or they may choose to contract to receive blood products from a blood center. For ease of discussion, it is assumed that the blood bank is divided into distinct areas, each with its own purpose and function. In reality, with the exception of very large transfusion services, these areas are not physically separated but overlap within the overall structure of the blood bank laboratory (Table 14–2). These areas include the following and are discussed in the following sections.

Component Preparation and Storage

Depending on the needs of a hospital, blood components may be acquired from external sources such as the American Red Cross or other regional blood centers, or components may be processed in-house.

Blood Banks with Collection Facilities

Blood banks that collect their own units of whole blood can use their blood resources more efficiently by separating them into a variety of components, including packed red blood cells (RBCs), platelets, fresh frozen plasma (FFP), and cryoprecipitate (Table 14–3) (also see Chapter 11).

To maximize the number of components derived from a unit of whole blood, processing must occur within 6 to 8

TABLE 14–1 Primary Government Agencies with Established Requirements for Blood Bank Operations	
Agency	**Authority**
Center for Medicare and Medicaid Services (CMS)	Regulates all aspects of human lab testing in the U.S. through the provisions of the Clinical Laboratory Improvement Amendments of 1988
Food and Drug Administration (FDA)	Regulates the collection, manufacture, transportation, and storage of blood products, as well as the tests and devices used to prepare the products through the provisions of the Federal Food, Drug and Cosmetic Act and the Public health Service Act
Occupational Safety and Health Administration (OSHA)	Regulates the workplace conditions and enforces safety standards through the provisions of the Occupational Safety and Health Act

TABLE 14–2 Blood Bank Areas and Functions	
Area	**Functions**
Component preparation and storage	• Separation of whole blood into packed RBCs, plasma, platelets, and cryoprecipitate • Storage of blood products at appropriate temperatures • Apheresis procedures

Donor processing	• Donor units tested for:
	  • ABO and Rh
	  • Antibody screen
	  • Serologic test for syphilis
	  • Transfusion-transmitted viruses

Main laboratory	• Patient samples tested for:
	  • ABO and Rh
	  • Antibody screen
	  • Crossmatch
	  • DAT
	  • Prenatal evaluation
	  • Postpartum evaluation
	  • Cord blood studies
	• Issue of blood products

Reference laboratory	• Resolution of:
	  • ABO and Rh discrepancies
	  • Antibody identification
	  • Positive DAT
	  • Warm autoantibodies
	  • Cold autoantibodies
	  • Transfusion reactions

hours of collection, depending on the anticoagulant used.[5] Within this period, the blood can be centrifuged to pack the RBCs by means of large, floor-model temperature-controlled centrifuges, and the plasma can be expressed and frozen. This is the process by which packed RBCs and FFP are made. If the unit of blood is maintained at room temperature throughout this process and the appropriate centrifugation times and speeds are observed, a platelet concentrate can also be derived from the expressed plasma before it is frozen. Additionally, through a controlled thawing process, the frozen plasma can be further manipulated to yield cryoprecipitate (Fig. 14–1).

Some blood components may also be prepared through a procedure known as apheresis. A donor's blood is removed in a sterile manner through tubing connected to an automated machine that processes the blood, removes the desired com-

TABLE 14–3 Components Made from Whole Blood and Processes of Component Preparation	
Component	**Processes of Preparation**
Granulocytes	Apheresis
RBCs	Leukoreduction filtration, centrifugation, apheresis
Platelets	In-line filtration, centrifugation, apheresis
Cryoprecipitated antihemophilic factor	Frozen plasma cryoprecipitation (slow thaw)
Fresh frozen plasma	Heavy spin centrifugation followed by freezing (−18°) or colder

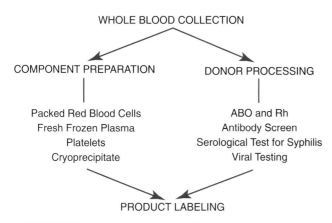

WHOLE BLOOD COLLECTION

COMPONENT PREPARATION   DONOR PROCESSING

Packed Red Blood Cells   ABO and Rh
Fresh Frozen Plasma   Antibody Screen
Platelets   Serological Test for Syphilis
Cryoprecipitate   Viral Testing

PRODUCT LABELING

■ **FIGURE 14–1**   Processing of whole blood units from collection to labeling. Note that component preparation and donor processing may occur concurrently.

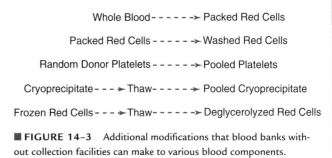

Whole Blood - - - - - → Packed Red Cells

Packed Red Cells - - - - - → Washed Red Cells

Random Donor Platelets - - - - - → Pooled Platelets

Cryoprecipitate - - - → Thaw - - - - - → Pooled Cryoprecipitate

Frozen Red Cells - - - → Thaw - - - - - → Deglycerolyzed Red Cells

■ **FIGURE 14–3**   Additional modifications that blood banks without collection facilities can make to various blood components.

ponent (platelets, plasma, granulocytes, RBCs), and returns the remainder of the components back to the donor. **(Fig. 14–2)** (also see Chapter 17).[6]

Blood Banks Without Collection Facilities

Blood banks that depend on an outside source for their blood supplies usually receive their products in component form.

However, situations do arise in which products must be modified **(Fig. 14–3)**. For example, a patient who is deficient in IgA may require washed RBCs. Automated cell washers are used to prepare this product. A unit of blood is introduced into a sterile disposable bowl that has tubing connected to a normal saline solution. A portion of this saline is added to the bowl, the cells and saline are mixed, the mixture is centrifuged, and the supernatant is removed through waste tubing. Multiple washes can be performed in this manner **(Fig. 14–4)**.

Blood components such as platelet concentrates and cryoprecipitate may be received as individual units but are more easily administered if pooled before infusion. Such product manipulation is common in most blood banks.

Sterile connecting devices (STCDs) have also become commonplace in some blood banks **(Fig. 14–5)**. These devices produce sterile welds between two pieces of compatible tubing. This procedure permits sterile connection of a variety of

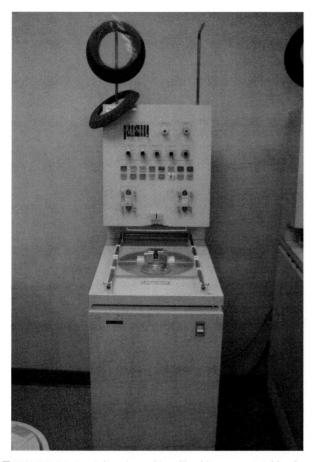

■ **FIGURE 14–2**   Apheresis machines like this one are capable of selectively removing blood components from a donor and returning the remaining ones to donor circulation.

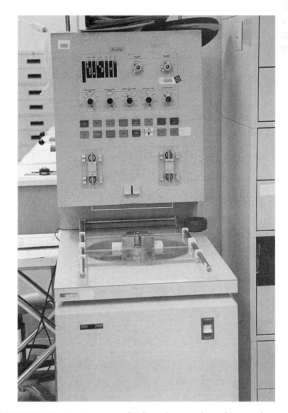

■ **FIGURE 14–4**   Automated cell washers such as this may be used to prepare washed RBCs or deglycerolize frozen RBCs. (Courtesy National Institutes of Health, Bethesda, MD.)

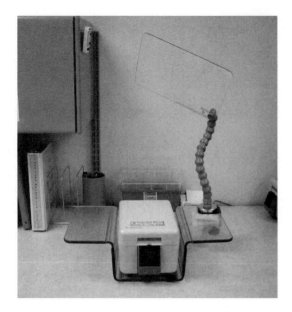

■ **FIGURE 14-5**   This sterile docking device allows for entry into donor units without affecting the expiration date of the product.

containers and tube diameters. Sterile connecting devices can be used in many settings; for example transplant patients often require a specific type of RBCs and a specific type of plasma depending on the ABO type of the donor and the recipient. If apheresis platelets are ordered for a transplant patient and the plasma contained in this product is incompatible, an STCD can be used to replace the incompatible plasma with sterile saline in the apheresis unit. Other applications of STCDs are listed in **Box 14-1**.

If freezers capable of maintaining temperatures at or below −65°C are available, blood banks may choose to freeze rare or autologous units in 40 percent glycerol for long-term storage. The same automated cell washers for washing cells for the patient deficient in IgA can be used to remove the glycerol from these units before transfusion by adding increasingly diluted concentrations of saline to thawed cells.

A patient who is immunosuppressed (e.g., bone marrow transplant recipient) may have a restriction in the record to irradiate all cellular products prior to transfusion. Irradiation renders donor lymphocytes nonfunctional and protects against graft-versus-host disease. Usually, irradiators are housed only in large transfusion services so that if such a product is required in a small hospital, an external resource is used. An irradiated product is usually labeled with an irradiation sticker showing the date and time of irradiation. The expiration date of the unit may change depending on the product irradiated (see Chapter 11).

Regardless of the method used to obtain blood and blood components, all blood banks must follow certain requirements for storing blood products.[4,5] Therefore, the following equipment is common to most blood banks:

1. Refrigerators maintained at 1° to 6°C for the storage of packed RBCs and whole blood
2. Freezers maintained at −18°C or lower for the storage of FFP and cryoprecipitate
3. Freezers maintained at −65°C or lower for the storage of RBCs frozen in 40 percent glycerol
4. Platelet rotators (**Fig. 14-6**) or flatbed agitators (**Fig. 14-7**) that provide constant gentle agitation at room temperature for the storage of apheresis and random donor platelets.

Donor Processing

Before a unit of blood can be placed into the general inventory (rendering it available to be used for crossmatching purposes), testing must be performed to determine its suitability for transfusion. This is the responsibility of the donor processing area. These tests must be performed at each donation regardless of the number of times a donor has previously donated. A separate tube of blood is collected from the donor at the time of donation for this purpose. **Box 14-2** lists the tests that are performed on blood after donation.

Automation has greatly increased the efficiency and productivity of this section of the blood bank.[6] Description of these tests and of the automation is provided in Chapter 11.

Product Labeling

Labeling of blood products may occur only after a careful review of all test results shows the unit to be suitable for transfusion. Suitability requirements include:

BOX 14-1
Applications of Sterile Connecting Devices

● Adding a fourth bag to a whole blood collection triple-pack for the production of cryoprecipitated AHF from FFP
● Connection of an additive solution to an RBC unit
● Addition of an in-line filter for leukocyte reduction
● Addition of a third storage container to a plateletpheresis harness
● Pooling of blood components
● Preparation of aliquots for pediatric transfusion
● Attachment of processing solutions
   ● Additive solutions for RBCs
   ● Glycerol for frozen RBCs
   ● Normal saline to replace incompatible plasma

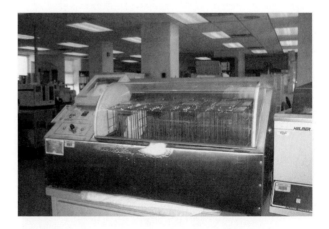

■ **FIGURE 14-6**   Platelet rotators prevent the formation of platelet aggregates and optimize the exchange of gases required for platelet survival.

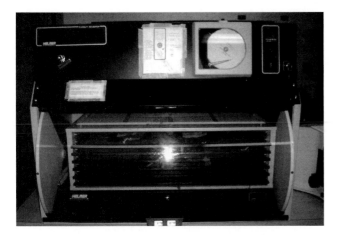

■ **FIGURE 14–7**   Flatbed agitators like this one provide optimal environmental conditions for platelet viability during storage.

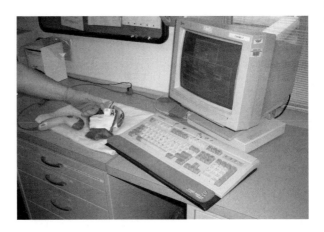

■ **FIGURE 14–8**   When all testing requirements are complete and discrepancies are resolved, a packed RBC unit is labeled prior to storage.

1. No discrepancies in the ABO and Rh testing
2. Absence of detectable antibodies in plasma-containing components
3. Nonreactive viral marker tests
4. Nonreactive syphilis test

When the established criteria are met, the RBCs and any other components are labeled with the appropriate ABO, Rh, and expiration date, and the products are stored at their proper temperatures **(Fig. 14–8)**.

Units received from outside sources would have undergone the required testing and been deemed suitable for transfusion by the shipping facility. However, according to AABB *Standards,* the blood bank to which this blood is shipped is required to reconfirm the labeled ABO of each RBC-containing product received.[5] As a cost containment measure, many blood banks confirm group O units using a commercially available mixture of monoclonal anti-A and anti-B in a single reagent (anti-A,B) and confirm other blood groups using separate anti-A and anti-B reagents **(Table 14–4)**. Because of the potential sensitization that may occur if Rh-

positive blood is transfused to an Rh-negative patient, the Rh type of all Rh-negative units must be reconfirmed.

Main Laboratory

Patient care is the primary mission of the main laboratory. Here the testing is performed that determines the compatibility between a patient requiring transfusion and the unit of blood to be transfused. Because of the severe adverse reaction that may occur if the wrong unit of blood is transfused, great care must be taken both in the testing performed and in specimen and unit identification and paperwork.[7] Common approaches are evident in the pretransfusion testing protocols that are established by different blood banks to ensure the orderly, timely, and accurate processing of patient samples **(Fig. 14–9)**.

Sample Acceptance

Proper patient identification is crucial for any specimen used in blood bank testing. Consequences may be fatal if a blood specimen is labeled with the wrong patient's name. Thus, each specimen and request form the blood bank receives are carefully examined for proper spelling of the patient's name, correct identification number, correct date of collection, and identity of the phlebotomist.

Routine Testing

Once a patient sample has been judged acceptable, the testing requested by the patient's physician can be performed

BOX 14–2
Testing of Donor Blood

Required Tests
- ABO and Rh
- Antibody screen
- Serologic test for syphilis
- Hepatitis B surface antigen (HBsAg)
- Antibodies to human immunodeficiency virus (Anti-HIV)
- Antibodies to human T-cell lymphotropic virus (Anti-HTLV-I/II)
- Antibodies to hepatitis C virus (Anti-HCV)
- Human immunodeficiency virus antigen (HIV-1-Ag)
- Antibodies to hepatitis B core antigen (Anti-HBc)
- Nucleic acid amplification testing (NAT)

TABLE 14–4   Abbreviated ABO and Rh Retype Protocol

Blood Type	Test Performed
A Positive	Anti-A, Anti-B
B Positive	Anti A, Anti-B
AB Positive	Anti A, Anti-B
O Positive	Anti-A,B
A Negative	Anti-A, Anti-B, Anti-D
B Negative	Anti A, Anti-B, Anti-D
AB Negative	Anti A, Anti-B, Anti-D
O Negative	Anti-A,B, Anti-D

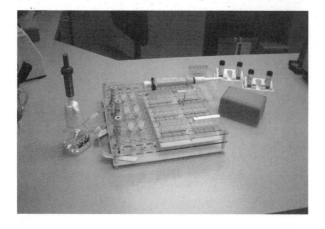

■ FIGURE 14–9 Patient samples received by the blood bank laboratory are identified, and a sample tube is carefully organized prior to testing.

shown to express a weak D antigen using an antiglobulin technique, many hospitals choose to contain costs and utilize time more efficiently by eliminating testing of patient samples for weak D and by determining patient Rh types based on immediate spin results only (see Chapter 7).

To increase the sensitivity of the antibody screen, some blood banks use a three-cell antibody screening set that provides homozygous antigen expression in all major blood group systems. In the absence of a positive antibody screen, if blood is needed on an emergency basis during surgery, it can be released using an abbreviated crossmatch if the patient has no history of significant antibodies. If an antibody is detected, identification of that antibody is performed, and compatible units are reserved for the patient.

Type and Crossmatch

When a physician orders units to be crossmatched for a patient, more testing is necessary than the order itself implies. ABO and Rh testing and antibody screening must be performed on a current patient specimen. The same specimen is also used to crossmatch with a segment of the unit intended for transfusion. In the absence of extreme emergency, the unit of blood can be issued for transfusion only if all testing discrepancies are resolved and the crossmatch is compatible. If the result of the antibody screen is positive, the antibody must be identified. If the antibody is clinically significant, antigen-negative units must be chosen for transfusion.

Abbreviated crossmatch protocols have been adopted by some blood banks for routine crossmatching and by others for emergency situations only. In these protocols, ABO and Rh testing and antibody screening are performed. In the absence of clinically significant antibodies, blood is issued after an immediate spin crossmatch that serves as a confirmation of ABO compatibility.

An electronic or computer crossmatch is another method of crossmatching donor and patient that is intended to replace serologic compatibility testing. Two separate ABO and

(Fig. 14–10). Tests are usually requested as a group, and for ease in ordering a "shorthand notation" designates a group. These may include:

1. Type and screen
2. Type and crossmatch
3. Prenatal evaluation, postpartum evaluation
4. Cord blood studies

Type and Screen

Many surgical procedures have a very low probability of requiring blood transfusion. To better utilize their blood supplies, blood bankers may choose not to crossmatch units of blood for these procedures but instead to use a type and screen protocol. ABO and Rh testing and antibody screening are performed using a current patient specimen.

Because only a small percentage of individuals who type as Rh-negative by means of an immediate spin technique are

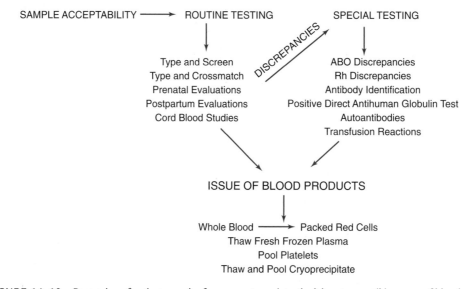

■ FIGURE 14–10   Processing of patient samples from acceptance into the laboratory until issuance of blood products.

Rh tests are performed on a patient's RBCs and entered into a validated computer system; the ABO confirmatory test on a unit of blood is also entered. At the time when the blood is to be issued to the patient for transfusion, the computer verifies the ABO compatibility between the donor unit and the patient and allows the release of the blood. If ABO incompatibilities between the recipient and the donor unit are discovered, the computer alerts the user to the discrepancy so that the blood will not be released (see Chapter 13).

Prenatal Evaluation

Accurate serologic testing of obstetric patients is an essential component in the prevention and treatment of hemolytic disease of the newborn (HDN). Maternal blood samples are evaluated during pregnancy to determine the ABO group and Rh type of the mother and the presence of serum antibodies that have the potential to cause HDN. If the woman is classified as Rh-negative after testing for D and weak D, she may be a candidate for antenatal Rh-immune globulin. If the result of the antibody screen is positive, the antibody must be identified. Serial titrations may be performed during the course of the pregnancy if the antibody is considered potentially harmful to the fetus. The obstetrician uses these laboratory results together with other methods for evaluating the fetal condition and the need for clinical intervention (see Chapter 20.)

Postpartum Evaluation

All women admitted for delivery are required to be tested to determine their Rh status. A test for weak D is performed on any specimen that shows a negative reaction on immediate spin. If the mother is Rh-negative and her baby is Rh-positive, the maternal sample is further evaluated to detect a fetomaternal hemorrhage (FMH) in excess of 30 mL of whole blood. (One 300-μg dose of RhIg prevents maternal Rh immunization from exposure of up to 30 mL of fetal whole blood.)[5] Commercial kits utilizing rosetting techniques are commonly used for this purpose. Once an FMH in excess of 30 mL of whole blood has been detected, quantification is performed using a Kleihauer-Betke test, flow cytometry, or enzyme-linked antiglobulin test. This may be performed in the blood bank or in a separate laboratory. If HDN is suspected, an antibody screen is performed on the mother's serum, and if the result is positive, attempts are made to identify the antibody.

Cord Blood Studies

Protocols to evaluate cord blood specimens can vary widely from blood bank to blood bank. Cord blood from infants born to Rh-negative mothers is tested for D and for weak D to determine the mother's candidacy for RhIg prophylaxis. ABO and Rh typing and DAT are performed on cord samples from infants born to women with clinically significant antibodies. Additional testing may also be performed. Many blood banks follow published guidelines stating that beyond these circumstances, routine testing of cord blood is not necessary unless the clinical situation warrants it. If an infant develops symptoms that suggest HDN, a full cord blood study is performed that may include ABO and Rh typing (including a weak test

for D), DAT and, if the DAT result is positive, an eluate and subsequent antibody identification are performed. Note that only forward testing is performed in the ABO test.

Requests for Other Blood Components

When components containing large amounts of RBCs (e.g., granulocyte concentrates) are requested, pretransfusion testing is identical to that performed for RBC requests. There are no such requirements for platelets or FFP, although for the latter some blood banks may perform reverse grouping once the ABO type of the recipient has been determined.

Issue of Blood Products

After all pretransfusion testing has been completed, blood components may be released for transfusion to the designated recipient. It is essential that all serologic discrepancies be resolved before issue of blood products, except in extreme emergency. The individual in the blood bank who will issue the blood product inspects the unit for any abnormal appearance (Box 14–3) and verifies that all required transfusion forms and labels are complete and that they adequately identify the transfusion recipient. If another individual is responsible for delivering the blood product to the appropriate location, he or she may also verify that all information is complete. A computer crossmatch may also be performed at this time, and if there are no discrepancies the component can be released for transfusion. Some form of documentation is used to record the transaction.

Some component preparation or modification may be necessary before the issue of blood products. FFP may be thawed in a constant-temperature (30°C-37°C) water bath, individual platelet concentrates may be pooled into a single bag for ease of transfusion, and a packed RBC may need to be irradiated (Fig. 14–11).[5] These modifications may shorten the expiration date of the products and must be reflected on the unit itself and in the computer system.

Reference Laboratory

Whether it is an entity separate from the main laboratory or, as in most cases, an integrated part, the reference laboratory is the problem-solving section of the transfusion service. The goal of the reference laboratory is to ensure that any discrepancies detected in routine testing are resolved in an accurate and time-efficient manner. Other chapters in this book discuss in depth the various problems encountered in serologic testing and the strategies for resolving them. Here is a brief

---

BOX 14–3
Reasons to Quarantine Blood Components Before Shipment or Transfusions

1. Plasma of RBC unit is brown, red, murky, or purple
2. Zone of hemolysis above RBC mass
3. Inadequate sealing of RBC segments in tubing
4. Hemolysis of RBCs
5. Grossly lipemic units

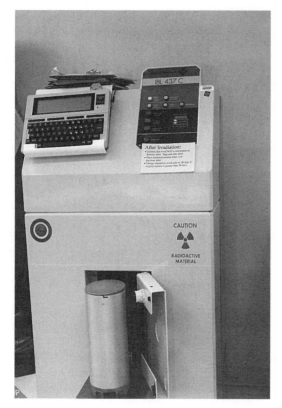

■ FIGURE 14–11   Irradiators are used to prevent lymphocytes in RBC products from causing graft-versus-host disease in susceptible patient populations. (Courtesy National Institutes of Health, Bethesda, MD.)

summary of some situations and common methods used in their investigation. It should be noted that before any serologic testing is performed, special testing should always include an investigation of patient's diagnosis, age, pregnancy, drug, and transfusion history.

ABO Discrepancies

All inconsistencies between forward and reverse grouping must be resolved before an ABO interpretation can be made (see Chapter 6). ABO investigations may include:

1. Variations in incubation times and temperatures
2. Testing with A_2 cells or anti-A_1 lectin
3. Room temperature antibody identification
4. Adsorption and elution using human sources of anti-A or anti-B
5. Autoadsorption
6. Removal of RBC-bound cold autoantibodies
7. Secretor studies

Rh Discrepancies

Problems in Rh typing may occur because of certain clinical conditions or inherited characteristics (see Chapter 7). Rh investigations may include:

1. Rh phenotyping
2. Adsorption and elution using Rh antisera
3. Isolation of cell populations
4. Use of rare antisera and RBCs

Antibody Identification

A positive antibody screen in the absence of a positive auto-control or DAT result indicates possible alloantibody immunization by means of blood transfusion or pregnancy (see Chapter 12). To establish the identity and clinical significance of an antibody and to provide appropriate blood for transfusion, antibody investigation may include:

1. Antibody identification panels using various enhancement media (albumin, low ionic strength solution, polyethylene glycol) and test systems (such as tubes, gel, or solid phase technologies)
2. Antibody identification panels pretreated with reagents such as enzymes, dithiothreitol (DTT), or 2-aminoethylisothiouronium bromide
3. Neutralization using such substances as plasma, saliva, urine, or human milk
4. Antigen typing
5. Titration
6. Adsorption and elution studies
7. Treatment of serum with DTT or 2-mercaptoethanol
8. IgG subclassing
9. Monocyte monolayer assay
10. Use of rare sera and cells

Positive DAT

A positive DAT may be the result of an immune reaction to a drug, a disease state, or a delayed hemolytic transfusion reaction (see Chapter 18). The investigation of a positive DAT may include:

1. Use of monospecific reagents (anti-IgG, anti-C3)
2. Elution techniques
3. Antibody identification
4. Removal of cell-bound antibody using chloroquine diphosphate
5. RBC phenotyping
6. Drug studies
7. Cell separation techniques

Warm Autoantibodies

In addition to causing a positive DAT, the presence of a warm autoantibody in a patient's serum may mask the presence of clinically significant alloantibodies (see Chapter 21). Tests performed in the investigation of warm autoantibodies may include:

1. Removal of RBC-bound autoantibody followed by serum autoadsorption
2. Heterologous or differential serum adsorptions
3. Elution techniques
4. Autoantibody identification
5. Reticulocyte enrichment or other cell separation techniques

Cold Autoantibodies

Potent cold autoantibodies may cause discrepancies in ABO testing as well as a positive DAT result and may mask the presence of clinically significant alloantibodies (see Chapter 21). The management of cold autoantibodies may include:

1. Removal of RBC-bound autoantibody using 37°C saline
2. Prewarmed technique
3. Antibody identification
4. Autoadsorption
5. Adsorption using rabbit erythrocyte stroma
6. Treatment of serum or cells with DTT or 2-ME

Transfusion Reactions

Any adverse reactions to transfusion must be investigated to determine if the reaction is antibody-mediated (see Chapter 18). The extent of transfusion reaction investigations varies widely, depending on the policies established by a particular blood bank and the result of initial testing. If there is strong evidence of an antibody-mediated transfusion reaction, further investigation may include:

1. Elution followed by antibody identification
2. Use of more sensitive techniques for antibody detection in serum and eluates, including enzymes, polybrene, polyethylene glycol, or enzyme-linked antiglobulin test
3. Cell separation techniques

Like laboratories at blood centers, hospital blood banks that collect their own units of blood process them to make a variety of components, including packed red blood cells (PRBCs), FFP, platelets, and cryoprecipitate. **Table 14–3** lists the common blood products made from a unit of whole blood and the processes used to make these components.

Personnel Requirements

The pursuit of quality begins with people. This is no less true for the blood bank laboratory, where the essence of service is all about quality: providing blood and blood products that are safe for transfusion. Like all complex organizations, the blood bank laboratory is staffed by a variety of individuals with various credentials and qualifications. Blood bank laboratory work centers on labor-intensive tasks and sophisticated analyses often performed under conditions of stress complicated by emergency requests for blood. Work demands like these can only be met by an educated, well-trained, and highly-skilled labor force.

In recognition that quality laboratory testing is in part a function of the people performing the analyses, the U.S. government included personnel requirements in the Clinical Laboratory Improvement Amendments of 1988 (CLIA '88). Subpart M of these regulations establishes personnel qualifications for laboratories performing certain types of testing. Blood bank laboratories are engaged in both moderately and highly complex testing. Manual tube testing has long been the standard method for the testing done in the blood bank laboratory. More recently, however, less labor-intensive methods have been employed. These include gel technologies **(Fig. 14–12)** and solid phase RBC adherence (see **Fig. 11–11**, chapter 11). These methods allow for workload consolidation and facilitate ease of cross-training testing personnel.

Under CLIA, blood bank laboratories must employ personnel who are qualified by education, training, and/ or experience.[4] In all cases, the blood bank laboratory must have a qualified director to manage the personnel and the operations. However, the director may delegate to a qualified supervisor the day-to-day work-related activities that include personnel management and reporting of test results.

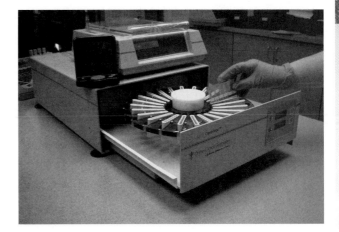

■ **FIGURE 14–12**   A gel card is loaded into a centrifuge. The gel test employs the principle of controlled centrifugation of RBCs through a dextran-acrylamide gel/reagent matrix contained in a specially designed microtube.

Standard Operating Procedures

Orientation to a blood bank laboratory begins with reading the standard operating procedure (SOP) manuals. These manuals, usually located at the workbench and accessible to all personnel, contain information outlining the operations of the laboratory; details on how, when and why particular activities are done; and procedures for all tests performed. SOP manuals are integral components of any blood bank laboratory's quality assurance program (see Chapter 24). They are reviewed at least annually and updated on a regular basis to reflect changes in operations and implementation of new regulations.

Summary

The modern blood bank laboratory is a dynamic workplace. It is here that donated blood undergoes rigorous testing to make sure it is safe for transfusion. These may include blood collection, component preparation and storage, and donor and recipient testing.

SUMMARY CHART:
Important Points to Remember (MT/MLT)

➤ The goal of every blood bank laboratory is to provide quality service and safe blood products.

➤ All blood bank laboratory operations are regulated by law.

➤ Personnel employed by blood bank laboratories must be qualified by education, training, and/or experience.

➤ A primary source of operational information is the SOP manual.

➤ Hemapheresis is a process that uses an apheresis machine to selectively remove components from donor blood.

➤ Blood and blood components must be stored and shipped under conditions that ensure their viability.

➤ Every donor unit is tested to determine ABO group and Rh type, including weak D when indicated. Units are also tested for select and viral markers.

➤ The type of Rh-negative units must be confirmed because of potential sensitization that may occur if Rh-positive blood is transfused to an Rh-negative recipient.

➤ Manual tube procedures are being replaced by emerging technologies, including gel-based methods and automation.

REVIEW QUESTIONS

1. What is the shipping temperature requirement for plasma?
   a. 1–6°F or higher
   b. 1–6°C or lower
   c. −18°F or higher
   d. −18°C or lower

2. Which test would not be included in a type and screen?
   a. ABO group
   b. Rh type
   c. Hepatitis A antibody quantitation
   d. Clinically significant antibody determination

3. This U.S. government agency regulates testing of human specimens through provisions of CLIA '88.
   a. OSHA
   b. FDA
   c. CMS
   d. AABB

4. A shipment of platelets has been received, but transfusion is delayed for 1 hour. What is the best course of action to ensure optimal viability of the product?
   a. Refrigerate the units subsequent to confirmation of ABO and Rh type
   b. Incubate at 37°C and perform compatibility testing
   c. Store at room temperature on a flatbed agitator
   d. Place the platelets in the −18°C freezer until transfused

5. Federal regulations and AABB *Standards* stipulate that blood bank laboratories must employ a _____ qualified by education, training, and/or experience to oversee all personnel and operations.
   a. Director
   b. Clinical consultant
   c. Quality representative
   d. Technical supervisor

6. Under what circumstances must the Rh type be confirmed?
   a. Donor unit previously typed as Rh-positive
   b. Donor unit previously typed as Rh-negative
   c. Donor unit previously typed as A-, B-, or O-negative
   d. Donor unit previously typed as A-, B- or O-positive

7. The process whereby selected blood components are directly collected from a donor using sterile technique is:
   a. Compatibility testing
   b. Hemapheresis
   c. Leukoreduction
   d. Phlebotomy

8. What factors determine the maximum number of components that may be derived from one unit of whole blood?
   a. Time and anticoagulant
   b. Time and collection container composition
   c. Temperature and collection container size
   d. Container composition and anticoagulant

REFERENCES

1. General Accounting Office, GAO-02–1095T (2002). Maintaining an adequate blood supply is key to emergency preparedness.
2. Goodman, C, et al: Ensuring blood safety and availability in the US: Technological advances, costs and challenges to payment-final report. Transfusion 2003; 43:3S.
3. Fridey, J: Standards for Blood Banks and Transfusion Services, 22nd ed. American Association of Blood Banks, Bethesda, MD, 2003.
4. Code of Federal Regulations. Title 42 CFR Parts 493 to end. Washington, DC: US Government Printing Office, 2001 (revised annually).
5. Brecher, ME, et al: Technical Manual, 14th ed. American Association of Blood Banks, Bethesda, MD, 2002.
6. Check, W: Order in the blood bank: Automation steps up. CAP Today 2002; 16:42.
7. Sazama, K: Best practices for reducing transfusion errors, deaths from transfusions: Sources of error. CBER 2002.

fifteen

Alternative Technologies and Automation in Routine Blood Bank Testing

**Denise M. Harmening, PhD, MT(ASCP), CLS(NCA), and
Phyllis S. Walker, MS, MT(ASCP)SBB**

OBJECTIVES

On completion of this chapter, the learner should be able to:

1. Define the principles of gel and solid-phase technology.
2. Describe the test reactions and methods of grading reactions for each technology.
3. List the advantages and disadvantages of each technology.
4. Compare the two technologies in terms of equipment, test reactions, procedures, sensitivity, and quality control.
5. Discuss the automated equipment that is available for each technology.

Introduction

Previous chapters have discussed ABO and Rh typing, direct antiglobulin testing (DAT), and antibody detection and identification procedures based on routine tube testing techniques. In response to the pressures of current good manufacturing practices, two alternative technologies, the gel test and solid-phase assays, have emerged to provide accurate, reproducible blood bank testing. These technologies offer increased safety provided by plasticware and decreased biohazardous waste. In addition, automation decreases the opportunities for human errors and frees laboratory personnel to perform other tasks. This chapter presents the history, basic principle, test reactions, and advantages and disadvantages of each technology and discusses the automation of the testing technology.

Gel Technology

History

In 1985 the gel test was developed by Dr. Yves Lapierre of Lyon, France.[1] Various media, including gelatin, acrylamide gel, and glass beads, were investigated in an attempt to trap agglutinates during a standardized sedimentation or centrifugation step. Gel particles appeared to be the ideal material for trapping agglutinates, and this discovery led to a patented process for the separation of red blood cell (RBC) agglutination reactions. In addition, it was discovered that antiglobulin testing could be performed without multiple saline washes to remove unbound immunoglobulin and that antiglobulin control cells were not needed to confirm the presence of antiglobulin reagent in negative tests. Compared with traditional tube technology, the gel test provides a more stable endpoint and a more reproducible result. This improvement reduces the variability associated with the physical resuspension of RBC buttons after centrifugation and the subsequent interpretation of hemagglutination reactions.

In 1988 Dr. Lapierre aligned with DiaMed A.G., Murten, Switzerland, for the commercial development and production of the gel test in Europe. In September 1994, Micro Typing Systems (MTS) Inc., Pompano Beach, Florida, an affiliated partner of DiaMed A.G., received a Food and Drug Administration (FDA) license to manufacture and distribute an antiglobulin anti-IgG gel card and a buffered gel card in the United States. In January 1995, Ortho Diagnostic Systems Inc. (ODSI) and MTS signed an agreement giving ODSI exclusive rights to distribute the gel test in North America. In March 2002, Ortho-Clinical Diagnostics, Inc. acquired MTS, which is now known as Micro Typing Systems, a wholly owned subsidiary of Ortho-Clinical Diagnostics, Inc. This gel-based test is named the ID-Micro Typing System™.[2]

Principle

The gel test, which is performed in a specially designed microtube, is based on the controlled centrifugation of RBCs through a dextran-acrylamide gel that contains predispensed reagents **(Fig. 15–1)**. Each microtube is composed of an upper reaction chamber that is wider than the tube itself and a long, narrow portion referred to as the column (see **Fig. 15–1)**. In the gel test, a plastic card with microtubes is used instead of test tubes **(Fig. 15–2)**. A gel card is approximately 5×7 centimeters and consists of six microtubes. Each microtube contains predispensed gel, diluent, and reagents if applicable. Measured volumes of serum or plasma and/or RBCs are dispensed into the reaction chamber of the microtube **(Fig. 15–3)**. If appropriate, the card is incubated **(Fig. 15–4)** and then centrifuged **(Fig. 15–5)**.

The reaction chamber is actually a miniature test tube, providing an area for the sensitization of RBCs (antigen-antibody binding) during incubation. The column of each microtube contains dextran-acrylamide gel particles suspended in a diluent or reagent. The shape and length of the column provides a large surface area for prolonged contact of the RBCs with the gel particles during centrifugation.

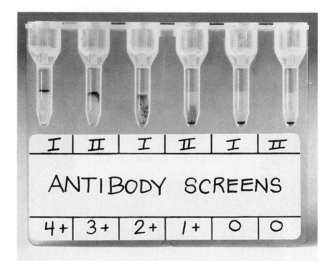

■ FIGURE 15–2   The gel card (microtubes are used instead of test tubes).

The gel particles are beads of dextran-acrylamide that make up 75 percent of the gel-liquid mixture that is preloaded into each microtube.[2] The gel particles are porous, and they serve as a reaction medium and filter, sieving the RBC agglutinates according to size during centrifugation. Large agglutinates are trapped at the top of the gel and are not allowed to travel through the gel during the centrifugation of the card **(Fig. 15–6)**. Agglutinated RBCs remain fixed or suspended in the gel, while unagglutinated RBCs travel unimpeded through the length of the microtube, forming a pellet at the bottom following centrifugation.

Unlike agglutination in the traditional test tube hemagglutination method, the gel test reactions are stable, allowing observation or review for up to 3 days.

Test Reactions

Agglutination reactions in the gel test are graded from 1+ to 4+ (including mixed field), just as the reactions in test tube hemagglutination technique are graded **(Fig. 15–7)**.[2]

In the gel test, a 4+ reaction is characterized by a

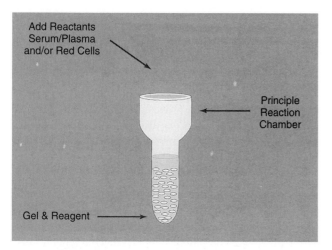

■ FIGURE 15–1   Illustration of gel microtube.

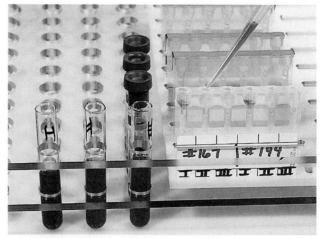

■ FIGURE 15–3   Pipetting into gel card microtubes.

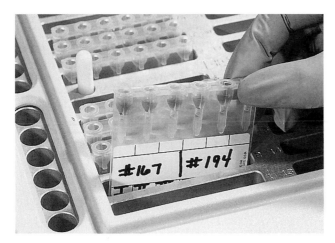

■ FIGURE 15–4   Incubation of gel cards.

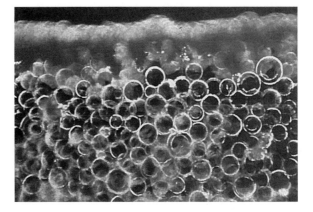

■ FIGURE 15–6   Magnified photograph of agglutinated RBCs trapped above the gel matrix.

solid band of agglutinated RBCs at the top of the gel column. Usually, no RBCs are visible at the bottom of the microtube.

A 3+ reaction is characterized by a predominant amount of agglutinated RBCs near the top of the gel column, with a few agglutinates staggered below the thicker band. The majority of agglutinates are observed in the top half of the gel column.

A 2+ reaction is characterized by RBC agglutinates that are dispersed throughout the gel column, with a few agglutinates at the bottom of the microtube. Agglutinates are distributed throughout the upper and lower halves of the gel.

A 1+ reaction is characterized by RBC agglutinates that are predominantly in the lower half of the gel column, with some RBCs at the bottom of the microtube. These reactions may be weak, with only a few agglutinates remaining in the gel area just above the RBC pellet at the bottom of the microtube.

In a negative reaction, the RBCs form a well-delineated pellet at the bottom of the microtube. The gel above the RBC pellet is clear and free of agglutinates.

Mixed-field reactions are characterized by a layer of agglutinated RBCs at the top of the gel accompanied by a pellet of unagglutinated cells at the bottom of the microtube. Negative reactions may appear mixed-field when incompletely clotted serum samples are used in the gel test. Fibrin strands in such sera may trap unagglutinated RBCs, forming a thin line at the top of the gel. Other unagglutinated cells pass through the gel during centrifugation and travel to the bottom of the microtube. Before interpreting reactions as mixed-field, the clinical history of the patient should be considered. For example, recently transfused patients or bone marrow transplant recipients are expected to have mixed populations of RBCs, and their RBCs commonly produce mixed-field reactions.

Tests Approved by the FDA

Gel technology is currently approved for ABO forward and reverse grouping, Rh typing, DAT, antibody screen, antibody identification, and compatibility testing. The ABO blood grouping card contains gels that include anti-A, anti-B, and anti-A,B for forward grouping. Microtubes with buffered gel are used for ABO reverse grouping.[3] The Rh typing card uses microtubes filled with gel containing anti-D.[4] The Rh phenotype card contains gels that contain anti-D, anti-C, anti-E, anti-c, anti-e, and a control.[5] Microtubes filled with gel containing anti-IgG are used for compatibility testing, antibody detection, and identification.[6]

Advantages and Disadvantages

Gel technology is applicable to a broad range of blood bank tests, and it offers several advantages over routine tube testing.[7] Standardization is one of the major advantages, inasmuch as there is no tube shaking to resuspend the RBC button. Tube shaking techniques vary among technologists, which results in variation in the reading, grading and interpretation of the test. The gel technique provides stable, well-defined endpoints of the agglutination reaction. It includes simple standardized procedures, no wash steps, and no need for antiglobulin control cells. These factors combine to produce more objective, consistent, and reproducible interpretation of the test results.

Because the gel technology offers objective, consistent results, it is ideally suited to individuals who have been cross-trained to work in the blood bank. Other advantages include the decreased sample volume needed for testing and the enhanced sensitivity and specificity of gel technology. Finally, gel technology offers improved productivity, standardization, and ability to meet regulatory requirements when compared with traditional tube testing.[8] **Table 15–1** describes these

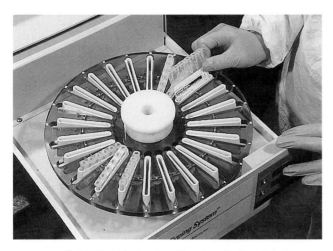

■ FIGURE 15–5   Centrifugation of gel cards.

ID-Micro Typing System™

Gel Technology Reaction Grading Chart

Agglutinated cells form a cell layer at the top of the gel media.

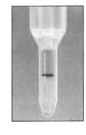

4+

Agglutinated cells disperse throughout the gel media and may concentrate toward the bottom of the microtube.

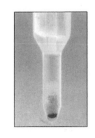

1+

Agglutinated cells begin to disperse into gel media and are concentrated near the top of the microtube.

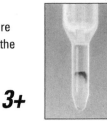

3+

All cells pass through the gel media and form a cell button at the bottom of the microtube.

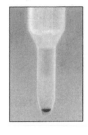

Negative

Agglutinated cells disperse into the gel media and are observed throughout the length of the microtube.

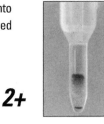

2+

Agglutinated cells form a layer at the top of the gel media. Unagglutinated cells pass to the bottom of the microtube.

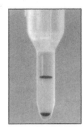

Mixed-Field

■ FIGURE 15–7   Gel technology reaction grading chart. Courtesy of Ortho Diagnostic Systems, Inc., Raritan, NJ, 1995

three advantages in more detail. The major disadvantage of the gel technology is the need to purchase special incubators and centrifuges to accommodate the microtube cards used for testing. In addition, a specific pipette must be used to dispense 25 μL of plasma or serum and 50 μL of a 0.8 percent suspension of RBCs into the reaction chambers of the microtubes.[9]

Solid-Phase Technology

History

Solid-phase immunoassays have been used for many years in immunology and chemistry laboratories. In these test sys-

tems (immunoassays), one of the test reactants (either antigen or antibody) is bound to a solid support (usually a microtiter well) before the test is started. The ability of plastics, such as polystyrene, to absorb proteins from solution and to bind them irreversibly made solid-phase serologic assays in plastic microplate wells possible. In 1978 Rosenfield and coworkers[10] were the first to apply the principle of solid-phase immunoassay to RBC typing and antibody screening tests. Other investigators were quick to follow with the solid-phase red cell adherence (SPRCA) technology. In 1984, Plapp and coworkers reported the use of SPRCA for the detection of RBC antigens and antibodies.[11,12]

SPRCA was developed commercially and manufactured

TABLE 15–1   Advantages of the Gel Technology in Terms of Productivity, Standardization, and Regulatory Issues

Improves Productivity	Increases Standardization	Addresses Regulatory Issues
Fewer procedural steps minimize hands-on time	Clearly defined endpoints promote uniform interpretation among technologists	Enhanced cGMP compliance attained through simplified training and standardized procedures
Standardized procedures simplify interpretation, reducing repeat and unnecessary testing	Use of precise measurements decreases test performance variability	Minimal handling of reagents and samples increases biosafety
Easy-to-perform testing enables optimal utilization of personnel	Elimination of technique-dependent steps improves consistency of test results	Test performance verification and NCCLS-formatted SOPs are provided to ensure easy implementation

cGMP = current good manufacturing practices; NCCLS = National Committee in Clinical Laboratory Standards; SOPs = standard operational procedures.

under the trade name of Capture® by Immucor for the detection of RBC- and platelet-related antibodies. In the Capture® technology, tests were adapted to microplate wells, either as full 96-well U-bottomed plates or as 1 × 8 or 2 × 8 strips of U-bottomed wells.[13] The first-generation SPRCA assays to be designed commercially included Capture-R® for the detection of RBC antibodies and Capture-P® for the detection of platelet antibodies.[13] To perform these tests, a laboratory centrifuge capable of holding 96-well microplates or strip wells was required, along with a microplate incubator and an illuminated reading surface or microplate reader (**Fig. 15–8**).

Solid-phase immunoassays are currently available to detect antibodies to RBCs, platelets, syphilis, and cytomegalovirus.[14]

Principle

As mentioned previously, the principle of solid-phase immunoassay is based on SPRCA.[11] The first-generation tests use chemically modified microplate test wells in which intact reagent RBCs are bound to the microwells before starting the test. Patient serum or plasma and low ionic strength saline (LISS) are added to the RBC-coated microwells and incubated at 37∞C. After incubation, the wells are washed free of residual serum proteins, an indicator of anti-IgG–coated RBCs is added, and the microwells are centrifuged. Centrifugation forces the indicator RBCs to contact the

immobilized sensitized reagent RBCs. Positive tests show adherence of indicator RBCs to part or all of the well bottom, depending on the strength of the reaction (**Figs. 15–9 and 15–10**).

In second-generation antibody screening tests, RBC membranes are bound to the microplate test wells and dried during the manufacturing process.

Capture-R® (Immucor) for the detection of RBC antibodies is a first-generation solid-phase test, and Capture-R® Ready-Screen/Capture-R® Ready-ID® (Immucor) are second-generation tests.[13]

Solidscreen® (Biotest) is a solid-phase test that detects antibody using microplate wells that are coated with polyspecific antihuman globulin (AHG).[13]

Test Reactions

In solid-phase technology, the target antigen (i.e., RBCs) is affixed to the bottom of the microplate wells. The test plasma or serum and LISS are added to the wells, and they are incu-

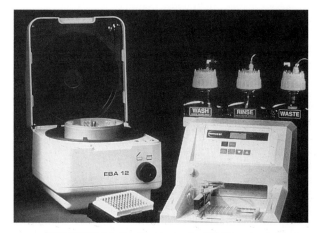

■ FIGURE 15–8   Equipment for SPRCA technology.

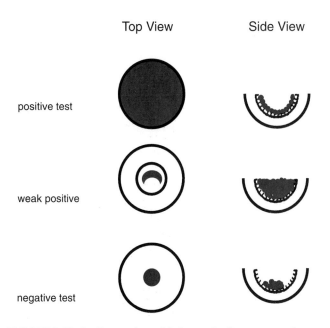

■ FIGURE 15–9   Test results: solid-phase cell adherence assay for the detection of antigens (illustration).

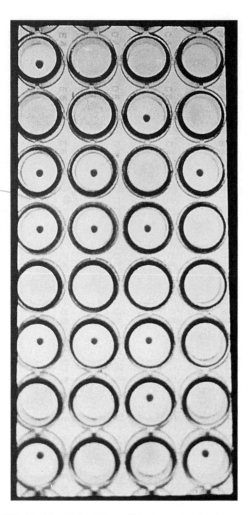

■ **FIGURE 15–10**   Test results: solid-phase red cell adherence assay for the detection of antigens.

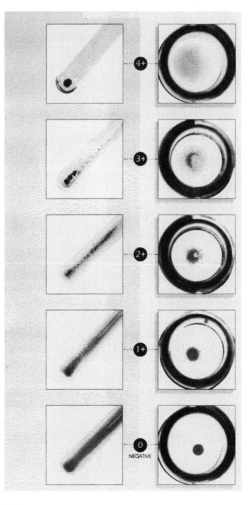

■ **FIGURE 15–11**   Comparison of traditional tube test reactions with solid-phase reactions.

bated at 37°C to allow time for possible antibodies to attach to the antigen in the well. The wells are washed with pH-buffered isotonic saline to remove unbound plasma or serum; indicator cells are added; and the microplates are centrifuged. The indicator cells are AHG-coated RBCs. If antibody has attached to the antigen, the indicator cells will form a mono-layer of RBCs. If no antibody is present, nothing is attached to the antigen, and the indicator cells form a clearly delineated button at the center of the microplate well following centrifugation. **Figure 15–11** compares test results from solid-phase technology with traditional tube testing reactions.

Solid-phase assays may be performed with either plasma or serum, but plasma is preferable. If a clotted sample is incompletely clotted, the serum is difficult to remove during the wash cycle. Residual unbound serum may clot and make the endpoint of the test unreadable. For best results, the manufacturer recommends adding a pH-stabilizing buffer to the isotonic saline that is used to wash the microplates. A suitable buffer is available from the manufacturer.[15]

Tests Approved by the FDA

Solid-phase technology is currently approved for antibody screening, antibody identification, and compatibility testing. Antibody screening cells are available as a two-cell (I and II)

screen, four-cell screens, or as a pool of two cells. The two-cell screen is recommended for antibody detection for transfusion recipients. Pooled cells are used for donor antibody detection when increased sensitivity is undesirable. A panel is available for RBC antibody identification.

Advantages and Disadvantages

As with gel technology, standardization is the major advantage of solid-phase technology. Solid-phase technology provides stable, well-defined endpoints of the reaction. Objective, consistent, reproducible test results facilitate technologist training or cross-training. Other advantages include ease of use. No predilution of reagents is required. It is possible to test hemolyzed, lipemic, or icteric samples, and the enhanced sensitivity makes the detection of weak alloantibodies easier. The Immucor Capture® technology has the added safety feature that a color change in the LISS ensures that the patient sample was added to the test system.

The major disadvantage of solid-phase technology is the need for a centrifuge that can spin microplates, a 37°C incubator for microplates, and a light source for reading the final results. In addition, the increased sensitivity may also be a disadvantage inasmuch as solid-phase may detect weak autoantibodies that other systems miss.

TABLE 15–2   Current Tests Available for the Two Alternative Technologies*

Test	Gel Test (Ortho)	Solid-Phase (Immucor)
ABO—Forward	Yes	No
ABO—Reverse	Yes	No
Rh typing	Yes	No
Antibody screen	Yes	Yes
Crossmatch	Yes	Yes
Antibody identification	Yes	Yes
Auto-control (IgG only)	Yes	Yes
DAT	No	No

*Gel test. (Ortho Clinical Diagnostics, Inc., Raritan, NJ); solid-phase, Immucor, Inc., Norcross, GA.

Comparison of Technologies

This section compares the two alternative technologies in terms of equipment needed, procedures, test reactions, sensitivity, quality control, and automation.[16] Table 15–2 lists the current tests available for both of the alternative technologies, and Table 15–3 compares the features of the two technologies for routine blood bank testing.

Equipment

The gel technology requires special incubators and centrifuges to accommodate the cards. The solid-phase technology requires a centrifuge that can spin microplates, a 37°C incubator for microplates, and a light source for reading the final results. Automated and semiautomated equipment approved by the FDA is currently available for the solid-phase and gel technology.

Both technologies improve safety and decrease hazardous waste, inasmuch as the use of plastic eliminates the danger associated with broken glass, and miniaturized reaction chambers reduce the quantity of hazardous waste.

Test Reactions and Procedures

Both technologies demonstrate reproducible endpoints. The gel test uses a special pipette to precisely measure the quantity of test cells and sera. The solid-phase technology uses drops of cells and sera. By standardizing the reactants in the assay and eliminating variation in the tube-shaking technique, it is possible to eliminate the subjectivity associated with interpreting the endpoint of test tube agglutination tests. Quantitation of these assays is also less subjective than in conventional test tube technology. The gel test is read as 4+, 3+, 2+, 1+, MF or negative, and it is based on agglutination reactions. The ease of quantitating reactions with the gel test is an advantage when evaluating an antibody identification for multiple antibodies or dosage effects. Similarly, the solid-phase assays are read as weak positive, positive, or negative.

Mixed-field agglutination produces a characteristic pattern in the gel technology. In this technology, the agglutinated population of RBCs is trapped in the gel, and the unagglutinated population is pelleted at the bottom of the microtube following centrifugation. The ability to recognize mixed-field reactions is particularly valuable in evaluating a possible transfusion reaction or the survival of a minor population of transfused cells.

The endpoints of the new technologies are extremely stable, and they can be read 2 to 3 days after the test is performed. Such stability is a distinct advantage when less experienced technologists are cross-trained to work in the transfusion service. When the interpretation of an assay is unclear, it is helpful to be able to retain the test results until a supervisor can review them.

TABLE 15–3   Routine Blood Bank Testing: Comparison of Traditional and Alternative Methods

	Traditional	Gel	Solid-Phase
Reaction chamber	Tube	Microtube card	Microplate wells
Reaction patterns	Agglutination	Agglutination	Solid-phase immune adherence
Reaction matrix	None (cells and serum/plasma)	Immunologically inert dextran-acrylamide gels	Chemically modified polystyrene microplate wells
Testing detection	AHG (antihuman globulin sera)	AHG (antihuman globulin sera)	Anti-IgG–coated red cells
Washing required	Yes	No	Yes
Centrifugation required	Yes	Yes	Yes
Reaction readings	Quantitative: 1+ to 4+, MF	Quantitative: 1+ to 4+, MF	Semiquantitative: strong pos, pos, neg, no MF
Stable reactions	No	Yes (2–3 days)	Yes (2 days)
Quality control	Positive and negative controls/ Coombs' check cells	Lot number of cards and diluent on day of use	LISS color change, pos and neg control
Special equipment	No	Yes	Yes
Automation (FDA-approved)	No	Yes	Yes

MF = mixed-field.

The procedures for both technologies parallel steps performed in routine blood bank tube testing, including pipetting, incubating, spinning, and reading. The washing cycle step has been eliminated with the gel technology. Because the endpoint of both assays detects IgG, it is possible to perform an auto-control to detect IgG-coated cells. An auto-control cannot be substituted for a DAT, however, because none of the technologies currently detects C3d complement–coated cells. Table 15–4 compares the procedural steps of the two technologies.

Sensitivity

Although both of the technologies are LISS-based, their sensitivity differ. The technologies have been shown to detect at least as many IgG antibodies as the conventional test tube methods using the LISS antiglobulin technique. The solid-phase technology is more sensitive than traditional serologic techniques. The sensitivity of all the technologies can be modified by pretreating the test cells or monolayer with enzymes, dithiothreitol, or chloroquine. Increased sensitivity is an advantage when a low-titered, clinically significant antibody is present, but it is a disadvantage when a low-titered warm autoantibody is present. Assays that detect only IgG avoid clinically insignificant IgM antibodies such as cold agglutinins; however, they also fail to detect clinically significant IgM antibodies that may be forming during a primary immune response. The alternative technologies detect IgG antibodies, including both clinically significant and insignificant IgG antibodies, such as high titer, low avidity antibodies. The gel technique may also detect IgM antibodies if incompatible cells form a lattice in the reaction chamber and are trapped at the top of the gel during centrifugation.

Quality Control

In addition to routine quality control (QC) for the 37°C incubator, centrifuge, pipette tips, and pipette dispenser used in testing, the technologies have other QC features. The gel test uses special dispensers to prepare the RBC suspensions and special pipettes to add a measured volume of plasma/serum and RBCs. Each lot number of cards and diluent should be tested on the day of use to confirm that the test cards and the diluted reagent RBCs are reacting as expected.

The manufacturer of the solid-phase technology recommends including a positive and a negative control with each batch of tests. In addition, in the solid-phase system, the LISS is formulated to detect the addition of plasma by a color change from purple to blue when plasma is added. This feature protects the user from failing to add plasma to a well.

Automation

Blood banks and transfusion services are the last areas of the clinical laboratory to move to automation. Chemistry, hematology, and immunology have been using automation for many years, but blood services have been hampered by the complexity of the testing and the subjectivity of the test interpretation. In recent years, new pressure has been applied to this area of the laboratory. Personnel shortages, turnaround time requirements, and the need for cost containment produced by increased managed care and greater regulatory demands have provided the incentive for blood services to seek automation. Automated equipment provides a partial solution to personnel shortages and turnaround requirements. By using walk-away automation, laboratory personnel are able to perform multiple tasks simultaneously. Automated equipment also provides the level of quality assurance required by new regulatory standards. Barcoding reduces identification errors by providing accurate patient and reagent identification. Standardized techniques reduce testing errors.

Automation in blood centers was first applied to infectious disease testing. These assays are easier to automate because they are less subjective than serologic tests. Although viral marker testing is performed in all blood centers, the equipment discussed in this chapter focuses on equipment that automates serologic testing in blood centers and transfusion services.

Gel Technology

Automated equipment for the gel test is being used successfully in Europe. Similar equipment (ProVue™) has received FDA approval in the United States. ProVue™ (Fig. 15–12) is a walk-away instrument with a capacity for 48 samples and 16 reagents. Instrument safety features include a bar-code tracking system and three cameras that record sample, reagent,

---

TABLE 15–4   Procedural Steps of Two Alternative Technologies

Procedural Steps	Solid-Phase		
	Preloaded Microwells	Selected Cells	Gel Test
1. Add RBCs to wells or tubes	N/A	Yes	Yes
2. Centrifuge plate to form monolayer	N/A	Yes	N/A
3. Wash away unbound RBCs	N/A	Yes	N/A
4. Add test serum/plasma	Yes	Yes	Yes
5. Incubation	15 min	15 min	15 min
6. Wash cycle	Yes	Yes	N/A
7. Add indicator cells	Yes	Yes	N/A
8. Centrifuge	2 min	2 min	10 min

* Solid-phase (Immucor, Inc., Norcross GA); gel test (Ortho Clinical Diagnostics, Inc., Raritan, NJ);
  RBC = red blood cells; N/A = not applicable.

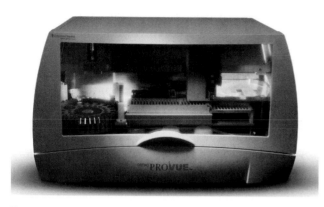

■ FIGURE 15–12   ProVue™ instrument. (Reprinted with permission from Ortho Clinical Diagnostics, Inc.)

and card identification. A camera in the instrument performs image analysis and uses a mathematical algorithm to interpret the results. The gel test can be performed semi-automated using the TECAN MEGAFlex, a robotic liquid sample processor **(Fig. 15–13)**. The TECAN MEGAFlex instrument, which contains detectors for the liquid level and for clots, adds the reactants in the assay to the reaction chamber in the top of the microtube. Following incubation, the operator moves the gel cards into the MTS reader, which centrifuges and reads up to 24 cards at one time. A picture of each card's results, with strength of reactivity and result interpretation, is displayed on a computer screen. The operator reviews the display and accepts or changes the data, and then exports the data to the laboratory information system.

Solid-Phase Technology

Solid-phase technology has been fully automated, and two models of equipment are FDA-approved: the ABS2000 and the ROSYS Plato. The ABS2000 (see **Fig. 11–11**) is a walk-away instrument that performs ABO, Rh and donor confirmations by microplate hemagglutination technique, and IgG antibody screens and compatibility tests by solid-phase technique. The ROSYS Plato (see **Fig. 11–12**) is a semiautomated instrument that performs ABO and Rh testing by hemagglutination technique and screens for antibodies to RBC antigens, cytomegalovirus, and syphilis by solid phase technique. The ROSYS Plato has an off-line centrifuge and a stand-alone reader. The reader, the IBG Multireader Plus, reads hemag-

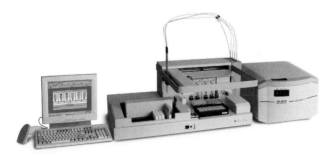

■ FIGURE 15–13   TECAN MEGAFlex liquid handing system and MTS Reader M. (Reprinted with permission from Ortho Clinical Diagnostics, Inc.)

glutination and solid-phase results, interprets the results using an algorithm, and transmits the results to an information system. The ABS2000 and the ROSYS Plato have bar code readers to ensure proper identification of samples and reagents. In addition, these instruments have liquid level sensors, clot detectors, controlled temperature settings, and incubation timers.

SUMMARY CHART:
Important Points to Remember (MT/MLT)

➤ The major advantages of these technologies over routine tube testing are:

➤ Standardization: There is no tube shaking or resuspension of an RBC button to cause subjectivity in the interpretation of the test.

➤ Stability: There are well-defined endpoints of the reaction.

➤ Decreased sample volume needed for testing

➤ Enhanced sensitivity and specificity

➤ The principle of the gel test is hemagglutination.

➤ In the gel test, RBCs and serum/plasma are allowed to incubate together in a reaction chamber.

➤ Following incubation, controlled centrifugation drives the RBCs through a specially designed microtube filled with beads of dextran-acrylamide gel.

➤ Agglutinated cells remain at the top of the tube or are trapped in the gel, depending on the size of the agglutinates.

➤ Unagglutinated cells move through the gel to the bottom of the tube.

➤ The gel test reactions are stable for observation or review for 2–3 days.

➤ Gel technology is currently approved for ABO forward and reverse grouping, Rh typing, DAT, antibody screening, antibody identification, and compatibility testing.

➤ The major disadvantage of the gel technology is the need to purchase special equipment: a centrifuge to accommodate the microtube cards used for testing and a pipettor and pipettes for dispensing plasma or serum and RBC suspensions into the reaction chambers of the microtubes.

➤ The principle of solid-phase technology is based on SPRCA.

➤ In solid-phase technology, the target antigen (RBCs) is affixed to the bottom of the microplate wells.

➤ If patient plasma contains antibodies to the antigen, the antibodies attach to the fixed antigen. Indicator cells detect attached antibodies by forming a monolayer of RBCs.

➤ If patient plasma contains no antibodies to the antigen, there is no attachment to the antigen, and the indicator cells form a clearly delineated button at the center of the microplate well.

➤ Solid-phase reactions are stable for observation or review for 2 days.

➤ Solid-phase technology is currently approved for antibody screening, antibody identification, and compatibility testing.

➤ Advantages of solid-phase technology include ease of use because no predilution of reagents is required and the ability to test hemolyzed, lipemic, or icteric samples. Enhanced sensitivity increases the detection of weak alloantibodies.

➤ The major disadvantage of solid-phase technology is the need to purchase special equipment: a centrifuge that can spin microplates, a 37°C incubator for microplates, and a light source for reading final results.

REVIEW QUESTIONS

1. The endpoint of the gel test is detected by:
   a. Agglutination
   b. Hemolysis
   c. Precipitation
   d. Attachment of indicator cells

2. The endpoint of the solid-phase test is detected by:
   a. Agglutination
   b. Hemolysis
   c. Precipitation
   d. Attachment of indicator cells

3. An advantage for both gel and solid-phase technology is:
   a. No cell washing steps
   b. Standardization
   c. Use of IgG-coated control cells
   d. Specialized equipment

4. A disadvantage for both gel and solid-phase technology is:
   a. Decreased sensitivity
   b. Inability to test hemolyzed, lipemic, or icteric samples
   c. Inability to detect C3d complement–coated cells
   d. Large sample requirement

5. A safety feature in the solid-phase test is:
   a. Air bubble barrier
   b. Viscous barrier
   c. Color change of the LISS
   d. Use of IgG-coated control cells

REFERENCES

1. Lapierre, Y, et al: The gel test: A new way to detect red cell antigen-antibody reactions. Transfusion 30:109, 1990.
2. ID-Micro Typing System™ Question and Answer Guide. Ortho Diagnostic Systems, Raritan, NJ, 1996.
3. Package insert for MTS Buffered Gel Card™. Pompano Beach, FL. Micro Typing Systems, 1995.
4. Package insert for MTS Anti-D Card™. Pompano Beach, FL. Micro Typing Systems, 1995.
5. Package insert for Rh Phenotype Card™. Pompano Beach, FL. Micro Typing Systems, 1995.
6. Package insert for MTS Anti-IgG Card™. Pompano Beach, FL. Micro Typing Systems, 1995.
7. Chan, A, et al: The impact of a gel system on routine work in a general hospital blood bank. Immunohematology 12:30, 1996.
8. A new era begins: Introducing ID-MTS, ID-Micro Typing System™ (Product brochure). Ortho Diagnostics Systems, Raritan, NJ, November 1995.
9. Package insert for ID-Pipetor FP-2™. Pompano Beach, FL. Micro Typing Systems, 1995.
10. Rosenfield, RE, Kochwa, SE, and Kaczera, Z: Solid phase serology for the study of human erythrocyte antigen-antibody reactions. Proceedings, Plenary Session, 25th Congress, International Society Blood Transfusion. Paris, 1978.
11. Plapp, FV, et al: Blood antigens and antibodies: Solid phase adherence assays. Lab Manage 22:39, 1984.
12. Moore, HH: Automated reading of red cell antibody detection tests by a solid phase antiglobulin technique. Transfusion 24:218, 1985.
13. Rolih, S, et al: Solid phase red cell adherence assays. La Transfusione del Sangue 36:4, 1991.
14. Haslam, GM, et al: A comparison of two solid phase systems for antibody detection. Immunohematology 11:8, 1995.
15. Capture-R® (solid phase technology). Package insert for Capture-R Ready Screen® and Capture-R Ready-ID®. Immucor, Norcross, GA, 1994.
16. Walker, PS: New technologies in transfusion medicine. Lab Med 28:258, 1997.

sixteen

Transfusion Therapy and Transfusion in Transplantation

Melanie S. Kennedy, MD, and
Haifeng M. Wu, MD

OBJECTIVES

On completion of this chapter, the learner should be able to:

1. Describe the blood components currently available for therapeutic use.
2. Discuss the indications for each blood component and product, including the approximate volume of each product.
3. Select the appropriate blood product for patients with specific disorders.
4. State the expected incremental increase of a patient's hematocrit level following transfusion of each unit of packed red blood cells (RBCs) and platelet count following transfusion of each unit of platelets.
5. List the required procedures to prepare each blood component for transfusion.
6. List the groups of recipients at highest risk of infection from transfusion of cytomegalovirus-positive RBCs or platelets.
7. Discuss the role of irradiation in the prevention of transfusion-associated graft-versus-host disease (GVHD).
8. Discuss selection of components by blood types with ABO mismatched bone marrow transplant.

9. List the four categories of transplantation.
10. Discuss transfusion requirements in liver transplantation.
11. List the types of tissues that can be harvested from a cadaveric donor.
12. State the purpose of the surgical blood order schedule.
13. State the main advantages and disadvantages of autologous transfusion.
14. Review the most important factors to consider when emergency transfusion is indicated.
15. Define massive transfusion.
16. Differentiate the various transfusion requirements of oncology patients.
17. Compare and contrast hemophilia A and von Willebrand's disease.
18. State the respective blood products of choice for treatment of von Willebrand's disease and hemophilia A.
19. Specify the steps involved in the proper administration of blood.

Blood Components

Blood and blood components are considered drugs because of their use in treating diseases. As with drugs, adverse effects may occur, necessitating careful consideration of therapy. The transfusion of blood cells is also transplantation, in that the cells must survive and function after transfusion to have a therapeutic effect. The transfusion of RBCs, the best tolerated form of transplantation, may cause rejection, as in a hemolytic transfusion reaction. The rejection of platelets, as shown by refractoriness to platelet transfusion, is relatively common in multiply transfused patients.

Transfusion therapy is used primarily to treat two conditions: inadequate oxygen-carrying capacity because of anemia or blood loss, and insufficient coagulation proteins or platelets to provide adequate hemostasis. Each patient requires an individualized plan reflecting the patient's changing clinical condition, anticipated blood loss, capacity for compensatory mechanisms, and laboratory results. Some patients do not require transfusion, even in anemia or thrombocytopenia, because their clinical conditions are stable and they have little or no risk of adverse outcomes. An example is a patient with iron-deficiency anemia with minor symptoms.

Component therapy is the transfusion of the specific blood component needed by the patient. By using blood components, several patients can be treated with the blood from one donor, giving optimal use of every donation of blood. **Table 16–1** is a summary of the blood components and products discussed in this chapter.[1,2]

Whole Blood

When compared with the circulating blood in the donor's blood vessels, the product whole blood is diluted in the proportion of eight parts circulating blood to one part anticoagulant. The citrate in the anticoagulant chelates ionized calcium, preventing activation of the coagulation system. The glucose, adenine, and phosphate (if present) serve as substrates for RBC metabolism during storage (see Chapter 1).

TABLE 16–1   Blood Components and Plasma Derivatives

Category	Major Indications	Composition	Volume
Whole blood	Symptomatic anemia with large-volume deficit	Approx. Hct 40%	570 mL
Red blood cells: RBCs, (adenine-saline added), RBC pheresis	Symptomatic anemia	Approx. Hct 55–70%	330 mL
Red blood cells: deglycerolyzed; Washed	Symptomatic anemia Severe allergic reactions	Approx. Hct 75%	180 mL
Red blood cells:Leukocyte-reduced	Symptomatic anemia Febrile reactions due to leukocyte antibodies Reduce CMV transmission Reduce HLA alloimmunization	$<5 \times 10^6$ WBC	330 mL
Platelets: Platelets pooled	Bleeding due to thrombocytopenia or platelet function abnormality Prevention of bleeding from marrow hypoplasia	$\geq 5.5 \times 10^{10}$ platelets/unit	60 mL/unit
Platelets pheresis	see Platelets Crossmatched and/or HLA-matched	$\geq 3.0 \times 10^{11}$ /unit	300 mL
Platelets leukocyte-reduced Platelets pheresis Leukocytes-reduced	see Platelets Prevention of febrile reactions Prevention of HLA-alloimmunization	see Platelets	300 mL
Granulocytes Pheresis	Neutropenia with infection unresponsive to appropriate antibiotics	$\geq 1.0 \times 10^{10}$ PMN/unit	220 mL
Fresh frozen plasma	Deficiency of labile and stable plasma coagulation factors; TTP	All coagulation factors	220 mL
Thawed plasma	Deficiency of stable coagulation factors; TTP	Reduced factors V and VIII	220 mL
Plasma Cryoprecipitate-reduced	TTP, HUS	Reduced fibrinogen, factors VIII and XIII, and vWF	200 mL
Cryoprecipitate	Hypofibrinogenemia Factor XIII deficiency	Fibrinogen, vWF, factors VIII and XIII	15 mL

Circular of information for the use of human blood and blood components, American Association of Blood Banks, America's Blood Centers, American Red Cross, Washington, DC, 2002.

The transfusion of whole blood is limited to a few clinical conditions. Whole blood should be used to replace the loss of both RBC mass and plasma volume.[1,2] Thus, rapidly bleeding patients can receive whole blood, although most commonly RBCs are used and are equally effective clinically.

A definite contraindication to the use of whole blood is severe chronic anemia. Patients with chronic anemia have a reduced amount of RBCs but have compensated by increasing their plasma volume to restore their total blood volume. Thus, these patients do not need the plasma in the whole blood and, in fact, may adversely respond to the unneeded plasma by developing pulmonary edema and heart failure because of volume overload. This is more likely to occur in patients with kidney failure or pre-existing heart failure.

For the typical 70-kg (155-lb) adult, each unit of whole blood should increase the hematocrit level 3 to 5 percent or hemoglobin 1 to 1.5 g/dL. After transfusion, the increase may not be apparent until 48 to 72 hours when the patient's blood volume adjusts to normal. For example, a patient with a 5000-mL blood volume and 25 percent hematocrit level has 1250-mL RBCs. With transfusion of 500-mL whole blood containing 200-mL RBCs, the blood volume will be 5500 mL and result in 26.4 percent hematocrit. When the patient's blood volume readjusts to 5000 mL, the hematocrit level will be 29 percent (1450 mL divided by 5000 mL). The increase is greater in a smaller person and less in a larger one.

In pediatric patients, a dose of 8 mL/kg will increase the hemoglobin about 1 g/dL or the hematocrit 3 percent to 4 percent.

RBCs

RBCs are indicated for increasing the RBC mass in patients who require increased oxygen-carrying capacity.[1,2] These patients typically have pulse rates greater than 100 beats per minute; respiration rates greater than 30 breaths per minute; and may experience dizziness, weakness, angina (chest pain), and difficulty thinking. The decreased RBC mass may be caused by decreased bone marrow production (leukemia or aplastic anemia), decreased RBC survival (hemolytic anemia), or surgical or traumatic bleeding.

The human body compensates for anemia by increasing plasma volume, increasing heart rate, increasing respiratory rate, and increasing oxygen extraction from the RBCs. Normally, only about 25 percent of the oxygen is extracted, but with increased demand at the organ and tissue level, up to 50 percent of the oxygen can be extracted. When the demand exceeds 50 percent of the oxygen content, the compensatory mechanisms fail, and the patient requires transfusion.

There are no set hemoglobin levels that indicate a need for transfusion. Although the level of 7 g/dL has been used for many years for surgical and leukemic patients, the critical level is 6.0 g/dL or less. Consensus committees suggest trigger values of hemoglobin of less than 6.0 g/dL in the absence of disease and between 7 and 8 g/dL with disease[3] for patients with heart, lung, or cerebral vascular disease.[4,5] Most renal dialysis patients can tolerate 6 g/dL. In fact, healthy individuals could tolerate hemoglobin levels as low as 5.0 g/dL with minimal effects,[5] especially if they are placed at bed rest or at decreased levels of activity and given supplemental oxygen.[6]

Transfusion of RBCs is contraindicated in patients who are well compensated for the anemia, such as those with chronic renal failure. RBCs should not be used to treat nutritional anemia, such as iron deficiency or pernicious anemia, unless the patient shows signs of decompensation (need for increased oxygen-carrying capacity). RBC transfusion is not to be used to enhance general well-being, promote wound healing, prevent infection, expand blood volume when oxygen-carrying capacity is adequate, or prevent future anemia.

Each unit of transfused RBCs is expected to increase the hemoglobin level 1 to 1.5 g/dL and the hematocrit level 3 to 5 percent in the typical 70-kg (154-lb) human, the same as whole blood. The increase in hemoglobin and hematocrit is evident more quickly than with 1 unit of whole blood, because the adjustment in blood volume is less. As in the example for whole blood, the RBC volume would be increased the same amount, to 1450 mL, but the blood volume is increased only 300 mL to 5300 mL. The hematocrit level is increased immediately to 27.2 percent.

RBCs prepared with additive solutions such as AS-1 or AS-3 have greater volume than with citrate-phosphate-dextrose (CPD) or citrate-phosphate-dextrose-adenine (CPDA-1), 330 mL versus 250 to 275 mL (see Chapter 1), but the additive solution units have less plasma. The RBC mass is the same. Therefore, the hematocrit differs from 70 to 80 percent for CPDA-1 RBCs to 55 to 70 percent for additive solution RBCs (see **Table 16–1**).

Leukocyte-Reduced RBCs

The average unit of RBCs contains approximately 2×10^9 leukocytes. Donor leukocytes may cause febrile nonhemolytic transfusion reactions, transfusion-associated graft-versus-host disease (TA-GVHD), and transfusion-related immune suppression. In addition, human leukocyte antigens (HLA) are responsible for alloimmunization. Leukocytes may harbor cytomegalovirus (CMV), Epstein-Barr virus, human immunodeficiency virus (HIV), or human T lymphotropic virus.

To reduce HLA alloimmunization and CMV transmission, the leukocyte content must be reduced to less than 5×10^6, which can be achieved by using one of several third-generation leukocyte reduction filters.[7] With these filters, most RBC units are less than 1×10^6; some are 1×10^4. In the United States,[8] the standard leukocyte content is less than 5×10^6; in Europe, the standard is less than 1×10^6. Controversial is the effect of leukocyte-reduced blood on length of hospital stay and postsurgical wound infection. However, febrile nonhemolytic transfusion reactions are decreased by the use of leukocyte-reduced RBCs and platelets[7] (**Table 16–2**).

Washed RBCs and Frozen/Deglycerolized RBCs

Patients who have severe allergic (anaphylactic) transfusion reactions to ordinary units of RBCs may benefit from receiving washed RBCs.[1] The washing process removes plasma proteins, the cause of most allergic reactions. Washed RBCs are used for the rare patient who has anti-IgA antibodies because of IgA deficiency.

Freezing RBCs allows the long-term storage of rare blood donor units, autologous units, and units for special purposes, such as intrauterine transfusion. Because the process needed to deglycerolize the RBCs removes nearly all the plasma, these units, although more expensive, can be used interchangeably with washed RBCs. The 24-hour outdate of

TABLE 16-2 Leukocyte-Reduced RBCs and Platelets

INDICATIONS	
Accepted	**Controversial**
Decrease febrile nonhemolytic transfusion reactions	Decrease hospital length of stay
Decrease alloimmunization to white blood cell antigens	Decrease postsurgical infections
Decrease transmission of CMV	Decrease incidence of cancer recurrence postsurgery

washed or deglycerolized RBCs severely limits the use of these components. The expected hematocrit increase for washed or deglycerolized RBCs is the same as that for regular RBC units.

Platelets and Plateletpheresis

Platelets are essential for the formation of the primary hemostatic plug and maintenance of normal hemostasis. Patients with severe thrombocytopenia (low platelet count) or abnormal platelet function may have petechiae, ecchymoses, and mucosal or spontaneous hemorrhage. The thrombocytopenia may be caused by decreased platelet production (e.g., after chemotherapy for malignancy) or increased destruction (e.g., disseminated intravascular coagulation [DIC]). Massive transfusion, which is discussed later in this chapter, may also cause thrombocytopenia because of the rapid consumption of platelets for hemostasis and the dilution of the platelets by resuscitation fluids and RBC transfusion.

Platelet transfusions are indicated for patients who are bleeding because of thrombocytopenia (**Box 16-1**) or, in a few cases, owing to abnormally functioning platelets.[9] In addition, platelets are indicated as prophylaxis for patients who have platelet counts under 5000 to 10,000/μL.[10]

Each unit of platelets (concentrate) must contain at least 5.5×10^{10} platelets[11] and should increase the platelet count 5000 to 10,000/μL in the typical 70-kg human. Pools of 4 to 6 units, then, will contain roughly 3×10^{11} platelets and should give a platelet increment of 20,000 to 60,000/μL. Massive splenomegaly, high fever, sepsis, disseminated intravascular coagulation, and platelet or HLA antibodies can cause less than expected platelet count increment and survival. The 10-minute to 1-hour post-transfusion platelet count increment is less affected by splenomegaly, high fever, and DIC than by the presence of platelet or HLA antibodies.[12] If the 10-minute increment is less than 50 percent of that expected on two occasions, the patient is considered refractory. Positive

BOX 16-1
Indications for Platelet Transfusion

- Thrombocytopenia
- Chemotherapy for malignancy (decreased production, <10,000/μL)
- Disseminated intravascular coagulation (increased destruction, < 50,000/μL)
- Massive transfusion (platelet dilution, < 50,000/μL)

platelet crossmatches and/or positive HLA antibody screen is considered evidence of alloimmunization. Platelet crossmatching with available inventory can speed the provision of platelets for transfusion, as HLA-typing the patient as well as recruiting HLA-compatible platelet donors can be time-consuming.

A plateletpheresis component is prepared from one donor and must contain a minimum of 3×10^{11} platelets.[11] One plateletpheresis is equivalent to one dose of platelets (e.g., a pool of 4 to 6 units). Components procured by apheresis can be given as random products, platelet crossmatched, or, because of their HLA types, as HLA-matched products. HLA-matched platelets should be irradiated.

A corrected count increment using a 10-minute to 1-hour post-transfusion platelet count can provide valuable information about patient response to a platelet component.[12] The platelet count increment is corrected for differences in body size so that more reliable estimates of expected platelet increment can be determined.[13] The expected corrected platelet increment is >10,000/μL per m². One formula for corrected count increment is:

$$\frac{\text{Absolute platelet increment/μL} \times \text{body surface area (m}^2)}{\text{Number of platelets transfused } (10^{11})}$$

in which the absolute platelet increment is the post-transfusion platelet count minus the pretransfusion platelet count, the body surface area is expressed as square meters, and the number of platelets transfused is 3.0 for plateletpheresis product or is determined by multiplying the number of units (bags) of platelets by 0.55 (the number of platelets in each unit expressed in 10^{11}).

For example, a patient with 10,000/μL platelet count has a body surface area of 1.3 m². Six units of platelets are given. The 1-hour post-transfusion platelet count is 50,000/μL. Put these into the formula:

$$\frac{(50,000/\text{μL} - 10,000/\text{μL}) \times 1.3}{6 \text{ units} \times 0.55/\text{unit}} = 15,758/\text{μL}$$

The answer shows that the patient has a good increment (>10,000/μL) and is not refractory to platelets. An answer less than 5000/μL indicates refractoriness. The formula can be used for plateletpheresis by using 3 (times 10^{11}) as the number of platelets in each unit.

In addition to HLA- and platelet-specific antigens, ABO antigens are also expressed on the platelet membrane. Sometimes platelets are selected for transfusion without regard to ABO; however, group O recipients may have a lower increment when given group A platelets than when group-identical platelets are selected.[14] Group A, B, and AB patients may also develop a positive direct antiglobulin test owing to passive transfer of anti-A, anti-B, or anti-A,B when several ABO-incompatible platelet transfusions are given.

Although platelet membranes do not express Rh antigens, platelet concentrates contain small amounts of RBCs and thus can immunize patients to Rh antigens. Rh-immune globulin can be given to girls and women of childbearing potential to prevent Rh sensitization. Each 300-μg vial of Rh immune globulin is adequate for 30 platelet concentrates or three plateletphereses.

For the same reasons as RBCs, platelet components may also be leukocyte-reduced or washed. Special filters are available. Washing platelet components removes some platelets as well as plasma proteins and is an open method, requiring a 4-hour expiration time. Therefore, platelet components should be washed only to prevent severe allergic reactions or to remove alloantibodies in cases of neonatal alloimmune thrombocytopenia.

Granulocytes Pheresis

Patients who have received intensive chemotherapy for leukemia or bone marrow transplant, or both, may develop severe neutropenia and serious bacterial or fungal infection. Without neutrophils (granulocytes), the patient may have difficulty controlling an infection, even with appropriate antibiotic treatment. Criteria have been developed to identify patients who are most likely to benefit from granulocyte transfusions: those with fever, neutrophil counts less than 500/µL, septicemia or bacterial infection unresponsive to antibiotics, reversible bone marrow hypoplasia, and a reasonable chance for survival.[1] Prophylactic use of granulocytes transfusions is of doubtful value for those patients who have neutropenia but no demonstrable infection.

Newborn infants may develop overwhelming infection with neutropenia because of their limited bone marrow reserve for neutrophil production. In addition, neonatal neutrophils have impaired function. Recent studies have shown granulocyte transfusions to be beneficial for these patients. For an adult, the usual dose is one granulocyte pheresis product daily for 4 or more days. For neonates, a portion of a granulocyte pheresis unit is usually given once or twice.

Granulocytes components should be administered as soon as possible and within 24 hours of collection.[15] In most instances, the granulocyte pheresis needs to be cross-matched because of significant content of RBCs.[15] The patient must be monitored for resolution of symptoms and clinical evidence of efficacy. The neutrophil count will increase to 1000/µL or more in response to infusion of granulocyte-colony stimulating factor (G-CSF)–mobilized granulocyte pheresis.

Fresh Frozen Plasma (FFP)

Fresh frozen plasma (FFP) contains all coagulation factors. FFP can be used to treat multiple coagulation deficiencies occurring in patients with liver failure, DIC, vitamin K deficiency, warfarin overdose, or massive transfusion.[16] Sometimes, FFP is used to treat patients with single factor deficiencies, such as factor XI deficiency.

Vitamin K deficiency or warfarin overdose should be treated with vitamin K orally, intravenously, or intramuscularly if liver function is adequate and with an adequate interval (4 to 24 hours) before a major or minor hemostatic challenge such as surgery. FFP is given if the patient is actively bleeding or if time is not available for warfarin reversal before surgery.

Patients with liver disease or liver failure frequently develop clinical coagulopathy due to impaired hepatic synthesis of all coagulation factors as well as antithrombotic factors. FFP is the product of choice for patients with multiple-factor deficiencies and hemorrhage or impending surgery. Usually 4 to 6 units of FFP effectively control hemostasis. Even so, FFP may not correct coagulation tests to normal range because of dysfibrinogenemia. Mild hemostatic abnormalities do not predict bleeding, so correction is not indicated for minor procedures, such as liver biopsy.[17] In addition, FFP is not a concentrate so that volume overload may be a serious complication of FFP transfusion.

Congenital coagulation factor deficiencies may also be treated with FFP, although the dose requirement for surgical procedures and serious bleeding may be so great as to cause pulmonary edema as a result of volume overload, even in a young individual with a healthy cardiovascular system. Factor concentrates (see discussions) currently offer more effective modes of therapy. Factor XI deficiency, however, is still treated by plasma infusion, requiring 20 percent to 30 percent factor XI levels for adequate hemostasis. This disease is milder than hemophilia A (factor VIII deficiency) or hemophilia B (factor IX deficiency). Factor XI also has a long half-life, so treatment is not needed on a daily basis.

A coagulation factor unit is defined as the activity in 1 mL of pooled normal plasma, so 100 percent activity is 1 unit/mL or 100 units/dL. About 30 percent activity of each of the coagulation factors is required for adequate hemostasis. Thus, less than half of the plasma volume, or about 4 to 6 FFP units, is required to correct a coagulopathy such as in liver disease or DIC. With continued hemorrhage, additional doses are usually needed if the prothrombin time is more than 1.5 normal or the international normalized ratio is greater than 1.8 to 2.0. Because several key clotting factors, such as factor VII, VIII, or IX, have half-lives less than 24 hours, repeated transfusions are required to control postoperative bleeding or to maintain hemostasis. For example, factor IX has a half-life of 18 to 24 hours, requiring daily transfusions.

FFP is sometimes used as a replacement fluid during plasma exchange (therapeutic plasmapheresis) (see Chapter 17). In cases of thrombotic thrombocytopenic purpura, FFP provides a metalloprotease and removes inhibitors, thus reversing the symptoms. The syndrome of hemolysis, elevated liver enzymes, and low platelets (HELLP)[18] occurs in a subgroup of pregnant women who have pre-eclampsia (pregnancy-induced hypertension and proteinuria) and usually occurs in the postpartum period. Plasmapheresis is used when the disease does not remit on its own.

FFP should not be used for blood volume expansion or protein replacement because safer products are available for these purposes—serum albumin, synthetic colloids, and balanced salt solutions—none of which transmit disease or cause severe allergic reactions or transfusion-associated acute lung injury.

FFP should be ABO-compatible with the recipient's RBCs, but the Rh type can be disregarded.

Thawed Plasma or Liquid Plasma

Thawed plasma is FFP that is stored 24 hours to 5 days after thawing. Thawed plasma contains decreased amounts of the labile coagulation factors V and VIII and thus is not recommended for treatment of patients who have a clinically significant deficiency of either or both of these clotting factors. The plasma can be used for treatment of stable coagulation deficiency, especially for warfarin overdose or reversal. The rare factor XI deficiency can also be treated with thawed plasma. Thawed plasma can be used for patients undergoing plasma exchange for thrombotic thrombocytopenic purpura (TTP), hemolytic-uremic syndrome, or HELLP.

Cryoprecipitate-Reduced Plasma

Large molecular weight von Willebrand's factor (vWF) multimers, decreased protease, or the presence of protease inhibitors may contribute to the development of TTP. Some patients apparently respond better to the use of the supernatant plasma from the preparation of cryoprecipitate (cryoprecipitate-reduced plasma, commonly called cryopoor plasma).[19]

Cryoprecipitate

Currently, cryoprecipitate is used primarily for fibrinogen replacement. The American Association of Blood Banks (AABB) has a requirement for at least 150 mg in each unit of cryoprecipitate.[15] Fibrinogen replacement may be required in patients with liver failure, DIC, or massive transfusion and in rare patients with congenital fibrinogen deficiency. A fibrinogen plasma level of about 80 mg/dL is recommended for adequate hemostasis with surgery or trauma.

For example, a patient's fibrinogen must be increased from 30 mg/dL to 100 mg/dL, or an increment of 70 mg/dL (100 – 30 mg/dL). To calculate the amount to be infused, first convert milligrams per deciliter to milligrams per milliliter by dividing by 100 (100 mL/dL). Multiplying this figure, 0.7 mg/mL, by the plasma volume, 3000 mL, we thus require 2100 mg (0.7 mg/mL × 3000 mL). To calculate the number of bags needed, divide 2100 mg by 250 mg/bag, which equals 14 bags (instead, plasma volume can be converted to deciliters by dividing by 100 mL/dL).

Cryoprecipitate can also be used as a source of fibrin sealant (or glue),[20] which consists of a unit of cryoprecipitate as the source of fibrinogen. Bovine thrombin is mixed with the contents of the bag of cryoprecipitate at the tip of a spray gun (atomizer). The fibrinogen, activated by the thrombin, acts as a fibrin sealant for the applied area. The glue is applied topically on prosthetic vascular grafts and vascular tissue planes in surgery. FDA-approved fibrin sealant, which has been treated to reduce viral transmission, is available.

Cryoprecipitate was originally prepared as a source of factor VIII. The components also contain fibrinogen, vWF, and factor XIII (Table 16–3). This product can be used to correct the deficiency of some of these coagulation factors. Each unit of cryoprecipitate must contain at least 80 units of factor VIII (Table 16–3). Currently, mild or moderate factor VIII deficiency (hemophilia A) is usually treated with desmopressin acetate (1-deamino-[8-D-arginine]-vasopressin [DDAVP]) or factor VIII, or both, whereas severe factor VIII deficiency is treated only with factor VIII.

Cryoprecipitate has been used to treat patients with von Willebrand's disorder, a deficiency of vWF. Cryoprecipitate is no longer considered the product of choice for factor VIII deficiency or von Willebrand's disorder. Virus-safe factor VIII with an assayed amount of factor VIII and vWF is available.

Factor VIII

Patients with hemophilia A or factor VIII deficiency have spontaneous hemorrhages that are treated with recombinant or human plasma source factor VIII replacement.[21] Plasma source factor VIII is prepared from plasma obtained from paid donors by plasmapheresis or from volunteer whole blood donors. Factor VIII is treated by different methods, such as pasteurization, nanofiltration, and solvent detergent, to ensure sterility for human immunodeficiency virus (HIV), hepatitis B virus, and hepatitis C virus (HCV).[22,23] Cases of hepatitis A have been reported but are rare. The recombinant human product (Table 16–4) is not derived from human plasma; therefore, it is virus-safe.

Both the plasma source and recombinant factor VIII are stored at refrigerator temperatures and are reconstituted with saline at the time of infusion. This ease of handling allows home therapy for individuals with hemophilia.

The following example illustrates the calculation of the dose of factor VIII:

A 70-kg hemophiliac patient with a hematocrit level of 30 percent has an initial factor VIII level of 4 percent (4 units/dL, 0.04 units/mL). How many units of factor VIII concentrate should be given to raise his factor VIII level to 50 percent?

{desired factor VIII (units/mL) − initial factor VIII (units/mL)} × plasma volume (mL) = units of factor VIII required

Blood volume = weight (kg) × 70 mL/kg, or 70 kg × 70 mL/kg = 4900 mL

Plasma volume = blood volume (mL) × (1.0 − Hct), or 4900 mL × (1.0 − 0.30) = 3430 mL

Putting into formula:

3430 mL × (0.50 − 0.04) = 1578 units

The assayed value on the label can be divided into the number of units required to obtain the number of vials to be infused.

Only factor VIII products labeled as containing vWF should be used for patients with von Willebrand's disease.

TABLE 16–3 Cryoprecipitate

Constituents	Amount
Factor VIII	80–120 U/concentrate
Fibrinogen	150–250 mg/concentrate
vWF	40–70% of original FFP
Factor XIII	20–30% of original FFP

American Association of Blood Banks, Arlington, VA, 1985, with permission.

TABLE 16–4 Recombinant Human Products (Purified)

Product	Indications
Factor VIII	Hemophilia A
Factor IX	Hemophilia B
Factor VIIa	Inhibitors in hemophilia A or B
	Factor VII deficiency
	Acquired factor VII deficiency*
	Liver disease
	Warfarin overdose

*Studies under way

Factor IX

Factor IX complex (prothrombin complex) is prepared from pooled plasma using various methods of separation and viral inactivation. The prothrombin complex contains factors II, VII, IX, and X; however, the product is recommended for factor IX–deficient patients (hemophilia B), patients with factor VII or X deficiency (rare), and selected patients with factor VIII inhibitors or reversal of warfarin overdose.[23] Activated coagulation factors present in prothrombin complex may cause thrombosis, especially in patients with liver disease. Recombinant human factor IX (see **Table 16–4**) is effective only in the management of factor IX deficiency.

The dose is calculated in the same manner as that for factor VIII concentrate, using the assayed value of factor IX on the label, with the caveat that half the dose of factor IX rapidly diffuses into tissues, and half remains within the intravascular space, so the initial dose must be doubled.

Antithrombin and Other Concentrates

Antithrombin is a protease inhibitor with activity toward thrombin. Heparin accelerates the binding and inactivation of thrombin by antithrombin. The hereditary deficiency of antithrombin is associated with venous thromboses, whereas the acquired deficiency is seen most frequently with DIC. Antithrombin concentrates are licensed for use in the United States for patients with hereditary deficiency of antithrombin. The product is pasteurized to eliminate the risk of HIV or HCV infections. Antithrombin has been shown to provide no significant clinical benefit in acquired deficiency. Thawed plasma and FFP are alternative sources of antithrombin I.

Protein C and protein S are vitamin K–dependent proteins synthesized in the liver. Protein S functions as a cofactor for activated protein C (APC), which, in turn, inactivates factors V and VIII, thus preventing thrombus formation. Deficiency (hereditary or acquired) leads to a hypercoagulable state (i.e., the tendency for thrombosis). Protein C concentrates are currently approved for use only in hereditary deficiency states. However, recent studies demonstrate APC therapy improves the clinical outcome of DIC.

Alpha$_1$-protease inhibitor concentrates are available for patients with α_1-antitrypsin deficiency. This inherited condition is associated with emphysema and liver disease. The product is heat-treated to decrease transmission of viruses.

C1-esterase inhibitor concentrates are not currently approved for use in the United States. Deficiency of C1-esterase inhibitor results in life-threatening angioedema of the mucosa and submucosa of the respiratory and gastrointestinal tracts.

Recombinant human activated factor VII (rFVIIa) (see **Table 16–4**) has been used reliably to control bleeding episodes in hemophilia A and B patients with inhibitors.[24,25] Studies of the use of rFVIIa in patients with factor VII deficiency or liver disease have been promising.[26]

Albumin

Albumin is prepared by chemical and physical fractionation of pooled plasma. Albumin is available as a 5 percent or a 25 percent solution, of which 96 percent of the protein content is albumin. The product is heat-treated and has proved to be virus-safe over many years of use.

Albumin may be used to treat patients requiring volume replacement. Whether albumin or colloids other than crystalloid (i.e., saline or electrolyte) solutions are better for treating hypovolemia with shock is controversial. Albumin is used routinely as the replacement fluid in many plasmapheresis procedures, replacing the colloid that is removed during the procedures. Albumin can be used in the treatment of burn patients for replacement of colloid pressure as well.

Albumin can be used with diuretics to induce diuresis in patients with low total protein because of severe liver or protein-losing disease. The 25 percent solution brings about five times its volume from extravascular water into the vascular space. Thus, patients receiving 25 percent albumin need to have adequate extravascular water and compensatory mechanisms to deal with the expansion of the blood volume.

Immune Globulin

Immune globulin prepared from pooled plasma is primarily IgG. Although small amounts of IgM and IgA may be present in some preparations, others are free of these contaminating proteins.[27] Products are available for intramuscular or intravenous administration. The intramuscular product must not be given intravenously because severe anaphylactic reactions may occur. The intravenous product must be given slowly to lessen the risk of reaction.

Immune globulin is used for patients with congenital hypogammaglobulinemia and for patients exposed to diseases such as hepatitis A or measles.[27] For hypogammaglobulinemia, monthly injections are usually given because of the 22-day half-life of IgG. The recommended dose is 0.7 mL/kg intramuscularly or 100 mg/kg intravenously. For hepatitis A prophylaxis, 0.02 to 0.04 mL/kg intramuscularly is recommended.

The intravenous preparation of immune globulin is used increasingly in the therapy of autoimmune diseases, such as immune thrombocytopenia[27] and myasthenia gravis. Various mechanisms of action have been postulated. Conceivably, the infused immune globulin blocks the reticuloendothelial system or mononuclear phagocytic system.

Various hyperimmune globulins are available for prevention of diseases such as hepatitis B, varicella zoster, rabies, mumps, and others. These are prepared from the plasma of donors who have high antibody titers to the specific virus causing the disease. The dose is recommended in the package insert. It should be noted that preparations such as hepatitis B hyperimmune globulin provide only passive immunity after an exposure. They do not confer permanent immunity and so must be accompanied by active immunization.

Rh immune globulin was developed to protect the Rh-negative female who is pregnant or delivers an Rh-positive infant (see Chapter 20). Much of the IgG in this preparation is directed against the D antigen within the Rh system. Administration of this preparation allows attachment of anti-D to any Rh-positive cells of the infant that have entered the maternal circulation. The antibody-bound cells are subsequently removed by the macrophages of the mother, preventing active immunization or sensitization (see Chapter 20).

An Rh immune globulin product, which can be administered intravenously or intramuscularly, is approved for use in idiopathic thrombocytopenic purpura patients who are Rh-positive.[28] The proposed mechanism of action is blockage of the reticuloendothelial system by anti-D–coated RBCs, thereby reducing the destruction of autoantibody-coated platelets.

For RBC transfusion accidents, the number of RhIg vials is calculated by dividing the volume of Rh-positive packed RBCs transfused by 15 mL, the amount of RBCs covered by one vial. The number of vials can be large, so the entire dose is often divided and administered in several injections at separate sites. The intravenous preparation may also be used. Another approach is to perform an exchange transfusion with Rh-negative blood and then calculate the dose based on the number of Rh-positive RBCs remaining in the circulation. For platelet concentrates, one vial is sufficient for 30 or more units (bags), because each unit contains fewer than 0.5 mL RBCs. The dose for leukocyte concentrates can be calculated by obtaining the hematocrit and volume of the product from the supplier.

Immune globulins may cause anaphylactic reactions (flushing, hypotension, dyspnea, nausea, vomiting, diarrhea, and back pain). Caution should be used in patients with known IgA deficiency and previous anaphylactic reactions to blood components.

Special Considerations for Transfusion

Leukocyte-Reduced Blood Components

Leukocyte-reduction filters are designed to remove more than 99.9% of leukocytes from RBCs and platelet products. The goal is fewer than 5×10^6 (1×10^6 in Europe) remaining in the RBC unit. Prestorage filtration in the laboratory, rather than at the bedside, is more reliable for reduction of leukocytes.

Leukocyte-reduced RBCs and platelets can be used to prevent febrile nonhemolytic transfusion reactions, prevent or delay the development of HLA antibodies, and reduce the risk of transmission of CMV. Controversial effects of leukocyte reduction include decreased mortality and length of hospital stay.[29,30]

CMV-Negative Blood Components

CMV is carried, in a latent or infectious form, in neutrophils and monocytes. Transfusion of these virus-infected cells in a cellular product such as RBCs or platelets can transmit infection. Infection of the patients can be reduced by using leukocyte-reduction filters[31,32] or by providing CMV antibody–negative blood. CMV-negative or leukocyte-reduced components are indicated for recipients who are CMV-negative and at risk for severe sequelae of CMV infections.[5] The risk is greatest for CMV-negative pregnant women (mainly for the benefit of the fetus), CMV-negative bone marrow and hematoprogenitor cell transplant recipients, and premature infants weighing less than 1200 g.

Irradiated Blood Components

Blood components are irradiated with gamma radiation to prevent GVHD, which requires three conditions to occur:

1. Transfusion or transplantation of immunocompetent T lymphocytes
2. Histocompatibility differences between graft and recipient (major or minor HLA or other histocompatibility antigens)
3. Usually, an immunocompromised recipient.[33]

Common after allogeneic bone marrow or hematopoietic progenitor cell transplantation, GVHD is a syndrome affecting mainly skin, liver, and gut.

TA-GVHD, occurring less frequently, is caused by viable T lymphocytes in cellular blood components (e.g., RBCs and platelets). The mortality rate is high[33,34]; therefore, prevention is key. Prevention centers on irradiation of cellular components before administration to significantly immunocompromised individuals. Irradiation doses range from 2500 to 5000 cGy, with the higher doses being more effective but more damaging to RBCs. Irradiation decreases or eliminates the mitogenic (blastogenic) capacity of the transfused T cells, rendering the donor T cells immunoincompetent.

At risk for TA-GVHD are transfusion recipients with congenital immunodeficiencies (severe combined immunodeficiency, DiGeorge's syndrome, Wiskott-Aldrich syndrome), Hodgkin's lymphoma, bone marrow transplants (allogeneic or autologous), intrauterine transfusion of fetuses, exchange transfusion of neonates, or donations from blood relatives and HLA-matched platelets.[33,34] In the last case, immunocompetent recipients have experienced TA-GVHD after receiving nonirradiated directed donations primarily from first-degree relatives. The related donor is homozygous for one of the patient's (host's) HLA haplotypes, so the patient is incapable of rejecting the donor's (graft's) T lymphocytes, which then can act against the HLA antigens encoded by the patient's other haplotype. The donor lymphocytes then reject the host.[35] The required level of immunosuppression for a recipient to develop TA-GVHD is unknown, although the severe immunosuppressive conditions listed previously are most at risk. In addition, the dose of lymphocytes needed for TA-GVHD to occur is unknown. For this reason, prevention is dependent on irradiation and *not* on reduction of lymphocytes by filtration.

Transfusion in Transplantation

Transplantation can be autologous, allogeneic (related or unrelated), syngeneic (twin), or xenogeneic (Table 16–5). An example of autologous transplantation is the harvest of hematopoietic progenitor cells (HPCs) from a patient with Hodgkin's disease for his or her own transplant. Allogeneic is the harvest of cells, organs, or tissues from one human to transplant into another. The donor may be related or unrelated. Syngeneic is the situation of identical twins, one of whom is healthy and the other with a disease treatable by transplantation. Xenogeneic is the use of organs or tissues from another species, such as the transplant of porcine heart valves.

Related donors may have HLA types identical to those of the recipients (Table 16–6) However, siblings have only a one

TABLE 16–5 Hematopoietic Progenitor Cell (HPC) Transplantation	
Types of Transplant	**Definition**
Autologous	Harvesting HPCs from self, "rescue"
Allogeneic	From one human to another Related or unrelated
Syngeneic	Identical twin or triplet
Xenogeneic	Another species

TABLE 16–6	Related Transplantation
Sibling—HLA	25% identical 50% one haplotype 25% mismatch
Parents—HLA	100% one haplotype

BOX 16–3
Donor Side Effects of G-CSF

- Bone pain
- Headaches
- Nausea, sometimes vomiting
- Thrombocytopenia

in four chance of being HLA-identical; parents and children have only one haplotype identical, unless they have the rare condition of homozygous haplotypes.

Bone Marrow and HPC Transplantation

HPCs can be obtained from bone marrow, peripheral blood, and cord blood.[36] HPC transplantation is used to treat patients with Hodgkin's disease, lymphoma, acute and chronic leukemia, congenital immune deficiencies, and aplastic anemia (Box 16–2). Allogeneic donors must be screened the same as blood donors. For the safety of the donor, a history and physical examination, EKG, and screening laboratory tests should be completed before donation.

Bone marrow for transplantation is being replaced, for the most part, with peripheral blood hematopoietic progenitor cells (PB-HPCs) collected by leukopheresis.[37] Collection of bone marrow from a donor involves general or local anesthetic, operating room time, a hospital stay, and recovery time. Bone marrow is harvested from the iliac crest, with multiple puncture sites and multiple aspirations into syringes. Depending on the size of the recipient, as much as 1.5 L can be collected. The bone marrow is filtered to remove clots, fat, and bone fragments.

PB-HPCs are collected by leukopheresis from normal donors for allogeneic transplant into a patient. The related or unrelated donor is administered G-CSF for 4 to 5 days to expand and mobilize HPCs from the bone marrow into the peripheral blood, increasing the white blood cell count to 20,000/μL or more. The donor may have bone pain from the expansion of the bone marrow. Other side effects may include headache, nausea, and vomiting. Commonly, the platelet count will decrease with G-CSF stimulation and HPC collection. A few donors have developed chronic thrombocytopenia **(Box 16–3)**. Collection of PB-HPC is usually accomplished in 1 to 2 days.

Autologous donors are generally given chemotherapy to take advantage of the rebound of the bone marrow in combination with G-CSF and/or granulocyte-macrophage colony-stimulating factor to stimulate the release of more HPC into the peripheral blood.[38,39] Collection of PB-HPCs

may need to be continued daily for 4 to 5 days to obtain sufficient yield.

Both the bone marrow and HPC products may need further processing. **(Box 16–4)** With ABO-incompatible bone marrow, the plasma or RBCs may be reduced to lessen the risk of a major or minor hemolytic transfusion reaction when the bone marrow is infused. With both products, the number of T lymphocytes may be reduced to lessen GVHD. Malignant cells can be reduced or eliminated. Selection of CD34 positive cells (early HPC) can also be accomplished.

The dose of cells to be transplanted can be expressed as nucleated cells per kg body weight of the recipient. Generally, $2–4 \times 10^8$ are required. As more centers have available CD34 enumeration by flow cytometry, the dose required is $2–6 \times 10^6$ CD34 positive cells per kg.[39]

Both products may be infused fresh or stored up to 24 hours at 20° to 24°C or 4°C, infusing as soon as possible. Both products can be frozen using 10% dimethyl sulfoxide (DMSO) as a cryoprotectant, storing at -80°C or in the vapor phase of liquid nitrogen. Thawing should be rapid, and the cells should be infused as soon as possible after thawing. These products must not be irradiated or infused through a leukocyte reduction filter.

Bone marrow and PB-HPC transplantation carry a high risk of morbidity and mortality for the recipients. Major ABO incompatibility may cause hemolysis of the donor RBCs, especially with bone marrow infusions if the RBCs are not reduced before infusion **(Table 16–7)**. Major ABO incompatibility may also delay engraftment of the erythropoietic line because of potent circulating ABO antibodies. Removing plasma from bone marrow with minor ABO incompatibility will lessen the chance of hemolysis of the patient's RBCs. A rare and often fatal condition is the rapid destruction of the patient's RBCs by antibody produced by passenger lymphocytes from the donor HPC product.

Allogeneic donors must be carefully matched for HLA antigens to reduce the risk of severe GVHD[37] **(Table 16–8)**. Acute GVHD occurs within a few days to 100 days post-transplantation. The GVHD may be mild, with a minor skin rash, or severe, with bullous skin lesions, jaundice, and unrelenting diarrhea. Chronic GVHD follows the acute phase or

BOX 16–2
Diseases Treated by BMT

- Congenital immune deficiencies
- Aplastic anemia
- Leukemia, acute or chronic
- Lymphoma
- Hodgkin's disease

BOX 16–4
Cell Populations of HPCs

- CD-34 positive MNCs
- RBCs
- T cells
- Malignant cells in oncology patients

TABLE 16–7	ABO Incompatibility		
	Donor	**Patient**	
Major	A	O	Hemolyze donor RBCs Delayed engraftment
Minor	O	A	Hemolyze patient RBCs Anti-A GVHD

BOX 16–5
DMSO Side Effects

- Nausea
- Diarrhea
- Flushing
- Bradycardia
- Hypertension
- Abdominal pain
- Hypotension

may occur months later. When severe, the scarring may lead to cirrhosis and systemic sclerosis. These recipients may develop veno-occlusive disease of the liver, infection, hemorrhage, and disease relapse. In addition, the recipients may not engraft or may have delayed engraftment. The infusion of DMSO may be accompanied by nausea, vomiting, diarrhea, chills, and anaphylactoid reaction (**Box 16–5**).

Autologous recipients generally have less severe complications than allogeneic recipients. However, they do not have the advantage of GVHD, which also exerts a graft-versus-leukemia effect. Engraftment may be delayed or not occur.

Cord blood, harvested from the delivered placenta, is rich in progenitor cells[40] (**Box 16–6**). About 100 mL is collected with a CD34 content of about 1.5×10^5 cells.[41] Cord blood has been used successfully in children weighing less than 45 kg, with failure of engraftment in some recipients weighing more than 45 kg. Platelet engraftment is frequently delayed. GVHD with cord blood transplantation is apparently less likely to occur than with bone marrow or PB-HPC transplants.

Considerable preparations are necessary before collection of the cord blood (**Box 16–7**). The mother must provide informed consent, the maternal and family history, all the items asked of blood donors, and the history of genetic disorders. ABO, Rh, and HLA type must be determined on the infant, and the RBC antibody screen is determined on the mother.

Donors of bone marrow or PB-HPC may be requested to donate lymphocytes for their recipients who have leukemia relapse. The donor lymphocytes exert a graft-versus-leukemia effect, which can be successful in controlling the recipient's disease.

Transfusion in recipients of HPC transplantation requires attention to selection of blood products. Cellular products (RBC and platelets) must be irradiated to prevent TA-GVHD. As the recipients are not completely immunologically reconstituted for months to years after transplant, they are susceptible to GVHD as well as infections. Patients with HPC transplants may develop severe CMV disease. CMV-negative allogeneic and autologous recipients should receive leukocyte-reduced or CMV-negative transfusions.

Patients with engraftment as expected will need blood product transfusions for 1 to 3 weeks. However, those with complications of delayed engraftment, GVHD, or infections

will require blood support for weeks to months. Platelets may need to be crossmatched and/or HLA-matched.

ABO mismatched transplants present interesting problems. RBCs and platelets/plasma will have separate preferred ABO blood groups in many cases (**Table 16–9**). The table is used by selecting the ABO compatible blood group(s) that are common to both donor and recipient. In the first example, both the donor and the recipient can receive group O RBCs and A or AB plasma or platelets. In the second example, the recipient should receive group O RBCs and AB plasma or platelets. However, if HLA matched platelets are required, the preferred ABO group may not be available.

In these examples, as the HPC cells engraft, the recipient will slowly become the donor's ABO group. In the first example, the anti-A in the recipient will become weaker over several weeks, eventually becoming undetectable. About that time, small proportions of group A cells will be detected as mixed field reactions. Eventually, the recipient will type as group A, both forward and reverse.

In the second example, the group A recipient has anti-B, so the group B donor RBCs in the HPC product may be hemolyzed during the infusion and cause an acute hemolytic reaction. In addition, the engraftment of the HPCs may be delayed because of the circulating anti-B.

In both cases, transfusing the blood group of choice for RBCS, plasma, and platelets is extremely important.

Solid Organ Transplantation

Each year, about 5000 cadaveric donors become available for harvest of solid organs (**Table 16–10**). Most of these donors will be eligible for kidney harvest, with each donor having two kidneys, thus, about 8000 kidneys will be available for transplantation. Kidneys are less susceptible to ischemia than the other organs listed in the table; therefore, fewer hearts and livers are available. Lungs have the most stringent criteria for transplantation acceptability.

ABO compatibility is important to organ transplantation. Major ABO incompatibility may lead to rapid organ injury and death of the organ.

TABLE 16–8	GVHD	
Acute		Few days to 100 days post-transplantation Stage or grade for severity Skin, liver, and gut involved
Chronic		Follows acute or months later "Scarring"—cirrhosis, systemic sclerosis

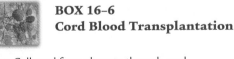

BOX 16–6
Cord Blood Transplantation

- Collected from placenta through cord
- HLA mismatches engraft
- Less frequent GVHD
- Volume limitations

BOX 16–7
Cord Blood Considerations

- Informed consent
- Maternal and family history and genetic disorders
- ABO & Rh—infant
- Antibody screen—mother
- HLA typing—infant

TABLE 16–10 Organ Transplants—6,000 Donors, 2002

Kidney	8500
Heart	2100
Liver	5000
Pancreas	600
Lung	1000

Organ Procurement and Transplantation Network (OPTN) data as of November 21, 2003.

Liver transplantation requires the most transfusion support as compared with other organs.[42] As the liver is the source of coagulation and antithrombotic factors, coagulation parameters may be severely abnormal. In addition, with portal hypertension, the spleen is enlarged and traps platelets, resulting in a decreased platelet count. Portal hypertension can also contribute to excessive bleeding during the operation. Each liver transplant requires 10 to 20 RBCs, several pools of platelets, 10 to 20 units of FFP, and sometimes several pools of cryoprecipitate. Plasma must be transfused judiciously because liver function is necessary to metabolize the citrate anticoagulant in the plasma. High citrate levels can result in hypocalcemia, causing heart conduction abnormalities and deteriorating heart function.

In liver transplantation, massive transfusion with several blood volume replacements may be required. In these situations, the ABO type of RBCs may need to be switched, such as an AB patient transfused with group A (Table 16–11). The Rh-negative type of patient may need to be disregarded and Rh-positive RBCs transfused. Occasional patients may have multiple RBC antibodies with limited compatible antigen(s)–negative RBC units. In these cases, the first 5 to 10 units can be antigen(s)-negative, and then transfusion of antigen-untested or -incompatible with one or more antigen, followed by the remaining antigen(s)-negative units. In these cases, close communication with operating room personnel (especially the anesthetist) can help predict the need for blood and the appropriate timing of the selection of units.

Heart and heart/lung transplantations usually require few units of blood, similar to other cardiopulmonary bypass procedures. However, if the patient is placed on a cardiac assist device to await the availability of a heart for transplant, platelets and RBCs may be needed to replace those damaged by the device. Renal and renal/pancreas transplants usually do not require blood components.

Tissue Transplantation

Various tissues can be harvested from cadaveric donors, as listed in Table 16–12. Each can donate two corneas, long bones, bone chips, multiple tendons, many square centimeters of skin, and multiple heart valves. Except for cornea and skin, the tissues can be processed, sterilized, and packaged for sale to hospitals and clinics for use in surgical procedures.

Transfusion Therapy in Special Conditions

Surgical Blood Order Schedule; Type and Screen

Reviews of blood transfusion practices have found that most surgical procedures do not require blood transfusion. Crossmatching for procedures with a low likelihood of transfusion increases the number of crossmatches performed, increases the amount of blood inventory in reserve and unavailable for transfusion, and contributes to the aging and possible outdating of the blood components. Patients can be better served by performing only a type and antibody screen. If the antibody screen is positive, antibody identification must be completed and compatible units found. However, if the antibody screen is negative, ABO- and Rh-type–specific blood may be released after an immediate spin crossmatch in those rare instances when transfusion is required (Box 16–8).

For a patient who is likely to require blood transfusion, the number of crossmatched units should be no more than twice those usually required for that surgical procedure. Thus, the crossmatch-to-transfusion (C/T) ratio will be between 2:1 and 3:1, which has been shown to be optimal practice. Although individual institutions may vary, general outlines are available concerning the surgical blood ordering schedule.[43]

Autologous Transfusion

Autologous (self) transfusion is the donation of blood by the intended recipient; the infusion of blood from another donor is homologous transfusion. The patient's own blood is the safest blood possible, reducing the possibility of transfusion reaction or transmission of infectious disease.[44,45]

TABLE 16–9 Selection of ABO Blood Component

	Can Receive	
	RBCs	Plasma
Donor A	A, O	A, AB
Recipient O	O	A, AB, O, B
Donor B	B, O	B, AB
Recipient A	A, O	A, AB

TABLE 16–11 Transfusion in Liver Transplant

Problem	Solution
ABO identical may not be possible	B patients switch to O AB patients switch to A
Multiple antibodies	Begin and end with antigen negative

TABLE 16–12	Tissue Transplantation, 2001	
	Harvest	**Transplantation**
Cornea	45,000	45,000
Bone	5000	300,000
Tendon	3000	6000
Skin	2000	3500
Heart valves	1500	2000
Dura mater	100	400

L. Jones, personal communication, 2002.

One type of autologous transfusion is the predeposit of blood by the patient (Fig. 16–1). Collected by regular blood donation procedure, the blood can be stored liquid or, for longer storage, frozen. Patients may donate several units of blood over a period of weeks, taking iron supplements to stimulate erythropoiesis. Predeposit autologous donation is usually reserved for patients anticipating a need for transfusion, such as scheduled surgery. However, patients with multiple RBC antibodies or antibodies to high-incidence antigens may store frozen units for unanticipated future need.

The use of recombinant erythropoietin may avoid the transfusion of homologous RBC products and allow more than the usual two to three units collected before surgery.[46]

Another type of autologous transfusion, intraoperative hemodilution, is the collection of one or two units of blood from the patient just before a surgical procedure, replacing the removed blood volume with crystalloid or colloid solution. Then, at the end of surgery, the blood units are infused into the patient. Care must be taken to label and to store the blood units properly and to identify the blood units with the patient before infusion.

Salvage of shed blood may be performed intraoperatively and/or postoperatively for autologous transfusion (see Fig. 16–1). Several types of equipment are available for collecting, washing, and filtering shed blood before reinfusion. Washing of intraoperative salvage blood is generally recommended to remove the cellular debris, fat, and other contaminants. Heparin or citrate solutions may be used for anticoagulation of the shed blood, although postoperative salvage of thoracotomy blood may not require anticoagulation. Blood exposed to serosal surfaces, such as the pleural lining, is defibrinated. Meticulous salvage of shed blood has allowed surgical procedures that once required many units of blood to be performed without the need for homologous blood.

BOX 16–8
Surgical Blood Order Schedule

- Purpose: Reduce unnecessary crossmatching
- Examples
- Type and screen
  - Exploratory laparotomy
  - Cholecystectomy
  - Two units crossmatched
  - Pulmonary lobectomy
  - Hemicolectomy

Emergency Transfusion

Patients who are rapidly or uncontrollably bleeding may require immediate transfusion. Group O RBCs are selected for patients for whom transfusion cannot wait until the ABO and Rh type of the patient can be determined.[47] Group O–negative RBC units should be used, especially if the patient is a female of childbearing potential. A male patient or an older female patient can be switched from Rh-negative to Rh-positive RBCs if few O-negative units are available and massive transfusion is required.

Patients should be resuscitated with crystalloid or colloid solutions, and transfusions should be reserved for those patients losing more than 20 percent of their blood volume. The condition of most patients allows determination of ABO and Rh type and selection of ABO- and Rh-type–specific blood for transfusion. Delaying blood transfusion in emergency situations may be more dangerous than the small risk of transfusing incompatible blood before the antibody screen and crossmatch are completed.[47] After issuing O blood or type-specific blood, the antibody screen can be completed, and decisions can then be made for the selection of additional units of blood. If the patient has been typed and screened for a surgical procedure and his or her antibody screen is negative, ABO- and Rh-type–specific blood can be selected and given after an immediate spin crossmatch.

Massive Transfusion

Massive transfusion is defined as the replacement of one or more blood volumes within 24 hours, or about 10 units of blood in an adult. The strategy for treatment of massive hemorrhage is outlined in Table 16–13. Analysis of the patient's clinical status and laboratory tests is essential for deciding appropriate transfusion therapy. Patients receiving less than one blood volume replacement rarely require platelet or plasma transfusion. Patients receiving two blood volumes usually require platelet and plasma transfusion.[48] If the patient is actively bleeding, platelets are required if the platelet count is less than 50,000/μL, and plasma is needed if the PT ratio is greater than 1.5, or the INR is greater than 1.8 to 2.0, or the activated partial thromboplastin time (PTT) exceeds 60 seconds. Fibrinogen levels should also be monitored because replacement by cryoprecipitate may be indicated when the fibrinogen level is less than 100 mg/dL.[6] Maintenance of the blood volume is of utmost importance in preventing tissue damage and worsening of thrombocytopenia and coagulopathy because of shock.[47] Extensive monitoring of PT, PTT, platelet count, fibrinogen, hemoglobin, and hematocrit can help direct the choice of the most indicated products during the duration of the massive transfusion.

A patient in critical condition and a limited supply of type-specific blood may require a change in ABO or Rh types. An Rh-negative male or postmenopausal female patient may be switched from Rh-negative to Rh-positive blood if there is concern about exhausting the inventory of Rh-negative blood. However, an Rh-negative potentially childbearing woman should receive Rh-negative RBC products as long as possible.

Neonatal and Pediatric Transfusion

Premature infants frequently require transfusion of small amounts of RBCs to replace blood drawn for laboratory

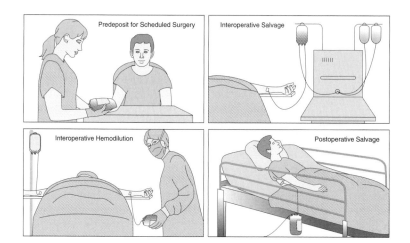

■ **FIGURE 16–1** Types of autologous transfusions. (From Kennedy,[55] with permission.)

tests. A dose of 8 to 10 mL/kg will increase the hemoglobin approximately 3 g/dL. Various methods are available for preparing small aliquots for transfusion. Small aliquots of donor blood can be transferred from the collection bag to a satellite bag or transfer bag, or blood can be withdrawn from the collection bag or transfer bag using an injection site coupler and needle and syringe or a sterile docking device and syringe.

The aliquot must be labeled clearly with the name and identifying numbers of the patient and donor. The blood must be fully tested, the same as blood for adult transfusion. Blood units less than 7 days old are preferred to reduce the risk of hyperkalemia and to maximize the 2,3-diphosphoglycerate levels, although in some instances CPDA-1 RBCs 14 to 21 days old are used routinely (Box 16–9).

For very low birth weight infants, the blood should be selected to be CMV-seronegative or leukocyte-reduced to prevent CMV infection, which can be serious in premature infants. Indeed, pregnant women should be given CMV-negative leukocyte-reduced cellular components if they test negative for CMV.

Irradiation of the blood is recommended to prevent possible TA-GVHD when blood is used for intrauterine transfusion, for an exchange transfusion, (see Chapter 20), or perhaps for transfusion of a premature (less than 1200g) neonate. Transfusions in a full-term newborn infant do not require routine irradiation.[33,34]

Infants who are hypoxic or acidotic should receive blood tested and negative for hemoglobin S.

Transfusion in Oncology

The bone marrow of oncology patients may function poorly because of chemotherapy, radiation therapy, or infiltration and replacement of the bone marrow with malignant cells. Repeated RBC and platelet transfusions may lead to the need for rare RBC units and/or HLA-matched plateletpheresis components because of incompatibility problems. Platelet use, as well, may necessitate a change from Rh-negative to Rh-positive products. RhIg may be given to a woman with childbearing potential to protect against immunization. There are less than 5 mL of Rh-positive RBCs present in each Rh-positive plateletpheresis component or pool of platelet concentrates. One 300-μg dose of RhIg can neutralize the effects of up to 15 mL of Rh-positive cells. Thus, one dose could be used for three doses or more of platelets.

In addition, some malignancies such as chronic lymphocytic leukemia and lymphoma are frequently complicated by autoimmune hemolytic anemia, increased destruction of RBCs, and pretransfusion testing problems.

Oncology patients with hematologic malignancies, such as Hodgkin's disease and lymphoma, are at increased risk of TA-GVHD because of the chemotherapy agents used for treatment. Therefore, these patients should receive irradiated blood components.

Coagulation Factor Deficiencies

Factor VIII is normally complexed with another plasma protein, vWF. Both proteins are necessary for normal hemostasis.

TABLE 16–13 Strategy for Massive Hemorrhage	
Condition	**Treatment**
Low blood volume*	Crystalloid or colloid
Low oxygen-carrying capacity*	RBCs
Hemorrhage owing to:	
Thrombocytopenia	Platelet concentrates
Coagulopathy	FFP, cryoprecititate (if fibrinogen is low)

Kennedy, MS (ed): Blood Transfusion Therapy: An Audiovisual Program. American Association of Blood Banks, Arlington, VA, 1985, with permission.
*If these occur simultaneously, whole blood may be indicated.

BOX 16–9
Neonatal RBC Transfusions

Aliquoted units

- Less than 7 days old, unless infused slowly
- O-negative or compatible with mother and infant
- CMV-negative or leukocyte-reduced
- Hemoglobin S–negative for hypoxic newborns

Dose

- 10 mL/kg over 2–3 hours

Patients with hemophilia A, or classic hemophilia, have factor VIII deficiency. Hemophilia A patients have factor VIII levels less than 50 percent, although clinical disease is generally not apparent unless the factor VIII level is less than 10 percent (normal 80 to 120) (Table 16–14). Individuals with a level less than 1 percent have severe and spontaneous bleeding, typically into muscles and joints. The vWF level is usually normal in patients with hemophilia A.

Von Willebrand's disease is defined by a deficiency of vWF. Type I von Willebrand's disease is characterized by a reduced amount of all sizes of vWF multimers and is milder than type III, in which little or no vWF is produced. Type IIA is distinguished by a deficiency of high molecular weight multimers, whereas type IIB is discriminated by abnormal high molecular weight multimers that have an increased avidity for binding to platelets. Type I patients have the ability to make the full spectrum of vWF multimers but do not produce them in normal amounts. DDAVP, a synthetic vasopressin analog, can stimulate release of the vWF from the vascular endothelium in type I patients. DDAVP, however, is contraindicated in type IIB von Willebrand's disease. Many factor VIII products are assayed for vWF and can be used for type III von Willebrand's disease or in type I disease when DDAVP treatment has failed.

Hemophilia B is the congenital deficiency of factor IX. Factor IX is activated by factors XIa and VIIa. The activated factor IX (IXa), along with factor VIII, ionized calcium, and phospholipid, activates factor X to Xa. Factor IX deficiency should be treated with recombinant factor IX or prothrombin complex concentrates. Factor IX concentrates are made virus-safe by various sterilization techniques.[23]

All coagulation factors except vWF are made in the liver. With severe liver failure, multiple coagulation factor deficiencies occur. In addition, some of the coagulation factors produced may be abnormal. The liver also produces many of the thrombolytic proteins, leading to imbalance between the coagulation process and the control mechanism. FFP, having normal amounts of all these proteins, can be used to treat these patients.

Vitamin K aids in the carboxylation of factors II, VII, IX, and X. With the absence of vitamin K or the use of drugs, such as warfarin, that interfere with vitamin K metabolism, the inactive coagulation proteins cannot be carboxylated to active forms. Vitamin K rather than FFP administration is recommended to correct vitamin K deficiency or warfarin overdose. Because several hours are required for vitamin K effectiveness, depending on route of administration, signs of hemorrhage or impending surgery may require transfusion of FFP.

DIC is the uncontrolled activation and consumption of coagulation proteins, causing small thrombi within the vascular system throughout the body. Treatment is aimed at correcting the cause of the DIC: sepsis, disseminated malignancy, certain acute leukemias, obstetric complications, or shock. In some cases, transfusion of FFP, platelets, or cryoprecipitate may be required. Monitoring of the PT, PTT, platelet count, fibrinogen, and hemoglobin and hematocrit levels helps direct the choice of the next component to be used.

Platelet functional disorders may be caused by drugs, uremia, or congenital abnormalities. Platelet transfusions in these patients should be reserved for the treatment of hemorrhage or the impending need for normal hemostasis (such as a surgical procedure) to decrease development of platelet refractoriness. In uremia, DDAVP may be beneficial as well as dialysis or RBC transfusions. DDAVP releases fresh, functional vWF from endothelial cells. Dialysis removes by-products of protein metabolism that degrade vWF and coat platelets, thus making both nonfunctional.

General Blood Transfusion Practices

Blood Administration

Blood must be administered carefully for patient safety (Fig. 16–2). The positive identification of the patient, patient's blood specimen, and blood unit for transfusion is essential. Careful identification procedures prevent a major cause of transfusion-related deaths: ABO incompatibility. Clerical errors represent the main cause of transfusion-related deaths and acute hemolytic transfusion reactions.[49] The identification process begins with positive identification of the patient; that is, asking patients to state or spell their name while you read their armband. A patient identification label is prepared at the bedside after the specimen is drawn. This prevents an empty specimen tube from being labeled with one patient's name and potentially being used for the collection of specimen from another patient. The labels are applied to the specimen tubes before leaving the bedside to avoid labeling the wrong tube.

Positive identification is carried out in the laboratory. Clerical check is performed as results are generated and as blood is issued from the blood bank. The final clerical check is performed at the patient bedside as the nurse compares the patient armband with the blood bank tag attached to the component to be transfused.

The patient with difficult veins should have the intravenous infusion device in place before the blood is issued from the transfusion service. All blood components must be filtered (170-μm filter) because clots and cellular debris

TABLE 16–14 Differential Diagnosis of Hemophilia A and von Willebrand's Disease		
	Hemophilia A	**von Willebrand's Disease**
Typical coagulation values	VIII < 50%, vWF 50%–150%	VIII 2%–50%, vWF <40%
Bleeding time	Usually normal	Prolonged
Clinical course	Bleeding into joints and muscles	Cutaneous/mucosal bleeding
	Bleeding with trauma	Bleeding with trauma or
	or surgery	surgery

Kennedy, MS (ed): Blood Transfusion Therapy: An Audiovisual Program. American Association of Blood Banks, Arlington, VA, 1985, with permission.

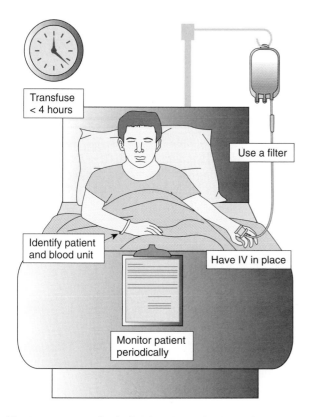

■ **FIGURE 16–2** Blood administration and patient safety. (From Kennedy,[55] with permission.)

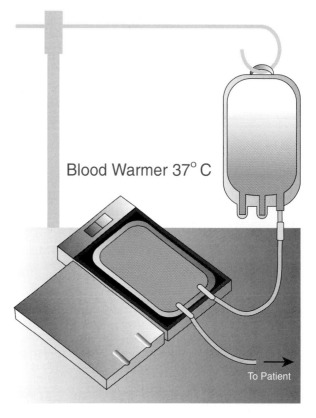

■ **FIGURE 16–3** Blood warming. (From Kennedy,[55] with permission.)

develop during storage. Blood components are infused slowly for the first 10 to 15 minutes while the patient is observed closely for signs of a transfusion reaction. The blood components should then be infused as quickly as tolerated or, at most, within 4 hours. The patient's vital signs (pulse, respiration, blood pressure, and temperature) should be monitored periodically during the transfusion to detect signs of transfusion reaction. Signs and symptoms are fever with back pain (acute hemolytic transfusion reaction), anaphylaxis, hives or pruritus (urticarial reaction), congestive heart failure (volume overload), and fever alone (febrile nonhemolytic transfusion reaction). A delayed hemolytic transfusion reaction (jaundice, decreasing hematocrit level) may be diagnosed only 7 to 10 days after transfusion and thus is not considered an immediate reaction.

In standard blood administration sets, the 70 to 170 μm filter is a "clot-screen" filter that removes gross clots and cellular debris. A standard blood administration filter must be used for transfusion of all blood components.

Rapid transfusion, including exchange transfusion, requires blood warming because the cold blood can cause hypothermia in the patient, which increases the possibility of cardiac arrhythmia and hemorrhage. A patient with paroxysmal cold hemoglobinuria or with potent cold agglutinins may also require blood warming. The blood warmer should have automatic temperature control set with an alarm that will sound if the blood is warmed over 42°C **(Fig. 16–3)**. Blood units must not be warmed by immersion in a waterbath or by a domestic microwave oven because uneven heating, damage to blood cells, and denaturation of blood proteins may occur.

Only isotonic (0.9 percent) saline or 5 percent albumin should be used to dilute blood components, because other intravenous solutions may damage the RBCs and cause hemolysis (dextrose solutions such as D_5W) or initiate coagulation in the infusion set (calcium-containing solutions such as lactated Ringer's solution). In addition, some drugs may cause hemolysis if injected through the blood infusion set.

Hospital Transfusion Committee

The Joint Commission on Accreditation of Healthcare Organizations (JCAHO) requires all blood transfusions to be reviewed for appropriate use. A hospital transfusion committee, although not required by JCAHO, may serve as the peer review group for transfusions. Blood usage review may also be performed prospectively if criteria are approved by the medical staff.[50] The blood bank director may interact and correspond directly with the chair of individual hospital departments concerning medical staff blood component usage patterns. Appropriate criteria for blood transfusion have been published **(Table 16–15)**, serving as a guide for review.[51–54] The results of the review can be used by the transfusion committee to recommend changes in practice by the hospital staff to improve patient care. The transfusion committee also reviews each transfusion reaction to ensure that adverse reactions are unavoidable. In addition, the transfusion committee ensures that appropriate procedures (such as for blood administration) are in place and are followed by hospital personnel.

The transfusion committee is most effective if the various groups who order and administer blood, such as surgeons, anesthesiologists, and oncologists, are represented on the

TABLE 16–15   Criteria for Transfusion Audit

All Blood Components

Review of patients with transfusion reactions of hemolysis, severe allergic signs or anaphylaxis, circulatory overload, or infection

Review of patients with abnormal liver function or diagnosis of hepatitis within 6 months of transfusion

Charts of patients with adverse reaction or transfusion-transmitted disease must contain physician evaluation

Whole Blood

Indications:	Actively bleeding *and* blood loss >25% total blood volume *or* actively bleeding and received 4 units RBCs
Outcome:	H/H < 24 hours after transfusion
	Surgical procedures: postoperative hemoglobin < preoperative hemoglobin

RBCs[52]

Indications:	Decreased oxygen-carrying capacity
	acute loss of >15% blood volume
	or hemoglobin <6 g/dL or hematocrit <18%
	or symptoms related to anemia
Exceptions:	Patients with hemoglobin >7 g/dL and coronary artery disease, chronic pulmonary disease, or cerebral vascular disease
Outcome:	H/H <24 hours after transfusion
	Surgical patients: postoperative hemoglobin < preoperative hemoglobin

Platelets

Indications:	Platelet count <5,000–10,000/μL without hemorrhage
	or hemorrhage and platelet count <50,000/μL
	or operative procedure in <12 hours and platelet count <50,000/μL
	Review of patients receiving platelets and with autoimmune thrombocytopenia purpura, thrombotic thrombocytopenia purpura, or hemolytic uremic syndrome
Outcome:	Platelet count immediately before and 10 minutes–1 hour post-transfusion

FFP

Indications:	Patients with bleeding or invasive procedure
	PTT >60 sec
	or INR >1.8
	or documented coagulation factor deficiency
Outcome:	PT, PTT, or coagulation factor assay immediately before and fewer than 4 hours after transfusion

Cryoprecipitate

Indications:	Fibrinogen deficiency or factor XIII deficiency
Outcome:	Fibrinogen or factor XIII determination after transfusion

Modified from the National Institutes of Health Consensus Conference. JAMA 257:1777, 1987, and JAMA 253:551, 1985; Silberstein, LE, et al: Strategies for the review of transfusion practices. JAMA 262:1993, 1989; Simon, TL, et al: Practice parameter for the use of red blood cell transfusions. Arch Pathol Lab Med 122:130, 1998,[54] and AuBuchon, JP, et al: Guidelines for blood utilization review, AABB, Bethesda, MD, 2001.[50]
H/H = hemoglobin hematocrit

committee. The transfusion committee must have a mechanism for reporting activities and recommendations to the medical staff and hospital administration. Optimally, the transfusion committee ensures that the most appropriate, efficient, and safe use of the blood supply is achieved.

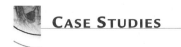

CASE STUDIES

Case 1

A 55-year-old man is contemplating surgery for severe arthritis in the right hip.

1. What should be known to determine how many units of RBCs should be crossmatched?

2. How can it be determined if the patient can donate blood (autologous predeposit) for use during surgery?

3. The patient has a history of bleeding after a tonsillectomy at age 7 years. What tests should be done to further study this potential problem?

4. If the patient is found to have von Willebrand's disease, which blood components might be necessary?

Answers

1. It is necessary to know the patient's hemoglobin and hematocrit levels, the surgeon's usual blood usage, whether this is the first surgical procedure on this hip (redo surgery uses more blood), and whether the patient has any pretransfusion compatibility problems.

2. Considerations should be the patient's general health, hemoglobin and hematocrit levels, amount of time

between request for donation and the time of surgery, and whether the patient has infectious diseases that might interfere (e.g., bacterial infections).

3. Tests should include PT, PTT, and platelet count. If these tests are normal and von Willebrand's disease is suspected, vWF workup should be considered.

4. If the patient has moderate to severe von Willebrand's disease, the patient may need either factor VIII concentrate known to contain vWF or cryoprecipitate.

Case 2

A 45-year-old woman complains of tiredness and weakness. She appears pale. Laboratory results are as follows: hemoglobin 6.2 g/dL, hematocrit 22%, MCV 75 fL, MCHC 28%. On further questioning, she reports excessive menstrual bleeding, sometimes lasting for several weeks.

1. Does this patient need a transfusion? Justify your answer.
2. If the intern decides to give two units of RBCs, what would be the resulting hemoglobin and hematocrit levels?

Answers

1. Yes, her hemoglobin is close to 6.0 g/dL, which is the criterion for RBC transfusion. She will be less tired and weak if she receives a transfusion. No, she is not in any acute distress. She is iron-deficient (from blood loss) and should be treated with iron replacement rather than with transfusion, which has higher risk of complications.

2. For adults, each unit of blood should increase the hemoglobin 1 g/dL and the hematocrit 3 percentage points. For accuracy, this is based on a hypothetical 70-kg man. For smaller men and women, the increase is greater; for larger ones, less.

Case 3

A 22-year-old woman presents with easy bruising and fatigue. A complete blood count reveals hemoglobin 9.0 g/dL, hematocrit 27%, WBC 15,000/μL, and platelet count 15,000/μL. The hematologist plans to perform a bone marrow biopsy and aspiration.

1. What blood component(s) is (are) indicated? Why?
2. Describe how the dose is calculated. What laboratory result is desired?
3. The patient receives chemotherapy, and 2 weeks later the hemoglobin is 7.0 g/dL and the hematocrit 21%. The patient complains of shortness of breath when hurrying to the bus stop. The physician decides to order RBC transfusion. What dose of RBCs is indicated? How is this determined?

Answers

1. The platelet count is below 50,000/μL; therefore, a platelet transfusion is indicated. Without the platelet transfusion, she would be at increased risk of bleeding from the site of the bone marrow biopsy. Although the hemoglobin and hematocrit levels are lower than normal for a woman of this age, an RBC transfusion is not indicated (hemoglobin >6.0 g/dL in an otherwise healthy young adult).

2. For an adult, each unit (bag) of platelet concentrate should increase the patient's platelet count by 5000–10,000/μL. The platelet count should be at about 50,000/μL because a

bone marrow biopsy is an invasive procedure. Thus, about four units of platelet concentrates would be indicated.

3. If it is anticipated that the patient will experience bone marrow recovery soon (after the chemotherapy), just one unit of RBCs is indicated. If, however, the bone marrow will be suppressed for several weeks, two units are indicated, with a recheck in a couple weeks for another possible transfusion. Each unit of RBCs is expected to increase the hemoglobin level about 1 g/dL.

Case 4

A 45-year-old man is diagnosed with non-Hodgkin's lymphoma. He types as B, Rh-positive. His brother is found to be HLA-matched, but is A, Rh-positive. The brother donates peripheral blood HPC, which is transplanted in the patient on April 25, 2003. The patient requires long-term transfusion support and receives 57 RBCs, 107 platelets apheresis, 30 FFP, and 6 cryoprecipitate.

1. Which blood group(s) should be selected for the RBC transfusions?
2. For FFP and platelets, which blood type(s) should be selected?

The patient's ABO testing for specific days post transplant is shown below.

3. What is the interpretation of his ABO group on day 147?
4. What is the blood group interpretation on day 200? On day 156?

Answers

1. The blood group for RBC transfusions is O, which is the only blood group compatible with both the donor and recipient. If A is chosen, the cells will be hemolyzed or have a shortened life span because of the preexisting anti-A in the patient. If B is chosen, engraftment will be difficult to determine.

2. Group AB should be selected for FFP and platelet transfusion. If group A is selected, the anti-B in the plasma is incompatible with the recipient's RBC and tissue antigens (B). The anti-A in group B products is incompatible with the donor RBCs and, if selected, may contribute to delayed engraftment of RBC precursors.

3. On day 117, the interpretation is B, as B cells and anti-A are present.

4. On day 200, the interpretation is group A, because A cells and anti-B are present, and B cells and anti-A are absent. On day 156, the forward type is group O (remember that the patient is receiving group O RBC transfusions), but the reverse type still has anti-A; thus, the interpretation is indeterminate.

Day Post-Transplantation	Anti-A	Anti-B	A cells	B cells
Day 117	0	1+ (mf)	1+	0
Day 147	0	wk (mf)	2+	0
Day 156	0	0	1+	0
Day 200	wk (mf)	0	0	1+

mf = mixed field

SUMMARY CHART:

Important Points to Remember (MT/MLT)

➤ Transfusion therapy is used primarily to treat two conditions: inadequate oxygen-carrying capacity because of anemia or blood loss and insufficient coagulation proteins to provide adequate hemostasis.

➤ A unit of whole blood or packed RBCs in an adult should increase the hematocrit level 3 percent or hemoglobin level 1.0–1.5 g/dL.

➤ RBCs are indicated for increasing the RBC mass in patients who require increased oxygen-carrying capacity.

➤ Platelet transfusions are indicated for patients who are bleeding because of thrombocytopenia. In addition, platelets are indicated prophylactically for patients who have platelet counts under 5000–10,000/μL.

➤ Each unit of platelets should increase the platelet count 5000–10,000/μL in the typical 70-kg human; each should contain at least 5.5×10^{10} platelets.

➤ A plateletpheresis product is prepared from one donor and must contain a minimum of 3×10^{11} platelets.

➤ FFP contains all coagulation factors and is indicated for patients with multiple coagulation deficiencies that occur in liver failure, DIC, vitamin K deficiency, warfarin overdose, and massive transfusion.

➤ Cryoprecipitate contains at least 80 units of factor VIII and 150 mg of fibrinogen, as well as vWF, and factor XIII.

➤ Factor IX is used in the treatment of persons with hemophilia B.

➤ Immunoglobulin (Ig) is used in the treatment of congenital hypogammaglobulinemia and patients exposed to hepatitis A or measles.

➤ Massive transfusion is defined as the replacement of one or more blood volume(s) within 24 hours, or about 10 units of blood in an adult.

➤ Emergency transfusion warrants group O RBCs when patient type is not yet known.

REVIEW QUESTIONS

1. Leukocyte-reduced filters can do all of the following *except*:
   a. Reduce the risk of CMV infection
   b. Prevent or reduce the risk of HLA alloimmunization
   c. Prevent febrile, nonhemolytic transfusion reactions
   d. Prevent TA-GVHD

2. Albumin should *not* be given for:
   a. Burns
   b. Shock
   c. Nutrition
   d. Plasmapheresis

3. Of the following, which blood type is selected when a patient cannot wait for ABO-matched blood?
   a. A
   b. B
   c. O
   d. AB

4. Which patient does not need an irradiated component?
   a. Bone marrow transplant recipient
   b. Neonate weighing less than 1200 g
   c. Healthy adult receiving an RBC transfusion
   d. Healthy adult receiving an RBC transfusion from a blood relative

5. RBC transfusions should be given:
   a. Within 4 hours
   b. With lactated Ringer's solution
   c. With dextrose and water
   d. With cryoprecipitate

6. Which type of transplantation requires all cellular blood components to be irradiated?
   a. Bone marrow
   b. Heart
   c. Liver
   d. Pancreas
   e. Kidney

7. Characteristics of deglycerolized RBCs include the following *except*:
   a. Inexpensive
   b. 24-hour expiration date after thawing
   c. Used for rare antigen-type donor blood
   d. Used for IgA-deficient recipients

8. Select the appropriate product for the indicated patient or need:

I. Hemophilia A	A. Factor VIII
II. Hemophilia B	B. Cryoprecipitate
III. Fibrinogen deficiency	C. FFP
IV. Bone marrow transplant patient with anemia unresponsive to iron and vitamin B_{12} therapy	D. Irradiated RBCs
V. Increase oxygen-carrying capacity	E. RBCs
VI. Vitamin K deficiency and hemorrhage	F. Granulocytes pheresis
VII. Factor XIII deficiency	G. Leukocyte-reduced RBCs
VIII. Directed donation from a blood relative	H. Washed or deglycerolized RBCs
IX. Repeated febrile transfusion reactions	I. Immune globulin
X. Anaphylaxis	J. Hepatitis B immune globulin
XI. Life-threatening neutropenia	K. 0.9 percent saline
XII. Needlestick accident with infectious blood (hepatitis B)	L. Lactated Ringer's solution

XIII. Immunodeficiency

XIV. Used for dilution of RBCs

M. 5 percent dextrose and water solution

N. Factor IX

REFERENCES

1. Triulzi, DJ (ed): Blood Transfusion Therapy: A Physician's Handbook, ed 7. American Association of Blood Banks, Bethesda, MD, 2002, p 2.
2. Circular of Information for the Use of Human Blood and Blood Products. American Association of Blood Bank, America's Blood Centers, American Red Cross, Washington, DC, July 2002.
3. Silberstein, LE, et al: Strategies for the review of transfusion practices. JAMA 262:1993, 1989.
4. Gould, SA, et al: The physiologic basis of the use of blood and blood products. Surg Annu 16:13, 1984.
5. Spence, RK, et al: Transfusion guidelines for cardiovascular surgery: Lessons learned from operations in Jehovah's witnesses. J Vascular Surg 16:825, 1992.
6. Weiskopf, RB, et al.: Oxygen reverses deficits of cognitive function and memory and increased heart rate induced by acute severe isovolemic anemia. Anesthesiology 96:871, 2002.
7. Triulzi, DJ (ed): Blood Transfusion Therapy: A Physician's Handbook, ed 7. American Association of Blood Banks, Bethesda, MD, 2002, p. 10.
8. Garlin JB, ed. Standards for Blood Banks and Transfusion Services, ed 21. American Association Blood Banks, Bethesda, MD, 2002, p. 29
9. National Institutes of Health Consensus Conference: Platelet transfusion therapy. JAMA 257:1777, 1987.
10. Heckman, KD, et al. Randomized study of prophylactic platelet transfusion threshold during induction therapy for adult acute leukemia: 10,000/µL versus 20,000/µL. J Clin Oncol 15:1143, 1997.
11. Triulzi, DJ (ed): Blood Transfusion Therapy: A Physician's Handbook, ed 7. American Association of Blood Banks, Bethesda, MD, 2002.
12. Daly, PA, et al: Platelet transfusion therapy: One-hour post-transfusion increments are valuable in predicting the need for HLA-matched preparations. JAMA 243:435, 1980.
13. McFarland, JG, Anderson, AJ, and Slichter, SJ: Factors influencing the transfusion response to HLA-selected apheresis donor platelets in patients refractory to random platelet concentrates. Br J Haematol 73:380, 1989.
14. Slichter, SJ: Algorithm for managing the platelet refractory patient. J Clin Apheresis 12:4, 1997.
15. Garlin JB, ed: Standards for Blood Banks and Transfusion Services, ed 21. American Association of Blood Banks, Bethesda, MD, 2002, p. 36.
16. Practice Guidelines Development Task Force: Practice parameter for the use of fresh-frozen plasma, cryoprecipitate, and platelets. JAMA 271:777, 1994.
17. McVay PA, and Toy, PTCY: Lack of increased bleeding after liver biopsy in patients with mild hemostatic abnormalities. Am J Clin Pathol 94:747, 1990.
18. Martin, JN, et al: Postpartum plasma exchange for atypical preeclampsia-eclampsia as HELLP (hemolysis, elevated liver enzymes, and low platelets) syndrome. Am J Obstet Gynecol 172:1107, 1995.
19. Rock, G, et al: Cryosupernatant as replacement fluid for plasma exchange in thrombotic thrombocytopenia purpura. Members of the Canadian Apheresis Group. Br J Haematol 94:383, 1996
20. Radosevich, M, Goubran, HA, and Burnouf, T: Fibrin sealant: Scientific rationale, production methods, properties, and current clinical use. Vox Sang 72:133, 1997.
21. Furie, B, Limentani, SA, and Rosenfield, CG: A practical guide to the evaluation and treatment of hemophilia. Blood 84:3, 1994.
22. Colvin, BT: Guidelines on therapeutic products to treat haemophilia and other hereditary coagulation disorders. Hemophilia 3:63, 1997.
23. Kasper, CK, Lusher, JM, and the Transfusion Practices Committee: Recent evolution of clotting factor concentrates for hemophilia A and B. Transfusion 33:422, 1993.
24. Roberts, HR: Recombinant factor VIIa (Novoseven) and the safety of treatment. Semin Hematol 38:48, 2001.
25. Kulkarni, R, et al: Therapeutic choices for patients with hemophilia and high-titered inhibitors. Am J Hematol 67:240, 2001.
26. Kositchaiwat, C, and Chuansumrit, A: Experiences with recombinant factor VIIa for the prevention of bleeding in patients with chronic disease undergoing percutaneous liver biopsies and endoscopic retrograde cholangiopancreatography (ERCP). Thromb Haemost 86:1125, 2001
27. National Institute of Health Consensus Conference: Intravenous immunoglobulin: Prevention and treatment of disease. JAMA 264:3189, 1990.
28. Bussel, BJ, et al: Intravenous anti-D treatment of immune thrombocytopenic purpura: Analysis of efficacy, toxicity, and mechanism of effect. Blood 77:1884, 1991.
29. Hebert, PC, et al: Clinical outcome following institution of the Canadian universal leukoreduction program for red blood cell transfusion. JAMA 289:1941, 2003.
30. Fergusson, D, et al: Clinical outcome following institution of the Canadian universal leukoreduction program for premature infants. JAMA 289:1950, 2003.
31. Bowden, RA, et al: A comparison of filtered leukocyte-reduced and cytomegalovirus (CMV) seronegative blood products for the prevention of transfusion-associated CMV infection after marrow transplant. Blood 86:3598, 1995.
32. Laupacis, A, et al: Prevention of posttransfusion CMV in the era of universal WBC reduction: a consensus statement. Transfusion 41:560, 2001.
33. Anderson, KC, and Weinstein, HJ: Transfusion-associated graft-versus-host disease. N Engl J Med 323:315, 1990.
34. Linden, JV, and Pisciotto, PT: Transfusion-associated graft-versus-host disease and blood irradiation. Transfus Med Rev 6:116, 1992.
35. Otsuka, S, et al: The critical role of blood from HLA-homozygous donors in fatal transfusion-associated graft-versus-host disease in immunocompetent patients. Transfusion 31:260, 1991.
36. Korbling, M, and Anderlini, P: Peripheral blood stem cell versus bone marrow allotransplantation: Does the source of hematopoietic stem cells matter? Blood 98:2900, 2001.
37. Bensinger, B, and Storb, R: Allogeneic peripheral blood stem cell transplantation. Rev Clin Exp Hematol 5:67, 2001.
38. Weaver, CH, et al: Collection of peripheral blood progenitor cells after the administration of cyclophosphamide, etoposide, and granulocyte-colony-stimulating factor: An analysis of 497 patients. Transfusion 37:896, 1997.
39. To, LB, et al: The biology and clinical uses of blood stem cells. Blood 89:2233, 1997.
40. Ballen, K, et al: Current status of cord blood banking and transplantation in the United States and Europe. Biol Blood Marrow Transplant 7:635, 2001.
41. Rubinstein P, et al: Outcomes among 562 recipients of placental-blood transplants from unrelated donors. N Engl J Med 339:1565, 1998.
42. Ramsey, G, and Sherman, LA: Transfusion therapy in solid organ transplantation. Hematol Oncol Clin North Am 8:1117, 1994.
43. Brecher ME (ed): Technical Manual, ed 14. American Association Blood Banks, Bethesda, MD, 2002, p 84.
44. Ibid., p 106.
45. Santrach, PJ (ed.) Standards for preoperative autologous blood collection and administration, ed 1. American Association of Blood banks, Bethesda, MD, 2001.
46. Goodnough, LT, Monk, TG, and Andriole, GL: Erythropoietin therapy. N Engl J Med 336:933, 1997.
47. Kruskall, MS, et al: Transfusion therapy in emergency medicine. Ann Emerg Med 17:327, 1988.
48. Leslie, SD, and Toy, TCY: Laboratory hemostatic abnormalities in massively transfused patients given red blood cells and crystalloid. Am J Clin Pathol 96:770, 1991.
49. Sazama, K: Reports of 355 transfusion-associated deaths: 1976 through 1985. Transfusion 30:583, 1990.
50. AuBuchon JP (ed): Guidelines for Blood Utilization Review. American Association of Blood Banks, Bethesda. MD, 2001.
51. Spence, RK: Surgical red blood cell transfusion practice policies. Am J Surg 170:3S, 1995.
52. American Society of Anesthesiologists Task Force on Blood Component Therapy: Practice guidelines for blood component therapy. Anesthesiology 84:732, 1996.
53. Stehling, L, et al: Guidelines for blood utilization review. Transfusion 34:438, 1994.
54. Simon, TL, et al: Practice parameter for the use of red blood cell transfusions. Arch Pathol Lab Med 122:130, 1998.
55. Kennedy, MS (ed): Blood Transfusion Therapy: An Audiovisual Program. American Association of Blood Banks, Arlington, VA, 1985.

seventeen

Apheresis

Francis R. Rodwig, Jr, MD, MPH

=== **OBJECTIVES** ===

On completion of this chapter, the learner should be able to:

1. Define apheresis, leukapheresis, plateletpheresis, plasmapheresis, erythrocytapheresis, and therapeutic apheresis.
2. Describe the procedures of continuous flow centrifugation and intermittent flow centrifugation.
3. Discuss the use of membrane technology in the separation of blood components.
4. State the American Association of Blood Banks requirements for apheresis donations.
5. State the shelf life of platelet concentrates and granulocyte concentrates.
6. List the therapeutic indications for apheresis, differentiating between conditions requiring plasma exchange and those necessitating cytapheresis.
7. Describe the different types of adsorbents and their clinical application.
8. Identify the factors that can be removed by plasmapheresis.
9. Discuss the possible adverse effects of apheresis.

History and Development

Apheresis (or hemapheresis) is a term of Greek derivation that means "to separate or remove." In an apheresis procedure, blood is withdrawn from a donor or patient and separated into its components. One (or more) of the components is retained, and the remaining constituents are recombined and returned to the individual. Any of the components of blood can be removed, and the procedures are specified by the component selected. Thus, the process of removing the plasma from the blood is termed plasmapheresis. Similar terms are given to the removal of the other blood components, including platelets (plateletpheresis or thrombocytapheresis), red blood cells (erythrocytapheresis), or leukocytes (leukapheresis)

When anticoagulated blood is centrifuged in a test tube, it separates into red blood cells (RBCs), white blood cells (WBCs), platelets, and plasma because of the different weights (specific gravities) of these components **(Fig. 17–1)**. When a pipette is placed at the appropriate level in the test tube, any of these components can be aspirated. The most widely used apheresis equipment applies the same concept, using a machine with a centrifuge bowl or belt. Blood is removed from an individual (usually with a large-bore needle), anticoagulated, and transported directly to the separation mechanism, where it is separated into specific components. Once the components have been separated, any component can be withdrawn. The remaining portions of the blood are then mixed and returned to the donor or patient **(Fig. 17–2)**.

Depending on the goal of the individual procedures (e.g., collecting platelets, removing plasma or RBCs), the instruments must be adjusted appropriately. The variables are

1. Centrifuge speed and diameter;
2. Duration of dwell time of the blood in the centrifuge;
3. Type of solutions added, such as anticoagulants or sedimenting agents; and
4. Cellular content or plasma volume of the patient or donor.

By manipulating these variables, the operator can harvest plasma, platelets, WBCs, or RBCs for commercial or therapeutic purposes. A computerized control panel allows the operator to select the desired procedure and collection parameters. The machines are equipped with optical sensors

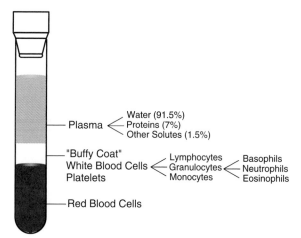

■ **FIGURE 17–1**   Sedimented blood sample. From Harmening, D.M. Clinical Hematology and Fundamentals, of Hemostasis, 4/e, Fig. 1-1, p.2, 2002 F.A. Davis.

that detect specific plasma-cell or cell-cell interfaces and divert components according to the preselected mode.

Methodology

Procedures for performing apheresis vary according to the particular component of the blood to be harvested and the equipment used. Manufacturers' instructions should always be consulted for specific techniques. The amount of time for a particular procedure can range from 45 to 120 minutes. Currently available machines use disposable equipment, which includes sterile bags, tubing, and collection chambers unique to the machine. Platelets collected using these systems are considered "closed," with a 5-day dating period.

The most commonly used instruments employ the centrifugation method of separation. This method can be divided into two basic categories:

1. Intermittent flow centrifugation (IFC)
2. Continuous flow centrifugation (CFC)

Apheresis by membrane filtration techniques is occasionally used.

Equipment

IFC procedures are performed in cycles (also called passes). Blood is drawn from an individual with the assistance of a pump. To keep the blood from clotting, an anticoagulant is added to the tubing. The blood is pumped into the separation

mechanism (in this case, a centrifuge bowl) through the inlet port. The bowl rotates at a fixed speed, separating the components according to their specific gravities. A rotary seal is used, resulting in a closed system. The RBCs, which have greater mass, are packed against the outer rim of the bowl, followed by the WBCs, platelets, and plasma. The separated component(s) flow from the bowl through the outlet port and are harvested as desired into separate collection bags (**Fig. 17–3**). The undesired components are diverted into a reinfusion bag and returned to the individual. Reinfusion completes one cycle. The cycles are repeated until the desired quantity of product is obtained (e.g., a plateletpheresis procedure usually takes 6 to 8 cycles to collect a therapeutic dose).

One of the advantages of the IFC procedure is that it can be done with only one venipuncture (one-arm procedure; that is, the blood is drawn and reinfused through the same needle). The amount of time for the process can be reduced if both arms are used: one for phlebotomy and one for reinfusion (two-arm procedure). The most widely used machines of this type are manufactured by the Haemonetics Corporation. The Mobile Collection Systems are versatile,

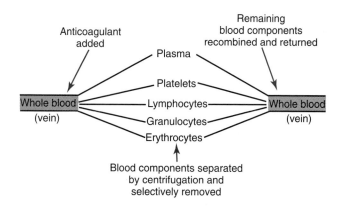

■ **FIGURE 17–2**   Principles of apheresis.

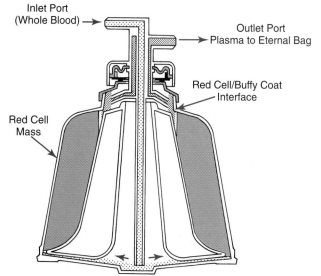

■ **FIGURE 17–3**   Cross-section of Haemonetics centrifuge bowl (IFC procedure). (Courtesy Haemonetics Corporation, Inc., Braintree, MA.)

portable, fully automated, and capable of efficient component collections **(Fig. 17–4)**. The Plasma Collection System (PCS2) is designed to collect plasma for transfusions or source plasma.

CFC procedures withdraw, process, and return the blood to the individual simultaneously. This is in contrast to IFC procedures, which complete a cycle before beginning the next one. Because blood is drawn and returned continuously during a procedure, two venipuncture sites are necessary. Occasionally, especially with therapeutic procedures, a dual-lumen central venous catheter is used. Blood is drawn from the phlebotomy site with the assistance of a pump, mixed with anticoagulant, and collected in a chamber or belt, depending on the machine. Separation of the components is achieved through centrifugation, and the specific component is diverted and retained in a collection bag. The remainder of the blood is reinfused to the individual via the second venipuncture site. The process of phlebotomy, separation, and reinfusion is uninterrupted, or continuous. Examples of machines employing this concept are the Baxter/Fenwal CS-3000 Plus and the newest model, the Amicus **(Fig. 17–5)**; the GAMBRO Spectra **(Fig. 17–6)**; and the Fresenius AS-104 **(Fig. 17–7)**.

The IFC and CFC machines have individual advantages and disadvantages.[1] The IFC equipment is usually smaller and more mobile. A single venipuncture may be used with the IFC procedures, whereas two venipunctures are usually required with the CFC procedures. New protocols have been developed to allow the CFC equipment to operate with single access (e.g,

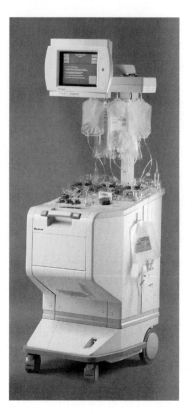

■ **FIGURE 17–5** Baxter/Fenwal Amicus (Courtesy Baxter Healthcare Corporation, Deerfield, IL.)

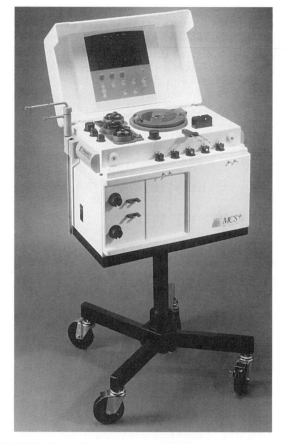

■ **FIGURE 17–4** The Haemonetics MCS Plus LN9000. (Courtesy Haemonetics Corporation, Inc., Braintree, MA.)

on the Amicus and Spectra). The extracorporeal volume (the amount of blood out of the individual in the centrifuge bowl and tubing) is usually greater with the IFC than with the CFC machines. This may be an important consideration in individuals with small blood volumes (e.g., children and older people). The extra volume removed may lead to difficulties in maintaining proper fluid volume in the individual and may cause adverse effects during the procedure. The choice of equipment should be based on the functions and needs of the institution and the requirements of the donor or patient.

In the last several years, improvements in technology have allowed the advantages of each system to be incorporated into a single platform. Examples of this platform are the GAMBRO Trima **(Fig. 17–8)** and the Baxter/Fenwal Alyx. These improvements in both hardware and software allow the collection of multiple components (e.g., each of these apheresis machines can collect two units of RBCs, and the Trima can also collect several different combinations of RBCs/plasma/platelets during a single apheresis procedure). Another important improvement allows these products to be leukoreduced at the time of collection.

Membrane filtration technology can also be used to separate blood components. Blood that passes over membranes with specific pore sizes allows passage of plasma through the membrane while the cellular portion passes over it. Filtration has several advantages over centrifugation, including the collection of a cell-free product and the ability to selectively remove plasma components by varying the pore size. However, the newer CFC equipment can perform most varieties of apheresis, whereas the membrane devices are usually limited to plasma collection. Another cell separation technology that combines centrifugation and membrane filtration for

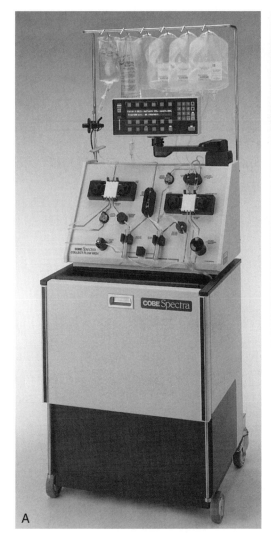

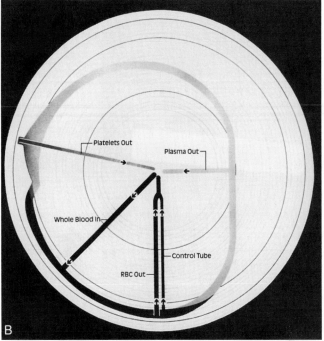

■ FIGURE 17–6.   A, The COBE (now GAMBRO) Spectra apheresis system. B, The separation chamber uses a unique asymmetric design to minimize contamination from RBCs and WBCs. (Courtesy GAMBRO BCT, Inc., Lakewood, CO.)

plasma collection is in the Fenwal Autopheresis-C. This intermittent flow machine collects blood in a small cylinder that rotates, forcing plasma through a polycarbonate membrane (Fig. 17–9).[2]

Apheresis products may be collected manually, using a refrigerated centrifuge and a specialized multiple plastic bag system. Procedures to ensure that the blood is reinfused to the right individual are required. Specific requirements are outlined in the AABB *Standards*.[3] With the automated technology currently available, the manual procedure is rarely utilized and is of historical interest only.

Fluids

All apheresis procedures use anticoagulants to prevent blood from clotting as it enters the separation mechanism. The most common anticoagulant is acid citrate dextrose, although heparin is occasionally used. Normal saline is used to prime the system, to keep the line open, and to help maintain fluid volume. For granulocyte collections, a sedimenting agent is usually added. The most commonly used agent is hydroxyethyl starch.[4] This solution induces rouleaux formation so that better separation between the WBCs and RBCs is achieved and greater efficiency of collection of the granulocytes is achieved.

In therapeutic plasmapheresis procedures, large volumes of a patient's plasma are retained. The fluid must be replaced to maintain appropriate intravascular volume and oncotic pressure. Several solutions are available, and the choice is determined by each institution. Crystalloids such as normal saline may be used. Because saline provides less oncotic pressure than plasma, two to three times the volume removed must be replaced. Normal serum albumin in a 5 percent solution (NSA) is the most commonly used replacement fluid and is usually replaced in a 1:1 ratio. These products provide the proper oncotic properties but increase the cost of the procedure. Mixtures of normal saline and NSA have also been used. Because NSA can be expensive and is subject to shortages, HES has recently been used successfully as a portion of the replacement fluid.[5,6] Fresh frozen plasma (FFP) contains all the constituents of the removed plasma and thus would appear to be the optimal replacement fluid. However, the disadvantages of FFP include possible disease transmission, ABO incompatibility, citrate toxicity, and sensitization to plasma proteins and cellular antigens. It has been implicated in fatal reactions and is now recommended primarily for the treatment of patients with thrombotic thrombocytopenic purpura (TTP), hemolytic uremic syndrome (HUS), and severe liver disease.

Publications suggest that TTP is caused by an antibody to a protease that cleaves the large von Willebrand factor (vWF) multimers. The large multimers then facilitate platelet aggregation, leading to the microangiopathic thrombi characteristic of this disease syndrome.[7,8]. It had been previously observed that these large vWF multimers were present in patients with TTP, which led to the use of cryopoor plasma (with its reduced vWF content) as a replacement fluid alternative.[9]

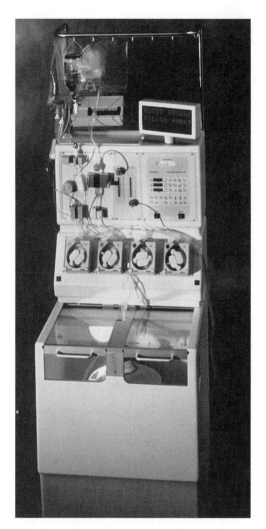

■ FIGURE 17–7　The Fresenius AS-104. (Courtesy Fresenius USA, Inc., Walnut Creek, CA.)

General Requirements

A qualified, licensed physician is responsible for all aspects of the apheresis program. Good equipment and a well-trained, motivated staff are essential. Operators of automated machines must be knowledgeable in all aspects of operation and troubleshooting. Individuals hired to perform these procedures may be medical technologists, nurses, or technicians trained on the job. Regardless of the professional background of the apheresis staff, operators must participate in an intensive orientation program and demonstrate continued competency in all aspects of apheresis.[10] This training should include machine operation and quality control; donor selection; familiarity with the standards of the American Association of Blood Banks (AABB),[3] Code of Federal Regulations (CFR),[11] and documentation; management of complications; and venous access. An apheresis operator should be friendly and outgoing. Because the procedures are often lengthy, complications may be avoided by the operator's ability to relieve the donor's or patient's boredom and anxiety. Although serious complications are unusual, it is essential to have another qualified individual immediately available to assist in case of emergencies. A physician does not have to be in the room but should be within reach if complications should occur.

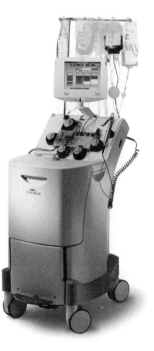

■ FIGURE 17–8　The GAMBRO Trima apheresis system. (Courtesy GAMBRO BCT, Inc. Lakewood, CO.)

Written, informed consent must be obtained from donors and patients. The procedure, possible risks and benefits, and alternative modes of therapy must be explained in understandable language. The individual must then be given the opportunity to accept or to reject the procedure.

The apheresis unit must contain an operator's manual with detailed instructions concerning the following:

1. Informed consent process
2. Standardized protocols and policies for component collection (donors) and therapeutic procedures (patients)

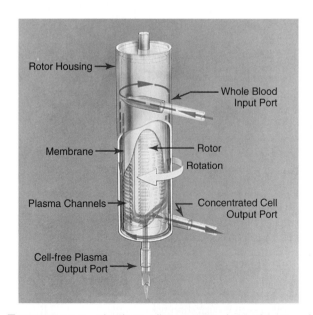

■ FIGURE 17–9　The Plasmacell-C separation device of the Fenwal Autopheresis-C. (Courtesy Baxter Healthcare Corporation, Deerfield, IL.)

3. Quality control of the equipment and apheresis products (component collections)
4. Management of adverse reactions
5. Postapheresis care
6. Proper record-keeping; documentation should comply with AABB *Standards* and the CFR

Applications

Blood banks were established for the primary purpose of providing compatible and viable RBCs to restore oxygen-carrying capacity to the tissues. Anticoagulant/preservative solutions and plastic bags were developed that allowed maximum storage of RBCs with acceptable post-transfusion survival and function. As advances were made in medicine—particularly in the area of chemotherapy—blood banks were faced with the demands for products to overcome the effects of bone marrow depression caused by these drugs. Patients needed platelets and WBCs to survive the period of intensive drug therapy. The doses of blood components required to treat such patients effectively could not be met by products prepared from single whole blood donations. New technology had to be developed to collect larger quantities of a component from a single donor. In addition, increasing concern about transfusion-transmitted diseases and alloimmunization led to the development of programs to reduce the number of donor exposures to the patient. Automated or semiautomated apheresis equipment was the answer to the new demands placed on the blood banks. Component collection thus became the primary application of apheresis equipment.

It was soon realized that the machines could also be used therapeutically to treat patients with certain diseases. The rationale for the procedure was to remove the pathologic component from the blood or patient. Therefore, the use of apheresis technology can be divided into two categories: component collections and therapeutic procedures.

Component Collections

In component collections, a normal, healthy donor undergoes a procedure to obtain a specific blood component that will be transfused to a patient. In general, most of the requirements for whole blood donations must be met. Apheresis donors must meet the requirements established by the AABB[3] *Standards* and FDA regulations.[11]

Replacement fluids other than normal saline are generally not required in component collections. However, careful monitoring of fluid volume in and out is required to prevent complications from shifts in blood volume. The extracorporeal blood volume (volume out of the donor) should not exceed 10.5 mL per kg of body weight at any time during the procedure.[3]

The donor's total blood volume may be obtained from a chart by using the height, weight, and sex of the individual. The extracorporeal volume is calculated from the volume of the apheresis chamber, the donor's hematocrit, and the total blood volume. Several of the modern apheresis machines perform these calculations automatically. If not, the manufacturer must be consulted for the formulas used for each specific machine.

Plateletpheresis

Platelet transfusions are indicated in patients who are bleeding or at increased risk for bleeding secondary to thrombocy-topenia or platelet dysfunction. Platelets for transfusion can be provided by platelet concentrates, which are harvested from routine whole blood donations, or by apheresis. In a plateletpheresis procedure, a portion of the donor's platelets and plasma is removed with the return of the donor's RBCs, WBCs, and remaining plasma. Sedimenting agents are not necessary for this procedure. The platelets are selectively separated from the whole blood and retained in a collection bag manufactured specifically for platelet storage. The platelet yield is related to the donor's initial platelet count, the amount of blood processed, and the volume of the product collected. If the plateletpheresis procedure is the individual's initial donation, or if 4 weeks have elapsed since the prior platelet donation, a platelet count is not required. If the plateletpheresis is performed more frequently than every 4 weeks, a platelet count should be obtained and must be more than $150,000/\mu L$ before performing subsequent plateletpheresis. If the donor's RBCs cannot be reinfused during a procedure, or if the participant donates a unit of whole blood, 8 weeks should elapse before a subsequent cytapheresis procedure, unless the RBC loss was less than 200 mL, the hemoglobin requirement is met, and the donor is found acceptable by a blood bank physician. The maximum amount of plasma that can be retained during each plateletpheresis procedure should not exceed 500 mL if the donor weighs less than 175 pounds, or 600 mL if the donor weighs more than 175 pounds.

Routinely, the number of platelets in an apheresis product is equivalent to 6 to 10 random platelet concentrates. AABB *Standards* requires that 75 percent of plateletpheresis products tested contain a minimum of 3×10^{11} platelets, a value approximately six times that of a random platelet concentrate.[3] An apheresis donor for platelets must not have taken aspirin-containing medication or nonsteroidal anti-inflammatory drugs within the last 36 hours.[3] These drugs, by inhibiting the enzyme cyclo-oxygenase in the prostaglandin pathway, prevent adequate platelet aggregation and the release of platelet adenosine diphosphate. Because an apheresis product would be the sole source of platelets for the patient, careful screening of potential donors is essential for obtaining therapeutically effective products. A routine plateletpheresis procedure typically takes 45 to 90 minutes. The product is usually prepared in a closed system, approved for 5 days' storage. If the product is prepared in a open system, it must be transfused within 24 hours. Platelets stored at room temperature (20° to 24°C) should be maintained with continuous, gentle agitation. The pH at the end of the storage period must be 6.2 or greater in more than 90 percent of units tested. If RBC contamination in the product is negligible (less than 2 mL), compatibility testing is not required, but it is recommended that the donor plasma be ABO-compatible with the recipient, especially with a neonate.[12]

Leukapheresis

Granulocytes are occasionally needed as a transfusion product for patients who are severely neutropenic and have infections that are unresponsive to traditional therapy. To collect the large numbers of cells needed, apheresis techniques are applied. Initially, this therapy showed great promise. However, the lack of consistent, significant data indicating the clinical benefit of granulocyte transfusions, the difficulties obtaining granulocytes, and their adverse effects have led to a decline in their popularity. The best successes have been found in septic infants. In some studies the limited success of granulocyte transfusions has been attributed to the inadequate dose of granulocytes obtained.[13] Several techniques have been used to enhance the yield of these cells.

Because the granulocyte layer interfaces with the RBC layer (see **Fig. 17–1**), the use of the sedimenting agent HES allows better separation and improved yield while minimizing RBC contamination. Although HES is largely removed by the reticuloendothelial system, residual HES has been reported in a donor up to 1 year after granulocytapheresis. However, long-term complications have not been identified. Although a lower molecular weight preparation of HES with improved urinary excretion has been used safely,[14] a report indicates that this product may be less efficient in collecting granulocytes.[15] Also, HES is a colloidal plasma volume expander and may lead to headaches and peripheral edema as a result of expanded intravascular blood volumes. Each facility should have a policy indicating the maximum cumulative dose of any sedimenting agent within a given time interval.[3] Less than 2 percent of the distribution of granulocytes in the body is present in the circulation, with a small fraction of the marginal pool, and the remainder is in the bone marrow. Corticosteroids, such as prednisone or dexamethasone, can increase the number of circulating granulocytes by release of the marginal pool and slow their departure from the intravascular space. The use of steroids in donors before a granulocyte collection may exacerbate certain medical conditions, such as diabetes or hypertension, and should be used under the guidance of the blood bank physician.[12] The use of recombinant hematopoietic growth factors (granulocyte-colony stimulating factor [G-CSF] and granulocyte-macrophage colony stimulating factor [GM-CSF]) in granulocyte donors has resulted in marked increases in the collection of granulocytes (up to 1×10^{11}). This is a significant improvement over the current standard dose of 1×10^{10}. Initial studies indicate significant recovery and survival of these granulocytes. Although several side effects have been reported with the use of these growth factors, these are usually well tolerated.[16] The use of this mobilization strategy, as well as a more critical evaluation of the efficacy of this product, has resulted in a resurgence of interest in granulocyte transfusions.[17]

The granulocyte concentrate must contain a minimum of 1.0×10^{10} granulocytes in at least 75 percent of the units tested. The product has a shelf life of 24 hours at 20 to 24°C but should be transfused as soon as possible after collection for optimal therapeutic effectiveness. The product should be stored at room temperature without agitation. Because of the large numbers of viable lymphocytes present, granulocyte preparations must be irradiated to prevent graft-versus-host disease (GVHD) in immunocompromised recipients or if the donor is related to the recipient. The function of the granulocytes is not affected by the irradiation. Leukocyte depletion filters must not be used. Contamination of granulocyte preparations with RBCs is extremely common. Compatibility testing is required in products containing greater than 2 mL of RBCs and should be ABO-compatible with the patient's plasma. Appropriate records of the procedure, yield of granulocytes, and donor information are required.[3]

Erythrocytapheresis

RBCs can now be collected by apheresis methods, either at two standard units of RBCs or one unit of RBCs collected concurrently with plasma and/or platelets. If two units of RBCs are collected by apheresis, the donor must wait 16 weeks before providing another donation that includes RBCs. The donor requirements for the donations are also more stringent than whole blood donation for height, weight, and hematocrit (females must be at least 5'5", weigh at least 150 pounds, and have a hematocrit level of 40%; males must be at least 5'1", weigh at least 130 pounds, and also have a hematocrit level of 40%).[3] These procedures may be performed on both allogeneic and autologous donors. There are several advantages to automated RBC collection, including:

1. Standardized RBC mass collection (180 to 200 mL);
2. Use of smaller needles for collection;
3. Use of saline compensation, which reduces the risk of hypovolemia;
4. On-line separation, eliminating secondary separation procedures;
5. Reduced costs of testing, data entry, and staffing

Plasmapheresis

In plasmapheresis, the plasma is separated from the cellular components in a collection bag and retained, and then the cells are reinfused to the donor. The procedure may be performed by a manual method, although plasma is most commonly collected by automated equipment. For the clinical setting, plasmapheresis may be used to increase the inventory of FFP of a particular ABO group, such as group AB. The procedure may be used to collect immune plasma from donors with increased concentrations of certain plasma immunoglobulins for patients who are immunosuppressed and have been exposed to varicella, herpes, or other diseases. Reference laboratories perform apheresis to collect rare RBC and WBC antibodies. Commercially, plasma centers use serial plasmapheresis to draw plasma for manufacturing into such products as plasma derivatives, hepatitis immune globulin, and Rh-immune globulin.

If the procedure is performed no more than once every 4 weeks, the criteria that apply to whole blood donation should be used. However, if the donor is participating in a serial plasmapheresis program (plasma is donated more frequently than once every 4 weeks), AABB *Standards* requires additional and continuous assessment of the donor's health.[3] At least every 4 months, all records and laboratory tests must be reviewed and evaluated by a physician, and a serum protein electrophoresis or immunoglobulin level must be determined. If the donor's RBCs during a procedure have not been reinfused, 8 weeks must elapse before the donor may be reinstated in the program.

Proper identification of the RBC reinfusion bag is essential, particularly during manual procedures when the bag is separated from the donor. The RBCs must be returned within 2 hours of the phlebotomy. RBC loss must not be greater than 25 mL per week. The volume of blood and plasma that can be processed and retained has been determined for each instrument by the FDA.[18] In manual procedures, the amount of whole blood that can be processed must not be greater than 500 mL at one time, not more than 1000 mL (1200 mL if the donor weighs at least 176 pounds) in any 48-hour period, and not more than 2000 mL (2400 mL if the donor weighs at least 176 pounds) in a 7-day period. If donor's weight exceeds 175 pounds, the amount of whole blood that can be processed at any one time must be less than or equal to 600 mL.

Hematopoietic Progenitor Cells

In the field of transfusion medicine there has been significant growth in the use of cytapheresis to collect hematopoietic progenitor cells. Bone marrow transplantation is used in the treatment of multiple disorders, including leukemia, solid tumors such as breast cancer, thalassemia, aplastic anemia, and sickle cell anemia, among others. Traditionally, autologous or allogeneic marrow, which includes the progenitor cells, is collected from the patient's or donor's bone marrow. Once harvested, the marrow undergoes extensive processing before storage. The processing can require cell separation, RBC removal, buffy coat concentration, and mononuclear cell purification. In addition, malignant cells in the marrow may be purged by monoclonal antibodies. Techniques have been developed using the currently available apheresis equipment to perform these tasks.[19] Following marrow ablation with myelosuppressive chemotherapy or radiation therapy, or both, the collected progenitor cells are infused to repopulate the marrow, which then begins to redevelop all cell lines.

The primitive progenitor cells that are capable of differentiation are also contained within the peripheral blood and are often termed peripheral blood stem cells. These cells can be collected by current apheresis techniques. Multiple collections by apheresis are usually needed, and the number and frequency of procedures are determined by the yield of progenitor cells obtained and the patient's condition. Similar to their use in the collection of granulocytes, hematopoietic growth factors are now frequently used to increase the number of circulating stem cells in the peripheral circulation and increase the yield.[20]

There are several advantages to using progenitor cells collected by apheresis over traditional bone marrow collection. Anesthesia is avoided, and the procedures can be performed safely in the outpatient setting. Patients with extensive infiltration of their marrow by a tumor or with myelofibrosis can still undergo progenitor cell collection. Other advantages include a shorter period of cytopenia, decreased transfusion requirements, fewer infectious complications, and decreased length of hospitalization. Disadvantages may include the complications of central venous access, including infection and thrombosis; length of time to collect an adequate dose; the increased volume of the product; and contamination with mature lymphocytes.[21]

There have been remarkable advances in the field of hematopoetic progenitor cell transplantation over the last several years. Because there is a considerable amount of information on donor/patient selection and care, laboratory testing, and collection, storage, and infusion of cells, there are FDA regulations[22] and standards published by the AABB[23] and the Foundation for the Accreditation of Cellular Therapy.[24]

The enormous complexity of this practice is beyond the scope of this chapter on apheresis; the regulations and standards as well as other relevant literature should be consulted.[25,26]

Therapeutic Procedures

Therapeutic apheresis, with the removal of any blood component, is an accepted and standard therapy for many diseases. However, the last decade has provided the medical field with sufficient data to evaluate apheresis as a form of therapy more realistically and to define its role in the treatment of disease. The AABB and the American Society for Apheresis have summarized the current indication categories, which have been published (Table 17–1).[27]

Apheresis can be very effective in alleviating the symptoms produced by an underlying disease state. Efficacy of the

TABLE 17–1 Indication Categories for Therapeutic Apheresis		
Disease	**Procedure**	**Indication Category**
Renal and metabolic diseases		
Anti-glomerular basement membrane antibody disease	Plasma exchange	I
Rapidly progressive glomerulonephritis	Plasma exchange	II
Hemolytic uremic syndrome	Plasma exchange	III
Renal transplantation	Plasma exchange	
Rejection	Plasma exchange	IV
Sensitization	Plasma exchange	III
Recurrent focal glomerulosclerosis	Plasma exchange	III
Heart transplant rejection	Plasma exchange	III
	Photopheresis	III
Acute hepatic failure	Plasma exchange	III
Familial hypercholesterolemia	Selective adsorption	I
	Plasma exchange	II
Overdose or poisoning	Plasma exchange	III
Phytanic acid storage disease	Plasma exchange	I
Autoimmune and rheumatic diseases		
Cryoglobulinemia	Plasma exchange	II
Idiopathic thrombocytopenic purpura	Immunoadsorption	II
Raynaud's phenomenon	Plasma exchange	III
Vasculitis	Plasma exchange	III
Autoimmune hemolytic anemia	Plasma exchange	III
Rheumatoid arthritis	Immunoadsorption	II
	Lymphoplasmapheresis	II
	Plasma exchange	IV
Scleroderma or progressive systemic sclerosis	Plasma exchange	III
Systemic lupus erythematosus	Plasma exchange	III

(Continued)

TABLE 17–1   Indication Categories for Therapeutic Apheresis *(continued)*

Disease	Procedure	Indication Category
Hematologic diseases		
ABO incompatible marrow transplant	RBC removal (marrow)	I
	Plasma exchange (recipient)	II
Erythrocytosis/polycythemia vera	Phlebotomy	I
	Erythrocytapheresis	II
Leukocytosis and thrombocytosis	Cytapheresis	I
Thrombotic thrombocytopenia purpura	Plasma exchange	I
Posttransfusion purpura	Plasma exchange	I
Sickle cell diseases	RBC exchange	I
Myeloma, paraproteins, or hyperviscosity	Plasma exchange	II
Myeloma or acute renal failure	Plasma exchange	II
Coagulation factor inhibitors	Plasma exchange	II
Aplastic anemia or pure RBC aplasia	Plasma exchange	III
Cutaneous T-cell lymphoma	Photopheresis	I
	Leukapheresis	III
HDN	Plasma exchange	III
PLT alloimmunization and refractoriness	Plasma exchange	III
	Immunoadsorption	III
Malaria or babesiosis	RBC exchange	III
Neurologic disorders		
Chronic inflammatory demyelinating polyradiculoneuropathy	Plasma exchange	I
Acute inflammatory demyelinating polyradiculoneuropathy	Plasma exchange	I
Lambert-Eaton myasthenic syndrome	Plasma exchange	II
Multiple sclerosis		
Relapsing	Plasma exchange	III
Progressive	Plasma exchange	III
	Lymphocytapheresis	III
Myasthenia gravis	Plasma exchange	I
Acute central nervous system inflammatory demyelinating disease	Plasma exchange	II
Paraneoplastic neurologic syndromes	Plasma exchange	III
	Immunoadsorption	III
Demyelinating polyneuropathy with IgG and IgA	Plasma exchange	I
	Immunoadsorption	III
Sydenham's chorea	Plasma exchange	II
Polyneuropathy with IgM (with or without Waldenström's)	Plasma exchange	II
	Immunoadsorption	III
Cryoglobulinemia with polyneuropathy	Plasma exchange	II
Multiple myeloma with polyneuropathy	Plasma exchange	III
POEMS syndrome*	Plasma exchange	III
Systemic (AL) amyloidosis	Plasma exchange	IV
Polymyositis or dermatomyositis	Plasma exchange	III
	Leukapheresis	IV
Inclusion-body myositis	Plasma exchange	III
	Leukapheresis	IV
Rasmussen's encephalitis	Plasma exchange	III
Stiff-Man syndrome	Plasma exchange	III
PANDAS†	Plasma exchange	II

The indication categories for therapeutic apheresis are as follows: **Category I.** Therapeutic apheresis is standard and acceptable, either as primary therapy or as a first-line adjunct to other initial therapies. Efficacy is based on controlled or well-designed clinical trials or a broad base of published experience. **Category II.** Therapeutic apheresis is generally accepted in a supportive role. **Category III.** Therapeutic apheresis is not clearly indicated based on insufficient evidence, conflicting results, or inability to document a favorable risk-to-benefit ratio. Applications in this category may represent heroic or last-ditch efforts on behalf of a patient. **Category IV.** Therapeutic apheresis has been demonstrated to have a lack of efficacy. Clinical applications should be undertaken only under an approved research protocol.
* POEMS symdrome = polyneuropathy, organomegaly, endocrinopathy, monoclonal gammopathy, and skin lesions.
†PANDAS = pediatric autoimmune neuropsychiatric disorders.

procedure is enhanced by concomitant drug therapy, particularly immunosuppressive therapy in immune-mediated problems. Duration of the effects of the procedure varies with the individual. The course of therapy may last from several days to several months and is based on the response and tolerance of the patient.

Therapeutic apheresis has placed blood banks in the position of direct medical care for the patient. This situation has necessitated a change in the perspective of the medical direc-

tor and the technical staff. Clearly defined policies must delineate the responsibility of the blood bank and the attending physician. Issues such as who makes the decision about vascular access, who orders laboratory tests to evaluate and to monitor the patient, and who chooses replacement fluids must be resolved. The medical director should be involved with the attending physician in deciding whether there are clinical indications for the procedure. The technical staff must be properly trained to care for very ill patients.

Confidence in handling emergency situations is essential. Attention must be given to the patient's medication schedule. Apheresis may dangerously lower plasma levels of medications given before the procedure. Proper documentation of all facets of the procedure is required. Written informed consent must be properly obtained from the patient.

The rationale of therapeutic apheresis is based on the following:

1. A pathogenic substance exists in the blood that contributes to a disease process or its symptoms.
2. The substance can be more effectively removed by apheresis than by the body's own homeostatic mechanisms.

The apheresis procedures that reduce the level of the substance involved and thereby improve the symptoms are classified by the component removed: cytapheresis if the component is cellular; plasma exchange (or immunoadsorption) if the substance circulates in the plasma. (It should be noted that this text is not intended to provide detailed information on the description or management of specific diseases. If needed, more thorough reviews should be consulted.[28,29])

Therapeutic Cytapheresis

Plateletpheresis (thrombocytopheresis) can be used to treat patients who have abnormally elevated platelet counts with related symptoms.[30] This condition has been reported in patients with myeloproliferative disorders such as polycythemia vera. Patients having platelet counts greater than 1,000,000/μL may develop thrombotic or hemorrhagic complications. During a routine apheresis procedure, the platelet count can be decreased by as much as one third to one half the initial value. The procedure can be repeated as frequently as necessary until drug therapy becomes effective and the symptoms disappear.

Leukapheresis has been used to treat patients with leukemia, usually of the myeloid lineage. This therapy is particularly indicated in patients with impending leukostasis, in which leukocyte aggregates and thrombi may interfere with pulmonary and cerebral blood flow. Leukocyte counts in excess of 100,000/μL are considered appropriate indications for instituting apheresis therapy. The greatest therapeutic benefits are seen in acute cases under the following conditions:

1. Drug therapy was just started and has not yet taken effect
2. Drug therapy is contraindicated
3. Patients have become refractory to drug treatment

Lymphocytapheresis (the removal of lymphocytes) and lymphoplasmapheresis have been investigated as a means of producing immunosuppression in conditions with a cellular immune mechanism such as rheumatoid arthritis, systemic lupus erythematosus, kidney transplant rejection, and autoimmune and alloimmune diseases. These procedures are not used routinely, and further studies are required to determine efficacy and to assess possible long-term complications from the procedures.

The therapeutic uses of cytapheresis involve depletion of cellular constituents without replacement. Erythrocytapheresis, however, is considered an exchange procedure. A predetermined quantity of RBCs is removed from the patient and replaced with homologous blood. The procedure has been used successfully to treat various complications of sickle cell disease, such as priapism, acute chest syndrome, and impending stroke.[31] Other indications are rare. Successful therapy has been reported in patients with severe parasitic infections from malaria and babesiosis.[32,33]

Therapeutic Plasmapheresis (Plasma Exchange)

Plasmapheresis is the removal and retention of the plasma, with return of all cellular components to the patient. This therapeutic procedure has become synonymous with the term "plasma exchange," which describes the protocol more accurately. The purpose is to remove the offending agent in the plasma causing the clinical symptoms. The larger volume of plasma that is removed must be replaced or exchanged. It has been postulated that beneficial effects of the procedure, particularly in diseases that involve malfunction of the immune system, may be attributed to the removal of the factors listed in **Box 17–1**.[34]

The efficiency of plasma exchange is related to the amount of plasma removed. The effect is diluted by the necessity to replace the plasma to maintain the patient's fluid volume. A procedure that removes an amount of plasma equal to the patient's plasma volume is called a one-volume exchange. The actual amount of plasma removed may vary from 2 to 4 L, depending on the patient's size. A one-volume exchange should reduce the unwanted plasma component to approximately 30 percent of its initial value. If a second plasma volume is removed as part of the same procedure, the procedure becomes less efficient, reducing the component from 30 percent to only 10 percent.[8] Because of the diminishing effect of increased plasma removal, it is recommended that approximately 1 to 1.5 plasma volumes be exchanged per procedure.[35]

Synthesis and catabolism of the pathologic component as well as its distribution between the extravascular and intravascular space are factors affecting the outcome of plasma exchange. If the antibody that causes the patient's symptoms is IgM, apheresis can be an effective therapeutic tool. IgM is primarily intravascular and is synthesized slowly, whereas IgG is distributed equally in the intravascular and extravascular spaces. Reappearance of IgG in the plasma occurs more quickly because of re-equilibration. Removal of IgG with apheresis can lead to increased antibody synthesis (rebound phenomenon). Because of this effect, therapeutic procedures performed to remove IgG antibodies are most effective when combined with immunosuppressive drugs.

BOX 17–1
Factors Removed by Plasmapheresis

1. Immune complexes (e.g., systemic lupus erythematosus)
2. Autoantibodies or alloantibodies (e.g., factor VIII inhibitors)
3. Antibodies causing hyperviscosity (e.g., Waldenström's macroglobulinemia)
4. Inflammatory mediators (e.g., fibrinogen and complement)
5. Antibody blocking the normal function of the immune system
6. Protein-bound toxins (e.g., barbiturate poisoning)
7. Lipoproteins
8. Platelet-aggregating factors (e.g., possible role in TTP)

Immunoadsorption

Immunoadsorption refers to a method in which a specific ligand is bound to an insoluble matrix in a column or filter. Plasma is then perfused over the column, with selective removal of the pathogenic substance and return of the patient's own plasma. The removal is usually mediated by an antigen-antibody or chemical reaction. Both off-line and on-line procedures have been developed using current apheresis equipment. A diagram of the process is shown in **Figure 17–10**.

A number of adsorptive matrices have been used with varying specificity. **Table 17–2** lists some of the adsorbents, the substance removed, and the clinical applications of each.

Staphylococcal protein A as an immunoadsorbent has gained greater acceptance in clinical use. This ligand has an affinity for IgG classes 1, 2, and 4 as well as IgG immune complexes. The immunoaffinity column currently has federal licensure to treat patients with acute and chronic idiopathic thrombocytopenic purpura.[36] The column has also shown promise in the treatment of a variety of other disease processes, including human immunodeficiency virus–associated thrombocytopenia,[37] chemotherapy-induced TTP/HUS,[38] and alloimmunization resulting in platelet refractoriness.[39] A number of adverse reactions, including fever, chills, rash, and a fatality, have been reported.[40]

The mechanism of action of these columns is not well established. Removal of IgG and immune complexes alone cannot explain the clinical benefit of the treatment. There appears to be a significant immunomodulatory effect of this treatment, with enhanced anti-idiotypic antibody regulation and activated cellular immune function.[41]

Familial hypercholesterolemia (homozygous type II), associated with abnormal metabolism of the low-density lipoprotein (LDL) and increased plasma cholesterol levels, is a significant cause of morbidity and mortality from premature

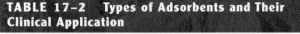

TABLE 17–2 Types of Adsorbents and Their Clinical Application

Adsorbent	Substance Removed	Application
Charcoal	Bile acids	Cholestatic pruritus
A and B antigens	Anti-A, anti-B	Transplantation
Anti-LDL, heparin	LDL	Hypercholesterolemia
DNA	ANA, immune complexes	Systemic lupus erythematosus
Protein A	IgG, immune complexes	ITP, cancer, HUS

ANA = antinuclear antibodies; HUS = hemolytic uremic syndrome; ITP = idiopathic thrombocytopenic purpura; LDL = low-density lipoproteins.

atherosclerotic cardiovascular disease. Plasma exchange therapy is only partially effective in this disorder. LDL-apheresis selectively removes LDL and very low density lipoprotein and has been associated with regression of cardiovasular disease.[42] The FDA has granted approval for the use of the Kaneka Liposorber adsorption system.

Photopheresis

Photopheresis is a specialized leukocytapheresis technique, requiring a special intermittent flow machine utilizing bowl technology. This treatment has been shown to be efficacious and has been approved by the FDA for cutaneous T-cell lymphoma, a malignant skin disorder characterized by an abnormal proliferation of CD4 lymphocytes. The patient is treated with the drug psoralen, which binds to the DNA of all nucleated cells. Following the leukocytapheresis, the

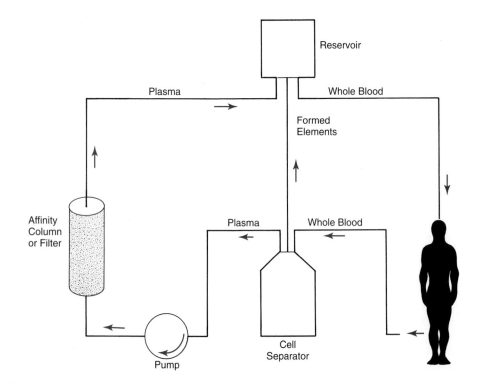

■ FIGURE 17–10 Perfusion of plasma over columns or filters. (From Berkman, EM, and Umlas, J [eds]: Therapeutic Hemapheresis: A Technical Workshop. American Association of Blood Banks, Washington, DC, 1980, p 142, with permission.)

collected WBCs are exposed to ultraviolet light, which activates the psoralen and prevents replication. These treated cells are then returned to the patient, inducing an immune response against the abnormal lymphocyte clone.[43] Photopheresis has been used in several other immunologically mediated conditions, including scleroderma,[44] rheumatoid arthritis,[45] chronic heart and lung transplant rejection,[46] and acute and chronic GVHD following allogeneic marrow transplant.[47]

Adverse Effects

Apheresis is accepted as a relatively safe procedure, but complications do occur. Adverse effects may be observed in component collections as well as in therapeutic procedures. In the latter case, it is sometimes difficult to evaluate whether the deleterious effects were caused by the procedure or by the underlying disease. Some of the problems encountered are listed in **Box 17–2**.

Citrate toxicity is usually observed during cytapheresis component collections when anticoagulated plasma is returned at a rapid rate. Citrate is the anticoagulant used in apheresis and is normally metabolized quickly in the liver. However, if the amount of citrate infused exceeds the body's ability to metabolize it, the level of ionized calcium may decrease, and the donor may feel numbness or tingling around the mouth. If FFP is used as replacement fluid during a therapeutic plasma exchange, this phenomenon is more likely to occur. Decreasing the reinfusion rate usually alleviates the symptoms, or the donor may be given exogenous calcium. Intravenous calcium is not recommended on a routine basis. If unattended, the symptoms can lead to tetany and cardiac arrythmia.

Complications of the vascular access needed for apheresis procedures are relatively common and include hematoma formation, localized or systemic infections, phlebitis, and neuropathies. Vasovagal reactions can often be avoided by attentive, receptive apheresis operators. Individuals undergoing these procedures require assurance from the operators. Hypovolemia is observed more frequently with IFC equipment. Careful monitoring of the volume in and out is necessary to prevent hypovolemia and hypervolemia. Allergic reactions are related to the replacement fluids. This is generally observed in cases in which FFP is administered, but it has

also been reported with albumin. Hemolysis is usually caused by a mechanical problem with the equipment, such as a kink in the plastic tubing. Observing the return line is critical in avoiding this problem. Air embolism and clotting factor deficiencies are not commonly observed.

Deaths resulting from therapeutic apheresis procedures have been reported.[48] The majority of these have been caused by circulatory (cardiac arrest or arrythmia) or respiratory complications (acute pulmonary edema or adult respiratory distress syndrome). Of the 50 cases reported, 25 had received plasma as part or all of the replacement fluid. Because plasma has been associated with fatalities, its use is recommended only in cases of TTP or HUS in which there is a specific indication for its use. Plasma is also capable of transmitting diseases such as hepatitis and the human immunodeficiency viruses.

Summary

The field of apheresis continues to evolve, as do all areas of transfusion medicine. Emerging technology has resulted in dramatic advances in the understanding of the immune response and the diseases associated with immune abnormalities. Also, innovative apheresis techniques, such as the collection of multiple components, including RBCs and leukocyte-reduced platelets, increase the ability to produce the optimal component for patients. Transfusion and transplantation practices, especially hematopoetic progenitor cell transplantation, have benefited from this knowledge and will continue to rely on the collection of cellular or plasma components by apheresis for transfusion or therapeutic purposes.

BOX 17–2
Adverse Effects of Apheresis

1. Citrate toxicity
2. Vascular access complications (hematoma, sepsis, phlebitis, neuropathy)
3. Vasovagal reactions
4. Hypovolemia
5. Allergic reactions
6. Hemolysis
7. Air embolus
8. Depletion of clotting factors
9. Circulatory and respiratory distress
10. Transfusion-transmitted diseases
11. Lymphocyte loss
12. Depletion of proteins and immunoglobulins

SUMMARY CHART:
Important Points to Remember (MT/SBB)

➤ In an apheresis procedure, blood is withdrawn from a donor or patient and separated into its components. One or more of the components is retained, and the remaining constituents are recombined and returned to the individual.

➤ The process of removing plasma from the blood is termed plasmapheresis; removal of platelets is termed plateletpheresis or thrombocytopheresis; removal of RBCs is termed erythrocytapheresis; removal of leukocytes is known as leukapheresis.

➤ The variables of automated apheresis instruments include (1) centrifuge speed and diameter, (2) length of dwell time of the blood in the centrifuge, (3) the type of solutions added (anticoagulants), and (4) the cellular content or plasma volume of the donor.

➤ Apheresis equipment that uses IFC requires only one venipuncture, in which the blood is drawn and reinfused through the same needle. Once the desired component is separated, the remaining components are reinfused to the donor, and one cycle is complete. Therapeutic procedures usually require many cycles to reach an acceptable dose.

➤ CFC procedures withdraw, process, and return the blood to the individual simultaneously. Two venipuncture sites are necessary. The process of phlebotomy, separation, and reinfusion is uninterrupted.

➤ Membrane filtration technology uses membranes with specific pore sizes, allowing the passage of plasma through the membrane while the cellular portion passes over it.

➤ The most common anticoagulant used in apheresis is acid citrate dextrose.

➤ In therapeutic plasmapheresis procedures, the replacement fluids used to maintain appropriate intravascular volume and oncotic pressure include normal saline, hydroxyethyl starch, FFP, and 5 percent serum albumin.

➤ Granulocyte concentrates must contain a minimum of 1.0×10^{10} granulocytes in at least 75% of units tested.

➤ Plateletpheresis products should contain a minimum of 3×10^{11} platelets, which is equivalent to 6 to 10 random platelet concentrates in 90% of units tested.

REVIEW QUESTIONS

1. American Association of Blood Bank *Standards* requires that plateletpheresis products:
   a. Prepared in a closed system be transfused within 24 hours
   b. Contain 3×10^{11} platelets in $\geq 90\%$ of the units tested
   c. Have a compatibility test performed before transfusion
   d. Have a pH of 6.2 or greater on the day of collection

2. Therapeutic cytapheresis is used in patients with:
   a. Sickle cell disease to reduce the number of crises
   b. Systemic lupus erythematosus to remove immune complexes
   c. Leukemia to help increase granulocyte production
   d. Myasthenia gravis to increase antibody production

3. The minimum interval allowed between plateletpheresis component collection procedures is:
   a. 24 hours
   b. 48 hours
   c. 7 days
   d. 8 weeks

4. In plasma exchange, the therapeutic effectiveness is:
   a. Greatest with the first plasma volume removed
   b. Affected by the type of replacement fluid used
   c. Enhanced if the unwanted antibody is IgG rather than IgM
   d. Independent of the use of concomitant immunosuppressive therapy

5. The replacement fluid indicated during plasma exchange for TTP or HUS is:
   a. Normal (0.9%) saline
   b. HES
   c. FFP
   d. ACD
   e. NSA (5%)

6. The most common adverse effect of plateletpheresis collection is:
   a. Allergic reactions
   b. Hepatitis
   c. Hemolysis
   d. Citrate effect
   e. Air embolism

7. Apheresis can be used to collect all of the following except:
   a. Leukocytes
   b. Macrophages
   c. Hematopoetic progenitor cells
   d. Platelets
   e. Lymphocytes

8. Platelets collected in a closed apheresis system have a shelf life of:
   a. 35 days
   b. 24 hours
   c. 5 days
   d. 21 days
   e. 7 days

9. Peripheral blood stem cells are:
   a. Responsible for phagocytosis of bacteria
   b. Removed during erythrocytapheresis
   c. Pluripotential hematopoietic precursors that circulate in the peripheral blood
   d. Immature RBCs used for transfusion in patients with thalassemia
   e. Lymphocytes involved with the immune response

10. Advantages of CFC over IFC include:
    a. Portability
    b. Greater extracorporeal volume
    c. Two venipunctures needed
    d. Single venipuncture needed
    e. Lower extracorporeal volume

REFERENCES

1. Price, TH: Centrifugal equipment for the performance of therapeutic hemapheresis procedures. In MacPherson, JL, and Kaspirisin, DO (eds): Therapeutic Hemapheresis, vol 1. CRC Press, Boca Raton, FL, 1985, p 123.
2. Rock, G, Tittley, P, and McCombie, N: Plasma collection using an automated membrane device. Transfusion 26:269, 1986.
3. Menitove, JE, ed: Standards for blood banks and transfusion services, 21st ed. American Association of Blood Banks, Bethesda, MD, 2002.
4. Heustis, DW, et al: Use of hydroxyethyl starch to improve granulocyte collection in the Latham blood processor. Transfusion 15:1559, 1975.
5. Brecher, ME, and Owen, HG: Washout kinetics of colloidal starch as a partial or full replacement for plasma exchange. J Clin Apheresis 11:123, 1996.
6. Brecher, ME, Owen, HG, and Bandarenko, N: Alternatives to albumin: Starch replacement for plasma exchange. J Clin Apheresis 12:146, 1997.
7. Furlan, M, et al: von Willebrand factor–cleaving protease in acute thrombotic thrombocytopenic purpura and the hemolytic-uremic syndrome. N Engl J Med 339:1578, 1998.
8. Tsai, HM, and Chun-Yet Lian E: Antibodies to von Willebrand factor–cleaving protease in acute thrombotic thrombocytopenic purpura. N Engl J Med 339:1585, 1998.
9. Rock, G, et al: Cryosupernatant as replacement fluid for plasma exchange in thrombotic thrombocytopenic purpura. Br J Haematol 94:383, 1996.
10. American Society for Apheresis: Organizational guidelines for therapeutic apheresis facilities. J Clin Apheresis 11:42, 1996.
11. Code of Federal Regulations. Title 21 CFR Part 640. Washington, DC. US Government Printing Office, 2002.
12. Brecher, ME (ed): Technical Manual, ed 14. American Association of Blood Banks, Bethesda, MD, 2002, p 127.

13. Vamvakas, EC, and Pineda, AA: Determinants of the efficacy of prophylactic granlocyte transfusions: A meta-analysis. J Clin Apheresis 12:74, 1997.

14. Strauss, RG, et al: Selecting the optimal dose of low-molecular-weight hydroxyethyl starch (pentastarch) for granulocyte collection. Transfusion 27:350, 1987.

15. Lee, JH, et al: A controlled study of the efficacy of hetastarch and pentastarch in granulocyte collections by centrifugal leukapheresis. Blood 86:4662, 1995.

16. Bandarenko, N, et al: Apheresis: New opportunities. Clin Lab Med 16:907, 1996.

17. Strauss, RG: Clinical perspectives of granulocyte transfusions: Efficacy to date. J Clin Apheresis 10:114, 1995.

18. Food and Drug Administration: Guidance for industry: Recommendations for collecting blood cells by automated apheresis methods. Rockville, MD: CBER Office of Communication, Training, and Manufacturers Assistance, January 2001.

19. Areman, EM, and Sacher, RA: Bone marrow processing for transplantation. Transfus Med Rev 5:214, 1991.

20. Bishop, MR, et al: High-dose therapy and peripheral blood progenitor cell transplantation: Effects of recombinant human granulocyte-macrophage colony-stimulating factor on the autograft. Blood 83:610, 1994.

21. Badarenko, N, et al: Apheresis: New opportunities. Clin Lab Med 16:907, 1996.

22. Food and Drug Administration: Current good tissue practice for manufacturers of human cellular and tissue-based products: Inspection and enforcement; proposed rule. 21 CFR 1271. Federal Register 66:1507, 2001.

23. Haley, NR, ed: Standards for Hematopoietic Progenitor Cell and Cellular Product Therapy Services, 3rd ed. American Association of Blood Banks, Bethesda, MD, 2002.

24. Warkentin, PI (ed): Standards for Hematopoietic Progenitor Cell Collection, Processing and Transplantation, 2nd ed. Foundation for the Accreditation of Cellular Therapy, Omaha, NE, 2002.

25. Brecher, ME, et al (eds): Hematopoietic Progenitor Cells: Processing, Standards, and Practice. American Association of Blood Banks, Bethesda, MD, 1995.

26. Areman, EM, Deeg, HJ, and Sacher, RA: Bone Marrow and Stem Cell Processing: A Manual of Current Techniques. FA Davis, Philadelphia, 1992.

27. Smith, JW, Weinstein, R, and Hillyer, KL: Therapeutic apheresis: A summary of current indication categories endorsed by the AABB and the American Society for Apheresis. Transfusion 43:820, 2003.

28. McLeod, BC (ed): Clinical application of therapeutic hemapheresis. J Clin Apheresis.1999; 14 (special issue): No. 4.

29. McLeod, BC, Price, TH, Drew MJ (eds): Apheresis: Principles and Practice. AABB Press, Bethesda, MD, 1997.

30. Taft, EG: Therapeutic apheresis. Hum Pathol 14:235, 1983.

31. Kleinman, SH, and Goldfinger, D: Erythrocytapheresis (ERCP) in sickle cell disease. In MacPherson, JL, and Kaspirisin, DO (eds): Therapeutic Hemapheresis, vol 2. CRC Press, Boca Raton, FL, 1985, p 129.

32. Yarrish, RL, et al: Transfusion malaria: Treatment with exchange transfusion after delayed diagnosis. Arch Intern Med 142:187, 1982.

33. Cahill, KM, et al: Red cell exchange: Treatment of babesiosis in a splenectomized patient. Transfusion 21:193, 1981.

34. Patten, E: Pathophysiology of the immune system. In Kilins, J, and Jones, JM (eds): Therapeutic Apheresis. American Association of Blood Banks, Arlington, VA, 1983, p 19.

35. Klein, HG: Effect of plasma exchange on plasma constituents: Choice of replacement solutions and kinetics of exchange. In MacPherson, JL, and Kaspirisin, DO (eds): Therapeutic Hemapheresis, vol 2. CRC Press, Boca Raton, FL, 1985, p 5.

36. Felson, DT, et al: The Prosorba column for treatment of refractory rheumatoid arthritis: A randmomized, double-blind, sham-controlled trial. Arthritis Rheum 42:2153, 1999.

37. Mittelman, A, et al: Treatment of patients with HIV thrombocytopenia and hemolytic uremic syndrome with protein A (Prosorba® Column) immunoadsorption. Semin Hematol 26 (Suppl 1):15, 1989.

38. Snyder, HW, Jr, et al: Successful treatment of cancer-chemotherapy–associated thrombotic thrombocytopenic purpura/hemolytic uremic syndrome (TTP/HUS) with protein A immunoadsorption. Blood 76(Suppl 1):4679, 1990.

39. Christie, DJ, et al: Protein A column therapy in the treatment of immunologic refractoriness to platelet transfusion. Blood 76 (Suppl 1):4679, 1990.

40. Heustis, DW, and Morrison, FS: Adverse effects of immune adsorption with staphylococcal protein A columns. Transfus Med Rev 10:62, 1996.

41. Pineda, AA: Immunoaffinity apheresis columns: Clinical applications and therapeutic mechanisms of action. In Sacher, RA, et al: Cellular and Humoral Immunotherapy and Apheresis. American Association of Blood Banks, Arlington, VA, 1991, p 31.

42. Gordon, BR, and Saal, SD: Low-density lipoprotein apheresis using the Liposorber dextran sulfate cellulose system for patients with hypercholesterolemia refractory to medical therapy. J Clin Apheresis 11:128, 1996.

43. Edelson, R, et al: Treatment of cutaneous T-cell lymphoma by extracorporeal photochemotherapy—Preliminary results. N Engl J Med 316:297, 1987.

44. Rook, AH, et al: Treatment of systemic sclerosis with extracorporeal photochemotherapy. Arch Dermatol 128:337, 1992.

45. Malawista, SE, Trock, DH, and Edelson, RL: Treatment of rheumatoid arthritis by extracorporeal photochemotherapy: A pilot study. Arthritis Rheum 34:646, 1991.

46. Constanza-Nordin, MR, et al: Successful treatment of heart transplant rejection with photopheresis. Transplantation 53: 808, 1992.

47. Rossetti F, et al: Extracorporeal photochemotherapy for the treatment of graft-vs-host disease. Bone Marrow Transplant 18(Suppl 2):175, 1996.

48. Heustis, DW: Risks and safety practices in hemapheresis procedures. Arch Pathol Lab Med 113:273, 1989.

eighteen

Adverse Effects of Blood Transfusion

Lloyd O. Cook, MD, MBA Scott C. Wise, MSA, MT(ASCP)SBB, and Patricia Joyce Larison, MA, MT(ASCP)SBB

OBJECTIVES

On completion of this chapter, the learner should be able to:

1. Define transfusion reaction.
2. Discuss risks of transfusions.
3. Compare and contrast immediate hemolytic transfusion reactions (IHTR) with delayed hemolytic transfusion reactions (DHTR).
4. List the types of IHTRs and DHTRs.
5. Differentiate the clinical signs and symptoms of of IHTRs and DHTRs.
6. List laboratory findings associated with IHTRs and DHTRs.
7. Discuss definition, pathophysiology, signs, symptoms, therapy, prevention, and clinical work-up of IHTRs and DHTRs.
8. List antibodies most associated with IHTRs and DHTRs.

9. Identify procedures to follow at a patient's bedside in the event of a suspected transfusion reaction.
10. Discuss the importance of the patient's history in relation to medications, transfusion history, and pregnancies.
11. List logical steps and procedures to follow in a laboratory investigation of transfusion reactions.
12. Discuss reporting of transfusion reaction work-ups.
13. List accreditation agencies involved in determining policies regarding transfusion reactions.
14. State regulatory record requirements and procedures to follow in reporting a fatal transfusion reaction.

Introduction

"Transfusion" is an irreversible event that carries potential benefits and risks to the recipient. A "transfusion reaction" is any unfavorable transfusion-related event occurring in a patient during or after transfusion of blood components. Proper recognition of, appropriate therapy for, and prevention of transfusion reactions require that the clinical and laboratory to staff understand various types of reactions. Transfusion reactions are divided into immune and nonimmune and are categorized according to the time of transfusion as immediate or delayed. By knowing the rapidity of onset and mechanism of action, transfusionists can better assess current and future risks along with proper treatment and preventive measures.

Risks of Transfusion

As with any medical or technical procedure, the act of blood component transfusion has the potential for both benefit and risk to the patient. Table 18–1 lists specific adverse consequences of transfusions.

The risk of fatality from noninfectious causes was analyzed using transfusion-associated death reports from registered blood establishments submitted to the Food and Drug Administration (FDA) from 1976 through 1985.[1] Box 18–1 lists typical causes of transfusion-associated deaths. Of the 256 immediate hemolysis deaths reported to be caused by noninfectious complications, clerical error was the prime factor determined as the fundamental flaw. Diseases that can cause red blood cell (RBC) hemolysis and might be misinterpreted for a hemolytic transfusion reaction (HTR) are listed in Box 18–2. These hemolytic episodes may be termed "pseudohemolytic" as the cause of hemolysis is a disease state in the patient and not an immune or nonimmune type of transfusion reaction.

BOX 18–1
Some Typical Causes of Transfusion-Associated Deaths

- Acute hemolysis (ABO-incompatible blood components)
- Acute pulmonary edema
- Bacterial contamination of product
- Delayed hemolytic reactions
- Anaphylaxis
- External hemolysis (e.g., temperature exceeded 40°C)
- Acute hemolysis; damaged blood component (e.g., nondeglycerolized, improper solution)
- Transfusion-associated graft-versus-host disease

Rates of Risks

Occurrence rates of the various transfusion reaction types, along with their signs and symptoms, are useful in determining the most probable type of reaction a patient may be experiencing.

A National Institutes of Health Consensus Conference panel[2] reviewed occurrence data for common immune transfusion reactions and assigned the following rates of occurrence per unit transfused:

1. Nonhemolytic febrile transfusion reaction (NHFTR), 1 to 2 percent
2. Allergic, 1 to 2 percent
3. Immediate hemolytic transfusion reaction (IHTR) and delayed hemolytic transfusion reaction (DHTR), 1:6000;
4. Fatal immediate, 1:100,000.

A review of rates of risk, including occurrence of reactions and fatality episodes, summarized the following frequencies:

1. Acute hemolytic reaction, 1:25,000
2. DHTR, 1:2500
3. Noncardiogenic pulmonary edema, 1:1000
4. Transfusion-associated graft-versus-host disease (TA-GVHD) and related donor, 1:7000
5. TA-GVHD and unrelated donor, 1:39,000[3]

Linden and coworkers[4] reviewed transfusion data collected by the New York State Department of Health for 1990 to 1995, along with comparison data collected by the FDA for 1994. These data were analyzed for the frequency of death resulting from various types of transfusion reactions. Some of the data compiled by Isbister and Linden and associates are collated in Table 18–2. General, everyday types of fatality risks, collected by Isbister, are included for perspective on degree of risk.

TABLE 18–1   Immediate and Delayed Noninfectious Transfusion Reaction Effects

Immediate	Delayed
Immune	
IHTR	DHTR
FNHTR	Alloimmunization
Allergic reaction	PTP
Anaphylaxis and anaphylactoid reactions	TA-GVHD
TRALI	Immunosuppression
Nonimmune	
Bacterial contamination	Iron overload
TACO	Air embolism
Physical or chemical RBC damage	
Depletion and dilution of coagulation factors and platelets	

IHTR = immediate hemolytic transfusion reactions, DHTR = delayed hemolytic transfusion reaction; FNHTR = febrile nonhemolytic transfusion reaction; PTP = post-transfusion purpura; TA-GVHD = transfusion-associated graft-versus-host disease; TACO = transfusion-associated circulatory overload; TRALI = transfusion-related acute lung injury

BOX 18–2
Diseases Simulating Transfusion Reactions

1. Paroxysmal nocturnal hemoglobinuria
2. Autoimmune hemolytic anemia
3. Glucose-6-phosphate dehydrogenase deficiency
4. Malignant hyperthermia
5. Hemoglobinopathies
6. RBC membrane defects

TABLE 18–2   Frequency of Death for Selected Transfusion Reactions

Type of Reaction	NYS/DOH*	FDA
Acute hemolytic	1:1,700,000	1:1,300,000
Delayed hemolytic	0	1:560,000
Noncardiogenic pulmonary edema	1:3,000,000	1:6,600,000
TA-GVHD	0	1:10,000,000

Risk of Death for Selected General Situations

Lifetime risk	1:1
Cancer	1:4
Coronary artery bypass surgery	1:33
Admission to a hospital	1:200
Driving a car	1:5000
Flying on a commercial airline	1:500,000

*NYS/DOH = New York State, Dept of Health

Error Analysis

An internal study of the 355 reports received by the FDA of transfusion-associated fatality cases for 1976 through 1982 sought to identify where errors occurred in preventable transfusion-associated deaths.[5] Box 18–3 identifies locations where errors associated with transfusion reactions have occurred. Four leading causes of preventable laboratory errors were the following:

1. Improper specimen identification
2. Improper patient identification
3. Antibody identification error
4. Crossmatch procedure error

For nursing, anesthesia, and medical staff errors, improper patient identification was by far the major cause of transfusion death. Thus, adherence to proper transfusion standards, policies, and procedures is essential to reduce transfusion-associated fatalities. Box 18–4 summarizes frequent error causes associated with transfusion reactions.

Some studies have demonstrated wide variability in the rate of occurrence of DHTR,[6] which can be attributed to reduced clinical recognition of DHTR and the nonspecific clinical evidence of DHTR in complicated patient cases of fever, jaundice, anemia, and so forth, which may be linked to other disease processes. Although rare, there have been single-case reports of death attributable to DHTR, with the incidence of DHTR fatalities about one-sixth (1:600,000) that of IHTR fatalities.[7]

Anaphylactic and anaphylactoid reactions are immediate immune reactions in which there are systemic symptoms including hypotension, loss of consciousness, shock and, in rare cases, death.[8] About 1 person in 700 healthy individuals in the general population is immunoglobin A (IgA)–deficient.

Anti-IgA

BOX 18–3
Locations of Preventable Transfusion-Associated Deaths, in Order of Occurrence

- Laboratory
- Nursing service
- Anesthesia service
- Clinical staff

BOX 18–4
Summary of Frequent Error Causes Associated with Transfusion Reactions

1. Patient misidentification
2. Sample error
3. Wrong blood issued
4. Transcription error
5. Administration error
6. Technical error
7. Storage error

Despite this relatively large risk group, anaphylactic and anaphylactoid reactions occur at very low rates, about 1 in 20,000 transfusions.[9] Errors in clinical diagnosis and case reporting do not allow calculation of an accurate risk rate.

Acute pulmonary injury accounted for 15 percent of the fatal transfusion-associated reports and was the third most reported cause of transfusion-associated deaths.[10] Bacterial contamination of blood components and nonimmune hemolysis accounted for the next largest number of cases reported to the FDA from 1976 to 1985.

Hemolytic Transfusion Reaction (HTR)

HTRs can occur either at the time of transfusion (immediate) or a few (3 to 7) days after transfusion (delayed). HTRs most often occur with the transfusion of incompatible RBCs but may also occur with the transfusion of ABO-incompatible plasma containing products such as plasma and platelets; they also may be chemically or physcially induced.

Immediate Hemolytic Transfusion Reaction (IHTR)

Definition

Most commonly, an IHTR occurs very soon after the transfusion of incompatible RBCs. The RBCs are rapidly destroyed, releasing hemoglobin and RBC stromata into the circulation. In an anesthetized patient, hemoglobinuria, abnormal bleeding at the surgical wound site, and hypotension may be the only warning signs of IHTR. The reaction period varies from 1 to 2 hours.[11] However, signs and symptoms can occur within minutes after starting the transfusion. ABO-incompatible transfusions may be life-threatening, causing shock, acute renal failure, and disseminated intravascular coagulation (DIC). Prompt diagnosis and treatment are essential.

Pathophysiology

The underlying cause of IHTR is transfusion of an incompatible whole blood or RBC product to a recipient. The four most commonly identified RBC antibodies causing IHTR are anti-A, anti-Kell, anti-Jk^a, and anti-Fy^a.[12] These four antibodies are traditionally considered binders of complement to RBC surfaces and have efficient in-vitro lytic properties. Immune-mediated IHTR can destroy RBCs by one of two mechanisms: intravascular or extravascular hemolysis. In both, the initial event is the binding of patient antibody to the transfused incompatible RBCs, which forms an antigen-antibody (Ag-Ab) complex on the RBC surface. Intravascular RBC lysis releases hemoglobin, RBC stromata, and intracellular enzymes, manifesting in hemoglobinemia and hemoglobinuria. In the kidney, damage to sclera of the glomerulus, cortex, and tubules may occur. In the liver, damage to the hepatic portals and hepatocytes may occur. **Figure 18–1** depicts the intravascular hemolysis pathway.

Extravascular IHTR is characterized by Ag-Ab complex formation on RBCs with incomplete activation of complement. Because RBC lysis does not occur intravascularly, there is no release into the circulation of free hemoglobin, RBC enzymes, or RBC stromata.

Signs, Symptoms, and Clinical Work-Up

The clinical signs and symptoms of IHTR may be profound. **Box 18–5** lists clinical signs and symptoms that can occur in IHTR and that can usually be observed in a conscious patient. Several important clinical findings include[13]:

1. 35 percent of patients with IHTR experience fever, with or without chills
2. 34 percent experience oliguria with complete recovery
3. 13 percent develop anuria
4. 10 percent die, with sustained hypotension being the primary clinical finding
5. 8 percent experience coagulopathy

Signs and symptoms associated with extravascular IHTR are usually mild and not life-threatening. Fever, chills, jaundice, unexpected anemia, and decreased haptoglobin are usual

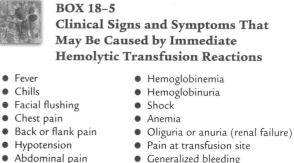

IHTR

BOX 18–5
Clinical Signs and Symptoms That May Be Caused by Immediate Hemolytic Transfusion Reactions

- Fever
- Chills
- Facial flushing
- Chest pain
- Back or flank pain
- Hypotension
- Abdominal pain
- Nausea
- Dyspnea
- Vomiting

- Hemoglobinemia
- Hemoglobinuria
- Shock
- Anemia
- Oliguria or anuria (renal failure)
- Pain at transfusion site
- Generalized bleeding
- Urticaria
- Diarrhea
- Disseminated intravascular coagulation

findings. Once an IHTR is suspected, immediate action is required. **Box 18–6** abbreviates the bedside procedure guidelines for handling suspected IHTR.

Therapy and Prevention

Patient care in IHTR is focused on prevention and supportive measures. The physician should monitor the patient closely for risk factors to DIC, hypotension, and acute renal failure.[14] Traditionally, mannitol has been the agent of choice to induce renal diuresis and to prevent renal failure. More recently, chemical agents such as ethacrynic acid and furosemide have been used to improve renal blood flow and induce diuresis.[15] Hypotension is treated with intravenous fluids and vasoactive drugs (e.g., dopamine) as necessary. Blood component therapy, such as fresh frozen plasma (FFP), cryoprecipitate, and platelet concentrates, should be used in patients having a bleeding diathesis or significant coagulation abnormalities. Extravascular IHTR usually does not require therapeutic intervention. To ensure the patient's welfare, vital signs, coagulation status, and renal output should be monitored.

Because most IHTRs are caused by clerical (i.e., human) error, they are potentially preventable. All policies and procedures should be followed to ensure proper patient identification, sample collection and labeling, unit identification, patient testing, handling, and correct transfusion at the bedside. **Box 18–7** lists preventive measures to minimize transfusion reactions.

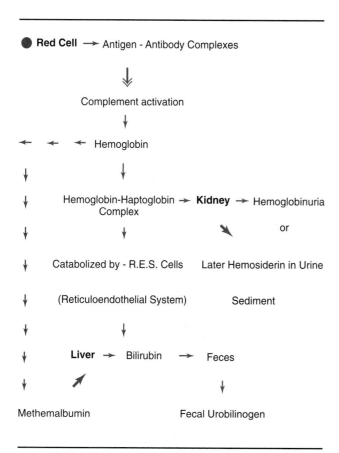

● Red Cell → Antigen - Antibody Complexes

↓↓

Complement activation

↓

← ← ← Hemoglobin

Hemoglobin-Haptoglobin → **Kidney** → Hemoglobinuria
Complex

or

Catabolized by - R.E.S. Cells   Later Hemosiderin in Urine

(Reticuloendothelial System)   Sediment

Liver → Bilirubin → Feces

Methemalbumin   Fecal Urobilinogen

■ **FIGURE 18–1**   Intravascular hemolysis pathway.

BOX 18–6
Immediate Transfusion Reaction Bedside Procedures

1. *Stop the transfusion.*
2. Keep intravenous line open with physiologic saline.
3. Notify patient's physician and transfusion service.
4. Take care of patient per physician's orders.
5. Perform bedside clerical checks.
6. Return unit, set, and attached solution to blood bank.
7. Collect appropriate blood specimens for evaluation.
8. Document reaction.

BOX 18-7
Preventive Transfusion Reaction Measures

- Store RBCs only in blood bank–monitored refrigerators.
- Never warm RBCs above 37°C for transfusion.
- Do not transfuse blood if patient or donor identification is not accurate.
- Never sign out blood by name only.
- Do not add medications to blood.
- Follow procedures for issuing blood components.
- Follow protocol for specimen collection, labeling, and testing.
- Follow transfusion policies and procedures.

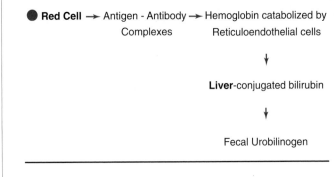

■ FIGURE 18-2   Extravascular hemolysis pathway.

Delayed Hemolytic Transfusion Reaction (DHTR)

Definition

DHTR is most often the result of an anamnestic response in a patient who has previously been sensitized by transfusion, pregnancy, or transplant and in whom antibody is not detectable by standard pretransfusion methods. Clinical signs and symptoms are usually mild; severe DHTR cases and fatalities are uncommon. Unexpected or unexplained decreases in hemoglobin or hematocrit values following transfusion should be investigated as a possible DHTR.

Pathophysiology

Two different types of DHTR have been identified:

1. Secondary (anamnestic) response to transfused RBCs
2. Primary alloimmunization

In DHTR caused by a secondary response, about 3 to 7 days from time of transfusion are necessary for enough antibody to be produced by the patient to cause clinical signs and symptoms of extravascular RBC hemolysis. In DHTR caused by primary alloimmunization, the patient has no past history of pregnancy, transfusion, or transplant. It should be noted that time from transfusion to onset of clinical signs and symptoms of hemolysis and detection of the causative antibody is longer for DHTR than for IHTR.

Extravascular hemolysis is the mechanism of RBC destruction for both types of DHTR. **Figure 18-2** depicts the extravascular hemolysis pathway. Patient antibody attaches to the specific foreign donor RBC antigen, causing sensitization of RBCs, which are removed by the reticuloendothelial system, commonly called the monocyte-macrophage system. **Table 18-3** groups common and uncommon antibodies implicated in DHTR.[16] DHTRs have also been associated with bone marrow transplantation and may be caused by human leukocyte antibodies (HLAs) in some cases.[17]

Signs, Symptoms, and Clinical Work-Up

Clinical signs and symptoms of DHTR are mild compared with those of IHTR because of the extravascular hemolysis and may be undetected clinically. In DHTR, complement is not activated; therefore, no intravascular hemolysis occurs, as observed in IHTR.[18] If clinically detected, DHTR is most commonly manifested by mild fever or fever with chills, and mod-

erate jaundice may be observed. Oliguria and DIC are rare.[19] **Table 18-4** lists signs and symptoms that have been observed in DHTR.

When DHTR is suspected, blood specimens (both clotted and anticoagulated) should be sent to the blood bank for post-transfusion reaction investigation. Other laboratory testing for DHTR may include hemoglobin, hematocrit, and coagulation studies and renal function tests. Sometimes it may not be possible to determine the clinical significance of an RBC antibody, or there may be evidence of an HTR in the absence of serological evidence. More specialized techiques such as RBC survival studies or the monocyte-monolayer assay can provide clues regarding the survival of RBCs in the circulation and clinical signficance of the antibody involved.[20] The patient should be observed closely for signs and symptoms indicating severe complications.

Therapy and Prevention

The goal of therapy is to prevent and, if necessary, treat severe complications of DHTR. Renal function can be supported with intravenous fluid therapy to maintain a normovolemic status.

Only symptomatic anemia should be treated with RBC transfusions. Clinical signs and symptoms of hemolysis or DIC should be monitored to reduce the risk of renal failure. Because DHTR is usually caused by an anamnestic response, a thorough medical history, including previous transfusions, pregnancies, transplants, and transfusion reactions, should be taken. The blood bank should be alerted to any previously reported complicating factors. Ideally, a type and screen should be performed at the time of admission on patients who may need transfusion, who have previously received blood, or who have known risk factors such as pregnancy or previous RBC exposure.

TABLE 18-3	Antibodies Implicated in DHTR
Common Antibodies	**Uncommon Antibodies**
Anti-Jk^a	Anti-A$_1$
Anti-E	Anti-P$_1$
Anti-D	
Anti-C	
Anti-K	
Anti-Fy^a	
Anti-M	

TABLE 18-4   Clinical Signs and Symptoms of DHTR

Common Signs and Symptoms	Unusual Signs and Symptoms
Fever	Hemoglobinemia
Anemia	Hemoglobinuria
Mild jaundice	Shock
	Renal failure

Immediate Nonhemolytic Transfusion Reactions

The common types of immediate nonhemolytic transfusion reactions are febrile and allergic. Anaphylaxis, anaphylactoid reaction, and TRALI occur less frequently. Although the immune system is a common pathway for each of these reactions, intravascular or extravascular RBC hemolysis does not occur.

Febrile Nonhemolytic Transfusion Reaction

Definition

Febrile nonhemolytic transfusion reaction (FNHTR) occurs in about 1 percent of transfusions. Along with allergic reactions, FNHTR is the most commonly encountered type of transfusion reaction. Several common definitions are used regarding FNHTR, based on increases in temperature after transfusion. The American Association of Blood Banks (AABB) *Technical Manual* defines FNHTR as a 1°C temperature rise associated with transfusion and having no medical explanation other than blood component transfusion.[21] Others[22] define FNHTR as:

1. Any 1°C or greater temperature increase above the patient's baseline temperature, during or within 24 hours after transfusion, with a minimum recorded temperature of 38°C; or
2. A 1°C temperature increase above the patient's baseline pretransfusion temperature during or within 8 hours after the end of the transfusion

Pathophysiology

FNHTRs are caused by leukocyte antibodies present in the patient's plasma. The leukocyte antibodies are commonly directed against antigens present on monocytes, granulocytes, or lymphocytes.[23] Alloimmunization by prior blood transfusion, tissue transplantation, or pregnancy is the causative stimulus for antibody formation. These antibodies are predominantly HLA or lymphocytotoxic antibodies.[24]

The febrile mechanism still has not been fully explained. The febrile reaction may follow activation of the complement system, producing C5a, which causes production and release of the pyrogen interleukin-1 (IL-1) from the patient's macrophages and monocytes.[25] IL-1 may initiate synthesis of prostaglandins (PGE_2) in the hypothalamic cells, resulting in an additional pyrogenic effect.[26] Release of pyrogens from the transfused white blood cells (WBCs) also plays a role in fever development and other clinical signs and symptoms.

Signs, Symptoms, and Clinical Work-Up

The most frequent expressions of FNHTRs are fever with or without chills and, rarely, hypotension. Most symptoms are mild and benign. Occasionally, a patient may briefly exhibit pronounced pallor. Severe reactions may include hypotension, cyanosis, tachycardia, tachypnea, dyspnea, cough, limited fibrinolysis, and transient leukopenia.[27]

FNHTR is a diagnosis of exclusion inasmuch as the nonspecific signs and symptoms can have many other causes. For example, fever can be caused by IHTR, bacteremia, drugs taken by the patient, or another underlying illness. Past medical history for transfusion, transplantation, pregnancy, and drug therapy is important for accurate diagnosis.

Tests to evaluate FNHTRs may vary from one laboratory to another. When an FNHTR is suspected, the transfusion should be stopped, but the intravenous line should be kept open with normal saline to support treatment in the event of a severe complication.

Therapy and Prevention

Because leukocyte antibodies are the primary cause of FNHTR, leukocyte-reduced blood components are indicated. A variety of methods have been developed that effectively remove enough leukocytes from blood components to prevent FNHTR, including laboratory or bedside filtration using leukoreduction blood filters, washed RBCs, deglycerolized RBCs, or centrifugation.

Because approximately one in eight patients reacts to the next unit transfused following an FNHTR, many recommend documenting two or more FNHTRs before ordering leukocyte-reduced blood components. Antipyretics such as aspirin or acetaminophen can be used to premedicate a patient before transfusion. Aspirin is contraindicated in patients with thrombocytopenia and thrombocytopathy.

Even with WBC reduction in blood components, not all FNHTRs can be prevented. Premedication may be beneficial to patients with documented histories of FNHTR. As leukoreduction filter costs decline, more aggressive use of them should reduce the incidence of FNHTR.

Allergic (Urticarial) Transfusion Reactions

Definition

Allergic, or urticarial, transfusion reactions are as commonly reported as FNHTRs. If clinical signs and symptoms appear within minutes of exposure, the allergic reaction is of the immediate hypersensitivity type. Anaphylactic and anaphylactoid reactions are also of the immediate hypersensitivity type but are clinically more severe and are discussed later.

Pathophysiology

Despite the fact that allergic reactions are one of the two most commonly reported transfusion reactions, the definitive causes are still not known. Two possible etiologies have been proposed,[27] based on the passive transfer of donor plasma to a patient after transfusion of a blood component:

1. The donor plasma has a foreign protein (allergen) with which immunoglobulin E reagin (IgE) or immunoglobin G (IgG), or both, antibodies in patient plasma react.

2. The donor plasma has reagins (IgE or IgG or both) that combine with allergens in the patient plasma.

Histamine appears to be the primary mediator of the allergic response.[28] Histamine is released when the allergen-reagin complex attaches to the surface of tissue mast cells. On release from mast cells, histamine increases vascular dilation and permeability, allowing vascular fluids to escape into tissues. This causes swelling and raised red welts that may itch (pruritus). Another group of mediators that may participate in allergic reactions is leukotrienes, which have been estimated to be about a thousand times more potent than histamine.[29]

Signs, Symptoms, and Clinical Work-Up

The majority of allergic reactions are mild and not life-threatening. Most common signs and symptoms include local erythema (redness), pruritus (itching), and hives (raised, firm, red welts). Fever may or may not be present. Rarely, allergic reactions can be severe, with angioneurotic edema, laryngeal edema, and bronchial asthma.

No reliable laboratory tests are available to identify the offending allergens or reagins causing an allergic reaction. Bedside observation focuses on identifying the manifestations of an allergic reaction, monitoring for severe effects, and instituting supportive care.

Therapy and Prevention

Treatment with an antihistamine such as diphenhydramine (Benadryl) is often sufficient for mild forms of allergic reactions. In patients with histories of repeated allergic reactions, plasma is often removed from blood components (washed RBCs; washed platelets). Premedication with antihistamines before transfusion is also common. For severe allergic reactions, aminophylline, epinephrine, or corticosteroids may be necessary. Some clinicians permit temporary cessation of blood component transfusion when a mild allergic reaction is observed, while antihistamine treatment is given. After antihistamine administration, the same component transfusion is resumed. Because some allergic reactions can be severe, some blood banks recommend following the same transfusion reaction protocol as in other transfusion reactions and observing the patient for any severe reaction effects.

Allergic reactions cannot be completely prevented. For patients with suspected or documented histories of allergic reactions, the usual prevention strategies are premedication, plasma-deficient blood components, or all three.

Anaphylactic and Anaphylactoid Reactions

Definition

Anaphylactic and anaphylactoid reactions are of the immediate hypersensitivity type of immune system response. Anaphylaxis can range from mild urticaria (hives) and pruritus to severe shock and death. Any organ of the body can be involved, such as the lungs, blood vessels, nerves, skin, and gastrointestinal tract.[30] Two significant features distinguish anaphylactic and anaphylactoid reactions from other types of transfusion reactions:

1. Fever is absent
2. Clinical signs and symptoms occur after transfusion of just a few milliliters of plasma or plasma-containing blood components

Pathophysiology

Anaphylactic and anaphylactoid reactions are attributed to IgA deficiency in patients who have developed anti-IgA antibodies by sensitization from transfusion or pregnancy.[31] Despite the fact that about 1 in 700 people have some level of IgA deficiency, anaphylactic and anaphylactoid reactions are quite rare.[32]

As discussed previously in allergic transfusion reactions, immune hypersensitivity reactions are mediated by histamines and leukotrienes.

Signs, Symptoms, and Clinical Work-Up

These hypersensitivity reactions have been divided into two categories:

1. Anaphylactic, in patients deficient in IgA who have class-specific IgA antibodies
2. Anaphylactoid, in patients having normal levels of IgA but a limited type-specific anti-IgA that reacts with light chain (kappa or lambda) of the donor's IgA.

Anaphylactic reactions are sudden in onset with pronounced symptoms that may include coughing, dyspnea, nausea, emesis, bronchospasm, flushing of skin, chest pain, hypotension, abdominal cramps, diarrhea, possible shock, loss of consciousness, and death. Anaphylactoid reactions are usually less severe and are characterized by urticaria, periorbital swelling, dyspnea, and perilaryngeal edema.

There is no predictive test to determine who is at risk for either anaphylactic or anaphylactoid reactions. If either type of reaction is suspected, a patient serum sample can be immunoelectrophoresed to determine IgA levels, or immunodiffusion techniques may identify subclass antibodies.

Therapy and Prevention

Treatment measures must be prompt:

1. Stop the transfusion, and do not restart transfusion of the blood component.
2. Keep the intravenous line open with normal saline.
3. Give epinephrine (usually about 0.5 mL of 1:1000 solution) immediately.
4. For severe reactions, corticosteroids or aminophylline, or both, may be indicated. Airway patency must be maintained, and vital signs must be stabilized by appropriate means.

The diagnosis of anaphylactic and anaphylactoid reactions is retrospective; therefore, special measures must be taken for patients with documented or suspected histories of these reactions. If a plasma-containing blood component has been implicated in the anaphylactic or anaphylactoid reactions and the patient requires transfusions, two approaches may be considered:

1. Remove all plasma from the blood component before transfusion, or
2. Transfuse blood components from donors lacking IgA.

Even a small amount of plasma found in fibrin glue preparation may cause anaphylactic reactions.[33] In a prospective study, colloid transfusion products also caused a risk of anaphylactoid reactions (plasma-protein solutions, 0.003 percent; hydroxyethyl starch (HES), 0.006 percent; dextran, 0.008 percent; and gelatin solution, 0.038 percent).[34] Therefore, any transfusible source of IgA antigenic material can precipitate anaphylactic or anaphylactoid reactions.

Noncardiogenic Pulmonary Edema Reactions (TRALI)

Definition

Several terms have been used to identify pulmonary complications associated with blood component transfusion: noncardiogenic pulmonary edema (NCPE), transfusion-related acute lung injury (TRALI), pulmonary hypersensitivity reaction, and allergic pulmonary edema. The clinical picture of these conditions are similar to that of adult respiratory distress syndrome (ARDS).

Pathophysiology

Although the cause of TRALI is not well understood, the most consistent finding is leukocyte antibodies in donor or patient plasma. Several mechanisms for lung injury have been postulated and include the following:

1. Antileukocyte antibodies in donor or patient plasma could initiate complement-mediated pulmonary capillary endothelial injury
2. Antileukocyte antibodies could react with leukocytes to trigger the complement system to produce C3a and C5a

This, in turn, would cause tissue basophils and platelets to release histamine and serotonin, resulting in leukocyte emboli aggregating in the lung capillary bed.[35] Whatever the mechanism, capillary damage induces interstitial edema and fluid in alveolar air spaces, causing decreased gas exchange and hypoxia.

Signs, Symptoms, and Clinical Work-Up

TRALI is usually characterized by chills, cough, fever, cyanosis, hypotension, and increasing respiratory distress shortly after transfusion of blood component volumes that usually do not produce hypervolemia. Clinical signs and symptoms may be mild, resolving after a few days, or severe, resulting in rapidly progressive pulmonary failure. Sera from both the donor and patient should be tested for antileukocyte antibodies. The diagnosis of TRALI is one of exclusion. Conditions that should be excluded are heart failure, volume overload, bacterial sepsis, and myocardial infarction.

Therapy and Prevention

If clinical signs and symptoms occur during transfusion, the transfusion should be discontinued and not restarted. Explicit procedures should be followed for handling the transfusion reaction. With adequate respiratory and hemodynamic supportive treatment, TRALI pulmonary infiltrates usually clear after several days.[35]

If TRALI is caused by patient antileukocyte antibodies, then leukoreduced blood component preparations should be used. If TRALI is caused by donor leukocyte antibodies, no special blood component preparations appear to be indicated for the patient in the future. Deferral of donors associated with TRALI cases is a complicated and controversial issue. At present, no standard has been set for acceptance or deferral of donors associated with TRALI cases.

Transfusion-Associated Circulatory Overload

Definition

Transfusion-associated circulatory overload (TACO) is a good example of an iatrogenic (physician-caused) transfusion reaction. Patients at significant risk include children, elderly patients, and patients with chronic normovolemic anemia, cardiac disease, thalassemia major, or sickle cell disease.[36]

Pathophysiology

The most frequent cause of TACO is transfusion of a unit at too fast a rate. Hypervolemia associated with transfusion leads to congestive heart failure and pulmonary edema (which may or may not be reversible).

Signs, Symptoms, and Clinical Work-Up

Clinical circulatory overload effects include dyspnea, coughing, cyanosis, orthopnea, chest discomfort, headache, restlessness, tachycardia, systolic hypertension (greater than 50mmHg increase), and abnormal electrocardiogram results.

The transfusion should be stopped immediately. If transfusion is critical to patient therapy, the slowest possible infusion rate must be used. The intravenous line should be maintained, and the patient may be placed in a sitting position. Electrocardiogram and chest x-ray examinations to assess cardiac and pulmonary status should be considered. If possible, central venous pressure and peripheral vital signs should be monitored closely.

Therapy and Prevention

Rapid reduction of hypervolemia and patient respiratory and cardiac support are primary goals. Oxygen therapy and intravenous diuretics should be used appropriately. If more rapid fluid volume reduction is necessary, therapeutic phlebotomy can be used. Cardiac arrhythmias or decreased myocardial function should be corrected.

The usual rate of transfusion is about 200 mL/hr. In patients at risk or with histories of circulatory overload, rates of 100 mL/hr or less are appropriate. Donor units should be split into aliquots to permit transfusion for longer periods. RBCs should be used instead of whole blood. Washed or frozen washed RBCs have been advocated to reduce plasma oncotic load to the patient.[37] In some patients with chronic normovolemic anemia who have hematocrit levels in the range of 10 to 20 percent, a therapeutic phlebotomy to reduce plasma volume equal to the intended transfusion volume should be considered.

Bacterial Contamination Reactions

Definition

Although the frequency of bacterial contamination of blood components is low, this type of septic reaction can have a rapid onset and lead to death. Of the deaths caused by bacterial contamination of blood components reported to the Centers for Disease Control (CDC), most are caused by blood components contaminated by *Yersinia enterocolitica*. Since 1987, 20 cases have been reported to the CDC, with 12 deaths caused by this organism. Cases have been reported with transfused RBCs, platelets,[38] and other blood components as well as with manufactured products such as intravenous solutions and HES.[39]

Pathophysiology

Transfusion reactions attributed to bacterial contamination reactions are commonly caused by endotoxin produced by bacteria capable of growing in cold temperatures (psychrophilic) such as *Pseudomonas* species, *Escherichia coli*, and *Y. enterocolitica*.[40]

Signs, Symptoms, and Clinical Work-Up

Clinical signs and symptoms of septic reactions usually appear rapidly during transfusion or within about 30 minutes after transfusion. Clinically, this type of reaction is termed warm and is characterized by dryness and flushing of the patient's skin. Additional manifestations include fever, hypotension, shaking, chills, muscle pain, vomiting, abdominal cramps, bloody diarrhea, hemoglobinuria, shock, renal failure, and DIC.

Rapid recognition of sepsis caused by bacterial contamination is essential. At the first sign of the reaction, the transfusion must be stopped immediately, the intravenous line kept open, and instructions for handling transfusion reactions followed. The blood component unit and any associated fluids and transfusion equipment should be sent immediately to the blood bank for visual inspection, Gram stain, and cultures. In addition, blood cultures should be drawn from the patient as soon as possible for detection of aerobic or anaerobic organisms.

Therapy and Prevention

Broad-spectrum antibiotics should be immediately administered intravenously. Therapy for shock, steroids, vasopressors such as dopamine, fluid support, respiratory ventilation, and maintenance of renal function may be indicated.

Bacterial contamination of blood components usually occurs at the time of phlebotomy, during the component preparation or processing, or during thawing of blood components in waterbaths. Strict adherence to policies and procedures regarding blood component collection, storage, handling, and preparation is essential to reducing risk. Visual observation of RBC units for color change at the time of issue for transfusion is required, but this step alone cannot guarantee that there is no bacterial contamination. Visual inspection of components before release from the transfusion service includes looking for the presence of brown or purple discoloration, visible clots, or hemolysis. However, gross observation is often inadequate in detecting the presence of bacterial contamination. One preventive measure is to make sure the blood components are infused within standard allowable maximum time limits (usually 4 hours). Adherence to good component production methods and prudent transfusion practices is currently the best strategy to reduce the risk of bacterial contamination and sepsis.

Physically or Chemically Induced Transfusion Reactions

Definition

Patients are at risk of experiencing a transfusion reaction caused by a broad range of physical or chemical factors that either affect a blood component or are a consequence of the transfusion event. Physically or chemically induced transfusion reactions (PCITRs) are a heterogeneous group and can include physical RBC damage, depletion and dilution of coagulation factors and platelets, hypothermia, citrate toxicity, hypokalemia or hyperkalemia (decreased or increased ionized serum potassium level in the patient), and air embolism. Because the clinical signs and symptoms of PCITR can be subtle, the transfusionist must be alert to identify and to correct these reaction effects. **Box 18–8** lists physical, mechanical, and inheritance induced nonhemolytic transfusion reaction examples.

Pathophysiology

RBCs are susceptible to membrane damage and intravascular lysis by hypertonic or hypotonic solutions, heat damage from blood warmers, freezing damage in the absence of a cryoprotective agent, and mechanical damage such as that caused by roller pumps in a blood pump. During massive transfusion (replacement of patient's total blood volume within 24 hours), rapid depletion and dilution of platelets and plasma coagulation factors can occur. Hypothermia, a core body temperature lower than 35°C, is usually associated with large volumes of cold fluid transfusions.

Excess citrate from transfusions can act on the patient's ionized calcium in the plasma and may result in hypocalcemia. Transfusion-associated hyperkalemia can be caused by the intracellular loss of potassium from RBCs during storage in the blood unit plasma. Transfusion-induced hypo-

---

BOX 18–8
Nonhemolytic Transfusion Reactions: Physically, Chemically, and Inherited Induced Examples

- *Physical Damage to RBCs*
  Intravascular lysis by hypertonic or hypotonic solutions.
  Heat damage from blood warmers, during shipping, in hot rooms.
  Freeze damage in absence of cryoprotective agent, during shipping.

- *Mechanical Damage*
  Blood pumps, roller pumps.
  Infusion under pressure through small-bore needles.

- *Patients with Intrinsic Abnormal Cells*
  Congenital hemolytic anemias such as G-6-PD deficiency.
  Patients in sickle cell crisis.
  Patients with paroxysmal nocturnal hemoglobinuria or autoimmune hemolytic anemia.

kalemia is most likely to be caused by infusion of intracellular potassium-depleted RBC blood components, such as washed RBCs or frozen washed RBCs.

Mechanical or chemical damage of transfused RBCs can result in intravascular hemolysis. The resulting free hemoglobin is rapidly cleared by the kidneys. Usually the resulting RBC stroma does not induce DIC, but DIC is a possibility.[41] Coagulation factors, especially factor VIII, decline in activity level during blood component storage, and factor levels can be reduced by use of fluid replacement solutions such as colloids and crystalloids during massive transfusions.[42]

Hypothermia inhibits the immune system function, intensifies lactic acidosis and cardiac arrhythmias, and can cause coagulopathies.[43] Citrate toxicity is caused by the rapid lowering of plasma-free calcium ions caused by chelation with citrate. Massive transfusion is seldom a cause of citrate toxicity, but automated apheresis procedures using large amounts of citrate anticoagulant are a more likely cause.[44] Hyperkalemia and hypokalemia can cause cardiac arrhythmias and seizures.

Signs, Symptoms, and Clinical Work-Up

Many of the clinical signs and symptoms of PCITR are nonspecific. The more common signs and symptoms include facial numbness, chills, generalized numbness, muscle twitching, cardiac arrhythmias, nausea, vomiting, perioral tingling, altered respirations, and anxiety. Laboratory tests for PCITR investigation may include electrolyte levels, serum ionized calcium, blood pH, blood glucose, urinalysis, hemoglobin, hematocrit, platelet count, prothrombin time, and activated partial thromboplastin time.

Therapy and Prevention

Treatment is directed at correcting the underlying cause of the signs and symptoms. For example, hypothermia could be treated by placing the patient on a warming blanket and giving supportive care to any cardiac arrhythmias or electrolyte imbalance. Heparin might be indicated for DIC caused by physical RBC lysis. Citrate toxicity is often rapidly self-correcting, but administration of a calcium-rich product such as milk or an antacid with calcium gluconate (e.g., Tums) is usually adequate.

Precautionary measures are the best strategies to avoid PCITR. Blood warmers can be used to avoid hypothermia. Prudent use of platelet concentrates and FFP may avoid rapid depletion and dilution of coagulation factors during massive transfusion. Monitoring the patient's mental status and vital signs may prove valuable in detecting rapid changes in levels of calcium and potassium. Close monitoring of RBCs transfused through blood pumps can avoid mechanical destruction. In general, attention to proper transfusion practices can greatly reduce the risk of PCITRs.

Delayed Nonhemolytic Transfusion Reactions

Alloimmunization

Definition

Alloimmunization may result from prior exposure to donor blood components. As an adverse effect of blood component transfusion, alloimmunization is a significant complication. Even very small amounts of donor antigenic RBCs can elicit an alloimmune response.[45] Adverse effects may include difficulty in finding compatible RBC units because of the presence of clinically significant RBC antibodies, transfusion reactions, or platelet refractoriness.[46]

Pathophysiology

Because no two humans (except identical twins) have the same genetic inheritance, exposure to foreign antigens by blood component transfusions, tissue transplantation, or pregnancy may cause a patient's immune system to produce alloantibodies.

With the first exposure to foreign antigen, lymphocyte memory is invoked. This results in a moderate production of IgM and IgG antibodies. Secondary exposure elicits rapid production of large amounts of IgG-class antibody, rising rapidly in the first 2 days after reexposure to the antigen. The antibody produced attaches to the antigenic surface and may interact with the complement system or reticuloendothelial system (RES) or monocyte phagocytic system (MPS).[47]

Signs, Symptoms, and Clinical Work-Up

Clinical signs and symptoms may be mild, including slight fever and falling hemoglobin and hematocrit levels; or severe, including platelet refractoriness with bleeding. To detect an alloimmunization state in a patient, several tests can be beneficial. The antibody screen test is used to detect clinically significant RBC antibodies. If HLA antibodies are suspected, lymphocyte panels and lymphocytotoxic antibody procedures can be performed on the patient's serum. However, a thorough patient history of past transfusions, transplantations, and pregnancies is important.

Therapy and Prevention

Treatment depends on the type and severity of the transfusion reaction. Most reactions are mild and often missed clinically. Severe reactions should be treated promptly, as appropriate. Alloimmunization cannot be prevented completely. With the advent of third-generation bedside leukocyte filters, delay—if not prevention—of antileukocyte antibody production is now possible.[48] The matching of donor and patient RBC phenotypes to avoid sensitization in chronically transfusion-dependent patient populations has also been recommended to prevent the patient's formation of RBC antibodies. **Table 18–5** lists occurrence of alloimmunization and other transfusion reactions.

Post-Transfusion Purpura

Definition

Post-transfusion purpura (PTP) is a rare complication of blood transfusion, usually involving platelet concentrates (PCs). PTP is characterized by a rapid onset of thrombocytopenia as a result of anamnestic production of platelet alloantibody. Post-transfusion purpura usually occurs in multiparous females. The lag time between transfusion and onset of thrombocytopenia is approximately 7 to 14 days.

TABLE 18–5 Relative Occurrence of Transfusion Reaction Effects

Type of Reaction	Common	Less Common	Unusual
Allergic reaction	×		
Alloimmunization	×		
Febrile reaction	×		
Depletion and dilution of coagulation factors and platelets		×	
DHTR		×	
TACO		×	
Anaphylaxis and anaphylactoid reactions			×
Bacterial contamination			×
Immediate hemolytic transfusion reactions			×
Iron overload			×
Noncardiogenic pulmonary edema			×
Physical RBC damage			×
Posttransfusion purpura			×
TA-GVHD			×

Pathophysiology

The platelet antibody specificity most frequently identified is HPA-1a (anti-PL^{A1}). About 2 percent of people are negative for the PL^{A1} platelet-specific antigen. Other implicated antibody specificities are HLA-A2 and lymphocytotoxic antibodies.

Platelet alloantibody attaches to the platelet surface, which permits extravascular destruction by the RES in the liver and spleen. The patient's autologous platelets are destroyed, enhancing the thrombocytopenia. The exact mechanism of platelet destruction has not been fully eplained.

Signs, Symptoms, and Clinical Work-Up

Purpura and thrombocytopenia occur about 1 to 2 weeks after transfusion. Thrombocytopenia can be severe, with platelet counts of less than 10,000/mm^3. Hematuria, melena, and vaginal bleeding have also been reported. Diagnosis is retrospective because the purpura and thrombocytopenia start a week or two after transfusion. Platelet counts and coagulation support should be considered. The thrombocytopenia is usually self-limited. Platelet transfusions should be reserved for severe cases inasmuch as they are usually not beneficial. Patient sera should be tested for platelet-specific antibodies, HLA antibodies, and lymphocytotoxic antibodies.

Therapy and Prevention

Three types of therapy have been advocated: corticosteroids, exchange transfusions, and plasmapheresis.[49] Intravenous immunoglobulin therapy has also been advocated.[50] Review of the PTP literature does not yield a strong consensus of opinion on treatment of PTP. In an acute, bleeding patient with concomitant lesions, the most likely therapeutic regimen would be moderate-dose corticosteroids (prednisone), intravenous IgG, and plasmapheresis (personal communication, L. Lutcher, MD). Exchange transfusions would be reserved for cases in which initial therapy was considered a failure. Platelet transfusion should be avoided as much as possible during the PTP treatment period. Furthermore, there are no good ways to prevent PTP. A thorough patient history of prior transfusion and any adverse reactions should be taken before all blood component therapy. In suspicious cases with possible risk, appropriate antibody studies should be considered.

Transfusion-Associated Graft-Versus-Host Disease (TA-GVHD)

Definition

Transfusion-associated graft-versus-host-disease (TA-GVHD) is a complication of blood component therapy or bone marrow transplantation. Although TA-GVHD is a rare complication of transfusion, significant populations of patients are at risk, and mortality is significant. Members of the at-risk groups include patients experiencing lymphopenia or bone marrow suppression, fetuses receiving intrauterine transfusions, newborn infants receiving exchange transfusions, individuals with congenital immunodeficiency syndromes, patients with certain hematologic and oncologic disorders, and patients receiving blood components from blood relatives.[51] The fatality rate for TA-GVHD has been documented at 84 percent, with a median survival period of 21 days posttransfusion.[52] Death is usually caused by infection or hemorrhage secondary to bone marrow aplasia.

Pathophysiology

TA-GVHD is caused by a proliferation of T-cell lymphocytes derived from the donor blood that is responding immunologically to major and minor histocompatibility antigens in the patient. Patients with cell-mediated immunodeficiency are at risk of not being able to reject transfused lymphocytes. Another risk group includes patients who have an HLA type that is haploidentical with that of the donor; these are usually first-degree relatives.[53] The mechanism of TA-GVHD has not been fully explained.

Signs, Symptoms, and Clinical Work-Up

Most clinical signs and symptoms of TA-GVHD appear in about 3 to 30 days after transfusion.[53] Pancytopenia is a clinically significant indication of TA-GVHD. Other effects include fever, elevated liver enzymes, copious watery diarrhea, erythematous skin rash progressing to erythroderma, and desquamation.

Tissue biopsies and laboratory tests assessing liver function status should be considered if histologic changes indicative of TA-GVHD are found in the liver, gastrointestinal tract, skin, or bone marrow. Close observation for infection or coagulation abnormalities should be monitored because these complications are responsible for most TA-GVHD fatalities. HLA cell typing to confirm the presence of donor cells in the patient's circulation is used to confirm diagnosis.[54]

Therapy and Prevention

Various therapeutic treatments have been used in patients with TA-GVHD, including corticosteroids, cyclosporine, methotrexate, azathioprine, and antithymocyte globulin. To date, the clinical efficacy of these and other experimental agents have not proved adequate in TA-GVHD. Because there is no adequate therapy for TA-GVHD, prevention is the only way to avoid potential fatalities.

Blood component gamma irradiation has been demonstrated as the best current technology to reduce the risk of TA-GVHD.[55] The usual dosage range is 25 Gray (Gy) to 35 Gy (1 Gray = 100 rads).[56] Irradiation of the blood component before transfusion results in inactivation of the lymphocytes in the blood components, inhibiting lymphocyte blast transformation and mitotic activity. **Box 18–9** details recipients who would be candidates for irradiated blood components before transfusion to reduce the risk of TA-GVHD.

Iron Overload

Definition

A long-term complication of RBC transfusion is iron overload, also known as transfusion hemosiderosis. Each unit of RBCs has about 225 mg of iron as part of the hemoglobin molecules. Patients with certain diseases are chronically dependent on RBC transfusion support as part of therapy. Some of these diseases include congenital hemolytic anemias, aplastic anemia, and chronic renal failure.

Pathophysiology

Accumulated iron begins to affect the function of heart, liver, and endocrine glands. The full mechanism of iron overload leading to hemosiderosis has not yet been fully explained. A likely pathologic effect is interference of mitochondrial function by excess iron accumulation.

Signs, Symptoms, and Clinical Work-Up

Clinical signs and symptoms of hemosiderosis may include muscle weakness, fatigue, weight loss, mild jaundice, anemia, mild diabetes, and cardiac arrhythmias. A long history of chronic RBC transfusion should be a strong clinical indicator for diagnosis of iron overload. Assessment of storage iron levels, such as ferritin levels and other iron studies, should be performed. Tissue stains specific for iron in tissue biopsies should be considered.

Therapy and Prevention

Removal of accumulated tissue iron stores without lowering patient hemoglobin levels is the treatment of choice. Subcutaneous infusion of desferrioxamine, an iron-chelating agent, has been tried with some success. Chronically transfusion-dependent patients should be exposed to as few units of RBCs as possible. One promising strategy is hypertransfusion using units rich in neocytes (young RBCs) to reduce the frequency of transfusion.[57]

Immunosuppression

Definition

Immunosuppression is a generalized, nonspecific effect that diminishes the activity of the recipient's immune system soon after blood component(s) transfusion. Since the early 1970s, immunosuppression of the transfusion recipient's immune system has been observed.[58] Individuals receiving RBC transfusions before renal transplantation were noted to have better graft survival than individuals who did not receive RBC transfusions. Some studies have linked postsurgical bacterial infections with blood component transfusions.[59,60] Also, transfusions have been associated with tumor recurrence in colorectal cancer patients. Thus, immunosuppression has a potentially wide range of effects on the transfusion recipient. However, a review of more than 60 articles reporting results on immunosuppression, some using a statistical tool called meta-analysis, did not define a post-transfusion immunosuppressive effect.[61] Obviously, this is an area of controversy that only further research will resolve as to the substance and degree of blood component immunosuppression.

Pathophysiology

To date, no specific mechanism or mechanisms have been definitely proved as the pathway for post-transfusion immunosuppression. Several theories have been put forward, such as rapid uptake of blood component cellular matter into the RES or MPS, but no supportive proof has been developed to identify a cause-and-effect relationship.

Signs, Symptoms, and Clinical Work-Up

No specific signs or symptoms have been attributed to immunosuppression. Given the generalized nature of the immunosuppressive response, no specific work-up has been defined. The importance is realizing that blood component transfusion may impart an increased risk of a suppressive effect on the transfusion recipient's immune system. The transfusionist must always keep in mind any potential as well as likely adverse effects of transfusion, with the goal to minimize such adverse effects, if possible.

Therapy and Prevention

Currently, because of limited knowledge about immunosuppression, no specific therapy regimen is available. Prevention centers around the basic principle of transfusing a patient only when necessary with the appropriate blood component(s) in the dosage amounts most likely to have a beneficial effect. Thus, benefit must exceed risk for the transfusion to be justifiable; the patient is properly required to assume this potential risk. **Table 18–6** identifies commonly transfused blood components, functions, and associated transfusion reaction complications.

Transfusion Reaction Investigation

Adverse clinical manifestations after transfusion of blood components must be evaluated promptly and to the extent

---

BOX 18–9
Blood Component Irradiation:
Clinical Indications for Transfusion
Recipients to Reduce the Risk of
GVHD

- Bone marrow or peripheral blood stem cell recipients
- Fetuses receiving intrauterine transfusions
- Selected immunocompromised or immunodeficient recipients
- Recipients of donor units known to be from a blood relative
- Recipients of HLA-selected platelets or platelets known to be HLA-homozygous
- Other—per physician order and transfusion service physician approval

TABLE 18–6   Commonly Transfused Blood Components, Functions, and Associated Transfusion Reaction Complications

Component	Function	Potential Reactions
RBCs	Carry oxygen to tissues and restore RBC mass following hemorrhage.	Allergic, febrile, hemolytic, bacterial contamination, alloimmunization, RGVHD, circulatory overload, iron overload, anaphylactic, metabolic complications, and immunosuppression.
Platelets	Treat bleeding thrombocytopenic patients with severely decreased or functionally abnormal platelets, or patients with dilutional thrombocytopenia, or some patients with platelet consumption (DIC).	Same as RBCs. After repeat transfusions, refractoriness to platelets may develop.
FFP	Patients requiring labile coagulation plasma factors, used in dilutional coagulopathy, and in plasma exchanges for TTP.	Allergic, anaphylactic, fever, bacterial contamination, circulatory overload, and metabolic complications.
Cryoprecipitate	Control of bleeding associated with factor VIII deficiency, for von Willebrand's disease, and replacement of fibrinogen or factor XIII.	Same as for RBCs. A positive DAT may develop if ABO-incompatible cyoprecipitate is given, rarely hemolysis.

GVHD = graft-versus-host disease; DIC = disseminated intravascular coagulation; TTP = thrombotic thrombocytopenic purpura; DAT = direct antiglobulin test.

considered appropriate by the medical director. The exceptions to this rule are circulatory overload and allergic reactions, which do not have to be evaluated to the same extent as HTRs. The transfusionist must first recognize that a transfusion reaction is occurring and then must take action immediately by initiating appropriate established procedures for transfusion reaction responses. Investigations of transfusion reactions are necessary for:

1. Diagnosis
2. Selection of appropriate therapy
3. Transfusion management
4. Prevention of future transfusion reactions

Investigation should include correlations of clinical data with laboratory results. Transfusion reaction protocols may vary according to the patient's clinical signs and symptoms, federal regulations, and assessment by the medical director and the patient's physician. In the investigation, one should remember that absence of evidence is not evidence of the absence of a transfusion reaction!

Any investigation of a suspected transfusion reaction must include investigation of clinical data to include the following:

1. Diagnosis
2. Medical history of pregnancies, transplants, and previous transfusions
3. Current medications
4. Clinical signs and symptoms of the reaction

The transfusion history may give clues as to the possible cause of the reaction. During the investigation, the following questions related to the transfusion and medical information may be included:

1. How many milliliters of RBCs or blood component were transfused?
2. How fast and for how long was the unit transfused?
3. Were RBCs given cold or warmed?
4. Was the transfusion given under pressure, and what size needle was used?

5. How was it given? Was a filter used, and if so, what type? What other solutions were given?
6. Were any drugs given at the time of transfusion?

A transfusion reaction form should be completed for each reaction and include the patient's pretransfusion and posttransfusion vital signs, type of reaction, time of occurrence, amount transfused, and other pertinent information.

The transfusion service must have a procedure manual detailing instructions to follow when a transfusion reaction occurs. Box 18–10 details standard operating transfusion reaction procedures to include in manuals. To investigate a suspected HTR, the transfusion service should receive promptly after the transfusion a clotted blood sample, properly collected (avoiding hemolysis) and labeled, along with a nonclotted ethylenediaminetetraacetic acid specimen. Tests considered appropriate for an investigation are determined by the transfusion service medical director, indicated by the patient's clinical signs and symptoms, or ordered by the patient's physician.

BOX 18–10
Standard Operating Procedures for Transfusion Reactions

● *Transfusion Service Manual*
 Detection, reporting, and evaluation SOPs.
 Specimen requirements.
 Clerical and technical check procedures.
 Return of bag, solutions, filter set, and intact tubing.
 Immediate and extended investigation procedures.
 Test procedures and record policies.
 Interpretations, reporting, and notification, procedures.

● *Nursing Manual*
 Recognition and response SOPs.
 Signs and symptom descriptions.
 Stop the transfusion instructions.
 Patient care responsibilities.
 Notification to physician and transfusion service.

SOPS = standard operating procedures

Depending on the preliminary investigation results, more specimens may be required:

1. A clotted blood specimen drawn 5 to 7 hours after transfusion for unconjugated indirect bilirubin determination.
2. The first voided post-transfusion urine collection.
3. Other specimens collected at various times that are considered appropriate to the transfusion reaction investigation.

Immediate Laboratory Investigation

Laboratory transfusion reaction investigative procedures vary, but all begin with immediate preliminary procedures. Based on the preliminary investigative results and the patient's clinical condition, further testing may be necessary. **Box 18–11** outlines immediate and extended procedures that may be performed in investigating HTRs.[62] Immediate transfusion reaction procedures include clerical checks, visual inspection, and direct antiglobulin test (DAT).

Clerical Checks

Because many of the transfusion reactions reported have resulted from clerical errors (mislabeling and misidentification), immediate investigation should always begin with clerical checks. Clerical checks should identify any possible errors or discrepancies in patient or donor identification. Clerical checks may include patient and specimen identification data; blood unit inspection; tubing, filter, and solution examina-

BOX 18–11
Laboratory Investigation Outline for HTR

- *Immediate Procedures*
  Clerical checks
  Visual inspection of serum and plasma for free hemoglobin (pretransfusion and post-transfusion)
  Direct antiglobulin test—posttransfusion EDTA sample

- *"As Required" Procedures*
  ABO grouping and RH typing, pretransfusion and post-transfusion
  Major compatibility test, pretransfusion and post-transfusion specimens
  Antibody screen test, pretransfusion and post-transfusion specimens
  Alloantibody identification
  Antigen typings
  Free hemoglobin in first-voided urine posttransfusion
  Unconjugated (indirect) bilirubin 5–7 hours posttransfusion

- *Extended Procedures (as indicated)*
  Gram stain and bacterial culture of unit(s)
  Quantitative serum hemoglobin
  Serum haptoglobin on pretransfusion and post-transfusion specimens
  Serial hemoglobin, hematocrit, and platelet counts
  Peripheral blood smear
  Coagulation and renal output studies
  Hemoglobin electrophoresis
  Urine hemosiderin

EDTA = ethylenediaminetetraacetic acid.

BOX 18–12
Post-transfusion Reaction Verifications

- Rule out the possibility that the patient received the wrong blood component.
- Verify the fact that the appropriate blood component was selected, accurately tested, and properly issued within expiration period.
- Verify accuracy of patient and donor ABO and Rh type.
- Verify accuracy of labels and records.
- Rule out the possibility that any other patient or blood component was involved.

tion; and label and record checks. **Box 18–12** itemizes post-transfusion verification procedures.

Visual Inspection

Observe the serum of the patient's pretransfusion and post-transfusion reaction blood specimens. The color of pretransfusion reaction serum and immediate post-transfusion recipient serum or plasma should be compared for evidence of RBC hemolysis. This is critical to investigation of an HTR. Normal serum or plasma appears pale yellow. If plasma or serum contains 0.2 g/L (20 mg/dL) of free hemoglobin, it will appear pink. If free hemoglobin exceeds 1 g/L (100 mg/dL), the plasma or serum will appear red.[63] During color observation, if only the post-transfusion specimen shows pink or red discoloration, a hemolytic process can be presumed. The post-transfusion plasma sample should be measured spectrophotometrically to quantitate the amount of free plasma hemoglobin. If the sample was not collected immediately after the transfusion, hemoglobin can be converted to bilirubin, which changes the plasma to a bright yellow. The maximum bilirubin concentration usually occurs 3 to 6 hours after a hemolytic transfusion episode.[64] Myoglobin can cause serum to appear pink. If crush injuries exist, differentiation of myoglobin from hemoglobin should be determined. In the absence of extensive muscle trauma, myoglobin is unlikely.[65] **Figure 18–3** depicts pretransfusion and post-transfusion reaction specimens from a patient with sickle cell disease experiencing a DHTR that demonstrates visually discernible free hemoglobin in the post-transfusion specimen.

A visual inspection of the return blood bag(s), solution(s), and attached tubing and filter set(s) may rule out hemolysis from nonimmunologic causes. RBC hemolysis has been reported from open-heart bypass surgery machines, blood pumps, infusion through small-bore needles, infusion of blood under high pressure, drugs or solutions added to blood lines, heating or freezing blood improperly, and bacterial contamination.

DAT

In suspected immediate or delayed hemolytic reactions, a DAT should be performed on the post-transfusion specimen. The DAT result may be negative if the incompatible transfused cells have been immediately destroyed. In both immediate and delayed reactions, the DAT result may be positive, show mixed-field reactions, or be negative. When the DAT result appears as mixed-field agglutination, there are mixtures of

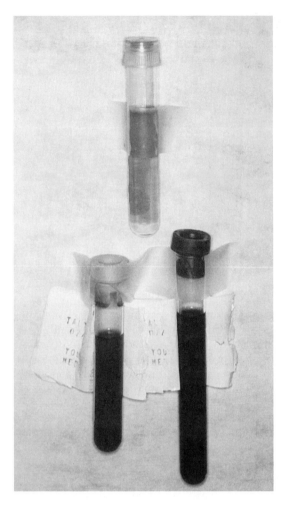

■ **FIGURE 18–3** Color comparison of pretransfusion (top tube) and post-transfusion (bottom tubes) blood specimens from a sickle cell patient experiencing a DHTR.

BOX 18–13
Approaches to DAT

● *DAT Result Positive*
   Perform an elution and determine specificity.
   Repeat DAT on several specimens to detect rising antibody titers.

● *DAT Result Negative*
   Perform an elution, if clinical hemolysis present.
   If there exist too few antibody molecules to detect, perform an elution and concentrate antibody.
   If all incompatible RBCs are destroyed, screen serum, perform clerical and technical checks, and repeat DAT later with new specimen.

DAT = direct antiglobulin test; RBC = red blood cell.

agglutinated transfused donor cells along with unagglutinated patient cells. **Box 18–13** summarizes some approaches to DAT testing.

Additional Testing

If the immediate procedures suggest hemolysis, or if the results are misleading or negative but the patient's signs and symptoms suggest immune hemolysis, then additional testing is necessary. Testing may include the following procedures.

ABO Grouping and Rh Typing

The recipient pretransfusion and post-transfusion reaction blood specimens and donor segments should be tested, and misidentification of any other patient sample or donor unit should be ruled out.

Compatibility Test

When indicated, testing should include the pretransfusion and post-transfusion reaction samples tested with RBCs from donor units involved. An incompatible crossmatch with the pretransfusion sample indicates an original error (clerical or technical) with recipient or donor specimens. Incompatibility with only the post-transfusion specimen indicates a possible anamnestic response (as seen in DHTR) or a patient sample identification problem.

Antibody Screen and Alloantibody Identification

To determine whether the transfusion reaction was the result of an antibody, the antibody screening tests should be repeated on the pretransfusion and post-transfusion reaction specimen and donor unit. **Box 18–14** identifies causes of false-negative antibody screen results that should be considered in transfusion reaction investigations. Unexpected alloantibodies found in the patient's serum should be identified and any post-transfusion reaction-positive DAT result investigated. If the pretransfusion or post-transfusion antibody screening tests are reactive, identification is essential to determine antibody specificity to avoid another reaction when the patient requires further transfusion. Once antibody specificity is determined, all donor units must be tested for the corresponding antigen before additional transfusions are performed.

Urine Test

The first-voided post-transfusion reaction specimen should be examined for the presence of free hemoglobin. Intact RBCs (hematuria) represent bleeding, not hemolysis. When unex-

BOX 18–14
Causes of False-Negative Antibody Screen Results

● Failure to detect antibody in original test procedure
● Test not sensitive enough to detect antibody
● Clerical or technical error
● Antibody screening cells represented a single dose of antigen (donor screen cells from a heterozygote)
● Antibody identified in post-transfusion specimen only (may represent anamnestic response or patient sample identification problem)

TABLE 18–7	**Urine Reagent Strip (Multistix) Chart for Suspected HTR**			
	Reaction	Identify Reason	Microscopic (Rule Out Intact RBCs)	Monitor Patient's Renal Function
Free hemoglobin	Positive	✓	✓	✓ Evaluate further
Urobilinogen (<1 Ehrlich unit* is normal)	Positive (pink-red)	✓		✓ Evaluate further

*1 Ehrlich unit = 1 mg/dL of urobilinogen

plained hemoglobinemia occurs, the urine can be examined for hemoglobinuria. Table 18–7 indicates responses when using reagent strips to test urine for free hemoglobin and urobilinogen in suspected HTRs.

A week or more after suspected HTR investigation, the patient's urine can be examined for hemosiderinuria. Hemosiderin can appear in urine when the level exceeds 0.25 g/L (25 mg/dL) as free hemosiderin.[66]

Bilirubin Test

A change from a pretransfusion normal pale yellow serum to a post-transfusion reaction bright or deep yellow serum should prompt an investigation for RBC hemolysis. The maximum concentration of bilirubin following hemolysis is not evident until approximately 3 to 6 hours after transfusion.[67] The post-transfusion result for indirect bilirubin should be compared with the pretransfusion result. Bilirubin excretion may return to normal within 24 hours.

Hemoglobin and Hematocrit

Hemoglobinemia occurs when large excesses of free hemoglobin are released into the blood. The hemoglobin and hematocrit can be monitored to detect a drop in hemoglobin or failure of the transfusion to raise the hematocrit. Box 18–15 summarizes laboratory evidence supporting a diagnosis of DHTR. Hemoglobinemia immediately after a transfusion reaction confirms hemolysis, provided that an acceptable blood specimen was collected. Serial hematocrits and hemoglobin testing may be necessary to demonstrate therapeutic or nontherapeutic responses. Table 18–8 lists suggested times when some tests may be performed when investigating a possible HTR.

Extended testing depends on analysis and interpretations of tests performed and the patient's clinical condition.

Reporting Transfusion Reaction Work-Ups

If the laboratory evaluation or test interpretations suggest an HTR or a bacterial contamination, the patient's physician and transfusion service medical director must be notified immediately. After the medical director of the transfusion service has evaluated the laboratory results, interpretations must be recorded in the patient's chart. The transfusion service must maintain the testing results, interpretations, and reaction classification for referral if the patient requires further transfusion therapy. The AABB *Standards* requires that transfusion records of patients with difficult blood typing, clinically significant antibodies, and adverse reactions to transfusions be retained indefinitely. They also require that before blood is issued for transfusion, the patient's current records with those of the past 12 months must be compared for ABO and Rh typings, clinically significant antibodies, and any severe adverse transfusion reactions; and the comparison must be documented.

Both federal regulatory and voluntary accreditation agencies require investigation and reporting of recipient adverse transfusion reactions. The FDA's *Code of Federal Regulations* states the requirements for transfusion reaction reporting. If a reaction results in a fatality, the Director of the Office of Compliance for the Center of Biologic Evaluation and Research must be notified by telephone or telegraph as soon as possible. A required written report to the director must follow within 7 days of the investigation. Other voluntary agencies requiring investigation and internal reporting of transfusion reactions include the College of American Pathologists and the AABB. These agencies require that written transfusion reaction policies and procedures include steps for detection, evaluation, and reporting of adverse transfusion reactions.

Summary

This chapter has outlined post-transfusion difficulties associated with blood components. The transfusion service should establish policies and procedures that optimize transfusion practices and provide safety to transfusion recipients with reduced risk of morbidity and mortality. Continuous quality improvement of transfusion practices for the patient's safety requires constant review and surveillance of procedures, practices, and standards. The summary chart lists key points to remember.

BOX 18–15
Laboratory Evidence Suggesting DHTRs

- Positive DAT result after transfusion; pretransfusion DAT result negative
- Post-transfusion indirect bilirubin elevation
- Post-transfusion hemoglobin decrease 2 g/dL or more
- Hemoglobinuria or hemosiderinuria
- Antibody present 3–5 days (or more) after transfusion, antibody absent before transfusion

DAT = direct antiglobulin test

TABLE 18–8   Times to Perform Laboratory Test to Investigate IHTRs and DHTRs

	Immediate	1–3 Hours	3–6 Hours	24 Hours	Days
Blood					
Antibody IHTR	✓	✓	✓	✓	✓
Antibody DHTR					✓
Direct Coombs IHTR	✓				May need to repeat
Direct Coombs					✓
DHTR					✓
Hemoglobinemia	✓	✓	✓		
Haptoglobin			✓	✓	✓
Bilirubin			✓ 3–12 hours		✓
Methemalbumin		✓	✓	✓	✓ 1–2 days
Urine					
Hemoglobin	✓	✓	✓		
Urobilinogen				✓	✓
Hemosiderin					✓

IHTR = immediate hemolytic transfusion reaction; DHTR = delayed hemolytic transfusion reaction.

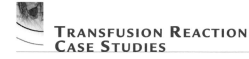

TRANSFUSION REACTION CASE STUDIES

Case 1

A 45-year-old man was admitted to the hospital with gastrointestinal bleeding from recurrent peptic ulcers. The patient had received a transfusion 4 months earlier for the same symptoms. The patient's hemoglobin on admission was 70 g/L (7 g/dL). Four units of RBCs were ordered and crossmatched, found to be compatible, and transfused. Five days after the transfusion, the patient appeared pale and mildly jaundiced and had a fever of 39°C. A complete blood count (CBC) and a blood culture were ordered by the physician.

1. The patient's 5-day post-transfusion hemoglobin was 50.0 g/L (5 g/dL); hematocrit 0.15 L/L (15%). Spherocytes were present on the peripheral blood smear. Because of the low hemoglobin, two units of RBCs were ordered by the patient's physician.
2. Five days after transfusion, two units of RBCs were crossmatched and found to be incompatible. The antibody screen was positive at this time. Five days previously, the antibody screen test result had been negative. A transfusion reaction work-up was initiated.
3. No clerical errors were revealed.
4. Repeat ABO and Rh typings on pretransfusion and post-transfusion reaction specimens confirmed original results. Repeat crossmatch tests on pretransfusion and post-transfusion patient specimens with donor units revealed no incompatibility. The pretransfusion DAT result was negative, but the post-transfusion DAT result was positive because of IgG sensitization. Panels completed on the patient's serum and eluate revealed the following antibody identification:
   a. Serum: Anti-Jkᵃ by enzyme technique
   b. Eluate: Anti-Jkᵃ by enzyme technique
   c. Phenotyping of patient's RBCs for Jkᵃ antigen (pretransfusion specimen)
   d. Patient's test results: Jkᵃ negative
5. Results of the patient's blood culture, Gram stain, and culture of the donor unit were negative.
6. This case illustrates the laboratory results of a DHTR. Anti-Jkᵃ is known for its transient properties of appearing and disappearing and for its enhancement by enzymes. The reaction occurred at a time when transfusion was least suspected as the cause. The transfusion caused a secondary immune stimulus, resulting in rise in antibody titer. In DHTR from transfused donor RBCs, destruction is usually gradual. The patient experienced anemia, fever, and mild jaundice 3–7 days after the transfusion. The post-transfusion compatibility test result was negative because enhancement by enzymes was needed to detect the anti-Jkᵃ. If the patient should require future transfusion, blood lacking Jkᵃ antigen would be required.
7. The patient had DHTR caused by Jkᵃ antibody.

Case 2

1. A 55-year-old man was hospitalized to have abdominal surgery for carcinoma. The patient had no previous history of transfusion.
2. The patient's admission hemoglobin was 100 g/L (10 g/dL). Two units of RBCs were ordered for the surgery. The patient was blood group O-positive. The antibody screen result was negative. Two units of RBCs were crossmatched and found compatible. During surgery, after receipt of the first unit of RBCs, the patient experienced oozing at the surgical site. His blood pressure fell from a pretransfusion level of 120/70 mmHg to 80/40 mmHg after the transfusion. The transfusion was immediately stopped, and the hypotension was treated. A new blood sample was sent to the blood bank, and four more units of RBCs were requested immediately.
3. The blood bank technologist, on typing the new post-transfusion sample, obtained the following results:

Reactions of Cells		Reaction of Serum with RBCs		
Anti-A	Anti-B	A₁	B	O
+mf	neg	++	+++	neg

mf = mixed field, + = positive, neg = negative

4. Repeat typing of the patient's pretransfusion blood specimen confirmed the blood group as originally designated O-positive. The post-transfusion reaction specimen revealed mixed-field agglutination when tested with anti-A antisera. The surgeon was notified by the medical director that a potential immune-hemolytic reaction may be in progress.

5. Clerical checks were performed in both the blood bank and the operating room. On completion of the clerical checks, it was determined that the wrong unit of blood had been selected for this patient. Two patients with similar names were undergoing surgery at the same time. The unit had been selected from the operating room refrigerator by name only and had not been checked to include hospital identification number before transfusion. It was additionally determined that two persons had not checked the unit before transfusion as required by the hospital transfusion policy. Investigation eliminated the possibility that any other patient was at risk for a similar incident at that time. The inadvertently transfused unit was determined to be group A-positive.

6. The postreaction DAT test result was negative, indicating rapid destruction of the incompatible transfused RBCs. The pretransfusion and post-transfusion antibody screen test results were negative. The crossmatch on the pretransfusion specimens with the original group O donor units revealed no incompatibility. Hemoglobinemia and hemoglobinuria were present, with free hemoglobin demonstrated in the first post-transfusion urine specimen. The patient developed a hemorrhagic coagulopathy with afibrinogenemia. His platelets decreased, with a concomitant increase in fibrinogen and fibrin degradation products. He soon became anuric, producing only 50 mL of urine in 12 hours. The patient's condition deteriorated despite attempts to control the hemorrhagic process, and he died. Autopsy findings 4 days post-transfusion revealed hemoglobin casts in the renal tubules of the patient's kidneys.

7. In an anesthetized patient the only symptoms of an HTR may be oozing, bleeding, or hypotension, as experienced by this patient. The erroneously transfused group A donor unit RBCs reacted with the patient's anti-A antibody, resulting in destruction of the transfused donor cells. The coagulation system was activated, resulting in a hemorrhagic diathesis with resultant acute renal failure and death. To prevent HTR, identity of the patient and donor blood component by two persons is essential to ensure that the appropriate blood component is transfused. Blood must never be released if it is identified by a patient's name. There must be not only verification policies but also monitoring to ensure that established policies are followed. At the first sign of a transfusion reaction, the transfusion must be stopped, a line left open for normal saline administration, the patient immediately attended, and an immediate investigation initiated. Most errors in ABO mismatch of blood transfusion are misidentification of either the patient or blood sample. Human errors resulting in serious or fatal transfusion reactions are often litigated, not excused.

8. This patient had an immune acute HTR caused by ABO incompatibility.

Case 3

1. A 45-year-old woman was admitted to the hospital for a hysterectomy. The patient had been pregnant four times and had no history of transfusions. She was taking no medications. The patient's admission CBC revealed a low hemoglobin of 70 g/L (7.0 g/dL). The physician ordered a unit of RBCs to be given before surgery to correct her anemia before an elective hysterectomy.

2. A unit of group O Rh-positive RBCs was crossmatched and found compatible. The patient's antibody screen test result was negative.

3. A transfusion of group O Rh-positive compatible RBCs was begun at 1:45 PM and given through a standard 170-μm blood infusion set. After receiving approximately half the RBCs, the patient experienced chills, and her temperature rose from a pretransfusion temperature of 37.2°C to 39.4°C. She had a severe headache and felt anxious and uncomfortable. The blood transfusion was stopped and the patient's physician notified. A transfusion reaction investigation was initiated.

4. No clerical errors were detected. Donor and patient identifications were verified.

5. Examination of the patient's pretransfusion and post-transfusion blood and urine specimens revealed no visible hemolysis. The DAT result on the post-transfusion blood specimen was negative. No RBC alloantibodies were detected in the serum of the patient or the donor. Repeat blood typings and crossmatch tests on the pretransfusion and post-transfusion specimens and donor unit confirmed the original test results. No incompatibility was demonstrated. Results of the serum bilirubin test 5 hours after the transfusion were normal. Bacterial contamination was ruled out by a negative culture and Gram stain.

6. Because serologic test results did not indicate a hemolytic reaction, blood group incompatibility, or bacterial contamination, other causes were considered. The patient's four pregnancies and transfusion reaction signs and symptoms suggested that a reaction to donor leukocytes had occurred. Leukocytes in RBC and platelet transfusions have been associated frequently with adverse effects (1 to 3%) when transfused to recipients who are alloimmunized from previous pregnancies, transfusions, or organ transplantation. The reactions are frequently associated with alloimmunization to HLA class I or leukocyte-specific antigens. RBC transfusions contain approximately 2 to 5×10^9 leukocytes. However, leukocyte reduction of up to 3-log (99.9%) can be achieved by using adsorption RBC filters. This reduction can prevent recurrent FNHTRs and delay of alloimmunization to leukocyte antigens in selected patients requiring long-term transfusion therapy.

7. This patient had an FNHTR. If she should experience two or more similar reactions, leukocyte-poor prepared blood or an in-line leukocyte reduction filter should be used. Although there are a number of ways to prepare leukocyte-poor blood, third-generation adsorption filters that remove leukocytes by adherence can achieve profound leukocyte reduction.

Case 4

1. A 38-year-old man arrived at the hospital emergency department (ED) complaining of abdominal pain. A CBC was ordered. His hemoglobin level was found to be 70 g/L (7 g/dL). The physician determined evidence of bleeding and ordered two units of RBCs immediately. The patient

had no history of prior transfusion and was taking no medications.

2. Two units of RBCs were crossmatched and found compatible. The patient's antibody screen test was negative. One compatible donor unit was released to the ED.

3. After proper identification of the unit of RBCs with the patient by two persons, vital signs were checked and recorded, and the transfusion was initiated. Thirty minutes after the transfusion had begun, the patient experienced a slight rash and itching. No other associated adverse effects were noted. The patient was given diphenhydramine (Benadryl). While the medication took effect, the transfusion was discontinued and normal saline transfused. Once the symptoms subsided (15–20 minutes), the transfusion was continued with no ill effects noted.

4. Urticarial reaction is the only immediate immunologic adverse effect of transfusion in which the transfusion can continue, provided that no other adverse effects occur. This type of reaction is likely to be caused by the passive transfer of IgE or IgG antiatopen (e.g., hay fever reaction to pollen), or both, from the donor plasma to the recipient. Histamine is presumed the mediator because it is released from antigen attached to the mast cell along with the IgE antibody. If the signs and symptoms are more severe (pulmonary edema, asthma, facial edema, hives over entire body) or become more severe after medicative treatment, the transfusion must be stopped immediately and investigated.

5. This patient had an urticarial reaction, which was treated effectively with Benadryl.

Case 5

1. A teenage girl undergoing chemotherapy for an adenosarcoma developed pancytopenia. The patient had a history of multiple transfusions of blood components.

2. On admission the patient was found to have small petechiae on her arms, face, mouth, chest, and conjunctiva. The admitting physician ordered an emergency platelet count and, on receiving the results, ordered eight irradiated pooled platelet concentrates immediately. Within several minutes of the platelet transfusion, the patient developed tightness in the chest, flushing of the skin, respiratory distress, coughing, and hypotension. The transfusion was stopped, and the patient was given epinephrine according to physician's order. The patient's physician consulted with the transfusion service medical director concerning a therapeutic approach for additional platelet transfusions.

3. The patient's platelet count at admission was 11.2×10^9/L, and the WBC count was 33.4×10^9/L.

4. No clerical errors were found.

5. Platelet studies after transfusion revealed no patient or donor antibodies to specific platelet or WBC antigens, and the patient's serum contained normal levels of IgA.

6. This patient experienced severe, immediate, and generalized reaction symptoms to transfused pooled platelet concentrates that were resolved by treatment with epinephrine. She also experienced a severe anaphylactoid reaction to plasma proteins in the platelet concentrates. After consultation with the transfusion service medical director, the patient was given irradiated washed platelet

concentrates prepared using the COBE 2991 blood cell processor.

7. After the washed irradiated platelets were transfused through a leukocyte reduction filter, the patient experienced no further adverse reactions to transfused platelets.

Case 6

1. A pregnant woman (primigravida) with a history of sickle cell disease had been monitored in the hospital clinic for over 11 years. She had had many past sickle cell crises requiring medical attention. The patient had previously received multiple transfusion of RBCs.

2. Two units of group O Rh-negative RBCs were ordered, crossmatched, and found compatible. The patient's antibody screen test result was negative.

3. At 22 weeks' gestation, the patient was given a prophylactic transfusion of two units of compatible RBCs in the clinic. Seven days later she received another transfusion of two additional compatible units of RBCs.

4. Sixteen days after transfusion of the initial two units, the patient returned to the clinic complaining of pain. She was afebrile but icteric and was admitted to the hospital. During days 16 to 23, the patient had a marked decrease in hemoglobin concentration.

5. Blood samples submitted to the transfusion service revealed that the patient had a positive DAT result. An elution test was performed. Antibody panel results of the elution study revealed that the patient had developed anti-Co^b antibody. Twenty-seven days after the initial transfusion of the two units of RBCs, the antibody screen test remained positive.

6. The patient's total hemoglobin concentration decreased from 11.0 g/dL to 6.0 g/dL during days 16 to 23. Her hemoglobin A concentration at 23 days was 2.0 g/dL. Urinalysis results 16 days after transfusion of the two initial RBC units showed an elevation of bilirubin.

7. After transfusion of the two RBC units, this patient developed anti-Co^b antibody. This antibody is usually IgG in nature and can cause hemolytic transfusion reactions. Approximately 11% of random donor units would be incompatible if a patient had detectable anti-Co^b. Co^b is a low-incidence antigen in the Colton blood group system.

8. This patient suffered a DHTR caused by anti-Co^b. She experienced a fall in hemoglobin concentration accompanied by a positive antibody screen and positive DAT test. Anti-Co^b was identified in the patient's serum and eluate, prepared from her RBCs.

SUMMARY CHART:
Important Points to Remember (MT/MLT)

➤ Transfusion reactions range from benign to fatal.

➤ Any suspected transfusion reaction must be evaluated promptly.

➤ If a death occurs as a consequence of transfusion, notify the FDA within 24 hours.

➤ At the first sign of a transfusion reaction, stop the transfusion.

➤ Rule out wrongly transfused blood in anesthetized patients with bleeding at the surgical site, hypotension, and hemoglobinuria.

➤ Recipients of any transfused blood component may produce alloantibodies.

➤ Alloimmunization and infection are major adverse transfusion complications.

➤ FNHTRs have undefined temperature increases greater than 1°C during or hours after transfusion.

➤ Fatal HTRs caused by errors in patient identification are associated with ABO incompatibility.

➤ TA-GVHD can be prevented by irradiating blood components before transfusion.

➤ TACO can be lessened by defined transfusion criteria and conservative fluid management.

➤ An anamnestic antibody response may be elicited about 7–10 days post-transfusion in DHTR patients who were previously immunized.

➤ Do not add drugs or incompatible solutions to RBCs to avoid hemolysis.

➤ Transfusions can save lives; however, one must be aware of transfusion risks; recognize reactions, causes, and means of management; and ensure proper identification and administration.

REVIEW QUESTIONS

1. Plasma that contains free hemoglobin in quantities of 100 mg/dL has a color that appears:
   a. Straw yellow
   b. Faint pink
   c. Deep, bright yellow
   d. Red
   e. Blue

2. Transfused plasma constituents resulting in immediate erythema, itching, and hives best typify which of the following transfusion reactions?
   a. HTR
   b. DHTR
   c. Allergic
   d. Iron overload
   e. Alloimmunization

3. Which listed transfusion reaction may result from an anamnestic response following a secondary exposure to donor RBCs?
   a. IHTR
   b. Alloimmunization
   c. Anaphylactoid reaction
   d. TACO
   e. TA-GVHD

4. Patients at greatest risk of developing TACO may include:
   a. Children
   b. Elderly people
   c. Patients with chronic normovolemic anemia
   d. Patients with sickle cell disease
   e. All of the above

5. Which listed transfusion reaction is most associated with transfused patients lacking IgA immunoglobulin?
   a. Anaphylactic
   b. Hemolytic
   c. Febrile
   d. TACO
   e. Allergic

6. The result of the DAT after a delayed transfusion reaction may be:
   a. Positive
   b. Mixed-field
   c. Positive because of complement coating only
   d. Negative
   e. All of the above

7. A transfusion reaction that usually appears rapidly during the transfusion termed "warm" and that may result in fever, shock, or death is which of the following?
   a. Hemolytic
   b. Bacterial contamination
   c. TACO
   d. Allergic
   e. FNHTR

8. After an IHTR, the recipient's serum bilirubin may return to normal in:
   a. 5 hours
   b. 12 hours
   c. 48 hours
   d. 3 hours
   e. 24 hours

9. Which of the following antibodies is most responsible for IHTR?
   a. Anti-Le^a
   b. Anti-N
   c. Anti-A
   d. Anti-M
   e. Anti-D

10. Fatal transfusion reactions are most frequently caused by:
    a. Clerical errors
    b. Improper refrigeration
    c. Overheated blood
    d. Mechanical trauma
    e. Filters

11. When a suspected hemolytic reaction occurs, the first thing to do is:
    a. Slow the transfusion rate and call the physician
    b. Administer medication to stop the reaction

c. Stop the transfusion but keep the intravenous line open with saline

d. First inform the laboratory to begin an investigation

e. Begin technical checks

12. Which of the following are symptoms of FNHTR?
    a. Shock, hemoglobinuria, hypotension
    b. Respiratory distress, vascular instability, shock
    c. DIC, renal failure, hemoglobinuria
    d. Temperature rise of 1°C with transfusion
    e. Temperature rise of 2°C or more with transfusion

13. If a patient experiences two or more FNHTRs, with each reaction becoming more severe, the easiest preventive approach for transfusion of RBCs is to:
    a. Administer the RBCs slowly
    b. Use specialized filters that remove most of the WBCs
    c. Use washed RBCs
    d. Administer smaller amounts of RBCs
    e. Use phenotypically matched RBCs

14. FNHTR is characterized by which of the following descriptions?
    a. Occurring in 50% of transfusions
    b. Rarely occurring after transfusions
    c. Occurring in about 1% of transfusions
    d. Occurring in 99% of transfusions
    e. Resulting from clerical errors

15. DHTRs from anamnestic responses usually occur within which time period?
    a. 5 hours
    b. 24 hours
    c. Several weeks after transfusion
    d. 3–7 days after transfusion
    e. 48 hours post-transfusion

16. Pretransfusion irradiation of all blood products in certain patients is done to prevent which of the following?
    a. CMV
    b. TA-GVHD
    c. FNHTR
    d. PNH
    e. HTR

17. If a fatality results directly from a transfusion complication, what organization must be notified within 24 hours of the fatality?
    a. FDA
    b. CAP
    c. AABB
    d. CDC
    e. JCAHO

18. The most common reason for transfusion of leukocyte-poor blood is that the recipient:
    a. Has RBC alloantibodies
    b. Has a positive DAT result
    c. Has been pregnant
    d. Has experienced an urticarial reaction
    e. Has had two or more FNHTRs

19. When a patient receiving platelet transfusion experiences purpura, the most likely cause is:
    a. RBC alloantibodies
    b. Platelet antigens
    c. Contaminating leukocytes in the platelet component
    d. Platelet antibodies
    e. Plasma proteins in the blood component

20. Symptoms of an IHTR in an anesthetized patient may present only as:
    a. Unexplained hypotension and abnormal bleeding
    b. Unexplained hypertension and thrombocytopenia
    c. Pale skin color
    d. Abdominal distention
    e. Respiratory distress

21. Of the transfusion reaction types listed, which results in thrombocytopenia owing to platelet alloantibody?
    a. IHTR
    b. TA-GVHD
    c. FNHTR
    d. PTP
    e. DHTR

22. Bacterial contamination of blood components can occur:
    a. At the time of phlebotomy
    b. During component preparation
    c. In components stored at room temperature
    d. During thawing in waterbaths
    e. All of the above

23. A patient was suspected of having an adverse reaction to a transfusion. The patient experienced urticaria. Which is the most likely associated etiology for urticaria?
    a. Plasma proteins
    b. Leukoagglutinins
    c. Platelet antibodies
    d. Antibody-induced intravascular hemolysis
    e. Antibody-induced extravascular hemolysis

24. A patient was suspected of having TA-GVHD as a result of transfusion therapy. What may cause TA-GVHD?
    a. Transfused contaminated blood components
    b. Functional T lymphocytes in cellular blood components
    c. Hypersensitivity reaction
    d. Results from platelet-specific antibody following transfusion
    e. Results from transfused serum proteins (IgE) reacting with recipient antibodies

25. IHTR reactions resulting from ABO-incompatible transfused RBCs are usually associated with which of the following findings?
    a. Intact RBCs in the urine
    b. Presence of leukoagglutinins
    c. Hemoglobinuria
    d. Extravascular hemolysis
    e. An increase in the serum haptoglobin concentration

26. RBC alloimmunization can result from:
    a. Pregnancy
    b. Platelet transfusions
    c. Leukocyte transfusions
    d. RBC transfusions
    e. All of the above

27. Transfusion reactions can be caused by:
    a. Citrate toxicity
    b. Hyperkalemia
    c. Overheated donor blood
    d. Adding drugs to donor unit
    e. All of the above

28. What electrolyte may fall in level as a result of citrate toxicity from massive transfusions?
    a. Calcium
    b. Phosphorus
    c. Sodium
    d. Potassium
    e. Magnesium

29. In looking at the first-voided postreaction urine specimen, hematuria (representing bleeding, not hemolysis) would be represented by the finding of:
    a. Free hemoglobin
    b. Hemosiderin
    c. Urobilinogen
    d. Intact RBCs
    e. All of the above

30. A patient was suspected of having an adverse reaction to a transfusion of RBCs. The patient experienced an FNHTR. Which is the most likely associated etiology?
    a. Plasma proteins
    b. Leukoagglutinins
    c. Platelet antibodies
    d. Antibody-induced intravascular hemolysis
    e. Antibody-induced extravascular hemolysis

REFERENCES

1. Sazama, K: Reports of 355 transfusion associated deaths: 1976 through 1985. Transfusion 30:583, 1990.
2. NIH Consensus Conference: Perioperative red cell transfusion. JAMA 260:2700, 1988.
3. Isbister, JP: Risk management in transfusion medicine. Transfus Med Rev 10:183, 1996.
4. Linden, JV, Tourault, MA, and Scribner, CL: Decrease in frequency of transfusion fatalities. Transfusion 37:243, 1997.
5. Pritchard, E: Transfusion-Associated Fatalities: Review of Bureau of Biologic Reports 1976–1982. Health Care Finance Administration Regional Office, Philadelphia, 1982.
6. Moore, SB, et al: Delayed hemolytic transfusion reactions: Evidence of the need for an improved pretransfusion compatibility test. Am J Clin Pathol 74:94, 1980.
7. Sazama, K, op cit, p 585.
8. Brecher, M.E. (ed): Technical Manual, ed 14. American Association of Blood Banks, Bethesda, MD, 2002, p 595–597.
9. Pineda, AA, and Taswell, HF: Transfusion reactions associated with anti-IgA antibodies: Report of four cases nd review of the literature. Transfusion 15:10, 1975.
10. Sazama, K, op cit, p 583.
11. Holland, PV: The diagnosis and management of transfusion reactions and other adverse effects of transfusion. In Petz, LD, and Swisher, SN (eds): Clinical Practice of Transfusion Medicine, ed 2. Churchill Livingstone, New York, 1989, p 714.
12. Taswell, HF: Hemolytic transfusion reactions: Frequency and clinical and laboratory aspects. In Bell, CA (ed): A Seminar on Immune Mediated Cell Destruction. American Association of Blood Banks, Washington, DC, 1981, p 71.Taswell, HF, op cit, p 76.
13. Pineda, AA, Brzica, SM, and Taswell, HF: Hemolytic transfusion reaction: Recent experience in a large blood bank. Mayo Clin Proc 53:378, 1978.
14. Popovsky, MA, Abel, MD, and Moore, SB: Transfusion-related acute lung injury associated with passive transfer of antileukocyte antibodies. Am Rev Respir Dis 128:185, 1983.
15. Hammerschmidt, DE, and Jacob, HS: Adverse pulmonary reactions to transfusion. Adv Intern Med 27:511, 1983.
16. Furling, MB, and Monaghan, WP: Delayed hemolytic episodes due to anti-M. Transfusion 21:45, 1981.
17. Panzer, S, et al: Haemolytic transfusion reactions due to HLA antibodies. Lancet 1:474, 1987.
18. Chaplin, H, Jr: The implication of red cell–bound complement in delayed hemolytic transfusion reactions. Transfusion 24:185, 1984.
19. Holland, PV, and Wallerstein, RO: Delayed hemolytic transfusion reaction with acute renal failure. JAMA 204:1007, 1968.
20. Popovsky, MA. Transfusion Reactions, AABB Press, Bethesda, MD, 2001, p 32.
21. Brecher, M.E., op cit, p 595–597.
22. Wenz, B: Microaggregate blood filtration and febrile transfusion reaction: A comparative study. Transfusion 23:95, 1983.
23. Gleichmann, H, and Greininger, J: Over 95% sensitization against allogenic leukocytes following single massive blood transfusion. Vox Sang 28:66, 1975.
24. Moore, SB, et al: Transfusion-induced alloimmunization in patients awaiting renal allografts. Vox Sang 47:354, 1984.
25. Okusawa, S, et al: C5a induction of human interleukin-1: Synergistic effect with endotoxin or interferon-[alpha]. J Immunol 139:2635, 1987.
26. Dinnarello, CA, and Wolff, SM: Molecular basis of fever in humans. Am J Med 72:799, 1982.
27. Wenz, B: Clinical and laboratory precautions that reduce the adverse reactions, alloimmunization, infectivity, and possibly immunomodulation associated with homologous transfusions. Tranfus Med Rev 4:3, 1990.
28. Seldon, TH: Untoward reactions and complications during transfusions and infusions. Anesthesiology 22:810, 1961.
29. Thompson, JS: Urticaria and angioedema. Ann Intern Med 69:361, 1968.
30. Bochner, BS, and Lichtenstein, LM: Anaphylaxis. N Engl J Med 324:1785, 1991.
31. Vyas, GN, et al: Serologic specificity of human anti-IgA and its significance in transfusion. Blood 34:573, 1969.
32. Mollison, PL, Englefriet, CP, and Contreas, M: Blood Transfusion in Clinical Medicine, ed 9. Blackwell Scientific, Oxford, 1993, p 690.
33. Milde, LN: An anaphylactic reaction to fibrin glue. Anesth Analg 69:684, 1989.
34. Ring, J, and Messmer, K: Incidence and severity of anaphylactoid reactions to colloid volume substitutes. Lancet 1:466, 1977.
35. Hammerschmidt, DE, et al: Association of complement activation and elevated plasma-C5a with adult respiratory distress syndrome. Lancet 1:947, 1980.
36. Holland, PV: Other adverse effects of transfusion. In Petz, LD, and Swisher, SN (eds): Clinical Practice of Blood Transfusion. Churchill Livingstone, New York, 1981, p 783.
37. Goldfinger, D, and Lowe, C: Prevention of adverse reactions to blood transfusion by the administration of saline washed red blood cells. Transfusion 21:277, 1981.
38. Wagner, SJ, et al: Transfusion-associated bacterial sepsis. Clin Microbiol Rev 7:290, 1994.
39. Wagner, SJ, et al: Comparison of bacteria growth in single and pooled platelet concentrates after deliberate inoculation and storage. Transfusion 35:298, 1995.
40. Klein, HG, et al: Current status of microbial contamination of blood components: Summary of a conference. Transfusion 37:95, 1997.
41. Mammen, E, and Walt, A: Eight years of experience with massive blood transfusion. J Trauma 11:275, 1971.
42. Quick, AJ: Influence of erythrocytes on the coagulation of blood. Am J Med Sci 239:101, 1960.
43. Barton, JC: Massive transfusion: Complications and their management. J Tenn Med Assoc 68:895, 1975.
44. Best, R, Syverud, S, and Novak, RM: Trauma and hypothermia. Am J Emerg Med 3:48, 1985.
45. Silberstein, LE, et al: Calcium homeostasis during therapeutic plasma exchange. Transfusion 26:151, 1986.
46. Wolfowitz, E, and Schechter, Y: More about alloimmunization by transfusion of fresh-frozen plasma. Transfusion 24:544, 1984.
47. Cox, JV, et al: Risk of alloimmunization and delayed hemolytic transfusion reactions in patients with sickle cell disease. Arch Intern Med 148:2488, 1988.
48. Salama, A, and Mueller-Eckhardt, C: Delayed hemolytic transfusion reactions: Evidence for complement activation involving allogeneic and autologous red cells. Transfusion 24:188, 1984.
49. Cimo, PL, and Aster, RH: Posttransfusion purpura: Successful treatment by exchange transfusion. N Engl J Med 287:290, 1980.
50. Mueller-Eckhardt, C, et al: High-dose intravenous immunoglobulin for posttransfusion purpura (abstract P12–21). Eighteenth Congress of the International Society of Blood Transfusion, 1984, p 194.
51. Brubaker, DB: Human posttransfusion graft-versus-host disease. Vox Sang 45:401, 1983.
52. Anderson, KC, and Weinstein, HJ: Transfusion-associated graft-versus-host disease. N Engl J Med 323:315, 1990.
53. Linden, JV, and Pisciotto, PT: Transfusion-associated graft-versus-host disease and blood irradiation. Transfus Med Rev 6:116, 1992.

54. Siimes, MA, and Hoskimies, S: Chronic graft-versus-host disease after blood transfusions confirmed by incompatible HLA antigens in bone marrow. Lancet 1:42, 1982.
55. Button, LN, et al: The effects of irradiation on blood components. Transfusion 21:419, 1981.
56. Anderson, KC, et al: Variation in blood component irradiation practice: Implications for prevention of transfusion-associated graft-versus-host disease. Blood 77:2096, 1991.
57. Propper, RD, Button, LN, and Nathan, DG: New approach to transfusion management of thalassemia. Blood 55:55, 1980.
58. Opelz, G, et al: Effect of blood transfusions on subsequent kidney transplants. Transplant Proc 5:253, 1973.
59. Graves, A, et al: Relationship of transfusion and infection in a burn population. J Trauma 29:948, 1989.
60. Heal, JM, and Cohen, HJ: Do white cells in stored blood components reduce the likelihood of posttransfusion bacterial sepsis? Transfusion 31:581, 1991.
61. Blumberg, N, and Heal, JM: Effects of transfusion on immune function: Cancer recurrence and infection. Arch Pathol Lab Med 118:371, 1994.
62. Bacon, JM, and Young, IF: ABO incompatible blood transfusion. Pathology 21:181, 1989.
63. Mollison, PL, op cit, p. 540.
64. Ibid, p 541.
65. Standards for Blood Banks and Transfusion Services, ed. 22. American Association of Blood Banks, Bethesda, MD, 1997. p 41.
66. Mollison, PL, op cit, p 518.
67. Mollison, PL, op cit, p 518.

BIBLIOGRAPHY

Ciavarella, D (ed): Symposium on leukocyte-depleted blood products. Transfus Med Rev (suppl 1) 4, 1990.
Dutcher, JP (ed): Modern Transfusion Therapy. CRC Press, Boca Raton, FL, 1990.
Miale, JB (ed): Laboratory Medicine: Hematology, ed 6. CV Mosby, St Louis, 1982.
Mollison, PL, Engelfriet, CP, and Contreras, M: Blood Transfusion in Clinical Medicine, ed 9. Blackwell Scientific, Boston, 1993.
Petz, LD, and Swisher, SN (eds): Clinical Practice of Transfusion Medicine, ed 6. Churchill Livingstone, New York, 1989.
Popovsky, MA: Transfusion Reactions. American Association of Blood Banks, Bethesda, MD, 1996.
Rutnam, RC, and Miller, WV (eds): Transfusion Therapy: Principles and Procedures. Aspen Systems Corporation, Rockville, MD, 1981.
Turgeon, ML: Fundamentals of Immunohematology: Theory and Technique. Lea & Febiger, Philadelphia, 1989.

nineteen

Transfusion-Transmitted Diseases

Elizabeth F. Williams, MHS, CLS (NCA), MT (ASCP) SBB, **Patsy C. Jarreau**, MHS, CLS (NCA), MT (ASCP), **and Michele B. Zitzmann**, MHS, CLS (NCA), MT (ASCP)

OBJECTIVES

On completion of this chapter, the learner should be able to:

1. Discuss the pathology, epidemiology, laboratory testing, and prophylaxis/treatment of the following diseases: hepatitis A-G, human immunodeficiency viruses 1 and 2, human T-cell lymphotropic viruses I and II, and West Nile virus (WNV).
2. Discuss the implication of the following diseases for blood transfusions: Epstein-Barr virus, cytomegalovirus (CMV),

parvovirus B19, herpesvirus 6 and 8, general bacterial contamination, syphilis, *Babesia microti*, *Trypanosoma cruzi*, malaria (*Plasmodium* species), and Creutzfeldt-Jakob disease and variant Creutzfeldt-Jakob disease.
3. Describe procedures for look-back and recipient follow-up.
4. Discuss pathogen inactivation for plasma and cellular components.

Introduction

Blood is a life-saving resource. In the United States, blood components are subjected to rigorous testing that makes them extremely safe and renders the likelihood of a transfusion-transmitted disease (TTD) very small. However, bacterial, viral, parasitic, and prion pathogens constantly evolve and, if not detected in the testing process, can cause harm and even death.

Donor Testing

Once a donor passes the medical screen and donor questionnaire, required serologic testing is performed for hepatitis B

surface antigen (HBsAg), antibody to hepatitis B core antigen (anti-HBc), antibody to hepatitis C virus (anti-HCV), antibodies to HIV (anti-HIV 1/2), antibody to human T-cell lymphotropic virus types I and II (anti-HTLV-I/II), and for syphilis. Nucleic acid amplification testing (NAT) was licensed in 2003 in the United States to test for HCV RNA and HIV RNA. In the 22nd edition of the AABB *Standards,*[1] HIV RNA replaced testing for the HIV-1 p24 antigen. Implementation of NAT testing for WNV was begun in June 2003 **(Table 19–1)**.[2]

As currently used test methods are extremely sensitive, confirmatory tests are used to detect false-positives. These tests, which vary by the disease, include: polymerase chain reaction (PCR), Western blot (WB), radioimmunoprecipitin

TABLE 19–1 Disease Transmission Prevention—Required Tests

Hepatitis B	HBsAg anti-HBc
Hepatitis C	anti-HCV HCV RNA
HIV	anti-HIV-1/2 HIV-1 RNA
HTLV	anti-HTLV-I/II
Syphilis	STS
West Nile Virus	WNV RNA

assay (RIPA), and recombinant immunoblot assay (RIBA), among others.

Surrogate markers (alanine aminotransferase [ALT] and anti-HBc) were used in the past to detect non-A, non-B hepatitis. Due to the sensitivity of the current testing for HCV, ALT is no longer required. However, most blood centers are continuing to perform both tests. ALT testing has continued because it is required by the European Union countries for recovered plasma. The U.S. Food and Drug Administration (FDA) recommends performance of anti-HBc in part because of cases of liver donors who were HBsAg-negative but anti-HBc–reactive and transmitted HBV to the recipients.[3]

Many other organisms may be transfusion-transmitted; however, tests for them are not routinely performed in the blood screening process. These include other viruses such as Epstein-Barr virus (EBV), CMV, parvovirus B19 (B19), bacteria (now considered to be the leading cause of death from transfusion),[4] parasites such as *Babesia microti* and *Trypanosoma cruzi,* malaria, and prion diseases.

Transfusion-Associated Hepatitis

Hepatitis is a generic term describing inflammation of the liver. Symptoms typically include jaundice, dark urine, hepato-megaly, anorexia, malaise, fever, nausea, abdominal pain, and vomiting. Clinically, hepatitis ranges from being asymptomatic to resulting in death.[5]

It can be caused by many things, including viruses, bacteria, noninfectious agents such as chemicals (including drugs and alcohol), ionizing radiation, and autoimmune processes.[5,6] EBV, CMV, parvovirus, and herpes simplex virus (HSV) can cause hepatitis as a complication, but because it is not the primary disease, these viruses are not considered hepatitis viruses.[6,7] The hepatitis viruses affect the liver as the primary clinical manifestation. Hepatitis viruses can be transmitted through the fecal/oral route or parenterally (through contact with blood and other body fluids).[5]

Hepatitis A (HAV) and hepatitis E (HEV) are mainly transmitted through the fecal/oral route. Hepatitis B (HBV), hepatitis C (HCV), hepatitis D (HDV), and hepatitis G (HB-C/HGV) are primarily transmitted parenterally.[5]

HAV

HAV belongs to the *Picornaviridae* family of viruses and is a small, nonenveloped, single-stranded enterovirus RNA virus. Of all the forms of hepatitis viruses, it is the most common.[5,8]

Clinical Manifestations and Pathology

Symptoms, if they occur at all, generally appear abruptly and last fewer than 2 months but may persist for as long as 6 months in some individuals. They may include nausea, vomiting, anorexia, fatigue, fever, and jaundice. Less than 10 percent of children under 6 years will develop jaundice. Jaundice is more common in older children and adults, occurring in 40 to 50 percent of children between 6 to 14 years and 70 to 80 percent of individuals older than 14 years. The disease is rarely fatal. Fulminant, cholestatic, or relapsing hepatitis may occur. There is no chronic state.[9,10]

Epidemiology and Transmission

Transmission is primarily through the fecal/oral route, spread through water, food, and person-to-person contact. Poor hygiene and poor sanitation contribute to the spread of HAV. Because young children are generally asymptomatic, the disease is predominantly spread from person-to-person within the household. Other areas of concern are individuals who are exposed in day-care centers, neonatal intensive care units, institutions for the mentally handicapped, or those who have sexual contact with infected individuals or illegal drug users.[5,8,11] A risk factor cannot be identified in 46 percent of cases.[10]

Transmission of HAV through blood or blood components has been reported.[12–15] HAV is not inactivated by solvent/detergent because it lacks a lipid envelope. However, transmission through transfusion is so rare that blood components are not screened for HAV. The viremia is very short and usually occurs around the time of onset of acute symptoms, which would prevent blood donation.

Seroprevalence rates approach 100 percent in some developing countries. Approximately 33 percent of individuals living in the United States are seropositive, with rates of infection in the western United States higher than the U.S. average. This number may be low due to underreporting of asymptomatic or unrecognized cases (Table 19–2).[10]

Laboratory Diagnosis

Most of the virus is shed in the feces during the incubation period and declines to low levels by the onset of symptoms. The presence of IgM anti-HAV antibody is required for diagnosis of hepatitis A. The IgM antibodies usually peak during the first month of illness and decline to undetectable levels over the next 6 to 12 months. Antibodies that confer lifelong immunity develop in response to infection (Fig. 19–1).[6,9]

Prophylaxis and Treatment

A vaccine to HAV was licensed in the United States in 1995 for anyone older than 2 years. The number of cases has been decreasing since then, especially in areas and populations where the vaccine has been routinely given to all children. By 1998 the levels had dropped to historic lows. Because the vaccine is produced from inactivated HAV, it is believed that the risk is low for pregnant women and that no special precautions should be taken for immunocompromised persons.[10] Other prevention methods include improvement in water purification, good hygiene, and improved sanitation. In May 2001, the FDA licensed a combined HAV/HBV vaccine for anyone 18 years or older.[16]

TABLE 19–2 Disease Burden from Hepatitis A, B, and C in the United States (8/11/01)*					
	Hepatitis A		**Hepatitis B**		**Hepatitis C**	
	2001	2000	2001	2000	2001	2000
Number of acute cases reported	10,616	13,397	7,844	8036	no data	
Estimated number of acute clinical cases	45,000	57,000	22,000	22,000	4,000	5,700
Estimated number of new infections	93,000	143,000	78,000	81,000	25,000	35,000
Number of persons with chronic infections	No chronic infection		1.25 million		2.7 million	
Estimated annual number of chronic liver disease deaths	No chronic infection		5,000		8,000 – 10,000	
Percent ever infected	31.3%		4.9%		1.8%	

*CDC: available at: http://www.cdc.gov/ncidod/diseases/hepatitis/resource/dz_burden02.htm

Immune globulin can be used pre-exposure to protect those traveling to high HAV-endemic areas or postexposure to prevent infection in those exposed within a family, after an outbreak at a day-care center, or from a common source of exposure such as a restaurant. Immune globulin should be used postexposure within 2 weeks for maximum protection.[9] It can be given concurrently with the vaccine for pre-exposure prophylaxis for travelers.[10]

HBV

HBV is a partially double-stranded circular DNA virus of the *Hepadnaviridae* family.[5]

Clinical Manifestations and Pathology

In the United States an estimated 300,000 persons are infected annually with HBV and there are approximately 750,000 to 1 million HBV carriers. Of these carriers, approximately 25 percent will progress to active hepatitis and possible cirrhosis of the liver. Four thousand will die of HBV-related cirrhosis, and 800 will die from HBV-related liver cancer (see **Table 19–2**).[4]

The clinical picture of HBV infection is highly variable. The individual may be completely asymptomatic or present with typical signs of disease, including jaundice, dark urine,

hepatomegaly, anorexia, malaise, fever, nausea, abdominal pain, and vomiting. For children younger than 5 years, fewer than 10 percent show signs of jaundice and clinical illness. However, infections acquired at birth or between ages 1 to 5 years result in a chronic infection 90 percent and 30 percent of the time, respectively. For those older than 5 years, up to 50 percent will have clinical illness, but only 2 to 10 percent will develop a chronic infection. Mortality rates in acute HBV are approximately 0.55 to 1 percent as compared with a 15 to 25 percent death rate following chronic HBV infection.[17]

Hepatocellular carcinoma (HCC) is epidemiologically linked to HBV. Risk for development of HCC is 12 to 300 times greater in HBsAg-positive individuals. Men have three to four times greater risk than women. In Taiwan, the number two cause of death in men older than 40 years is HCC.[18]

Epidemiology and Transmission

HBV is transmitted through exposure to bodily fluids containing the virus from an infected individual. Concentrations of the virus are at high levels in blood, serum, and wound exudates; at moderate levels in semen, vaginal fluids, and saliva; and at low levels in urine, feces, sweat, tears, and breast milk. Transmission may be sexual, parenteral and perinatal.[17] Percutaneous transmission may occur through needle stick (drug use, occupational hazard, acupuncture, tattooing, or body piercing), hemodialysis, human bite, transfusion of unscreened blood or blood products, or sharing razors. Permucosal transmission can occur through sexual intercourse, vertically from mother to infant (transplacental or through breast milk), or through contact with infected household objects (toothbrush or razor).[5] Virus on enviromental surfaces remains infectious for up to 1 week.[18]

The National Notifiable Diseases Surveillance System and the Viral Hepatitis Surveillance Program collated all causes for acute HBV reported from 1990 to 2000. Although 32 percent of cases had no identified risk factor, 36 percent had a sexual risk factor, 14 percent were intravenous (IV) drug users, and 18 percent had other risk factors.[18]

Laboratory Diagnosis

HBV consists of several proteins or antigens to which the body can make antibodies (**Fig. 19–2**). A surface antigen protein, HBsAg, is on the outer envelope of the virus. It can also be found floating free in the plasma. Antibodies can be

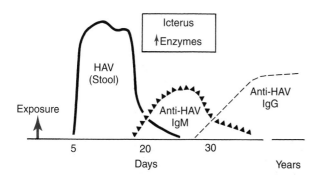

■ FIGURE 19–1   Markers in acute HAV infection. The typical pattern of HAV infection includes early shedding of virus in the stool, appearance of IgM anti-HAV, and immunity on recovery.

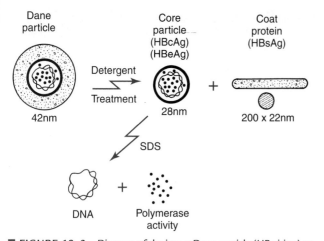

■ FIGURE 19–2   Diagram of the intact Dane particle (HB virion) as seen by electron microscopy. Detergent treatment disrupts the particle, releasing DNA (double- and single-standed) and DNA polymerase activity.

produced to two proteins within the core, hepatitis B core antigen (HBcAg) and hepatitis Be antigen (HBeAg). Viral replication levels of these markers along with the host's production of IgM or IgG antibodies are all used to make an initial diagnosis and follow the course of infection **(Table 19–3)**.[6]

HBV DNA is the first marker to appear and can be detected by polymerase chain reaction (PCR) testing before HBsAg reaches detectable levels.[3] However, NAT testing for HBV is not performed routinely in blood centers. The level of HBV DNA is so low before the appearance of HBsAg that only a few individuals would be detected by the current NAT pooling techniques used.[19] HBsAg is detectable 2 to 12 weeks postexposure during the acute stage and becomes undetectable in 12 to 20 weeks after development of anti-HBsAg **(Fig. 19–3)**. If the patient develops chronic HBV, the level of HBsAg remains high. HBsAg can be used to monitor the stages of HBV from the acute, active infection to recovery or a chronic infection. It is also used to screen donor blood.[6]

HBeAg appears after the HBsAg and, in recovering patients, disappears before HBsAg. In chronic patients, it remains elevated. HBeAg is present during the time of active replication of the virus and is considered a marker of high infectivity.[6]

HBcAg is present in the serum but is undetectable. However, IgM anti-HBc is the first antibody to appear, and it persists for about 6 months. Appearance of this antibody indicates current or recent acute infection.[6]

ALT testing is no longer required in the United States. However, it continues to be performed because it is required by the European Union countries for recovered plasma.[3]

Prophylaxis and Treatment

The donor questionnaire is used to identify individuals at risk for HBV infection. For those who are not eliminated by that process, testing for HBsAg and anti-HBc can be performed.

An HBV vaccine was licensed in 1981 and introduced in 1982. Once the screening of all pregnant women in the late 1980s and vaccinations of infants and adolescents in the early 1990s became widespread, the number of cases dropped to approximately 20 per 100,000 persons by 1995.[18] By 2000, the AABB[20] listed the frequency of post-transfusion HBV as 1 in 137,000 units of blood. Further decline is expected. Currently, the vaccine can be given alone on in combination with HAV. The combined HAV/HBV vaccine was licensed in 2001.[16]

Gamma globulin injections (HBIG) and the vaccine given soon after exposure or within 12 hours of birth, if the mother is infected, may prevent infection. Three other treatments licensed by the FDA are interferon (IFN)-α-2b,[21] lamivudine, and adefovir dipivoxil.[22] Once a patient has been diagnosed, family members should be tested. If uninfected, they should be vaccinated. If infected, they should be treated.

HCV

HCV is a member of the *Flaviviridae* virus family. It is a small, lipid-enveloped, single-stranded RNA virus.[5] HCV was discovered in 1989 and was soon recognized as the primary cause of post-transfusion non-A, non-B hepatitis. It is now considered the most frequent cause of chronic hepatitis, cirrhosis, and HCC in the United States.[23]

Clinical Manifestations and Pathology

The incubation period of HCV is 2 to 26 weeks. The average is 6 to 7 weeks, followed by seroconversion occurring in 8 to 9 weeks. Of all HCV cases, 60 to 70 percent are asymptomatic, with an additional 10 to 20 percent having nonspecific symptoms such as anorexia, malaise, fatigue, or abdominal pain. Most symptomatic cases are very mild. Of HCV-infected individuals, 75 to 85 percent become chronic carriers, with 20 percent developing liver cirrhosis and 10 to 15 percent developing HCC.[5] Most cases of cirrhosis do not develop within the first 20 to 25 years of disease.[24,25]

HCV is the leading cause of liver transplants in the United States. HCV-associated chronic liver disease kills between 8,000 to 10,000 individuals each year.[5] For those individuals with chronic HCV, alcohol, even in moderate amounts, should be avoided because it is known to exacerbate chronic hepatitis and lead to fibrosis and cirrhosis.[25]

Epidemiology and Transmission

Because most HCV cases are asymptomatic, the worldwide incidence is unknown (see **Table 19–2**). However, it is estimated that there are 170 million chronic carriers worldwide.[26] The risk of post-transfusion HCV has declined dramatically since the introduction of testing.

HCV can be transmitted percutaneously through needle stick, hemodialysis, human bite, transplant or transfusion, and/or by acupuncture, tattooing, or body piercing. It can also be transmitted permucosally through sexual intercourse, contact with infected toothbrush or razor, or perinatally. Individuals most at risk are IV drug users, those with an occupational exposure, or hemodialysis patients. Up to 40 percent of cases are not associated with an identified risk.[5,26]

Laboratory Diagnosis

Diagnosis of HCV is difficult. Not only are symptoms so mild in acute cases as to make separation of acute HCV from chronic HCV difficult, but separating HCV from other forms of liver disease is not easy. Diagnosis depends on biochemical

TABLE 19-3   Molecular and Serologic Tests in the Diagnosis of Viral Hepatitis

Virus	Test Reactivity							Interpretation
HBV	DNA	HBsAg	anti-HBc Total	anti-HBc IgM	Anti-HBs	HBeAg	Anti-HBe	
	+	+	+/−	+/−	−	+/−	−	Early acute HBV infection/chronic carrier
	+	+	+	+	−	+	−	Acute infection
	+/−	−	+	+	−	+/−	+/−	Early convalescent infection/possible early chronic carrier
	+/−	+	+	−	−	+/−	+/−	Chronic carrier
	−	−	+	−	+	−	+/−	Recovered infection
	−	−	−	−	+	−	−	Vaccination or recovered infection
	−	−	+	−	−	−	−	Recovered infection? False-positive?
	+	−	−	−	−	−	−	Window period
HDV	RNA	HBsAG	anti-HBc		Anti-HBs		anti-HDV	
	+	+	+		−		+	Acute or chronic HDV infection
	−	−	+		+		+	Recovered infection
HCV	RNA	Anti-HCV Screening EIA	5-1-1	Recombinant Antigens c100-3	c33c	c22-3		
	+/−	+	Not available					Possible acute or chronic HCV infection
	−	+	−	−	−	−		False-positive
	+/−	+	+	+	−	−		Possible false-positive (if RNA is negative); possible acute infection (if RNA is positive)†
	+/−	+	−	−	+	+		Early acute or chronic infection (if RNA is positive); false-positive or late recovery (if RNA is negative)†
	+	+	+	+	+	+		Acute or chronic infection
	−	+	+/−	+/−	+	+		Recovered HCV†
HAV	RNA	anti-HAV Total	IgM					
	+	+	+					Acute HAV
	−	+	−					Recovered HAV/vaccinated
HEV	RNA	anti-HEV Total	IgM					
	+	+	+					Acute HEV
	+	+	−					Recovered HEV

AABB Technical Manual, 14th edition, 2002, pp. 616–17.

HBsAg=hepatitis B surface antigen; anti-HBc=antibody to hepatitis B core antigen; anti-HBs=antibody to HBsAg; HBeAg=hepatitis B e antigen; anti-HDV=antibody to hepatitis D virus; anti-HAV=antibody to hepatitis A virus; anti-HCV=antibody to hepatitis C virus; anti-HEV=antibody to hepatitis E virus.

*Those with HBeAg are more infectious and likely to transmit vertically.

†Anti-5-1-1 and anti-c100-3 generally appear later than anti-c22-3 and anti-c33c during seroconversion and may disappear spontaneously, during immunosuppression or after successful antiviral therapy.

changes suggestive of HCV, detection of HCV RNA or anti-HCV in serum, and/or a known exposure to the virus.

Anti-HCV was the first FDA licensed test for HCV.[23] Currently, the AABB[20] requires serological screening tests be performed for anti-HCV and NAT testing for HCV RNA for all blood products. Only about 0.21 percent of U.S. donors are repeatedly reactive by enzyme assay (EIA), and these donations cannot be used for transfusion (see **Table 19–3**).[3]

Recombinant immunoblot assays (RIBA), licensed by the FDA, can be used for confirmation of anti-HCV tests. Seventy to 90 percent of all RIBA-positive tests are also positive for HCV by NAT methods. Those units that are positive for HCV RNA approach 100 percent infectivity. The repeatedly reactive EIA tests that are RIBA-negative or indeterminant (approximately 37 percent of EIA repeatedly reactive donors) are rarely infectious.[3]

In 1999, under the FDA-sanctioned Investigational New Drug status, NAT for HCV RNA was implemented for donor screening. This testing reduced the window period to 10 to 30 days. NAT has since received FDA approval for donor testing. NAT testing is performed in mini-pools of 16 to 24 samples. Once automated procedures are available, NAT can be performed on single samples. As of July 2001, 113 cases of HCV-RNA–positive, anti-HCV–negative units had been detected by NAT out of more than 25 million units screened.[27]

Prophylaxis and Treatment

Currently there is no HCV vaccine. Prevention consists of worldwide screening of blood and blood products; destruction or sterilization of needles, surgical, or dental instruments; universal precautions; and education about the risks as recommended by the World Health Organization.[5]

Antiviral therapies consist of IFN-α or pegylated IFN-α2a or -α2b monotherapy or in combination with ribavirin.[24,26] Optimal therapy is now considered to be pegylated IFN and ribavirin combination for chronic HCV.[23,26] It appears that IFN alone may work well in acute cases.[23] In a small study by

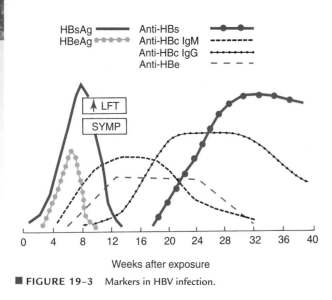

HBsAg ——— Anti-HBs ●——●
HBeAg ●●●●● Anti-HBc IgM --------
Anti-HBc IgG ·-·-·-·
Anti-HBe -- -- --

LFT
SYMP

Weeks after exposure

■ **FIGURE 19–3**   Markers in HBV infection.

Gerlach et al,[26] 50 percent of patients with acute HCV spontaneously and permanently cleared the virus within the first 3 to 4 months. Patients who were still viremic at 3 months and were treated at that point had an 80 percent clearance rate. However, most cases were not symptomatic and therefore were not noticed and treated until the patient was in the chronic phase. Treatment with INF-α and ribavirin in these chronic cases achieved only a 30 to 54 percent sustained viral clearance.[26] There is considerable debate on whether to treat immediately or wait to see if the individual spontaneously recovers and avoid the side effects of INF treatment.[23,24,26]

HDV

HDV is a defective, single-stranded RNA virus that is found only in the patients with HBV infection. It requires HBsAg in order to synthesize an envelope protein. It was previously called the delta antigen. If HBV and HDV are contracted concurrently, this co-infection, as compared with HBV alone, appears to cause a more severe acute disease, with a higher risk of fulminant hepatitis (2 to 20 percent) but a lesser risk of developing chronic hepatitis. Individuals with chronic HBV who contract HDV can develop a superinfection.[6,28] Approximately 15 to 30 percent of individuals with chronic HBV develop chronic liver disease with cirrhosis as compared with 70 to 80 percent of individuals with HBV and HDV superinfection.

Those at highest risk of infection are IV drug users. This infection can also be transmitted sexually. Perinatal HDV transmission is rare.[28]

HDV is detected by testing for IgM and/or IgG anti-HDV and/or HDAg and HDV RNA in the serum. However, tests for HDV are not required for blood donations.[28] If a donor has HBV, the unit will not be used for transfusion. As HDV cannot exist without HBV, testing for HBV will eliminate any infections with HDV.

HEV

HEV is a member of the *Calciviridae* family of nonenveloped RNA viruses. It is rare in the United States, and there are no recorded cases of transfusion transmission.[5] As in HAV, HEV is spread through the fecal/oral route, usually through contaminated drinking water in developing countries. A carrier state does not develop after the acute, usually self-limiting, illness.[6]

Clinical Manifestations and Pathology

Symptoms are the same as for any hepatitis. Generally, these cases are short-lived but can be prolonged. During outbreaks, cases of fulminant liver failure are seen more frequently among pregnant women, and the mortality rate in this group is high (15 to 25 percent).[5,29,30]

Epidemiology and Transmission

HEV usually occurs in developing countries and is responsible for acute, sporadic cases of infection that can be short-lived or prolonged. The fecal/oral route is the most common form of transmission. Most cases in the United States are found in travelers returning from an endemic country.[31] HEV does not progress to a chronic state. Very rare person-to-person transmission has been documented but parenteral or sexual transmission has not. It is most commonly seen in young adults.[32]

Laboratory Diagnosis

Both IgM and IgG antibody to HEV (anti-HEV) may occur following HEV infection. The titer of IgM anti-HEV declines rapidly during early convalescence; IgG anti-HEV persists and appears to provide at least short-term protection against disease (see **Table 19–3**). Due to its rarity, there are no commercially available serological tests available in the United States to diagnose HEV infection.[6] However, research laboratories are capable of detecting:

1. IgM and IgG anti-HEV in serum using EIAs and WB
2. HEV-RNA in serum and stool using PCR
3. HEV antigen in serum and liver by immunofluorescent antibody blocking assays.[31]

Prophylaxis and Treatment

Water supplies must be cleaned and sewage disposal handled properly to prevent the spread of HEV. Administration of immune globulin pre- or postexposure in endemic areas has not reduced the number of cases.[33] Immunization has not proved effective, but work is under way to develop recombinant vaccines. No treatment is currently available for HEV.[31,32]

Hepatitis G Virus

GB virus C (GBV-C) and hepatitis G virus (HGV) are two genotypes of the same enveloped RNA virus that belongs to the *Flaviviridae* family.[34,35] Approximately 1 to 2 percent of U.S. donors have tested positive for HGV, making this virus more common than HCV.[36] However, recent reports do not implicate GBV-C/HGV as a cause of hepatitis.

Clinical Manifestations and Pathology

Although acute, chronic, and fulminant hepatic failure cases have been associated with GBV-C/HGV, there are other studies that do not implicate GBV-C/HGV. One article showing a strong association with fulminant hepatitis dealt with a certain mutated strain of GBV-C/HGV.[37] In another article by Halasz[38], 33 GBV-C/HGV individuals were identified who had no co-infection with other known hepatitis viruses. No evidence of liver disease, clinical or biochemical, was found. In fact, there is some evidence that patients with HIV who have a co-infection with HGV have a slower progression to AIDS.[35] Overall data do not support GBV-C/HGV as a major cause of liver failure.

Epidemiology and Transmission

HGV is thought to be transmitted parenterally,[39] and transmission through clotting factor concentrates[40] has been noted in the literature. However, there appears to be a greater risk of infection due to risky sexual behavior rather than through parenteral transmission.[38,41,42] It has been found in 20 to 24 percent of intravenous drug users and in higher rates among people with HIV.[35] Vertical/perinatal transmission from mother to child has been documented.[38,43]

Most adult infections appear to be transient, with viral clearance followed by antibody to the viral envelope (E2) production. Vertical/perinatal infections and other infections established early in life can last for years but do not cause liver disease.[38,44]

Laboratory Diagnosis

Reverse transcription polymerase chain reaction (RT-PCR) for GBV-C/HGV-RNA is used to diagnose a current, ongoing infection. Anti-E2 along with a negative PCR for GBV-C/HGV-RNA indicates a past infection and recovery. Individuals who never develop the GBV-C/HGV E2 antibody are still infected.[42,45] These assays are first-generation, and the evaluation has not been completed on the sensitivity and specificity of these assays.[38]

Prophylaxis and Treatment

Interferon-α treatment has been used with conflicting results. In most cases, the level of the GBV-C/HGV-RNA returned to normal levels once therapy was discontinued. Only a small percentage of cases with low pretreatment viral loads had a predictable sustained response.[46]

Other Possible Hepatitis Viruses

In the search for causes of the non-A-E hepatitis, other viruses have been studied. These include TT virus (TTV), SANBAN virus, TTV-like minivirus (TLMV), SEN virus (SENV), and Sentinel virus (SNTV). Findings on these viruses are reviewed in an article by Ira K. Mushahwar[47] and briefly discussed below.

TTV has a high prevalance in the general population and has been found in blood and blood products.[48] Evidence linking it to liver damage, hepatocellular carcinoma, or non-A-E hepatitis has not been demonstrated.[49,50] Very little is known about SANBAN virus or any disease association with the virus. It was discovered in one human serum also positive for TTV. TLMV resembles TTV, and only four isolates have been identified. One article discussed transmission through transfusion with no adverse effects to the recipient.[51] The SEN virus appears to have eight genotypes, SENV-A to H, three of which, SENV-C, SENV-D, and SENV-H, may have an association with post-transfusion hepatitis. SENV is transmissible through

blood transfusions[52] and in a study was found to be present in significantly higher number of hemodialysis patients than in controls. However, there was no evidence to suggest any pathogenicity due to the SENV.[53] SNTV has also been isolated in non-A-E hepatitis cases.[47]

All of these viruses appear to have a close evolutionary relationship. But because they, for the most part, lack pathogenicity and all of the criteria to be classified as a hepatitis virus, there is debate whether they should be considered candidates for hepatitis viruses. "These criteria include replication in hepatocytes and subsequent damage to the livers of infected hosts, transmission to naive chimpanzees with concomitant elevation in serum ALT levels, and abnormal liver pathology as well as evidence for development of acute and/or chronic hepatitis."[47]

HIV Types 1 and 2

HIV-1 and HIV-2 are well recognized as the etiologic agents of AIDS. AIDS was first diagnosed in 1981, but the causative agent was not identified until 1984. Soon after the discovery of the disease, it became evident that an association existed between the blood supply and its transmission.[54,55]

HIV is a retrovirus that is spherical in shape, with an approximate diameter of 100 nm. It consists of an envelope of glycoproteins, core proteins, and an inner core of viral RNA and reverse transcriptase. Infection with the virus causes a slowly progressing immune disorder. The causative viruses, HIV-1 and HIV-2, are similar in structure, varying primarily in the envelope proteins (**Fig. 19–4** and **Table 19–4**). Almost all cases in the United States result from infection with the HIV-1 virus. HIV-2 is prevalent in West Africa but very rarely diagnosed in the United States and usually linked to an association with West Africa.

Profile

Clinical Manifestations and Pathology

Primary infection with HIV may be asymptomatic or result in a mild, chronic lymphadenopathy with symptoms similar to those seen in infectious mononucleosis. Symptoms may occur within 6 to 12 weeks of infection and persist for a few days to 2 weeks. HIV enters the cell by the binding of the virus glycoprotein 120 with cell surface receptors. Cells possessing these receptors include CD4+ lymphocytes, macrophages, and other antigen-presenting cells. The disease may have a long, clinical latency period with the absence of clinical symptoms. During this period, antibody concentration and viral load reach equilibrium. As the viral load increases and the

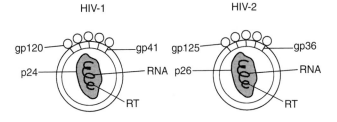

■ **FIGURE 19–4** Schematic representation of human immunodeficiency virus genomes, HIV-1, and HIV-2. RT= reverse transcriptase.

TABLE 19–4   Components of the HIV Virus

| Gene | Bands Observed | | Protein |
	HIV-1	HIV-2	
Gag	p18, p24, p15	p16, p26, p55	Core
Pol	p31		Endonuclease
	p51, p65	p68	Reverse transcriptase
Env	gp41	gp36	Transmembrane protein
	gp120, gp160	gp140, gp125	Envelope unit

p = protein; gp = glycoprotein (number indicates molecular weight).

CD4 count decreases, the patient progresses toward clinical AIDS. When the CD4 count is less than 200/μL, the patient is classified as having clinical AIDS. The resultant immunodeficiency allows the onset of opportunistic infections such as *Pneumocystis carinii* pneumonia, Kaposi's sarcoma, fungal infections, and a host of others. About 50 percent of patients do not progress to clinical AIDS for 10 years or more.[56]

Epidemiology and Transmission

The number of cases of HIV infection rose rapidly in the 1980s after identification of the disease. From 1981 to 2001, approximately 1.3 to 1.4 million persons were infected with HIV,[57] and more than 800,000 cases of AIDS were reported to the CDC. After the incorporation of combination retroviral drug therapy in treatment protocols in the late 1990s, there was a significant reduction in the reported numbers of new AIDS cases and deaths. Reduction of death rates has resulted in an increased number of persons living with AIDS. Since 1998 the number of new cases in the United States has remained stable at about 40,000 per year.[58] It is estimated that 850,000 to 950,000 persons are infected with HIV and that 180,000 to 250,000 (25 percent) are unaware of their positive serostatus.[57]

HIV is transmitted through sexual contact with an infected person, use of contaminated needles during drug use, and very rarely through transfusion of blood or blood components. Congenital transmission may also occur. No scientific evidence has been found that HIV is transmitted environmentally or through contact with saliva, sweat, or tears.[59] High-risk populations include men who have sex with men and IV drug users. The blood supply is most at risk from those individuals who have been recently infected with the virus but have not yet produced antibodies.

It was recognized over a decade ago that transfusion of blood and components from HIV-infected individuals may result in HIV infection in the recipient and development of transfusion-associated AIDS. HIV infection may occur after receiving a single contaminated unit of whole blood or its components. Albumin and immune globulins have not been reported to transmit HIV. Blood donor screening practices have dramatically reduced the incidence of transfusion-related transmission, but the possibility of transmission of HIV remains when the donor has not yet seroconverted and the level of virus in the blood is low. This subpopulation of HIV-infected persons who are unaware of their positive serostatus may pose the greatest risk to the blood supply.

Laboratory Diagnosis

The use of very sensitive serologic testing in screening the blood supply has resulted in an extremely low risk of HIV transmission. The pattern of serologic markers detected in HIV infection is shown in **Figure 19–5**. The window period is that time after infection but before antibody or antigen is detectable by currently available testing procedures. Only a very small number of donors donate in the window period, about 1 in 4 million.[60] It is possible for a donation to be infectious but to test negative for HIV-1/HIV-2 antibodies when the donor is in the window period. Antibodies are detectable at about 22 days after infection. Beginning in 1985, screening of all blood donations for antibodies to HIV-1 using an EIA was instituted. Testing for HIV-2 was initiated in 1992. An EIA technique is now used to test simultaneously for HIV-1 and HIV-2. Positive screening tests are repeated in duplicate, and if at least one of the duplicates also tests positive, WB or immunofluorescent antibody assay is used for confirmation. Interpretation of HIV antibody results related to blood donations is described in **Figure 19–6**.[3] Expansion of donor screening protocols in 1996 to include p24 core antigen testing reduced the window period from an estimated 22 days to 16 days. Using HIV antigen and antibody screening, the estimated risk of transmission of HIV through a single antibody negative component is 1 in 676,000.[61]

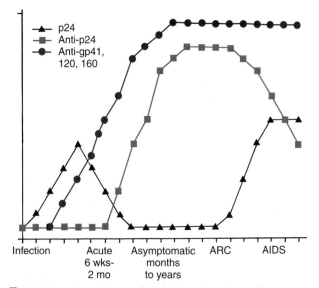

■ **FIGURE 19–5**   Pattern of serologic markers detected in HIV infection. ARC = AIDS-related complex.

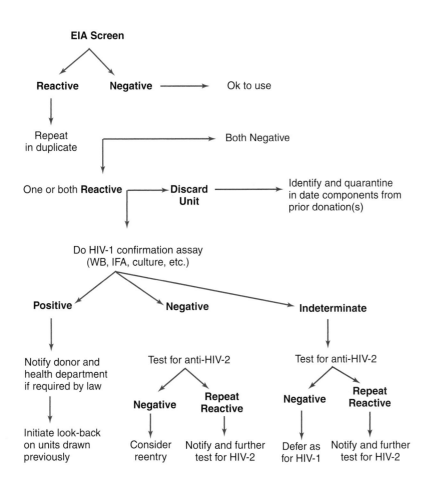

FIGURE 19–6   Decision tree for anti-HIV-1/HIV-2 testing of donor blood. IFA=immunofluorescence assay; WB=Western blot. (From American Association of Blood Banks Technical Manual, 14th ed., 2002, p 627, with permission.)

The FDA approved the use of NAT HIV-1 RNA testing under its investigational new drug exemptions policy in 1999. Screening of donations using NAT testing was implemented nationwide. NAT testing has reduced the window period to about 12 days, according to the FDA.[62] The first NAT test procedure was licensed in February 2002. As of 2004, p24 antigen testing has been removed from donor protocols due to the increased sensitivity of NAT testing for genetic material.[1] Blood donations may be tested for HIV-1 RNA by single donor or minipool using NAT. Mini-pool testing involves pooling of 16 donations and testing for evidence of HIV infection. As automated procedures are not available, pooling allows implementation of NAT testing by reducing costs and time involved for required testing. This procedure is limited due to the dilution effect of HIV-negative donations in the pool. It is possible to obtain a negative NAT test on a pool that includes a positive donor. If the viral copies present in the positive donation are low, dilution resulting from pooling with negative donations may produce a negative result.[63] Upon availability of automation, minipool testing will be replaced by single-donor NAT testing. NAT testing has reduced the risk of HIV transmission to about 1 in 1.9 million.[64]

The FDA approved a waived rapid diagnostic test kit for HIV-1 in early 2003. Many individuals who are tested for HIV never return to their health-care provider for the results. The rapid test can be performed on whole blood in 20 minutes and can be performed outside traditional laboratory or clinical settings. Positive results must be confirmed by a more specific test procedure. It is hoped that the availability of this test and the rapidity of results will reduce the number of infected individuals who are unaware of their serostatus and thus reduce the number of HIV-positive donors.

Prophylaxis and Treatment

Programs to prevent HIV infection are aimed primarily at reducing high-risk behaviors. It is hoped that continued education of the public about methods of transmission and increased availability of HIV testing will further reduce the spread of HIV/AIDS.[65] The CDC recommends routine HIV testing of all pregnant women and screening of all neonates whose mothers have not been tested to reduce perinatal transmission.

Treatment with highly active antiretroviral therapy has lengthened life and improved quality of life for those infected with HIV. Use of this therapy has resulted in stable HIV morbidity and mortality rates since 1998.[58]

Human T-Cell Lymphotropic Viruses Types I/II (HTLV-I and II)

HTLV-I and HTLV-II are RNA retroviruses. HTLV-I causes a T-cell proliferation with persistent infection.[66] Once the RNA has been transcribed into DNA, it is integrated randomly into the host cell's genome.[6,67] Once integrated into the DNA, the provirus can either complete its replication cycle or remain latent for many years.

Profile

Clinical Manifestations and Pathology

HTLV-I was the first retrovirus to be associated with a human disease. That association was with adult T-cell lymphoma/leukemia (ATL), a highly aggressive, mature T-cell non-Hodgkin's lymphoma with a leukemic phase.[3,66–68] ATL does not respond well to chemotherapy, and mean survival time with acute ATL is less than 1 year. Immunodeficiency similar to that of patients with AIDS develops, making the ATL patient susceptible to other hematologic malignancies.[67] HTLV-I is also associated with the progressive neurologic disorder known as HTLV-I-associated myelopathy/tropical spastic paraparesis (HAM/TSP). A few case reports in the literature suggest that HTLV-II may have an impact on the development of neurologic diseases, including HAM, but subsequent studies have failed to support this with convincing evidence.[68]

Epidemiologic data suggest blood donors infected with HTLV-I or HTLV-II have an excess of infectious syndromes, such as pneumonia, bronchitis, and urinary infections.[69] HTLV-I is associated with uveitis and infective dermatitis of children, Sjögren's syndrome, polymyositis, and facial nerve palsy.[6,66,68]

Epidemiology and Transmission

HTLV-I is transmitted vertically (breast-feeding), sexually (transmission from male to female more common), and parenterally (blood transfusion or IV drug abuse).[6,68] Because recipients of RBCs, platelets, and whole blood, but not fresh frozen plasma, have seroconverted, it is believed that transmission requires introduction of infected living white blood cells (WBCs).[66,67] This theory is supported by the fact that units stored for at least 7 days before transfusion are less likely to transmit the virus.

There appears to be a strong correlation between disease development and host factors such as cytotoxic T lymphocytes and HLA types. Susceptibility to ATL seems to correlate with polymorphisms of the tumor necrosis factor α (TNF-α) that result in an increased production of TNF-α.[67] In individuals with HAM/TSP, both cellular and humoral immune responses are increased as compared with those of asymptomatic carriers and seronegative controls.[68] However, ATL seems to occur in persons who were infected as infants, with a latent period of approximately 67 years, whereas HAM/TSP is generally seen in individuals who are infected in childhood or as an adult, with a variable latency as short as weeks to months. There is a 40 to 60 percent probability of seroconversion within 51 days following an infected blood transfusion.[66] For both diseases, the ability of the host to keep the proviral load low correlates with asymptomatic carriers.[67,68]

Worldwide, it is estimated that 10 to 20 million people are infected with HTLV-I and HTLV-II.[67,68] It is endemic in parts of southern Japan, central and West Africa, the Caribbean, the Middle East, Melanesia, Papua New Guinea, the Solomon Islands, and among Australian aborigines. In the United States, HTLV-I and HTLV-II are seen in primarily in IV drug users. HTLV-I is also seen in immigrants from endemic areas, whereas HTLV-II is seen in some Native American populations.[66,68] Indications from the high numbers of carriers and low numbers of individuals diagnosed with actual disease are that most carriers are asymptomatic their entire lives.[66,67]

Laboratory Diagnosis

Because the majority of carriers are asymptomatic, diagnosis is based on seroconversion after exposure. In the United States, FDA-licensed EIA using whole virus lysates from both viruses is used to detect both anti-HTLV-I and anti-HTLV-II.

With 60 percent homology between the HTLV-I and HTLV-II, antibody cross reactivity causes difficulty in distinguishing between the two viruses. Results are reported as reactive or negative for HTLV-I/II. No licensed confirmatory test is currently available, but most blood centers perform a confirmatory test under the Investigational New Drug (IND) protocol. Confirmatory tests are not performed until the test is repeatedly reactive and retested by EIA from a different manufacturer (Fig. 19–7).[70] All donated blood is currently screened by EIA to remove units positive for HTLV-I or HTLV-II from the donor pool. The AABB[70] and FDA[71] have published guidelines on the use of the unit for transfusion and donor notification as shown in Figure 19–7. The guidelines state that if the donor is repeatedly reactive by the test of record (original EIA) but negative by the second licensed EIA of a different type (different manufacturer), the donor is still eligible for donation. The donor can continue to donate as long as the test-of-record EIA is negative on the next donation. If the donor is repeatedly reactive by test of record on two separate occasions or on the same donation by the test-of-record assay and the different manufacturer's EIA, the donor is indefinitely deferred.

Prophylaxis and Treatment

ATL does not respond well to treatment. However, early treatment with corticosteroids appears to have some effect on HAM/TSP. There is no treatment for chronic or advanced disease.[66] The best prophylaxis is to prevent exposure. However, as the majority of infected individuals are asymptomatic, it is difficult to prevent spread to an uninfected individual vertically or sexually. Infected mothers should not breast-feed.

WNV

WNV is a member of the *Flavivirus* family and is a human, avian, and equine neuropathogen.[72] It is a single-stranded RNA lipid-enveloped virion[73] that is common in Africa, West Asia, and the Middle East. WNV is a member of the Japanese encephalitis virus antigenic complex that includes St. Louis encephalitis virus prevalent in the Americas, Japanese encephalitis virus prevalent in East Asia, and Murray Valley encephalitis virus and Kunjun virus prevalent in Australia.[74] WNV was first documented in the western hemisphere when 149 cases were reported in New York in 1999. In the United States in 2002, a total of 4156 human cases of WNV-associated illness with 284 fatalities were reported in 44 states and the District of Columbia.[75] With the report of one human case in California, the virus crossed the continent in 3 years, substantially expanding its geographic area. The CDC reported it as the largest WNV epidemic documented in the Western hemisphere.[76] In the United States, as of September 2003, there were 4827 human cases, with 93 deaths.[77]

Profile

Clinical Manifestations and Pathology

WNV is usually subclinical but may cause a mild flu-like disease. However, the strain in the United States is often associated with more severe disease. Outbreaks in 2002 determined by antibody screening that 20 to 30 percent of infected individuals exhibited symptoms ranging from mild fever and

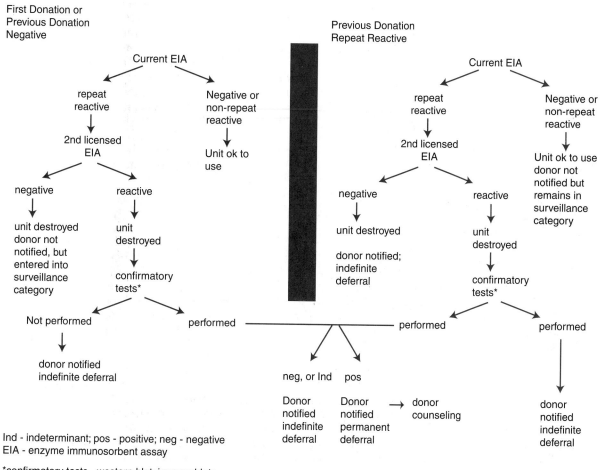

First Donation or
Previous Donation
Negative

Current EIA

repeat reactive → Negative or non-repeat reactive

2nd licensed EIA

Negative or non-repeat reactive → Unit ok to use

negative → reactive

unit destroyed donor not notified, but entered into surveillance category

unit destroyed → confirmatory tests*

Not performed → performed

Not performed → donor notified indefinite deferral

Previous Donation
Repeat Reactive

Current EIA

repeat reactive → Negative or non-repeat reactive

2nd licensed EIA

Negative or non-repeat reactive → Unit ok to use donor not notified but remains in surveillance category

negative → reactive

unit destroyed donor notified; indefinite deferral

unit destroyed → confirmatory tests*

performed → performed

neg, or Ind → pos

Donor notified indefinite deferral

Donor notified permanent deferral → donor counseling

donor notified indefinite deferral

Ind - indeterminant; pos - positive; neg - negative
EIA - enzyme immunosorbent assay

*confirmatory tests - western blot; immunoblot; recombinant immunoprecipitation assay

■ **FIGURE 19-7** Flowchart for HTLV-I/II testing.[70,71]

headache, through an extensive rash, eye pain, vomiting, inflamed lymph nodes, prolonged lymphocytopenia, muscle weakness, and disorientation, to an acute flaccid paralysis and poliomyelitis.[73] The association of paralysis and poliomyelitis with WNV is recent. It is a peripheral demyelinating process similar to Guillain-Barré syndrome.[78] WNV is capable of crossing the blood brain barrier and can cause what is known as "West Nile encephalitis, West Nile meningitis, or West Nile meningoencephalitis."[79] Approximately 1 in 150 infections results in severe neurologic disease that may cause permanent neurologic impairment, with encephalitis reported more often than meningitis. The risk of severe neurologic disease increases markedly for anyone over the age of 50 years,[80–82] with fatalities occurring more often in those older than 65 years who present with encephalitis.[72] Case fatalities range between 4 and 18 percent. In the United States in 2002, 9 percent of patients who developed meningoencephalitis died, with advanced age being an important risk factor.[74]

Epidemiology and Transmission

Birds are the primary amplifying hosts in a mosquito-bird-mosquito cycle. Incidentally, mosquitoes feed off infected birds and then bite humans. Although at least 16 species of misquotes have been found to carry WNV, the genus *Culex* is the chief vector.[72–74] The infection in humans has an incubation period of approximately 3 to 14 days following the mosquito bite, with symptoms lasting 3 to 6 days. Other animals can become infected, including horses, cats, dogs, bats, chipmunks, skunks, squirrels, and domestic birds and rabbits. Other than humans and birds, only horses seem to be severely affected by the disease.[83,84] Although mosquito bites are the most common route of infection, there is a slight risk of contracting WNV from blood components,[85] donated organs,[86,87] and breast milk.[85,88] During the epidemic outbreak of 2002, 23 persons were reported to have been infected through transfusion.[2] Other routes being investigated are transplacental and laboratory-acquired WNV through percutaneous inoculation.[89,90]

Laboratory Diagnosis

Viremia usually lasts approximately 6 days and peaks around the onset of symptoms. Once clinical symptoms occur, the IgM WNV-specific antibody titer increases, and the virus concentration in the blood stream decreases. Until July 2003, diagnosis depended on the clinical findings and specific laboratory tests. IgM antibody-capture enzyme-linked immunosorbent assay (ELISA) was the method used to detect IgM antibody to the WNV in serum and cerebrospinal fluid (CSF). In the 1999 and 2000 outbreak in New York, 95 percent of all infected patients for whom CSF was tested had a demonstrable IgM antibody. However, because all *Flaviviruses* are antigenically similar, cross reactivity has been observed in testing persons who have been vaccinated for a *Flavivirus*, such as yellow fever or Japanese encephalitis, or recently infected with another *Flavivirus,* such as St. Louis encephalitis or dengue fever. The plaque reduction neutralization test is the most specific test for arthropod-borne flaviviruses and helps to distinguish false-positive IgM antibody-capture ELISA from cross reactivity.[80] In fatal cases, immunohistochemistry can be used by testing brain tissue with virus-specific monoclonal antibodies.[91]

Clinically, the serologic tests for IgM antibodies to WNV using ELISA can be used for testing symptomatic patients. Because the virus is in the bloodstream before either symptoms or antibodies develop, blood screening tests for WNV that identify the virus itself were needed. In June 2003, two commercial WNV-screening NATs were distributed, and implementation of donor blood testing began "under phase III investigationl new drug (IND) FDA approval."[2,92] As of July 14, 2003, all civilian blood donations were being screened by NAT. Units are initially screened individually or in pools of 6 or 16, depending on the kit manufacturer. Individual samples are tested only if the pool is positive with NAT.[2,92]

If an individual donor tested NAT-positive, all current blood components were discarded, and any unused components donated within the last 14 to 28 days by that individual were retrieved. Additional NAT tests were performed by another laboratory for confirmation, using a different amplification technique or different primers. The original sample collected from the donor was assayed for WNV-specific IgM antibody. The donor was questioned again about "recent travel history, other exposure history, and review of symptoms compatible with WNV illness before or after illness."[93] Donors were classified as viremic if the initial donor sample was NAT-positive by pool and by individual testing, and the individual sample was repeatedly reactive using alternate NAT protocols.[2] With the implementation of NAT testing, approximately 2.5 million units were screened for WNV from June to mid-September, 2003. Only 1285 (0.50 percent) were WNV-positive by NAT. Of the positive units, 601 (0.02 percent) were considered viremic, and results are pending for an additional 209.[2]

The sensitivity of the testing using pooled samples is still under investigation. In a retrospective study by a large blood donor center, all previous samples that had tested negative in a pool were retested individually. Components were immediately retrieved and quarantined if positive. Recipients were notified if the component had already been transfused. Two cases of transfusion-associated WNV transmission were identified; both recipients were recovering as of September 16, 2003. Currently, it is not logistically feasible for all units to be tested individually.[93]

Prophylaxis and Treatment

Individuals should avoid mosquitoes and wear mosquito repellant and appropriate clothing if they are going to be in a mosquito-infested area. Once infected, there is no licensed treatment, only supportive therapy. Research is ongoing for the use of ribavirin, interferon-α,[73] and West Nile immune globulin in treatment for WNV. Having survived the illness, a person is immune for life.

Other Viruses

CMV

CMV is a member of the herpesvirus group[94] and is found in all geographic locations and socioeconomic groups, with a higher prevalence in developing countries. In areas with lower socioeconomic conditions, the prevalence approaches 100 percent. Of adults in the United States, 50 to 85 percent have been exposed to CMV by the age of 40 years.

Clinical Manifestations and Pathology

When exposure occurs after birth to an individual with a competent immune system, there are generally few symptoms. Rarely, mononucleosis-like symptoms with fever and mild hepatitis occur. Once an individual is exposed, CMV can remain latent in the tissues and leukocytes for years, with reactivation occurring due to a severe immune system impairment.[94]

Those at the highest risk of a CMV infection are individuals receiving allogeneic marrow transplants and the fetus. CMV-seronegative recipients transplanted with CMV-seronegative allogeneic marrow are at risk if they receive untested and non-WBC-reduced blood components. The risk of seroconversion and serious disease is 20 to 50 percent. CMV-seronegative women who become infected in the first 2 trimesters have a 35 to 55 percent chance of delivering an affected infant, many of which will have clinically apparent disease. Intrauterine transfusions with CMV-positive components is also a high risk to the fetus.[95]

Individuals at moderate risk are recipients of solid organ transplants, persons with HIV, and individuals who may require an allogeneic marrow transplant in the future. When the individual becomes immunosuppressed, a reactivation of a latent infection is possible, resulting in a clinically apparent infection.[95]

Low birth-weight neonates and autologous marrow recipients are considered to be at low risk. Preterm, multitransfused neonates weighing less than 1200 grams are currently considered to be at a lower risk than once considered, as a result of better transfusion techniques and management of their condition. However, leukocyte-reduced or CMV-negative units reduce the risk of CMV infection in these low birth-weight neonates.[3] The neonate may be exposed at the time of delivery, through breast-feeding, or on contact with seropositive individuals. Approximately 1 percent of all newborns are infected with CMV, but most are asymptomatic at birth.[96] The fetus that is exposed to the mother's reactivation of the virus during pregnancy rather than a primary exposure rarely has any damage.[96] The autologous marrow recipient is not as immunosuppressed as the allogeneic marrow recipient, and therefore CMV infection does not present a problem.[95]

Epidemiology and Transmission

Transmission occurs from person to person through contact with infected body fluids, which may include urine, semen, saliva, blood, cervical secretions, and breast milk. CMV is the most frequently transmitted virus from mother to fetus.[96]

Seronegative individuals who are recipients of an organ transplant or hematopoietic progenitor cells from a seronegative donor and AIDS patients who are not currently infected with CMV are also at risk.[3] The rate of transmission of CMV to bone marrow recipients or to neonates has been documented at 13 to 38 percent.[97] In one study, five of the six patients who contracted CMV after organ transplantation died.[98]

Laboratory Diagnosis

Antibodies formed to CMV last a lifetime and can be detected by ELISA. Other laboratory tests include fluorescence assays, indirect hemagglutination, and latex agglutination. If the patient is symptomatic, active infection can be detected by viral culture of urine, throat swabs, and tissue samples.[94]

CMV DNA tests are currently being investigated for use in detecting blood donors who have been exposed but have not yet seroconverted. Tests for anti-CMV would be negative for these individuals when, in fact, their blood might be capable of transmitting the disease. In one study by Roback et al, previously described CMV PCR assays were compared. The performances of the seven assays varied greatly in sensitivity, specificity, and reproducibility.[97]

Prophylaxis and Treatment

Currently, there is no treatment for CMV for a healthy individual; vaccines are still in the research and development stage. Infants are being evaluated using antiviral drug therapy, and ganciclovir is being used for patients with depressed immunity.

Blood and blood components are not universally screened for CMV because of the generally benign course of this disease and the high percentage of carriers of the virus. To prevent CMV transmission, leukocyte-reduced blood or blood from seronegative donors may be used. Leukoreduction using high-efficiency filters such that the final level of leukocytes is less than or equal to 5×10^6 leukocytes per component appears to work well with high-risk neonates (weighing less than 1200 grams) and transplant recipients.[3] In an AABB bulletin, prestorage leukoreduction was encouraged rather than bedside leukoreduction.

EBV

EBV is a ubiquitous member of the herpesvirus family. As many as 95 percent of the adult population in the United States have been exposed to the virus by the age of 40 years and maintain an asymptomatic latent infection in B lymphocytes for life. Infections occurring in infants or young children are usually asymptomatic. In adolescence and young adulthood, EBV causes infectious mononucleosis in 30 to 50 percent of patients.[99]

Although transfusion transmission is rarely an individual's first exposure to the virus and reactivation usually occurs only in immunocompromised individuals, there are a few cases in the literature of transfusion-associated EBV. EBV is not detected by current practices and could cause severe consequences in immunocompromised patients, particularly organ transplant patients.[100]

EBV has been called the "kissing disease" because the virus usually replicates in the cells of the oropharynx, possibly in infected B cells. The virus is shed in the saliva and is most frequently associated with infectious mononucleosis.

EBV was first discovered in 1964 in Burkitt's lymphoma cells.[101] Since then it has been associated with many illnesses besides infectious mononucleosis and cancers such as nasopharyngeal carcinoma,[102] non-Hodgkin's lymphoma and oral hairy leukoplakia in AIDS patients,[103] T-cell lymphomas,[104] and Hodgkin's disease.[105]

Antiviral drugs are generally not effective, except for oral hairy leukoplakia,[106] with treatment being mainly supportive for whatever the illness, complication, or cancer displayed by the patient.[107]

Parvovirus B19

Human B19 parvovirus (B19) is a small, single-stranded DNA nonenveloped virus[108] and is the only known pathogenic human parvovirus.[109] It causes a common childhood illness called "fifth disease" and is usually transmitted through respiratory secretions. Fifth disease presents with a mild rash described as "slapped cheek" when occurring on the face and a lacy red rash when occurring on the trunk and limbs. Approximately 50 percent of adults have been exposed as children or adolescents and have protective antibodies. Primary infection in an adult is usually asymptomatic, but a rash and/or joint pain and swelling may occur transiently.[110,111]

As in all viral infections, the virus must enter the cell through a specific cell receptor. B19 parvovirus enters the red blood cell (RBC) via the P antigen and replicates in the erythroid progenitor cells. The cytotoxicity of erythroid precursors can lead to serious illness in individuals with chronic hemolytic anemia, such as sickle cell disease and thalassemia, who may have a transient aplastic crisis. Severe RBC aplasia or chronic anemia may manifest in patients with chronic or acquired immunodeficiency, malignancies, or organ transplant recipients. Hydrops fetalis and fetal death can occur when the virus is transmitted during pregnancy.[108,109]

The viremic stage occurs shortly after infection. A donor would be asymptomatic but capable of transmitting the virus during this period. This is a concern for donor centers because the rate of seroconversion is high after exposure. In one study, B19 DNA was found in approximately 1 out of 800 donations. B19 is very resistant to heat and detergent and has been found through PCR to be present in plasma components. Because of the lack of inactivation in the manufacturing process, B19 has been implicated in several studies, with transmission through factor concentrates, solvent/detergent-pooled plasma, fibrin sealant[112] and, in one study, through an antithrombin III concentrate.[113] There are also rare reports of transmission through RBCs[114] and one through platelets transfused after a bone marrow transplant.[115] B19 DNA has also been detected by PCR in albumin and immunoglobulin samples[112] with at least one case of transmission being attributed to IV immune globulin.[116]

In a study by Weimer et al,[113] plasmas were tested for B19 DNA levels by PCR, and those with high titers were eliminated from the pool used in the manufacture of antithrombin III (ATIII). After the manufacturing process, PCR was used to compare ATIII concentrates made from a pool in which high titers were excluded and ATIII concentrates that were made from a pool that had not been tested for B19 DNA. None of the concentrates manufactured with high-titer plasma eliminated from the pool were PCR-positive, whereas 66 percent of the concentrates that were not tested prior to manufacturing were PCR-positive. This indicates the effectiveness of eliminating high-titer plasmas in reducing the B19 DNA to undetectable levels.

In December 2002, the FDA 75th Blood Products Advisory Committee met to compile issues on B19 for which it was "seeking advice." The three main issues put forth in the document, "Parvovirus B19 NAT for Whole Blood and Source Plasma," were whether the risks of transfusing high-titer (more than 10^6 geq/mL) B19 NAT-positive units were sufficiently high to withhold the components from use, temporarily defer the donor, and should these donors be notified to protect their close contacts.[117] All four major fractionators are currently addressing the issue by performing in-process controls to keep high-titer plasmas out of the pool.[118]

Human Herpesvirus 6 (HHV-6) and 8 (HHV-8)

Human herpesvirus 6 (HHV-6) is a very common virus that causes a lifelong infection. Seroprevalence approaches 100 percent in some populations. After infection, the virus replicates in the salivary gland and then remains latent in lymphocytes, monocytes, and perhaps other tissues, without obvious pathology.[119]

In childhood, HHV-6 causes roseola infantum, also known as exanthem subitum or sixth disease. Symptoms are those of a mild, acute febrile disease. In immunocompetent adults, it is very rare to find infection or reaction from sites other than the salivary gland where secretions from saliva are a known source of transmission. Side effects are not common; they can include lymphoadenopathy and fulminant hepatitis. Primary infection or viral reactivation can have devastating results such as bone marrow suppression, encephalitis, hepatitis, organ rejection, and death in immunosuppressed persons.[119]

HHV-6 has been associated with a number of diseases other than roseola infantum, i.e., multiple sclerosis and lymphoproliferative and neoplastic disorders. However, these findings are still controversial.[119] There is no evidence to support a TTD association; with the high level of seropositivity in the population, blood components are not being tested for HHV-6.[3]

HHV-8 is another human herpesvirus. Unlike HHV-6, it is not common in the population. Only 3 percent of donors are seropositive in the United States.[120] It is associated with several diseases that generally affect the immunosuppressed patient. These include Kaposi's sarcoma (KS), primary effusion lymphoma, and multicentric Castleman's disease.[121] Spread is generally through sexual contact. However, in KS patients, 30 to 50 percent have circulating lymphocytes harboring HHV-8, which lends support to the premise that exposure to HHV-8 could be transfusion-associated. There has been no evidence to support this to date.[120] In post-transplant patients who develop KS, it appears to be due to reactivation. However, there is strong evidence for transmission through organ transplantation in at least two cases.[121] Currently, as with HHV-6, blood components are not being screened for HHV-8.

Bacterial Contamination

In General

As the infection risk for other diseases has decreased due to better donor testing, bacterial contamination has come to the forefront. Currently, the AABB considers bacterial contamination to be the "most significant current infectious threat from blood transfusion."[122] Although the incidence of transfusion-associated bacterial sepsis is low, the morbiditiy and mortality rates are high. According to the FDA, the most common cause of death from transfusion-transmitted infectious diseases is bacterial sepsis.[123]

Clinical Manifestations and Pathology

The most common signs and symptoms of transfusion-associated sepsis are rigors, fever, and tachycardia.[124] Other symptoms may include shock, low back pain, disseminated intravascular coagulation (DIC), and an increase or decrease in systolic blood pressure.[3] The mortality rate from sepsis and toxemia due to bacterially contaminated RBC units is greater than 60 percent.[3] Although the number of contaminated platelet units is much greater, the mortality rate is not as high as it is for RBCs. However, platelet contamination is considered to be underreported. Sepsis due to platelets can occur hours after the transfusion, and the connection may be unrecognized. This may be due to the fact that many patients who receive platelets are already immunosuppressed because of their condition or treatment, and the sepsis may be attributed to the immunosuppression.[3]

Epidemiology and Transmission

Bacterial contamination usually originates with the donor, either through skin contamination at the phlebotomy site or an asymptomatic bacteremia. It may also occur through contamination during processing.[3,125] Contamination rates in the United States have been estimated to be 0.2 percent for RBCs and as high as 10 percent for platelets. It is estimated that a febrile transfusion reaction caused by contaminated blood occurs once for every 10 to 20,000 units and that a death occurs once for every six million units.[126]

According to the CDC,[125] Yersinia enterocolitica is the most common isolate found in RBC units, followed by Pseudomonas species. Together, these two account for more than 80 percent of all bacterial infections transmitted by RBCs. In a study by Kunishima,[127] Propionibacterium acnes, a common isolate of human skin, was the most common bacterial contaminant in RBCs. It is a slow-growing anaerobic bacteria that can go unrecognized if tested in aerobic conditions or by using short-term bacterial cultural methods. Although P. acnes has been implicated in only a few cases of transfusion-related sepsis, studies are needed to confirm long-term safety as it has been associated with sarcoidosis.

Staphylococcus epidermidis, Staphylococcus aureus, and Bacillus species, all normal skin flora, are the most common organisms found in platelets. Salmonella and Serratia species are also common in contaminated platelets.[126]

Laboratory Diagnosis

Before the unit of RBCs or platelets is issued, the unit should be inspected for discoloration (dark purple or black), which strongly indicates contamination.[126] The unit may have no visible evidence of contamination at the time of issue. However, clots in the unit and hemolysis may also indicate contamination. Because the bacteria in the unit consume the oxygen, the cells may lyse, resulting in discoloration in the unit as compared with the segments that remain normal in color.[3]

To detect bacterial contamination, both the donor blood component and the recipient's blood should be tested. It is better to test the component itself and not the segments as they may be negative.[3] Two culture methods have been cleared by the FDA for quality control monitoring of bacterial contamination in platelets. Both methods can be used for leukocyte-reduced apheresis platelets, whereas only one can be used for leukocyte-reduced whole-blood derived platelets. However, the FDA will not allow either method to be cited in product labeling.[128]

Culture techniques are capable of detecting one bacterial organism per milliliter (1 CFU/mL) but require time for the bacteria to grow. These FDA-approved methods require less validation than the other methods that do not have FDA approval. If Gram stain, acridine orange, or Wright's stain is used, it should be performed as close to the time of transfusion as possible to reflect current conditions. Multireagent strips detect most of the contaminated units by monitoring glucose and pH, but the bacterial levels must be greater than 10^7 CFU/mL for these to work.[128]

One of the reasons for mandated component outdate is based on the fact that storage conditions can contribute to bacterial growth. In 1983, the FDA allowed a 7-day limit for platelets, but the limit was reduced to 5 days when bacterial contamination was reported in 7-day platelets. The current 5-day outdate is a precaution against bacterial growth in platelets stored at room temperature. Once pooled, this 5-day outdate is reduced to 4 hours. Currently, there is no practical, economical way to test all units. However, in March 2003, the AABB presented its position to the Blood Products Advisory Committee, encouraging the FDA to allow prestorage pooling of platelets using sterile connection devices with testing performed on the pooled unit. Because culture testing will necessitate some delay in release of the platelets, the Committee also recommends that these pooled products have a 7-day outdate to prevent wasting units.[129] As of September 2003, no change had been made to the 7-day outdate.

Prophylaxis and Treatment

One of the best ways to avoid contamination is careful donor selection. The selection process is facilitated by the medical history questionnaire and physical, followed by a careful phlebotomy using a cleansed site that is not scarred or dimpled as these areas may harbor bacteria in increased amounts.[128]

The 22nd edition of the AABB *Standards* states that "the blood bank or transfusion service shall have methods to limit and detect bacterial contamination in all platelet components."[1] Use of apheresis platelets, careful phlebotomy technique, and phlebotomy diversion are listed by the AABB as methods to limit bacterial comtamination of platelets; culture, staining, and dipstick methods can be used to detect bacteria.[128] Currently, there is no single strategy that will both prevent and detect bacterial contamination of platelets.

Use of apheresis platelets rather than pooled whole blood–derived platelets from multiple donors reduces the incidence of contamination occuring during phlebotomy. However, apheresis platelets cannot meet all platelet transfusion needs, and whole blood–derived platelets are still needed. Therefore, arm preparation for phlebotomy is of paramount importance. Standard 5.6.2 in the 22nd edition of the *Standards* states that the use of green soap will no longer be allowed.[1] Improved bacterial disinfection has been correlated with the use of an iodine-based scrub. Alcohol and chlorhexidine is recommended for donors allergic to iodine.[128]

Phlebotomy diversion consists of collecting the first 20 to 30 mL of blood in a separate container to be used for testing. This reduces the quantity of skin contaminants entering the unit during phlebotomy and appears to be very effective in reducing *Staphylococcus* species contamination.[130] Several blood bag manufacturers have developed systems with a diversion pouch.

Leukodepletion of units can be helpful in removing phagocytized bacteria along with the leukocytes. Some advocate this for RBCs to reduce *Yersinia* contamination. Other methods under consideration listed in the AABB *Technical Manual* include endotoxin assays, detection of by-products of bacterial metabolism, NAT, and pathogen inactivation methods.[3]

Waterbaths used in a blood bank can have high bacterial counts unless disinfected frequently. An overwrap is recommended for any components placed in the waterbath, with inspection of the outlet ports before use.

If transfusion-associated sepsis is suspected, treatment should begin immediately without waiting for laboratory confirmation. Treatment should include IV antibiotics and necessary therapy for whatever symptoms are present, such as shock, renal failure, and DIC.[3]

Syphilis

Treponema pallidum, the causative agent of syphilis, is a spirochete. It is usually spread through sexual contact but can be transmitted through blood transfusions. A transfusion-associated case has not occurred in the United States in over 30 years.[131] Reasons include the facts that syphilis is rare in the United States; the spirochetemia phase is short—it does not tolerate heat, cold, or drying out so the storage of blood at 4°C quickly destroys any spriochetes; and the donor questionnaire has improved donor selection.[3,132]

The standard serologic tests for syphilis (STSs) usually do not detect a donor in the spirochetemia phase who has not yet seroconverted. Spirochetemia is short, and seroconversion usually occurs after this phase.[3] However, the STS is still required for blood donors despite the fact that in 1978 a federal advisory panel recommended that this requirement be eliminated. In 1985 the recommendation to drop STS testing was published but, because of the AIDS epidemic and the possibility that syphilis could be a marker for AIDS,[133] the FDA withheld the proposed rule to drop STS from donor testing. In 1999 a proposal was published by the FDA questioning the continued testing for syphilis and seeking scientific evidence that would support a decision to continue or to stop testing.[132] The 22nd edition of the AABB *Standards* continues to require the STS.[1]

Polymerase chain reaction followed by Southern blotting and a labeled probe have been used to confirm the presence of treponemal antigen. The test is capable of detecting as few as one treponeme in CSF.[131] However, in a study using NAT for detecting spirochetemia in 82 blood donors, all results were negative.[134] In another study with a different NAT assay, the results were conflicting. Further studies on blood donors should be done to evaluate this technology for use in detecting syphilis.[135]

Tick-Borne Bacterial Agents

Lyme disease, Rocky Mountain spotted fever (RMSF), and ehrlichioses are all bacterial diseases spread by a tick bite. Lyme disease is caused by the spirochete *Borrelia burgdorferi* and RMSF (*Rickettsia rickettsii*) and ehrlichioses (*Ehrlichia* species) are caused by bacteria that are obligate intracellular pathogens. There has been only one case of transfusion-transmitted RMSF, no confirmed cases of Lyme disease, and only one possible case of ehrlichiosis.[136]

Transfusion-Associated Parasites

At least three parasites have been associated with transfusion-associated infections:

1. *Babesia microti*
2. *Trypanosoma cruzi*
3. Malaria (*Plasmodium* species)

Several additional parasites have been identified in association with transfusion-associated disease. These include *Leishmania* species, other *Trypanosoma* species, *Toxoplasma gondii*, and the microfilarial parasites. Most of these infections occur on rare occasions and typically involve patients who are severely immunocompromised. The risk for acquiring a blood transfusion containing these parasites may be underreported in endemic areas but has always been very low in the United States. However, in October 2003, the AABB put forth a recommendation to blood collection facilities that all individuals who had been in Iraq should be deferred for 1 year from the last date of departure. This was done after cases of leishmaniasis were reported in personnel stationed in Iraq.

Babesia microti

Babesiosis, a zoonotic disease, is usually transmitted by the bite of an infected deer tick. Infection is caused by the protozoan parasite, *Babesia*, which infects the RBCs. *Babesia microti* is the most commonly reported species of *Babesia* to cause human infection in the United States.[137] Recently, the M01-type, WA1-type, and CA1-type *Babesia* species have been identified as causing clinical disease.[137–139]*Babesia* infection may also be acquired by blood transfusion and solid organ transplant. More than 40 cases of transfusion-transmitted *B. microti* have been reported in the United States.[140,141]

Clinical Manifestations and Pathology

Most cases of babesiosis are asymptomatic. Symptomatic patients usually develop a malaria-type illness characterized by fever, chills, lethargy, and hemolytic anemia. The risk for developing severe complications, which include renal failure, DIC, and respiratory distress syndrome, increases for elderly, asplenic, or immunocompromised patients. Reported incubation periods for symptomatic patients range from 1 to 8 weeks after transfusion; therefore it is important that physicians consider babesiosis when diagnosing a febrile illness following a transfusion.[3,142]

Epidemiology and Transmission

Babesia is most prevalent in the northeastern United States, including New York, Massachusetts, and Connecticut.[3,142,143]

The incidence is higher during the spring and summer months, which corresponds to the increase in tick activity and outdoor recreation of humans. Persons infected with *Babesia* may not have clinical signs of illness for an extended time. Infected persons who donate blood during the asymptomatic period pose the greatest risk to the blood supply, as they probably have infectious organisms circulating in their bloodstreams. Units of packed RBCs (liquid stored and frozen deglycerolized) and platelet units, which contain RBCs, have been associated with transmission.[136,140,144] *B. microti* can survive in refrigerated, uncoagulated blood for 21 to 35 days.[3,136]

Laboratory Diagnosis

Prompt diagnosis is essential, as *Babesia* responds well to antibiotic therapy but can be fatal in certain risk groups if not properly treated. There is no specific test to diagnose an infection with *B. microti*. Thick- and thin-blood smears stained with Giemsa or Wright stain can be examined for intra-erythrocytic organisms. A single negative smear does not rule out an infection. Serologic tests are available, but cross-reactivity with other species of *Babesia* and *Plasmodium* can occur.[145] The indirect fluorescent antibody test is the serologic test most often performed to diagnose uncertain or suspected chronic infections.[146]

Prophylaxis and Treatment

Babesiosis can be effectively treated with antibiotic therapy. There is no specific drug of choice, but quinine and clindamycin are very effective. In addition, the combination of atovaquone and azithromycin can be as effective in patients without a life-threatening illness.[137] Apheresis has also been successful in patients who fail to respond to antibiotic therapy.[147,148]

There is no test currently available to screen for asymptomatic carriers of *Babesia*. Many blood banks have added questions to their donor questionnaire that address topics such as living in an endemic area and previous *Babesia* infection. Some blood banks have chosen to defer individuals that reside in areas that are heavily tick-infested in the summer months.[149] This practice may have little value as donors may remain asymptomatic for months after exposure to the organism. Donors with a history of babesiosis should be deferred from donating blood.[3,140] Because *B. microti* can be transmitted by blood donated from asymptomatic donors, effective measures for preventing transmission are needed.

Trypanosoma cruzi

Trypanosoma cruzi is a flagellate protozoan that is the etiologic agent of Chagas disease (American trypanosomiasis). It is estimated that 16 to 18 million people are infected with Chagas disease and that another 100 million are at risk.[145,150,151] The disease is naturally acquired by the bite of a reduviid bug, thus making it a zoonotic infection. However, the risk for transfusion-transmitted infection does exist.

Clinical Manifestations and Pathology

The acute phase of Chagas disease is initiated when the organism enters the host. The reduviid bug bite produces a localized nodule, referred to as a chagoma. The chagoma is usually painful and may take up to 3 months to heal. Clinical symptoms may be mild or absent; therefore, many cases are not diagnosed until the chronic phase of the disease. Symptoms include anemia, weakness, chills, intermittent fever, edema, lymphadenopathy, myocarditis, and gastrointestinal symptoms. Death may occur within a few weeks or months after initial infection.

Following the acute phase, the disease may enter a latent phase, which can last up to 40 years.[150] During this phase, the patient is usually asymptomatic but has parasites circulating in the bloodstream. Transfusion-associated Chagas disease is most likely to occur during this phase.

Chagas disease usually progresses to the chronic phase years or decades after the acute phase.[145,150,152,153] In the chronic phase, the organism begins to cause damage to cardiac tissue, thus causing cardiomyopathy. Since Chagas disease is not very common in the United States, it can be easily misdiagnosed. One study revealed that 72 percent of Chagas disease patients in the United States had been treated for other cardiomyopathies for as long as 9 years before Chagas' disease was diagnosed.[150,154]

Epidemiology and Transmission

Chagas disease is endemic in Central and South America and some areas of Mexico.[3,144,145,150,152,155,156] Infection with *T. cruzi* in the United States is rare because of the low number of infected bugs and high standards for housing. However, because of the large number of immigrants living in the United States, there is an increased incidence of transfusion-associated Chagas disease. It is estimated that there may be 50,000 to 100,000 immigrants with *T. cruzi* infection living in the United States.[150,152,153,155,156] These infected individuals pose a risk of infecting recipients of their donated blood. There have been four reported cases of *T. cruzi* infection acquired by blood transfusion in North America.[3,150,155,157–159] All cases occurred in immunocompromised patients. This number could be higher if we consider there may be other cases not detected in immunocompetent patients receiving blood. *T. cruzi* can survive in platelets stored at room temperature, RBC units at 4°C, and during cryopreservation and thawing.[150] In addition to blood transfusions, Chagas disease can be transmitted congenitally, transplacentally, or through solid organ transplantation.[144,145,150,156,157]

Laboratory Diagnosis

Acute Chagas disease is diagnosed by detecting the organism in the patient's blood. Blood smears stained with Giemsa or Wright stain may be examined for the characteristic C- or U-shaped trypomastigote **(Fig. 19–8)**. Anticoagulated blood or the buffy coat may also be evaluated for motile organisms.

Chronic Chagas disease is diagnosed serologically. Such testing includes complement fixation, immunofluorescence, and ELISA. False-positive reactions are common; therefore it is recommended that patient specimens be analyzed using more than one assay. Trypomastigotes are rare or absent in the peripheral blood during the chronic phase, so examination of blood smears is not useful.

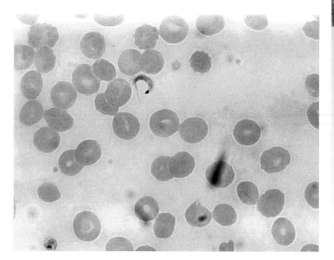

■ **FIGURE 19–8**   *T. cruzi* trypomastigote.

Prophylaxis and Treatment

Several blood centers with a large immigrant population from endemic areas have found a seroprevalence of 0.1 to 0.2 percent among donors identified as at-risk by a questionnaire.[3,155,160] Although a questionnaire may seem to be a cost-effective approach to prevention of transfusion-associated Chagas disease, it is not able to identify all at-risk donors. Comprehension skills, compliance, and vertical transmission to second-generation immigrants are issues that must be considered.[3]

Currently, routine screening for anti–*T. cruzi* antibodies in the blood bank is not available, as there is not a recommended assay that is highly sensitive and specific. There is also no evidence that routine screening would adequately improve the safety of the blood supply in the United States.[3] Many ethical and legal questions will emerge if a screening procedure is implemented.

Nifurtimox and benznidazole are the drugs of choice to treat Chagas disease.[145,153] Both drugs must be administered over a prolonged period and often cause serious side effects. Allopurinol is an alternative treatment, which usually causes fewer side effects.[145,160] Drug therapy is only beneficial to patients with acute Chagas' disease. Once the infection progresses to the chronic phase, there is no appropriate therapy.

Malaria (*Plasmodium* Species)

Malaria, another intraerythrocytic protozoan infection, may be caused by several species of the genus *Plasmodium* (*P. malaria*, *P. falciparum*, *P. vivax*, and *P. ovale*). Natural transmission occurs through the bite of a female *Anopheles* mosquito, but infection may also occur following transfusion of infected blood. Malaria is very rare in the United States, but it is the most common parasitic complication of transfusion.[3] At least 103 cases of transfusion-transmitted malaria in the United States have been reported to the CDC.[3,161]

Clinical Manifestations and Pathology

Symptoms include fever, chills, headache, anemia, hemolysis, and spenomegaly. There may be variations in symptoms among the different species of *Plasmodium*. Malaria often mimics other diseases, and its diagnosis is often delayed due to lack of suspicion in nonendemic areas.

Epidemiology and Transmission

Malaria is endemic in tropical and subtropical areas as well as in West Africa. More than 250 million people throughout the world are infected with malaria.[145] Many people associate malaria with a history of traveling to an endemic area. However, other transmission modes are possible, including blood transfusions and congential infection.

Transfusion-associated malaria is acquired by receiving blood products from an asymptomatic carrier. *Plasmodium* can survive in blood components stored at room temperature or 4°C for at least a week, and deglycerolized RBCs can transmit disease.[3]

Laboratory Diagnosis

Examination of thick- and thin-blood smears is performed to diagnose infection with malaria. Although each species of *Plasmodium* varies morphologically, diagnosis can be quite difficult. Depending on the species of *Plasmodium* and the stage of the parasite's life cycle, timing is crucial when evaluating the blood smear. A single negative smear does not rule out a diagnosis of malaria.

Prophylaxis and Treatment

A practical or cost-effective serologic test to screen asymptomatic donors does not exist. According to AABB *Standards,* persons who have traveled to an endemic area are deferred for 1 year, and those who have had malaria, immigrated from, or lived in an endemic area are deferred for 3 years.[1,3,149]

Chloroquine is generally effective for chemoprophylaxis and treatment of all four species of *Plasmodium*. Therapy has become more complicated due to the increase in resistance of *P. falciparum* and, more recently, *P. vivax* to chloroquine. It is important for the physician to carefully evaluate the species of *Plasmodium* causing the illness, the estimated parasitemia, and the travel history of the patient. This information is necessary to prescribe appropriate therapy and decrease the chance of resistance by the organism.

Some individuals have a natural immunity to certain species of malaria, caused by a genetic alteration in their RBCs. These include persons who have sickle cell anemia or trait, G6PD deficiency, or RBCs that lack the Duffy blood group antigen. There is also research being performed toward development of a vaccine that would provide protection against malarial infections.[145,162,163]

Prion Disease

Creutzfeldt-Jakob Disease (CJD)

Creutzfeldt-Jakob Disease (CJD) is one of the transmissible spongiform encephalopathies (TSE). These are rare diseases characterized by fatal neurodegeneration resulting in spongelike lesions in the brain. Although a definitive diagnosis can be made only at autopsy, neurologic signs and symptoms and disease progression are used to make a preliminary diagnosis. Animals, such as sheep, goats, cattle, cats, minks, deer, and

elk, and humans can be affected by TSE. In humans, sporatic CJD is the most common form, representing 85 to 90 percent of all human cases, generally occurring in late middle age (average age 60 years). An inherited form due to a gene mutation accounts for another 5 to 10 percent of cases, and iatrogenic CJD acquired through contaminated neurosurgical equipment, cornea or dura mater transplants, or human-derived pituitary growth hormones accounts for less than 5 percent of cases. The sporadic, inherited, and iatrogenic CJD are considered the classic CJD.[164–166] In 1996 a variant form of CJD (vCJD) affecting younger individuals was noted, and epidemiologic evidence linked vCJD to bovine spongiform encephalopathy, possibly from eating contaminated beef. Of the 129 cases reported from 1996 to 2002, most were in the United Kingdom.[165]

The causative agent of all TSEs is believed to be a "prion," which is described as a self-replicating protein. It does not contain nucleic acid but is formed when the normal cell surface glycoprotein, the prion protein, is conformationally changed to an abnormal form. This abnormal form accumulates in the brain and makes the brain tissue highly infectious. It is resistant to inactivation by heat, radiation, and formalin.[167]

Once symptoms are noted, death usually occurs within a year.[166] However, the incubation period in humans varies from 4 to 20 years and may eventually prove to be longer in some cases.

There is no epidemiologic evidence linking classic CJD to TTD. However, in vCJD cases, prion particles have been found in lymphoreticular tissues, including the tonsils, spleen, and lymph nodes. As blood is intimately involved with the lymphoreticular system, concerns arose regarding the ability of vCJD individuals to transmit the prion to recipients of blood or blood products.[164,166] In February 2004, an article in Lancet reported the first possible case of transfusion-transmitted vCJD.[168]

Currently, there is no reliable diagnostic test that can detect asymptomatic individuals. Therefore, donor deferral policy of high-risk individuals is used for prevention.[164,165]

Pathogen Inactivation

The safety of the blood supply in the United States has improved greatly over the years, with improved screening of donors and testing of the blood product. However, pathogen inactivation methods have been developed to account for residual risks associated with serologic window periods, virus variants, laboratory errors, and for organisms for which testing is not performed routinely.[169] The possibility of newly emerging pathogens also exists as evidenced by WNV that can be transmitted by blood.

Plasma Derivatives

Heat inactivation, the first pathogen inactivation intervention, has been used since 1948 to treat albumin.[3] Even before the introduction of third-generation testing for HBsAg, heat inactivation prevented the transmission of HBV. Albumin has never transmitted HIV or HCV, even though plasma was collected, processed, and used before the availability of tests for HIV and HCV. Both viruses are heat-labile.[170]

In 1973 third-generation assays for HBsAg were licensed.

Only one case of HBV transmission by immune globulin was ever documented before then. Intramuscular immune globulin has never transmitted HIV or HCV. All immunoglobulin plasma pools were screened for HBsAg, and only those that were negative were used. Viral inactivation included cold-ethanol (Cohn-Oncley) fractionation and anion-exchange chromotography (for one IV immunoglobulin). However, in 1994 the FDA required viral clearance processing or proof of absence of HCV by NAT testing because of outbreaks of HCV from anion-exchange chromatography in Ireland and Germany that did not use a viral clearance procedure. NAT is now used in the processing of all source plasmas.[3]

Coagulation factors had a high rate of viral transmission until the early 1980s. Chronic hepatitis was the biggest problem until HIV emerged. More than 50 percent of all hemophiliacs receiving concentrates became infected with HIV. Since 1987 these clotting factors have become very safe with implementation of a variety of virus inactivation steps, and there have been no cases of HIV transmission. Today, all manufacturers use methods that either remove the virus or inactivate it. The lipid-enveloped viruses, HIV, HBV, HCV, HTLV, EBV, CMV, HHV-6 and HHV-8, are all inactivated by use of organic solvents and detergents. This process is not effective with non-lipid-enveloped viruses such as HAV and parvovirus B-19.[3,170]

The current risk of enveloped virus transmission is very low because of the combination of treatments such as heat-treatment, solvent/detergent treatment, and purification with monoclonal antibodies. With the exception of one case of HCV transmission in IV immune globulin in 1994, there have been no cases of HBV, HCV, or HIV since 1985 by any U.S. licensed plasma derivative.[170]

Cellular Components

Pathogen inactivation using psorlen activated by ultraviolet light has been tested with platelet concentrates. It has been shown to inactivate cell-associated viruses, cell-free viruses, and selected prokaryotic organisms. Whether this process will work against intracellular bacterial organisms has not been established. Questions related to toxicity and damage to platelet function have not been answered.[171]

PEN110 (INACTINE, V.I. Technologies, Watertown, MA) is a water-soluble cation that can diffuse through the cell membrane. Once PEN110 enters the cell, it uses nucleic acids as a substrate for both activation and reaction and disrupts transcription and replication of the pathogen genome.[169] Toxicity appears to be low enough for human use, but saline washings ensure low levels of the compound. In clinical trials, tested RBCs survived normally after 28 days of storage and subjects exposed to small volumes of PEN110-treated RBCs tolerated them well.[172] In recent studies, PEN110 was found to be capable of effectively inactivating WNV, enveloped and nonenveloped viruses, bacteria, and parasites.[173–175]

Quarantine and Recipient Tracing (Look Back)

All blood banks and transfusion services are required to have a process to detect, report, and evaluate any complication of transfusion including recipient development of HBV, HCV,

HIV, and/or HTLV. There must be an established method to notify donors of any abnormality with the predonation evaluation, laboratory testing, or recipient follow-up. A report should be submitted to the collecting agency when the recipient of a blood component develops a TTD.[1]

Current donations that test positive for HBV, HCV, HIV, and/or HTLV cannot be used for transfusion.[1] All prior donations from these donors become suspect. The timeline and standards using the look-back procedure for identification of recipients of a component from the implicated donation or other donations by the same donor differ depending on the disease. Any prior components still in date must be quarantined, and the disposition depends on results of licensed supplemental tests.[3,176–180]

If on recipient follow-up, it is noted that a patient developed HBV, HCV, HIV, or HTLV after receiving a single unit from one donor, that donor is permanently deferred. If the recipient received donations from several donors, all donors do not have to be excluded. These implicated donors may be called in for retesting. If a donor has been implicated in more than one case of TTD, this donor should be retested and possibly permanently deferred.[3] Once a donor has been implicated in a TTD, other recipients of a component from the suspected donor should be contacted. The donor must be placed on the appropriate donor deferral list if subsequent tests are positive.[3]

Autologous donations positive for HBV, HCV, HIV, HTLV, and/or syphilis can be used. If they are not transfused at the collecting facility, the collecting facility must notify the transfusion service. Testing must be repeated every 30 days on at least the first unit to be shipped. Information about abnormalities must be transmitted to the patient and the patient's physician.[1]

Any fatalities due to a TTD must be reported to the Director of the Center for Biologics Evaluation and Research within 1 working day, followed by a written report within 7 days.[176]

SUMMARY CHART:
Important Points to Remember (MT/MLT)

➤ The first and most important step in ensuring that transfused blood will not transmit a pathogenic virus is careful selection of the donor.

➤ HAV is usually spread by the fecal/oral route in communities where hygiene is compromised.

➤ On infection with HBV, the first serologic marker to appear is HBsAg, followed by HBeAg and IgM anti-HBc within the first few weeks of exposure.

➤ HBIG is an immune globulin prepared from persons with a high titer of anti-HBs and is used to provide passive immunity to health-care workers and others who are exposed to patients with HBV infection.

➤ A combined vaccine for HAV and HBV is available to provide immunity.

➤ HDV infection is common among drug addicts and can

occur simultaneously with HBV infection; diagnosis depends on finding anti-HDV or HDV RNA in the serum.

➤ Of all HCV infections, 60 to 70 percent are asymptomatic. With the implementation of NAT testing for HCV, the window period has been reduced to 10 to 30 days.

➤ HCV is the leading cause of liver transplants in the United States.

➤ Diagnosis of HIV-1 and HIV-2 infection is dependent on the presence of antibodies to both envelope and core proteins; HIV-positive persons with fewer than 200 CD4+ T cells per μL are considered to have AIDS in the absence of symptoms.

➤ Transfusion-associated CMV infection is a concern for seronegative allogeneic organ transplant recipients and the fetus. Reactivation of a latent infection can occur when an individual becomes severly immunocompromised.

➤ The risk of CMV infection to low birth-weight neonates is not as great as it was in the past due to better transfusion techniques and management of their conditions.

➤ The WB confirmation test detects the presence of anti-HIV and determines with which viral proteins the antibodies react.

➤ The window period for HIV can be shortened by use of the polymerase chain reaction, which detects HIV infection before tests for antigen or antibody are positive.

➤ There are no proven cases of transfusion transmitted classical CJD; vCJD may be transmitted by eating contaminated beef, and one case of transfusion-transmission has been reported

➤ Bacterial contamination is the most frequent cause of transfusion-transmitted infection.

➤ Because routine screening for parasitic infections is not currently available, many blood banks have added questions to their donor questionnaire that address topics associated with risk for parasitic infection.

➤ Pathogen inactivation methods are under development to remove the residual risk of transfusion–associated disease due to the window period, virus variants, laboratory mistakes, and new, emerging diseases.

➤ Look-back is a process mandated by the FDA that directs collection facilities to notify donors who test positive for viral markers, to notify prior recipients of components of the possibility of infection, and to quarantine or discard implicated components currently in inventory.

REVIEW QUESTIONS

1. The fecal/oral route is common in transmission of which of these hepatitis viruses?
   a. HAV
   b. HBV
   c. HDV
   d. HCV

2. Which of the following is the component of choice for a low birth-weight infant with a hemoglobin of 8 g/dL if the mother is anti-CMV negative?
   a. Whole blood from a donor with anti-CMV
   b. RBCs from a donor who is anti-CMV negative
   c. Leukoreduced platelets
   d. Solvent detergent–treated plasma

3. Which of the following tests is useful to confirm that a patient or donor is infected with HCV?
   a. ALT + anti-HBc
   b. Anti-HIV 1/2
   c. Lymph node biopsy
   d. RIBA

4. Currently, which of the following does the AABB consider to be the most significant infectious threat from transfusion?
   a. Bacterial contamination
   b. CMV
   c. Hepatitis
   d. HIV

5. Which of the following is the most frequently transmitted virus from mother to fetus?
   a. HIV
   b. Hepatitis
   c. CMV
   d. EBV

6. Jaundice due to HAV is seen most often in the:
   a. adolescent
   b. adult
   c. child younger than 6 years old
   d. newborn

7. Currently, steps taken to reduce transfusion-transmitted CMV include:
   a. plaque reduction neutralization test
   b. NAT testing
   c. leukoreduction
   d. mini-pool screening

8. HBV remains infectious on environmental surfaces for 1:
   a. day
   b. week
   c. month
   d. year

9. HBV is transmitted most frequently:
   a. by needle sharing among IV drug users
   b. through blood transfusions
   c. by unknown methods
   d. by sexual activity

10. Which of the following is the most common cause of chronic hepatitis, cirrhosis, and hepatocellular carcinoma in the United States?
    a. HAV
    b. HBV
    c. HCV
    d. HDV

11. The first retrovirus to be associated with human disease was:
    a. HCV
    b. HIV
    c. HTLV-I
    d. WNV

12. All of the following statements are true concerning WNV except:
    a. 1 in 500 infections results in severe neurologic disease.
    b. Severe disease occurs most frequently in the over-50 age group.
    c. Deaths occur more often in those over 65 years who present with encephalitis.
    d. Fatalities occur in approximately 38 percent of infected individuals.

13. The primary host for WNV is:
    a. birds
    b. horses
    c. humans
    d. bats

14. Tests for WNV include all of the following except:
    a. ELISA
    b. NAT
    c. Plaque reduction neutralization test
    d. immunofluorescent antibody assay

15. Individuals exposed to EBV maintain an asymptomatic latent infection in:
    a. B cells
    b. T cells
    c. all lymphocytes
    d. monocytes

16. Fifth disease is caused by:
    a. CMV
    b. EBV
    c. parvovirus B19
    d. HTLV-II

17. Transient aplastic crisis can occur with:
    a. parvovirus B19
    b. WNV
    c. CMV
    d. EBV

18. Reasons why syphilis is so rare in the United States blood supply include all of the following except:
    a. 4°C storage conditions
    b. donor questionnaire
    c. short spirochetemia
    d. NAT testing

19. Nucleic acid amplification testing for HIV was instituted in donor testing protocols to:
    a. identify donors with late-stage HIV who lack antibodies
    b. confirm the presence of anti-HIV in asymptomatic HIV-infected donors
    c. reduce the window period by detecting the virus earlier than other available tests
    d. detect antibodies to specific HIV viral proteins including anti-p24, anti-gp41, and anti-gp120

20. Screening for HIV is performed using the following technique:
    a. Enzyme immunoassay
    b. WB
    c. Immunofluorescent antibody assay
    d. NAT

21. The first form of pathogen inactivation was:
    a. chemical
    b. heat
    c. cold-ethanol fractionation
    d. anion-exchange chromotography

22. What is the most common parasitic complication of transfusion?
    a. *Babesia microti*
    b. *Trypanosoma cruzi*
    c. *Plasmodium* species
    d. *Toxoplasma gondii*

23. Which organism has a characteristic C- or U-shape on stained blood smears?
    a. *Trypanosoma cruzi*
    b. *Plasmodium vivax*
    c. *Plasmodium falciparum*
    d. *Babesia microti*

24. Which transfusion-associated parasite may have asymptomatic carriers?
    a. *Babesia microti*
    b. *Trypanosoma cruzi*
    c. *Plasmodium* species
    d. All of the above

25. Which disease is naturally caused by the bite of a deer tick?
    a. Chagas disease
    b. Babesiosis
    c. Malaria
    d. Leishmaniasis

REFERENCES

1. American Association of Blood Banks: Standards for blood banks and transfusion services, ed 22, 2003.
2. Centers for Disease Control and Prevention: Detection of West Nile virus in blood donations—United States, 2003. MMWR 52:769, 2003.
3. Brecher, ME (ed): Technical manual, ed 14. American Association of Blood Banks, Bethesda, MD, 2002.
4. Goodman, C et al: Ensuring blood safety and availability in the US: Technological advances, cost, and challenges to payment—final report. Transfusion 43 (8 suppl):3S, 2003.
5. Abbott Diagnostics Educational Services: Hepatitis learning guide. Abbott Diagnostics, Abbott Park, IL, 1998.
6. Miller, LE. Serology of viral infections. In: Stevens CD (ed): Clinical immunology and serology: A laboratory perspective, ed 2. FA Davis Company, Philadephia, 2003, p 324.
7. Halasz R, et al: GB virus C/hepatitis G virus. Scand J Infect Dis 33:572, 2001.
8. Koff RS: Hepatitis A. Lancet 351:1643, 1998.
9. Centers for Disease Control and Prevention: Frequently asked questions. Available from http://www.cdc.gov/ncidod/diseases/hepatitis/a/faqa.htm [accessed August 12, 2003].
10. Centers for Disease Control and Prevention. Viral hepatitis: historical perspec-

tive. Available from http://www.cdc.gov/ncidod/diseases/hepatitis/slideset/index.htm [accessed August 18, 2003.]

11. Lemon, SM: Type A viral hepatitis: Epidemiology, diagnosis, and prevention. Clin Chem 43;8:1494, 1994.

12. Lemon, SM: The natural history of hepatitis A: The potential for transmission by transfusion of blood or blood products. Vox Sang 67 (suppl 4):19, 1994.

13. Soucie, JM, et al: Hepatitis A virus infections associated with clotting factor concentrates in the United States. Transfusion 38:573, 1998.

14. Hollinger, FB, et al: Post transfusion hepatitis type A. JAMA 250:2312, 1983.

15. Mannucci, PM, et al: Transmission of hepatitis B to patients with hemophilia by factor VIII concentrates treated with organic solvent and detergent to inactivate viruses. Ann Intern Med 120:1, 1994.

16. Centers for Disease Control and Prevention: Notice to readers: FDA approval for a combined hepatitis A and B vaccine. MMWR 50: 806, 2001. Available at http://www.cdc.gov/mmwr/preview/mmwrhtml/mm5037a4.htm [Accessed September 24, 2003].

17. Centers for Disease Control and Prevention: Hepatitis B virus. Available at http://www.cdc.gov/ncidod/diseases/hepatitis/slideset/index.htm [Accessed September 24, 2003].

18. Centers for Disease Control and Prevention. Hepatitis B and refugees: A clinical perspective. Available at http://www.cdc.gov/ncidod/diseases/hepatitis/slideset/index.htm [Accessed September 21, 2003].

19. Busch MP, et al: Nucleic acid amplification testing of blood donors for transfusion-transmitted diseases: Report of the interorganizational task force on nucleic acid amplification testing of blood donors. Transfusion 40:143, 2000.

20. American Association of Blood Banks: All about blood. Available at http://www.aabb.org/All_About_Blood/FAQs/aabb_faqs.htm [Accessed September 24, 2003].

21. Lox, ASF, and McMahon, BF: AASLD practice guidelines: Chronic hepatitis B. Hepatology 34:1225, 2001.

22. Marcellin, P, et al: Adefovir dipivoxil for treatment of hepatits B antigen-positive chronic hepatitis B. N Engl J Med. 348:808, 2003.

23. Hoofnagle, JH: Therapy for acute hepatitis C. N Engl J Med 345:1495, 2001..

24. Hofer, H, et al: Spontaneous viral clearance in patients with acute hepatitis C can be predicted by repeated measurements of serum viral load. Hepatology 37:60, 2003.

25. Rigamonti, C, et al: Moderate alcohol consumption increases oxidative stress in patients with chronic hepatitis C. Hepatology 38:42, 2003.

26. Gerlach, JT: Acute hepatitis C: High rate of both spontaneous and treatment-induced viral clearance. Gastroenterology 125:80, 2003.

27. Delwart, E, et al: First case of HIV transmission by an RNA-screened blood donation. Presented at the 9th Conference on Retroviruses and Opportunitic Infections, Seattle, 2–14–02. Available at http://www.retroconference.org/2002/Posters/13519.pdf [Accessed September 17, 2003].

28. Centers for Disease Control and Prevention: Hepatitis D virus. Available at http://www.cdc.gov/ncidod/diseases/hepatitis/slideset/index.htm [Accessed September 21, 2003].

29. Khuroo, MS, et al: Incidence and severity of viral hepatitis in pregnancy. Am J Med 70:252, 1981.

30. Tsega, E, et al: Acute sporadic viral hepatitis in Ethiopia: Causes, risk factors, and effects on pregnancy. Clin Infect Dis 14: 961, 1992.

31. Centers for Disease Control and Prevention: Hepatitis E virus. Available at http://www.cdc.gov/ncidod/diseases/hepatitis/slideset/index.htm [Accessed September 21, 2003].

32. Krawczynski, D, et al: Hepatitis E. Infect Dis Clin North Am. 14: 669, 2000.

33. Arankalle, VA, et al: Role of immune serum globulins in pregnant women during an epidemic of hepatitis E. J Viral Hepat 5:199, 1998.

34. Leary, TP, et al: Sequence and genomic organization of GBV-C: A novel member of the Flaviviridae associated with human non A-E hepatitis. J Med Virol 48:60, 1996.

35. Nunnari, G, et al: Slower progression of HIV-1 infection in persons with GB virus C coinfection correlates with an intact T-helper 1 cytokine profile. Ann Intern Med 139: 26, 2003.

36. Alter, H, et al: The incidence of transfusion associated hepatits G vrus infection and its relation to liver disease. N Engl J Med 336: 747, 1997.

37. Heringlake, S, et al: Association between fulminant hepatic failure and a strain of GB virus C. Lancet 348: 1626, 1996.

38. Halasz, R, et al: GB virus C/hepatitis G virus. Scand J Infect Dis 33: 572, 2001.

39. Linnen, J, et al: Molecular cloning and disease association of hepatitis G virus: A transfusion-transmissible agent. Science 271: 505, 1996.

40. Alonso-Rubiano, E, et al: Hepatitis G virus in clotting factor concentrates. Haemophilia 9:110, 2003.

41. Scallan, MF, et al: Sexual transmission of Gb virus C /hepatitis G virus. J Med Virol 55, 203, 1998.

42. Sathar, MA, et al: GB virus C/hepatitis G virus (GBV-C/HGV): Still looking for a disease. Int J Exper Pathol 81: 305, 2000.

43. Inaba, N, et al: Maternal-infant transmission of hepatitis G virus. Am J Obstet Gynecol 177:1537, 1997.

44. Zanetti, AR, et al: Multicenter trial on mother-infant transmission of GBV-virus. J Med Virol 54: 107, 1998.

45. Tacke, M, et al: Humoral immune response to the E2 protein of the hepatitis G virus is associated with long-term recovery from infection and reveals a high frequency of hepaitis G virus exposure among healthy blood donors. Hepatology 26:1626, 1997.

46. Jarvis, LM, et al: The effect of treatment with alpha-interferon on hepatitis G/GBV-C viraemia. The CONSTRUCT Group. Scand J Gastroenterol 33:195, 1999.

47. Mushahwar, IK: Commentary: Recently discovered blood-borne viruses: Are they hepatitis viruses or merely endosymbionts? J Med Virol 62:399, 2000.

48. Simmonds, P, et al: Detection of a novel DNA virus (TTV) in blood donors and blood products. Lancet 352:191, 1998.

49. Yoshida, H, et al: Poor association of TT virus viremia with hepatocellular carcinoma. Liver 20:247, 2000.

50. Sugiyama, K, et al: Prevalence to TTV DNA among children with a history of transfusion or liver disease. J Med Virol 60:172, 2000.

51. Takahashi, K, et al: Identification of a new human DNA virus (TTV-like minivirus, TLMV) intermediately related to TT virus and chicken anemia virus. Arch Virol 145:979, 2000.

52. Canada Communicable Disease Report: Is there an association between SEN virus and liver disease? Reviewing the evidence. Available from http://www.hc-sc.gc.ca/pphb-dgspsp/publicat/ccdr-rmtc/02vol28/dr2807ea.html [Accessed August 15, 2003].

53. Kobayashi N, et. Al: Clinical significance of SEN virus infection in patients on maintenance haemodialysis. Nephrol Dial Transplant 18:348, 2003.

54. Centers for Disease Control: Pneumocystis carinii pneumonia among persons with hemophilia A. MMWR 31:652, 1982.

55. Ragni, MV et al: 1986 update of HIV seroprevalence, seroconversion, AIDS incidence, and immunologic correlates of HIV infection in patients with hemophilia A and B. Blood 70:786, 1987.

56. Turgeon, ML: Immunology and Serology in Laboratory Medicine, ed 3. Mosby, St. Louis, 2003, p. 331.

57. Fleming, P, et al: HIV prevalence in the United States, 2000. [Abstract]. In Program and Abstracts of the 9th Conference on Retroviruses and Opportunitic Infections, Seattle, 2–14–02.

58. Centers for Disease Control and Prevention: HIV/AIDS surveillance report. 13:6, 2001.

59. Centers for Disease Contol and Prevention: HIV and its transmission. Available at www.cdc.gov/hiv/pubs/facts/transmission.htm [Accessed September 25, 2003].

60. American Red Cross: Nucleic acid testing: Investigations to detect blood viruses more effectively fact sheet. Available at www.redcross/services/biomed/blood/supply/nucleic.html [Accessed September 25, 2003].

61. Goodnough, LT, et al: Transfusion medicine. First of two parts—blood transfusion [comment]. NEJM 340:438, 1999.

62. FDA approves first nucleic acid test (NAT) system to screen whole blood donors for infections with human immunodeficiency virus (HIV) and hepatitis C virus (HCV). Rockville (MD):FDA 2002 Feb 28. Available at http://www.fda.gov/

63. Ling AE, et al: Failure of routine HIV-1 tests in a case involving transmission with preseroconversion blood components during the infectious window period [comment]. JAMA 284: 210, 2000

64. Bush, M: FDA NAT implementation workshop. Rockville, MD, FDA; 2001 Dec.

65. Centers for Disease Control: Advancing HIV prevention: New strategies for a changing epidemic—United States, 2003. MMWR 52:229, 2003.

66. Manns, A, Hisada, M, and La Grenade, L: Human T-lymphotropic virus type I infection. Lancet 353:1951, 1999.

67. Matsuoka, M: Human T-cell leukemia virus type I and adult T-cell leukemia. Oncogene 22:5131, 2003.

68. Nagai, M, and Osame, M: Human T-cell lymphotropic virus type I and neurological diseases. J Neurovirol 9:228, 2003.

69. Murphy, EL, et al: Increased prevalence of infectious diseases and other adverse outcomes in human T lymphotropic virus types I- and II-infected blood donors. J Infect Dis 176:1468, 1997.

70. American Association of Blood Banks: Dual enzyme immuno assay (EIA) approach for deferral and notification of anti-HTLV-I/II EIA reactive donors. Association Bulletin #99–9. Available at http://www.aabb.org/members_only/archives/association_bulletins/ab99–9.htm. [Accessed on September 25, 2003].

71. FDA, Center for Biologics Evaluation and Research: Guidance for industry: donor screening for antibodies to HTLV-II, August 1997. Available at http://www.fda.gov/cber/gdlns/htlv-ii.pdf [Accessed September 25, 2003].

72. Campbell, GL, et al: West Nile virus. Lancet of Infectious Disease Nile 2:519, 2002.

73. Prowse, CV: An ABC for West Nile virus. Transfus Med 13:1, 2003.

74. Petersen, LR, Marfin, AA, and Gubler, DJ: West Nile virus. JAMA 290:524, 2003.

75. Centers for Disease Control and Prevention: West Nile virus 2002 case count. Available at http://www.cdc.gov/ncidod/dvbid/westnile/surv&controlCaseCount02.htm [Accessed September 25, 2003].

76. Centers for Disease Control and Prevention: Provisional surveillance summary of the West Nile virus epidemic—United States, January–November 2002. MMWR 51:1129, 2002

77. Centers for Disease Control and Prevention: West Nile virus 2003 human cases as of September 24, 2003, 3am MDT.Available at http://www.cdc.gov/ncidod/dvbid/westnile/surv&controlCaseCount03.htm [Accessed September 25, 2003].

78. Centers for Disease Control and Prevention: Acute flaccid paralysis snydrome associated with West Nile virus infection—Mississippi and Louisiana, July–August 2002. MMWR 51: 825, 2002.

79. Centers for Disease Control and Prevention: West Nile virus: Overview of West Nile virus. Available at http://www.cdc.gov/ncidod/dvbid/westnile/qa/overview.htm [Accessed September 25, 2003].

80. Petersen, LR, Marfin, AA: West Nile virus: A primer for clinicians. Ann Intern Med 137:173, 2002.

81. Centers for Disease Control and Prevention: West Nile virus: West Nile virus is

a risk you can do something about with a few simple steps. Available at http://www.cdc.gov/ncidod/dvbid/westnile/brochure.htm [Accessed September 20, 2003].

82. Huang, C, et al: First isolation of West Nile virus from a patient with encephalitis in the United States. Emerg Infect Dis 8:1367, 2002.

83. FDA, guidance for industry, recommendations for the assessment of donor suitability and blood and blood product safety in cases of known or suspected West Nile virus infection. Available at http://www.fda.gov/cber/gdlns/wnvguid.htm [Accessed September 20, 2003].

84. FDA Consumer Magazine, Jan–Feb 2003. Available at http://www.fda.gov/fdac/features/2003/103_virus.html [Accessed September 20, 2003].

85. Centers for Disease Control and Prevention: Public health dispatch: Investigations of West Nile virus infections in recipients of blood transfusion. MMWR 51:973, 2002.

86. Centers for Disease Control and Prevention: Public health dispatch: West Nile virus infection in organ donor and transplant recipients—Georgia and Florida, 2002. MMWR 51:790, 2002.

87. Centers for Disease Control and Prevention: Investigations of West Nile virus infections in recipient or organ transplantation and blood transfusion. MMWR 51:833, 2002.

88. Centers for Disease Control and Prevention: Possible West Nile virus transmission to an infant through breast feeding—Michagan, 2002. MMWR 51:877, 2002

89. Centers for Disease Control and Prevention: Intrauterine West Nile virus infection—New York, 2002. MMWR 51:1135, 2002.

90. Centers for Disease Control and Prevention: Laboratory-acquired West Nile virus infections—United States, 2002. MMWR 51:1133, 2002.

91. Centers for Disease Control and Prevention: Epidemic/Epizootic West Nile virus in the United States: guidelines for surveillance, prevention, and control, rev 3, 2003. Available at: http://www.cdc.gov/ncidod/dvbid/westnile/lab_guidance.htm [Accessed September 20, 2003].

92. American Association of Blood Banks: Recommended guidance for reporting West Nile viremic blood donors to state and/or local public health departments and reporting donors who subsequently develop West Nile virus illness to blood collection facilities. AABB Association Bulletin 03–08, June 25, 2003. Available at http://www.aabb.org/members_only/archives/association_bulletins/ab03–8.htm [Accessed September 21, 2003].

93. Centers for Disease Control and Prevention: Dispatch: Update: Detection of West Nile virus in blood donations—United States, 2003. MMWR 52:2003.

94. Centers for Disease Control and Prevention: Cytomegalovirus (CMV) infection. October 26, 2002. Available at http://www.cdc.gov/ncidod/diseases/cmv.htm [Accessed September 25, 2003].

95. Laupacis, A, et.al: Conference report: Prevention of posttransfusion CMV in the era of universal WBC reduction: A consensus statement. Transfusion 41:560, 2001.

96. Ely, JW, Yankowitz, J, and Bowdler, NC: Evaluation of pregnant women exposed to respiratory viruses. Available at http://www.aafp.org/afp/20000515/3065.html [Accessed September 25, 2003].

97. Roback, JD, et al: Multicenter evauation of PCR methods for detecting CMV DNA in blood donors. Transfusion 41:1249, 2001.

98. Roback, JD, Bray, RA, and Hillyer, CD. Longitudinal monitoring of WBC subsets in packed RBC units after filtration: Implications for transfusion transmission of infections. Trasnfusion 40:500, 2000.

99. Centers for Disease Control and Prevention: Epstein-Barr virus and infectious mononucleosis. November 26, 2002. Available at http://www.cdc.gov/ncidod/diseases/ebv.htm [Accessed September 25, 2003].

100. Tattevin, P, et al: Transfusion-related infectious mononucleosis. Journal of Infectious Disease 34:777, 2002.

101. Epstein, MA, Achong, BG, and Barr, YM: Virus particles in cultured lymphoblasts from Burkitts's lymphoma. Lancet 1:702, 1964.

102. zur Hausen H, et al: EBV DNA in biopsies of Burkitt tumours and anaplastic carcinomas of the nasopharynx. Nature 228:1056, 1970.

103. Greenspan JS, et al: Replication of Epstein-Barr virus within the epithelial cells of oral "hairy" leukoplakia, an AIDS-associated lesion. N Engl J Med 313:1564, 1985.

104. Jones JF, et al: T-cell lymphomas containing Epstein-Barr viral DNA in patients with chronic Epstien-Barr virus infections. N Engl J Med 318:733, 1988.

105. Weiss, LM, et al: Detection of Epstein-Barr viral genomes in Reed-Sternberg cells on Hodgkin's disease. N Engl J Med: 320-502, 1989.

106. Resnick, L, et al: Regression of oral hairy leukoplakia after orally administered acyclovir therapy. JAMA 259:384, 1998.

107. Straus, SE, et al: Epstein-Barr virus infections: Biology, pathogenesis, and management. Ann Intern Med 118:45, 1993.

108. Brown, KE, Young, NS, and Barbosa, LH: Parvovirus B19: Implications for transfusion medicine. Transfusion 41:130, 2001.

109. Brown, KE, et al: Resistance to parvovirus B19 infection due to lack of virus receptor (erythrocyte P antigen). New Engl J Med 330:1192, 1994.

110. Centers for Disease Control and Prevention: Parvovirus B19 (Fifth Disease). Available at http://www.cdc.gov/ncidod/diseases/parvovirus/B19.htm [Accessed September 25, 2003].

111. Centers for Disease Control and Prevention: Parvovirus B19 infection and pregnancy. Available at http://www.cdc.gov/ncidod/diseases/parvovirus/B19&preg.htm [Accessed September 25, 2003].

112. Kawamura, M, et. al: Frequency of transmission of human parvovirus B19 infection by fibrin sealant used during thoracic surgery. Ann Thoracic Surg 73:1098, 2002.

113. Weimer, T, et al: High-titer screening PCR: A successful strategy for reducing the parvovirus B19 load in plasma pools for fractionation. Transfusion 41:1500, 2001.

114. Koenigbauer, UF, Eastlund, T, and Day, JW: Clinical illness due to parvovirus B19 infection after infusion of solvent/detergent-treated pooled plasma. Transfusion 40:1203, 2000.

115. Cohen BJ, et al: Chronic anemia due to parvovirus B19 infection in a bone marrow transplant patient after platelet transfusion. Transfusion 37:947, 1997.

116. Hayakawa, F, et al: Life-threatening human parvovirus B19 infection transmitted by IV immune globulin. Br J Haematol 118:1187, 2002.

117. Blood Products Advisory Committee: 75th Meeting, December 12, 2002. Parvovirus B19 NAT for whole blood and source plasma. Available at http://www.fda.gov/ohrms/dockets/ac/02/briefing/3913b1_Parvovirus%20B19%20NAT%20Dec%202002%20Yu.htm [Accessed September 25, 2003].

118. Tabor, E, and Epstein, JS: NAT screening of blood and plasma donations: Evolution of technology and regulatory policy. Transfusion 42:1230, 2002.

119. Campadelli-Fiume, G, et al: Synopses: Human herpesvirus 6: An emerging pathogen. Emerg Infect Dis 5:353 1999.

120. Pellett, PE, et al: Multicenter comparison of serologic assays and estimation of human herpesvirus 8 seroprevalence among US donors. Transfusion 43:1260, 2003.

121. Luppi M, et al: Molecular evidence of organ-related transmission of Kaposi sarcoma-associated herpesvirus or human herpesvirus-8 in transplant patients. Blood 96:3279, 2000.

122. AABB Comments Before the Blood Products Advisory Committee: Bacterial contamination of platelet components, December 12, 2002. Available at http://www.aabb.org/Members_Only/Archives/Regulatory_and_Legislative_Services/bactcontbpac121202.htm. (Accessed on Oct. 4, 2004).

123. Lee, J-H: Bacterial contamination of platelets workshop. Sept. 1999. Available at http://www.fda.gov/cber/minutes/bact092499.pdf [Accessed on September 25, 2003].

124. Kuehnert, MJ, et al: Transfusion-transmitted bacterial infection in the United States, 1998 through 2000. Transfusion:41;1493, 2001

125. Centers for Disease Control: Red blood cell transfusions contaminated with *Yersinia enterocolitica*—United States, 1991–1996, and initiation of a national study to detect bacteria-associated transfusion reactions. MMWR 46:553, 1997.

126. Centers for Disease Control: The BaCon study: Bacterial contamination. Available at http://www.cdc.gov/ncidod/hip/bacon/ [Accessed September 3, 2003].

127. Kunishima, S, et al: Presence of *Propionibacterium acnes* in blood components. Transfusion 41:1126, 2001.

128. Dodd, R, and Lipton, KS: Guidance on implementation of new bacterial reduction and detection standards. Available at http://www.aabb.org/members_only/archives/association_bulletins/ab03–10.htm [Accessed September 4, 2003].

129. AABB Comments Before the Blood Products Advisory Committee: Platelet pooling. May 14, 2003. Available at http://www.aabb.org/Members_Only/Archives/Regulatory_and_Legislative_Services/ppbpac031403.htm [Accessed September 26, 2003].

130. de Korte, D, et al: Diversion of first blood volume results in a reduction of bacterial contamination for whole blood collections. Vox Sang 83:13, 2002.

131. Stevens, CD. Spirochete diseases. In Clinical Immunology and Aerology: A Laboratory Perspective, ed 2. FA Davis Company, Philadephia, 2003: p 294.

132. Current utility of screening blood donors for antibodies to syphilis: The FDA framework. 67th BPAC Meeting, September 15, 2000. Available at http://www.fda.gov/ohrms/dockets/ac/00/backgrd/3649b2c/sld001.htm [Accessed September 5, 2003].

133. BPAC Atatement of the American Association of Blood Banks Before the Blood Products Advisory Committee, September 14, 2000. Available at http://www.aabb.org/pressroom/press_releases/prbpacsyph091400.htm [Accessed September 5, 2003].

134. Orton, S, et al: Prevalence of circulating T. pallidum in STS+/FTA-Abs+ blood donors (abstract). Transfusion 39 (suppl):2S, 1999.

135. Markowitz ,L: Presentation to the FDA Blood Products Advisory Committee, September 15, 2000. Available at http://www.fda.gov/ohrms/dockets/ac/00/backgrd.1364962.htm. (Accessed 10/4/04)

136. McQuiston, JH, et al: Transmission of tick-borne agents of disease by blood transfusion: A review of known and potential risks in the United States. Transfusion 40:274, 2000.

137. Lux, JZ, et al: Transfusion-associated babesiosis after heart transplant. Emerg Infect Dis 9:116, 2003.

138. Herwaldt, BL, et al: Transfusion-transmitted babesiosis in Washington state: First reported case caused by a WA1-type parasite. J Infect Dis 175:1259, 1997.

139. Kjemtrup, AM, et al: Investigation of transfusion transmission of a WA1-type babesial parasite to a premature infant in California. Transfusion 42:1482, 2002.

140. Herwaldt, BL, et al: Transmission of *Babesia microti* in Minnesota through four blood donations from the same donor over a 6-month period. Transfusion 42:1154, 2002.

141. Cable, RG, and Trouern-Trend, J. Tickborne Infections: Blood Safety and Surveillance. Marcel Dekker, New York, 2001, p 399.

142. Linden, JV, et al: Transfusion-associated transmission of babesiosis in New York state. Transfusion 40:285, 2000.

143. Spiess, BD, et al: Perioperative transfusion medicine. Williams & Wilkins, Baltimore, 1998, p 101.

144. Lettau, LA. Nosocomial transmission and infection control aspects of parasitic and ectoparasitic diseases part II. Infect Control Hosp Epidemiol 12:111, 1991.

145. Garcia, LS, and Bruckner, DA: Diagnostic Medical Parasitology, ed 2. American Society for Microbiology, Washington, D.C., 1993, p 113; p 169.
146. Pantanowitz, L, et al: Laboratory diagnosis of babesiosis. Lab Med 32:84, 2001.
147. Jocoby, GA, et al: Treatment of transfusion-transmitted babesiosis by exchange transfusion. New Engl J Med 303:1098, 1980.
148. Evenson, DA, et al: Therapeutic apheresis for babesiosis. J Clin Apher 13:32, 1998.
149. McCullogh, J: Transfusion Medicine. McGraw-Hill, New York, 1998, p 377.
150. Pan, AA, and Winkler, MA: The threat of Chagas' disease in transfusion medicine. Lab Med 28:269, 1997.
151. Leiby, DA, et al: Prospective evaluation of a patient with *Trypanosoma cruzi* infection transmitted by transfusion. New Engl J Med 341:1237, 1999.
152. Moraes-Souza, H, and Bordin JO: Strategies for prevention of transfusion-associated Chagas' disease. Transfus Med Rev 10:161, 1996.
153. Kirchhoff, LV: Is *Trypanosoma cruzi* a new threat to our blood supply? Ann Intern Med 111:773, 1989.
154. Hagar, JM, and Rahimtoola, SH: Chagas' heart disease in the United States. New Engl J Med 325:763,1991.
155. Leiby, DA, et al: Seroepidemiology of *Trypanosoma cruzi,* etiologic agent of Chagas' disease, in US blood donors. J Infect Dis 176:1047, 1997.
156. Kirchhoff, LV: American trypanosomiasis (Chagas' disease): A tropical disease now in the United States. New Engl J Med 329:639, 1993.
157. Leiby, DA, et al: *Trypanosoma cruzi* in a low-to-moderate-risk blood donor population: Seroprevalence and possible congenital transmission. Transfusion 39:310, 1999.
158. Grant, IH, et al: Transfusion-associated acute Chagas' disease acquired in the United States. Ann Intern Med 111:849,1989.
159. Nickerson, P, et al: Transfusion-associated *Trypanosoma cruzi* infection in a non-endemic area. Ann Intern Med 111:851, 1989.
160. Markell, EK, et al: Medical Parasitology, ed 8. W.B. Saunders, Philadelphia, 1999, p 90. p 134.
161. Centers for Disease Control and Prevention: Transfusion-transmitted malaria—Missouri and Pennsylvania, 1996–1998. MMWR 48:253, 1999.
162. Hoffman, SL, et al: Progress toward malaria pre-erythrocytic vaccines. Science 252:520, 1991.
163. Siddiqui, WA: Where are we in the quest for vaccines for malaria? Drugs 41:1,1991.
164. Cervenakova L, et al: Factor VIII and transmissible spongiform encephalopathy: The case for safety. Haemophilia 8(2),63–75.
165. World Health Organization: Variant Cruetzfeldt-Jakob disease. Fact Sheet No. 180. Revised November 2002. Available at http://www.who.int/mediacentre/factsheets/fs180/en/print.html [Accessed September 26, 2003].
166. Centers for Disease Control and Prevention: Bovine spongiform encephalophthy and Creutzfeldt-Jakob disease. Questions and answers regarding Creutzfeldt-Jakob disease infection-control practices. Available at http://www.cdc.gov/ncidod/diseases/cjd/cjd_inf_ctrl_qa.htm [Accesssed September 26, 2003].
167. McKnight, C: Clinical implications of bovine spongiform encephalopathy. Clin Infect Dis 32:1726, 2001.
168. Llewelyn, CA, et al: Possible transmission of variant Creutzfeldt-Jakob disease by blood transfusion. Lancet 363: 417, 2004.
169. Purmal, A, et al: Process for the preparation of pathogen-inactivated RBC concentrates by using PEN110 chemistry: Preclinical studies. Transfusion 42:139, 2002.
170. Tabor, E: The epidemiology of virus transmission by plasma derivatives: Clinical studies verifying the lack of transmission of hepatitis B and C viruses and HIV type 1. Transfusion 39:1160, 1999.
171. Belanger, KJ, et al: Psoralen photochemical inactivation or *Orientia tsutsugamushi* in platelet concentrates. Transfusion 40:1503, 2000.
172. AuBuchon, JP, et al: Production of pathogen-inactivated RBC concentrates using PEN110 chemistry: A phase I clinical study. Transfusion 42:146, 2002.
173. Lazo, A, et al: Broad-spectrum virus reduction in red cell concentrates using INACTINE™ PEN110 chemistry. Vox Sang 83:313, 2002.
174. Ohagen, A, et al: Inactivation of HIV in blood. Transfusion 42:1308, 2002.
175. Zavizion, B, et al: Prevention of *Yersinia enterocolitica, Pseudomonas fluorescens,* and *Pseudomonas putida* outgrowth in deliberately inoculated blood by a novel pathogen-reduction process. Transfusion 43:135- 2003.
176. Food and Drug Administration: Notification process for transfusion related fatalities and donation related Deaths, May 15, 2002. Available at http://www.fda.gov/cber/transfusion.htm. [Accessed September 18, 2003].
177. Food and Drug Administration: Memorandum: Recommendations for the quarantine and disposition of units from prior collections from donors with repeatedly reactive screening tests for hepatitis B virus (HBV), hepatitis C virus (HCV), and human T-lymphotropic virus type I (HTLV-I), July 19, 1996. Available at http://www.fda.gov/cber/memo.htm [Accessed September 18, 2003].
178. Food and Drug Administration. Draft guidance for industry: Current good manufacturing practice for blood and blood components: (1) quarantine and disposition of units from prior collections from donors with repeatedly reactive screening tests for antibody to hepatitis C virus (HCV); (2) supplemental testing and the notification of consignees and blood recipients of donor test results for anti-HCV, June 17, 1999. Available at http://www.fda.gov/cber/blood/bldguid.htm [Accessed September 18, 2003].
179. Food and Drug Administration: Guidance for Industry: Donor screening for antibodies to HTLV-II, August 15, 1997. Available at http://www.fda.gov/cber/blood/bldguid.htm [Accessed September 18, 2003].
180. Food and Drug Administration: Current good manufacturing practice for blood and blood components: Notification of consignees receiving blood and blood components at increased risk for transmitting HIV infection, July 19, 1996. Available at http://www.fda.gov/cber/bldmem/mem71996.pdf [Accessed September 18, 2003].

twenty

Hemolytic Disease of the Newborn and Fetus

Melanie S. Kennedy, MD, and Dave Krugh, MT(ASCP)SBB, CLS, CLCP (NCA)

OBJECTIVES

On completion of this chapter, the learner should be able to:

1. State the definition and characteristics of hemolytic disease of the newborn and fetus (HDN).
2. Describe the role of the technologist in the diagnosis and clinical management of HDN.
3. Compare and contrast ABO versus Rh HDN in terms of:
   - Pathogenesis
   - Incidence
   - Blood types of mother and baby
   - Severity of disease
   - Laboratory data: anemia, direct antiglobulin test (DAT), and bilirubin
   - Prevention and treatment
4. Define Rh-immune globulin and describe its function.
5. Identify the indications and contraindications for administration of Rh-immune globulin.
6. List the tests used for detection of fetomaternal hemorrhage.
7. Outline the protocol for testing of maternal and cord blood in cases of suspected HDN.
8. Given maternal and infant ABO blood group phenotypes, state the possible ABO donor blood group(s) that would be selected for an exchange transfusion. Be specific as to donor blood groups for both the plasma and red blood cells (RBCs).
9. State the blood components and the maximum age of the donor unit preferred for intrauterine or exchange transfusions.
10. State with whom (mother and child) the crossmatch for a neonate must always be compatible.

HDN is the destruction of the RBCs of the fetus and neonate by antibodies produced by the mother. The mother can be stimulated to form the antibodies by previous pregnancy or transfusion and sometimes during the second and third trimester of pregnancy. Previously, about 95 percent of the cases were caused by antibodies in the mother directed against the Rh antigen D. The incidence of the disease caused by anti-D has steadily decreased since 1968 with the introduction of Rh immune globulin (RhIg). Rh(D) incompatibility is common, although other RBC incompatibilities are surpassing D in frequency at referral centers.[1] Because Rh(D) incompatibility was the major concern for many years, the diagnosis and treatment of HDN caused by anti-D has been the emphasis of much investigation. These findings can be applied to other clinically significant RBC antibodies causing HDN, except for ABO antibodies, which will be discussed separately.

In addition to the use of RhIg, many other advances have been made in the diagnosis and treatment of HDN. Ultrasonography, Doppler assessment of middle cerebral artery peak velocity,[2] percutaneous umbilical blood sampling, allele-specific gene amplification studies on fetal cells in amniotic fluid, and intrauterine transfusion have greatly increased the success of accurately diagnosing and adequately treating this disease.

Etiology

Historical Overview

Although the changes in the fetus and newborn were noted as early as the 17th century, it was not until 1939 that Levine and Stetson reported a transfusion reaction from transfusing the husband's blood to a postpartum woman. They postulated that the mother had been immunized to the father's antigen through a fetal maternal hemorrhage. The antigen was later found to be Rh(D).

Disease Mechanism

HDN is caused by the destruction of the RBCs of the fetus by antibodies produced by the mother. Only antibodies of the immunoglobulin G (IgG) class are actively transported across the placenta; other classes, such as IgA and IgM, are not. Most IgG antibodies are directed against bacterial, fungal, and viral antigens, so the transfer of IgG from the mother to the fetus is beneficial. However, in HDN, the antibodies are directed against those antigens on the fetal RBCs that were inherited from the father.

Rh HDN

Usually in Rh(D) HDN, the Rh-positive firstborn infant of an Rh-negative mother is unaffected because the mother has not yet been immunized. During gestation, and particularly at delivery when the placenta separates from the uterus, variable numbers of fetal RBCs enter the maternal circulation (see **Color Plate 15**). These fetal cells, carrying D antigen inherited from the father, immunize the mother and stimulate the production of anti-D. Once the mother is immunized to D antigen, all subsequent offspring inheriting the D antigen will be affected. The maternal anti-D crosses the placenta and binds to the fetal Rh-positive cells **(Fig. 20–1)**. The sensitized RBCs are destroyed by the fetal reticuloendothelial system, resulting in anemia.

Factors Affecting Immunization and Severity

Antigenic Exposure

Fetomaternal hemorrhage during pregnancy can cause significant increases in maternal antibody titers, leading to increasing severity of HDN. Transplacental hemorrhage of fetal RBCs into the maternal circulation occurs in up to 7 percent of women during gestation as determined by the acid-elution method for fetal hemoglobin.[3] Using molecular

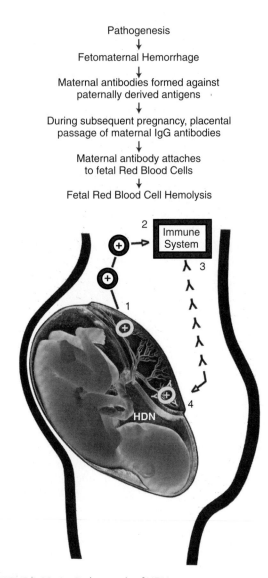

Pathogenesis
↓
Fetomaternal Hemorrhage
↓
Maternal antibodies formed against paternally derived antigens
↓
During subsequent pregnancy, placental passage of maternal IgG antibodies
↓
Maternal antibody attaches to fetal Red Blood Cells
↓
Fetal Red Blood Cell Hemolysis

■ FIGURE 20–1   Pathogenesis of HDN.

biology techniques, 50[4] to 65 percent[5] of pregnant women have nucleated fetal cells in their peripheral blood. In addition, interventions such as amniocentesis and chorionic villus sampling, as well as trauma to the abdomen, may increase the risk of fetomaternal hemorrhage. At delivery, the incidence is more than 50 percent. In the majority of cases, the volume of fetomaternal hemorrhage is small; however, as little as 1 mL of fetal RBCs can immunize the mother.

The number of antigenic sites on the fetal RBCs corresponds to heterozygous RBCs, because all fetal antigens incompatible with the mother have been inherited from the father, who can give only one set of genes to the fetus.

Host Factors

The ability of individuals to produce antibody in response to antigenic exposure varies, depending on complex genetic factors. In Rh-negative individuals who are transfused with 200 mL of Rh-positive RBCs, about 85 percent form anti-D.[6] Nearly all the nonresponders will fail to produce anti-D even with repeated exposures to Rh-positive blood. On the other hand, the risk of immunization is only about 9 percent for an Rh-negative mother after an Rh-positive pregnancy if RhIg is not administered.

Immunoglobulin Class

Immunoglobulin class and subclass of the maternal antibody affect the severity of the HDN. Of the immunoglobulin classes (IgG, IgM, IgA, IgE, and IgD), only IgG is transported across the placenta. The active transport of IgG begins in the second trimester and continues until birth. The IgG molecules are transported via the Fc portion of the antibodies.

Of the four subclasses of IgG antibody, IgG_1 and IgG_3 are more efficient in RBC hemolysis than are IgG_2 and IgG_4. Therefore, the subclass(es) in the mother can affect the severity of the hemolytic disease. All subclasses are transported across the placenta.

Antibody Specificity

Of all the RBC antigens, D is the most antigenic. For this reason, only Rh-negative blood is transfused to Rh-negative females of childbearing potential. Other antigens in the Rh system, such as C, E, and c, are also potent immunogens (although less than D) (Table 20–1). These other Rh antibodies have been associated with moderate to severe cases of HDN. Anti-E and anti-c have caused severe HDN requiring intervention and treatment.

Of the non–Rh-system antibodies, anti-Kell is considered the most clinically significant in its ability to cause HDN. Kell antigens are present on immature erythroid cells in the bone marrow, so severe anemia occurs not only from destruction of circulating RBCs but also from precursors. Almost any IgG RBC antibody is capable of causing HDN, although the disease caused by these antibodies is usually mild to moderate in severity. Nevertheless, all pregnant women with IgG RBC antibodies should be followed closely for HDN. Vengelen-Tyler[7] lists and discusses 64 different RBC antibody specificities reported to cause HDN.

Influence of ABO Group

When the mother is ABO-incompatible with the fetus (major incompatibility), the incidence of detectable fetomaternal hemorrhage is decreased. Investigators noted many years ago that the incidence of D immunization is less in mothers with major ABO incompatibility with the fetus. The ABO incompatibility protects somewhat against Rh immunization apparently by the hemolysis in the mother's circulation of ABO-incompatible D-positive fetal RBCs before the D antigen can be recognized by the mother's immune system.

Pathogenesis

Hemolysis, Anemia, and Erythropoiesis

Hemolysis occurs when maternal IgG attaches to specific antigens of the fetal RBCs (see Fig. 20–1). The antibody-coated cells are removed from the circulation by the macrophages of the spleen. The rate of destruction depends on antibody titer and specificity as well as on the number of antigenic sites on the fetal RBCs. Destruction of fetal RBCs and the resulting anemia stimulate the fetal bone marrow to produce RBCs at an accelerated rate, even to the point that immature RBCs (erythroblasts) are released into the circulation. The term "erythroblastosis fetalis" was used to describe this finding. When the bone marrow fails to produce enough RBCs to keep up with the rate of RBC destruction, erythropoiesis outside the bone marrow is increased in the hematopoietic tissues of the spleen and liver. The spleen and liver become enlarged (hepatosple-nomegaly), resulting in portal hypertension and hepatocellular damage.

Severe anemia along with hypoproteinemia caused by decreased hepatic production of plasma proteins leads to the development of high-output cardiac failure with generalized edema, effusions, and ascites, a condition known as hydrops fetalis. In severely affected cases, hydrops can develop at 18 to 20 weeks' gestation. In the past, hydrops fetalis was almost uniformly fatal; currently, most fetuses with this condition can be treated successfully.[1,8]

The process of RBC destruction goes on even after such an infant is delivered alive—in fact, as long as maternal antibody persists in the newborn infant's circulation. The rate of RBC destruction after birth decreases because no more maternal antibody is entering the infant's circulation through the placenta. However, IgG is distributed both extravascularly and intravascularly and has a half-life of 25 days, so antibody binding and hemolysis of RBCs continue for several days to weeks after delivery.

Bilirubin

The RBC destruction releases hemoglobin, which is metabolized to bilirubin (Fig. 20–2). This bilirubin is called "indirect" because indirect methods are required to measure the bilirubin in the laboratory. The indirect bilirubin is transported across the placenta and conjugated in the maternal liver to "direct" bilirubin. The conjugated bilirubin is then excreted by the mother. Although levels of total bilirubin in the fetal circulation and in the amniotic fluid may be elevated, these do not cause clinical disease in the fetus. However, after birth, accumulation of metabolic by-products of RBC destruction can become a severe problem for the newborn infant. The newborn liver is unable to conjugate bilirubin efficiently, especially in premature infants. With moderate to severe hemolysis, the unconjugated or indirect bilirubin can reach levels toxic to the infant's brain (generally, more than 18 to 20 mg/dL) and, if left untreated, can cause kernicterus or permanent damage to parts of the brain.

TABLE 20–1   ANTIBODIES IDENTIFIED IN PRENATAL SPECIMENS

	Cause of HDN	
Common	**Rare**	**Never**
anti-D	anti-Fy[a]	anti-Le[a]
anti-D + C	anti-s	anti-Le[b]
anti-D + E	anti-M	anti-I
anti-C	anti-N	anti-IH
anti-E	anti-S	anti-P₁
anti-c	anti-JK[a]	
anti-e		
anti-K		

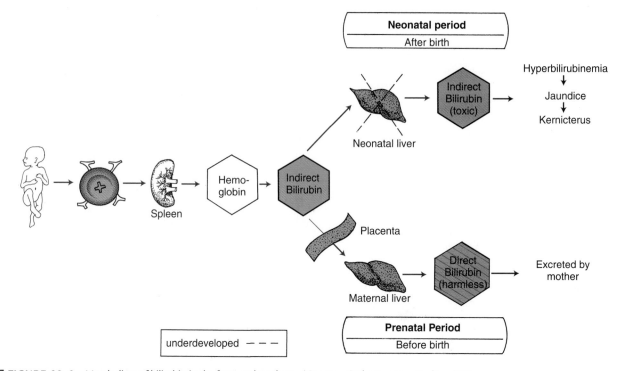

■ FIGURE 20–2 Metabolism of bilirubin in the fetus and newborn. (Courtesy Ortho Systems, Raritan, NJ.)

Diagnosis and Management

The diagnosis and management of HDN require close cooperation among the pregnant patient, her obstetrician, her spouse or partner, and the personnel of the clinical laboratory performing the serologic testing. Serologic and clinical tests performed at appropriate times during the pregnancy can accurately determine the level of antibody in the maternal circulation, the potential of the antibody to cause HDN, and the severity of RBC destruction during gestation (**Fig. 20–3**). If clinical and serologic data indicate that the fetus is becoming severely anemic, interventions such as intrauterine transfusion can be used to treat the anemia and prevent the development of severe disease.

Serologic Testing

The recommended obstetric practice is to perform a type-and-antibody screen at the first prenatal visit, preferably during the first trimester. At that time, the pregnant woman can be asked about previous pregnancies and their outcomes and prior transfusions. Previous severe disease and poor outcome predict similar findings in the current pregnancy. Although antibody titers are useful in assessing the extent of intrauterine fetal anemia during the first affected pregnancy, antibody titers are less predictive in subsequent pregnancies.

ABO and Rh Testing

The testing of the specimen should include ABO and Rh testing for D antigen. The Rh test may include weak D if no immediate reaction with anti-D occurs. The patient's RBCs should also be tested simultaneously with Rh control reagent while testing for weak D to avoid false-positive reac-

tions due to spontaneous agglutination of RBCs. If the patient is weak D–positive, the patient can be considered Rh-positive. In rare cases, weak D phenotype is caused by missing a part of the Rh antigen (see Chapter 7). Such patients may produce anti-D as an alloantibody, which has been reported to cause HDN.

Antibody Screen

The test conditions must be able to detect clinically significant IgG alloantibodies that are reactive at 37°C and in the antiglobulin phase. At least two separate reagent screening cells, covering all common blood group antigens (preferably homozygous), should be used. An antibody-enhancing medium such as polyethylene glycol (PeG) or low ionic strength saline solution (LISS) can increase sensitivity of the assay. Many prenatal patients produce clinically insignificant antibodies, such as anti-Le^a and/or anti-Le^b. Therefore, many experts in prenatal and perinatal immunohematology recommend omitting immediate spin and room temperature incubation phases and using anti-IgG rather than polyspecific antiglobulin reagent. These steps reduce detection of IgM antibodies, which cannot cross the placenta.

If the antibody screen is nonreactive, repeat testing is recommended before RhIg therapy in Rh-negative prenatal patients and in the third trimester if the patient has been transfused or has a history of unexpected antibodies.[9]

Antibody Identification

If the antibody screen is reactive, the antibody identity must be determined. Follow-up testing will depend on the antibody specificity. Cold reactive IgM antibodies such as anti-I, anti-IH, anti-Le^a, anti-Le^b, and anti-P_1 can be ignored. As

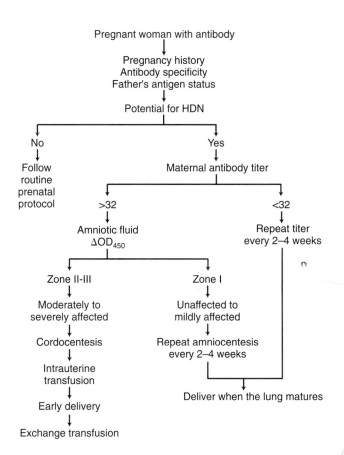

Pregnant woman with antibody

Pregnancy history
Antibody specificity
Father's antigen status

Potential for HDN

No → Follow routine prenatal protocol

Yes → Maternal antibody titer

>32 → Amniotic fluid ΔOD$_{450}$

<32 → Repeat titer every 2–4 weeks

Zone II-III → Moderately to severely affected → Cordocentesis → Intrauterine transfusion → Early delivery → Exchange transfusion

Zone I → Unaffected to mildly affected → Repeat amniocentesis every 2–4 weeks

Deliver when the lung matures

■ **FIGURE 20–3** Diagnosis and management of HDN. (Modified from Kennedy, MS: Essentials of immunohematology and blood therapy. In Zuspan, FP, and Quilligan, EJ (eds): Practical Manual of Obstetrical Care. CV Mosby, St Louis, 1982, p 119, with permission.)

mentioned earlier, Lewis system antibodies are rather common in pregnant women but have not been reported to cause HDN.

Antibodies such as anti-M and anti-N can be IgM or IgG or a combination of both. Both anti-M and anti-N can cause mild to moderate HDN, although rarely. To establish the immunoglobulin class, the serum can be treated with sulfhydryl reagents such as dithiothreitol or 2-mercaptoethanol and then retested with appropriate controls. The J-chain of IgM antibodies will be destroyed by this treatment; IgG antibodies will remain reactive.

Many Rh-negative pregnant women have weakly reactive anti-D, particularly during the third trimester. Most of these women have received RhIg (see subsequent text), either after an event with increased risk of fetomaternal hemorrhage or at 28 weeks' gestation (antenatal). The passively administered anti-D will be weakly reactive in testing and will remain demonstrable for 2 months or longer. This must be distinguished from active immunization. A titer higher than 4 almost always indicates active immunization. With a titer under 4, active immunization cannot be ruled out but is less likely.

If the antibody specificity is determined to be clinically significant and the antibody is IgG, further testing is required. Other than anti-D, the most common and most significant antibodies are anti-K, anti-E, anti-c, anti-C, and anti-Fy^a (see **Table 20–1**).

Paternal Phenotype

A specimen of the father's blood should be obtained and tested for the presence and zygosity of the corresponding antigen. If the mother has anti-D and the father is D-positive, a complete Rh phenotype can help determine his chance of being homozygous or heterozygous for the D antigen by determining the most probable genotype. The information is helpful in determining further testing of the mother and in counseling her about potential treatment plans and complications of HDN.

In cases of antibody specificity other than D, testing the father can save a great deal of time, expense, and worry if he is shown to lack the corresponding antigen. For example, only 10 percent of the random population is positive for the Kell antigen. The mother must be counseled in private as to the paternity of the fetus to assure accurate paternal phenotyping.

Amniocyte Testing

If the mother has anti-D and the father is most likely to be heterozygous for the D antigen, amniocentesis can be done as early as 10 to 12 weeks' gestation to determine whether the amniocytes carry the gene for the D antigen. Amniocytes can be similarly tested for the genes coding c, e, C, E, K, Fy^a, Fy^b, Jk^a, Jk^b, and M.

Antibody Titers

The relative concentration of all antibodies capable of crossing the placenta and causing HDN must be determined by antibody titration. The patient serum is serially diluted and tested against appropriate RBCs to determine the highest dilution at which a reaction occurs. The method must include the indirect antiglobulin phase using anti-IgG reagent. The result is expressed as either the reciprocal of the titration endpoint or as a titer score.

The titration must be performed exactly the same way each time the patient's serum is tested. The recommended method is the saline antiglobulin test, with 60-minute incubation at 37°C and the use of anti-IgG reagent. The RBCs used for each titration should have the same genotype (preferably from the same donor and homozygous for the antigen of interest), approximately the same storage time, and the same concentration. The first serum specimen should be frozen and run in parallel with later specimens. Only a difference of greater than 2 dilutions, or a score change of more than 10, is considered a significant change in titer.

Each laboratory should develop its own critical titer levels by reviewing the outcome of a number of pregnancies complicated by HDN. In general, a titer of 16 to 32 is considered significant. If the initial titer is 16 or higher, a second titer should be done at about 18 to 20 weeks' gestation. A titer reproducibly and repeatedly at 32 or above represents an indication for amniocentesis or percutaneous umbilical blood sampling between 18 and 24 weeks' gestation.

When the titer is less than 32, the titer should be repeated at 4-week intervals, beginning at 18 to 20 weeks' gestation, and every 2–4 weeks during the third trimester. The last determination should be made within a week of the expected date of delivery.

Antibody titer alone cannot predict severity of HDN.[9] In some sensitized women, the antibody titer may remain moderately high throughout pregnancy while the fetus is becoming more severely affected. Similarly, a previously sensitized woman may have consistently high antibody titer whether pregnant or not and, if pregnant, whether the fetus is Rh-positive or Rh-negative. In others, the titer may rise rapidly, which portends increasing severity of HDN. However, antibody titers consistently below the laboratory's critical titer throughout the pregnancy reliably predict an unaffected or mild-to-moderately affected fetus.

Titration studies at time of delivery are not recommended as they provide no clinically useful information.

Amniocentesis and Cordocentesis

At about 18 to 20 weeks' gestation, further diagnosis and treatment are begun. Patients with a history of a severely affected fetus or early fetal death may require earlier intervention. Under ultrasound guidance, amniocentesis is done to assess the status of the fetus. The concentration of bilirubin pigment in the amniotic fluid correlates with the extent of fetal anemia. The amniotic fluid is subjected to a spectrophotometric scan at steadily increasing wavelengths, so that the change in the optical density ($\triangle$OD) at 450 nm (the absorbance of bilirubin) can be calculated.[10] The measurement is plotted on the Liley graph **(Fig. 20–4)** according to gestational age. The optical density of the amniotic fluid is high in the second trimester and steadily decreases until delivery. An increasing or unchanging $\triangle$OD 450 nm as pregnancy proceeds predicts worsening of the fetal hemolytic disease and the need for frequent monitoring and intervention if indicated. Values in zone III indicate severe and often life-threatening hemolysis (fetal hemoglobin less than 8 g/dL) and require urgent intervention. In zone II, most fetuses have moderate disease that may require intervention. Values in zone I predict mild or no disease, which do not require intervention.

Amniotic fluid analysis, although a useful tool, represents an indirect prediction of the severity of fetal anemia. Recent advances in sonography have allowed clinicians to obtain a sample of the fetal blood through a procedure called percutaneous umbilical blood sampling, or cordocentesis. Using high-resolution ultrasound with color Doppler enhancement of blood flow, the umbilical vein is visualized at the level of the cord insertion into the placenta **(Fig. 20–5)**. A needle is inserted into the umbilical vessel, and a sample of the fetal blood is obtained. The fetal blood sample can then be tested for hemoglobin, hematocrit, blood type, antigen phenotype, and DAT.

Intrauterine Transfusion

Intervention in the form of intrauterine transfusion becomes necessary when one or more of the following conditions exists:

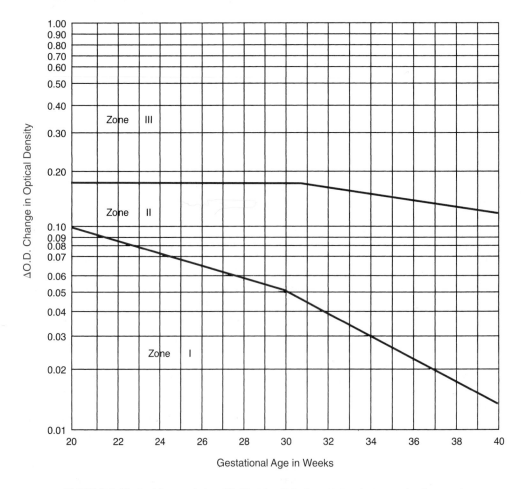

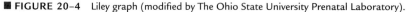

■ **FIGURE 20–4**   Liley graph (modified by The Ohio State University Prenatal Laboratory).

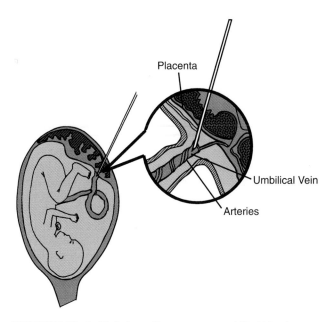

■ FIGURE 20–5 Technique of percutaneous umbilical blood sampling (cordocentesis). (From Ludomirski,[8] p 91, with permission.)

1. Amniotic fluid △OD 450 nm results are in high zone II or in zone III.
2. Cordocentesis blood sample has hemoglobin level less than 10 g/dL.
3. Fetal hydrops is noted on ultrasound examination.

Intrauterine transfusion can be performed intraperitoneally by injecting the RBCs into the fetal peritoneal cavity where the RBCs can be absorbed into the circulation. More recently, cordocentesis has been used to inject donor RBCs directly into the fetal umbilical vein.[8] The goal of intrauterine transfusion is to maintain fetal hemoglobin above 10 g/dL. Once intrauterine transfusion is initiated, the procedure is repeated every 2 to 4 weeks until 34 to 36 weeks' gestation or until the fetal lungs are mature, when early delivery can be performed. The initial intrauterine transfusion is rarely performed after 34 weeks' gestation. Intrauterine transfusion can suppress the fetal bone marrow from producing RBCs. During the first weeks after birth, the infant may require RBC transfusion.

Amniocentesis and cordocentesis have several risks, among them trauma to the placenta, which may cause increased antibody titers because of antigenic challenge to the mother through fetomaternal hemorrhage.

Early Delivery

Early delivery was used for many years for moderate-to-severe disease to interrupt the transport of maternal antibody to the fetus and to allow exchange transfusion. With the use of repeated and frequent IV transfusions in the fetus, delivery before the lungs are mature can usually be avoided.

Phototherapy

After delivery, phototherapy with ultraviolet light can be used to change unconjugated bilirubin to biliverdin. In infants with mild-to-moderate hemolysis, the use of phototherapy

may avoid the need for exchange transfusion to treat hyper-bilirubinemia and anemia.

Serologic Testing of the Newborn Infant

ABO Grouping

ABO antigens are not fully developed in newborn infants and thus may give weaker reactions than in older children and adults. In addition, the infant does not have his or her own isoagglutinins but may have those of the mother, so reverse grouping cannot be used to confirm the ABO group.

Rh Typing

Rarely, the infant's RBCs can be heavily antibody-bound with maternal anti-D causing a false-negative Rh type, or what has been called blocked Rh. An eluate from these RBCs will reveal anti-D, and typing of the eluted RBCs will show reaction with anti-D.

DAT

The most important serologic test for diagnosis of HDN is the DAT with anti-IgG reagent. The positive test result indicates antibody is coating the infant's RBCs; however, the strength of the reaction does not correlate well with the severity of the HDN. A positive test result may be found in infants without clinical or other laboratory evidence of hemolysis (e.g., mother received RhIg). A positive DAT may invalidate Rh typing.

Elution

The routine preparation of an eluate of all infants with a positive DAT result is unnecessary. Elution in cases of known HDN and post-natal ABO incompatibility (see discussion later) is not needed, because eluate results do not change therapy. The preparation of an eluate may be helpful when the cause of HDN is in question. As noted earlier, the resolution of a case of blocked Rh will require an eluate.

Newborn Transfusions

The newborn infant may receive small aliquot transfusions or exchange transfusions, or both. Small aliquots can be used to correct anemia when the bilirubin level is not high enough to warrant an exchange transfusion. Exchange transfusions are used primarily to remove high levels of unconjugated bilirubin and thus to prevent kernicterus. Premature newborn infants are more likely than full-term infants to require exchange transfusions for elevated bilirubin because their livers are less able to conjugate bilirubin. Other advantages of exchange transfusion include the removal of part of the circulating maternal antibody, removal of sensitized RBCs, replacement of incompatible RBCs with compatible RBCs, and suppression of erythropoiesis (**Box 20–1**). All of these help interrupt the bilirubin production caused by hemolysis; however, the suppression of erythropoiesis by small aliquot or exchange transfusions may cause anemia to occur after the immediate neonatal period.

Although full-term newborn infants normally have rather high hemoglobin levels (14 to 20 g/dL), a level below 12 g/dL

BOX 20–1
Beneficial Effects of Exchange Transfusion

- Removal of bilirubin
- Removal of sensitized RBCs
- Removal of incompatible antibody
- Replacement of incompatible RBCs with compatible RBCs
- Suppression of erythropoiesis (reduced production of incompatible RBCs)

is considered anemia that may require transfusion. Lower than 8 g/dL is considered severe anemia and corresponds to zone III of the Liley graph, whereas 8 to 12 g/dL corresponds to zone II. A cord blood sample closely correlates with the levels during gestation. If the obstetrician infuses placenta blood after delivery, the infant's hemoglobin level will be higher than that of the cord blood sample.

Selection of Blood

Most centers treating HDN use group O RBCs for intrauterine as well as neonatal transfusions. The RBCs must be antigen-negative for the respective antibodies. Donors are usually cytomegalovirus (CMV)-negative as well. Physicians in these centers are usually transfusing neonates for other indications, such as RBC replacement for blood samples taken for laboratory tests. This allows a small inventory of group O CMV-negative donor units to be set aside for intrauterine and neonatal transfusions. Rh-negative units are selected for fetuses and neonates whose blood types are unknown or are Rh-negative.

For intrauterine transfusion, the hematocrit level of the RBCs should be greater than 70 percent, because of the small volume transfused and the need to correct severe anemia.

For exchange transfusions, one practice is to prepare RBCs from whole blood units and then replace the plasma with group AB plasma to reduce the amount of blood group antibodies transfused. This procedure may be avoided if both the neonate and the mother are the same ABO group.

Blood transfused to the fetus and premature infant should also be irradiated to prevent graft-versus-host disease (see Chapter 16). It is also recommended that blood for exchange transfusion not contain hemoglobin S, because the decreased oxygen tension that may occur early in the neonatal period may cause hemoglobin S–containing blood to sickle. Traditionally, blood units less than 7 days from collection from the donor are selected. Special circumstances, such as the need for units of mother's blood when high-incidence

BOX 20–2
Additional Indications for RhIg

- Amniocentesis
- Chorionic villus sampling
- Abortion (spontaneous and induced)
- Ectopic pregnancy
- Abdominal trauma
- Accidental or inadvertent transfusion
- Abdominal trauma
- Greater than 40 weeks gestation

antibodies are involved, have shown that older blood units can be safe and effective for the newborn.

RhIg

Active immunization induced by RBC antigen can be prevented by the concurrent administration of the corresponding RBC antibody. This principle has been used to prevent immunization to D antigen by the use of high-titered RhIg.

During pregnancy and delivery, mixing of fetal and maternal blood occurs. If the mother is Rh-negative and the fetus is Rh-positive, the mother has up to a 9 percent chance of being stimulated to form anti-D[3]. As little as 1 mL of fetal RBCs can elicit a response. Before delivery, the risk of sensitization is 1.5 to 1.9 percent of susceptible women, indicating that a significant amount of fetal RBCs can enter the maternal circulation during pregnancy.[1] However, the greatest risk of immunization to Rh is at delivery.

Mechanism of Action

The administered RhIg attaches to the fetal Rh-positive RBCs in the maternal circulation (Color Plate 16). The antibody-coated RBCs are removed by the macrophages in the maternal spleen. The RBC antigens are thus unavailable for dendritic cells to present antigen to T helper cells.[11] The amount of antibody necessary to prevent alloimmunization has been determined experimentally and is known to be less than that required to saturate all D antigen sites.

Indications

Antenatal

Because of the known risk of Rh immunization during pregnancy, RhIg should be given early in the third trimester, or at about 28 weeks' gestation. The dose does not pose a risk to the fetus, inasmuch as this amount will cause a titer of only 1 or 2 in the mother.[1] However, a positive DAT result may be observed in the newborn. **Box 20–2** lists additional indications.

Postpartum

The Rh-negative nonimmunized mother should receive RhIg soon after delivery of an Rh-positive infant. Based on experiments conducted many years ago, the recommended interval is within 72 hours after delivery. Even if more than 72 hours have elapsed, RhIg should still be given, inasmuch as it may be effective and is not contraindicated.

The mother should be D-negative **(Fig. 20–6)**. The infant should be D-positive or weak D-positive. If the type of the infant is unknown (e.g., if the infant is stillborn), RhIg should also be administered. Antibody titers are not recommended because the amount of circulating RhIg does not correlate with effectiveness of the immune suppression or with the amount of fetomaternal hemorrhage.[12]

The half-life of IgG is about 25 days, so only about 10 percent of the antenatal dose will be present at 40 weeks' gestation. It is essential that the anti-D from antenatal RhIg present at delivery not be interpreted erroneously as active rather than passive immunization. Omission of the indicated dose after delivery may lead to active immunization.

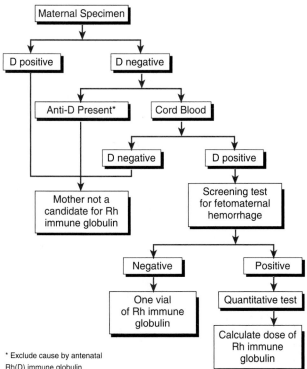

* Exclude cause by antenatal
Rh(D) immune globulin

■ **FIGURE 20–6**   Decision tree for the indications and dose of RhIg as determined by laboratory test results. If the cord or neonatal blood specimen is unavailable, assume the fetus is D-positive. (Modified from Kennedy,[13] p 235, with permission.)

Dose and Administration

The regular-dose vial in the United States contains sufficient anti-D to protect against 15 mL of packed RBCs or 30 mL of whole blood. This is equal to 300 μg of the World Health Organization (WHO) reference material. The regular-dose vial in the United Kingdom contains about 100 μg, which appears to be adequate for postpartum prophylaxis. The total fetal blood volume is estimated to be less than 5 mL at 12 weeks. The microdose can be used for abortions and ectopic pregnancies before the 12th week of gestation.[13]

An IV preparation of RhIg is approved for use in the United States. This product also contains 300 μg in each vial and can be administered either intramuscularly or intravenously. Additional manufacturing steps are required to allow IV use, so the product is more expensive.

Massive fetomaternal hemorrhages of more than 30 mL of whole blood occur in less than 1 percent of deliveries. These massive hemorrhages can lead to immunization if adequate RhIg is not administered. A maternal sample should be obtained within 1 hour of delivery to test for massive fetomaternal hemorrhage by a screening test, such as the rosette technique. If positive, quantitation of the hemorrhage must be done by Kleihauer-Betke or similar test or by flow cytometry. In the Kleihauer-Betke test, a maternal blood smear is treated with acid and then stained with counterstain. Fetal cells contain fetal hemoglobin (Hgb F) that is resistant to acid and will remain pink. The maternal cells will appear as ghosts. After 2000 cells are counted, the percentage of fetal cells is

determined, and the volume of fetal hemorrhage is calculated using the formula:

$$\frac{\text{Number of fetal cells} \times \text{Maternal blood volume}}{\text{Number of maternal cells}} =$$

Volume of fetomaternal hemorrhage

The calculated volume of fetomaternal hemorrhage is then divided by 30 to determine the number of required vials of RhIg. A simpler way to calculate the dose is to multiply the fetal cell percentage by 50, which gives the volume of fetomaternal hemorrhage in milliliters. If needed, additional vials of RhIg should be administered within 72 hours of delivery or as soon as possible.

The RhIg must be injected according to the product label. The IV product can also be given intramuscularly. The intramuscular form must be given intramuscularly only. IV injections of intramuscular preparations can cause severe anaphylactic reactions because of the anticomplementary activity of these products. RhIg also contains IgA and may be contraindicated in patients with anti-IgA and IgA deficiency who have had anaphylactic reactions to blood products.

Other Considerations

RhIg is of no benefit once a person has been actively immunized and has formed anti-D. Care must be taken, however, to distinguish women who have been passively immunized by antenatal administration of RhIg from those who have been actively immunized by exposure to Rh-positive RBCs.

Care must also be taken so that fetal Rh-positive RBCs in the maternal circulation are not interpreted as maternal, because then the mother would be assumed erroneously to be weak D-positive. The difference is distinguished by a quantitative test such as the Kleihauer-Betke.

RhIg is not indicated for the mother if the infant is found to be D-negative and weak D-negative. The blood type of fetuses in abortions, stillbirths, and ectopic pregnancies usually cannot be determined; therefore, RhIg should be administered in these circumstances. RhIg must not be given to the newborn infant.

There is no risk of transmission of the viral diseases hepatitis A and B and human immunodeficiency virus.[14] RhIg has been reported to contain antibody to hepatitis A and B and thus may cause false-positive hepatitis serology.[15]

ABO HDN

ABO incompatibility between the mother and newborn infant can cause HDN. Maternal ABO antibodies that are IgG can cross the placenta and attach to the ABO-incompatible antigens of the fetal RBCs. However, destruction of fetal RBCs leading to severe anemia is extremely rare. More commonly, the disease is manifested by the onset of hyperbilirubinemia and jaundice within 12 to 48 hours of birth. The increasing levels of bilirubin can be treated with phototherapy. Severe cases requiring exchange transfusion are extremely rare. A comparison of ABO versus Rh HDN is shown in **Table 20–2**.

As the incidence of HDN caused by Rho(D) has declined, ABO incompatibility has become the most common cause of

TABLE 20–2   Comparison of ABO Versus Rh HDN

Characteristic	ABO	Rh
First pregnancy	Yes	Rare
Disease predicted by titers	No	Yes
Antibody IgG	Yes (anti-A,B)	Yes (anti-D, etc.)
Bilirubin at birth	Normal range	Elevated
Anemia at birth	No	Yes
Phototherapy	Yes	Yes
Exchange transfusion	Rare	Sometimes
Intrauterine transfusion	None	Sometimes
Spherocytosis	Yes	Rare

HDN. Statistically, mother and infant are ABO-incompatible in one of every five pregnancies.

Factors Affecting Incidence and Severity

ABO antibodies are present in the sera of all individuals whose RBCs lack the corresponding antigen. These antibodies, the result of environmental stimulus, occur more frequently as high-titered IgG antibodies in group O individuals than in group A or B individuals. Hence, ABO HDN is nearly always limited to A or B infants of group O mothers with potent anti-A,B. Most occur in group A infants in white populations. In the black population, however, group B infants are more often affected, and the overall incidence of ABO HDN is several times greater than in other groups.

The mother's history of prior transfusions or pregnancies seems unrelated to the occurrence and severity of the disease. Thus, ABO HDN may occur in the first pregnancy and in any, but not necessarily all, subsequent pregnancies. However, tetanus toxoid administration and helminth parasite infection during pregnancy have been linked to the production of high-titered IgG ABO antibodies and severe HDN.

Even high-titered IgG antibodies that are transported across the placenta seem incapable of causing significant RBC destruction in an ABO-incompatible fetus. These infants are delivered with mild anemia or normal hemoglobin levels. The mild course of ABO HDN is related more to the poor development of ABO antigens on fetal RBCs than the characteristics of the maternal antibody. ABO antigens are not fully developed until after the first year of life. Group A infant RBCs are serologically more similar to A_2 adult cells, with group A_2 infant RBCs much weaker. The weakened A antigen on fetal and neonatal RBCs is more readily demonstrable with human than with monoclonal anti-A reagents. As expected, group A_2 infants are less likely to have ABO HDN.

The laboratory findings in ABO HDN differ from those in **Table 20–2** for Rh disease. Microspherocytes and increased RBC fragility in the infant are characteristic of ABO HDN but not of Rh HDN. The severity of the disease is independent of the presence of a positive DAT result or demonstrable anti-A, anti-B, or anti-A,B in the eluate of the infant's RBCs.

The bilirubin peak is later, at 1 to 3 days. Phototherapy is usually sufficient for slowly rising bilirubin levels. With rapidly increasing bilirubin levels, exchange transfusion with group O RBCs may be required. The serious consequences of Rh and other blood groups causing HDN, such as stillbirth, hydrops fetalis, and kernicterus, are extremely rare in ABO HDN.

Prenatal Screening

Many workers have tried to use the immunoglobulin class and titer of maternal ABO antibodies to predict ABO HDN. These tests are laborious and at best demonstrate the presence of IgG maternal antibody but do not correlate well with the extent of fetal RBC destruction. Consequently, detection of ABO HDN is best done after birth.

Postnatal Diagnosis

No single serologic test is diagnostic for ABO HDN. When a newborn infant develops jaundice within 12 to 48 hours after birth, various causes of jaundice need to be investigated, and ABO HDN is only one. The DAT on the cord or neonatal RBCs is the most important diagnostic test. In all cases of ABO HDN requiring transfusion therapy, the DAT result has been positive.[16] On the other hand, the DAT result can be positive even in the absence of signs and symptoms of clinical anemia in the newborn infant. However, these infants may have compensated anemia, or the RBCs may not be destroyed by the reticuloendothelial system.

Collecting cord blood samples on all delivered infants is highly recommended. The sample should be collected by venipuncture to avoid contamination with Wharton's jelly and maternal blood and should be anticoagulated for storage. If the neonatal infant develops jaundice, ABO, Rh, and DAT results can be assessed. The DAT result is neither strongly nor consistently positive, although 90 percent of the cases complicated by jaundice are positive.[17] When the DAT result is negative but the infant is jaundiced, other causes of jaundice should be investigated. In the rare cases in which ABO incompatibility can be the only cause of neonatal jaundice but the DAT result is negative, the eluate of the cord RBCs always reveals ABO antibodies. The eluate can also be helpful when the mother's blood specimen is not available.

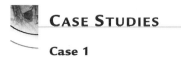

CASE STUDIES

Case 1

Mother: gravida 1 para 0
Current pregnancy:
ABO/Rh(D) typing: O-negative
Today's antibody screen: Positive
Antibody identification: Anti-D
4 weeks ago antibody screen: Negative
6 months ago antibody screen: Negative
Gestational age: 32 weeks
What is the most probable cause of anti-D in this mother?

Answer

The most probable cause is that the mother received prophylactic Rh immune globulin at 28 weeks' gestation. The antibody screen was negative at 28 weeks' gestation prior to the administration of Rh immune globulin. The antibody titer of anti-D due to Rh immune globulin is typically less than 1:4 (4).

After delivery, is this mother an Rh immune globulin candidate?

Answer

Yes, unless the newborn infant is Rh(D)-negative.

Case 2

Mother: gravida 4 para 2
History:
Firstborn child unaffected
Secondborn child mildly affected, positive DAT at birth and required no treatment
Third child stillborn
Mother had anti-D during second and third pregnancies
Current pregnancy:
ABO/Rh(D) typing: O-positive
Antibody screen: Positive
Antibody identification: Anti-D
Antibody titer:
Saline: negative
AHG: 1:128 (128)
Gestational age: 8 weeks
Same father as the three previous pregnancies (he is homozygous for the D antigen)
What is the most likely Rh(D) type of the fetus?

Answer

The maternal history, the same father, and the father homozygous for the D antigen suggest that the infant is Rh(D)-positive.

When should the titer be repeated?

Answer

The titer should be repeated in 6 weeks (16 weeks' gestation).
Is there any intervention that should be done now? Why?

Answer

The infant is only 8 weeks' gestational age, so it is too early in the pregnancy to perform any intervention (cordocentesis, intrauterine transfusion). The earliest an intervention can take place is 18 to 20 weeks.

When should amniocentesis be performed?

Answer

The patient should be scheduled for an amniocentesis at 16 to 18 weeks' gestation to determine the $\triangle$OD 450.

Case 3

Mother: gravida 3 para 2
History:
Firstborn child unaffected, mother's antibody screen negative
Secondborn child mildly affected, ABO/Rh(D) typing A-positive, positive DAT, jaundice, mother O-positive, antibody screen negative
Current pregnancy:
ABO/Rh(D) typing: O-positive
Antibody screen: Positive
Antibody identification: Anti-Le^a
Gestational age: 32 weeks

What is the most probable cause of the second-born child being mildly affected?

Answer

The most probable cause is ABO HDN. Group O mothers produce IgG anti-A, which can cross the placenta.

Is the antibody identified in the current pregnancy clinically significant? Why?

Answer

No. Anti-Le^a does not cause HDN because Lewis antigens are poorly developed at birth.

Case 4

At a rural hospital near a migrant farm camp, a 32-year-old Hispanic woman has just delivered a severely anemic infant. At 6 weeks' gestation, the mother had been typed as A-negative, with positive antibody screen. The antibody was identified as anti-D, titer 256. A report stated that she had an intrauterine transfusion 3 weeks earlier at a university hospital in another state. The cord blood collected at delivery was typed as A-negative. On a heelstick specimen, the infant's hemoglobin was reported as 4.3 g/dL and bilirubin as 3.9 mg/dL. Typing results of this specimen are as follows:

| Anti-A | Anti-B | Anti-A,B | Anti-D | Anti-D | DAT |
| 0 | 0 | 0 | (IS)0 | (AHG)+ | +/− |

IS=immediate spin; AHG=antihuman globulin

What is the infant's blood type? Why is the infant so anemic? What further testing is indicated?

Answer

The blood types of the cord blood and heelstick specimens are different—A negative versus O weak D-positive. The severely anemic infant could have HDN, although the cord blood results do not indicate severe disease (DAT +/−). On the other hand, a large fetomaternal hemorrhage could have occurred. Further testing showed the following:

	Cord Blood	Heelstick
Anti-I	4 +	3 +
Kleihauer-Betke	0/1000	23/1000

The results indicate the cord blood specimen is all adult blood and the heelstick specimen is nearly all adult blood. How could that happen?

Answer

Cord blood should be collected by needle and syringe from the umbilical cord vein. Collecting the specimen by allowing blood from the placenta or cord to drip into the tube can contaminate the specimen with maternal blood. In this case, the tube marked "cord blood" could have been a mislabeled maternal sample. The heelstick is nearly all adult blood because of the recent intrauterine transfusion. Group O blood is usually used. As discussed in this chapter, transfusion causes suppression of erythropoiesis and therefore the production of few fetal RBCs. The cells produced are being hemolyzed by the high-titered maternal antibody. This leads to anemia, in this case quite severe, with elevated bilirubin levels indicating that hemolysis is occurring. Further testing was done on the heelstick specimen:

	Anti-A	Anti-B	RBC Eluate
4°C	0	+	Anti-D

These results indicate that the infant is probably B-positive and has HDN caused by anti-D.

SUMMARY CHART:
Important Points to Remember (MT/MLT)

➤ HDN is the destruction of the RBCs of the fetus and neonate by IgG antibodies produced by the mother.

➤ Only antibodies of the IgG class are actively transported across the placenta.

➤ In Rh HDN, the Rh-positive firstborn infant of an Rh-negative mother is unaffected because the mother has not yet been immunized; in subsequent pregnancies fetal cells carrying the Rh antigen immunize the Rh-negative mother and stimulate production of anti-D.

➤ In ABO HDN, the firstborn infant may be affected as well as subsequent pregnancies in which the mother is group O and the newborn is group A or B; the IgG antibody, anti-A,B in the mother's circulation, crosses the placenta and attaches to the ABO-incompatible antigens of the fetal RBCs.

➤ Erythroblastosis fetalis describes the presence of immature RBCs or erythroblasts in the fetal circulation because the splenic removal of the IgG-coated RBCs causes anemia; the term commonly used now is HDN.

➤ Although anti-D is the most antigenic of the Rh antibodies, anti-Kell is considered the most clinically significant of the non–Rh-system antibodies in the ability to cause HDN.

➤ Prenatal serologic tests for obstetric patients include an ABO, Rh, and antibody screen during the first trimester of pregnancy.

➤ A cord blood workup includes tests for ABO and Rh as well as DAT; the most important serologic test for diagnosis of HDN is the DAT with anti-IgG reagent.

➤ RhIg administered to the mother within 72 hours following delivery is used to prevent active immunization by the Rh(D) antigen on fetal cells; RhIg attaches to fetal Rh-positive RBCs in maternal circulation, blocking immunization and subsequent production of anti-D.

➤ A Kleihauer-Betke test or flow cytometry is used to quantitate the number of fetal Rh-positive cells in the mother's circulation as a result of a fetomaternal hemorrhage.

REVIEW QUESTIONS

1. HDN is characterized by:
   a. IgM antibody
   b. Nearly always anti-D
   c. Different RBC antigens between mother and father
   d. Antibody titer less than 32

2. The main difference between the fetus and the newborn is:
   a. Bilirubin metabolism
   b. Maternal antibody level
   c. Presence of anemia
   d. Size of RBCs

3. Kernicterus is caused by the effects of:
   a. Anemia
   b. Unconjugated bilirubin
   c. Antibody specificity
   d. Antibody titer

4. The advantages of cordocentesis include all of the following except:
   a. Allows measurement of fetal hemoglobin and hematocrit levels
   b. Allows antigen typing of fetal blood
   c. Allows direct transfusion of fetal circulation
   d. Decreases risk of trauma to the placenta

5. Amniocentesis is used to:
   a. Measure bilirubin in mg/dL
   b. Determine fetal blood type
   c. Determine change in optical density
   d. Measure hemoglobin in g/dL

6. Blood for intrauterine transfusion should be all of the following except:
   a. More than 7 days old
   b. Screened for CMV
   c. Gamma-irradiated
   d. Compatible with maternal serum

7. RhIg is indicated for:
   a. Mothers who have anti-D
   b. Infants who are Rh-negative
   c. Infants who have anti-D
   d. Mothers who are Rh-negative

8. RhIg is given without regard for fetal Rh type in all of the following conditions except:
   a. Ectopic pregnancy rupture
   b. Amniocentesis
   c. Induced abortion
   d. Full-term delivery

9. A Kleihauer-Betke test indicates 10 fetal cells per 1000 adult cells. For a woman with 5000 mL blood volume, the proper dose of RhIg is:
   a. One regular-dose vial
   b. Two regular-dose vials
   c. One microdose vial
   d. Two microdose vials

10. RhIg is indicated in which of the following circumstances?
   a. Mother weak D-positive, infant D-positive
   b. Mother D-negative, infant weak D-positive
   c. Mother weak D-positive, infant D-negative
   d. Mother D-negative, infant D-negative and weak D-negative

11. ABO HDN is usually mild because:
   a. ABO antigens are poorly developed in the fetus
   b. ABO antibodies prevent the disease
   c. ABO antibodies readily cross the placenta
   d. ABO incompatibility is rare

12. The Liley graph is used to plot amniotic fluid $\triangle$OD 450. A value in zone III indicates:
   a. The fetal hemoglobin is <12.5 g/dL
   b. The fetus is severely affected with HDN
   c. The gestational age is at least 34 weeks
   d. The fetus has a hereditary hemoglobinopathy

13. A woman without prenatal care delivers a healthy term infant. A cord blood sample shows the infant is A-positive with a positive DAT. The workup of the unexpected finding should include:
   a. Anti-C3 antiglobulin test
   b. Retest of the infant ABO
   c. Antibody screen on the mother's specimen
   d. ABO and Rh typing of the father

REFERENCES

1. Geifman-Holtzman, O, et al: Female alloimmunization with antibodies known to cause hemolytic disease. Obstet Gynecol 89:272, 1997.
2. Mari, G, et al. Noninvasive diagnosis by Doppler ultrasonography of fetal anemia due to maternal red-cell alloimmunization. Collaborative group for Doppler assessment of the blood velocity in anemic fetuses. N Eng J Med 342:9, 2000.
3. Mollison, PL, Engelfriet, CP, and Contreras, M: Blood Transfusion in Clinical Medicine, ed 10. Blackwell Scientific, London, 1997, p 395.
4. Dennis, YM, et al: Two-way cell traffic between mother and fetus: Biologic and clinical implications. Blood 88:4390, 1996.
5. Little, M-T, et al: Frequency of fetal cells in sorted subpopulations of nucleated erythroid and CD34+ hematopoietic progenitor cells from maternal peripheral blood. Blood 89:2347, 1997.
6. Mollison, PL, Engelfriet, CP, and Contreras, M: Blood Transfusion in Clinical Medicine, ed 10. Blackwell Scientific, London, 1997, p 169.
7. Vengelen-Tyler, V: The serological investigation of hemolytic disease of the newborn caused by antibodies other than anti-D. In Garratty, G (ed): Hemolytic Disease of the Newborn. American Association of Blood Banks, Arlington, VA, 1984, p 145.
8. Ludomirski, A: The anemic fetus: Direct access to the fetal circulation for diagnosis and treatment. In Kennedy, MS, Wilson, S, and Kelton, JG (eds): Perinatal Transfusion Medicine. American Association of Blood Banks, Arlington, VA, 1990, p 89.
9. Judd, WJ: Practice guidelines for prenatal and perinatal immunohematology, revisited. Transfusion 41:1445, 2001.
10. Williams, J, et al: Management of hemolytic disease of the newborn. Lab Med 33:467, 2002.
11. Mollison, PL, Engelfriet, CP, and Contreras, M: Blood Transfusion in Clinical Medicine, ed 10. Blackwell Scientific, London, 1997, p 169.
12. Ness, PM, and Salamon, JL: The failure of postinjection Rh immune globulin titers to detect large fetal-maternal hemorrhages. Am J Clin Pathol 85:604, 1986.
13. Kennedy, MS: Rho(D) immune globulin. In Rayburn, W, and Zuspan, FP (eds): Drug Therapy in Gynecology and Obstetrics, ed 3. CV Mosby, St. Louis, 1991, p 297.
14. Lack of transmission of human immunodeficiency virus through Rho(D) immune globulin (human). MMWR 36:728, 1987.
15. Tabor, E, Smallwood, LA, and Gerety, RJ: Antibodies to hepatitis A and B virus antigen in Rho(D) immune globulin. Lancet 1:322, 1986.
16. Issitt, PD, and Anstee, DJ: Applied Blood Group Serology, ed 4. Montgomery Scientific, Durham, NC, 1998, p 1045.
17. Walker, RH: Relevancy in the selection of serologic tests for the obstetric patient. In Garratty, G (ed): Hemolytic Disease of the Newborn. American Association of Blood Banks, Arlington, VA, 1984, p 173.

twenty-one

Autoimmune Hemolytic Anemias

Denise M. Harmening, PhD, MT(ASCP), CLS(NCA),
Nancy B. Steffey, MT(ASCP)SBB, **Lee Ann Prihoda,** MA Ed., MT(ASCP), SBB, **and**
Ralph E.B. Green, B. App. Sci, FAIMS, MACE

═══════════════════ **OBJECTIVES** ═══════════════════

On completion of this chapter, the learner should be able to:

1. Define autoantibody and compare the types of immune hemolytic anemias with respect to thermal amplitude, red blood cell (RBC) destruction, and the type of protein (antibody or complement) coating the RBCs.
2. Characterize autoantibodies that react at temperatures below 37°C and identify the common specificities of benign cold autoagglutinins.
3. Discuss problems encountered in laboratory testing of specimens containing cold autoagglutinins and outline testing procedures that can differentiate between specificities.
4. Discuss pathologic cold autoagglutinins, including laboratory testing and treatment.
5. Differentiate between idiopathic warm autoimmune

hemolytic anemia (WAIHA) and drug-induced immune hemolytic anemia.
6. Describe procedures used to investigate serologic findings and detect underlying clinically significant alloantibodies in the presence of cold autoantibodies.
7. Illustrate the clinical and laboratory findings in WAIHA, including RBC hemolysis, difficulties in serologic testing, and selection of blood for transfusion.
8. Describe procedures used to investigate serologic findings and detect underlying clinically significant alloantibodies in the presence of warm autoantibodies.
9. Compare the three classic mechanisms for drug-induced hemolysis and give examples of medications causing each type.

"Immune hemolytic anemia" is defined as shortened RBC survival mediated through the immune response, specifically by humoral antibody. Immune hemolysis is destruction of the RBC as a result of antibody production and is an acquired abnormality of the RBC membrane associated with demonstrable antibodies, as opposed to intracorpuscular defects such as enzyme deficiencies and hemoglobinopathies, which represent intrinsic abnormalities of the patient's RBCs.

The three broad categories of immune hemolytic anemias are:

1. Alloimmune
2. Autoimmune
3. Drug-induced

In an alloimmune response, the patient produces alloantibodies to foreign or non-self RBC antigens introduced into the circulation, most often through transfusion or pregnancy. For a discussion of alloantibody production, refer to Chapters 18 and 20 of this text.

This chapter focuses on the latter two categories of immune hemolytic anemias: autoimmune hemolytic anemia and drug-induced hemolytic anemia. An autoimmune response occurs when a patient produces antibodies against his or her own RBC antigens. A drug-induced hemolytic anemia is the result of a patient's production of antibody to a particular drug or drug complex, with ensuing damage to the patient's RBCs.

Autoantibodies

Definition

Antibodies that are directed against the individual's own RBCs are autoantibodies or autoagglutinins. Most autoantibodies react with high-incidence RBC antigens. They may agglutinate, sensitize, or lyse RBCs of most random donors as well as their own RBCs. RBC survival may be shortened by this circulating humoral antibody. However, many individuals will produce an autoantibody that readily attaches to their own RBCs but does not cause RBC destruction. Often, healthy blood donors will have a positive direct antiglobulin test (DAT), but do not exhibit evidence of increased RBC destruction or survival.

Studies in animal models indicate that production of antibodies against self occurs because of a failure of the mechanisms regulating the immune response.[1,2] Briefly, under normal circumstances, immunoglobulins are made by B lymphocytes. Another type of lymphocyte, the T lymphocyte, modulates the activity of the antibody-producing cells. Helper T cells assist immunocompetent B cells in making antibody against foreign antigens. Another population of T lymphocytes, suppressor T cells, has the opposite effect on B-cell activity; they prevent excessive proliferation of B cells and overproduction of antibodies. Suppressor T cells are thought to act through a feedback mechanism. An increasing concentration of antibody activates these T cells and suppresses further antibody production.[3]

Autoantibody production may be prevented through a similar mechanism. Suppressor T cells induce tolerance to self antigens by inhibiting B-cell activity. Conversely, loss of suppressor T-cell function could result in autoantibody production. Support for this concept comes from animal studies[2] and patients taking the drug alpha-methyldopa.[4] The cause of

dysfunction of the regulatory system is not understood, but microbial agents and drugs have been suggested.[5] For further discussion of the immune response, the reader is referred to Chapter 3 of this text.

Recognition and detection of autoantibodies in routine serologic investigations are extremely important. Identification of an autoantibody may explain decreased RBC survival in vivo and offer an explanation for an otherwise unexplained anemia. In serologic investigations, it is important to recognize the presence of an autoantibody in routine testing, including ABO/Rh typing, antibody screening, and compatibility testing. If a patient's RBCs are coated with autoantibody, it may be difficult to accurately determine the ABO/Rh type of the individual. If the patient's serum contains autoantibody, RBC antibody screening procedures, compatibility testing, and serum (reverse) ABO typing of the individual may present difficulty. It is likely that the patient's serum will be incompatible with all random donors, and potentially there will be an ABO discrepancy in the serum and cell ABO typing. The effect of autoantibodies on routine testing and techniques that can be used to resolve these difficulties are discussed in greater detail below. Serologic and clinical problems can be found separately or together.

Characterization

In individuals who have not been recently transfused, the presence of a positive DAT, a positive autocontrol, or serum autoantibody does not confer the diagnosis of autoimmune hemolytic anemia (AIHA). In themselves, these findings merely indicate the presence of autoantibody. Before the presence of an AIHA is established, it is important to verify the presence of immune-mediated RBC destruction. Evidence of increased RBC destruction is not always accompanied by decreased hemogloblin and hematocrit levels. These are only evident when the individual is no longer able to compensate for increased RBC destruction. However, before decreases in hemoglobin/hematocrit occur, there will be evidence of increased RBC destruction, which includes an increased reticulocyte count, unconjugated bilirubin levels, and lactate dehydrogenase (LDH) levels, and haptoglobin levels will be greatly decreased.

The individual who experiences immune RBC destruction may experience either compensated or uncompensated anemia. In compensated anemia, the rate of RBC production will nearly equal the rate of RBC destruction. These individuals will demonstrate an increased reticulocyte count but may experience a mild decrease in hemoglobin/hematocrit levels, depending on the rate of RBC production. Those individuals with uncompensated anemia demonstrate a rate of RBC destruction that exceeds the rate of RBC production. Hemolytic anemia is often demonstrated in a blood smear by macrocytosis, evidence of a young cell population, and spherocytosis, reflecting cell membrane damage. The reticulocyte count of these individuals is generally greater than 3 percent,[6] and the unconjugated bilirubin levels and LDH levels are also increased; however, the haptoglobin levels are remarkably decreased. With intravascular RBC destruction, hemoglobinemia and hemoglobinuria may occur. Because there are other causes of hemolysis (e.g., hereditary spherocytosis, hemoglobinopathies, and RBC enzyme defects), AIHA must be confirmed by additional serologic testing. Diagnostic tests include:

1. DAT, using polyspecific and monospecific antiglobulin reagents
2. Characterization of the autoantibody in the serum and/or eluate, using standard antibody detection and identification procedures

Based on these results and the clinical evaluation of the patient, AIHA may be diagnosed and classified as cold reactive, warm reactive, or drug-induced. The expected laboratory findings for each type are discussed in the following section. Petz and Garratty[7] devote a chapter in their book, *Acquired Immune Hemolytic Anemias*, to the diagnosis of the hemolytic anemias and another to drug-induced immune hemolytic anemia. The reader is referred to that text for a complete discussion.

It should be noted that individuals may have autoantibodies in their sera and on their RBCs but display no evidence of decreased RBC survival. All normal RBCs have a small amount of IgG and complement on their surface. Studies have shown that there may be 5 to 90 molecules of IgG/RBC and 5 to 500 molecules of complement/RBC in the average individual. Because standard laboratory tube testing will normally detect 100 to 500 molecules of IgG/RBC and 400 to 1100 molecules of complement/RBC, these individuals are not routinely identified as DAT-positive.[8] It should be noted that the recently implemented column agglutination (gel) testing appears to have an increased sensitivity in the detection of IgG-coated RBCs. Therefore, with the increase in the use of gel technology, a greater number of individuals may be found to be DAT-positive, with or without detectable evidence of RBC destruction. For example, the incidence of positive DATs in normal blood donor populations has been reported to be as high as 1 in 1000 in the U.S. population,[9] whereas the incidence in hospitalized patients ranges from 0.3 to 1.0 percent (using anti-IgG antiglobulin reagent)[10,11] and up to 15 percent (using polyspecific antiglobulin reagent).[12] Many of the latter group have only anticomplement bound to the RBCs. The differences between individuals who are affected (i.e., have AIHA) and those who are unaffected by autoantibodies are not clearly understood. Among the possibly significant factors are:

1. Thermal amplitude of antibody reactivity[13]
2. IgG subclass of the antibody[14]
3. Amount of antibody bound to the RBCs[14]
4. Ability of the antibody to fix complement in vivo[15]
5. Activity of the individual's macrophages[7]
6. Quantitative or qualitative change in band 3 and proteins 4.1 and 4.2 in the RBC membrane structure[16]

The opposite situation also occurs; in some patients with hemolytic anemia, autoantibodies cannot be demonstrated by routine techniques. Some patients have more IgG on their RBCs than normal but less than the amount detectable by the routine antiglobulin test.[17] In other cases, the patient's RBCs are sensitized with anti-IgA or anti-IgM.[18–20] Because polyspecific antihuman globulin (AHG) reagents must contain only anti-IgG and anti-C3d,[21] antibodies to other immunoglobulins are not consistently present, and cells sensitized with IgA or IgM may not give a positive test. Finally, prior to current requirements for polyspecific antiglobulin reagents, many commercial reagents did not routinely agglutinate cells coated with complement components.[22] Therefore, a negative DAT was not an unusual finding in patients with cold agglutinin hemolytic anemia. The reader is cautioned, however, to note the date of a publication in which AIHA associated with a negative DAT is reported.

As earlier stated, autoantibodies can be divided into two main groups, dependent on the optimal temperature of reactivity. About 70 percent of the reported cases of AIHA are those that react best at warm temperatures (37°C), and cold reactive (4° to 30°C) autoagglutinins account for about 18 percent. Drug-induced autoagglutinins are present in about 12 percent of the reported cases of AIHA. Characterization of autoantibodies is important because treatment of the patient and resolution of the serologic problems differ according to the optimal temperature of reactivity. The remainder of this chapter details clinical and laboratory aspects of cold reactive, warm reactive, and drug-induced autoantibodies.

Cold Reactive Autoantibodies

Benign Cold Autoantibodies

When testing is performed at 4°C, the most commonly encountered autoantibody is a benign cold agglutinin that is demonstrable in the serum of most normal, healthy individuals. Normally these antibodies present no serologic problem, because routine antibody detection tests are not performed at this temperature. The typical cold agglutinin has a relatively low titer: at 4°C it is less than 64. Occasionally, the antibody has increased thermal amplitude and will agglutinate cells at room temperature (20° to 24°C). However, even in this situation strongest reactivity is found at 4°C. **Table 21–1** compares the characteristics of benign (normal) cold autoantibodies with those of pathologic cold autoagglutinins. Most cold agglutinins react best with enzyme-treated cells; therefore, cold agglutinins are quite likely to be detected when ficin-treated cells are tested at immediate spin. Cold autoantibodies are IgM immunoglobulins and therefore can activate complement in vitro. In serum testing, reactivity may be seen in the antiglobulin phase, when polyspecific antihuman

TABLE 21–1 Characteristics of Normal (Benign) Cold and Pathologic Cold Autoantibodies

Characteristic	Normal (Benign)	Pathologic
Thermal range	Generally below 20–24°C	May be reactive at ≥30°C
Titer at 4°C	≤64	≥1000
Reactivity	Marginally enhanced with albumin	Strongly enhanced with albumin
Common specificity	Anti-I	Anti-I
Capable of binding complement	Yes	Yes
Clinically significant	No	Yes
Associated with disease	No	Yes—May be secondary to viral infections or *M. pneumonia*.

TABLE 21–2   Typical Reactivity Observed with Auto-Cold-Agglutinins

Test Phase	Autologous Cells	Group O Adult Cells
Saline 4°C	3+ to 4+	3+ to 4+
Saline 15°–18°C	1+ to 2+	1+ to 2+
Saline RT (20°–24°C)	0 to 1+	0 to 1+
Enzyme-treated cells (RT)	1+ to 4+	1+ to 4+
Saline 37°C	0	0
IgG antiglobulin	0	0

serum is used in antiglobulin testing. **Table 21–2** shows reactions typical of cold autoagglutinins.

Laboratory Tests Affected by Cold Autoagglutinins

Cold agglutinins sometimes interfere with routine serum and cell testing performed at room temperature. The extent to which they cause problems depends on how strongly the antibody reacts at this temperature (i.e., the concentration and thermal amplitude of the antibody). Although the normal cold autoantibodies found in the serum of most people do not typically interfere with testing, they are one of the more common causes of serologic problems. Therefore, one should be able to recognize these circumstances and identify methods to resolve problems associated with these antibodies.

ABO Typing

If an individual's RBCs are heavily coated with cold agglutinins, they may demonstrate spontaneous agglutination. Consequently, false-positive reactions can be obtained with routine ABO reagents. In most cases, valid results can be obtained by using patient's cells that have been washed once or twice with normal saline warmed to 37°C. The cold autoantibody is eluted from the cells during washing. For example, group O cells coated with cold autoantibody might show the following reactions before and after washing:

	Anti-A	Anti-B
Serum-suspended RBCs	+	+
Washed, saline-suspended RBCs	0	0

If more potent autoagglutinins are present, the specimen can be kept at 37°C after collection and the cells washed with saline at 37° to 45°C to remove the autoantibody.[23] In the rare situation in which washing with warm saline is not effective, thiol reagents (e.g., dithiothreitol) can be used to disperse the autoagglutination.[24] (See Procedure A in the Procedural Appendix of this chapter.) Because serum ABO grouping is performed at room temperature, cold autoagglutinins frequently cause discrepancies in the serum ABO (reverse) typing also. In the following example, the cell typing results indicate the cells are group AB. Therefore, one does not expect the serum to agglutinate either the A_1 or B cells. Although a number of explanations for this discrepancy exist, a cold agglutinin is a likely cause. Group O and autologous

cells should also be tested in the investigation of this apparent discrepancy. If a cold autoagglutinin is present, the autologous and group O cells will most likely be positive:

	Anti-A	Anti-B		
RBCs	+	+		

	A_1 cells	B cells	Autologous cells	Group O cells
Serum	+	+	+	+

Such a discrepancy is easily resolved if the cold reactive autoantibody is removed by an autoadsorption technique, and the tests with the A_1 and B cells are repeated with autoadsorbed serum. (See Procedure B in the Procedural Appendix.) Although it may be possible to resolve this discrepancy with prewarmed testing, one must remember that not all ABO isoagglutinins are reactive at 37°C, and erroneous test results may be obtained; therefore, autoadsorption procedures are preferred.

	A_1 cells	B cells	Autologous cells	Group O cells
Autoadsorbed serum	0	0	0	0

Rh(D) Typing

As in ABO cell grouping, false-positive reactions can be found with Rh reagents when RBCs coated with cold autoagglutinins are tested. This was previously a common problem encountered in typing with high-protein anti-D reagent where the anti-D and the Rh control were positive, rendering the test invalid. Today, the reagents in common use are monoclonal or a blending of monoclonal and low-protein anti-D reagent, which normally yields valid results. When a monoclonal reagent is used, many manufacturers consider a negative reaction with any of the ABO reagents as a control for the D typing; however, an Rh control serum is available from some manufacturers. As stated previously, if a discrepancy exists in the ABO typing, washing the cells in warm saline usually gives acceptable results. This also holds true when testing with low-protein anti-D. Thiol reagents may be used when washing with warm saline is ineffective; however, false-negative reactions may be found when using monoclonal antisera with thiol-treated cells.

Cold reactive IgM autoagglutinins can activate the complement cascade in vitro, causing complement components to be bound to the RBC surface, which can lead to false-positive reactions in the weak D (antiglobulin) test if cells from a clotted sample and polyspecific antihuman serum are used. In this instance, the Rh control test will also be positive. The use of monospecific anti-IgG for weak D testing or RBCs collected into ethylenediaminetetra-acetic acid (EDTA) can eliminate the problem of complement-binding cold agglutinins in D typing. The following examples illustrate these results:

Testing	Anti-D	Rh Control	Comments
Immediate spin	0	0	
Antihuman serum (polyspecific)	+	+	Detects complement components

Antihuman serum (anti-IgG)	0	0	Does not detect complement
RBC collected in EDTA	0	0	Complement not bound

Similar problems can be encountered in other antisera used in RBC phenotyping (e.g., K, Fy^a) that require the use of an antiglobulin test. The use of an anti-IgG antiglobulin reagent and/or a sample collected in EDTA is recommended when cold autoagglutinins are present.

Direct Antiglobulin Test

When a properly collected specimen is used (EDTA-anticoagulated RBCs), the DAT of a patient with benign cold autoagglutinins is negative. However, one frequently obtains a positive result using polyspecific antihuman serum if a clotted specimen is used, because complement can be activated in vitro. If monospecific reagents are used, these cells are agglutinated by anti-C3d but not by anti-IgG. As discussed in the previous section, false-positive antigen typings can be obtained when clotted specimens and polyspecific antihuman serum are used.

Antibody Detection and Identification

The frequency with which cold autoagglutinins interfere with detection and identification of RBC alloantibodies depends to a large extent on the routine procedures used in patient testing. As shown in **Table 21–2**, cold agglutinins react best at 4°C but are not detected because routine testing is not performed at this temperature. Room temperature–reactive autoantibodies will not usually be detected if the laboratory no longer performs routine antibody detection at this phase. Antibodies reactive only at room temperature are usually considered to be of no clinical significance. Benign cold autoagglutinins do not react at 37°C, but they may interfere with testing at the antiglobulin phase if polyspecific antihuman reagent is used, inasmuch as they may bind to cells at lower temperatures when the serum and cells are mixed together initially or during centrifugation following the 37°C incubation, and complement may be activated. Although the antibody elutes from the cell surface during the incubation or washing phases, the complement remains attached. Polyspecific antihuman serum will agglutinate the cells coated with C3. When enzyme-treated cells are used, reactions in all phases may be stronger.

Because most clinically significant antibodies capable of causing accelerated RBC destruction are detected by the antiglobulin test, reactions in this phase may be significant and must be investigated. The reactions caused by a cold autoagglutinin can mask the presence of clinically significant alloantibodies. Although the use of anti-IgG antiglobulin reagents will eliminate most problems with cold autoagglutinin reactivity in the AHG phase, it is often nessary to remove the cold reacting autoantibody by adsorption procedures to thoroughly investigate the reactivity observed in antiglobulin testing.

Other techniques useful in differentiating between cold autoantibodies and alloantibodies are prewarming tests or testing with autoadsorbed serum.[23] By prewarming the cells and serum prior to mixing, avoiding room temperature centrifugation after 37°C incubation and washing with saline at 37° to 45°C, the reaction between the cold autoagglutinin and RBC antigens can be prevented, thus avoiding complement activation. However, alloantibodies that are reactive at 37°C can bind to the cells and cause agglutination at the antiglobulin phase. (See Procedure C in the Procedural Appendix.) An example of the results of testing a serum that contains a cold autoagglutinin and anti-Fy^a using routine antiglobulin testing with polyspecific antiglobulin and testing with the prewarmed technique is shown in **Table 21–3**. Reactions are present in routine antiglobulin tests with both Fy^a(+) and Fy^a(−) cells. In a prewarmed test, only the reactions expected of the anti-Fy^a are evident. The weak reactions of the cold autoagglutinin are eliminated by prewarming the test. The prewarming technique is simple and successful in most cases. However, if the autoantibody is very potent, it may be difficult to maintain the cells and serum at 37°C to avoid the antigen-antibody interaction and complement activation.

Although prewarmed testing is very helpful in resolving problems caused by cold autoagglutinins, this technique should not be used indiscriminately. Cases have been reported in which clinically significant alloantibodies have been missed after prewarming.[25] Prewarming should be used only when the reactions obtained indicate the likely presence of a cold autoagglutinin (i.e., autocontrol-positive and reactions noted below 37°C). Because there is no immediate spin, room temperature, or 37° testing in the prewarmed procedure, IgM immunoglobulin components of a newly forming alloantibody may not be detected in this testing. Therefore, this testing must not be performed with patients transfused within the previous 3 months or patients without an accurate transfusion history. A cold autoagglutinin is not apt to be the answer if only weak reactions are present in the antiglobulin phase with anti-IgG and there is no evidence of reactivity at immediate spin or room temperature.

TABLE 21–3   Typical Reactivity Observed with a Patient Serum Containing a Clinically Significant Alloantibody (anti-Fy^a) and an Auto Cold-Agglutinin

RBCs tested	Standard Antiglobulin Testing with Polyspecific AHG	Prewarmed Antiglobulin Testing with Polyspecific AHG	Standard Antiglobulin Testing with Anti-IgG AHG
0, Fy(a+b−)	1+	1+	1+
0, Fy(a+b+)	1+	1+	1+
0, Fy(a−b+)	1+^{W}	0	0
Autologous cells	1+^{W}	0	0

When strong cold autoantibodies are present or if one wishes to identify a room temperature–reactive alloantibody, adsorption must be performed to remove the autoantibody. Autologous adsorption, described in Procedure B in the Procedural Appendix, may be performed if the patient has *not* been transfused within 3 months. In autoadsorption procedures, an aliquot of patient cells is incubated with an equal aliquot of the patient's serum at 4°C. Autoantibody is adsorbed onto the cells, and alloantibody remains in the serum. It may be necessary to repeat the adsorption several times if the autoantibody is a high-titer antibody. In order to enhance the adsorption process, the patient's RBCs may be treated with enzymes before adsorption to increase the amount of autoantibody removed by the adsorption. However, enzyme pretreatment should not be performed without confirming that the serum antibody is reactive with enzyme-treated cells. Autologous adsorption is not recommended if a patient has been recently transfused, because donor RBCs will be present in the patient's circulation. Alloantibodies as well as autoantibodies will be adsorbed if an autoadsorption is performed. In this situation, it is best to use allogeneic adsorption or adsorption using rabbit erythrocyte stroma. (See Procedure D in the Procedural Appendix.)

If anti-IgG antiglobulin reagent is used, the problems caused by most cold agglutinins can be avoided. The use of anti-IgG reagents is an attractive alternative when prewarming is not effective and there is not enough time to adsorb the serum.

Compatibility Testing

The difficulties encountered in antibody detection and identification tests are also found in compatibility tests because the most commonly encountered autoantibody (autoanti-I) is directed against an antigen that is found on the RBCs of most random donors as well as on most reagent RBCs. Compatibility tests, like antibody identification tests, can be performed with prewarmed or autoadsorbed serum, allogeneic adsorbed serum, or anti-IgG antiglobulin reagent.

Two other common cold agglutinins, anti-IH and anti-H, distinguish between group O reagent RBCs and random group A, B, or AB donor cells. Because these antibodies require the H antigen that is only weakly expressed on the RBCs of group A, B, or AB individuals, they are rarely encountered as an autoantibody. As discussed in the following section on specificity, anti-IH and anti-H react best with group O cells; they react less well with group A_1 and A_1B cells. Anti-IH and anti-H are found most often in the serum of group A_1 and A_1B persons; therefore, the units selected for compatibility testing (group A or AB) are those that give the weakest, if any, reactivity. On the other hand, group O cells (antibody screening cells) give the strongest reactions.

Specificity of Cold Autoagglutinins

Anti-I, Anti-i

Most cold reactive autoantibodies have anti-I specificity. The I antigen is fully expressed on the RBCs of virtually all adults, whereas it is only weakly expressed on cord RBCs. At birth, an infant's RBCs express the i antigen. As an infant matures, the antigen expressed is converted from the i antigen to the I antigen; the amount of I antigen increases until the adult levels are reached at about 2 years of age.[23] Very rarely do adult

RBCs lack the I antigen; if they do, they are termed "i adults" and may produce alloanti-I.

The reactivities of several examples of anti-I are given in **Table 21–4**. As shown, anti-I specificity may be apparent when a serum is tested with adult and cord cells. Benign cold autoantibodies, for example, react with adult cells but not with cord cells. Pathologic cold autoantibodies react with both adult and cord cells, but the preference for the adult cells is still obvious. Alloanti-I is frequently present in the serum of i adults.[26]

Anti-i is a relatively uncommon autoantibody. As shown in **Table 21–5**, this antibody reacts in an antithetical manner to anti-I. Cord cells and i adult cells have the strongest expression of the i antigen; adult I cells have the least.

Anti-H, Anti-IH

Cold agglutinins found in the serum of group A_1 and A_1B individuals (and, although rarely, group B) may have anti-H specificity. This antibody distinguishes between cells of various ABO groups. Group O and A_2 cells react best because they have the strongest expression of the H antigen. Group A_1 and A_1B cells have the least H antigen so they react weakly. Because the A_1 and A_1B individual's own cells demonstrate a very weak expression of the H antigen, anti-H and anti-IH are rarely found to be autoantibodies but rather alloantibodies that can be easily managed by the selection of type-specific RBCs. The pattern of reactivity seen with anti-H is shown in **Table 21–5**. See Chapter 6 for a discussion of the ABO system and H substance.

It is very important not to confuse cold reactive anti-H with the anti-H found in the serum of O_h (Bombay) individuals who lack the H antigen. Cold reactive anti-H is most often an alloantibody, but it may be found in A_1 or A_1B individuals as an autoantibody even though the cells of the antibody maker (A_1 or A_1B) may give considerably weaker reactions. The anti-H in the O_h person is a potent alloantibody, which reacts at 4° to 37°C with all cells except the rare O_h cell, and is capable of causing rapid intravascular RBC destruction.

Anti-IH, another of the usually harmless cold autoagglutinins, is also found more commonly in the serum of A_1 and A_1B individuals. This antibody agglutinates only RBCs that have both the I and the H antigens. As with anti-H, group O and group A_2 cells react best. The difference between these two antibodies is that group O i_{cord} cells and group O i_{adult} cells react as strongly as group O I_{adult} cells with anti-H but not with anti-IH (see **Table 21–5**).

TABLE 21–4 Typical Reactivity Observed with Serum Containing Auto-Anti-I with Adult and Cord Cells			
Serum	**Serum Dilution**	**Adult Cells**	**Cord Cells**
Benign Cold	Neat	3+	1+[w]
	1:2	1+	0
	1:4	1+[w]	0
	1:8	0	0
Pathologic Cold	Neat	4+	3+
	1:2	4+	2+
	1:4	4+	1+
	1:8	3+	1+

TABLE 21–5   Reactivity of Cold Autoagglutinins at 4°C with ABO-Compatible Cells

RBC Phenotype	Anti-I	Anti-i	Anti-H	Anti-IH	Anti-Pr*
O, I+ adult	4+	0 to 1+	4+	4+	4+
A₁, I+ adult	4+	0 to 1+	0–1+	0–1+	4+
A₂, I+ adult	4+	0 to 1+	2+	2+	4+
Oₕ, I+ adult	4+	0 to 1+	0	0 to 2+	4+
O, i+ adult	0 to 1+	4+	4+	0 to 1+	4+
O, i+ cord	0 to 1+	4+	4+	0 to 1+	4+
A₁, i+ adult	0 to 1+	4+	0–1+	0	4+
A₂, i+ adult	0 to 1+	4+	2+	0 to 2+	4+
Oₕ, i+ adult	0 to 1+	4+	0	0	4+
O, I+ adult ficin-treated	4+	1+–2+	4+	4+	0

*Anti-Pr is a less uncommonly encountered cold autoagglutinin that frequently mimics auto-anti-I.

Other Cold Reactive Autoagglutinins

A number of other less commonly encountered cold autoagglutinins have been described, such as anti-Pr, anti-Gd, and anti-Sdˣ (anti-Rₓ).[27] Cold autoantibodies with the specificity of anti-M have also been described.[28] Most researchers agree that specificity of cold reactive autoantibodies is primarily of academic interest and usually not clinically important. However, development of autoantibodies with specificities for integral components of the RBC membrane, such as the glycophorins or band 3, may be precursors for development of other autoimmune disorders such as systemic lupus erythematosus or rheumatoid arthritis.[29]

Pathologic Cold Autoagglutinins

Cold Hemagglutinin Disease (Idiopathic Cold AIHA)

Most cold autoagglutinins do not cause RBC destruction, but in some patients they can cause hemolytic anemia that varies in severity from mild to life-threatening intravascular lysis. Cold reactive immune hemolytic anemia may be a chronic, idiopathic (no identifiable cause) condition or an acute, transient disorder often associated with an infectious disease such as *Mycoplasma pneumoniae* pneumonia or infectious mononucleosis. Cold agglutinin syndrome, also called cold hemagglutinin disease (CHD) or idiopathic cold AIHA, represents approximately 18 percent of the cases of AIHA. A moderate chronic hemolytic anemia is produced by a cold autoantibody that optimally reacts at 4°C but also reacts at between 25° and 31°C. The antibody is usually an IgM immunoglobulin, which quite efficiently activates complement.

Clinical Picture

CHD occurs predominantly in older individuals, with a peak incidence in those over 50 years of age. Antibody specificity in this disorder is almost always anti-I, less commonly anti-i, and rarely anti-Pr. It is rarely severe and is usually seasonal, because the winter months often precipitate the signs and symptoms of a chronic hemolytic anemia. Acrocyanosis of the

hands, feet, ears, and nose is frequently the patient's main complaint along with a sense of numbness in the extremities. Changes take place when the person is exposed to the cold, because the cold autoantibody agglutinates the patient's RBCs as they pass through the skin capillaries, resulting in localized blood stasis. During cold winter weather, the temperature of an individual's blood falls to as low as 28°C in the extremities, activating the cold autoantibody in these patients. The antibody then agglutinates the RBCs and fixes complement as the cells flow through the capillaries of the skin, causing autoagglutination and signs of acrocyanosis. These patients may also experience hemoglobinuria, because the complement fixation may result in intravascular hemolysis. **Figure 21–1** illustrates the relation between LDH concentration, a reflection of the severity of hemolysis, and ambient temperature in these patients over a period of 18 months.[30] However, this intravascular hemolytic episode is not associated with fever, chills, or acute renal insufficiency, any one of which is characteristic of patients with paroxysmal cold hemoglobinuria (PCH) or severe WAIHA.

Patients usually display weakness, pallor, and weight loss, which are characteristic symptoms of a chronic anemia. CHD usually remains quite stable; however, if it does progress in severity, it is insidious in intensity. Physical findings such as hepatosplenomegaly are infrequent because of the mechanism of hemolysis. Other clinical features of CHD include jaundice and Raynaud's phenomenon (symptoms of cold intolerance, such as pain and bluish tinge in the fingertips and toes as a result of vasospasm). Patients with severe CHD usually live more comfortably in warmer climates.

Laboratory Findings

Laboratory findings in CHD include reticulocytosis and a positive DAT resulting from complement coating only. It is suggested that a simple serum screening procedure be performed initially to test the ability of the patient's serum to agglutinate autologous saline-suspended RBCs at 18 to 20°C. If this test result is positive, further steps may be taken to determine the titer and thermal amplitude of the patient's cold autoantibody. If it is negative, the diagnosis of CHD is unlikely. The

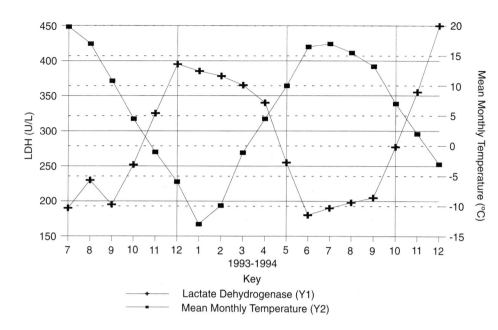

■ FIGURE 21–1 Seasonal hemolysis in cold agglutinin disease. As the ambient temperature decreases, the amount of hemolysis (reflected in serum lactate dehydrogenase levels) increases. During warmer months, LDH levels return to normal.

peripheral smear of a patient with CHD may show agglutination, polychromasia, mild to moderate anisocytosis, and poikilocytosis **(Color Plate 5)**. Autoagglutination of anticoagulated whole blood samples is characteristic of CHD and occurs quickly as the blood cools to room temperature, causing the binding of cold autoantibodies to the patient's RBCs. As a result of this autoagglutination, performance of automated blood counts and preparation of blood smears are extremely difficult with these patient samples. Leukocyte and platelet counts are usually normal. **Box 21–1** summarizes the clinical criteria for diagnosis of CHD.

Selection of Blood for Transfusion

Most patients with CHD do not require transfusion; however, when they do, it is sometimes difficult to select blood. As previously described, potent cold autoantibodies interfere with most routine tests. Perhaps the most difficult problem is to detect and identify alloantibodies. Procedures to manage these problems were described earlier in this chapter. It is important to provide RBCs compatible with any clinically sig-

nificant alloantibodies. Most patients receive transfusion of blood that is positive for the autoantibody. Units of i_{adult} RBCs are extremely rare and should be reserved for the rare i_{adult} patient with alloanti-I.

The issue of transfusion in CHD patients is most relevant in patients undergoing surgical procedures that use hypothermia (lowering of the body temperature to 22° to 30°C), such as cardiac procedures. For patients with CHD, blood for transfusion can be warmed by an approved blood warmer, or the operative procedures can be performed without subjecting the patient to hypothermia.[31]

Cold Autoantibodies Related to Infection (Secondary Cold AIHA)

CHD can also occur as a transient disorder secondary to infection. Episodes of cold AIHA often occur after upper respiratory infections. Approximately 50 percent of patients suffering from pneumonia caused by *M. pneumoniae* have cold agglutinin titer levels higher than 64. In the second or third week of the patient's illness, CHD may occur in association with the infection, and a rapid onset of hemolysis is observed. Pallor and jaundice are characteristically present. Acrocyanosis and hemoglobinuria are uncommon and not consistently present. Usually, resolution of the episode occurs within 2 to 3 weeks because the hemolysis is self-limiting. The offending cold autoantibody is an IgM immunoglobulin with a characteristic anti-I specificity. Very high titer levels of cold autoagglutinins are seen almost exclusively in patients with *M. pneumoniae*. It has been reported that the cold agglutinin produced in this infection is an immunologic response to the mycoplasma antigens, and this antibody cross-reacts with the RBC I antigen.

The antibodies produced in primary CHD and in this disorder secondary to *M. pneumoniae* both have anti-I specificity, and the RBCs are sensitized with complement components. If the complement cascade does not proceed to C9 (cell death by lysis), the macrophages of the reticuloendothelial system can still clear the sensitized RBCs through their receptors for C3b fragments, thereby causing hemolysis.

BOX 21–1
Clinical Criteria for the Diagnosis of CHD

- Clinical signs of an acquired hemolytic anemia, with a history (which may or may not be present) of acrocyanosis and hemoglobinuria on exposure to cold
- A positive DAT result using polyspecific antihuman sera
- A positive DAT result using monospecific anti-C3 antisera
- A negative DAT result using monospecific anti-IgG antisera
- The presence of reactivity in the patient's serum due to a cold autoantibody
- A cold agglutinin titer of 1000 or greater in saline at 4°C with visible agglutination of anticoagulated blood at room temperature

Adapted from Harmening, DM: Clinical Hematology and Fundamentals of Hemostasis, ed 4. FA Davis, Philadelphia, 2002, p 210, with permission.

TABLE 21-6   Secondary Cold AIHA

Type of Infection	Cold Autoantibody Specificity
Mycoplasma pneumoniae	Anti-I
Infectious mononucleosis	Anti-i

Infectious mononucleosis also may be associated with a hemolytic anemia resulting from a cold autoantibody. Although infrequent, it has been well documented that a high-titered IgM anti-i with a wide thermal range plays a major role in hemolytic anemia associated with this viral infection. Acute illness with a sore throat and a high fever, followed by weakness, anemia, and jaundice, is a characteristic feature of infectious mononucleosis. Lymphadenopathy and hepatosplenomegaly are common findings. A larger percentage of patients with infectious mononucleosis has been reported to develop anti-i, but only a small number of these patients develops the antibody of sufficient titer and thermal amplitude to induce in-vivo hemolysis. **Table 21–6** reviews the cold autoantibody specificity most commonly found in the infections that cause secondary CHD.

Treatment

Therapy for CHD is generally unnecessary. Most patients require no treatment and are instructed to avoid the cold, keep warm, or move to a milder climate. Patients with moderate anemia are given the same instructions and are urged to tolerate the symptoms rather than to use drugs on a therapeutic trial basis. There is some advantage to the use of plasma exchange in more severe cases, inasmuch as IgM antibodies have a predominantly intravascular distribution. However, response to plasma exchange is still variable in this patient population, and repeated plasma exchanges are often required on a frequent basis to maintain low plasma levels of autoagglutinating antibodies.

Corticosteroids also have been used but generally have a poor effect. In some patients whose RBCs are strongly coated with C3, successful results have been reported with corticosteroids. Some favorable responses also have been reported with the alkylating drug chlorambucil. Splenectomy is generally considered ineffective.

PCH (Paroxysmal Cold Hemoglobinuria)

PCH is the least common type of AIHA, with an incidence between 1 and 2 percent. It is, however, more common in children in association with viral illnesses such as measles, mumps, chickenpox, infectious mononucleosis, and the ill-defined flu syndrome. Originally, PCH was described in association with syphilis, with an autoantibody formed in response to the *Treponema pallidum* infection. However, with the effective treatment of syphilis with antibiotics, PCH is no longer commonly reported in relation to syphilis.

RBC destruction is caused by a cold autoantibody referred to as a biphasic autohemolysin, which binds to the patient's RBCs at low temperatures and fixes complement. Hemolysis occurs when the body temperature rises to 37°C and the sensitized cells undergo complement-mediated intravascular lysis. In contrast to the other cold reactive autoagglutinins,

the antibody in PCH is an IgG immunoglobulin with biphasic activity. The classic antibody produced in PCH is called the Donath-Landsteiner antibody and has the specificity of an autoanti-P. Other specificities have been reported, including anti-i[32] and anti-Pr-like.[33]

To confirm the diagnosis of PCH, the Donath-Landsteiner test is performed in the laboratory. This test involves the collection of a fresh blood sample from the patient. The serum is then separated from collected blood sample at 37 °C. Three sets of three test tubes, labeled A1–A2–A3, B1–B2–B3, and C1–C2–C3, are used to mix serum with washed group O RBCs that expresses the P antigen. In this test, tubes 1 and 2 of each set contain 10 drops of patient's serum, and tubes 2 and 3 of each set contain 10 drops of fresh normal serum. One volume of 50 percent suspension of washed P-positive RBCs is added to each tube, and all tubes are mixed. After mixing, the three A tubes are then placed in a melted ice bath for 30 minutes and then 1 hour at 37°C. The three B tubes are placed in melted ice bath for 90 minutes. The three C tubes are kept at 37°C for 90 minutes. After the appropriate time has passed, the tubes are centrifuged, and supernatant fluids are examined for hemolysis. **Table 21–7** summarizes the reactions of a positive Donath-Landsteiner test.

As the name PCH implies, paroxysmal or intermittent episodes of hemoglobinuria occur on exposure to cold. These acute attacks are characterized by sudden onset of fever, shaking chills, malaise, abdominal cramps, and back pain. All the signs of intravascular hemolysis are evident, along with hemoglobinemia, hemoglobinuria, and bilirubinemia, depending on the severity and frequency of the attack **(Fig. 21–2)**. This results in a severe and rapidly progressive anemia with hemoglobin levels frequently around 4 to 5 g/dL. Polychromasia, nucleated RBCs, and poikilocytosis are demonstrated in the peripheral smear, findings that are con-

TABLE 21-7   Donath-Landsteiner Test

	Tubes 1 Patient Serum (Tubes A1, B1, C1,)	Tubes 2 Patient Serum and Normal Serum(Tubes A2, B2, C2)	Tubes 3 Normal Serum[†] (Tubes A3, B3, C3)
Ice bath and 37°C (all A tubes)	+	+	0
Ice bath only (all B tubes)	0	0	0
37°C only (all C tubes)	0	0	0

+ = with hemolysis

0 = without hemolysis

† Tubes with normal serum are used as control

Note: The patient's blood should be clotted at 37°C and the serum separated at this temperature to avoid the loss of the autoantibody by cold autoadsorption prior to testing. Fresh normal serum should be included in the reaction medium as a source of complement as PCH patients may have low levels of serum complement. Omit the patient serum–only tubes (A1, B1, C1) if a limited amount of blood is available (i.e., a young child).

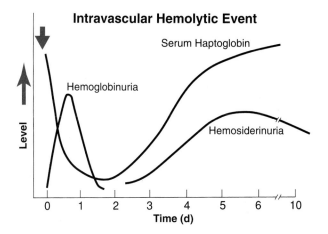

Intravascular Hemolytic Event

■ **FIGURE 21–2**   Indicator of acute intravascular hemolysis. Within a few hours of an acute hemolytic event, free hemoglobin is cleared from plasma, and the serum haptoglobin falls to undetectable levels. Hemoglobinuria ceases soon after this. If no further hemolysis occurs, the serum haptoglobin level recovers and methemalbumin disappears within several days. The urinary hemosiderin can provide more lasting evidence of the hemolytic event. (From Hillman, RS, and Finch, CA: Red Cell Manual, ed 7. FA Davis, Philadelphia, 1996, p 112, with permission.)

sistent with hemolytic anemia. These signs and symptoms, as well as hemoglobinuria, may resolve in a few hours or persist for days. Splenomegaly, hyperbilirubinemia, and renal insufficiency may also develop.

PCH is an acute hemolytic anemia occurring almost exclusively in children and young adults and almost always repre-

sents a transient disorder. Table 21–8 compares and contrasts PCH with CHD.

Treatment

For chronic forms of PCH, protection from cold exposure is the only useful therapy. Acute postinfection forms of PCH usually terminate spontaneously after resolution of the infectious process. Steroids and transfusion may be required, depending on the severity of the attacks.

Paroxysmal nocturnal hemoglobinuria (PNH) is often confused with PCH because of the similarity of the names and acronyms. An autoantibody has not been implicated in PNH; a membrane defect is thought to be involved. RBC destruction in PNH is complement-mediated because of the absence or reduced amounts of some complement regulatory proteins.[34] The only reason for this comment is to alert the reader to a common error in relating PCH and PNH.

Warm Reactive Autoantibodies

Autoantibodies that react best at 37°C are not found as often in the random population as the almost universal cold autoanti-I. However, many more of the true AIHAs are of the warm type (70 percent) than of the cold reactive type (18 percent).[7] As with the cold reactive autoantibodies, some individuals have apparently harmless warm autoantibodies. However, the harmless autoantibodies are serologically indistinguishable from the harmful ones. There are no diagnostic tests to determine which autoantibodies will cause RBC destruction. When a warm reactive autoantibody is encountered, it should be characterized as such and reported to the patient's physician. The presence of the antibody may alert the physician to an underlying autoimmune disease.

TABLE 21–8   Comparison of PCH and CHD

	PCH	CHD
Patient population	Children and young adults	Elderly or middle aged adults
Pathogenesis	Following viral infection	Idiopathic, lymphoproliferative disorder; following *M. pneumoniae* infection
Clinical features	Hemoglobinuria, acute attacks upon exposure to cold (symptoms resolve in hours to days)	Acrocyanosis; autoagglutination of blood at room temperature
Severity of hemolysis	Acute and rapid	Chronic and rarely severe
Site of hemolysis	Intravascular	Extravascular/intravascular
Autoantibody class	IgG (anti-P specificity; biphasic hemolysin)	IgM (anti-I/i) monophasic
DAT	2–3+ polyspecific AHG; neg. IgG 3–4+ monospecific C3 AHG	2–3+ polyspecific AHG; negative IgG; 3–4+ monospecific C3 AHG
Thermal range	Moderate (<20°C)	High (up to 30°–31°C)
Titer	Moderate (<64)	High (>1000)
Donath-Landsteiner test	Positive	Negative
Treatment	Supportive (disorder terminates when underlying illness resolves)	Avoid cold

Harmening DM: Clinical Hematology and Fundamentals of Hemostasis, ed 4. FA Davis, Philadelphia, 2002, p 212, with permission.

Clinical Findings

Patients with WAIHA present a different problem to the blood bank than those with cold AIHA. A significant percentage of cases suffers from an anemia of sufficient severity to require transfusion. The extent of anemia is variable; however, hemoglobins less than 7 g/dL are not uncommon. The onset of WAIHA is usually insidious and may be precipitated by a variety of factors such as infection,[35] trauma, surgery, pregnancy,[36] or psychological stress. In other patients, the onset is sudden and unexplained. WAIHA may be idiopathic with no underlying disease process or secondary to a pathologic disorder. **Box 21–2** lists the disorders commonly associated with AIHA.

Signs and symptoms appear when a significant anemia has developed. Pallor, weakness, dizziness, dyspnea, jaundice, and unexplained fever are occasionally presenting complaints. Hemolysis is usually acute at onset and may stabilize or continue to accelerate at a variable rate.

The peripheral blood smear usually displays polychromasia, reflecting reticulocytosis, which is characteristic of a hemolytic anemia **(Color Plate 6)**. Spherocytosis and occasionally RBC fragmentation, indicating extravascular hemolysis, can be demonstrated along with nucleated RBCs. An uncommon manifestation of WAIHA is reticulocytopenia. This may be associated with a hypoplastic marrow that is secondary to an underlying disease state. Because antigenic determinants on erythrocyte precursors can also react with the patient's RBC autoantibodies, reticulocytes can be destroyed as they are released from the bone marrow. Reticulocytopenia at the time of intense hemolysis, therefore, is associated with a high mortality rate. Products of hemolysis, such as bilirubin (particularly the unconjugated or indirect fraction) and urinary urobilinogen, are increased. In severe cases, depleted serum haptoglobin, hemoglobinemia, hemoglobinuria, and increases in LDH may be demonstrated.

RBC Hemolysis

In 80 percent of cases of WAIHA, the antibody causing the hemolysis is an IgG immunoglobulin, with IgG subclasses 1 and 3 found in patients demonstrating clinical signs of hemolytic anemia. In general, IgG3 antibodies are the most destructive to RBCs, followed by IgG1. IgG2 antibodies are less destructive, and IgG4 shows little or no RBC destruction.[37] The subclasses or isotypes of IgG are distinguished by the number of disulfide bonds present in the hinge region of the molecule, accounting for their different electrophoretic mobility and biologic properties. Refer to Chapter 3 for a complete discussion of the properties of the IgG subclasses. All IgG subclasses, except IgG4, possess the ability to bind complement via the classic pathway of activation, with IgG3 being more efficient than IgG1, which in turn is more efficient than IgG2. Macrophages possess receptors for the Fc region of IgG1 and IgG3.

Immune RBC destruction resulting from sensitization with IgG antibody is primarily extravascular, taking place in the fixed reticuloendothelial system (RES) cells of the liver and spleen. However, the spleen is 100 times more efficient in removal of IgG-sensitized RBCs. Macrophages are equipped with two important biologic receptors on their membranes:

1. Receptors for the Fc fragments of IgG1 and IgG3 immunoglobulins
2. Receptors for the C3b fragment of complement

Sensitized RBCs are phagocytized by interaction with RES mononuclear phagocytes, depending on which protein coats the erythrocytes. If only IgG coats the RBCs, gradual phagocytosis of the erythrocytes occurs. If both IgG and C3b coat the RBCs, there is a rapid phagocytosis, because the C3b fragment augments the action of IgG, enhancing sequestration and phagocytosis of the coated erythrocytes. If only C3b coats the RBCs, transient immune adherence occurs. It has been estimated that more than 100,000 molecules of the complement fragment would be required to induce phagocytosis. Therefore, the activity of the macrophages and the severity of hemolysis via phagocytosis of sensitized RBCs depend on various factors, summarized in **Box 21–3**.

Serologic Characteristics

Because warm reactive autoantibodies are typically IgG immunoglobulins, they react best by the antiglobulin technique. As a rule, they do not agglutinate saline-suspended RBCs after 37°C incubation. However, if albumin or another agglutination potentiator is added to the reaction mixture, agglutination may be observed in this phase. The antibodies may activate complement and are usually enhanced by enzyme techniques. Most of these autoantibodies react with a

---

BOX 21–2

Disorders Reported to be Frequently Associated with WAIHA Hemolytic Anemia

- Reticuloendothelial neoplasms, such as chronic lymphocytic leukemia, Hodgkin's disease, non-Hodgkin's lymphomas, thymomas
- Collagen disease, such as systemic lupus erythematosus, scleroderma, and rheumatoid arthritis
- Infectious diseases, such as viral syndromes in childhood and adults
- Immunologic diseases, such as hypogammaglobulinemia, dysglobulinemia, and other immune-deficiency syndromes
- Gastrointestinal diseases, such as ulcerative colitis
- Benign tumors, such as ovarian dermoid cysts
- Pregnancy

Adapted from Petz, LD, and Garratty, G: Acquired Immune Hemolytic Anemias. Churchill Livingstone, New York, 1980, p 32, with permission.

BOX 21–3

Factors Affecting Activity of Macrophages

- Subclass of IgG, especially IgG1 and IgG3
- Presence of complement (C3b) fragments
- Quantity of immunoglobulin or complement
- Number and activity of helper T cells (CD4)
- Number and activity of suppressor T cells (CD8)

Adapted from Pittiglio, D, and Sacher, RA: Clinical Hematology and Fundamentals of Hemostasis. FA Davis, Philadelphia, 1987, p 153, with permission.

high-incidence RBC antigen and often have a general specificity within the Rh blood group system, but there are reports of autoantibodies associated with most of the other blood group systems. Identification of autoantibodies is discussed in the following section. The typical reactions of warm autoantibodies are shown in **Table 21–9**.

Laboratory Tests Affected by Warm Reactive Autoantibodies

Warm reactive autoantibodies can interfere with most routine blood bank tests, and they may present more of a dilemma than cold autoagglutinins. Most cold autoantibodies can be avoided if testing is performed at 37°C or if anti-IgG antiglobulin is used. In the case of WAIHA, however, significant alloantibodies and the autoantibodies react best at 37°C. Therefore, more complicated and time-consuming procedures for resolving the problems may have to be used.

ABO Typing

Because warm reactive autoantibodies are not direct agglutinins, ABO grouping is usually not affected. Even though the patient's cells may be heavily coated with antibody, the antibodies normally do not agglutinate spontaneously when reagent anti-A and anti-B are added. Similarly, warm autoantibodies in the serum usually do not agglutinate saline-suspended A_1 and B cells.

Rh(D) Typing

False-positive Rh typing can be a problem, when the patient's cells are coated with warm reactive autoantibodies. The high-protein Rh antisera previously available for Rh testing demonstrated numerous testing problems. The agglutination potentiators that were added to many high-protein Rh typing reagents demonstrated direct agglutination with RBCs strongly coated with IgG immunoglobulins. For this reason, a control serum, consisting of patient cells and the matching Rh diluent, had to be tested in parallel with the D typing. The results of the D antigen typing were valid only when the control test result was negative. However, the current reagents available for D typing are monoclonal antisera containing no more than 7 percent protein additive. This antiserum demon-

strates a low incidence of false positive test results. Depending on the manufacturer of the antiserum, an Rh control serum may be recommended to be tested in parallel with the anti-D serum. Often the manufacturer will indicate that a negative test with an antiserum of a similar protein concentration (including ABO antisera) is sufficient to detect a false-positive reaction. However, because the autoantibody coating the patient's cells is an IgG immunoglobulin, it is not possible to detect individuals with a weak D phenotype using an antiglobulin test procedure. If a patient types as group AB, Rh D-positive (all tubes in the ABO cell typing and the D typing are positive), a separate Rh control (matched diluent or 6 percent albumin) must be tested along with the anti-D to ensure that the D antigen typing is valid (see Chapter 7). In an extreme situation, it may be necessary to pretreat the cells using the EDTA/glycine acid (EGA) method to remove coating-IgG immunoglobulins from the RBCs. (See Procedure J in the Procedural Appendix.) If DAT testing of the EGA pretreated cells is negative, it is possible to use these cells for weak D testing; however, an Rh control serum or 6 percent albumin should be tested in parallel to detect false-positive reactivity. *Note:* Although pretreatment of the RBCs with chloroquine diphosphate solution will remove a significant quantity of coating IgG immunoglobulins, it is not recommended that these cells be used for Rh(D) typing with monoclonal antiserum.[38] Another technique to detect a weak D type is the rosette test (see Chapter 20), which is commonly used in the detection of fetal-maternal hemorrhage. This screening test, used to detect fetal D-positive cells in the circulation of the D-negative mother, will also detect D-positive cells in any cell population. If the patient's cells are D-positive, the rosette test will be strongly positive. Because the rosette test does not incorporate an antiglobulin phase, a patient with a positive DAT can be accurately typed for the D antigen by this method. It is not absolutely necessary to determine the correct weak D typing of a patient with WAIHA, because D-negative RBCs can be transfused if necessary.

DAT

A positive DAT is expected in association with warm reactive autoantibodies. As autoantibody is produced, it adsorbs onto the antigen of that defined specificity present on the patient's own RBCs. The RBCs may then be coated with IgG alone (20 percent), IgG and complement (67 percent), or complement alone (13 percent).[7] In rare cases, the DAT may be negative or cells may be coated only with IgA or IgM.[18–20]

Antibody Detection and Identification

The serum of a patient with warm autoagglutinins may contain only autoantibody or a mixture of autoantibody and alloantibody if the patient has been previously transfused or pregnant. When smaller amounts of autoantibody have been produced, all of the autoantibody may be adsorbed onto the patient's cells in vivo, and no free autoantibody will be detectable in the serum. However, if the amount of antibody produced exceeds the number of RBC antigen sites available, serum antibody will be detected in antiglobulin phase testing. When warm reactive autoantibodies are present in the serum or on the patient's cells, the extent of the testing should be based on the patient's history. It must be confirmed that the antibody coating the patient's cells is an autoantibody,

TABLE 21–9 Serologic Reactions of Typical Warm Autoantibodies			
Test Phase	Reagent RBCs	Autologous Cells	Enzyme-Treated Reagent RBCs
Room temperature	Negative	Negative	Negative
37°C	Negative	Negative	Negative
IgG antiglobulin test	2+ to 4+	4+	4+
Polyspecific antiglobulin test	2+ to 4+	4+	4+
C3 antiglobulin test	0 to 2+	0 to 3+	0 to 2+

TABLE 21–10 Possible Risk of Clinically Significant Underlying Alloantibody in the Presence of Warm Autoantibody

Risk	HX of Transfusion	HX of Pregnancy	HX of HDN or HTR
Low	None	None	None
Moderate	≤3	≤2	None
High	≥4	≥3	Yes

HX = history; HDN = hemolytic disease of the newborn; HTR = hemolytic transfusion reaction

and limited testing should be performed to determine the specificity. Efforts must be made to detect and identify all clinically significant alloantibodies that might be masked by the autoantibody. If the patient has had a previous transfusion or has been pregnant, there is an inherent risk of previous alloimmunization. **Table 21–10** shows the likelihood that an underlying alloantibody may be present in the serum of patients with autoantibody on their RBCs and in their serum.

Evaluation of Autoantibody

A positive DAT can result from RBC alloantibodies coating recently transfused donor cells or drug-induced antibodies as well as RBC autoantibodies. IgG immunoglobulins will most likely be present on the cells in each case; however, antibody may not be present in the serum. It is important to differentiate the origins of a positive DAT because selection of RBCs for transfusion and treatment protocols differ. To make the distinction between these causes, one must have the patient's medical history, including an accurate history of previous transfusions and pregnancies, diagnoses, and medications. If a patient has had a recent transfusion, the possibility that alloantibodies and not autoantibodies are coating the remaining transfused donor cells must be considered. In most cases, by examining the DAT microscopically for mixed-field agglutination (which indicates a mixed-cell population) and by determining the specificity of the antibody in the eluate, it is possible to establish alloantibodies as the cause (see Chapter 18). Because warm autoantibodies are frequently associated with certain diseases, such as systemic lupus erythematosus,

and with medications, such as Aldomet, the patient's diagnosis and drug history are informative tools in helping establish autoantibodies as the cause of the positive DAT. As discussed below, the specificity of the antibody may be helpful in differentiating between autoantibody and alloantibody.

To identify the specificity of a warm reactive autoantibody, an eluate prepared from the patient's RBCs must be tested, in addition to the patient's serum, with a panel of reagent RBCs. (See Procedure F in the Procedural Appendix for instructions in preparing a digitonin acid eluate. *Note:* A commercial kit is also available for the preparation of acid eluates.) If the patient has a well-documented history that he or she has not been transfused within the past 3 months, it may be assumed that antibody activity in the eluate is autoantibody. However, if the patient has a history of transfusion or pregnancy, the serum may contain alloantibody in addition to autoantibody.

The specificity of an autoantibody may be different in the serum and in the eluate. Warm autoantibodies may have an apparent autoanti-e specificity in the serum but may show pan-agglutination of RBCs tested with the eluate. This difference may be qualitative or quantitative. The concentration of antibody removed from the cells in the elution process may be greater than that in the serum. **Table 21–11** illustrates an example of such reactivity. It should also be noted that elution procedures vary in their ability to remove coating immunoglobulins (i.e., a heat or freeze/thaw eluate generally reacts less strongly than an acid eluate or one of the chemical eluates, such as dichloromethane or ether).

A majority of the IgG antibodies detected in eluates prepared from the WAIHA patient's RBCs or in the patient's serum has a complex Rh-like specificity, similar to those shown in **Table 21–12**. Occasionally, an autoantibody may have what is termed "simple anti-e specificity" and reacts with all normal cells, except R_2R_2 (D+C−E+c+e−) cells. Much more frequently, reactivity is observed with all RBCs of normal Rh phenotype. In order to identify the specificity of a complex Rh-like autoantibody, one must have an extensive library of rare cells, which includes Rh_{null} and D-- cells. Testing of these cells should allow one to categorize the antibody as: anti-nl (normal), which reacts with all cells of common/normal Rh phenotypes, but not those that are partially deleted or Rh_{null}; anti-pdl (partially deleted), which reacts with all cells except Rh_{null}; and or anti-dl (deleted), which reacts with all cells.[39] However, it should be noted that this level of antibody identification is of academic interest rather than of practical application in the selection of donor units for transfusion.

TABLE 21–11 Typical Serologic Reactivity of Serum and Eluates Containing Warm Autoantibody

Reagent RBC Rh Type	Serum Warm Autoantibody IgG AGT	Acid Eluate Warm Autoantibody IgG AGT	Heat Eluate Warm Autoantibody IgG AGT	Serum Auto-Anti-e IgG AGT
R_0r (D+C−E−c+e+)	2+−3+	4+	2+	2+−3+
R_1R_1 (D+C+E−c−e+)	2+−3+	4+	2+	2+−3+
R_2R_2 (D+C−E+c+e−)	2+−3+	4+	2+	0
rr (D−C−E−c+e+)	2+−3+	4+	2+	2+−3+

IgG = monospecific anti-IgG; AGT = antiglobulin test

TABLE 21-12 Typical Serologic Reactions of Warm Autoantibodies with RBCs of Selected Rh Phenotypes

	Auto-Anti-e	Anti-nl	Anti-pdl	Anti-dl
R_1R_1 (normal)	+	+	+	+
R_2R_2 (normal)	0	+	+	+
rr (normal)	+	+	+	+
D-- (partially deleted)	0	0	+	+
Rh$_{null}$ (fully deleted)	0	0	0	+

nl = normal pdl = partially delected dl = fully deleted

There are numerous reports of autoantibodies with specificities other than Rh, many of which appear to be directed against RBC antigens of high incidence or a null phenotype. Among the other specificities are autoanti-U, -Wr[b], -En[a], -Kp[b],[40] -Vel,[41] and -Ge.[42] The reader is referred to Chapter 7 of Petz and Garratty[7] for a detailed discussion of autoantibody specificity. Apparent specificities such as these can cause confusion, especially when the patient has had a recent transfusion.

Determination of the patient's phenotype is one of the most valuable tools used to classify the antibody as "auto" or "allo." Most researchers agree that it is not necessary to do extensive studies to identify autoantibodies. However, it is recommended that a thorough investigation be conducted to identify alloantibody activity, including testing of at least one RBC that is phenotypically similar to those of the patient. By testing a commercial RBC panel, an antibody of simple specificity can be identified. Testing of phenotypically similar RBCs makes it possible to determine if the antibody activity is the result of multiple alloantibodies (the phenotypically similar cell will be nonreactive) or an autoantibody (the phenotypically similar cell will be reactive). There can be, however, many exceptions to these interpretations. The need to consider the medical history cannot be overemphasized.

Specificity of the autoantibody may be helpful in selecting blood for transfusion. Some practitioners prefer to transfuse RBCs that are compatible with the autoantibody, if simple specificity can be assigned, such as anti-e, and if there are no preexisting circumstances that would prevent this transfusion. (One would never select Rh-positive e-negative RBCs for an Rh-negative patient with auto-anti-e.) However, selecting donor units that are compatible with the patient's autoantibody cannot guarantee RBC survival, because the transfused cells are most likely going to be destroyed as rapidly as the patient's own cells, regardless of phenotype. It is best to reserve e-negative donor units for those patients with alloanti.

Detection and Identification of Alloantibodies

All researchers agree that detection and identification of all alloantibodies is of primary concern when one must give a transfusion to a patient with WAIHA, especially when the patient has had a previous transfusion or pregnancy. When autoantibody is found in the serum, it will typically mask any alloantibodies present. In this situation one can use several techniques:

1. If the autoantibody demonstrates a specificity, such as anti-e, test a panel of cells negative for the corresponding antigen (e-negative, in this case) and positive for all common clinically significant RBC antigens (Kell, Duffy, Kidd, S, and s) to exclude the presence of underlying alloantibodies.

2. If the patient has not had a recent transfusion (within the past 3 months), determine the patient's RBC phenotype using either monoclonal antisera, which does not require antiglobulin testing, or patient RBCs treated with an agent known to remove coating IgG immunoglobulins. The cells may be treated with chloroquine diphosphate solution or the EDTA/EGA procedure prior to phenotyping. (The EDTA/EGA procedure will remove all Kell system antigens.) If there is a sufficient quantity of patient RBCs available, prepare autologous cells for autoadsorption procedures. Pretreat the cells to remove coating autoantibody, using either of the methods described above or a similar reagent such as ZZAP. (See Procedure G.B in the Procedural Appendix.) This treatment will free antigens sites for adsorption of autoantibody.

3. If autoadsorption studies are not possible because the patient was recently transfused, and there is evidence of reticulocyte production, it may be possible to determine the patient's phenotype using a reticulocyte harvesting procedure. (See Procedure K of the Procedural Appendix.) This phenotyping information can be used to select RBCs that are phenotypically similar to those of the patient by matching the common RBC antigens: Rh, Kell, Kidd, Duffy, M, N, S, and s. Allogeneic adsorptions performed using this method to select phenotypically similar donor or reagent RBCs will remove autoantibody, but it will also adsorb an alloantibody to a common high incidence RBC antigen.

4. If it is not possible to determine the patient's RBC phenotyping, multiple allogeneic adsorptions may be performed by selecting three donor units that are known to lack common RBC antigens and are of all possible Rh antigen combinations. Typically, these cells include each of the following Rh types: D+C+E−c−e+, D+C−E+c+e−, and D−C−E−c+e+. Allogeneic adsorptions performed using this method will remove autoantibody but will also adsorb an alloantibody to a common high-incidence RBC antigen.

In typical warm autoadsorption procedures, the patient's serum and the patient's cells are incubated at 37°C, allowing the autoantibody to bind to antigen sites on the autologous cells, leaving alloantibody in the serum. To improve the uptake of autoantibody, the patient's RBCs should be pretreated with a reagent such as ZZAP or chloroquine diphosphate or the EDTA/EGA procedure to remove autoantibody and free RBC antigen sites for adsorption of autoantibody. The number of adsorptions needed to prepare the serum for alloantibody detection procedures depends on the amount of autoantibody present in the patient's serum and the test procedure used. By titering the patient's serum using simple doubling dilutions of the serum in 6 percent albumin and

TABLE 21–13   Antibody Detection Using Unadsorbed and Autoadsorbed Serum

	Unadsorbed		Adsorbed XI		Adsorbed X2	
	Serum A	Serum B	Serum A	Serum B	Serum A	Serum B
Reagent RBCs	AGT	AGT	AGT	AGT	AGT	AGT
Screening Cell I	3+	3+	1+	1+	0	0
Screening Cell II	3+	3+	1+	2+	0	2+

Serum A contains autoantibody with no underlying alloantibody
Serum B contains autoantibody with underlying alloantibody
AGT = antiglobulin test

testing the diluted serum with reagent RBCs or a phenotypically similar RBC using the enhancement solution that will be used in antibody detection, it is possible to estimate the amount of autoantibody present. If there is a large amount of autoantibody in the serum and/or gel testing or polyethylene glycol enhancement solution is used in testing, more than one absorption will be necessary. (See Procedure G in the Procedural Appendix.) **Table 21–13** gives an example of antibody detection tests using unadsorbed, once-adsorbed, and twice-adsorbed serum. In this example, one adsorption failed to remove all the autoantibody, but two adsorptions were effective. No underlying alloantibodies are evident in serum A of this example, but serum B shows a probable alloantibody in the adsorbed serum.

When performing adsorption procedures, the following circumstances must be considered. First, if the patient has been transfused recently, even small amounts of donor RBCs in the patient specimen may remove alloantibody during the absorption procedure. Autoadsorption procedures are never recommended in patients who have been transfused within the previous 3 months. Second, if the patient is severely anemic, it may not be possible to obtain autologous cells for multiple adsorptions. Third, whenever an adsorption is performed, whether with autologous or allogeneic cells, the serum is diluted to some extent. Some saline remains in "packed" RBCs. A weakly reactive alloantibody could be diluted and missed if multiple adsorptions are performed. Fourth, if allogeneic adsorptions are performed, it is possible to adsorb an alloantibody to a high-frequency RBC antigen that is present on the allogeneic cells that is not present on the patient's own cells.

When the patient has had a recent transfusion or is severely anemic, cells of selected phenotypes for adsorption can be used. If the patient's phenotype is unknown and cannot be determined, adsorptions can be performed using a trio of selected cells (R_1R_1, R_2R_2, and rr). These cells should also lack one or more antigens for the more commonly encountered clinically significant alloantibodies (e.g., Kell, Duffy, Kidd, Ss). As shown in **Table 21–14**, if the patient's serum is adsorbed with cells from donors of selected phenotypes and then the adsorbed sera are tested, many important alloantibodies can be detected.

Alternatively, if a pretransfusion phenotype is available for the patient, phenotypically matched RBCs can be used for adsorption. (See discussion of antigen typing the patient with a positive DAT in this chapter.) For example, examine the patient's RBC phenotype in **Table 21–15**. The patient should not form alloantibodies to RBC antigens that he or she possesses; therefore, we are concerned only with the antigens the patient lacks. The patient is negative for the following antigens: c, E, Fy^b, Jk^a, K, and S. If donor cells are selected that are also negative for c, E, K, and Jk^a and then they are enzyme-treated to destroy the Duffy and MNSs antigens, we can adsorb the autoantibody and leave the common alloantibodies that the patient might form. In this example, the patient has an underlying alloanti.

It is impossible to detect all clinically significant alloantibodies using allogeneic adsorptions, like those directed against high-incidence antigens. For example, an anti-K2 (Cellano) would be adsorbed onto virtually all random donor cells, because the K2 antigen is present on the cells of more than 99 percent of the population (such as the R_1R_1 and R_2R_2 adsorption cells in **Table 21–14** and the phenotypically matched donor in **Table 21–15**). An antibody such as this

TABLE 21–14   Differential Adsorption Technique for Detecting Alloantibodies in the Serum of a Patient with Warm-Reacting Autoantibodies

RBC	Phenotyping of Adsorbing RBC	Antibody Removed by Adsorption	Antibody Remaining in Serum
R_1R_1 (D+C+E−c−e+)	K−k+, Fy(a+b−), Jk(a−b+), S+s+	D,C,e,k,Fy^a,Jk^b, S,s	E,c,K,Fy^b,Jk^a
R_2R_2 (D+C−E+c+e−)	K−k+, Fy(a−b+), Jk(a+b−), S−s+	D,E,c,k,Fy^b,Jk^a, s	C,e,K,Fy^a,Jk^b,S
rr (D−C−E−c+e+)	K+k−, Fy(a−b+), Jk(a+b+), S+s−	c,e,K,Fy^b, Jk^a,Jk^b,S	D,C,E,k,Fy^a,s

TABLE 21-15   Adsorption of Autoantibody Using Phenotypically Similar Donor Cells. Patient's serum demonstrates 3+ agglutination with all cells including his own in antiglobulin testing.

Patient's RBC Phenotype	Phenotyping of Adsorbing RBC Prior to Ficin Treatment*	Antibody that May Be Removed by Adsorption	Antibody That May remain in Serum Note: *Ficin Treatment Denatures Fyᵃ, Fyᵇ,S,s
R₁R₁ (D+C+E−c−e+), K−k+, Fy(a+b−) Jk(a−b+), S−s+	R₁R₁, K−k+, Fy(a+b+), Jk(a−b+) S+s+	D,C,e,k,Jkᵇ	E,c,K,Fyᵃ, Fyᵇ,Jkᵃ, S,s

Testing below was performed with serum-adsorbed X2 with phenotypically similar ficin-treated cells described above.

Cell	D	C	E	c	e	K	k	Fyᵃ	Fyᵇ	Jkᵃ	Jkᵇ	S	s	AGT
#1	+	+	−	−	+	−	+	+	+	+	+	+	−	0
#2	+	+	+	−	+	−	+	−	+	−	+	+	+	0
#3	−	−	+	+	+	+	+	+	−	+	−	−	+	2+
#4	−	−	−	+	+	−	+	+	−	+	−	+	−	0
#5	−	−	−	+	+	+	+	−	−	+	+	+	+	2+
#6	−	−	+	+	+	−	+	+	−	+	+	+	+	0
#7	−	−	−	+	+	−	+	−	+	+	−	−	+	0

Result: The patient's serum contains an underlying alloanti-K.

would be differentiated from the autoantibody only if a cell negative for the high-incidence antigen happened to be present among the cells used for adsorption.

When alloantibodies are detected in the serum of a patient with WAIHA, it is necessary to test the patient's untrasfused RBCs for the absence of the corresponding antigen. When the patient has a positive DAT, usually with IgG coating the cells, antigen typing using an antiglobulin test (such as typing for Kell, Duffy, and Kidd antigens) will be invalid. Pretreatment of the patient's cells with chloroquine diphosphate solution to remove coating IgG immunoglobulins may permit valid RBC antigen typings. The EDTA/EGA procedure can also be used to remove coating IgG immunoglobulins; however, all Kell system antigens are destroyed. In all cases, careful attention should be paid to the pretreatment procedure, following instructions in the procedure or in the package insert of commercially available reagents to ensure that certain antigens will not be destroyed or weakened. The recent development of monoclonal antisera for all the common Rh antigens, the K1 (Kell) antigen, and the Kidd antigens (Jkᵃ and Jkᵇ) has facilitated RBC phenotyping. These antisera do not require antiglobulin phase testing and do not typically show falsepositive agglutination with RBCs strongly coated with IgG immunoglobulins.

Selection of Blood for Transfusion

Many patients with WAIHA never require transfusion; they can be managed with medical treatment. Occasionally, however, the anemia is so severe that transfusion cannot be avoided.[7] In addition, patients who have a nonhemolytic WAIHA pose problems when blood is needed for a surgical procedure. In these cases, after thorough serologic investigation the primary concern is to ensure compatibility with any alloantibodies in the patient's serum.

Compatibility with the autoantibody is controversial. If the autoantibody shows a simple specificity, such as anti-e, local practice may be to select donor units that are negative for the corresponding antigen. However, it must be ensured that the cells selected do not possess an antigen that is likely to result in stimulation of the patient to form alloantibodies. For example, because virtually all Rh-negative (D−) cells are e-positive, an Rh-negative (D−) patient with auto-anti-e specificity should not receive a transfusion of Rh-positive (D+) RBCs that lack the e antigen.[43] Singh and colleagues[44] report hemoglobin increments in patients with AIHA comparable to the expected increment even when e-positive units are transfused to patients with an apparent auto-anti-e. Finding compatible units for patients with a broad-specificity warm autoagglutinin is virtually impossible. "Least incompatible" RBCs may be selected for transfusion. However, the selection of in-vitro least incompatible RBCs may not translate to invivo most compatible RBCs. In all cases, the transfused donor cells are likely to be destroyed as rapidly as the patient's own RBCs. It is much more important that donor units be selected that are compatible with any alloantibodies detected using the techniques described in the previous section.

Treatment

Therapy is generally aimed at first treating the underlying disease, if one is present. General measures to support cardiovascular function are important for patients who are severely anemic. Transfusion should generally be avoided, if possible, because this may only accelerate hemolysis instead of ameliorating the anemia. However, transfusion should not be avoided in situations of life-threatening anemia. In many cases, even small amounts of transfused RBCs (one-half to one unit) are sufficient to relieve the symptoms of the anemia.[45]

The forms of treatment described in the discussions following are generally used, depending on the severity of the disorder.

Corticosteroid Administration and Use of Intravenous Immunoglobulin

One form of therapy involves the use of corticosteroids, such as prednisone. Initially, high doses of 100 to 200 mg of prednisone are maintained until the patient's hematocrit level stabilizes. Patients who have not had transfusions respond to steroid therapy more rapidly than those who are transfused.

Several mechanisms have been proposed for the action of prednisone, including:

1. Reduction of antibody synthesis
2. Altered antibody activity
3. Alteration of macrophage receptors for IgG and C3, which reduces the clearance of antibody-coated RBCs[46]

The dosage of prednisone should be reduced when the hematocrit begins to rise and the reticulocyte count drops. Finally, the steroids are withdrawn slowly over 2 to 4 months. A beneficial response to the administration of prednisone is demonstrated in 50 to 65 percent of all cases of WAIHA. An androgenic steroid, danazol, has also been beneficial in prednisone-resistant cases.[46] The use of intravenous immune globulin in patients unresponsive to corticosteroid treatment is controversial and appears to have limited efficacy.[47]

Splenectomy

If steroid therapy fails, or if a patient requires large doses of steroids to control hemolysis, splenectomy is usually recommended. The decision to perform a splenectomy requires clinical evaluation and judgment. There are three reasons for performing a splenectomy:

1. Failure of steroid therapy
2. Need for continuous high-dose steroid maintenance
3. Complications of steroid therapy

Splenectomy results in decreased production of antibody and removes a potent site of RBC damage and destruction. Patients who had a good initial response to steroids respond better with splenectomy than do those who failed initial steroid therapy.

It has been reported that as many as 60 percent of patients with WAIHA benefit from splenectomy if steroid dosages greater than 15 mg per day are also used to maintain remission.

Immunosuppressive Drugs

This is usually the last approach used in management of WAIHA. Azathioprine (Imuran) and cyclophosphamide are examples of immunosuppressive drugs that interfere with antibody synthesis by destroying dividing cells.

Experience with this therapy is limited. The most detrimental side effect that threatens the common use of these drugs is a potential for neoplastic growth as a result of the defective immune surveillance of immunosuppressed patients.

Mixed-Type Autoantibodies

Individuals demonstrating antibody activity that appears to have both "warm" and "cold" components are considered to have a mixed-type AIHA. Serologic testing will show autoantibody components typical of both warm and cold AIHA. Table 21–16 reviews and compares the characteristics of cold and warm AIHAs. Although the cold autoagglutinin in these individuals may react weakly at 4°C, it is usually reactive up to 30°C or above. The cold agglutinin is an IgM hemagglutinin capable of binding complement. The warm component is an IgG antibody; therefore, the patient will typically demonstrate a positive DAT with IgG and complement on the RBCs. Patients with mixed-type AIHA often present with extremely acute hemolysis and frequently require transfusion. Because there are two separate autoantibodies present, adsorption procedures must include both cold and warm adsorptions to completely remove autoagglutinins. In routine adsorption procedures, the patient's serum or plasma will be first adsorbed at 4°C with one or more aliquots of selected cells and then adsorbed at 37°C with additional aliquots of selected cells, using the procedures previously described. It has been found that corticosteroid treatment is most often effective in treating individuals with mixed-type AIHA.[48]

Drug-Induced Sensitization and Immune Hemolytic Anemia

Drugs can cause a variety of side effects, including immune destruction of RBCs, white blood cells (WBCs), and platelets, although the incidence is rare. Hemolytic anemia, leukopenia, and thrombocytopenia can occur separately, but in some patients more than one cell line can be affected. The cells may be coated with antibody, antibody and complement, or complement alone. The discussion in this section is limited to RBC problems, but many of the same principles also apply to platelets and leukocytes.

Drug-mediated problems may come to the attention of the blood bank technologist in one of two ways:

TABLE 21–16	Comparison of Warm and Cold AIHA	
	Warm AIHA	**Cold AIHA**
Optimal reaction temperature	>32°C	<30°C
Immunoglobulin classification	IgG	IgM
Complement activation	May bind complement	Binds complement
Site of hemolysis	Usually extravascular (no cell lysis)	Extravascular/ intravascular (cell lysis)
Frequency	70–75% of cases	16% of cases (PCH 1–2%)
Specificity	Frequently broad Rh-like	Ii system (PCH autoanti-P)

Adapted from Harmening, DM: Clinical Hematology and Fundamentals of Hemostasis, ed 4. F.A. Davis, Philadelphia, 2002, p 213, with permission.

1. A request for diagnostic testing on a patient with a possible hemolytic anemia
2. Unexpected results in routine testing; for example, a positive autologous control in the antiglobulin phase of antibody screening or compatibility testing or a positive DAT

Drugs should be suspected as a possible explanation for immune hemolysis or a positive DAT when there is no other reason for the serologic and hematologic findings and if the patient has a history of taking drugs. Because, with the exception of Aldomet-induced problems, drug-induced positive DATs and hemolytic anemia are relatively rare, other potential causes should be considered and investigated first. Petz and Garratty[7] review the four classic mechanisms proposed to account for drug-induced problems: immune complexes, drug adsorption, membrane modification, and autoantibody formation. Specific drugs have been commonly associated with one particular mechanism but may work by another.[49,50] Other theories postulate combining aspects of these earlier proposed mechanisms.[39] Drug-related positive DATs may be additionally classified as "drug-dependent" or "drug-independent." A discussion of the classic categories of drug-induced hemolytic anemias follows, including elements of these new hypotheses. Representative drugs associated with each mechanism as well as those known to act by multiple mechanisms are listed in **Table 21–17**.

Drug-Dependent or Immune Complex ("Innocent Bystander") Mechanism

Although the occurrence is rare, many drugs have been implicated in causing immune-mediated problems by the immune complex mechanism. This mechanism was first described in the early 1960s, and it was thought that drugs operating through this mechanism combine with plasma proteins to form immunogens.[51] The antibody (IgG or IgM) produced recognizes determinants on the drug. If the patient ingests the same drug (or a drug bearing the same haptenic group) after immunization, the formation of a drug-antidrug com-

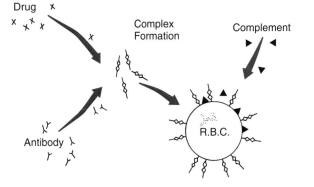

■ **FIGURE 21–3**   Immune complex mechanism. (From Petz and Garratty,[7] p 272, with permission.)

plex may occur. The complement cascade may be activated because of this antigen-antibody interaction. RBCs are thought to be involved in this process only as "innocent bystanders."[52] The soluble drug-antidrug complex nonspecifically adsorbs loosely to the RBC surface. Complement, when activated, sensitizes the cell and may cause lysis **(Fig. 21–3)**.

More recently, however, the concept of "neoantigen" formation has been proposed. In this model, the drug interacts in a noncovalent manner with a specific membrane component and forms a new determinant consisting of both drug and membrane components.

Because complement activation is involved in the immune complex, clinically affected patients frequently present with acute intravascular hemolysis.[23] When other causes for hemoglobinemia and hemoglobinuria have been excluded (e.g., ABO hemolytic transfusion reactions or cold AIHA), a drug-antidrug reaction should be considered. When obtaining the drug history, it is important to realize that this group of patients needs to take only small doses of the drug to be affected. The patient recovers rapidly once the drug is withdrawn.

TABLE 21–17 Examples of Some of the Drugs Implicated in Causing a Positive DAT			
Immune Complex:			
Sulfonamides	Cefotaxime	Hydralazine	Methotrexate
Quinine	Ceftriaxone	Zomax	Cephalosporins
Quinidine	Acetaminophen	Carbimazole	Fluorouracil (5-FU)
Nalidixic Acid	Teniposide (VM-26)	Zomepirac	Phenacetin
Aminopyrine	Probenecid	Tolmetin	Diclofenac
Drug Adsorption:			
Penicillin	Cefazolin	Cisplatin	Carbromal
Cephalothin	Cefamandole	Tetracycline	Cephaloridine
Cefoxitin	Erythromycin	Ceftriaxone	Streptomycin
Drug-Independent:			
Alpha-methyldopa	Levadopa	Ibuprofen	Procainamide
Mefenamic Acid	Chlorpromazine	Phenacetin	Ponstel
Tolmetin	Chlorpromazine	Nomifensine	Cephalosporins

It should be noted that some drugs may act using more than one proposed mechanism.

TABLE 21–18   Serologic Reactions Observed with Drug-Induced Positive DATs

Mechanism	Immunoglobulin on RBC	Serum and Eluate React with:
Immune complex	C3—Occasionally IgG and IgM	Cells, only if serum was **incubated with the drug** prior to testing. Routine testing with reagent RBCs is negative.
Drug adsorption	IgG—rarely C3 may be present	Cells only if they are **coated with the specific drug** prior to testing. Routine testing with reagent RBCs is negative.
Drug-independent	IgG	All "normal" RBCs. Routine testing with reagent RBCs is positive
Membrane modification	IgG, IgM, IgA, C3	No cells tested. The mechanism is nonimmunologic protein adsorption.

If polyspecific antihuman serum is used in DAT testing, the patient's DAT will usually be positive. If monospecific reagents are used, agglutination usually occurs with anticomplement but not with anti-IgG. Tests with anti-IgG are negative, even when the antibody is of the IgG class, because the drug-anti-drug complex is thought to elute from the cell during the washing procedure before the antiglobulin test.[53,54] Other routine blood bank tests are negative in all phases; the antibody is directed against a drug or the drug-RBC membrane "neoantigen," not a true RBC antigen. Therefore, the antibody screening procedures and compatibility tests are negative, unless an alloantibody is also present. An eluate tested with reagent RBCs will also be negative. A summary of typical serologic results is given in **Table 21–18**.

To confirm that a positive DAT is caused by a drug-antidrug reaction through the drug-dependent mechanism, the antibody in the patient's serum must be demonstrated. The patient's serum is incubated with a solution of the drug in question and ABO-compatible RBCs, which lack RBC antigens recognized by any alloantibodies detected in the patient's serum. Complement activation is the usual indicator of an antigen-antibody reaction; therefore, one should observe for hemolysis after incubation and use reagents containing anti-C3 activity for the antiglobulin test. A general procedure for demonstrating antibodies reacting by the immune complex mechanism, suggested by Garratty,[55] is given in Procedure H of the Procedural Appendix.

For the test results to be interpreted correctly, adequate controls must be performed. The patient's serum must not react with the cells when saline or the diluent used to dissolve the drug is substituted for the drug solution, and the drug solution must not hemolyze the suspension of cells nonspecifically. Examples of typical reactions with the patient's serum and control are given in **Table 21–19**.

An eluate from the patient's cells is usually nonreactive even if the drug and a source of complement are added. Very little antibody, if any, remains on the cells after washing.

In most blood banks, confirmatory testing is done only when the patient has hematologic complications and not when the patient simply has a history of taking the drug and a positive DAT. Some of the drugs known to cause immune complex–mediated problems are in frequent use and there is a large number of patients with a positive DAT and no evidence of hemolysis. Therefore, a full workup is only of academic interest and is not required before release of RBCs for transfusion.

Treatment involves discontinuing the use of the drug. Although hemolysis by this mechanism is rare, the onset is usually sudden and may be characterized by intravascular hemolysis and renal failure. Therefore, immediate cessation of the drug is essential. Steroid treatment may also be given.

Drug-Adsorption (Hapten) Mechanism

Unlike drugs acting through the immune complex mechanism, drugs operating through the drug-adsorption mechanism bind firmly to proteins, including the proteins of the RBC membrane (**Fig. 21–4**). Presumably because of their

TABLE 21–19   Test Results Observed in the Presence of Antidrug-Antibody Reactive by the Immune Complexing Mechanism:

Test	Patient	Fresh Serum*	Drug	RBCs	Results
Patient serum control	X	—	—	X	If negative, indicates no alloantibody to RBC present.
Fresh serum control	—	X	X	X	If negative, indicates no alloantibody to RBC or drug present.
Drug/RBC control	—	—	X	X	If negative, indicates drug solution will not cause agglutination alone.
Patient test	X	X	X	X	If agglutination is present and controls are all negative, indicates the presence of antidrug antibody. If negative no antidrug present.

*Fresh serum is the source of complement in this test.

X = sample added to tube. — = no sample added to tube.

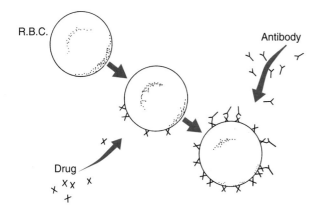

R.B.C.

Antibody

Drug

■ **FIGURE 21–4**   Drug adsorption mechanism. (From Petz and Garratty,[7] p 280, with permission.)

ability to bind to proteins, these drugs are better immunogens. For example, antibodies to penicillin, the drug most commonly associated with this mechanism, are found in about 3 percent of hospitalized patients receiving large doses of penicillin; of these, fewer than 5 percent develop a hemolytic anemia.[23] Even with the relatively high incidence of antipenicillin antibodies and the ability of the drug to bind to the RBC membrane, penicillin-induced positive DATs are rare.[12] The low incidence may reflect the fact that the patient must receive massive doses (10 million units per day) of penicillin for the cells to be coated adequately. Also, most penicillin antibodies are IgM and therefore not detected by the antiglobulin test. The penicillin antibody responsible for a positive DAT is most often IgG, less often IgM, IgA and/or IgD, and rarely complement.[39]

Laboratory test results are consistent with this description of the mechanism (see **Table 21–18**). Cells from patients with a positive DAT are usually coated with IgG alone. However, sometimes both IgG and complement are present on the cells. The patient's serum and eluate are nonreactive with reagent RBCs and random donor cells. Therefore, the antibody screen is negative, and crossmatches are compatible in all phases. However, if the serum and eluate are tested with penicillin-coated cells, agglutination does occur in the antiglobulin phase. The procedure for preparing the penicillin-coated cells is given in Procedure I of the Procedural Appendix.[55]

Because many patients have penicillin antibodies, Garratty emphasizes that when tested with drug-coated cells the serum antibody must be high titered and that the eluate must be positive before the findings are definitive.[7] Interpretation of the confirmatory tests to demonstrate antidrug antibody reactive by the drug adsorption method is outlined in **Table 21–20**.

Only a small percentage of those patients with penicillin-induced positive DATs exhibit hematologic complications. The clinical features of such a hemolytic episode differ from those of immune complex–mediated problems in several ways. Because the complement cascade is usually not activated, cell destruction is predominantly extravascular rather than intravascular. Therefore, the anemia develops more slowly and is not life-threatening unless the cause for the hemolysis is not recognized and the penicillin therapy is continued. Penicillin-induced hemolysis occurs only when the patient receives massive doses of the antibiotic, in contrast to the small amounts of drug that are necessary for hemolysis due to immune complexes. The patient improves once the drug is withdrawn, but hemolysis continues at a decreasing rate until cells heavily coated with penicillin are removed. The DAT may remain positive for several weeks. Mixed-field agglutination will be seen in the DAT because some cells are penicillin-coated but others are not. Anti-penicillin antibody may cross-react with ampicillin and methicillin.

Other drugs that cause a positive DAT and hemolytic anemia by this mechanism are most notably the cephalosporins (see **Table 21–17**). Distinguishing between cephalosporin-induced problems and penicillin-induced problems is technically difficult because the drugs have antigenic determinants in common, and anti-penicillin is frequently in the serum. Anti-penicillin reacts with Keflin-treated cells, anti-Keflin with penicillin-coated cells. Garratty[55] suggests that comparing the strength of the reactivity of the serum or eluate (titer or score) with penicillin-coated and Keflin-coated cells may be of value.

Reports of severe hemolytic episodes associated with the newer second- and third-generation cephalosporins appear to be increasing.[39,56–58] Several of these cases appear to involve aspects of both the immune complex and the drug-adsorption mechanisms. Immune-mediated hemolysis has occurred rapidly after administration of only a small amount of the drug. Because these antibiotics are routinely used in both adult and pediatric populations, any evidence of intravascular hemolysis should be noted and evaluated.

TABLE 21–20   Test Results Observed in the Presence of Antidrug Antibody Reactive by the Drug Adsorption Mechanism

Test	Patient Serum/Eluate	Drug-Coated RBCs	Uncoated RBCs	Results
Patient serum control	X	—	X	If negative, indicates no alloantibody to RBC present.
Drug/RBC control	—	X	—	If negative, indicates drug-coated cells will not spontaneously agglutinate.
Patient test	X	X	—	If agglutination is present and controls are all negative, indicates the presence of antidrug antibody. If negative, no antidrug present.

X = sample added to tube. — = no sample added to tube.

Membrane Modification (Nonimmunologic Protein Adsorption)

It is hypothesized that the cephalosporins, especially cephalothin (Keflin), both operate through the drug-adsorption mechanism and are able to modify RBCs so that plasma proteins (e.g., IgG, IgM, IgA, and complement) can bind to the membrane **(Fig. 21–5)**.[59] Consequently, RBCs from approximately 3 percent of patients receiving Keflin may exhibit a positive DAT with polyspecific and monospecific reagents. The uptake of immunoglobulins or complement components is not the result of a specific antigen-antibody reaction, so this mechanism is nonimmunologic. Because antibodies with blood group specificities are not involved, tests with the patient's serum and eluate are negative (see **Table 21–18**). Numerous cases of cephalosporin-associated hemolytic anemia have been reported but, as stated earlier, RBC destruction seems to have been mediated through the drug adsorption or immune complex mechanism rather than the membrane modification mechanism. There is no treatment approach because hemolytic anemia associated with the ingestion of these drugs has not been described in relation to membrane modification.

Autoantibody Formation

Unlike the drugs acting through the previously described mechanisms that induce production of an alloantibody against a determinant on a drug or on a combination of the drug and RBC membrane, alpha-methyldopa (Aldomet) induces the production of an autoantibody that recognizes RBC antigens.[60,61] The antibodies produced are serologically indistinguishable from those seen in patients with WAIHA (see previous section). Presence of the drug is not required to obtain positive reactions. Positive DATs are encountered in approximately 10 to 20 percent of patients receiving Aldomet as an antihypertensive. However, very few (0.5 to 1.0 percent) of this group of patients subsequently develop significant immune hemolytic anemia.[7,62] Other drugs that also cause autoantibody production are L-dopa, mefenamic acid, procainamide, and diclofenac[62,63] (see **Table 21–17**).

Several mechanisms by which Aldomet causes the production of autoantibodies have been proposed **(Box 21–4)**.[3,54,61] Kirtland, Horwitz, and Mohler[4] propose that methyldopa alters the function of T-suppressor cells and suggest that this

upset in the immune system would allow production of antibody against self. Worlledge and associates[61] suggest that the drug alters RBC membrane components, similar to the theory of "neoantigen" formation. However, at this time there is little evidence to support either of the theories. Much more work is needed to determine the true mechanisms involved in the production of drug-induced autoantibodies.

The serologic features of this type of drug-induced problem are very different from those of the other drug-related immune hemolytic anemias. As shown in **Table 21–18**, the antibody in the eluate *does* react with normal RBCs in the absence of the drug. Antibody of similar specificity and reactivity may be found in the serum. The patient's RBCs are usually coated with IgG, rarely with complement components.

Because the serology of Aldomet-induced positive DAT/immune hemolytic anemia is identical to that of the idiopathic WAIHA, one cannot establish in the laboratory that Aldomet is the cause of the problem. However, if the patient is receiving the drug, one should be highly suspicious. If Aldomet is withdrawn, autoantibody production will eventually stop, but it may be several months before the DAT is negative.

Treatment

Discontinuation of the drug is the treatment of choice for patients with a drug-induced hemolytic anemia. However, the presence of a positive DAT result does not necessarily imply that the drug must be discontinued if the effects of the drug are of therapeutic benefit and significant hemolysis is not present. In general, other drugs should be substituted, and the patient should be observed for resolution of the anemia to confirm a drug-induced hemolytic process. If the patient has a positive DAT without hemolysis, continued administration of the drug is optional.

Generally, the prognosis for patients with drug-induced hemolytic anemia is excellent. In **Table 21–21**, the four recognized mechanisms leading to the development of drug-related antibodies are compared.[64] **Table 21–22** contrasts the antibody characteristics of the various types of AIHAs.[64]

By understanding the mechanisms by which drugs can cause a positive DAT or immune hemolytic anemia, it can quickly be decided which laboratory tests are most likely to be

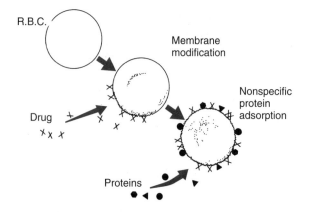

■ **FIGURE 21–5** Membrane modification mechanism. (From Petz and Garratty,[7] p 284, with permission.)

TABLE 21–21   **Mechanisms Leading to Development of Drug-Related Antibodies**

Mechanism	Prototype Drugs	Ig Class	DAT Results	Eluate	Frequency of Hemolysis
Immune complex	Quinidine Phenacetin	IgM or IgG	Positive—often C3 only, but IgG may be present	Often negative	Small doses of drugs may cause acute intravascular hemolysis with hemoglobinemia/hemoglobu-linuria; renal failure common.
Drug adsorption	Penicillins Streptomycin Cephalosporin	IgG	Strongly positive	Often negative	3–4% of patient on large doses (10,000,000 U) of penicillin, which is one of the most common causes of immune hemolysis, usually extravascular.
Membrane modification	Cephalosporins	Many plasma proteins	Positive because of variety of serum proteins	Negative	No hemolysis; however, 3% of patients receiving the drug develop a positive DAT.
Methyldopa-induced	Methyldopa (Aldomet)	IgG	Strongly positive	Positive—warm autoantibody identical to that found in WAIHA	0.8% develop a hemolytic anemia that mimics a warm AIHA. 15% of patients receiving methyldopa develop a positive DAT.

Adapted from Harmening, DM: Clinical Hematology and Fundamentals of Hemostasis, ed 4. FA Davis, Philadelphia, 2002, p 215, with permission.

informative. Many other drugs have been cited as a cause for hemolytic anemia; however, the majority of these have only one reported case, and the association between the hemolytic anemia and the drug may be unclear. Before any special testing is done, proceed in the following manner:

1. Obtain the patient's medical history, including transfusions, pregnancies, medications, and diagnosis.
2. Perform a DAT using RBCs collected in EDTA. Test the cells with a polyspecific antihuman serum and monospecific reagents.
3. Screen the patient's serum for RBC alloantibodies.
4. Prepare and test an eluate for RBC alloantibodies, if the patient has been recently transfused.

After evaluating this information, one can decide whether drugs are a possible cause of the problem and which of the mechanisms is involved. It is wise to also note that many

TABLE 21–22   **Summary of Antibody Characteristics in AIHA**

	Warm Reactive Autoantibody	Cold Reactive Autoantibody	Paroxysmal Cold Hemoglobinuria	Drug-Related Autoantibody
Immunoglobulin characteristics	Polyclonal IgG—occasionally IgM and IgA may be present	Polyclonal IgM in infection monoclonal kappa chain IgM in cold agglutinin disease	Polyclonal IgG	Polyclonal IgG
Complement activity	Variable	Always	Always	Depends on the mechanism of drug, antibody, and RBC interaction
Thermal reactivity	20°–37°C (optimum 37°C)	4°–32°C, rarely to 37°C (optimum 4°C)	4°–20°C biphasic hemolysin	20°–37°C (optimum 37°C)
Titer of free antibody	Low to moderate(<32), may be detectable only with enzyme-treated cells	High (>1000 at 4°C)	Moderate to low (<64)	Depends on the mechanism of drug, antibody, and RBC interaction
Reactivity of eluate with antibody screening cells	Usually pan-reactive	Nonreactive	Nonreactive	Pan-reactive with methyl-dopa type; nonreactive in all other cases
Most common specificity	Anti-Rh precursor; anti-common Rh; anti-LW; anti-U	Anti-I, anti-i, anti-Pr	Anti-P	Anti-e-like, methyldopa antidrug
Site of RBC destruction	Predominantly spleen with some liver involvement	Predominantly liver, rarely intravascular	Intravascular	Intravascular and spleen

Adapted from Harmening DM: Clinical Hematology and Fundamentals of Hemostasis, ed 4. FA Davis, Philadelphia, 2002, p 217, with permission.

drugs cause an immunologic reaction by both drug-dependent and drug-independent mechanisms. When other causes (e.g., transfusion reaction) have been excluded and the clinical situation warrants additional testing, drug-coated cells or solutions of the drug can be prepared for confirmatory tests. Testing procedures for the investigation of drug-induced AHIA require a library of control serum and cells and expertise in this testing. Without appropriate controls, it is possible to misinterpret test results and report either false-positive or false-negative results.

Summary

Distinguishing AIHAs, drug-induced as well as cold reactive and warm reactive, from a transfusion reaction caused by an alloantibody is of the utmost importance. Extensive workup of autoimmune antibodies is usually unnecessary. The most important concern in evaluation of autoantibodies is detection and identification of underlying clinically significant alloantibodies.

CASE STUDIES

Case 1

Part A

A 67-year-old woman was admitted to the coronary care unit for treatment of a severe upper respiratory infection and irregular heart rate. Her past medical history indicated the patient had a triple bypass 3 years ago but has enjoyed good health in the last 2 years. Twelve days before admission, she developed "a bad cold." Her symptoms have grown progressively worse until today, when she felt weak and very short of breath. Upon admission, it was noted that she was slightly jaundiced. She had three uneventful pregnancies and normal deliveries, and she "thinks" she had a transfusion during her heart surgery but nothing in the last 2 years. Her admission laboratory results follow:

Hemoglobin:	7.5 g/dL	Hematocrit:	23.2%
WBC count:	15.3 × 10³/mm³	Platelet count	125,000/ mm³

The physician has ordered a crossmatch for three units of packed RBCs to be given ASAP. The initial transfusion service results are given below:

Antisera Cells

Anti-A	Anti-B	Anti-D	A₁ cells	B cells
4+	Negative	4+	2+	4+

Cells tested	Immediate Spin (IS)	37°C	IgG/AGT
Immediate screening cell I	2+	0	0
Screening cell II	2+	0	0
x-match #1	2+	0	0
x-match #2	2+	0	0
x-match #3	2+	0	0

1. What problem do you note in the initial testing results?
2. What are possible explanations for these results?
3. What further testing must be performed before release of blood for transfusion?
4. Does the patient history give any clues as to the cause of the testing results?

Part B

An autocontrol was tested with screening cells at IS:

Cells tested	IS
Screening cell I	2+
Screening cell II	2+
Auto-control	2+

A DAT is also tested to obtain more information about this apparent autoantibody:

Polyspecific AHG: 3+
Anti-IgG: Negative
Anti-C3d: 3+

The reverse grouping, antibody screen, and compatibility testing are repeated using the patient's serum adsorbed one time at 4°C with her own RBCs. The immediate spin results are shown below:

Cells tested	IS
Screening cell I	0
Screening cell II	0
Auto cells	0
A₁ cells	0
B cells	4+
x-match #1	0
x-match #2	0
x-match #3	0

1. What is the patient's true ABO type and the result of the antibody screen?
2. What conclusions can you draw regarding the clinical significance of this antibody?
3. Is this antibody likely to cause hemolysis of the transfused RBCs?

Case 1 Answers

Part A

1. The forward and reverse typing do not match. The forward result is that typical of a group A, but the reverse is that of a group O (with weaker reactivity with the patient's serum and the A₁ cells). There is also an unexpected reaction in the immediate spin phase of the antibody screening test and the compatibility testing.
2. The patient may be a subgroup of A with anti-A₁ in the serum. However, the presence of anti-A₁ would not explain the reactions with the antibody screening cells. The patient may have an alloantibody reactive at room temperature, such as anti-Leᵃ or -Leᵇ, -M, -N, or -P₁. The reverse grouping cells are quite likely to be positive for any of these antigens, because these cells are prepared from random donors selected by ABO group and not RBC phenotype for common antigens. An RBC panel must be tested to

determine whether one of the antibodies might be responsible for the reactions. The patient may have a cold autoantibody that reacts with the reverse grouping cells as well as with the antibody screening cells and the donor units. An autocontrol would be helpful in determining if this might be the case. If the autocontrol is positive, a DAT is indicated to determine the nature of the protein coating the patient's RBCs.

3. As described in Question 2, an autocontrol, tested at immediate spin, and possibly an antibody identification panel must be performed in order to resolve the discrepancy. If the autocontrol is positive, cold autoadsorption procedures should be performed to obtain valid reactions without interference from the cold autoantibody.

4. The patient has an upper respiratory infection. It is known that infections with *Mycoplasma pneumoniae* are associated with CHD due to anti-I. The patient's clinical symptoms and laboratory evidence of anemia would also be consistent with CHD.

Part B

1. The patient is confirmed to be group A, D-positive, and the antibody screen performed with autoadsorbed serum is negative for clinically significant antibodies.

2. This antibody is most likely an autoanti-I, possibly produced in response to infection by *M. pneumoniae*. The antibody will cause hemolysis of the autologous cells, on some occasions resulting in clinical anemia. Because the antibody is IgM, causing sensitization of the cells with complement, there is no reaction in the antibody screen or compatibility testing with anti-IgG reagent. In this case, the use of autoabsorbed serum eliminated all aberrant reactions and allowed the provision of crossmatch-compatible RBCs for transfusion if needed.

3. If it is determined that this patient truly needs a transfusion, the RBCs may be administered through a blood warmer. If the RBCs are transfused at 30°–37°C, there should be minimal hemolysis. In this case, the hemolytic process is most likely transient and will resolve within 2–3 weeks with treatment of the primary disease. Supportive care and avoiding cold are the best therapy.

Case 2

Part A

A 45-year-old man was admitted with complaints of extreme fatigue and back pain. Admission test results are as follows:

Hemoglobin: 4.5 g/dL
Hematocrit: 14%
Reticulocyte count: 15%
Total bilirubin: 6.8 mg/dL

The attending physician orders four units of packed RBCs for transfusion as soon as possible. Records indicate that 3 years ago the patient received a transfusion of four units of leukoreduced RBCs following an automobile accident. No serologic problems were noted at that time. Initial pretransfusion testing follows:

Antisera Cells

Anti-A	Anti-B	Anti-D	A₁ cells	B cells
4+	Negative	4+	Negative	4+

Cells tested	IS	37°C	IgG/AGT
Screening cell I	0	0	2+
Screening cell II	0	0	2+
x-match #1	0	0	2+
x-match #2	0	0	2+
x-match #3	0	0	2+
x-match #4	0	0	2+

1. In light of the patient history and results, what kind of problems might be present in this patient?
2. What further information or testing would be helpful?

Part B

DAT was performed on the patient's cells:
Anti-IgG: 4+
Anti-C3b: Negative

A panel was performed on the patient's serum and all cells reacted (3+). An autocontrol was also 4+, as expected. The patient's history was investigated and the following points were noted: (1) The only known transfusions were the three units given 3 years ago and documented on the admission history. (2) Patient's medication history showed that he has had problems with hypertension and has taken methyldopa for the past 21 months.

1. What explanation for the serologic problems can you now propose?
2. What additional testing must be done to provide blood for this patient if the physician decides to transfuse?
3. What advice would you give the patient's physician regarding transfusion?

Part C

Because the patient has not been recently transfused, his cells were treated with ZZAP reagent, and his serum was adsorbed twice at 37°C. The antibody screen and crossmatches repeated with the adsorbed serum showed only agglutination (2+) with screening cell II in antiglobulin testing. A reagent RBC panel showed the following results, when tested with the adsorbed serum:

Cell	D	C	E	c	e	K	k	Fyᵃ	Fyᵇ	Jkᵃ	Jkᵇ	M	N	S	s	AGT
#1	+	0	+	+	0	0	+	+	0	+	0	+	+	+	+	2+
#2	+	+	0	0	+	0	+	0	+	0	+	0	+	0	+	0
#3	+	0	0	+	+	+	+	+	+	+	+	+	0	+	+	0
#4	+	+	+	+	0	+	+	0	+	0	+	+	+	0	2+
#5	0	0	0	+	+	0	+	+	0	+	0	+	+	+	0	0
#6	0	0	0	+	+	+	0	0	+	0	+	0	+	0	+	0
#7	0	0	0	+	+	0	+	+	0	+	0	+	0	+	0	0
#8	0	0	0	+	+	+	+	+	+	+	+	0	+	0	+	0
Auto																0

1. What antibody specificity(ies) is(are) evident?
2. What further testing must be done before release of blood for transfusion?
3. What additional tests might be helpful in providing blood for this patient in the future?

Case 2 Answers

Part A

1. The significantly decreased hemoglobin and increased reticulocyte count are indicative of a hemolytic episode.

The serologic results reveal a panagglutinin reactive with all cells tested at the antiglobulin phase. This patient may have a WAIHA.

2. A DAT should be performed to determine whether the antibody in the serum is autoantibody or alloantibody. If positive, anti-IgG and anti-C3 should be tested to identify the protein coating the cells. It is known that the patient has not had a recent transfusion. Information about his diagnosis and any medications he has been taking is needed. A panel should be performed to determine if the antibody shows a specificity.

Part B

1. From the serologic results and the history of methyldopa therapy, it is evident that the patient most likely has methyldopa-associated WAIHA.
2. Because the patient has had transfusions in the past, it is essential to ensure that he has no underlying alloantibodies before providing blood for transfusion. A warm autoadsorption can be performed because he has not been recently transfused. This will remove the autoantibody, leaving any alloantibodies to be identified.
3. If at all possible, transfusion should be delayed until any alloantibodies that may be present are detected. Transfusion will complicate the serologic picture and make it difficult to provide additional compatible RBCs. The transfused cells will be destroyed as rapidly as the patient's own cells. An alternative therapy for his hypertension should be started. After the patient stops taking the methyldopa, his clinical status will improve, although not rapidly. The autoantibody may be present in the patient's serum for up to 2 years.

Part C

1. An alloanti-E is present in this patient.
2. Any units released for transfusions should be verified as E-negative. The patient should also be typed for E to prove that the antibody is truly an alloantibody.
3. To prepare for future transfusions, it would be helpful to determine the patient's complete RBC phenotype using chloroquine-treated cells, EGA-treated cells, or monoclonal antisera. The patient can only make alloantibodies to the antigens he lacks; therefore, this information would be valuable in future antibody identification. When using the chloroquine method of removing IgG from RBCs, keep in mind that some antigens may be weakened by chloroquine treatment. Cells should be treated according to manufacturer's directions if using a commercially prepared reagent or an approved procedure.

Case 3

A 56-year-old male, complaining of urinary frequency and back pain, was seen by his physician. A urine analysis showed WBC casts, traces of blood, bacteria, WBCs, and nitrates. He was diagnosed as having a severe urinary tract infection (UTI). Because the patient had responded well to ceftriaxone during a previous UTI, the physician prescribed a 10-day course of ceftriaxone. On day 4, the patient returned, complaining of weakness on exertion and dark urine. His hemoglobin and hematocrit values were 7.4 g/dL and 22%, respectively. The physician ordered direct and indirect antiglobulin tests. The DAT was 2+ with anti-

IgG and 1+ with anti-C3. The antibody screen was negative at all phases.

1. What is the most likely explanation for the patient's symptoms and for the serologic results?
2. What further testing is necessary?
3. What therapy is needed at this time?

Case 3 Answers

1. This patient is most likely experiencing a drug-induced hemolytic episode. The third-generation cephalosporins (of which ceftriaxone is an example) are known to cause rapid hemolysis in some patients, especially if the patient was previously exposed to the drug. Cephalosporins have been shown to cause a positive DAT by formation of immune complexes, by drug adsorption, and by membrane modification. Most likely this hemolytic event is caused by a combination of immune complex formation and drug adsorption. The presence of both complement and IgG on the cells supports this assumption.
2. No additional testing is required. Testing with drug-coated cells or determination of the presence of immune complexes would be purely academic and not essential to treatment.
3. Ceftriaxone should be stopped immediately and another antibiotic substituted. The patient should recover after the drug is ceased. If the physician believes that transfusion is necessary, there should be no problems with compatibility testing.

SUMMARY CHART:
Important Points to Remember (MT/MLT)

➤ Immune hemolytic anemia is defined as shortened RBC survival mediated through the immune response, specifically by humoral antibody.

➤ In AIHA, patients produce alloantibodies to foreign RBC antigens introduced into their circulation, most often through transfusion or pregnancy.

➤ AIHA is self-limiting; when the foreign RBCs are cleared from circulation, RBC destruction stops.

➤ In AIHA, patients produce antibodies against their own RBC antigens.

➤ In AIHA the autoantibody is directed against the patient's own RBCs; therefore, there is a consistent source of antibody and antigen present for continuous RBC destruction.

➤ In drug-induced hemolytic anemia, patients produce antibody to a particular drug or drug complex, with subsequent damage to RBCs.

➤ AIHA may be classified as cold reactive (18 %), warm reactive (70%), or drug-induced (12%); diagnostic tests include the DAT and characterization of the autoantibody in the serum and/or eluate.

➤ In AIHA, serum antibody will not be detected until the amount of antibody produced exceeds the number of RBC antigen sites available on the patient's own RBCs.

➤ The common antibody specificity in both benign and pathologic cold autoagglutinins is anti-I.

➤ In CHD, the DAT will be positive because of complement coating of the RBCs; an antibody titer greater than 1000 may cause visible agglutination of anticoagulated blood.

➤ The classic antibody produced in PCH is called the Donath-Landsteiner antibody, and it has the specificity of autoanti-P. This biphasic antibody binds to patient RBCs at low temperatures and fixes complement. Hemolysis occurs when coated cells are warmed to 37°C and complement-mediated intravascular lysis occurs.

➤ In 80% of WAIHA, the antibody causing the hemolysis is an IgG immunoglobulin with IgG subclasses 1 and 3 found in association with most cases of hemolytic anemia.

➤ Warm reactive autoantibodies may activate complement, are generally enhanced by enzyme techniques, and often react with a general specificity within the Rh blood group system.

➤ When transfusing a patient with WAIHA, the primary concern is detection and identification of all alloantibodies that are masked by the warm autoantibody.

➤ In the immune complex drug mechanism, the soluble drug-antidrug complex nonspecifically adsorbs loosely to the RBC surface, yielding a positive DAT with polyspecific AHG and anti-C3.

➤ In the drug-adsorption (hapten) mechanism, drugs such as penicillin bind firmly to proteins of the RBC membrane. The DAT will show reactivity with polyspecific AHG and anti-IgG.

➤ In the membrane modification drug mechanism, drugs such as the cephalosporins modify the RBCs so that plasma proteins can bind to the membrane nonimmunologically. The DAT will demonstrate reactivity with both anti-IgG and anti-C3.

➤ In the autoantibody drug mechanism, the drug alphamethyldopa (Aldomet) induces production of an autoantibody that recognizes RBC antigens. Both the autoantibody and eluate are reactive with normal RBCs. The DAT is reactive with polyspecific AHG and anti-IgG.

REVIEW QUESTIONS

1. Immune hemolytic anemias may be classified in which of the following categories?
   a. Alloimmune
   b. Autoimmune
   c. Drug-induced
   d. All of the above

2. When preparing cells for a cold autoadsorption procedure, it is helpful to pretreat the cells with which of the following?
   a. Dithiothreitol
   b. Ficin
   c. Phosphate-buffered saline at pH 9.0
   d. Bovine albumin

3. The blood group involved in the autoantibody specificity in PCH is:
   a. P
   b. ABO
   c. Rh
   d. Lewis

4. Which of the following blood groups reacts best with an anti-H or anti-IH?
   a. A_1B
   b. B
   c. A_2
   d. A_1

5. With cold reactive autoantibodies, the protein coating the patient's cells and detected in the DAT is:
   a. C3
   b. IgG
   c. C4
   d. IgM

6. Problems in routine testing caused by cold reactive autoantibodies can usually be resolved by all of the following *except*:
   a. Prewarming
   b. Washing with warm saline
   c. Using anti-IgG antiglobulin serum
   d. Collecting clotted blood specimens

7. Pathologic cold autoagglutinins differ from common cold autoagglutinins in:
   a. Immunoglobulin class
   b. Thermal amplitude
   c. Antibody specificity
   d. DAT results on EDTA specimen

8. Cold AIHA is sometimes associated with infection by:
   a. *Staphylococcus aureus*
   b. *Mycoplasma pneumoniae*
   c. *Escherichia coli*
   d. Group A *Streptococcus*

9. Many warm reactive autoantibodies have a broad specificity within which of the following blood groups?
   a. Kell
   b. Duffy
   c. Rh
   d. Kidd

10. Valid Rh typing can usually be obtained on a patient with WAIHA using all of the following reagents or techniques *except*:
    a. Slide and modified tube anti-D
    b. Chloroquine-treated RBCs
    c. Rosette test
    d. Monoclonal blend anti-D

11. In pretransfusion testing for a patient with WAIHA, the primary concern is:
    a. Treating the patient's cells with chloroquine for reliable antigen typing

b. Adsorbing out all antibodies in the patient's serum to be able to provide compatible RBCs

c. Determining the exact specificity of the autoantibody so that compatible RBCs can be found

d. Discovering any existing significant alloantibodies in the patient's circulation

12. Penicillin given in massive doses has been associated with RBC hemolysis. Which of the classic mechanisms is involved in the hemolytic process?

a. Immune complex

b. Drug adsorption

c. Membrane modification

d. Autoantibody formation

13. Which of the following drugs has been associated with complement activation and rapid intravascular hemolysis?

a. Penicillins

b. Quinidine

c. Alpha-methyldopa

d. Cephalosporins

14. A patient is admitted with a hemoglobin of 5.6 g/dL. Initial pretransfusion workup appears to indicate the presence of a warm autoantibody in the serum and coating his RBCs. He received 6 U of RBCs in transfusion 2 years ago after an automobile accident. Which of the following would be most helpful in performing antibody detection and compatibility testing procedures?

a. Adsorb the autoantibody using the patient's enzyme-treated cells.

b. Perform an elution and use the eluate for compatibility testing.

c. Crossmatch random units until compatible units are found.

d. Collect blood from relatives who are more likely to be compatible.

15. A patient who is taking Aldomet has a positive DAT. An eluate prepared from his RBCs would be expected to:

a. React only with Aldomet-coated cells

b. Be neutralized by a suspension of Aldomet

c. React with all normal cells

d. React only with Rh_{null} cells

16. One method that can be used to separate patient cells from recently transfused donor cells is:

a. Chloroquine diphosphate treatment of the RBCs

b. Reticulocyte harvesting

c. EDTA/EGA treatment

d. Donath-Landsteiner testing

17. Monoclonal antisera is valuable in phenotyping RBCs with positive DATs because:

a. Both polyspecific and monospecific antihuman serum can be used in antiglobulin testing

b. Anti-C3 serum can be used in antiglobulin testing

c. It does not require antiglobulin testing

d. It does not require enzyme treatment of the cells prior to antiglobulin testing

18. Autoabsortion procedures to remove either warm or cold autoantibodies should not be used with a recently transfused patient. Recently means:

a. 3 days

b. 3 weeks

c. 6 weeks

d. 3 months

REFERENCES

1. Izui, S: Autoimmune hemolytic anemia. Curr Opin Immunol 6:926, 1994.
2. Barthold, DR, Kysela, S, and Steinberg, AD: Decline in suppressor T cell function with age in female NZB mice. J Immunol 112:9, 1974.
3. Banacerraf, B, and Unanue, ER: Textbook of Immunology. Williams & Wilkins, Baltimore, 1979.
4. Kirtland, HH, Horwitz, DA, and Mohler, DN: Inhibition of suppressor T cell function by methyldopa: A proposed cause of autoimmune hemolytic anemia. N Engl J Med 302:825, 1980.
5. van Loghem, JJ: Concepts on the origin of autoimmune diseases: The possible role of viral infection in the etiology of idiopathic autoimmune diseases. Semin Hematol 9:17, 1965.
6. Hillman, RS, and Finch, GA: Red Cell Manual, ed 5. FA Davis, Philadelphia, 1985, p 91.
7. Petz, LD, and Garratty, G: Acquired Immune Hemolytic Anemias. Churchill Livingstone, New York, 1980.
8. Brecher, ME (ed): Technical Manual, ed 14. American Association of Blood Banks, Bethesda, MD, 2002, p 422.
9. Allan, J, and Garratty, G: Positive direct antiglobulin tests in normal blood donors (abstract). Proceedings of the 16th Congress of the International Society of Blood Transfusion, Montreal, 1980.
10. Okuno, T, Germino, F, and Newman, B: Clinical significance of autologous control (abstract). American Society Clinical Pathologists 16, 1984.
11. Lau, P, Haesler, WE, and Wurzel, HA: Positive direct antiglobulin reaction in a patient population. Am J Clin Pathol 65:368, 1976.
12. Judd, WJ, et al: The evaluation of a positive direct antiglobulin test in pretransfusion testing. Transfusion 20:17, 1980.
13. Garratty, G, Petz, LD, and Hoops, JK: The correlation of cold agglutinin titrations in saline and albumin with haemolytic anaemia. Br J Haematol 35:587, 1977.
14. Engelfriet, CP, et al: Autoimmune hemolytic anemias: Serological studies with pure anti-immunoglobulin reagents. Clin Exp Immunol 3:605, 1968.
15. Rosse, WF: Quantitative immunology of immune hemolytic anemia: The relationship of cell-bound antibody to hemolysis and the effect of treatment. J Clin Invest 50:734, 1971.
16. De Angelis, V, et al: Abnormalities of membrane protein composition in patients with autoimmune haemolytic anaemia. Br J Hematol 95:273, 1996.
17. Gilliland, BC, Baxter, E, and Evans, RS: Red cell antibodies in acquired hemolytic anemia with negative antiglobulin serum tests. N Engl J Med 285:252, 1971.
18. Garratty, G: Autoimmune hemolytic anemia. In Garratty, G (ed): Immunobiology of Transfusion Medicine. Marcel Dekker, New York, 1994, p 493.
19. Stratton, F, et al: Acquired hemolytic anemia associated with IgA anti-e. Transfusion 12:197, 1972.
20. Sturgeon, P, et al: Autoimmune hemolytic anemia associated exclusively with IgA of Rh specificity. Transfusion 19:324, 1979.
21. Hoppe, PA: The role of the Bureau of Biologics in assuring reagent reliability. In Considerations in the Selection of Reagents. American Association of Blood Banks, Washington, DC, 1979, p 1.
22. Garratty, G, and Petz, LD: An evaluation of commercial antiglobulin sera with particular reference to their anticomplement properties. Transfusion 11:79, 1971.
23. Vengelen-Tyler, V (ed): Technical Manual, ed 12. American Association of Blood Banks, Bethesda, MD, 1996, p 379.
24. Reid, ME: Autoagglutination dispersal utilizing sulfhydryl compounds. Transfusion 18:353, 1978.
25. Judd, WJ: Controversies in transfusion medicine: Prewarmed tests: Con. Transfusion 35:271, 1995.
26. Chaplin, H, et al: Clinically significant allo-anti-I in an I-negative patient with massive hemorrhage. Transfusion 26:57, 1986.
27. Marsh, WL: Aspects of cold-reactive autoantibodies. In Bell, CA (ed): A Seminar on Laboratory Management of Hemolysis. American Association of Blood Banks, Washington, DC, 1979, p 79.
28. Combs, MR, et al: An auto-anti M causing hemolysis in vitro. Transfusion 31:756, 1991.
29. Garratty, G: Target antigens for red-cell-bound autoantibodies. In Nance, ST (ed): Clinical and Basic Science Aspects of Immunohematology. American Association of Blood Banks, Arlington, VA, 1991, p 33.
30. Lyckholm, LJ, and Edmond, MB: Seasonal hemolysis due to cold-agglutinin syndrome. N Engl J Med 334:437, 1996.
31. Aoki, A, et al: Cardiac operation without hypothermia for the patient with cold agglutinin. Chest 104:1627, 1993.
32. Shirey, RS, et al: An anti-i biphasic hemolysin in chronic paroxysmal cold hemoglobinuria. Transfusion 26:62, 1986.

33. Judd, WJ, et al: Donath-Landsteiner hemolytic anemia due to an anti-Pr-like biphasic hemolysin. Transfusion 26:423, 1986.
34. Reid, M: Association of red blood cell membrane abnormalities with blood group phenotype. In Garratty, G (ed): Immunobiology of Transfusion Medicine. Marcel Dekker, New York, 1994, p 257.
35. Salloum, E, and Lundberg, WB: Hemolytic anemia with positive direct antiglobulin test secondary to spontaneous cytomegalovirus infection in healthy adults. Acta Hematol 92:39, 1994.
36. Benraad, CEM, Scheerder, HAJM, and Overbeeke, MAM: Autoimmune haemolytic anaemia during pregnancy. Eur J Obstet Gynecol Reprod Biol 55:209, 1994.
37. Brecher, ME (ed): Technical Manual, ed 14. American Association of Blood Banks, Bethesda, MD, 2002, p427.
38. Edwards, JM, Moulds, JJ, and Judd, WJ: Chloroquine dissociation of antigen-antibody complexes: A new technique for typing red blood cells with a positive direct antiglobulin test. Transfusion 22:59, 1982.
39. Issitt, P, and Anstee, D: Applied Blood Group Serology, ed. 4. Montgomery Scientific Publications, Durham, NC, 1998, p 1021.
40. Win, N, et al: Autoimmune haemolytic anaemia in infancy with anti-Kp^b specificity. Vox Sang 71:187, 1994.
41. Becton, DL, and Kinney, TR: An infant girl with severe autoimmune hemolytic anemia: Apparent anti-Vel specificity. Vox Sang 51:108, 1986.
42. Reynolds, MV, Vengelen-Tyler, V, and Morel, PA: Autoimmune hemolytic anemia associated with auto anti-Ge. Vox Sang 41:61, 1981.
43. Wilkinson, SL: Serological approaches to transfusion of patients with allo- or autoantibodies. In Nance, ST (ed): Immune Destruction of Red Blood Cells. American Association of Blood Banks, Arlington, VA, 1989, pp 227.
44. Singh, M, Thompson, H, and Pallas, C: Response to transfusions in autoimmune hemolytic anemia. Abstracts of South Central Association of Blood Banks Annual Meeting, Tucson, AZ, 1997.
45. Jeffries, LC: Transfusion therapy in autoimmune hemolytic anemia. Hematol Oncol Clin North Am 8:1087, 1994.
46. Anderson, DR, and Kelton, JG: Mechanisms in intravascular and extravascular cell destruction. In Nance, ST (ed): Immune Destruction of Red Blood Cells. American Association of Blood Banks, Arlington, VA, 1989, p 39.
47. Flores, G, et al: Efficacy of intravenous immunoglobulin in the treatment of autoimmune hemolytic anemia: Results in 73 patients. Am J Hematol 44:237, 1993.
48. Brecher, ME (ed): Technical Manual, ed 14. American Association of Blood Banks, Bethesda, MD, 2002, p 433.
49. Kerr, RO, et al: Two mechanisms of erythrocyte destruction in penicillin-induced hemolytic anemia. N Engl J Med 298:1322, 1972.
50. Ries, CA, et al: Penicillin-induced immune hemolytic anemia. JAMA 233:432, 1975.
51. Shulman, NR: Mechanism of blood cell destruction in individuals sensitized to foreign antigens. Trans Assoc Am Physicians 76:72, 1963.
52. Dameshek, W: Autoimmunity: Theoretical aspects. Ann N Y Acad Sci 124:6, 1965.
53. Petz, LD, and Mueller-Eckhardt, C: Drug-induced immune hemolytic anemia. Transfusion 32:02, 1992.
54. Garratty, G: Drug-induced immune hemolytic anemia. In Garratty, G (ed): Immunobiology of Transfusion Medicine. Marcel Dekker, New York, 1994, p. 523.
55. Garratty, G: Laboratory Investigation of Drug-Induced Immune Hemolytic Anemia and/or Positive Antiglobulin Tests. American Association of Blood Banks, Washington, DC, 1979.
56. Eckrich, RJ, Fox, S, and Mallory, D: Cefotetan-induced immune hemolytic anemia due to the drug-adsorption mechanism. Immunohematology 10:51, 1994.
57. Bernini, JC, et al: Fatal hemolysis induced by ceftriaxone in a child with sickle cell anemia. J Pediatr 126:813, 1995.
58. Lascari, AD, and Amyot, K: Fatal hemolysis caused by ceftriaxone. J Pediatr 126:816, 1995.
59. Spath, P, Garratty, G, and Petz, LD: Studies on the immune response to penicillin and cephalothin in humans: Immunohematologic reactions to cephalothin administration. J Immunol 107:860, 1971.
60. Carstairs, KC, et al: Incidence of a positive direct Coombs' test in patients on alpha-methyldopa. Lancet 2:33, 1966.
61. Worlledge, SM, Carstairs, KC, and Dacie, JV: Autoimmune hemolytic anemia associated with methyldopa therapy. Lancet 2:135, 1966.
62. Petz, LD: Drug-induced hemolytic anemia. Transfus Med Rev 7:242, 1993.
63. Lopez, A, et al: Autoimmune hemolytic anemia induced by diclofenac. Ann Pharmacother 29:787, 1995.
64. Harmening, DM: Clinical Hematology and Fundamentals of Hemostasis, ed 3. FA Davis, Philadelphia, 1997, pp 221–243.

BIBLIOGRAPHY

Calvo, R, et al: Acute hemolytic anemia due to anti-i; frequent cold agglutinins in infectious mononucleosis. J Clin Invest 44:1033, 1965.
Carter, P, Koval, JJ, and Hobbs, JR: The relation of clinical and laboratory findings to the survival of patients with macroglobinaemia. Clin Exp Immunol 28:241, 1977.
Chaplin, H, and Avioli, LV: Autoimmune hemolytic anemia. Arch Intern Med 137:346, 1977.
Dacie, JV: Autoimmune hemolytic anemia. Arch Intern Med 135: 1293, 1975.
Dameshek, W: Alpha-methyldopa red cell antibody: Cross reaction or forbidden clone. N Engl J Med 276:1382, 1967.
Evans, RS, Baxter, E, and Gilliland, BC: Chronic hemolytic anemia due to cold agglutinins: A 20-year history of benign gammopathy with response to chlorambucil. Blood 42:463, 1973.
Forbes, CD, Craig, JA, and Mitchell, R: Acute intravascular hemolysis associated with cephalexin therapy. Postgrad Med J 48:186, 1972.
Frank, MM, Atkinson, JP, and Gadek, J: Cold agglutinins and cold agglutinin disease. Ann Rev Med 28:291, 1977.
Freedman, J, and Lim, FC: An immunohematologic complication of isoniazid. Vox Sang 35:126, 1978.
Garratty, G: Drug-induced immune hemolytic anemia and/or positive direct antiglobulin tests. Immunohematology 2:6, 1985.
Garratty, G: Target antigens for red-cell-bound autoantibodies. In Nance, ST (ed): Clinical and Basic Science Aspects of Immunohematology. American Association of Blood Banks, Arlington, VA, 1991, pp 33–72.
Gottlieb, AJ, and Wurzel, HA: Protein-quinone interaction: In vivo induction of indirect antiglobulin reactions with methyldopa. Blood 43:85, 1974.
Gralnick, HR, McGinniss, MH, and Elton, W: Hemolytic anemia associated with cephalothin. JAMA 217:1193, 1971.
Habibi, B: Drug induced red blood cell autoantibodies co-developed with drug specific antibodies causing haemolytic anaemias. Br J Haematol 61:139, 1985.
Harmening, DM: Modern Blood Banking and Transfusion Practices, ed 4. FA Davis, Philadelphia, 1999.
Harmening-Pittiglio, DM: Warm auto immune hemolytic anemia: A review of clinical and laboratory considerations. Immunohematology 1, 1984.
Hendry, EG: Osmolarity of human serum and of chemical solutions of importance. Clin Chem 7:156, 1961.
Jeannet, M, et al: Cephalothin-induced immune hemolytic anemia. Acta Haematol 55:109, 1976.
Kaplan, K, Reisburg, B, and Weinsteins, L: Cephaloridine studies of therapeutic activity and untoward effects. Arch Intern Med 121:17, 1968.
Kickler, TS, et al: Probenecid induced immune hemolytic anemia. J Rheumatol 13:208, 1986.
Kramer, MR, Levine, C, and Hershko, C: Severe reversible autoimmune haemolytic anaemia and thrombocytopenia associated with diclofenac therapy. Scand J Haematol 36:118, 1986.
Leddy, JP, and Swisher, SN: Acquired immune hemolytic disorders (including drug-induced immune hemolytic anemia). In Samter, M (ed): Immunological Diseases, ed 3, vol 2, 1978, p 1187.
Marchand, A: Charting a course for hemolytic anemia. Diagn Med 1981.
Marchand, A: Immune hemolytic anemia. Part I: Classification, manifestations and mechanism of destruction. Diagn Med 1982.
Marchand, A: Immune hemolytic anemia. Part II: Test procedures and strategy. Diagn Med 1983.
Petz, LD, and Branch, DR: Immune Hemolytic Anemias. Churchill Livingstone, Edinburgh, 1985.
Seldon, MR, et al: Ticarcillin-induced immune haemolytic anaemia. Scand J Haematol 28:459, 1982.
Silberstein, LE (ed): Autoimmune Disorders of Blood. American Association of Blood Banks, Bethesda, MD, 1996.
Tafani, O, et al: Fatal acute immune haemolytic anaemia caused by nalidixic acid. Br Med J 285:936, 1982.
Tanowitz, HB, Robbins, N, and Leidich, N: Hemolytic anemia: Associated with severe *Mycoplasma pneumoniae* pneumonia. N Y State J Med 78:2231, 1978.
Tuffs, L, and Mancharan, A: Flucloxacillin-induced haemolytic anaemia. Med J Aust 144:559, 1986.
Vengelen-Tyler,V (ed): Technical Manual, ed 13. American Association of Blood Banks, Bethesda, MD, 1999.
Wallace, ME, and Green, TS (eds): Selection of Procedures for Problem Solving. American Association of Blood Banks, Arlington, VA, 1983.
Wallace, ME, and Levitt, JS: Current Applications and Interpretations of the Direct Antiglobulin Test. American Association of Blood Banks, Arlington, VA, 1988.
Worlledge, SM: Immune drug-induced haemolytic anemias. Semin Hematol 6:181, 1969.

PROCEDURAL APPENDIX

A—Use of Thiol Reagents to Disperse Autoagglutination*

Application

Thiol reagents, which cleave the intersubunit disulfide bonds of pentameric IgM molecules, can be used to disperse agglutination caused by cold reactive autoantibodies. Treating spontaneously agglutinated RBCs with 2-mercaptoethanol (2-ME) or dithiothreitol (DTT) provides a nonagglutinated specimen for use in blood grouping tests.

Materials

1. 0.01 M DTT or 0.1 M 2-ME
2. Phosphate-buffered saline (PBS) at pH 7.3
3. Packed RBCs to be treated, washed three to four times

Method

1. Dilute washed RBCs to a 50% concentration in PBS.
2. To the RBCs, add an equal volume of 0.01 M DTT in PBS or 0.1 M 2-ME in PBS.
3. Mix and incubate at 37°C for 15 minutes for DTT or 10 minutes for 2-ME.
4. Wash RBCs three times.
5. Dilute the treated RBCs to a 3%–5% concentration in saline and use in blood grouping tests.

B—Cold Autoadsorption*

Application

Autoadsorption can be used to remove cold reactive autoantibodies, allowing detection of clinically significant alloantibodies.

Materials

1. 1% ficin or 1% papain
2. 2 mL of serum to be adsorbed
3. 3 mL of packed autologous RBCs

Method

1. Wash the RBCs four times in warm saline and divide into three equal aliquots in 13 × 100 mm test tubes. Completely remove supernatant after last wash.

2. Add an equal volume of 1% ficin or 1% papain to each aliquot of washed cells.
3. Mix and incubate at 37°C for 15 minutes.
4. Wash the RBCs three times in saline. Centrifuge the last wash for 5 minutes at 1000 × g, and remove as much of the supernatant saline as possible (see note).
5. To one tube of enzyme-treated RBCs, add 2 mL of the autologous serum.
6. Mix and incubate at 4°C for 30–60 minutes.
7. Centrifuge at 1000 × g for 5 minutes, and transfer the serum into a second tube of enzyme-treated autologous RBCs.
8. Mix and incubate at 4°C for 30–40 minutes.
9. In most cases, two adsorptions are sufficient to remove the autoantibody. If the autoantibody is particularly strong, repeat Steps 7 and 8 using the third tube of enzyme-treated RBCs.
10. After the final adsorption, test the serum for alloantibody activity.

Notes:

1. To avoid dilution of the serum and possible loss of weak alloantibody activity during the adsorption process, remove as much of the residual saline as possible in Step 4. Placing a narrow strip of filter paper into the packed RBCs helps remove saline that surrounds the packed cells.
2. Autoadsorption should not be used when the patient has recently received a transfusion. Adsorption with rabbit erythrocyte stroma may be used in this situation.

C—Prewarmed Technique for Testing Serum Containing Cold Agglutinins*

Application

The reactivity of IgM cold autoantibodies can be reduced or eliminated by performing prewarmed tests. Most problems encountered in compatibility testing, antibody detection, and identification tests that are caused by cold agglutinins can be resolved with the use of this technique. By preventing the reaction between the cold agglutinin and the RBC at room temperature (during centrifugation and testing), complement activation is prevented. The anti-C3 in polyspecific AHG reagent reacts with the remaining C3, making detection of significant AHG-reactive antibodies difficult. Prewarm-

*Adapted from Reid, ME: Autoagglutination dispersal utilizing sulfhydryl compounds. Transfusion 18:353, 1978.
*Adapted from Beattie, K, et al: Immunohematology Methods. American Red Cross, Rockville, MD, 1993.

*Adapted from Vengelen-Tyler, V (ed): Technical Manual, ed 13. American Association of Blood Banks, Bethesda, MD, 1999, p 671.

ing of the serum, cells, and additive will hinder the binding of the cold autoantibody and the resulting complement activation.

Materials

1. Normal saline, warmed to 37°C
2. Patient's serum
3. Additive solution (bovine albumin, low ionic strength solution, polyethylene glycol, etc.), if any
4. Cells to be tested (screening or panel cells, donor cells)
5. Antihuman globulin (AHG) anti-IgG

Method

1. Label one tube for each reagent or donor cell sample to be tested.
2. Add one drop of the appropriate 2%–4% cell suspension to each tube.
3. Place the tubes containing the RBCs, a tube containing a small amount of patient's serum, and a tube containing the additive solution, if any, at 37°C for 5–10 minutes.
4. Transfer two drops of prewarmed serum into each tube containing prewarmed RBCs; mix without removing the tubes from the incubator. Additive will be added according to manufacturer's insert.
5. Incubate at 37°C for at least 30 minutes with no additive, or the appropriate time for the additive used.
6. Without removing the tubes from the incubator, fill all tubes with prewarmed saline (37°C). Centrifuge and wash two to three more times with warm saline.
7. Add anti-IgG antiglobulin reagent, centrifuge, and record reactions. *Note:* Do not prewarm the anti-IgG reagent.

Notes:

1. Use of the anti-IgG antiglobulin reagent ensures that positive reactions caused by cold autoagglutinins with complement binding only will not be detected. Most significant antibodies react in the antiglobulin phase with anti-IgG reagent.
2. A prewarmed technique should be used only in situations in which a true cold autoagglutinin appears to be present and only if the patient has not been recently transfused.

D—Adsorption of Cold Autoantibodies with Rabbit Erythrocyte Stroma*

Application

Autoadsorption procedures are not recommended when a patient has recently received a transfusion. Rabbit erythrocytes are known to possess the I antigen, and stromata made from rabbit erythrocytes are commercially available for use in adsorption techniques.

*Adapted from Waligora, SK, and Edwards, JM: The use of rabbit red blood cells for the adsorption of cold autoagglutinins. Transfusion 23:328, 1983.

Materials

1. Rabbit erythrocyte stroma (REST[R], BCA, a division of Biopool International, West Chester, Pa)
2. Patient's serum containing cold autoantibodies

Method

1. Centrifuge for at least 2 minutes to pack the rabbit stroma and completely remove the supernatant.
2. Add 1 mL of the serum to be adsorbed.
3. Stopper and mix well using a vortex mixer.
4. Incubate at 4°C for 15–60 minutes, mixing occasionally.
5. Centrifuge for at least 2 minutes, and transfer the adsorbed serum to a clean tube.
6. Perform antibody screening, antibody identification, or compatibility testing according to routine procedures.

Notes:

1. In addition to the I antigen, rabbit erythrocyte stroma carries the B antigen, P system antigens, and H antigens. Therefore, serum adsorbed with rabbit RBC stroma should not be used for ABO reverse typing.
2. Some alloantibodies, including anti-D, anti-E, and anti-Le[b], have been reported to be adsorbed onto the rabbit RBC stroma.

E—Dissociation of IgG by Chloroquine

Application*

RBCs with a positive DAT cannot be used directly for blood grouping with antisera, such as anti-K1, anti-Fy[a], and -Fy[b] and others, that require the use of an indirect antiglobulin technique. Under controlled conditions, chloroquine diphosphate dissociates IgG from RBCs with little or no damage to the RBC membrane. Use of this procedure permits complete phenotyping of DAT-positive RBCs, including tests with antisera solely reactive by the indirect antiglobulin test.

Materials

1. Chloroquine diphosphate solution prepared by dissolving 20 g of chloroquine diphosphate in 100 mL of saline (pH 5.1)
2. RBCs with a positive DAT due to IgG coating
3. Control RBCs heterozygous for the antigen for which the test sample is to be phenotyped
4. Anti-IgG antiglobulin reagent

Method

1. To 1 volume of washed, packed IgG-coated test RBCs, add 4 volumes of chloroquine diphosphate solution. Treat the control sample similarly.
2. Mix and incubate at room temperature for 30 minutes.

*Adapted from Beaumont, AE, et al: An improved method for removal of red-cell-bound immunoglobulin using chloroquine solution. Immunohematology 10:22, 1994.

3. Remove a small aliquot (e.g., one drop) of the treated RBCs, and wash four times with saline.
4. Test the washed cells with anti-IgG.
5. If nonreactive with anti-IgG, wash the entire sample of treated test RBCs and the control sample three times in saline, and use for phenotyping with antiglobulin-reactive antisera. Use an anti-IgG reagent when testing these cells.
6. If the treated RBCs react with the anti-IgG after the 30-minute incubation, repeat steps 3 and 4 at 30-minute intervals (for a maximum incubation of 2 hours), until the RBCs are nonreactive with anti-IgG. Proceed as described in Step 5.

Notes:

1. Chloroquine diphosphate does not dissociate complement components from RBCs. If cells are coated with both IgG and C3 in vivo, test performed after chloroquine treatment should be done using anti-IgG.
2. Incubation of RBCs in chloroquine diphosphate should not be extended beyond 2 hours. Prolonged incubation at room temperature, or incubation at 37°C, may result in hemolysis and damage to or loss of RBC antigens. An alternate procedure described by Beaumont and associates recommends incubation at 30°C for 90 minutes or 37°C for 30 minutes. The reader is referred to this article for details. See footnote.
3. Some denaturation of Rh antigens may occur. This is most often noted when RBCs have hemolyzed following incubation with chloroquine diphosphate. NOTE: Monoclonal antisera should not be used in testing chloroquine-treated cells.
4. Include an inert control reagent when phenotyping chloroquine-treated RBCs.

F—Digitonin-Acid Elution*

Application

Removal of antibodies bound to RBC antigens is performed in investigation of a positive DAT associated with warm reactive (IgG) autoantibodies or alloantibodies and for the separation of mixtures of IgG antibodies.

Materials

1. Digitonin (0.5% w/v), prepared by dissolving 0.5 g of digitonin in 100 mL of distilled water. Store at 4°C.
2. Glycine (0.1 M, pH 3.0), prepared by dissolving 3.754 g of glycine in 500 mL of distilled water. Adjust pH to 3.0 with 12 N HCl. Store at 4°C.
3. Phosphate buffer (0.8 M, pH 8.2), prepared by dissolving 109.6 g of Na_2HPO_4 and 3.8 g of KH_2PO_4 in approximately 600 mL of distilled water. Adjust pH, if necessary, with

either 1 N NaOH or 1 N HCl. Dilute to a final volume of 1 L with distilled water. Store at 4°C.
4. Bovine serum albumin, 30%.
5. Packed RBCs (1 mL), washed six times in saline.
6. Supernatant saline from last wash.

Method

1. Warm reagents to 37°C before use and mix well.
2. Mix 1 mL of washed packed RBCs and 9 mL of saline in a 16 × 100 mm test tube.
3. Add 0.5 mL of digitonin, and mix by inversion until all RBCs are hemolyzed (at least 1 minute).
4. Centrifuge at $1000 \times g$ for 5 minutes, and discard the supernatant.
5. Wash the RBC stroma at least five times, or until it appears white. Centrifuge for at least 2 minutes during the washing process.
6. Discard the final supernatant wash solution, and add 2 mL of glycine to the stroma.
7. Mix by inversion for at least 1 minute.
8. Centrifuge the tube at $1000 \times g$ for 5 minutes.
9. Transfer the supernatant eluate to a clean test tube, and add 0.2 mL of phosphate buffer.
10. Mix and centrifuge at $1000 \times g$ for 2 minutes.
11. Transfer the supernatant into a clean test tube, and add one-third volume of 30% bovine serum albumin. Test in parallel with the last wash saline.

Notes:

1. The low pH of the acid buffer enhances elution of antibody from the RBC stroma. Phosphate buffer is added to restore neutrality to the acidic eluate. Persisting acidity may cause lysis of RBCs added to the eluate. Adding bovine albumin to the eluate protects against hemolysis.
2. Ensure that digitonin is well mixed and warmed to 37°C before use.
3. Use centrifugation times of at least 2 minutes when washing stroma.
4. Phosphate buffer will crystallize on storage at 4°C. Redissolve at 37°C before use.

G—Autologous Adsorption of Warm Reactive Autoantibodies

Application

Warm reactive autoantibodies may mask the presence of coexisting alloantibodies in a serum. Adsorbing the serum with autologous RBCs can remove autoantibody from the serum, permitting detection of underlying alloantibodies. Circulating autologous cells, however, are already coated with autoantibody. Some of the autoantibody must be removed from the surface of the autologous RBCs in order to achieve maximum removal of autoantibody by the adsorption process. Autoadsorption should not be performed if a patient has recently received a transfusion because the circulating transfused cells may absorb out alloantibodies.

*Adapted from Jenkins, DE, and Moore, WH: A rapid method for the preparation of high-potency auto- and alloantibody eluates. Transfusion 17:110, 1977.

A. Heat and Enzyme Method*

Materials

1. 6% bovine albumin, prepared by diluting 22% or 30% bovine albumin with saline
2. 1% ficin or 1% cysteine-activated papain
3. Blood sample containing warm reactive autoantibodies

Method

1. Wash 2 mL of RBCs four times in saline, and discard the final supernatant.
2. Add an equal volume of 6% albumin to the packed RBCs. Mix and incubate at 56° C for 3–5 minutes. Gently agitate the mixture during this time.
3. Centrifuge at 1000 × g for 2 minutes, and harvest the supernatant. This may be used for eluate if the patient's cells are in short supply.
4. Wash the cells three times in saline, and discard the final supernatant.
5. Add 1 mL of 1% ficin or papain to the RBCs. Mix and incubate at 37° for 15 minutes.
6. Wash the RBCs three times in saline. Centrifuge the last wash for at least 5 minutes at 1000 × g. Use suction to remove as much of the supernatant as practical.
7. Divide the RBCs into two equal aliquots.
8. To 1 aliquot add 2 mL of patient's serum. Mix and incubate at 37° C for 30 minutes.
9. Centrifuge at 1000 × g for 2 minutes, and transfer the serum to the second aliquot of enzyme-treated RBCs. Mix and incubate at 37° C for 30 minutes.
10. Centrifuge at 1000 × g for 2 minutes, and harvest the adsorbed serum.
11. Test the adsorbed serum for antibody activity using an indirect antiglobulin technique.

B. ZZAP Method†

Materials

1. 1% cysteine-activated papain
2. Phosphate-buffered saline (PBS) at pH 7.3
3. 0.2 M dithiothreitol (DTT) prepared by dissolving 1 g of DTT in 32.4 mL of pH 6.5 PBS. Dispense into 2.5 mL aliquots and store at or below −20°C
4. Blood samples containing warm reactive autoantibodies

Method

1. Prepare ZZAP reagent by mixing 0.5 mL of 1% cysteine-activated papain with 2.5 mL DTT and 2 mL pH 7.3 PBS.

Alternatively, use 1 mL of 1% ficin, 2.5 mL DTT, and 1.5 mL pH 6.5 PBS.
2. To two tubes, each containing 1 mL of packed RBCs, add 2 mL of ZZAP reagent. Mix and incubate at 37°C for 30 minutes.
3. Wash the RBCs three times in saline. Centrifuge the last wash at least 5 minutes at 1000 × g. Use suction to remove as much of the supernatant as practical.
4. Proceed from Step 8 in Procedure A above.

Interpretation

A two-fold autologous adsorption usually removes sufficient autoantibody from the serum so that alloantibody, if present, is readily apparent. Occasionally, two adsorptions are insufficient. If the patient's RBCs can be shown to have a negative DAT following heat treatment (Procedure A), ZZAP treatment (Procedure B), or chloroquine diphosphate treatment, such RBCs may be used to check the efficacy of the adsorption process. For example, if Procedure A was used and the heat-treated cells obtained after Step 4 have a negative DAT, the autoadsorbed serum should be tested against them and two group O RBC samples (screening cells). Results can be interpreted as follows:

1. When there is no reactivity against the group O reagent RBCs, it is unlikely that alloantibody is present.
2. If there is reactivity against both the patient's heat-treated RBCs and the group O cells, further adsorptions are necessary to remove the autoantibody.
3. When the adsorbed serum reacts with one or both of the group O reagent RBCs and not with the autologous RBCs, the serum contains alloantibody, and antibody identification studies should be undertaken on the adsorbed serum.

Notes:

1. ZZAP reagent should be prepared immediately before use.
2. ZZAP treatment destroys all Kell system antigens except Kx in addition to M, N, S, s, Fy^a, Fy^b, and other receptors that are destroyed by protease.
3. There is no need to wash RBCs before treatment with ZZAP.

H—Demonstration of Drug-Induced Immune Complex Formation*

Application

Certain drugs and their respective antibodies form immune complexes and attach weakly to RBCs. These nonspecifically

---

*Morel, PA, Bergren, ML, and Frank, BA: A simple method for detection of alloantibody in the presence of autoantibody (abstract). Transfusion 18:388, 1978.
†Branch, DR, and Petz, LD: A new reagent (ZZAP) having multiple applications in immunohematology. Am J Clin Pathol 78:161, 1982.

*Adapted from Garratty, G: Laboratory Investigation of Drug-Induced Immune Hemolytic Anemia and/or Positive Direct Antiglobulin Tests. American Association of Blood Banks, Washington, DC, 1979.

bound immune complexes activate complement, which may lead to hemolysis in vivo. This procedure provides a means to demonstrate in vitro the immune complex formation associated with drug-antidrug interactions.

Materials

1. Drug under investigation, in the same form (tablet, solution, capsules) that the patient is receiving
2. Phosphate-buffered saline (PBS) at pH 7.0–7.4
3. Patient's serum
4. Fresh normal serum known to lack unexpected antibodies as a source of complement
5. Group O RBCs, both untreated and treated with a proteolytic enzyme

Method

1. Prepare a 1 mg/mL suspension of the drug in PBS. Centrifuge and adjust the pH of the supernatant fluid to 7.0 with either 1 N NaOH or 1 N HCl, as required.
2. Using 0.2 mL of each reactant, prepare the following test mixtures: (a.) patient's serum + drug; (b) patient's serum + complement (normal serum) + drug; (c) patient's serum + complement (normal serum) + PBS; (d) normal serum + drug; and (e) normal serum + PBS
3. To three drops of each test mixture, add one drop of a 5% saline suspension of group O RBCs. To another three drops of each test mixture, add one drop of a 5% saline suspension of enzyme-treated group O reagent RBCs.
4. Mix and incubate at 37°C for 1–2 hours with periodic gentle mixing.
5. Centrifuge and examine for hemolysis/agglutination.
6. Wash the RBCs four times in saline, and test with a polyspecific antiglobulin reagent.

Interpretation

Hemolysis, agglutination, or coating can occur. Such reactivity in any of the tests containing patient's serum to which the drug was added and absence of reactivity in the corresponding control tests containing PBS instead of the drug indicate a drug-antidrug interaction.

Notes:

1. The use of a mortar and pestle (if the drug is in tablet form), incubation at 37°C, and vigorous shaking of the solution may help dissolve the drug.
2. Many drugs will not dissolve completely, but enough may be dissolved to react in serologic tests. Other methods, obtained from the manufacturer or other publications, may be needed to dissolve adequate quantities of some drugs.

I—Detection of Antibodies to Penicillin or Cephalothin*

Application

RBCs can be coated with penicillin or cephalosporins and tested to investigate a positive DAT associated with these antibiotics.

Materials

1. Barbital-buffered saline (BBS) at pH 9.6, prepared by dissolving 20.6 g of sodium barbital in 1 L of saline. Adjust to pH 9.6 with 0.1 N HCl. Store at 4°C.
2. Penicillin (1×10^6 U per 600 mg)
3. Cephalothin sodium (Keflin)—400 mg
4. Washed, packed group O RBCs (2 mL)
5. Serum or eluate to be tested

Method

1. Prepare penicillin-coated RBCs by incubating 1 mL of RBCs with 600 mg of penicillin in 15 mL BBS for 1 hour at room temperature. Wash three times in saline, and store in Alsever's solution at 4°C.
2. Prepare cephalothin-coated RBCs by incubating 1 mL of RBCs with 400 mg of cephalothin sodium in 10 mL of BBS for 2 hours at 37°C. Wash three times in saline, and store in Alsever's solution at 4°C.
3. Mix two or three drops of serum or eluate with one drop of a 5% suspension of drug-coated cells. Dilute serum 1:20 with saline for tests with cephalothin-coated cells.
4. Test in parallel uncoated RBCs from the same donor.
5. Incubate the tests at 37°C for 30–60 minutes. Centrifuge and examine macroscopically for agglutination. Grade and record results.
6. Wash the RBCs four times in saline and test by the indirect antiglobulin technique using polyspecific or anti-IgG reagent.

Interpretation

Antibodies to penicillin or cephalothin will react with drug-coated cells but not with uncoated cells. Antibodies to either drug may cross-react with RBCs coated with the other drug (e.g., antipenicillin antibodies cross-react with cephalothin-coated RBCs and vice-versa).

Notes:

1. Phosphate-buffered saline at pH 7.3 may be substituted for BBS in the preparation of cephalothin-coated RBCs.
2. All normal sera react with cephalothin-coated RBCs because such RBCs absorb all proteins nonimmunologi-

---

*Adapted from Garratty, G: Laboratory Investigation of Drug-Induced Hemolytic Anemia and/or Positive Direct Antiglobulin Tests. American Association of Blood Banks, Washington, DC, 1979.

cally. This reactivity does not occur with incubation times as short as 15 minutes or if the serum is diluted 1:20 with saline before testing.

3. Eluates do not contain enough protein to be absorbed non-immunologically by cephalothin-coated RBCs. Reactivity of an eluate with cephalothin-coated RBCs indicates antibody to cephalosporins, which may cross-react with penicillin-coated RBCs.

J—EDTA/Glycine Acid Method to Remove Antibodies from RBCs*

Application

EDTA/glycine acid can be used to dissociate antibody molecules from RBC membranes. This procedure is routinely used for blood typing tests or adsorption procedures. All common RBC antigens can be detected after treatment with EDTA/glycine acid except Kell system and Ev^a antigens. Thus, cells treated in this manner cannot be used to determine these phenotypes.

Specimen

RBCs with a positive DAT

Reagents

1. 10% EDTA, prepared by dissolving 2 g of disodium ethylenediamine tetraacetic acid (Na_2EDTA) in 20 mL of distilled or de-ionized water.
2. 0.1 M glycine-HCl buffer (pH 1.5), prepared by diluting 0.75 g of glycine to 100 mL with isotonic (unbuffered) saline. Adjust the pH to 1.5 using concentrated HCl.
3. 1.0 M TRIS-NaCl, prepared by dissolving 12.1 g of TRIS (hydroxymethyl aminomethane) and 5.25 g of sodium chloride (NaCl) to 100 mL with distilled or deionized water.

Procedure

1. Wash the RBCs to be treated six times with isotonic saline.
2. In a test tube, mix together 20 volumes of 0.1 M acid glycine-HCl (pH 1.5) with five volumes of 10% EDTA. This is the EDTA/glycine acid reagent.
3. Place 10 volumes of washed RBCs in a clean tube.
4. Add 20 volumes of EDTA/glycine acid.
5. Mix the contents of the tube thoroughly.
6. Incubate the mixture at room temperature for no more than 2 minutes.
7. Add one volume of 1.0 M TRIS-NaCl, and mix the contents of the tube.
8. Centrifuge at 900 to 1000 $\times$ g for 1–2 minutes, then aspirate, and discard the supernatant fluid.

9. Wash the RBCs four times with saline.
10. Test the washed cells with anti-IgG; if nonreactive with anti-IgG, the cells are ready for use in blood typing or adsorption procedures. If the DAT is positive, additional treatment can be performed.

Notes:

1. Overincubation of RBCs with EDTA/acid glycine causes irreversible damage to cell membrane.
2. Include a parallel control reagent, such as 6% bovine albumin, when typing treated RBCs.
3. Use anti-IgG, not a polyspecific antiglobulin reagent, in Step 10.
4. If a commercial kit is used, follow manufacturer's instructions for testing and controls.

K—Separation of Transfused from Autologous RBCs by Simple Centrifugation: Reticulocyte Harvesting*

Application

Newly formed autologous RBCs generally have a lower specific gravity than transfused cells and may be separated from the transfused cell population by simple centrifugation. The newly formed autologous cells concentrate at the top of the column of RBCs when blood is centrifuged in a microhematocrit tube, providing a simple method for recovering autologous cells in a blood sample from recently transfused patients. *Note*: RBCs from patients with hemoglobin S or spherocytic disorders are not effectively separated by this method.

Specimen

RBCs from whole blood collected into EDTA

Materials

1. Microhematocrit centrifuge
2. Plain (not heparinized) glass or plastic hematocrit tubes.
3. Sealant

Procedure

1. Wash the RBCs three times in saline. For the last wash, centrifuge the cells at 900–1000 g for 5 to 15 minutes.Remove as much of the supernatant fluid as possible without disturbing the buffy coat. Mix thoroughly.
2. Fill 10–12 microhematocrit tubes to the 60 mm mark with well-mixed washed RBCs.

*Adapted from Vengelen-Tyler, V (ed): Technical Manual, ed 13. American Association of Blood Banks, Bethesda, MD,1999.

*Adapted from Vengelen-Tyler, V (ed): Technical Manual, ed 13. American Association of Blood Banks, Bethesda, MD, 1999, p 665.

3. Seal the ends of the tubes by heat or with sealant.
4. Centrifuge all tubes in a microhematocrit centrifuge for 15 minutes.
5. Cut the microhematocrit tubes 5 mm below the top of the column of RBCs. This 5 mm segment contains the least dense, hence youngest, circulating RBCs.
6. Place the cut microhematocrit tubes into larger test tubes (10 or 12 × 75 mm), add saline, mix well and flush the RBCs from the microhematocrit tubes. Then either (a) centrifuge at 1000 × g for 1 minute and remove the empty microhematocrit tubes, or (b) transfer the saline-suspended RBCs to a clean test tube.
7. Wash the separated RBCs three times in saline before resuspending them to 2%–5% in saline for testing.

Notes:

1. Separation is better if 3 or more days have elapsed from the last RBC transfusion.
2. The RBCs should be mixed continuously while the microhematocrit tubes are being filled.
3. Separation techniques are only effective if the patient is producing normal or above normal numbers of reticulocytes. This method will be ineffective in patients with inadequate reticulocyte production.
4. Some RBC antigens may not be as strongly expressed on reticulocytes as on older cells. Particular attention should be given to determination of the E, e, c, Fy^a, Jk^a, and Ge antigens.

twenty-two

The HLA System

Donna L. Phelan, BA, CHS(ABHI), MT(HEW)

OBJECTIVES

On completion of this chapter, the learner should be able to:

1. Define the abbreviations HLA, MLR, SSO, SSP, SBT, and MHC.
2. Describe the three regions of the HLA complex located on the short arm of chromosome 6.
3. List the important characteristics of the HLA genes.
4. List the three exceptions to the practice of naming all serologic specificities on the basis of correlation with an identified sequence that eliminates the need for a provisional w designation.
5. Describe the current nomenclature for HLA genes.
6. Define the term "haplotype."
7. Describe the difference between HLA phenotype and HLA genotype.
8. List the characteristics of HLA class I and class II gene products.
9. Describe the characteristics of HLA antibodies.
10. Define linkage disequilibrium, a characteristic of HLA antigens.
11. Describe the techniques used for HLA antigen and allele detection.
12. Describe the techniques for HLA antibody detection.
13. Describe the role of HLA typing in paternity testing, disease association, platelet transfusion, and transplantation.

Introduction

Human leukocyte antigen (HLA) is a specialized branch or division of immunology for human histocompatibility testing. The laboratory discipline supports a number of clinical specialties in transplantation, transfusion, and immunogenetics. Because of its specialized nature, HLA is given relatively little attention in most training programs such as nursing or medical technology.

This chapter is intended to serve as an introduction to basic concepts of HLA and clinical applications of HLA testing. It is written for the reader with some training in the biomedical sciences and familiarity with general immunology concepts.

The emphasis of the chapter is on principles and concepts of HLA structure and function, HLA procedures, and the clinical application of HLA testing to immunogenetics (paternity and disease association), transfusion practices, and transplantation. Inasmuch as it is an overview of a technologically complex area, it lacks a great deal of detail. References are for further information.

Historical Perspective

Evidence for human leukocyte blood groups was first advanced in 1954 by Dausset,[1] who observed that patients whose sera contained leukoagglutinins had received a larger number of blood transfusions than other patients. He observed that these agglutinins were not autoantibodies as had been thought previously but, rather, alloantibodies produced by the infusion of cells bearing alloantigens not present in the recipient.

Dausset[2] also observed that the sera from seven patients with multiple transfusions agglutinated leukocytes from about 60 percent of the French population but not the leukocytes of the seven patients. He termed the leukocyte antigen defined by leukoagglutination techniques as MAC, derived from the first initials of three individuals who volunteered their time for the experiments. Family studies showed that leukocyte antigens were determined genetically. At about the same time, Payne[3] showed that the sera of patients with febrile nonhemolytic transfusion reactions often contained leukoagglutinins.

The microdroplet lymphocytotoxicity test was introduced by Terasaki and McClelland[4,5] at the First International Histocompatibility Workshop as a means to define MAC specificity clearly. The microdroplet technique was adopted as the standard method of typing because of the unreliability of the leukoagglutination test. In various modifications, this test is still the major HLA-typing serologic technique. The development of HLA typing was further aided by the introduction of computer analysis programs by van Rood and van Leeuwen[6] to study the serologic complexities. Despite numerous false-positive and false-negative serologic reactions, certain specificities could be discerned by computer analysis.

Van Rood applied computer analysis techniques to define specific HLA alleles. He tested approximately 66 sera containing leukoagglutinating antibodies against a random panel of 100 cells. Using two-by-two chi-square analysis, he compared reactivity of each serum with that of every other serum. In this way he was able to identify several groups of sera that were detecting common specificities. In addition, one group of sera having high chi-square values with each other but low values with other serum groups suggested products of allelic genes. Van Rood called this diallelic system 4, with 4[a] and 4[b] as alleles.

After the discovery of the first leukocyte antigens and a suitable test system, the number of defined serologic specificities increased rapidly. By 1967, they were all clearly shown to belong to the same genetic system, and the term HL-A (human leukocyte antigen, or HLA—the hyphen has since been deleted) was approved by the World Health Organization (WHO) Committee on Nomenclature.[7] The WHO Committee was formed to establish worldwide uniform nomenclature for the HLA antigens. The Committee meets after each international workshop and uses the data from the workshop to update and to assign new names for antigens. These workshops, which are collaborative efforts to advance the field of histocompatibility, are held approximately every 2 to 3 years **(Table 22–1)**. Standardized name assignments aid the rapid but orderly development in this field.

By 1967, it was generally accepted that the HLA antigens were coded by two closely linked loci, each coding for a multiple number of alleles.[8,9] Antigens were assigned to one of the loci, based on large population studies and segregation analysis within families. In 1970, the existence of a third locus was defined, which codes for only 10 different serologic antigens (to date).[10] Additional research disclosed that the lymphocytes from two different individuals would undergo blast transformation and divide when mixed and cultured in vitro. This cellular response is known as the mixed lymphocyte reaction (MLR).[11,12] In 1967, Bach and Amos[13] discovered that the MLR was negative when leukocytes from a pair of

TABLE 22–1   International Workshops

Year	Location	Advances
1964	Durham, North Carolina	Test techniques
1965	Leiden, The Netherlands	Antigens and transplantation
1967	Turin, Italy	Family typing studies
1970	Los Angeles, California	Common serum sets
1972	Evian, France	Population studies
1975	Arhus, Denmark	MLC, class II antigens
1977	Oxford, United Kingdom	Class II genetics
1980	Los Angeles, California	DR serology, haplotype analyses
1984	Munich, Germany, and Vienna, Austria	HTC, DNA technology
1987	Princeton, New Jersey, and New York, New York	RFLP, cellular typing
1991	Yokohama, Japan	DNA technology
1996	Paris, France	Molecular nomenclature typing techniques
2002	Seattle, Washington	

HLA identical siblings were mixed together, indicating that HLA gene products were responsible for the MLR activity. The technique used to test for MLR activity is the mixed lymphocyte culture (MLC). Mixed lymphocyte culture data revealed that there might be a fourth locus (D) very closely linked with the HLA complex. The Seventh International Histocompatibility Workshop in 1977 clearly established the D locus and also a new DR locus defined by serologic methods.[14] Most significantly, the typing of B lymphocytes for their DR specificities was accomplished. The letter *R* in DR indicates "related"; this locus was found to be either identical with or similar to the D locus identified by the MLC technique.

Evidence suggests that a separate HLA-D locus, defined only by MLR, does not exist. HLA-D assignments are the result of the combined effect of the HLA-DR, HLA-DQ, and HLA-DP determinants, subregions on the class II molecule.

Nomenclature

The HLA genetic region is a series of closely linked genes that determine major histocompatibility factors; that is, surface antigens or receptors that are responsible for the recognition and elimination of foreign tissues. The region is also referred to as the major histocompatibility complex (MHC). The HLA complex contains an estimated 35 to 40 genes physically grouped into three regions located on the short arm of chromosome 6 **(Fig. 22–1)**. The class I region encodes genes for the classic transplantation molecules, HLA-A, HLA-B, and HLA-C. It also encodes for additional nonclassic genes, including HLA-E, HLA-F, and HLA-G. The class II region encodes genes for the molecules HLA-DR, HLA-DP, and HLA-DQ composed of both α and β chains. DP molecules are the product of DPA1 and DPB1 alleles **(Fig. 22–2)**; DPB2 and DPA2 are pseudogenes, genes with mutations that prevent gene activation or transcription. DQ molecules are the product of DQA1 and DQB1 alleles. DR molecules use DRA but can use alleles coded by DRB1 (the classic DR specificities), DRB3 (DR52 molecules), DRB4 (DR53), and DRB5 (DR51).

The class III region encodes structurally and functionally

Human Chromosome 6

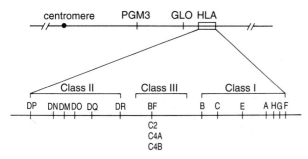

■ **FIGURE 22–1**   The HLA complex on the short arm of chromosome 6.

Class II

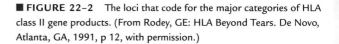

■ **FIGURE 22–2**   The loci that code for the major categories of HLA class II gene products. (From Rodey, GE: HLA Beyond Tears. De Novo, Atlanta, GA, 1991, p 12, with permission.)

diverse molecules, including C2, C4, Bf (the complement factors), 21-hydroxylase, and tumor necrosis factor. In addition, two other genes, glyoxalase-1 (GLO) and phosphoglucomutase-3 (PGM-3), are linked with the HLA complex.

One very important characteristic of HLA genes is that they are highly polymorphic, and several alleles exist at each locus. The antigenic specificities are designated by numbers following the locus symbol (e.g., HLA-A1, HLA-A2, HLA-B5, HLA-B7, and so on). Before the 1991 International Workshop, provisionally identified or tentative specificities carried the initial letter w (for "workshop") inserted between the locus letter designation and the temporary antigen specificity number. The w specificities required further definition and confirmation. For example, HLA-Bw53 indicated that the definition of the Bw53 specificity was not fully agreed upon by the WHO Committee on HLA nomenclature. After the 1991 Workshop, however, the WHO Committee agreed that all serologic speci-

ficities with the letter w indicating provisional status would, with three exceptions, drop the letter.[15] In the future, all serologic specificities will be named on the basis of correlation with an identified sequence, eliminating the need for a provisional w designation. The three exceptions are:

1. Bw4 and Bw6, to distinguish them as epitopes different from other B locus alleles
2. The C locus specificities where the w is retained to maintain distinction between HLA-C locus alleles and the complement components
3. The D and DP specificities defined by MLR and primed lymphocyte typing

Table 22–2 lists the current specificities of the HLA system recognized by the WHO Ccommittee. Note that specificities within the A and B loci are not numbered consecutively, as are those within the C, DR, DQ, and DP loci. This is because many

---

TABLE 22–2   HLA Serologic and Cellular Specificities Recognized by the Twelfth International Histocompatibility Workshop

A	B	C	D	DR	DQ	DP
A1	B5	Cw1	Dw1	DR1	DQ1	DPW1
A2	B7	Cw2	Dw2	DR103	DQ2	DPW2
A203	B703	Cw3	Dw3	DR2	DQ3	DPW3
A210	B8	Cw4	Dw4	DR3	DQ4	DPW4
A3	B12	Cw5	Dw5	DR4	DQ5 (1)	DPW5
A9	B13	Cw6	Dw6	DR5	DQ6 (1)	DPW6
A10	B14	Cw7	Dw7	DR6	DQ7 (3)	
A11	B15	Cw8	Dw8	DR7	DQ8 (3)	
A19	B16	Cw9 (w3)	Dw9	DR8	DQ9 (3)	
A23 (9)	B17	Cw10 (w3)	Dw10	DR9		
A24 (9)	B18		Dw11 (w7)	DR10		
A2403	B21		Dw12	DR11 (5)		
A25 (10)	B22		Dw13	DR12 (5)		
A26 (10)	B27		Dw14	DR13 (6)		
A28	B2708		Dw15	DR14 (6)		
A29 (19)	B35		Dw16	DR1403		
A30 (19)	B37		Dw17 (w7)	DR1404		
A31 (19)	B38 (16)		Dw18 (w6)	DR15 (2)		
A32 (19)	B39 (16)		Dw19 (w6)	DR16 (2)		
A33 (19)	B3901		Dw20	DR17 (3)		
A34 (10)	B3902		Dw21	DR18 (3)		
A36	B40		Dw22			
A43	B4005		Dw23	DR51		
A66 (10)	B41			DR52		
A68 (28)	B42		Dw24	DR52		

(continued)

TABLE 22-2   HLA Serologic and Cellular Specificities Recognized by the Twelfth International Histocompatibility Workshop (continued)

A	B	C	D	DR	DQ	DP
A69 (28)	B44 (12)	Dw25				
A74 (19)	B45 (12)	Dw26	DR53			
A80	B46					
	B47					
	B48					
	B49 (21)					
	B50 (21)					
	B51 (5)					
	B5102					
	B5103					
	B52 (5)					
	B53					
	B54 (22)					
	B55 (22)					
	B56 (22)					
	B57 (17)					
	B58 (17)					
	B59					
	B60 (40)					
	B61 (40)					
	B62 (15)					
	B63 (15)					
	B64 (14)					
	B65 (14)					
	B67					
	B70					
	B71 (70)					
	B72 (70)					
	B73					
	B75 (15)					
	B76 (15)					
	B77 (15)					
	B78					
	B81					
	Bw4					
	Bw6					

of the A and B specificities were established before the discovery of the latter loci and, to avoid renumbering, the existing numbers for the A and B loci were retained.

Also note in **Table 22–2** that many of the broad specificities are subdivided into two or more different specificities because of the detection of discrete gene products by monospecific antisera. Monospecific antisera by definition react only with antigenic determinants unique to the specific antigen. This process of splitting previously recognized antigens is still going on. **Table 22–3** lists the broad specificities and their designated split specificities. Also listed are associated antigens (#), which are variants of the original broad specificity and not splits as previously defined.

There are no 4 or 6 allelic assignments within the A and B loci, because these numbers were reserved for the leukocyte antigen systems under active investigation at the time the nomenclature was established. The antigens originally called 4 and 6 are now termed Bw4 and Bw6. Every HLA-B locus molecule and some HLA-A locus molecules carry either the Bw4 or the Bw6 antigenic determinant. The distribution of Bw4 and Bw6 determinants on HLA-A and HLA-B locus gene products is found in **Table 22–4**.

Current nomenclature was recommended during the Tenth International Histocompatibility Workshop in 1987; minor modifications were made in 1990, and total implementation was achieved after the Eleventh International Workshop in 1991. Many HLA allelic variants were discovered by nucleotide and amino acid sequence data that are not detectable by traditional serologic techniques. This complexity necessitated the development of the following nomenclature for HLA genes:

1. HLA- designates the MHC.
2. A capital letter indicates a specific locus (A, B, C, D, etc.) or region. All genes in the D region are prefixed by the letter D and followed by a second capital letter indicating the subregion (DR, DQ, DP, DO, DN, etc.).
3. Loci coding for the specific class II alpha and beta peptide chains are identified next (A1, A2, B1, B2).
4. Specific alleles are designated by * followed by a two-digit numeral defining the unique allele. The following two, two-digit numeral defines the variant of the specific allele. For example, the serologically defined HLA-B27 specificity is actually made up of seven distinct allelic variations. These alleles are now defined as HLA-B *2701 through *2707. The nomenclature of certain alleles contains a fifth digit, such as HLA-Cw *02021 and *02022. The fifth digit indicates that the two variants differ by a silent nucleotide substitution but not in amino acid sequence.

Some examples of current HLA genetic nomenclature are provided in **Table 22–5**.

TABLE 22–3 Broad Specificities, Their Splits, and Associated Antigens

Original Broad Specificities	Splits and Associated Antigens (#)
A2	A203#, A210#
A9	A23, A24, A2403#
A10	A25, A26, A34, A66
A19	A29, A30, A31, A32, A33, A74
A28	A68, A69
B5	B51, B52, B5102#, B5103#
B7	B703#
B12	B44, B45
B14	B64, B65
B15	B62, B63, B75, B76, B77
B16	B38, B39, B3901#, B3902#
B17	B57, B58
B21	B49, B50, B4005#
B22	B54, B55, B56
B27	B2708#
B40	B60, B61
B70	B71, B72
Cw3	Cw9, Cw10
DR1	DR103#
DR2	DR15, DR16
DR3	DR17, DR18
DR5	DR11, DR12
DR6	DR13, DR14, DR1403#, DR1404#
DQ1	DQ5, DQ6
DQ3	DQ7, DQ8, DQ9
Dw6	Dw18, Dw19
Dw7	Dw11, Dw17

TABLE 22–5 Examples of Current HLA Nomenclature

Serologic Specificity	Gene Locus	Allelic Variation	Number of Gene Products
HLA-A3	HLA-A	A*0301, A*0302, A*0303	3
HLA-B14	HLA-B	B*1401, B*1402	2
HLA-DR15	HLA-DRB1	DRB1*15011 DRB*1503 DRB1*15012 DRB1*1504 DRB1*15021 DRB1*1505 DRB1*15022 DRB1*1506	8
HLA-DQ2	HLA-DQB1	DQB1*0201 DQB1*0202 DQB1*0203	3

gous. If both alleles on that locus are the same, the person is homozygous.

Inheritance

The entire set of A, B, C, DR, DQ, and DP antigens located on one chromosome is called a haplotype. Genetic crossovers and recombination in the HLA region are uncommon (less than 1 percent), and thus a complete set of alleles located on a chromosome is usually inherited by children as a unit (haplotype).

Figure 22–3 illustrates the segregation of HLA haplotypes in a family. The two haplotypes of the father are labeled a and

Antigens and Antibodies

It is necessary to evaluate the HLA antigen composition in prospective donor-recipient pairs before organ transplantation and in candidates for platelet therapy refractory to random donor platelets. Even more important is the evaluation and identification of HLA antibodies in the serum of recipients before transplantation and transfusion. Evidence clearly indicates that presensitization to HLA antigens may cause rapid rejection of transplanted tissue or poor platelet survival following transfusion.[16] HLA-antigen testing is also used in disease correlation, paternity testing, and anthropologic studies.

Each person has two alleles for each locus. Both alleles or gene products of a locus are expressed codominantly; that is, there is equal expression of both alleles. The presence of one allele does not suppress the expression of the other. If there are two different alleles on one locus, the person is heterozy-

TABLE 22–4 Bw4 and Bw6 Associated Specificities

Bw4:	B5, B5102, B5103, B13, B17, B27, B37, B38 (16), B44 (12), B47, B49(21), B51(5), B52 (5), B53, B57 (17), B58(17), B59, B63(15), B77 (15) and A9, A23(9), A24(9), A2403, A25 (10), A32 (19)
Bw6:	B7, B703, B8, B14, B18, B22, B2708, B35, B39(16), B3901, B3902, B40, B4005, B41, B42, B45(12), B46, B48, B50 (21), B54 (22), B55 (22), B56 (22), B60(40), B61(40), B62 (15), B64 (14), B65 (14), B67, B70, B71 (70), B72 (70), B73, B75 (15), B76 (15), B78, B81

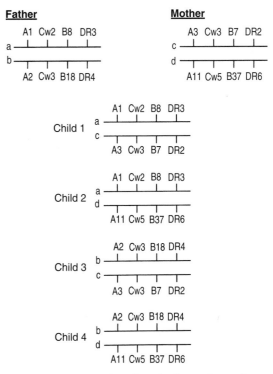

■ FIGURE 22–3 Segregation of HLA haplotypes in a pedigree. (From Tiwari, JL, and Terasaki, PI: HLA and Disease. Springer-Verlag, New York, 1985, p 8, with permission.)

b, and the mother's haplotypes are c and d. Each offspring inherits two haplotypes, one from each parent. Thus, only four possible haplotypes—ac, ad, bc, and bd—can be found in the offspring. It can be calculated that 25 percent of the offspring will have identical HLA haplotypes, 50 percent will share one HLA haplotype, and 25 percent will share no HLA haplotypes. An important corollary is that a parent and child can share only one haplotype, making an identical match between the two unlikely. It should also be apparent that uncles, grandparents, and cousins are very unlikely to have identical haplotypes with any given child. These are important factors when looking for a well-matched organ or blood donor.

The HLA phenotype, then, represents the surface markers or antigens detected in histocompatibility testing of a single individual. The HLA genotype represents the association of the alleles on the two chromosomes as determined by family studies, and the term haplotype refers to the allelic makeup of a single chromosome, illustrated in **Figure 22–4**.

HLA Gene Products

Structure

HLA gene products are globular glycoproteins, each composed of two noncovalently linked chains. Class I (HLA-A, HLA-B, and HLA-C) molecules consist of a heavy chain with a molecular weight of 45,000 daltons associated noncovalently with β_2-microglobulin, a nonpolymorphic protein of 12,000 dalton molecular weight found in serum and urine. The heavy chain folds into three domains and is inserted through the cell membrane via a hydrophobic sequence.[17]

Class II (HLA-DR, HLA-DQ, and HLA-DP) molecules consist of two similar-sized chains of a molecular weight of 33,000 (α) and 28,000 (β) daltons associated noncovalently throughout their extracellular portions. In these molecules, both chains are inserted through the membrane via hydrophobic regions. The extracellular portions of these chains fold into two domains.[18,19]

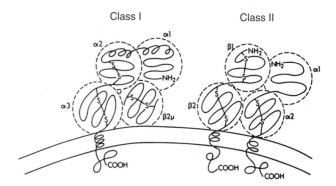

■ **FIGURE 22–5** Three-dimensional configurations of class I and II molecules. $\beta2\mu$ = B_2-microglobulin. (From Rodey, GE: HLA Beyond Tears. DeNovo, Atlanta, 1991, p 17, with permission.)

Class I molecules are present on all nucleated cells, dendritic cells, and platelets, whereas class II molecules have a much more restricted distribution. They are found only on B lymphocytes, activated T lymphocytes, macrophages, monocytes, and endothelial cells. Although class I and class II molecules have some obvious structural differences, they are thought to be very similar in overall three-dimensional configuration **(Fig. 22–5)**. Class I and class II molecules are also alike in that most of the polymorphism is expressed in the portion of the molecule farthest from the cell membrane.[20]

Early structural models of class I molecules indicated that the α-1 and α-2 domains consisted of stretches of amino acids that were arranged into helical structures rather than sheets typical of globular proteins. The crystallography studies of Bjorkman and colleagues[21] elucidated the three-dimensional structure of the class I, HLA-A2 molecule. The α_1 and α_2 domains form a platform overlaid by two helical structures to form the peptide binding site **(Fig. 22–6)**. This groove holds processed peptides for presentation to T cells.

The surface topography, created by the folding of globular proteins into three-dimensional configurations, is large and irregular, containing multiple, nonrepeating sites (antigenic

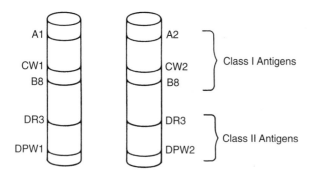

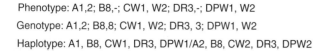

Phenotype: A1,2; B8,-; CW1, W2; DR3,-; DPW1, W2

Genotype: A1,2; B8,8; CW1, W2; DR3, 3; DPW1, W2

Haplotype: A1, B8, CW1, DR3, DPW1/A2, B8, CW2, DR3, DPW2

■ **FIGURE 22–4** Schematic representation of the HLA loci on the short arm of chromosome 6. (From Miller, WV, and Rodey, G: HLA Without Tears. American Society of Clinical Pathologists, Chicago, 1981, p 10, with permission.)

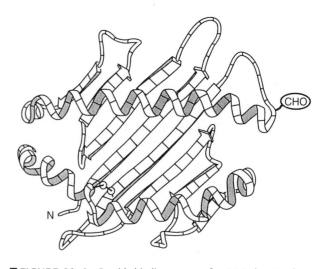

■ **FIGURE 22–6** Peptide-binding groove of an HLA class I molecule. CHO = attached carbohydrate unit; N = amino terminus. (The author thanks Dr. Peter Parham for providing this illustration.)

determinants or epitopes) that are potentially immunogenic. It is possible that the entire surface of the HLA molecule consists of these multiple, overlapping epitopes. An epitope is estimated to involve a minimum of five to six amino acid residues, but larger sequences are often necessary to construct the appropriate conformation.

Epitopes that differ among individual members of the same species are alloepitopes. HLA alloepitopes are defined with well-characterized alloantibodies and cloned T lymphocytes. Serologically defined epitopes are located primarily in and around the peptide groove and are finite in number. The epitopes recognized by T lymphocytes are less precisely mapped, very numerous, and distinct from the serologically defined ones.[22]

Function

The primary role of the adaptive arm of the immune system is to recognize and to eliminate foreign antigens. An essential feature of this function is the ability to discriminate between self and nonself, or foreign, antigens. Major histocompatibility complex class I and II molecules play a crucial role in the process of discrimination at the molecular, cellular, and species levels between self and nonself elements.

Antibodies

The majority of HLA alloantibodies are IgG. Antibodies to HLA molecules can be divided into two groups:

1. Those that detect a single HLA gene product ("private" antibodies binding to an epitope unique to one HLA gene product)
2. Those that detect more than one HLA gene product

These may be "public" (binding to epitopes shared by more than one HLA gene product) or cross-reactive (binding to structurally similar HLA epitopes).[23]

The monoclonal HLA antibody (MoAb) is produced by fusing HLA antibody-producing B cells with plasmacytoma lines.[24] Plasmacytoma cells arise from the malignant transformation of plasma cells or differentiated B cells. These cells continue to secrete antibody after transformation. MoAbs detect a broader range of epitopes because they are derived through xenoimmunization—immunization across different species.

Crossing Over

An event that infrequently complicates HLA-typing interpretation and haplotype determination is crossing over (or recombination). During meiosis, exchange of material between the paired chromosomes can occur. During chromosomal replication, replicated chromosomes often overlay each other, forming x-shaped chiasmata (Fig. 22–7). When the

chromosomes are pulled apart during meiotic division, breaks can occur at the crossover site, resulting in complementary exchange of genetic material. The further apart two loci are on a given chromosome, the more likely it is that genetic exchanges will take place. For example, recombination between HLA-A and HLA-DP occurs commonly, whereas recombination between HLA-DQ and HLA-DR is a rare event. Crossing over has the effect of rearranging the genes on the chromosome to produce new haplotypes in the general population.

Linkage Disequilibrium

An important characteristic of HLA antigens is the existence of linkage disequilibrium between the alleles of the loci. Linkage disequilibrium is the occurrence of HLA genes more frequently in the same haplotype than would be expected by chance alone. In the Rh system, the blood groups C, D, and e are found together more often than would be expected based on their individual gene frequencies. This is commonly found within the HLA system. In a randomly mating population at Hardy-Weinberg equilibrium,[25] the occurrence of two alleles from closely linked genes will be the product of their individual gene frequencies. If the observed value of the joint frequency is significantly different from the expected frequency (the product of the individual allele frequencies), the alleles are said to be in linkage disequilibrium. For example, if HLA-A1 and HLA-B8 gene frequencies are 0.16 and 0.1, respectively, in a population, the expected occurrence of an HLA haplotype bearing both A1 and B8 should be $0.16 \times 0.1 \times 100$, or 1.6 percent. In certain white populations, however, the actual occurrence of this haplotype is as high as 8 percent, far in excess of the expected frequency. The HLA alleles frequently associated through disequilibrium are listed in Table 22–6. Disequilibrium between the B and DR loci alleles may

TABLE 22–6   HLA Alleles Frequently Associated Through Disequilibrium in Different Populations

HLA-A, HLA-C, HLA-B	HLA-A, HLA-B, HLA-DR
White	
A1, Cw7, B8	A1, B8, DR3
A3, Cw7, B7	A3, B7, DR2
A2, Cw5, B44	A29, B44, DR7
A1, Cw6, B57	A3, B35, DR1
A11, Cw4, B35	A1, B17, DR7
A30, Cw6, B13	A30, B13, DR7
Black	
A36, Cw4, B53	A1, B8, DR3
A1, Cw7, B8	A30, B42, DR3
A11, Cw2, B35	A28, B64, DR7
A24, Cw4, B35	A2, B58, DR11
A2, Cw2, B72	A28, B58, DR14
A2, Cw7, B58	A3, B7, DR3
Asian	
A30, Cw6, B13	A24, B52, DR2
A2, Cw1, B46	A33, B44, DR14
A24, Cw1, B54	A24, B7, DR1
A33, Cw3, B58	A33, B44, DR13
A24, Cw7, B7	A30, B13, DR7
A11, Cw4, B62	A24, B54, DR4

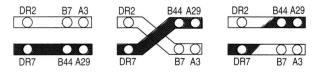

■ FIGURE 22–7   Schematic of a recombination event between HLA-B and HLA-DR.

account for problems in correlating B locus serotyping with allograft survival and disease associations, inasmuch as matching or typing for B locus alleles would, by disequilibrium, often result in matching or typing for DR locus alleles, which have been found to be clinically significant to allograft survival.

Cross Reactivity

Cross reactivity is a phenomenon in which an antiserum directed against one HLA antigenic determinant reacts with other HLA antigenic determinants as well. Cross-reactive antigens share important structural elements with one another but retain unique, specific elements. HLA serologists recognized very quickly that many of the HLA alloantibodies were serologically cross-reactive with HLA specificities.[26–28] Dausset and colleagues[29] suggested in 1967 that these antibodies might detect public specificities shared by multiple HLA gene products. The broadly reactive antibodies used in van Rood and von Leeuwen's original computer-derived HLA clusters also defined many of the currently defined major cross-reactive groups (CREGs).

The majority of cross-reactive alloantibodies detect HLA specificities of allelic molecules coded by the same locus. On the basis of these reactions, most specificities can be grouped into major CREGs (Figs. 22–8 and 22–9).[30,31] For example, the HLA-A locus antigens A2, A23, A24, and A28 share a common determinant and therefore make up the A2 CREG, or A2C. HLA-A28 also shares a common determinant with A26, A33, and A34, defining the A28 CREG. There are also at least three interlocus cross reactions detected by alloantisera and MoAbs that occur between the HLA-A and HLA-B loci: HLA-

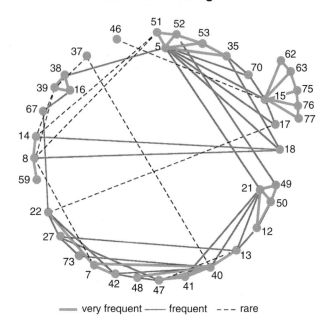

HLA-B Locus Cregs

— very frequent —— frequent - - - rare

■ **FIGURE 22–9** Cross-reactions within the HLA-B locus. (From Bender, K: The HLA System. Biotest Diagnostics, 1991, p 22, with permission.)

A23, HLA-A24, HLA-A25, and HLA-A32 with HLA-Bw4[32–35]; HLA-A11 with HLA-Bw6[36]; and HLA-A2 with HLA-B17.[37–39] Recently, cross-reactive groups have been defined molecularly using amino acid residues. Table 22–7 lists the residues identified and their correlative HLA-A,B antigens and representative CREGs.

Techniques of Histocompatibility Testing

The principles used in histocompatibility testing are basically similar to those used for red blood cell (RBC) testing; that is, known sera are used to type HLA antigens on test cells; recip-

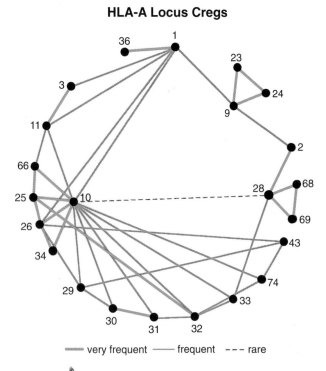

HLA-A Locus Cregs

— very frequent —— frequent - - - rare

■ **FIGURE 22–8** Cross reactions within the HLA-A locus. (From Bender, K: The HLA System. Biotest Diagnostics, 1991, p 21, with permission.)

TABLE 22–7 HLA-A,B Residues and Corresponding CREGs

Residue	A, B Antigens	CREG
R114	A1, A3, A11, A29, A36	A1C
K127	A2, A9, A23, A24, A28, A68, A69	A2C
A71–D74	B7, B22, B27, B42, B46, B54, B55, B56, B67	B7C
T69–S77	B8, B14, B16, B39, B64, B65, B78	B8C
T41	B12, B13, B21, B40, B41, B44, B45, B47, B49, B50, B60, B61	B12C
R83	A9, B5, A23, A24, A25, A32, B12, B13, B17, B21, B27, B37, B38, B44, B47, B49, B51, B52, B53, B57, B58, B59	Bw4
N80	B7, B8, A11, B14, B15, B16, B18, B22, B35, B39, B40, B41, B42, B45, B46, B48, B50, B54, B55, B56, B60, B61, B62, B64, B65, B67, B70, B71, B72, B75, B76, B78, B79	Bw6

ient serum is screened for the presence of HLA antibodies; and crossmatching of donor cells and recipient sera determines compatibility.

Preformed antibodies to tissue of donor and recipient may cause significant complications in transplantation or transfusion. Recipient lymphocytotoxic HLA antibodies to donor antigens have been associated with accelerated graft rejection and with poor response to platelet transfusion. Antibody in donor plasma to recipient leukocytes has been associated with severe pulmonary infiltrates and respiratory distress following transfusion. Thus, the clinical management of patients, pre- and post-transplant, includes screening for and determination of the specificity of anti-HLA class I and II antibodies that may be present.

Crossmatching involves serologic and cellular procedures. Serologic crossmatching is performed by cytotoxicity and flow cytometric techniques.[39] Enzyme-linked immunoadsorbent crossmatch assays (ELISA) are in development. Lymphocyte-defined compatibility is determined by the mixed-lymphocyte reaction or one of its modifications.

Over the past 10 years, practical techniques have been developed to characterize gene structure and specific alleles. The techniques of molecular genetics have revolutionized molecular biology. The three most common molecular assays employed in the clinical laboratory are sequence-specific oligonucleotides (SSO), sequence-specific primers (SSP), and sequence-based typing (SBT).

HLA Antigen Detection

The agglutination methods initially used to define the HLA complex have been succeeded by a precise microlymphocytotoxicity test.[40] Cytotoxicity techniques require only 1 to 2 μL of serum and are sensitive and reproducible.

Acid-citrated dextrose or phenol-free heparinized blood is used for testing. A purified lymphocyte suspension is prepared by layering whole blood on a Ficoll-Hypaque gradient and centrifuging. Residual RBCs and granulocytes are forced to the bottom of the gradient, and platelets remain in the supernatant. Lymphocytes collect at the gradient's interface and can be harvested, washed, and adjusted to appropriate test concentrations **(Fig. 22–10)**. HLA-A, HLA-B, and HLA-C typing is performed on this lymphocyte suspension. HLA-DR typing requires a purified B-lymphocyte suspension.

B-lymphocyte suspensions were generally prepared in two ways:

1. Nylon wool separation[41,42]
2. Fluorescent labeling[43]

The nylon wool separation of B lymphocytes was based on the observation that B cells adhere preferentially to nylon wool, from which they can be eluted, whereas T lymphocytes do not adhere to wool. Fluorescent labeling involved the incubation of lymphocytes with fluorescein isothiocyanate–labeled anti-immunoglobulin. B lymphocytes developed distinct fluorescent caps because of the binding of the labeled anti-immunoglobulin to the cell surface immunoglobulin found on B cells and not on T cells. A major advantage of the fluorescent labeling technique was that it did not involve the physical separation of T and B cells, in contrast to nylon wool separation.

Techniques currently used are immunomagnetic beads to positively select (target cells rosetted on beads) lymphocyte subpopulations for use in HLA typing, both for class I and II antigens.[44] These techniques provide rapid isolation of cells with a high degree of purity and use immunofluorescence lymphocytotoxicity. The technique for isolation of either T or B cells depends on the MoAb for bead coating.

HLA testing is performed in 60-well or 72-well microtiter trays. Antiserum test trays are prepared by dispensing 1 μL of serum into the bottom of each well, which contains mineral oil. Mineral oil is used to prevent evaporation of antisera during test incubations. Antiserum trays are frozen at −70°C until just before use. Upon use, they are removed from the freezer and thawed for 3 to 5 minutes.

Every laboratory performing HLA typing uses some form of complement-dependent microlymphocytotoxicity (CDC) **(Fig. 22–11)**. In this procedure, 1 μL of antisera is mixed with 1 μL of cells and incubated at room temperature for 30 minutes. Rabbit serum (5 μL) is added as a source of complement, and the cells are further incubated at room temperature for 60 minutes. Complement-mediated cell membrane injury that is induced in cells binding HLA antibody is visualized by the uptake or release of eosin-Y or trypan blue dye. The test is a tertiary binding assay that depends heavily on many factors—time, temperature, antibody strength—that influence the efficiency with which the antibodies will activate the complement cascade.

Trays are usually read on inverted phase contrast micro-

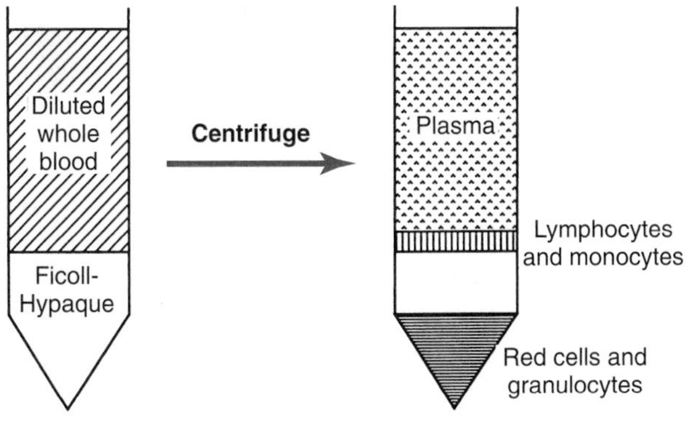

■ **FIGURE 22–10**   Lymphocyte separation.

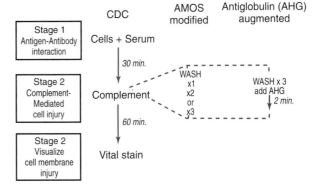

■ **FIGURE 22–11**   Complement-dependent microlymphocytotoxicity assay with two variations: three-wash AMOS and antiglobulin.

scopes. In properly adjusted phase, cells that have not been injured appear small, bright, and refractile. Injured cells that have taken up eosin-Y or trypan, blue owing to antibody and complement-mediated damage, flatten and appear large, dark, and nonrefractile. The percent of cell death is coded numerically: the number 8 is used for a strong positive with essentially all cells killed; the number 1 is used for a negative reaction in which cell viability is the same as in the negative control. By scoring the reaction of each known serum with test cells, a phenotype can be assigned. Antigen assignment is made by looking at the specificity of the defined HLA antibody in the positive wells. For example, if all wells containing HLA-A3 antibody are positive (eight reactions), the A3 antigen is assigned to the phenotype.

HLA-D Typing

Because allografted tissue is rejected by a lymphocyte-mediated immune response as well as by antibody response, tests have been developed that use a biologic response of lymphocytes to foreign antigens as a measure of histocompatibility. The MLR test provides an in-vitro model in which lymphocytes can be used both as responders (recipient cells) to foreign HLA-alloantigens and as stimulators (donor cells) carrying those antigens.[11] For example, lymphocytes of the recipient are mixed with lymphocytes of the donor, after donor lymphocytes have been treated with mitomycin C or x-irradiation to inhibit DNA synthesis. The response of the recipient cells to these treated donor cells in the MLR is measured by the incorporation of radioactive thymidine into the responding cells during cell division. If the responding cells have been stimulated, large amounts of labeled thymidine are incorporated into the newly synthesized DNA. This incorporation can be quantitated in a liquid scintillation counting device. Appropriate controls and replicate samples must be tested. The MLR reaction recognizes the antigenic differences on stimulator cells; therefore, cells bearing the same antigens as the responding cell will cause no stimulation. This indicates that the stimulator and the responder cells have the same HLA-D type.

HLA Antibody Detection Techniques

Detection and identification techniques of HLA antibodies are similar to those for RBC antibodies. The unknown serum is tested against a panel of cells or soluble antigen of known HLA phenotype. Targets from a large panel of donors must be selected if antibodies to all HLA specificities are to be detected. A panel of at least 30 carefully selected targets is required for initial screening in the determination of panel reactive antibody (PRA), and a panel of at least 60 cells is required for accurate antibody identification.

Microlymphocytotoxicity

The method depends on the purpose of the screen. When seeking alloantisera as typing reagents, it is essential to screen using the method for the typing procedure, the standard CDC being the most common. When screening recipient serum samples, a more sensitive technique—Amos-modified, extended incubation, or antihuman globulin—should be employed. The Amos-modified technique introduces a wash step after the initial serum-cell incubation. The wash step removes anticomplementary activity: aggregated immunoglobulin in the serum that can activate complement, making it unavailable for binding on the cell membranes. Standard CDC tests rarely detect 100 percent of the antigen-binding specificities of cross-reactive antibodies.[45,46] Sensitivity of the CDC test can be greatly enhanced by the addition of an antihuman globulin reagent following serum and cell incubation.[45] The addition of goat antihuman kappa chain increases the likelihood of complement binding and subsequent cell injury, especially in circumstances in which the amount of HLA-antibody binding is below the threshold of detection in the standard technique. The antihuman globulin test functions like a complement-independent technique with respect to HLA alloantibodies. If antibodies to class II molecules (DR and DQ) are to be identified, then separated or labeled B-lymphocyte suspensions of known phenotype must be used. Serum can be screened using freshly prepared lymphocytes or lymphocytes frozen in bulk or in trays. Lymphocytes frozen in trays have the advantage of rapid preparation, enabling serum to be screened in just a few hours.

The lymphocytotoxicity assay has several disadvantages. First, viable T and B lymphocytes are essential for an accurate assessment of the presence of antibody. Many laboratories routinely use frozen cells to maintain a consistent, representative panel of antigens. The process of freezing renders lymphocytes more fragile and susceptible to cell lysis, resulting in false positives. A second problem is the necessity to maintain a reliable and consistent antigen panel that reflects the ethnic composition of the patient population; HLA antigen frequencies are known to vary among different races. The requirement for activation of complement in the cytotoxicity assay results in a third disadvantage, the inability to detect non-complement-fixing antibodies. Differentiation between HLA-specific and non–HLA-specific antibodies and between IgG and IgM antibodies is not possible with the standard cytotoxicity assays. Two new techniques have been introduced as alternatives to the lymphocytoxicity assay for the detection of anti-HLA antibodies. These techniques overcome many of the pitfalls of the standard cytotoxicity assays. They employ ELISA and flow cytometry.

ELISA

The ELISA test uses purified HLA antigens, instead of lymphocytes or cells, as targets for antibodies that may be present in the patient's sera. The increased specificity of the assay, due to use of purified HLA antigens, offers the advantage of recognizing false-positive non-HLA reactions as well as distinguishing class I and II specificities. In addition, this method also differentiates between IgG and IgM antibody isotypes by the use of appropriate secondary detection antibody. ELISA can be used as a screening assay for the detection of anti-HLA antibodies as well as a method to determine antibody specificity. The screening assay utilizes a pool of purified HLA antigens. Results are interpreted as either positive or negative. The specificity determination assay utilizes a panel of purified antigens, rather than a pool, permitting the evaluation of PRA and HLA antibody specificity.

HLA class I and II antigens are purified from either transformed cell lines or from platelets with known HLA phenotypes. The affinity-purified HLA antigens, either pooled or specific, are bound directly to wells of microtiter plates. The specific binding of antibody from the test serum sample with any of the antigens is detected by subsequent incubation with alkaline phosphatase-conjugated antibody that recognizes human IgG. A quantitative measure of the reaction is obtained by spectrophotometry following addition of the appropriate enzyme substrate.

Flow Cytometry

The flow cytometric antibody screen detects antibody binding directly. Therefore, complement activation is not necessary as in the case of the lymphocytotoxicity assay. As with ELISA, flow screening can distinguish between IgG and IgM antibodies with the use of either anti-IgG or anti-IgM secondary antibodies. Flow screening can also detect noncomplement-fixing antibodies, because binding of the antibodies rather than complement fixation is measured. Flow cytometric antibody screens utilize T and B lymphocytes as targets or, in a newer technique, employ purified HLA antigens coated onto microparticles 2 to 4 μm in diameter.

Flow cytometry may be used to screen for the presence of HLA antibodies and determine antibody specificity in the same manner as the ELISA assays by utilizing either pooled or specific HLA antigen-coated microparticles as targets. Lymphocytes as targets have two problems:

1. Difficulty in distinguishing between HLA-specific and non-HLA antigens on lymphocytes
2. Inability to distinguish class I or II antibody specificity as B lymphocytes express both class I and II markers

The use of microparticles/beads coated with purified class I or II antigens circumvents these problems. HLA antibodies present in patient sera react specifically with the beads. After incubation of serum with beads, followed by staining with a fluorescently labeled anti-human IgG antibody, the anti-HLA IgG-positive serum shows a fluorescent channel shift as compared with the negative serum. Percent PRA is represented by the percentage of pooled beads that react positively with the serum.

HLA Crossmatch Techniques

Numerous techniques have been described and applied as crossmatch procedures for transplantation and transfusion. Lymphocytotoxicity is the most widely used technique because the assays are rapid and reproducible, and they use small volumes of recipient antisera and small numbers of donor cells. The primary purpose of crossmatching before transplantation or transfusion is to identify antibodies in the serum of the potential recipient to antigens present on donor tissues.

To facilitate detection of low levels of antibodies in potential recipients, sensitive techniques must be used, as in recipient serum screens. The correlation between hyperacute rejection and the presence of serum antibody against donor tissue is well established.[16] Cases of irreversible rejection during the first days after transplantation may be a result of low levels of antibody undetected by less sensitive techniques.[47-48] Bray and colleagues[49] observed that crossmatches performed with an immunofluorescence flow cytometric technique are highly sensitive in detecting donor HLA antibodies in potential allograft recipients, which were undetected by standard

serologic techniques (Amos and antihuman globulin). The flow cytometry crossmatch is performed by incubating donor cells with recipient sera, followed by a fluoresceinated goat antihuman immunoglobulin. A phycoerythrin-labeled antibody to detect either T or B cells is used to discriminate between the two subpopulations of lymphocytes. Cells are analyzed, and results are expressed as positive or negative, based on the shift in fluorescence intensity of the test serum with respect to negative serum (**Fig. 22–12**). To achieve good graft survival rates, centers are investigating more sensitive crossmatch techniques for the detection of donor-specific HLA alloantibodies.

The two newer detection methods for the presence of anti-HLA antibodies, ELISA and flow cytometry, were developed to overcome disadvantages inherent in the traditional lymphocytotoxicity assay. Both new assays are more sensitive than lymphocytoxicity and can differentiate between antibodies to HLA and non-HLA antigens. Furthermore, these assays can discriminate between IgG and IgM isotypes.

Both the ELISA and flow cytometry assays for detection of anti-HLA antibodies are relatively new. The clinical correlation between the presence of antibodies detected by these sensitive assays and graft survival is not yet established. For this reason, PRA and antibody specificity determined by the newer methods are considered only as initial tests and are not used as the sole basis for clinical decision-making. A final crossmatch with specific donor targets is required prior to transplant because not all HLA antigens are represented in the pools or panels of targets utilized in either of the assays.

HLA Molecular Techniques

HLA class II (HLA-DR, HLA-DQ, HLA-DP) typing is performed in most laboratories by DNA hybridization techniques.[50] These procedures have replaced serologic typing in many laboratories. HLA class I (HLA-A, HLA-B, HLA-C) typing is also

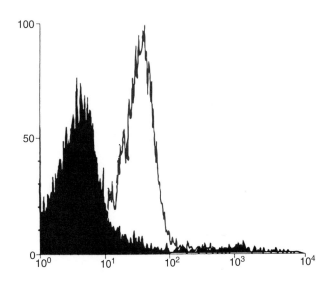

■ **FIGURE 22–12** Flow cytometry histogram illustrating the shift in fluorescence light intensity emitted by a cell population coated with fluorescein-labeled antibody. The horizontal abscissa represents increasing cell numbers and the y-axis represents increasing fluorescence. (From Rodey, GE: HLA Beyond Tears. DeNovo, Atlanta, 1991, p 17, with permission.)

performed by DNA techniques but in a restricted number of laboratories. Molecular typing for class I and II alleles is required in hematopoietic stem cell transplantation. Methods of HLA typing at the DNA level bypass the requirement of HLA protein expression and are possible because of the polymerase chain reaction (PCR) technology.

Sequence Specific Oligonucleotides (SSO)

SSO typing involves PCR amplification of a chosen sequence using primers flanking that sequence. The amplified DNA is immobilized on a membrane and hybridized with selected, labeled oligonucleotide probes. The reverse of this technique is utilized in laboratories with low throughput, where oligonucleotide probes are immobilized on membranes and hybridized with amplified DNA.

All known HLA alleles can be identified with one or a combination of allele-specific oligonucleotide probes. Different strategies are used, depending on the extent of resolution required. **Figure 22–13** illustrates a basic strategy for oligonucleotide typing. Although SSO is a powerfully reliable and accurate technology, it has been superseded by the more rapid technique of PCR-SSP.

SSP

In the SSP technique, oligonucleotide primers are designed to obtain amplification of specific alleles or groups of alleles. The typing method is based on the principle that a completely matched primer will be more efficiently used in the PCR reaction than a primer with one or more mismatches. The specificity of the typing system is part of the PCR reaction. Assignment of alleles is based on the presence or absence of amplified product normally detected by agarose gel electrophoresis and transillumination.

SBT

Direct nucleotide sequencing of HLA genes is utilized for high-resolution typing and is required in the definition of a new allele. Detection is not based on the use of sequence-specific oligonucleotide probe and prior knowledge of the

nucleotide sequences.[51,52] Therefore, previously undefined alleles can be detected. Sequencing methods can be diffentiated by the template, cloned or genomic DNA, and by the technique, automated or manual. Software, which aligns the derived sequences against established libraries, facilitates the analysis and assignment of alleles.

Clinical Significance of the HLA System

The identification of HLA antigens was driven by their potential clinical application to transplantation. The HLA system is still of primary clinical importance in transplantation, but it has recently become of great interest to individuals in the field of human genetics and to investigators of disease associations. HLAs are associated with disease susceptibility to a greater extent than any other known genetic marker in humans, and the HLA system has the highest exclusion probability of any single system in resolving cases of disputed paternity.[53]

Paternity

Paternity testing involves the analysis of genetic markers from the mother, child, and alleged father to determine whether the tested man could be the biologic father of a child. To accomplish this, the laboratory uses a number of techniques to accurately identify the polymorphic genetic markers in a paternity trio. Combinations of various genetic markers are used, including RBC markers and enzymes, serum proteins, HLA typing, and DNA testing. Previously, the most common combination of testing included RBC markers together with HLA typing. Owing to increased costs of HLA typing reagents and the significantly high power of exclusion when testing multiple DNA loci, DNA methodologies are used increasingly more than HLA typing.

Disease Association

It has been determined that HLA antigens are associated with disease susceptibility to a greater extent than any other known genetic marker.[54] Many genetic markers have been suspected to be associated with disease, the most extensively studied being blood groups, enzymes, and serum proteins. Data from these studies[55] show weak association of disease and relative risks of less than 2. Relative risk indicates how many times more frequently the disease occurs in individuals positive for the marker than in individuals negative for the marker. In contrast, the association between HLA-B27 and ankylosing spondylitis has a relative risk ranging from 60 to 100, depending on the population studied. Although many diseases associated with HLA have a relative risk value greater than 2, none exceed the strength of the association of HLA-B27 with ankylosing spondylitis. To date, 530 diseases have been studied.[54] A list of the most significant HLA/disease associations is given in **Table 22–8**.

The exact cause for the association of HLA to disease is unclear. There is no question that genetic factors coded within or near the HLA complex confer susceptibility for a variety of diseases. This susceptibility may somehow be related to altered immunologic responsiveness in many cases. It is also probable that the diseases in question may be a result of both multiple gene interactions and environmental factors. Although the study of HLA and disease associations is very

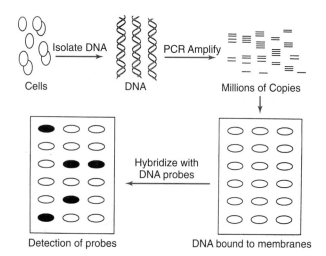

■ **FIGURE 22–13** Strategy for allele-specific oligonucleotide typing.

TABLE 22–8 Significant HLA Disease Associations

Disease	HLA	Relative Risk*
Narcolepsy	DR2	129.8
Ankylosing spondylitis	B27	69.1
Reiter's syndrome	B27	37.1
Dermatitis herpetiformis	DR3	17.3
	B8	9.8
Pemphigus vulgaris	DR4	14.6
	A26	4.8
	B38	4.6
Goodpasture's syndrome	DR2	13.8
Celiac disease	DR3	11.6
	DR7	7.7
	B8	7.6
Acute anterior uveitis	B27	8.2
Psoriasis vulgaris	Cw6	7.5
	B17	5.3
	B13	4.1
	B37	3.9
	DR7	3.2
Idiopathic hemochromatosis	A3	6.7
	B7	2.9
	B14	2.7
Sjögren's syndrome	Dw3	5.7
	B8	3.3
Juvenile rheumatoid arthritis	B27	3.9
	DR5	3.3
Behçet's disease	B5	3.8
Rheumatoid arthritis	DR4	3.8
	B27	2.0
Grave's disease	DR3	3.7
	B8	2.5
Juvenile diabetes mellitus	DR4	3.6
	DR3	3.3
	B8	2.5
	B15	2.1
Myasthenia gravis	B8	3.3
Multiple sclerosis	DR2	2.7
	B7	1.8

*Relative risk of the disease in the white population. Frequencies for other races can be found in Tiwari, JL, and Terasaki, Pl: HLA and Disease. New York, Springer-Verlag, 1995, p 33.

important in understanding disease susceptibility and manifestation, HLA alone is not clinically useful as a diagnostic tool.

Platelet Transfusion

Hematopoietic stem cell transplantation and more aggressive use of chemotherapy in the treatment of malignancies have led to a dramatic increase in platelet transfusions in the past decade. Human leukocyte class I antigens are expressed variably on platelets.[56–60] Alloimmunization to the HLA results in refractoriness to random donor platelet transfusions. Refractoriness is manifested by the failure to achieve a rise in the circulating platelet count 1 hour after infusion of adequate numbers of platelets. The refractory state is often associated with lymphocytotoxic HLA antibodies.

Considering the highly polymorphic nature of the HLA system, it is impossible to obtain sufficient numbers of HLA-typed donors to provide HLA-matched platelets for all alloimmunized patients. Duquesnoy and associates[61] demonstrated that platelet transfusions from donors mismatched only for cross-reactive antigens can effectively provide hemostasis for

refractory patients. For example, an HLA-A1,B7; -A11,B22 recipient might benefit from the platelets of an A1,B7; A3,B27 donor because A3 and A11 and B27 and B22 are cross-reactive. Table 22–9 lists the major cross-reactive groups and the private specificities associated with each. As a result of these observations, the donor pool necessary to sustain an HLA-matched platelet program can be reduced from 8000 to 10,000 to manageable numbers of 2000 to 5000.

Good platelet survival and HLA matching are not absolute. For example, poor transfusion results are sometimes obtained despite a perfect HLA match. Poor recovery may be a result of sensitization to non-HLA antigens, such as platelet-specific antigens. In contrast, excellent transfusion results are at other times obtained in the presence of complete HLA mismatch. Good recovery may be a function of:

1. A restricted pattern of alloimmunization—private versus public antibodies
2. Variable expression of HLA antigens on the platelet surface

Leukocytes are more immunogenic than platelets, and refractoriness is probably initiated by HLA antigens on the contaminating leukocytes. Evidence for this is based on a study by Brand and others,[62] in which they demonstrated a decreased rate of alloimmunization to random donor platelets when contaminating leukocytes were removed before transfusion. Herzig and colleagues[63] were also able to improve the transfusion response to HLA-matched platelets by removing the leukocytes. This type of approach might be useful for those patients who are unable to produce a response to HLA-matched platelets.

Transplantation

Clinical transplant immunology is a difficult field. Unlike animal experimentation, in which studies are performed under controlled conditions in selected inbred strains, transplant immunology deals with actual patients with different medical histories and backgrounds. Individuals working in transplant immunology must determine how best to select recipients and donors, when to increase or decrease immunosuppressive treatment, and how to precondition potential recipients so that their immune systems will accept a graft. Decisions are based on the relative merits of laboratory findings viewed against complex medical histories. Differences of opinion exist from center to center about the significance of immunologic test results and their considerations in clinical treatment protocols.

TABLE 22–9 Major CREGs and Their Private Specificities

Major CREG	Associated Private Specificities
A1 CREG	A1, 36, 3, 9 (23, 34), 10 (25, 26, 34, 66), 11, 19 (29, 30, 31, 32, 33), 28 (68, 69), 74
A2 CREG	A2, 9 (23, 24), 28 (68, 69), B17
B5 CREG	B5 (51, 52), 15 (62, 63, 75, 76, 77), 17 (57, 58), 18, 35, 49, 53, 70 (71, 72), 78
B7 CREG	B7, 42, 22 (54, 55, 56), 27, 40 (60, 61), 13, 41, 47, 48, 81
B8 CREG	B8, 14 (64, 65), 16 (38, 39), 18, 55
B12 CREG	B12, (44, 45), 21 (49, 50), 13, 40 (60, 61), 41, 48
4c CREG	A9 (23, 24), A25, A32, Bw4
6c CREG	Bw6, Cw1, Cw3, Cw7

Hematopoietic Stem Cell Transplantation

Hematopoietic stem cell transplantation (HSCT) is used to treat patients with severe aplastic anemia, immunodeficiency disease, and various forms of leukemia. Since 1980, there has been a change in the proportion of patients treated with bone marrow transplantation for malignant versus nonmalignant diseases.[64] Before 1980, 72 percent of bone marrow transplants were performed for nonmalignant diseases. Since 1980, 77 percent have been performed for malignant diseases.

Before 1980, bone marrow transplantation was performed only between HLA-identical siblings. This restricted transplantation to 35 to 40 percent of individuals eligible for transplant. Since then, an increasing number of transplants has been performed using family members or unrelated donors who are fully or partially HLA-matched with the recipient when no HLA-identical sibling is available.

Data on unrelated and related donor transplantation from the Fred Hutchinson Cancer Research center as of February 2003[65] indicate that the risk of graft rejection, graft-versus-host disease (GVHD), and death increase with one serologically defined "antigen"mismatch, multiple allele mismatches, lower marrow cell doses, and positive serum crossmatch. Data on unrelated donor transplantation from the National Marrow Donor Program (NMDP) and the Japanese Marrow Donor Program are similar.[66,67] Mismatching for HLA-A, -B, -DR, and -C was associated with statistically worse survival. Mismatching for HLA-DQ and -DP was not. When mismatches for HLA-A, -B, and -C are considered together, mismatching for HLA class I clearly has a deleterious effect on GVHD and mortality.

Because of the continuous difficulty of finding well-matched related (1/3) and unrelated (<50 percent) donors for HSCT, umbilical cord blood transplantation (UCBT) has increased over the past 15 years. UCBT is an accepted alternative to HSCT because the functional and phenotypic immaturity of UCB lymphocytes and/or the reduced T-cell dose contribute to UCB reduced alloreactivity. Therefore, limited HLA mismatches are better tolerated, and there is a decreased incidence of GVHD. The most limiting factor of UCBT is cell dosage in that quite frequently there are insufficient hematopoietic stem/progenitor cells in one UCB unit. UCB dose is of paramount importance in engraftment and survival after unrelated UCBT.

NMDP

The single most important factor for the potential increase of HSCT is expanding the donor pool to include both related and unrelated individuals. To meet the needs of patients who do not have a matched, related donor, the U.S. Congress authorized a federal contract in 1986 to establish a national marrow donor registry.

In response to a request for proposal, the NMDP was formed with cosponsorship of the American Association of Blood Banks, American Red Cross, and the Council of Community Blood Centers. The goals were to recruit a large number of informed HLA-typed volunteers to be listed as potential marrow donors, to combine all available donor HLA data into a centralized registry, and to establish a national coordinating center for facilitating donor searches and communication between donor and transplant centers. As of December 31, 2002, the NMDP had facilitated 15,556 unrelat-

ed marrow transplants throughout the world, 2,332 of which have been for minority patients. The NMDP registry contains information on 4,890,973 volunteers willing to donate their marrow/stem cells to patients needing unrelated donors. Recruiting minorities to be volunteer donors continues to be a focus for the NMDP, inasmuch as minorities represent only 1,288,786 (25%) volunteers on the registry. At any given time, there is an average of 3,000 patients searching the NMDP registry for a compatible donor.

Kidney

Kidney transplantation is used to treat end-stage renal disease. Transplantation is preferred over dialysis in treating patients with chronic renal failure because it is more cost-effective, and it usually returns patients to a state of relatively normal health. The best graft survival rates are obtained when kidneys are obtained from HLA-identical, ABO-compatible siblings, but such donors are available for relatively few patients.[68,69] Three general strategies are used by transplantation surgeons and immunologists to minimize graft rejection:

1. Immunosuppressive agents
2. Reduction of graft "foreignness"
3. Induction of tolerance

Immunosuppressive agents such as azathioprine, prednisone, thymoglobulin, cyclosporine, and tacrolimus are used to diminish the destructive immunologic responses to the graft. These agents are nonselective and carry risks of serious side effects, especially life-threatening infection.[70]

Extensive efforts are used to minimize graft "foreignness" through matching of donor and recipient antigens. Antigen disparities that most influence graft rejection include the ABO blood group antigens and the HLA antigens. Although it is still not clear what combinations of HLA gene products promote optimal graft survival rates, it is evident that 0 and 1 antigen mismatches result in increased graft survival.[71] In highly sensitized recipients, it is necessary to match for HLA-A and HLA-B because of the presence of class I HLA antibodies. Sanfilippo and colleagues[72] found that matching based on public cross-reactive antigens can provide the same association with graft outcome as private antigens. Matching for public antigens also promotes and increases the transplantation of minority patients. When matching for highly sensitized recipients, by either private or public antigens, identification of HLA serum antibodies is important. Oldfather and others[73] observed that crossmatch results can be predicted in highly sensitized recipients based on careful analysis of serum HLA-antibody specificities.

The third strategy is based on the induction of tolerance to donor-specific antigens. The evidence that transfusion of blood products before transplantation promotes graft acceptance suggests that tolerance induction may be feasible. In 1973, Opelz and coworkers[74] reported that blood transfusion might promote renal allograft survival in patients receiving kidneys from crossmatch-negative donors. In their retrospective study, graft survival rates at 1 year were significantly improved in patients who had received more than 10 transfusions (66 percent), compared with patients who had received 1 to 10 units (43 percent) or no transfusions (29 percent). Salvatierra and colleagues[75] applied this observation to the potential benefits of donor-specific blood transfusions and transplants between living related individuals. The effects of blood transfusion on the success of renal transplantation are complex and paradoxical. Transfusion of blood usually leads to HLA alloimmunization, and when this leads to HLA antibody production it is difficult to find compatible donors. Yet graft survival rates are improved when pretransplant blood is given to the recipient with no resulting sensitization. Data on the blood transfusion effect were obtained from recipients treated with azathioprine. There is a question whether blood transfusion is or will be necessary with new drug therapies such as cyclosporine and tacrolimus. Indications are that the transfusion effect will be lost with the newer immunosuppressive agents.

Two modalities, plasmapheresis and intravenous immune globulin (IVIG), are used in the treatment of rejection posttransplant and in the pretransplant desensitization of the patient.[76] Plasmapheresis has been demonstrated to remove HLA-specific antibody in many different clinical settings.[77,78] IVIG has been used to modulate immune responses and supress alloantibody. Several groups have had success using IVIG to decrease levels of anti-HLA antibody and to lower panel-reactive antibody among highly sensitized patients awaiting transplantation.[79,80]

Heart

Heart transplantation is used to treat cardiomyopathies and end-stage ischemic heart disease. Because of the organ's extremely short total ischemic time (3 hours for hearts, compared with 72 hours for kidneys), HLA matching is not feasible. Total ischemic time is the amount of time during which there is no blood flow through the organ. The single most important HLA pretransplant test is the HLA-antibody screen. Recipients with no preformed HLA antibodies receive transplants without crossmatching. Those with preformed HLA antibodies require pretransplant crossmatches to determine recipient-donor compatibility.

In a retrospective study by Yacoub et al,[81] an additive effect of class I and II matching on graft survival was observed. Matching for class II antigens had a marked influence on increased graft survival, whereas matching for class I antigens alone had no influence on the outcome. The Collaborative Transplant Study (CTS) data demonstrate similar findings: that the analysis of HLA-DR mismatches and the combined analysis of HLA-A, -B, and -DR shows correlations of graft outcome and matching.[82] It is now necessary to study methods for increasing the total ischemic time.

Liver

Orthotopic liver transplantation has become an established and successful therapeutic modality for patients with end-stage liver disease. Immunologic factors in recipient/donor matching for liver transplantation and recipient presensitization have largely been ignored in the past. The consequences of HLA presensitization and ABO incompatibility were recently underlined in two reports.[83–85] In the first, a retrospective analysis of preformed HLA antibodies demonstrated 1-year graft survivals of 40 percent in the presensitized individuals as compared with 83 percent in the nonsensitized individuals. In the second, survival of patients with emergency ABO-incompatible transplants was 30 percent compared with 76

percent in patients with emergency ABO-compatible grafts and 80 percent in patients with elective ABO-compatible grafts. In a third study on pediatric living-related liver transplantation, there was no evidence of a beneficial effect with HLA matching. However, a beneficial effect of matching was noted in the reduction protocol for immunosuppression. The CTS substantiated these findings of no effect on HLA matching in first transplants but found an effect of HLA-DR matching on retransplants.[82]

Lung

An overall review of the indications for lung transplantation during the past several years reveals that emphysema and cystic fibrosis account for the majority of double-lung transplants. The major indications for single-lung transplantation include pulmonary fibrosis (33 percent) and emphysema (41 percent). In addition, single-lung transplants for primary hypertension are being performed instead of heart-lung transplantation.

Short cold ischemic times for lungs, as with hearts, preclude prospective histocompatibility testing. However, the HLA matching between donor and recipient may play an important role in live-donor lung transplantation (2 to 3 percent) in an attempt to improve post-transplant conditions and graft survival rates.[86]

Pancreas and Islet Cell

The primary indication for pancreas transplantation is diabetes. The majority of pancreas transplants performed are simultaneous pancreas/kidney transplants (81 percent), with pancreas following kidney (12 percent) and pancreas alone (5 percent).

HLA matching, as reported by one of the largest pancreas transplant centers, has a major effect on graft survival,[87] particularly in the pancreas after kidney and pancreas alone transplants.

Because of increased risks of myocardial complications with pancreas transplantation, islet cell transplantation has been actively pursued. Although islet cell transplantation is technically simple, difficulty has been encountered in the achievement of sustained engraftment in humans due to insufficient cell numbers. To address this issue, a protocol was initiated in Alberta, Edmonton,[88] to transplant islets from multiple donors to attain sufficient islet mass. Sufficient islet mass was attained by transplanting islets from two donor pancreases in 6/7 patients. To date, the effect of HLA matching has not been studied, but data are being stored for future analyses.

United Network for Organ Sharing

In an effort to provide a rare commodity equitably, solid organs, the United Network for Organ Sharing (UNOS) was established in 1986. This organization received the federal contract to operate the National Organ Procurement and Transplantation Network (OPTN) and to develop an equitable scientific and medically sound organ allocation system. The OPTN is charged with developing policies that maximize use of organs donated for transplantation, ensuring quality of care for transplant patients, and addressing medical and ethical issues related to organ transplantation in the United States.

SUMMARY CHART:

Important Points to Remember (MT/SBB)

➤ The HLA genetic region is a series of closely linked genes located on the short arm of chromosome 6 that determine major histocompatibility factors; that is, surface antigens or receptors that are responsible for the recognition and elimination of foreign tissues.

➤ The HLA class I region encodes genes for the classic transplantation molecules HLA-A, HLA-B, and HLA-C; the class II region encodes genes for the molecules HLA-DR, HLA-DP, and HLA-DQ; the class III region encodes genes for C2, C4, Bf (complement factors), 21-hydroxylase, and tumor necrosis factor.

➤ The HLA genotype represents the association of the alleles on the two C6 chromosomes as determined by family studies, and the term haplotype refers to the allelic makeup of a single C6 chromosome.

➤ The majority of HLA alloantibodies are IgG and can be grouped into private antibodies (binding to an epitope unique to one HLA gene product), public antibodies (binding to epitopes shared by more than one HLA gene product), or cross-reactive (binding to structurally similar HLA epitopes) antibodies.

➤ Techniques of histocompatibility testing include antigen and allele typing; HLA antibody detection and identification, in which recipient serum is tested against a panel of cells; and crossmatching, in which specific donor cells and recipient sera are tested for compatibility.

➤ The general strategies employed by transplantation immunologists include use of immunosuppressive drugs, reduction of graft "foreignness," and induction of tolerance.

➤ Platelet refractoriness is manifested by the failure to achieve a rise in circulating platelet count 1 hour after infusion of adequate numbers of platelets.

REVIEW QUESTIONS

1. The HLA genes are located on which chromosome?
   a. 2
   b. 4
   c. 6
   d. 8
   e. 10

2. The majority of HLA antibodies belongs to what immunoglobulin class?
   a. IgA
   b. IgD
   c. IgE
   d. IgG
   e. IgM

3. What is the test of choice for HLA antigen testing?
   a. Agglutination
   b. Inhibition
   c. Cytotoxicity
   d. Fluorescent antibody test
   e. ELISA

4. Of the following diseases, which one has the highest relative risk in association with an HLA antigen?
   a. Ankylosing spondylitis
   b. Dermatitis herpetiformis
   c. Juvenile diabetes
   d. Narcolepsy
   e. Rheumatoid arthritis

5. Why is HLA matching not feasible in cardiac transplantation?
   a. No HLAs are present on cardiac cells
   b. No donors ever have HLA antibodies
   c. Total ischemic time is too long
   d. Total ischemic time is too short
   e. None of the above

6. DR52 molecules are the product of which alleles?
   a. DRA and DRB1
   b. DRA and DRB2
   c. DRA and DRB3
   d. DRA and DRB4
   e. DRA and DRB5

7. What is the molecular technique that detects undefined alleles?
   a. Restriction fragment length polymorphism
   b. Allele-specific oligonucleotide typing
   c. Sequence-specific primer typing
   d. Sequence-specific oligonucleotide typing
   e. Direct nucleotide sequencing

8. What represents the association of the alleles on the two C6 chromosomes as determined by family studies?
   a. Haplotype
   b. Genotype
   c. Phenotype
   d. Allotype
   e. Xenotype

REFERENCES

1. Dausset, H: Leukoagglutinins: Leukoagglutinins and blood transfusion. J Vox Sang 4:190, 1954.
2. Dausset, J: Iso-leuco-anticorps. Acta Haematol 20:156, 1958.
3. Payne, R: The association of febrile transfusion reactions with leukoagglutinins. J Vox Sang 2:233, 1957.
4. Terasaki, PI, and McClelland, JP: Microdroplet assay of human serum cytotoxins. Nature 204:998, 1964.
5. Terasaki, PI, et al: Microdroplet testing for HLA-A, -B, -C, and -D antigens. Am J Clin Pathol 69:103, 1978.
6. van Rood, JJ, and van Leeuwen, A: Leukocyte grouping: A method and its application. J Clin Invest 42:1382, 1963.
7. World Health Organization: Nomenclature for factors of the HL-A system. Bull WHO 39:483, 1968.
8. Dausset, J, et al: Le deuxieme sublocus du systeme HL-A. Nouv Rev Fr Hematol 8:861, 1968.
9. Singal, DP, et al: Serotyping for homo-transplantation: Preliminary studies of HL-A subunits and alleles. Transplantation 6:904, 1968.
10. Sandberg, L, et al: Evidence for a third sub-locus within the HLA chromosomal

region. In Terasaki, PI (ed): Histocompatibility Testing 1970. Munksgaard, Copenhagen, 1970, p 165.

11. Bach, FH, and Hirschhorn, K: Lymphocyte interaction: A potential histocompatibility test in vitro. Science 143:813, 1964.
12. Bain, B, and Lowenstein, L: Genetic studies on the mixed leukocyte reaction. Science 145:1315, 1964.
13. Bach, FH, and Amos, DB: Hu-1: Major histocompatibility locus in man. Science 156:1506, 1967.
14. Bodmer, WF, et al (eds): Histocompatibility Testing 1977. Munksgaard, Copenhagen, 1977.
15. Bodmer, JG, et al: Nomenclature for factors of the HLA system. Hum Immunol 53:1, 1997.
16. Kissmeyer-Nielson, F, et al: Hyperacute rejection of kidney allografts associated with preexisting humoral antibodies against donor cells. Lancet 1:662, 1966.
17. Orr, HT, et al: Complete amino acid sequence of a papain-solubilized human histocompatibility antigen, HLA-B7: Sequence determination and search for homologies. Biochem 18:5711, 1979.
18. Kaufman, JF, and Strominger, JL: Both chains of HLA-DR bind to the membrane with a penultimate hydrophobic region and the heavy chain is phosphorylated at its hydrophilic carboxy terminus. Proc Natl Acad Sci USA 76:6304, 1979.
19. Kaufman, JF, and Strominger, JL: The extracellular region of light chains from human and murine MHC class II antigens consists of two domains. J Immunol 130:808, 1983.
20. Figueroa, F, and Klein, J: The evolution of class II genes. Immunol Today 7:78, 1986.
21. Bjorkman, PJ, et al: Structure of the HLA class I histocompatibility antigen, HLA-A2. Nature 329:506, 1987.
22. Bjorkman, PJ, et al: The foreign antigen binding site and T cell recognition regions of class I histocompatibility antigens. Nature 329:512, 1987.
23. Rodey, GE, and Fuller, TC: Public epitopes and the antigenic structure of HLA molecules. Crit Rev Immunol 7:229, 1987.
24. Kohler, G, and Milstein, C: Derivation of specific antibody producing tissue culture and tumor lines by cell fusion. Eur J Immunol 6:611, 1976.
25. Lee, CC: Population Genetics. University of Chicago Press, Chicago, 1955.
26. Dausset, J, et al: Un nouvel antigene du systeme HL-A (Hu-1), 1' antigene 15 allelle possible des antigenes 1, 11, 12. Nouv Rev Fr Hematol 8:398, 1968.
27. Kissmeyer-Nielsen, F, Svejgaard, A, and Hange, M: Genetics of the HL-A transplantation system. Nature 291:1116, 1968.
28. Svejgaard, A, and Kissmeyer-Nielsen, F: Crossreactive human HL-A isoantibodies. Nature 219:868, 1968.
29. Legrand, L, and Dausset, J: Histocompatibility Testing 1972. Munksgaard, Copenhagen, 1972, p 441.
30. Rodey, G, et al: ASHI HLA class I public epitope workshop: Phase I report. Transpl Proc 19:872, 1987.
31. Colombani, J, Colombani, M, and Dausset, J: Cross-reactions in the HL-A system with special reference to Da 6 cross-reacting group. In Terasaki, PI (ed): Histocompatibility Testing 1970. Munksgaard, Copenhagen, 1970, p 79.
32. Legrand, L, and Dausset, J: The complexity of the HLA gene product: Possible evidence for a "public" determinant common to the first and second HLA series. Transplantation 19:177, 1975.
33. Scalamogne, M, et al: Crossreactivity between the first and second segregant series of the HLA system. Tissue Antigens 7:125, 1976.
34. Kostyu, DD, Cresswell, P, and Amos, DB: A public HLA antigen associated with HLA-A9, Aw32, and Bw4. Immunogenetics 10:433, 1980.
35. Muller, C, et al: Monoclonal antibody (Tu 48) defining alloantigenic class I determinants specific for HLA-Bw4 and HLA-Aw23, -Aw24 as well as -Aw32. Hum Immunol 5:269, 1982.
36. Belvedere, M, Mattiuz, PL, and Curtoni, ES: An antibody cross-reacting with LA and four antigens of the HLA system. Immunogenetics 1:538, 1975.
37. McMichael, AJ, et al: A monoclonal antibody that recognizes an antigenic determinant shared by HLA-A2 and B17. Hum Immunol 1:121, 1980.
38. Ahern, AT, et al: HLA-A2 and HLA-B17 antigens share an alloantigenic determinant. Hum Immunol 5:139, 1982.
39. Claas, F, et al: Alloantibodies to an antigenic determinant shared by HLA-A2 and B17. Tissue Antigens 19:388, 1982.
40. Troup, CM, and Walford, RL: Cytotoxicity test for the typing of human lymphocytes. Am J Clin Pathol 51:529, 1969.
41. Eisen, SA, Wedner, HJ, and Parker, CW: Isolation of pure human peripheral blood T-lymphocytes using nylon wool columns. Immunol Commun 1:571, 1972.
42. Lowry, R, et al: Improved B cell typing for HLA-DR using nylon wool column enriched B lymphocyte preparations. Tissue Antigens 14:325, 1979.
43. van Rood, JJ, van Leeuwen, A, and Ploem, JS: Simultaneous detection of two cell populations by two-color fluorescence and application to the recognition of B cell determinants. Nature 262:795, 1976.
44. Vartdal, F, et al: HLA class I and II typing using cells positively selected from blood by immunomagnetic isolation: A fast and reliable technique. Tissue Antigens 28:301, 1986.
45. Fuller, TC: Antigenic specificity of antibody reactive in the antiglobulin-augmented lymphocytotoxicity test. Transplantation 34:24, 1982.
46. Fuller, TC, and Rodey, GE: Specificity of alloantibodies against antigens of the HLA complex. In Theoretical Aspects of HLA: A Technical Workshop. American Association of Blood Banks, Arlington, VA, 1982, p 51.
47. Lucas, ZG, et al: Early renal transplant failure associated with subliminal sensitization. Transplantation 10:522, 1970.
48. Patel, R, and Briggs, WA: Limitation of the lymphocyte cytotoxicity crossmatch test in recipients of kidney transplants having preformed anti-leukocyte antibodies. N Engl J Med 284:1016, 1971.
49. Bray, RA: Flow cytometry in the transplant laboratory. Ann NY Acad Sci 677:138, 1993.
50. Tiercy, JM, Jannet, M, and Mach, B: A new approach for the analysis of HLA class II polymorphism: HLA oligo typing. Blood Rev 4:9, 1990.
51. Zemmour, J, and Parham, P: HLA class I nucleotide sequences. Hum Immunol 31:195, 1991.
52. Marsh, SGE, and Bodmer, J: HLA class II nucleotide sequences. Hum Immunol 31:207, 1991.
53. Polesky, HF: New concepts in paternity testing. Diagn Med 1981.
54. Tiwari, JL, and Terasaki, PI: HLA and Disease. New York, Springer-Verlag, 1985.
55. Mourant, AE, Kopec, AC, and Domaniewska-Solczak, K: Blood Groups and Diseases. New York, Oxford University Press, 1978.
56. Colombani, J: Blood platelets in HL-A serology. Transpl Proc 3:1078, 1971.
57. Svejgaard, A, Kissemeyer-Nielson, F, and Thorsby, E: HL-A typing of platelets. In Terasaki, PI (ed): Histocompatibility Testing 1970. Munksgaard, Copenhagen, 1970, p 160.
58. Leibert, M, and Aster, RH: Expression of HLA-B12 on platelets, on lymphocytes, and in serum: A quantitative study. Tissue Antigens 9:199, 1977.
59. Aster, RH, Szatkowski, N, and Liebert, M: Expression of HLA-B12, HLA-B8, W4, and W6 on platelets. Transpl Proc 9:1965, 1977.
60. Duquesnoy, RJ, Testin, J, and Aster, RH: Variable expression of W4 and W6 on platelets: Possible relevance to platelet transfusion therapy of alloimmunized thrombocytopenic patients. Transpl Proc 9:1827, 1977.
61. Duquesnoy, RJ, Filip, DJ, and Rody, GE: Successful transfusion of platelet "mismatched" for HLA antigens to alloimmunized thrombocytopenic patients. Am J Hematol 2:219, 1977.
62. Brand, A, van Leeuwen, A, and Eernisse, JG: Platelet immunology with special regard to platelet transfusion therapy. Excerpta Medica International Congress 415:639, 1978.
63. Herzig, RH, Herzig, GP, and Biell, MI: Correction of poor platelet transfusion responses with leukocyte-poor HLA-matched platelet concentrates. Blood 46:743, 1975.
64. Bortin, MM, and Rimm, AA: Increasing utilization of bone marrow transplantation. Transplantation 42:229, 1986.
65. Petersdorf, E, et al: Major-histocompatibility-complex class I alleles and antigens in hematopoietic cell transplantation. N Engl J Med 345:1794, 2001.
66. Flomenburg, N, et al: Impact of class I and class II high resolution matching on outcomes of unrelated donor bone marrow transplantation. Blood 104 (7):1923, 2004.
67. Morishima, RA, et al: For the Japanese Marrow Donor Program. Blood 99:4200, 2002.
68. Siegler, HF, et al: Comparisons of mixed leukocyte skin graft survival in families genotyped for HLA-A. Transpl Proc 3:115, 1971.
69. Hamburger, J, et al: The value of present methods used for the selection of organ donors. Transpl Proc 3:260, 1971.
70. Alexander, JW: Impact of transplantation on microbiology and infectious diseases. Transpl Proc 12:593, 1980.
71. Cecka, JM: The UNOS scientifc renal transplant registry 2000. Clin Transpl 1, 2001.
72. Sanfilippo, F, Vaughn, WK, and Spees, EKL: The effect of HLA-A, -B matching on cadaver renal allograft rejection comparing public and private specificities. Transplantation 38:483, 1984.
73. Oldfather, JW, et al: Prediction of crossmatch outcome in highly sensitized dialysis patients based on the identification of serum HLA antibodies. Transplantation 42:267, 1986.
74. Opelz, G, et al: Effect of blood transfusions on subsequent kidney transplants. Transpl Proc 5:253, 1973.
75. Salvatierra, O, Jr, et al: Deliberate donor-specific transfusions prior to living related renal transplantation: A new approach. Ann Surg 192:543, 1980.
76. Montgomery, RA, et al: Plasmapheresis and intravenous immune globulin provides effective rescue therapy for refractory humoral rejection and allows kidneys to be successfully transplanted into cross-match positive patients. Transplantation 70:887, 2000.
77. Ross, CN, et al: Renal transplantation following immunoadsorption in highly sensitized recipients. Transplantation 55: 785, 1993.
78. Hodge, EE, et al: Pretransplant removal of anti-HLA antibodies by plasmapheresis and continued suppression on cyclosporine-based therapy after heart-kidney transplant. Transpl Proc 26: 2750, 1994.
79. Kickler T, et al: A randomized, placebo-controlled trial of intravenous gamma globulin in alloimmunized thrombocytopenic patients. Blood 75:313, 1990.
80. Tyan DB, et al: Intravenous immunoglobulin suppression of HLA alloantibody in highly sensitized transplant candidates and transplantation with a histoincompatible organ. Transplantation 57:553, 1994.
81. Yacoub, M, et al: The influence of HLA matching in cardiac allograft recipients receiving CyA and Imuran (abstract). 11th International Congress of the Transplantation Society 1:S7, 1986.
82. Opelz, G: HLA matching in non-renal transplantation. CTS Newsletter 1, 1996.
83. Karuppan, S, Ericzon, BG, and Moller, E: Relevance of a positive crossmatch in liver transplantation. Transpl Int 4:18, 1991.

84. Gugenheim, J, Samuel, D, and Reynes, M: Liver transplantation across ABO blood group barriers. Lancet 336:519, 1990.

85. Mathew, J, et al: Biochemical and immunological evaluation of donor-specific soluble HLA in the circulation of liver transplant recipients. Transplantation 62:217, 1996.

86. Shaw, LR, Miller, JD, and Slutsky, AS: Ethics of lung transplantation with live donors. Lancet 338:461, 1991.

87. Gruessner, AC, and Sutherland, DER: Analysis of United States (US) and non-US pancreas transplants reported to UNOS and the International Pancreas Transplant Registry as of October, 2001. Clin Transpl 2001:41, 2002.

88. Shapiro, AMJ, et al: Islet transplantation in seven patients with type 1 diabetes mellitus using a glucocorticoid-free immunosuppressive regimen. N Engl J Med 2000.

Parentage Testing

Chantal Ricaud Harrison, MD

================ **OBJECTIVES** ================

On completion of this chapter, the learner should be able to:

1. State the goals of parentage testing.
2. List criteria used in choosing a genetic system for parentage testing.
3. Briefly describe the testing technologies used for the different types of genetic systems.
4. Briefly discuss the advantages and disadvantages of the different types of genetic systems.

5. Define and give examples of false direct and indirect exclusions.
6. List three causes of false direct and indirect exclusions.
7. Define paternity index (PI), probability of paternity (PP), and power of exclusion.
8. List organizations involved and resources available in quality improvement for parentage testing laboratories.

Introduction

Definition

Parentage testing refers to the testing of genetic markers that are inherited to determine the presence or absence of a biologic relationship. This is most commonly applied to answer the question whether a man is the biologic father of a child, but it can also be applied to the determination of maternity or siblingship.

History

The scientific basis for parentage testing can be traced back to the statistical analysis published by Bernstein[1] in 1924 demonstrating that the ABO blood group frequency distribu-

tion in Austria was most compatible with a three-allele theory. The ABO blood group testing results were first used in establishing nonpaternity in Vienna in 1926. As other blood groups were described and their inheritance established, they were used in paternity studies. Then, in 1955, Smithies[2] described the polymorphism of haptoglobin, opening the door to a new type of genetic system: enzymes and proteins. The next step occurred in 1972, when the extreme polymorphism of the human leukocyte antigen (HLA) system was demonstrated at the Evian workshop organized by Dausset.[3] All these genetic systems were expressed on different elements of the blood (red blood cells [RBCs], proteins, and leukocytes), but they had one important aspect in common: they were all dependent on a complex biochemical expression of the original genes. This group of genetic systems is often termed the "classic systems." The molecular genetics technology developed in the next decade laid the foundation for a revolution in parentage testing, heralded by the description by Jeffreys[4] in 1985 of a new type of polymorphism in human DNA: hypervariable minisatellites often referred to as variable number tandem repeats (VNTR). New genetic systems, tested by technologies that directly assess the variability of DNA, have become the norm. These are called DNA polymorphisms.

Over the past decade, there has been a rapid evolution of the DNA polymorphism testing technologies used in parentage testing and forensic analysis. Early on, VNTR systems were tested by treatment of the extracted DNA, with restriction enzymes followed by Southern blotting. This is called restriction fragment length polymorphism (RFLP) testing. After dominating the field for several years, RFLP testing ceded precedence to polymerase chain reaction (PCR) technology. Originally, PCR was often used to detect polymorphisms caused by point mutations or sequence specific polymorphisms (SSP) but soon was used to analyze a type of variable-number tandem repeats called short tandem repeats (STR).

Goals of Testing

The ultimate goal of parentage testing is to confirm a specific biologic relationship between the individual in question and another, usually a father or a mother or sometimes a sibling. When applied to the usual trio (mother, child, and alleged father), the goals are to exclude all falsely accused men and to provide sufficient inclusionary evidence if a man is not excluded.

Criteria for Selection of Genetic Systems

In selecting genetic systems to use in parentage testing, consider the following:

1. The system should be polymorphic; that is, it should have multiple alleles, ideally in Hardy-Weinberg equilibrium.
2. Inheritance pattern should be well established and follow Mendel's rules.
3. Mutation rate should be known to be low.
4. Possible genotypes should be easily deducible from the phenotype.
5. Testing methodology should be reliable, reproducible, and available in more than one laboratory.
6. Markers tested should be stable and not affected by environmental factors, age, disease, reagents, or methodology employed.
7. Databases of allele frequencies should be available for all ethnic groups that may be tested.
8. Allelic distributions should be able to provide a high probability of excluding a falsely accused man.
9. Each genetic system should be known to be genetically independent (e.g., no linkage disequilibrium) of all other genetic systems selected by the laboratory.

Types of Genetic Systems and Technology Used

Box 23–1 lists the most common classic genetic systems that have been widely used in the past. In the last few years, there

---

BOX 23–1
List of Classic Genetic Systems Used in Parentage Testing

RBC antigens

- ABO
- Rh
- MNSs
- Kell
- Duffy
- Kidd

RBC enzymes/Serum proteins

- PGM1
- ACP
- ESD
- Hp
- Gc

Immunoglobulin allotypes

- Gm
- Km
- Am

HLA

- A and B locus

---

has been an almost entire reliance on DNA polymorphism testing, specifically those based on STR systems using PCR technology. Table 23–1 lists the most common STR loci in current use.

RBC Antigens

Six blood groups have been routinely used in paternity testing: ABO, Rh, MNSs, Kell, Duffy, and Kidd. These systems have been in use for a very long time, and their potential pitfalls in interpretation are well known from the vast, worldwide experience accumulated. Phenotype determination is

---

TABLE 23–1 Chromosomal Location of Most Common STR Genetic Systems in Current Use

Locus	Chromosomal Location
D2S1338	2
D3S1358	3p21
D5S818	5q21–q31
D7S820	7q
D8S1179	8q24.1–24.2
D13S317	13q22–q31
D16S539	16q22–24
D18S51	18q21.3
D19S433	19
D21S11	21p11.1
CSF1PO	5q33.3–34
FGA	4q28
HUMTHO1	11p15–15.5
TPOX	2p23–2pter
VWA	12p12–pter

based on standard RBC agglutination techniques with regulated reagents and, with some extra built-in quality control steps, is indistinguishable from testing performed daily in most blood bank or transfusion services. This is why, until recently, the majority of laboratories performing parentage testing were associated with a blood bank or a transfusion service. Duplicate testing of each specimen is required. It is recommended that this be done independently by two individuals using two different sources of antisera. This will minimize the occurrence of inaccurate phenotypes as a result of reagent variability or technical error. Careful attention should be given when selecting positive control cells to ensure that the reagent antiserum can detect weak expressions of the antigen. An example is anti-C, which often contains mostly anti-Ce (rh$_i$) and may not react with the CcDE phenotype. This phenotype is not uncommon in Mexican-Americans, Native Americans, and Asian-Americans, and a false-negative reaction could lead to an erroneous interpretation of exclusion.

Only a few laboratories still include RBC antigen testing in their testing panel. However, on occasion it is still necessary to interpret previous results or perform testing on new individuals, the results of which need to be interpreted in light of previous testing performed with classic systems on persons who are now unavailable for additional testing (e.g., an additional child with a now-deceased but previously tested alleged father). Any blood center or transfusion service associated with a parentage testing laboratory could perform these tests without significant difficulty.

RBC Enzymes and Serum Proteins

RBC enzyme and serum protein genetic systems testing is infrequently performed with only two laboratories currently reporting proficiency testing results. Testing methodology consists of separating the different allelic proteins by electrophoresis, followed by staining. Subtyping of the *PGM1* and *Gc* alleles may be done using isoelectric focusing, which allows separation of molecules of similar size, thereby increasing the extent of polymorphism of the system. When isoelectric focusing is used, it is customary to refer to the system with a subscript letter *i* (e.g., $PGM1_i$ or Gc_i).

Phenotypes are identified by the number and respective position of the bands detected and comparison with control specimens expressing at least two known allotypes that are tested in parallel with the unknown specimens. Interpretation of the band patterns must be performed independently by two observers. Rare variants exist in most systems, and the laboratories should maintain a file of variants to permit identification of rare phenotypes.

Immunoglobulins

Three immunoglobulin chains demonstrate a polymorphism that has been applied to paternity testing. The gamma heavy chain expresses the Gm polymorphism; the kappa light chain expresses Km (also termed Inv); and the alpha heavy chain expresses Am. Determination of the phenotype is done by hemagglutination inhibition using indicator RBCs coated with antibodies of known phenotype and reagent anti-Gm, anti-Km, or anti-Am. Reagents are not widely available; genetic interpretation is complex; and phenotypic interpretation is often not possible in infants younger than 6 months of

age because of interference with maternal immunoglobulins. For these reasons, few laboratories in the world now use these genetic systems. They are mentioned solely for the sake of completion and historic perspective.

HLA

The HLA complex represents the most polymorphic genetic system in the human genome. As discussed in the previous chapter, it comprises multiple linked loci expressed as class I and class II antigens. In parentage testing with classic methodology (non-DNA), only antigens expressed by the A and the B loci are considered.

The usual method is termed "microlymphocytotoxicity." It depends on the evaluation of the reactions of live lymphocytes with a panel of cytotoxic antibodies of known specificity in the presence of complement. Testing is performed in 60 or 72 microwell trays preloaded with reagent antisera. A sufficient number of antisera should be used so that all HLA-A and HLA-B specificities recognized by the 1980 HLA Nomenclature Committee of the World Health Organization can be reliably identified. Additional antigens should be tested, if appropriate antisera can be obtained. The larger the number of antigens that can be defined, the more powerful the system becomes; that is, the better it is able to exclude falsely accused men. Because of the large number of existing antigens, no single tray can identify all relevant antigens. Some antigens occur more frequently in specific racial groups, and specially designed trays are available for African Americans and Asians. Such trays should be selected when appropriate.

Antisera are either of human origin or monoclonal, and monospecific sera are not available for a large number of antigens. It is required that each antigen be defined by at least two different operationally monospecific sera, by one monospecific and two multispecific sera, or by three multispecific sera. Phenotypes must be verified by reading two independent trays or tray sets. Each tray or tray set must be read independently.

In interpreting phenotypes, a certain amount of expertise is needed, requiring knowledge of cross reactivity between antigens and splits of broader reactivity (e.g., A9 splitting into A23 and A24) and familiarity with the unexpected reactivity of the antisera used (false-negative or extra reactions). Because of the variability of HLA antisera, it is recommended that all individuals in a parentage case be tested in the same laboratory.

DNA Polymorphisms: RFLP

RFLP refers to polymorphisms of the DNA that can be detected by restriction enzymes. These enzymes are endonucleases that recognize specific DNA sequences of 4 to 6 bases and cut the double-stranded DNA at that site. These enzymes have been isolated from bacteria and are named after the bacteria from which they were isolated (e.g., Eco RI from *Escherichia coli* RY13; Hae III from *Haemophilus aegyptius*). After the isolated DNA is incubated with the restriction enzyme (digestion step), it is electrophoresed on a gel to separate the DNA fragments according to length. The DNA is then denatured to dissociate the complementary strands, transferred by blotting (Southern blotting) to a membrane, and hybridized with a labeled probe to reveal the DNA fragments corresponding to the locus tested. Probes used to be labeled with radioactive P^{32}, but current detection is often achieved by a colorimetric or chemiluminescent method. Phenotypes are assigned as the length of the DNA fragments in kilobases (kb), measured by comparison with a sizing ladder consisting of DNA fragments of known size. Some variability in migration may occur within a gel, depending on the position of the electrophoretic lane (band shifting), and it is recommended that mixtures of DNA of each alleged father with each child be electrophoresed together in a single lane to observe for such band shifting and to confirm a match or mismatch in fragment size. **Figure 23–1** illustrates this process.

The DNA polymorphisms detected by RFLP may be of three types. The first type results from mutations, insertions, or deletions between restriction sites. The second type results from single-base mutations causing a new cutting site for the restriction enzyme or deleting a cutting site. The third type relates to the presence throughout the genome of noncoding DNA segments consisting of a variable number of repeats of a core-base sequence. These areas are called VNTRs. They are also called minisatellites, when the size of the core sequence typically ranges from 9 to 80 base pairs. It is this latter type of polymorphism that is widely applied to parentage testing.

As illustrated in **Figure 23–2**, the fragment size of VNTR loci depends on the number of repeats and on the restriction enzyme utilized. This is an important concept: the phenotype of the same individual at the same locus will differ between two laboratories if each uses a different restriction enzyme. This is why, when reporting RFLP results, it is mandatory to identify not only the locus and probe tested but also the restriction enzyme used. In the United States, the most common restriction enzymes used are Hae III and Pst I, whereas in Europe Hinf I is more popular. **Table 23–2** illustrates the different band sizes obtained on the same indi-

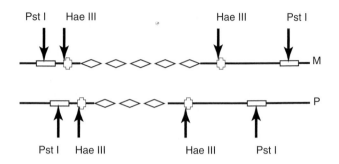

■ **FIGURE 23–2** RFLP fragment lengths depend on the number of tandem repeats and on the restriction enzyme used. The maternal allele has five repeat units, whereas the paternal allele has three. The fragments cut by Pst I are larger than the fragments cut by Hae III.

viduals at the same locus when using different restriction enzymes.

Another important concept with VNTR polymorphisms tested by RFLP has to do with the fact that the allele designation is a quantitative entity: a length of DNA in kilobase. As in any quantitative measurement there is a variability, which is referred to as sigma (σ). Another variable is the ability to distinguish between two close alleles (alleles differing by only a few repeats). This ability may vary greatly among laboratories, depending on the methodology used, especially the technical conditions during electrophoresis. This variability is referred to as delta (δ). Because of these two sources of variability, the allele frequency distribution for VNTR polymorphisms tested by RFLP is a continuous distribution, as opposed to the discrete distribution of allele frequencies in the classic genetic systems. For example, in most laboratories a DNA fragment measured at 1.60 kb cannot be considered different from a fragment measured at 1.57 kb or 1.63 kb. Each laboratory must decide, for each allele size, the range of allele sizes that are considered within matching criteria of the one measured. This range is called a "bin." The allele frequency used in the statistical calculations is actually the frequency of all the alleles falling into the bin for the allele size measured. Inasmuch as the size of the bin varies with the technical characteristics of the laboratories, the final statistical evaluation result (PI, PP, or probability of exclusion) may differ between two laboratories for the same locus with the same restriction enzyme, even if their band sizes are identical.

These VNTR loci are very polymorphic and thus are very powerful in excluding falsely accused men and in providing inclusionary evidence in true biologic relationships. However, their mutation rate can be up to 2 per 1000, which is small but not negligible.[5]

The number of laboratories performing testing of VNTR genetic systems by RFLP has decreased significantly in the last few years.

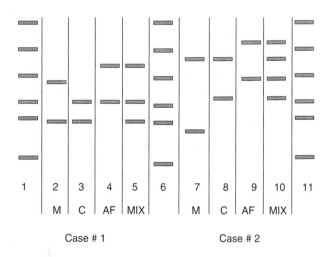

■ **FIGURE 23–1** Schematic representation of RFLP results from two paternity testing trios. Lanes 1, 6, and 11 represent sizing standards of known length used to measure the band size of each individual. Both cases consist of a mother (M), a child (C), an alleged father (AF), and a mixed lane with the child's and alleged father's DNA. In the first case, on the left, the paternal band of the child matches one of the bands of the alleged father, and the mixed lane contains only three bands; the alleged father is included. In the second case, none of the alleged father bands match the child's paternal band, and the mixed lane clearly demonstrates four bands; this is a mismatch.

TABLE 23–2   DNA-RFLP Results on a Parentage Testing Trio at the D2S44 Locus

	Hae III	Hinf I	Pst I
Mother	3.43, 4.25	4.55, 5.36	12.68, 13.53
Child	2.91, 3.43	4.03, 4.55	12.16, 12.68
Alleged father	2.91, 3.13	4.03, 4.25	12.16, 12.46

DNA Polymorphisms: PCR

This technology has seen a striking increase in popularity for parentage testing since 1994. The DNA fragment of interest is amplified several million times by the PCR technique, and the resulting alleles are identified by hybridization with a set of labeled probes, by the location on a gel after electrophoresis, or by the time of detection after capillary electrophoresis. The exact section of DNA that is amplified is defined by a pair of primers. The variation detected in the amplified products is caused by either DNA sequence polymorphisms or by fragment-length polymorphisms. The sequence-specific DNA polymorphism can be defined by a variety of techniques: hybridization of the PCR product with sequence-specific oligonucleotide probes (SSOP), presence of a product after amplification by SSP, or actual DNA sequencing, also referred to as sequence-based typing. These last two techniques are commonly used in testing for HLA polymorphisms with regard to matching for bone marrow or organ transplantation, but are not widely applied to parentage testing.

SSOP

Sequence-specific polymorphisms are the result of specific nucleotide differences at the locus tested. The phenotype is determined by dot blot using SSOPs. SSOP-based genetic systems that have been popular are the *DQA1* locus, which codes for the alpha chain of the HLA class II antigen DQ, and a group of five loci tested together: *LDLR, GYPA, HBGG, D7S8,* and *GC*. It is important to realize that *GYPA* is the locus coding for glycophorin A, which is the RBC transmembrane protein carrying the MN antigens, and that *GC* is the locus coding for the serum protein Gc. A laboratory should not test for these two loci by PCR technology and by classic techniques without realizing that the same genetic system is being investigated. In other words, in the final interpretation they should not be considered as different systems. Similarly, there is very strong linkage between *DQA1* and the *HLA-A* and *HLA-B* loci; thus, they cannot be considered genetically independent when calculating overall PP.

Amplified Fragment Length Polymorphisms (AmpFLPs)

The fragment length polymorphisms detected by PCR are similar to those detected by RFLP in that they consist of a variable number of repeats of noncoding DNA sequences. However, the core sequence is usually shorter. When the core sequence ranges from 2 to 5 base pairs (bp) and the overall length of the fragment sizes remains less than 350 bp, they are called microsatellites, or STRs. If the core sequence is greater than 5, they are called long tandem repeats (LTRs). Only one LTR locus has been widely used, D1S80. The almost exponential growth in the use of DNA polymorphisms by PCR for parentage testing is entirely caused by the interest in the STR systems, and new genetic systems are being described and put into use every year.

Although STR genetic systems are significantly less powerful than RFLP-based VNTR systems in excluding wrongly accused men or providing inclusionary evidence, they have distinct advantages that have put them forward as the foremost systems in current use. The main advantages of PCR-based STR testing, both for parentage and forensic testing, are as follows. First, discrete alleles can be identified, and current separation techniques can resolve fragments of DNA differing by only one base. Second, the quantities of DNA needed are minute and can easily be extracted from a few epithelial cells obtained from buccal swabs. Thus, the sample collection does not require a venipuncture. This is a great advantage, especially when testing small infants. In addition, there is almost no danger of parenteral exposure of infectious agents to the collector. Third, the technology allows simultaneous testing of several loci by multiplex amplification and very fast allele identification by capillary electrophoresis. This is conducive to automation and brief turnaround time.

The panels of STR loci currently in use consist mostly of repeats with core sequences of four bases (tetranucleotide repeats), although a few loci based on core sequences of five bases (pentanucleotides) have recently been introduced. A group of 12 loci dominates the field in conjunction with a 13th locus, amelogenin, that determines only sex and not inheritance. This group has been selected by the FBI as the core testing panel for a nationwide databank of crime-scene DNA evidence material. **Box 23–2** lists the STR loci included in the FBI Combined DNA Index System (CODIS) database. Readily available commercial kits provide convenient multiplex amplification for loci selected to match the CODIS STR core loci. A group of STR loci located on the Y chromosome has become available and has shown success in delineating male lineage. It can be used in paternity testing if the child is male.

Phenotypes should be reported following the recommendations of the International Society for Forensic Genetics, which means that alleles are identified by the repeat number. Variants that have additional bases to an exact repeat number are identified by the repeat number followed by a period and the number of additional bases (e.g., a common allele of TH01 is 9.3, which means that it has 9 tetranucleotide repeats and 3 additional bases).

Mitochondrial DNA

Noncoding hypervariable segments (the displacement loop) of mitochondrial DNA (mtDNA) are amplified by PCR and then sequenced. The sequence is then compared with a published reference sequence. Any deviation from the published sequence should be inherited from mother to child.

BOX 23–2
STR Systems Included in CODIS

- D3S1358
- D5S818
- D7S820
- D8S1179
- D13S317
- D16S539
- D18S51
- D21S11
- CSF1PO
- FGA
- THO1
- TPOX
- VWA
- Amelogenin

Inasmuch as mitochondria are passed on with the cytoplasm of the oocyte and not by spermatozoa, mitochondrial DNA can verify only maternal lineage. Mitochondrial DNA appears to be stable for extremely long periods (thousands of years). These genetic systems have been applied to anthropologic studies aimed at solving human evolution questions. Preserved mitochondrial DNA has been isolated from mummies and fossils.[6] This technique is very useful in demonstrating maternal lineage in long-distance relatives such as grandmother to grandchild or great-granduncle to great-grandnephew, and it was recently applied to the authentification of the remains of the family of Tsar Nicholas II of Russia, who were assassinated during the Bolshevik uprising.[7]

Interpretation of Results

In interpreting the testing results on a classic trio (mother, child, and alleged father), it is always assumed that the mother is the biologic mother. The results are first analyzed to determine whether the alleged father is excluded as the biologic father of the child. If he is not excluded, a statistical analysis is performed to determine his relative probability of being the biologic father of the child as compared with a random man unrelated to him or to the mother.

Terminology

In the past, when using the classic genetic systems, it was customary to interpret the results in one genetic system as an exclusion, direct or indirect, when the expected inheritance pattern was not observed. It was customary to accept a single direct exclusion as evidence of nonpaternity, whereas an indirect exclusion only suggested the possibility of nonpaternity and required confirmation by additional testing. However, as soon as some experience was accumulated with the newly introduced DNA polymorphisms, it became evident that mutations, which were extremely rare in the classic systems (less than one in a million), were being recognized in these new systems at a higher frequency. There appears to be a significant number of crossover mutations at the level of the tandem repeats. It is also likely that a number of single nucleotide mutations that can be detected at the DNA level may not result in a recognizable change in the final expression product when tested by classic technologies. When an inconsistency in the inheritance pattern is detected in a genetic system result concerning a DNA polymorphism, the term "exclusion" is not used; instead, the term "mismatch" is used to refer to the fact that the bands between the child and the alleged father do not match. The term exclusion is reserved for the final interpretation of the entire set of genetic systems tested. A minimum of two mismatches is required before an opinion of nonpaternity (or nonmaternity) is rendered.

In the following section, the terms "direct" and "indirect" exclusion are used for the interpretation of results in the classic genetic systems.

Direct Exclusion

A direct exclusion occurs when a marker is detected in the child but is absent in the mother and the alleged father. For example, the child has blood group B, the mother has group A, and the alleged father has group O. The B antigen on the child's RBCs is the result of the expression of the B gene, which is not present in the mother and thus must have been passed to the child by the child's biologic father. The tested man does not have it. Therefore, a direct exclusion is present.

Another situation that is interpreted as a direct exclusion occurs when the alleged father's phenotype demonstrates two markers and the child has neither one. For example, the alleged father's blood group is AB and the child's is O. The alleged father's phenotype implies that he has both the A gene and the B gene and thus must pass on either one of them to any of his children. The child has neither one.

Direct exclusions are considered very strong evidence of nonpaternity because they rely on direct observation of a marker with a known pattern of inheritance, which was not inherited as expected. As discussed later, false direct exclusions in classic genetic systems can occur but are extremely rare. Thus, a single direct exclusion in these systems is considered sufficient to render an opinion of nonpaternity as long as appropriate controls have been put in place to rule out rare situations.

Indirect Exclusion

An indirect exclusion occurs when a single marker is detected in the child and a different single marker is detected in the alleged father. For example, the child is Jk(a+b−), and the alleged father is Jk(a−b+). The indirect exclusion is based on the assumption that if a person expresses only one marker, he must be homozygous for the allele coding for the marker. In the example, the child types as Jk(a+b−) and is thus assumed to be homozygous for the Jk^a gene, but the alleged father is assumed to be homozygous for the Jk^b gene. This is interpreted as an indirect exclusion, because the man should pass on a Jk^b gene to any offspring, and the child does not have it. This situation is termed "apparent opposite homozygosity." The term "apparent" is very important. The homozygosity is assumed and not directly proved. A different allele not detected by the testing performed could be present, and the individual could actually be heterozygous. In fact, a silent allele does exist in the Kidd system, called Jk, which has no detectable product. Thus, the child could possibly be heterozygous for the Jk and the Jk^a alleles, and the alleged father could be heterozygous for the Jk and the Jk^b alleles. In this case, there would be no inconsistency in the inheritance pattern and no exclusion. However, this Jk gene is very rare and is seen almost only in populations originating in the Western Pacific Islands. Thus, if the individuals tested were North American whites or blacks, these results would be interpreted as an indirect exclusion.

Causes of False Exclusions

False direct exclusions can occur as the result of mutations that are significant enough to alter the final product, lack of precursor substance, suppressor activity at a locus unlinked to the one tested, or chimeric state of one of the tested individuals.

A classic example of the lack of a precursor substance is the Bombay phenotype, in which an individual is homozygous for the h gene and cannot produce H substance, the precursor substance for the A and B antigens. This person may have the A or B genes (or even both) and pass it on to an offspring, but he or she cannot express them and will have a phenotype of O. The offspring, more than likely, will inherit an *H* gene from the other parent inasmuch as the *h* gene is very rare, and thus he or she will be able to express the *A* or *B* gene inherited from the first parent. Thus, a Bombay phenotype in either parent can explain a trio: mother O, child A, alleged father O. However, Bombay phenotypes are extremely rare and can easily be detected by testing the O individuals with anti-H or by performing a reverse typing with O cells, inasmuch as all Bombay phenotypes have strong anti-H activity in their serum.

An example of an erroneous direct exclusion caused by a suppressor gene is illustrated in the following trio: alleged father Rh-negative, mother Rh-negative, child Rh-positive. In the Rh system, a null phenotype, although extremely rare, does exist. Rh_{null} individuals produce no Rh substances; that is, no D, C, c, E, or e antigens. Most Rh_{null} phenotypes are caused by a suppressor gene at an unknown but unlinked locus. Thus, a person typing D-negative may actually have a *D* gene at the Rh locus and pass it to an offspring without passing on the suppressor gene. However, this is a problem only if the trio is tested with anti-D, only because a complete Rh phenotype would immediately reveal that one of the Rh-negative individuals is actually Rh_{null}.

False indirect exclusions can occur secondary to the presence of silent alleles, alternative alleles that are not tested for, or weak variants not detected with the reagents or technique used. Silent or alternate alleles exist in almost all classic genetic systems, as is evident by the list in **Table 23–3**. This is why a single indirect exclusion is not sufficient evidence for an interpretation of nonpaternity. In some ethnic groups, a silent allele may be very common and should be taken into account in the statistical evaluation of inclusion, without even considering the situation as an indirect exclusion. This is the case for the Duffy system in African Americans. A third allele *Fy* exists that does not produce Fy^a or Fy^b substance. Over 60 percent of African Americans are Fy(a−b−), thus homozygous for the *Fy* gene. The frequency of this *Fy* gene in African Americans is 0.82. Thus, an Fy(a+b−) in an African American is more likely to be the result of an Fy^aFy phenotype than $Fy^a Fy^a$. A child with an Fy(a+b−) phenotype and an alleged father with an Fy(a−b+) phenotype should not lead to an interpretation of indirect exclusion but to a calculation of a PI, taking into account the relative probability of the Fy^b Fy^b versus $Fy Fy^b$ genotypes in the alleged father. This *Fy* gene also exists, but not at such a high frequency, in Hispanics, Arabs, and other populations of the Middle East. It is very rare in other whites, and if the tested individual were white, this combination of phenotypes could be interpreted as an indirect exclusion. This example illustrates the importance of having expertise in the existence of alternate alleles and their relative frequency in various populations when interpreting parentage testing results in the classic genetic systems.

Inclusionary Calculations

Three types of statistical evaluations can be calculated when the alleged father is not excluded: the PI, the PP, and the probability of exclusion. All these calculations are based on the assumption that the "random man" with whom the tested man is compared is biologically unrelated to him or to the mother. The standard calculations are not valid if a brother, father, uncle, or other close biologic relative of the tested man is a possible biologic father of the child. Another important aspect of the calculations is the need to have accurate allele frequencies for each genetic system tested, estimated from databases drawn from a sufficiently large sample population of the appropriate ethnic group.

Paternity Index (PI)

The PI is a likelihood ratio. It is calculated one genetic system at a time and is sometimes referred to as the system index (SI). If all the genetic systems tested are genetically independent from each other, the overall final PI is the product of all the system indices calculated. When the PI is greater than 100, the evidence for paternity is considered very strong.

This likelihood ratio is the ratio of the chance (X) that the tested man can contribute the obligatory gene or genes to any offspring to the chance (Y) that a random unrelated man of the appropriate ethnic background can contribute the same gene or genes to an offspring. An example of testing results on a trio is given in **Table 23–4**. In the first genetic system listed, the mother and child share the 11 allele, thus the obligatory gene (paternal allele in the child) is 12. The alleged father is heterozygous for this allele; thus, his chance of passing it on to an offspring is 0.5. The frequency of this allele in the general population is 0.330; thus, the SI is X/Y = 0.5/0.330 = 1.52. In the second system listed, the alleged father is homozygous for the obligatory gene 17; thus, his chance of passing it on is 1, and the SI is 1/0.212 = 4.72. In the third system, the mother and child are identical; thus, there are two possible paternal alleles in the child. The mother's chance of passing the 6 allele is 0.5, and it is also 0.5 for the 9.3 allele. If the mother passes the 6 allele, the corresponding paternal allele is 9.3. The alleged father's chance of passing this allele is 0, and the random man's chance is 0.335. If the mother passes on the 9.3 allele, the corresponding paternal allele is 6. The alleged father's chance of passing this allele is 0.5, and the random man's chance is 0.239. Thus X = 0.5 × 0 + 0.5 × 0.5 = 0.25, and Y = 0.5 × 0.335 + 0.5 × 0.239 = 0.287, and SI = X/Y = 0.25/0.287 = 0.87. The overall PI is the product of the three systems indices, or 1.52 × 4.72 × 0.87 = 6.24. This means that the tested man is 6.24 times more likely to pass on the appropriate genes to a child in all three genetic systems simultaneously than a random unrelated man.

Probability of Paternity (PP)

The probability is calculated from the PI. It is based on a statistical theory developed by Bayes and requires an estimate of

TABLE 23–3 Alternative Alleles at Classic Genetic Systems Loci		
Genetic System	**Null or Weak Alleles**	**Other Alleles**
ABO		cis AB
Rh	Rh null (amorph), −D−, CDE, ©D (E)	e Bantu, C^w
MNSs	S^u, En, Mk	M^g
Kell	K_0, McLeod	
Duffy	Fy, Fy^x	
Kidd	Jk	
Hp	Hp°	

TABLE 23–4   Calculation Results on a Paternity Testing Trio

	Mother	Child	Alleged Father	X	Y	SI	RMNE
CSF1PO	10, 11	11, 12	10, 12	0.5	0.330	1.52	0.551
D3S1358	15, 17	17	17	1	0.212	4.72	0.379
TH01	6, 9.3	6, 9.3	6, 9	0.25	0.287	0.87	0.819
Allele frequencies:							
CSF1PO	12: 0.330						
D3S1358	17: 0.212						
TH01	6: 0.239 9.3: 0.335						

the prior PP; that is, the probability that the tested man is the father of the child based on nongenetic evidence (e.g., social evidence, such as access to the woman at the right time, whether the man is fertile, etc.). Inasmuch as a parentage testing laboratory cannot evaluate such type of evidence, it is customary to assign the value of 0.5 to the prior probability. In other words, this means that before testing, the tested man and another untested man are given equal probability of being the biologic father of the child. If the prior probability is 0.5, the PP after testing becomes PP = PI/(PI + 1). In the case illustrated, the PP would be 6.24/7.24 = 0.862 or 86.2 percent. This result in most states would be considered too low to shift the burden of proof to the man, and additional testing in other genetic systems would be needed.

Probability of Exclusion

The probability of exclusion is the probability of excluding a falsely accused man, given the phenotypes of the mother and the child. This probability is entirely dependent on the mother-and-child phenotype combination and does not require knowledge of the alleged father's phenotype. It is evaluated by first calculating the proportion of men who would not be excluded; this number is called random men not excluded (RMNE). The probability of exclusion is 1−RMNE. If p is the sum of all the possible paternal alleles, then RMNE = p (2−p) for each genetic system. The overall RMNE for all the genetic systems tested is the product of all the RMNE, and the overall probability of exclusion is 1−overall RMNE. In the case illustrated in **Table 23–4**, the overall RMNE is 0.551 × 0.379 × 0.819 = 0.171, and the probability of exclusion is 0.829. The probability of exclusion represents the proportion of untested men who would have been excluded by the extent of testing performed (82.9 percent in this case) and is more easily understood by a layperson, such as a jury member or a judge. The PP is a more accurate way to quantify the situation, inasmuch as it includes all the genetic information available, whereas the probability of exclusion does not take into account the phenotype of the alleged father.

Nonclassic Situations

The majority of parentage testing cases consist of the classic trio of mother, child, and alleged father. However, nonclassic cases are more and more frequently encountered. This may be

because the newer technologies are better able to give reliable answers in these situations. It is not unusual to attempt to establish the presence or absence of a biologic relationship between an alleged father and a child when the mother is unavailable for testing. Special calculation formulas have been developed to apply to such cases.[8] Occasionally, the alleged father is dead, and a reconstruction of his possible genetic makeup is attempted by testing all available parents, siblings, and other children of the alleged father. Other biologic relationships, such as siblingship, may be in question in adoption, immigration, or inheritance cases.

Advantages and Disadvantages of the Different Types of Genetic Systems

The classic systems have the advantage of the vast experience accumulated over the decades during which they have been in place in many countries. Phenotypes are well recognized and consistently reproducible from laboratory to laboratory. Potential pitfalls have been thoroughly studied, gene frequency distributions are available for almost every population in the world, and the mutation rate has been shown to be extremely low (less than one in a million). Statistical analyses in inclusion cases give extremely consistent results between laboratories. However, they do have some serious drawbacks when compared with the newer technologies testing DNA polymorphisms. In particular, each genetic system, except for the HLA A and B antigens, has a relatively low average power of exclusion. The highest power of exclusion is achieved by $PGM1_i$ at 0.32, followed by MNSs and Gc_i at 0.31 and Rh 0.27, respectively. Virtually all other systems have a power of exclusion below 0.20. In contrast, the HLA A and B antigens, analyzed as a haplotype, have a power of exclusion of 0.87. By testing all the classic systems, a high power of exclusion can be achieved, but it is almost impractical to go beyond 0.99. In addition, to get the full benefit of these systems, one must be competent with a multiplicity of techniques. Fairly rigid restrictions exist on the type, amount, and quality of samples needed. Because of the small number of alleles existing in each system, often no more than two or three, the alleles lack efficacy in nonclassic cases.

The DNA polymorphisms by RFLP are extremely powerful genetic systems with average powers of exclusion almost always above 0.50 and often reaching above 0.90 per genetic system. Thus, testing only four different loci by DNA-RFLP ensures very high levels of PP in nonexcluded men. The sample required is any tissue or body fluid from which sufficient DNA can be extracted. Peripheral blood, buccal smears, amniotic fluid, chorionic villi, and tissue biopsies can be analyzed. Once extracted, DNA can be kept frozen for an indefinite period. However, the technique is time-consuming and labor-intensive, and turnaround times are long. The main drawback, however, may be the lack of precise correlation in the final PI value between laboratories testing the same loci. This is because, as previously discussed, the phenotypes consist of measured band sizes, with the unavoidable difficulties caused by a built-in incertitude in measurement. This can be very confusing when results from a case tested in several different laboratories are compared, and the results may give a false impression of unreliability to someone who is unfamiliar with the limitations of the methodology.

The DNA polymorphisms by PCR avoid this difficulty because they return to a discrete allele distribution. Even when identifying alleles of a genetic system depending on fragment length polymorphisms, one can actually identify the number of repeats and not a length of DNA subject to an imprecision in measurement. This technique has the least restriction in the amount and type of sample needed but the highest requirement in environmental controls to prevent sample contamination, inasmuch as it is based on high amplification of a very small amount of DNA. A great advantage of DNA-PCR technology is the ability to amplify as many as 10 or even more loci in a single amplification reaction. Current instrument technology allows the resolution of 10 STR loci in real-time analysis within 2 to 5 hours. However, these systems are not as powerful as DNA-RFLP systems, and two to three times the number of genetic systems need to be operated to achieve the same level of probability as with DNA-RFLP systems. Both types of DNA polymorphisms have in common a significantly higher mutation rate than the classic systems have. As previously discussed, this has resulted in abandoning the concept of direct and indirect exclusion that has been so effective in classic systems. A mismatch observed in a DNA polymorphism system should lead to the calculation of a system index, which takes into account the rate of mutation for that system. A single mismatch should never lead to an interpretation of nonpaternity but rather to the testing of additional systems.

Social and Legal Issues

Currently, more than 300,000 cases of parentage testing are performed every year in the United States. The majority of these cases are done to establish paternity for children, with the aim of obtaining child support. Child support enforcement agencies in all states actively pursue the identification of the biologic father of children who are eligible for their Aid to Families with Dependent Children for the purpose of seeking child support from the biologic father. Contracts with child support agencies account for most of the activity of many parentage testing laboratories. The majority of cases outside the child support enforcement agencies contracts also have a legal implication, such as child support or custody in divorce cases, inheritance rights, or immigration. Occasionally, cases have criminal implications relating to incest or statutory rape.

Every step in the collection, storage, processing, and testing of the samples must be carefully documented as to time of occurrence and person performing the task. An unbroken chain of custody must be maintained. The individuals tested must be carefully verified, and procedures must be in place to ensure that unauthorized persons do not have access to the samples or test results. Without careful attention to these aspects, the results may not be valid in court. If called to testify on the validity and significance of the testing results, the laboratory director must be able to re-create from the documented evidence every step in the handling of the case.

Accreditation and Quality Issues

Approximately 30 years ago, the American Association of Blood Banks (AABB) took the lead in promoting the establishment of standardization and quality in the field of paternity testing and created a standing committee on parentage testing. This committee offered educational opportunities such as workshops and publications. With the participation of the American Medical Association, the American Bar Association, and the Office of Child Support Enforcement, the Committee on Parentage Testing organized an international conference in 1982 at Airlie, Virginia, where a group of international experts established a common base to interpret inclusionary evidence. An accreditation program for parentage testing laboratories was implemented, and the first edition of *Standards for Parentage Testing Laboratories* was published in 1990. A complementary *Accreditation Requirements Manual* followed in 1991. The College of American Pathologists, with joint sponsorship by the AABB, initiated a proficiency testing program for parentage testing laboratories in 1993. The American Society for Clinical Pathology regularly offers educational activities in the form of workshops, teleconferences, and other continuing education activities.

Continuing involvement by professional organizations in the promotion of quality improvement and in the provision of opportunities for continuing education in the field of paternity testing is essential to the maintenance of a high level of accuracy and consistency in ascertaining biologic relationships.

CASE STUDIES

Case 1

An African American trio consisting of a mother, child, and alleged father is tested to establish paternity. The following results are obtained:

Genetic System	Mother	Child	Alleged Father
ABO	O	B	A
Rh	Dce	Dce	DCe
MNSs	MSs	MNs	Ns
Duffy	Fy(a+b−)	Fy(a+b−)	Fy(a−b+)
Kidd	Jk(a+b+)	Jk(a−b+)	Jk(a+b−)
HLA	A2, 30 B12, 42	A30 B17, 42	A2,B7,35

1. Which of the genetic systems tested reveal a direct exclusion?
   a. Rh and MNSs
   b. ABO and HLA

c. Rh and Kidd
d. Rh, Duffy, and Kidd
e. ABO, Rh, Duffy, Kidd, and HLA

2. Which of the genetic systems tested reveal an indirect exclusion?
   a. Rh and MNSs
   b. ABO and HLA
   c. Rh and Kidd
   d. Rh, Duffy, and Kidd
   e. ABO, Rh, Duffy, Kidd, and HLA

3. What is the best interpretation for the results in the Duffy system?
   a. This is a direct exclusion.
   b. This is an indirect exclusion.
   c. In this African American trio, this is consistent with the transmission of a silent allele by the alleged father.
   d. In this African American trio, this is consistent with the transmission of a silent allele by the mother.
   e. Whatever the racial background of the trio, there is no suspicion of exclusion in this genetic system.

Case 2

A white trio consisting of a mother, child, and alleged father is tested to establish paternity. The following results are obtained:

Genetic System	Mother	Child	Alleged Father
ABO	A	0	B
MNSs	MNs	MNs	NSs
GYPA	AB	AB	B
D2S44/ Hae III	3.42, 4.24	2.90, 3.42	2.90, 3.11
D3S1358	15, 16	15, 17	14, 18
FGA	21, 22	22, 25	20, 25
TH01	6, 9.3	9, 9.3	7, 9

4. The fourth genetic system tested (D2S44/Hae III) represents a(n):
   a. RBC antigen system tested by agglutination
   b. RBC enzyme system
   c. DNA polymorphism tested by RFLP
   d. SSP-DNA polymorphism tested by PCR
   e. STR-DNA polymorphism tested by PCR

5. The fifth genetic system tested (D3S1358) represents a(n):
   a. RBC antigen system tested by agglutination
   b. RBC enzyme system
   c. DNA polymorphism tested by RFLP
   d. SSP-DNA polymorphism tested by PCR
   e. STR-DNA polymorphism tested by PCR

6. Among the following statements relating to the interpretation of these results, choose the one that is true:
   a. The alleged father is excluded due to a direct exclusion at D3S1358.
   b. The alleged father is excluded due to an indirect exclusion at D3S1358.
   c. A mutation may have occurred at D3S1358.
   d. The alleged father is excluded due to a direct exclusion in the ABO system.
   e. The final PI can be obtained by multiplying the paternity indices of each of the seven systems tested.

Answers to Case Studies

Case 1:

1. b
2. c
3. c

In African Americans, the silent *Fy* alleles constitute 82 percent of the gene pool; thus, an Fy(a−b+) individual is much more likely to be heterozygous Fy^bFy than homozygous $Fy^b Fy^b$ and has a high probability of passing on an *Fy* gene.

Case 2:

4. c
5. d
6. c

In DNA polymorphisms, the mutation rate can be as high as 2 per 1000; thus, a single mismatch, when all other systems are consistent with paternity, may represent a mutation. A minimum of two mismatches is necessary before an interpretation of exclusion is rendered.

The MN RBC antigens tested by agglutination are a product from the same locus as the *GYPA* locus tested by PCR-SSP; thus, the PI from each of these two systems cannot be multiplied together. The best option is to choose the system giving the greatest PI and to ignore the PI of the other system.

SUMMARY CHART:

Important Points to Remember (SBB)

➤ Parentage testing refers to the testing of genetic markers that are inherited to determine the presence or absence of a biologic relationship.

➤ The ultimate goal of parentage testing is to confirm a specific biologic relationship with the individual in question, usually a father or a mother or sometimes a sibling.

➤ The blood group systems used most often in paternity testing are ABO, Rh, MNSs, Kell, Duffy, and Kidd.

➤ The HLA complex represents the most polymorphic genetic system in the human genome; only antigens expressed by the *A* and *B* loci are considered for parentage testing with non–DNA-based typing.

➤ RFLP refers to polymorphisms of the DNA that can be detected by restriction enzymes; polymorphisms detected in parentage testing relate to the presence of VNTR.

➤ In PCR, the DNA fragment of interest is amplified several million times, and the resulting product is identified either by hybridization with a set of labeled probes or by its location on a gel after electrophoresis.

➤ STRs have repeats that are 2 to 5 bp long.

➤ STR present on the Y chromosome can verify only male lineage.

➤ Mitochondrial DNA can verify only maternal lineage.

➤ The term mismatch refers to the fact that the bands between the child and the alleged father do not match; a minimum of two mismatches is required before an opinion of nonpaternity (or nonmaternity) is rendered.

➤ A direct exclusion occurs when a marker is detected in the child, whereas it is absent in the mother and the alleged father, or when the alleged father's phenotype demonstrates two markers and the child has neither one of them.

➤ An indirect exclusion occurs when a single marker is detected in the child and a different single marker is detected in the alleged father.

➤ False direct exclusions can occur as the result of mutations that are significant enough to alter the final product, lack of precursor substance, suppressor activity at a locus unlinked to the one tested, or chimeric state of one of the tested individuals.

➤ False indirect exclusions occur secondary to the presence of silent alleles (e.g., *Fy*).

REVIEW QUESTIONS

1. Among the combinations of attributes described below, select the one that would *not* be suitable for a genetic system used in parentage testing analysis.
   a. The system has multiple alleles in Hardy-Weinberg equilibrium.
   b. The system has a high mutation rate.
   c. Databases of allele frequencies are available for all ethnic groups tested by the laboratory.
   d. All systems selected are genetically independent from each other.
   e. Testing methodology is available in several laboratories.

2. In which of the following genetic systems is the allele frequency distribution continuous (not discrete)?
   a. DNA polymorphisms by RFLP
   b. DNA polymorphisms by PCR
   c. RBC antigens
   d. RBC enzymes
   e. Serum proteins

3. A false direct exclusion in RBC antigen genetic systems can be caused by:
   a. A silent allele
   b. A lack of precursor substance
   c. An alternate untested allele
   d. A weakly expressed variant
   e. Weak reagents

4. Among the following organizations, which one offers an accreditation program for parentage testing laboratories?
   a. AABB
   b. ASCP
   c. CAP
   d. FDA
   e. HCFA

REFERENCES

1. Bernstein, F: Ergebnisse einer biostatischen zusammenfassenden Betrachtung über die erblichen Blutstrukturen des Menschen. Klin Wschr 3:1495, 1924.
2. Smithies, O: Zone electrophoresis in starch gels: Group variations in the serum proteins of normal human adults. Biochem J 61:629, 1955.
3. Histocompatibility Testing 1972. Proceedings of the 5th International Conference. Evian. Munksgaard, Copenhagen, 1973.
4. Jeffreys, AJ, Wilson B, and Thein, SL: Hypervariable "minisatellite" regions in human DNA. Nature 314:67, 1985.
5. Brinkman B, et al: Mutation rate in human microsatellites: Influence of the structure and length of the tandem repeat. Am J Hum Genet 62:1408, 1998.
6. Krings, M, et al: Neanderthal DNA sequences and the origin of modern humans. Cell 90:19, 1997.
7. Ivanov, P, et al: Mitochondrial DNA sequence heteroplasmy in the grand duke of Russia: Giorgig Romanov establishes the authenticity of remains of Tsar Nicholas II. Nat Genet 12:417, 1996.
8. Brenner, CH: A note on paternity computation in cases lacking a mother. Transfusion 33:51, 1993.

BIBLIOGRAPHY

Allen, RW, Wallhermfechtel, M, and Miller, WV: The application of restriction fragment length polymorphism mapping to parentage testing. Transfusion 30:552, 1990.
Committee on DNA Forensic Science: The Evaluation of Forensic DNA Evidence: An Update. National Academic Press, Washington, DC, 1996, pp 53–54.
Guidance for Standards for Parentage Testing Laboratories, ed 5. American Association of Blood Banks, Bethesda, MD, 2002.
Polesky, HF: Parentage testing: Use of DNA polymorphisms and other genetic systems. In Henry, JB (ed): Clinical Diagnosis and Management by Laboratory Methods, ed 20. WB Saunders, Philadelphia, 2001, pp 1390–1401.
Standards for Parentage Testing Laboratories, ed 5. American Association of Blood Banks, Bethesda, MD, 2001.
Walker, RH: Molecular biology in paternity testing. Lab Med 23:752, 1992.

twenty-four

Quality Management in the Blood Bank

Lucia M. Berte, MA, MT(ASCP)SBB, DLM, CQA(ASQ)CQMgr

OBJECTIVES

On completion of this chapter, the learner should be able to:

1. Describe the difference between compliance and quality management.
2. List three building blocks of quality.
3. Describe the framework of a quality system for the blood bank and the medical laboratory.
4. List 10 quality system (QS) essentials and the blood bank operations to which they are applied.
5. Use a flowchart to describe a process.
6. State the role of validation in introducing a new process.
7. Name at least five blood bank process controls.
8. Explain the causes of variation in a process.

9. Describe the difference between a form and a record.
10. Explain the importance of document control for procedures.
11. State the difference between remedial and corrective action.
12. Describe the role of auditing in a QS.
13. Identify at least six sources of input for helping processes improve.
14. Define the activities in a problem-solving process.
15. Explain how to transition the QS of a blood bank into a whole laboratory.

Introduction

Several dictionaries define *quality* as "the degree of excellence." Blood banks must provide quality to their customers in many forms, including:

- Safe, satisfying donation experiences for blood donors
- Accurately labeled and tested blood components provided to transfusion services
- Timely, accurate transfusion services provided to physicians and other health care personnel
- Safe and efficacious blood transfusions to patients

For blood centers, hospital blood banks, and transfusion serv-

ices to provide a high degree of assurance of safe blood donation and transfusion practices to regulatory agencies, accrediting agencies, blood donors, physicians, patients, and patients' families, the following quality philosophy must be embraced:

- Quality, safety, and effectiveness are built into a product.
- Quality cannot be inspected or tested into a product.
- Each step in the process must be controlled to meet quality standards.[1]

The method of bringing this quality philosophy into all operations is for each facility to develop the building blocks of quality: quality control (QC), quality assurance (QA), and quality system (QS). When the building blocks are assembled, and the facility's management staff is actively involved in the monitoring and maintenance of the QS, quality management (QM) has been achieved. **Figure 24–1** demonstrates the building blocks of quality and their internationally accepted definitions.[2]

Compliance Versus Quality Management (QM)

Blood bank compliance with federal regulations and accreditation standards is required by the following organizations:

- United States Food and Drug Administration (FDA)[3,4]
- Joint Commission on Accreditation of Healthcare Organizations (JCAHO)[5,6]
- College of American Pathologists (CAP)[7]
- American Association of Blood Banks (AABB)[8]

Compliance programs are designed to evaluate how effectively the facility meets the requirements by detecting errors, deficiencies, and deviations. Compliance inspections measure the state of the facility's program with respect to the applicable standards at a single point in time and are usually conducted every 1 to 2 years. Although this process may seem logical, compliance programs alone are inadequate to find and to prioritize a facility's problems. Compliance simply requires the correction of identified deviations and deficiencies and usually leaves the facility with the false sense that it has solved its problems and has been brought into compliance. It should be no surprise that subsequent inspections often reveal the same deviations and deficiencies. That is because the facility's current QC and QA programs do not identify the underlying structural problems. Remember that quality cannot be inspected into a process. Facilities must design work processes in a way that *prevents* deficiencies and errors from occurring in the first place.

QM, on the other hand, is actively and continuously practiced by the blood bank's leaders, managers, and staff throughout all blood bank operations. With QM, the blood bank is always ready for an inspection because it has validated its processes; monitors process performance; knows where the problems are; continuously takes action to determine root causes of problems and remove them; and documents its actions. In QM organizations, quality is everyone's job all the time. Quality is not something we do in addition to our jobs—it's built *into* our jobs!

Quality Building Blocks

Quality Control (QC)

Most blood bank technologists are familiar with routine blood bank QC procedures such as daily testing of the reactivity of blood typing reagents; calibration of serologic centrifuges; and temperature monitoring of refrigerators, freezers, and thawing devices. Requirements for the type and frequency of QC are determined in regulations and accreditation standards, manufacturers' operator manuals and package inserts, and state and local requirements. Regular performance of QC reveals when a method, piece of equipment, or procedure is not working as expected.

Quality Appearance (QA)

QA is a set of planned actions to provide confidence that systems and elements that influence the quality of the product or service are working as expected, individually and collectively.[2] QA looks beyond the performance of a test method or piece of equipment; it addresses how well an entire process—sequence of activities—is functioning. This is particularly important in those processes that cross functional or departmental lines. For example, a blood center could monitor the number of times and reasons why a set of collected whole blood units transported from the collection site to the component processing site did not arrive in time or was not in an acceptable condition to make blood components. In the transfusion service, it is important to monitor the source, number of times, and reason why specimens collected for compatibility testing do not meet predetermined acceptance criteria. **Table 24–1** lists common QC and QA activities practiced by most blood banks.[9]

Quality Systems (QSs) in Blood Banking

Beginning with a quality guideline published for blood banks by the FDA,[10] there was a change in meaning, emphasis, and organization of quality activities. Accrediting agencies such as the JCAHO and AABB modified their quality requirements to resemble the quality models used in international manufacturing and service industries. These companies developed and maintain QSs that are both more comprehensive and more coordinated than either QC or QA. A QS provides a framework for applying quality principles and practices uniformly across all blood bank operations, starting with donor selection and proceeding through transfusion outcomes.

In its *Standards for Blood Banks and Transfusion Services*,[8] the AABB defined 10 quality system essentials (QSEs) for blood collection and transfusion service facilities and the blood bank operations to which they are applied. **Table 24–2** is a list of the QSEs and blood bank operations on which the AABB assesses blood banks in its accreditation program.

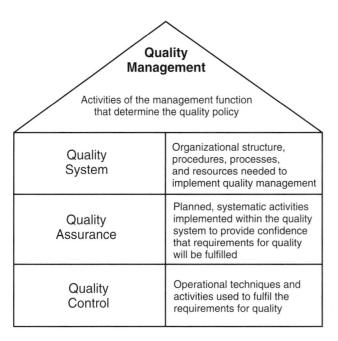

Quality Management	
Activities of the management function that determine the quality policy	
Quality System	Organizational structure, procedures, processes, and resources needed to implement quality management
Quality Assurance	Planned, systematic activities implemented within the quality system to provide confidence that requirements for quality will be fulfilled
Quality Control	Operational techniques and activities used to fulfil the requirements for quality

■ **FIGURE 24–1**   The building blocks of quality.

TABLE 24–1 Common Blood Bank QC Activities and QA Indicators

QC Activities	QA Indicators
Collection equipment Microhematocrit instrument Hemoglobin instrument Apheresis equipment Blood-weighing scales *Blood components* Red blood cell hematocrit Cryoprecipitated antihemophilic factor Platelet counts in platelet units Residual leukocyte counts in leukocyte- reduced components *Reagents* Copper sulfate Reagent red blood cells Reagent antisera Test kits for infectious disease testing *Laboratory equipment* Heating instruments Water baths Thawing devices for blood components pH meters Cell counters Centrifuges, refrigerated and serologic Cell washers Blood irradiators Refrigerators Freezers Platelet incubators Blood warmers Shipping containers	• Number of donor forms with incomplete or incorrect information • Number and types of unusable units and blood components • Number of blood typing discrepancies in donors and patients • Number of and reasons for invalid tests • Number of and reasons for labeling check failures • Number and source of improper and incomplete requests for blood components • Number and location of patients without proper identification at time of specimen collection or transfusion • Number of, source of, and reasons for unacceptable specimens • Number of times wrong component or ABO was selected for crossmatch or use • Number and type of transfusion complications • Number of and reasons for turnaround time failures

The next sections of this chapter discuss the blood bank's role and responsibilities in fulfilling QS essentials. It should become apparent that the essentials of a QS extend far beyond historic QC and QA practices. **Figure 24–2** demonstrates that the QS essentials are the foundation for blood bank operations in the path of workflow for both donor centers and transfusion services.

Quality Systems (QS) Essentials

Organization

The type and size of the organization determine the configuration of the blood bank's QS. In hospitals, there is usually an organization-wide quality function or department that prioritizes and coordinates quality projects, approves resources,

TABLE 24–2 QS Essentials and Blood Bank Operations

QS Essentials	Blood Bank Operations
Organization	Donor qualification
	Autologous donor qualification
Personnel	Apheresis donor qualification
	Blood collection
Equipment	Cytapheresis collection
	Preparation of components
Purchasing and inventory	Testing of donor blood
	Final labeling
Process control	Final inspection before distribution
	Patient samples and requests
Documents and records	Pretransfusion recipient testing
	Crossmatch
Occurrence management	Selection of blood components
	Special considerations for neonates
Assessments	Selection in special circumstances
	Final inspection before issue
Process improvement	Administration of blood and components
	Rh-immune globulin
Facilities and safety	Dispensing and use of tissue

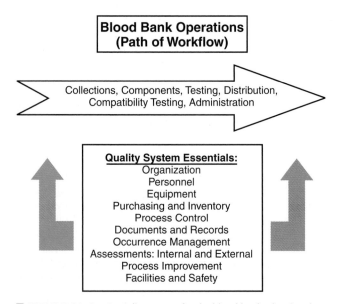

■ **FIGURE 24–2** A quality system for the blood bank, showing the relationship of QSEs to blood bank operations.

and receives reports and information from all hospital departments. The hospital-based blood bank or transfusion service must participate in blood bank quality-related activities, laboratory-wide quality initiatives, and the hospital's quality improvement program. The blood bank should state in writing its goals, objectives, and policies for each of the QSEs and relate them to the bigger laboratory and hospital quality goals. There should be an organization chart showing:

- All relationships among blood bank personnel
- The blood bank's link to the laboratory
- The blood bank's link to the hospital
- How the blood bank links to the hospital's quality function

A free-standing blood center must develop and manage the entirety of its QS. There may be a quality council represented by top-level management from the various departments. The council develops the blood center's quality goals, objectives, and policies; develops the strategies for QS implementation; provides resource support; prioritizes identified improvement projects; and provides support for cross-functional process improvements. There may also be a quality steering committee composed of senior managers and department staff who operationalize the quality strategies and implement process improvements. The blood center must also have written policies for QS essentials.

Personnel

Quality begins and ends with people. However, a quality problem is seldom an individual employee's fault. Rather, a quality problem is almost always due to a faulty process. All the quality goals, objectives, and policies in the world do not ensure safe and effective blood components and transfusions unless the people involved in blood banking know how their job fits into the organization, are trained to know the work processes and procedures, and do it right the first time every time. Blood bank management must work with the human resources departments in blood centers and hospitals to define qualifications for all blood bank jobs and to write job descriptions that include educational qualifications, experience, and federal, state, and local licensing requirements, where applicable, so that qualified persons can be hired. Table 24–3 shows the major types of training that personnel should receive once they are hired. This training extends significantly beyond just the task specifics of a particular job. The competence of personnel to continue to perform their assigned job functions and tasks must also be periodically evaluated and documented. Competence assessment challenges can include direct observation of job task performance, review of records, and written, verbal, or practical tests.

Equipment

There should be a process for installing new equipment and ensuring its proper functioning before it is used in daily operations. There must be schedules for calibration, preventive maintenance, and QC, with frequencies determined by regulations, accreditation requirements, manufacturers' written instructions, usage, testing volume, and equipment reliability. In addition to temperature-controlled equipment (e.g., refrigerators, freezers, incubators), instruments such as automated analyzers, readers, pipettors, and washers must also be installed and functioning properly before routine use. Defective equipment and instruments must be identified and

TABLE 24–3	Training for New Employees
Orientation	*Safety Training*
Organization	Emergency preparedness
Department	Accident reporting
Section	Chemical hygiene program
	Hazardous waste disposal program
	Infection control (including universal precautions, bioterrorism)
	Radiation safety, where applicable
Quality Training	*Work Processes and Procedures Training*
cGMP*	
QS	Work processes performed the job
Team skills	
Problem-solving skills	Procedures performed
	New work processes and procedures
	Revised work processes and procedures
Computer Training	*Medicare Compliance Training*
Hospital information system	Medicare necessity requirements
Department information system (e.g., laboratory)	Fraud and abuse reporting
Personal computers	
• e-mail	
• scheduling	
• on-line documentation	

*cGMP = Current Good Manufacturing Practice

repaired when necessary. Records must be kept of all installation, calibration, maintenance, and repair activities.

Purchasing and Inventory

In hospital-based blood banks and transfusion services, contract and purchasing issues are usually handled by the hospital's purchasing department. Blood bank personnel may or may not have control over the specific vendors with which the organization has agreements to purchase blood components, reagents and kits for testing, equipment, and other important supplies and materials. At a minimum, hospital-based blood banks and transfusion services need to have a process by which incoming blood components and critical supplies are inspected and tested, where required. In addition, blood banks and transfusion services need to have effective processes for managing inventories of reagents, supplies, and blood components.

Blood centers need to have specified processes for selecting vendors of equipment, supplies, and services, and for entering into and amending agreements. In addition, blood centers must also have processes for receipt, inspection, and testing (where required) of incoming critical materials (such as blood bags and infectious disease testing kits), blood components (such as leukocyte-reduced platelets), and blood products (such as albumin, clotting factor concentrates, and immune globulins).

Process Control

A *process* can be defined as a set of interrelated resources and activities that transforms inputs into outputs. *Process control* is a set of activities that ensures that a given work process will keep operating in a state that is continuously able to meet process goals without compromising the process itself. *Total process control* is the evaluation of the performance of a process, comparison of actual performance to a goal, and action taken on any significant difference. Process control is a means to build quality, safety, and effectiveness into the product or service from the beginning. It is important to understand the sequence of activities in a process, develop and write procedures, validate the process to ensure that it works as expected before actual use, measure the process to see that it stays in control, and understand when and why the process has variations.

The FDA has published its requirements for process control as the current *Good Manufacturing Practices* (cGMP) that are cited in the Code of Federal Regulations.[3,4] The cGMP requires that facilities design their processes and procedures to ensure that blood components are manufactured consistently to meet the quality standards appropriate for their intended use.

Flowcharting

Figure 24–3 is a stepwise flow of the elements of total process control. The best tool for understanding a process is to flowchart it. Flowcharting graphically represents the sequence of activities in a process and shows how the inputs are converted into outputs. Flowcharts help to develop a common understanding of a process. Mapping current work processes reveals bottlenecks, missing actions, decision points, dead ends, and choices that can lead to errors, delays, and unnec-

essary work. Mapping a new process facilitates understanding of where human and other resources will be needed for successful accomplishment. Flowcharting can be done on paper or with commercially available software programs. **Figure 24–4** is a basic flowchart for modifying a unit of whole blood collected in a main bag that has a satellite container. It illustrates different decision points and production choices.

Standard Operating Procedures

A work process involves a number of people who perform a sequence of actions over a period of time. A process flowchart describes in a visual manner what happens. From a process flowchart, specific procedures can be identified that answer the question of how to do the action depicted in the process. Procedures are the steps taken by one person who performs just one action in the larger process. For example, the process

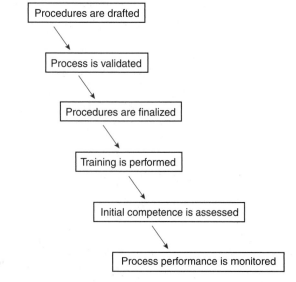

Total Process Control

■ FIGURE 24–3   The activities within total process control.

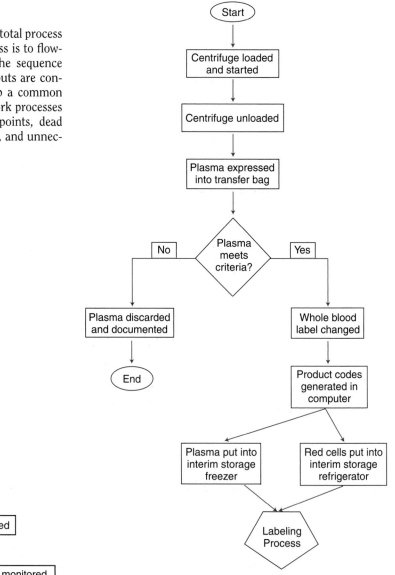

■ FIGURE 24–4   An example of a flowchart for processing a unit of whole blood collected in a double bag.

to provide a physician with a patient's ABO and Rh type involves ordering the test, collecting an appropriate specimen, delivering it to the laboratory, performing the test, and reporting the results. Across a span of time, different people order the test, collect the specimen, perform the ABO/Rh test, and deliver the results. In this process, there needs to be specific written procedures for ordering tests manually or on the computer system, collecting and labeling the specimen, delivering the specimen to the laboratory, performing the ABO/Rh testing, and reporting the results.

Validation

To ensure that new processes will work as needed, they must be validated before being put into use. Validation tests all elements of a new process to provide a high degree of assurance that the process will work as intended. For example, when a new test for a transfusion-transmitted disease is added to those performed on donated blood units, the new test method—with its associated instruments, test kits, computer functions, and procedures—must be validated in each blood bank that will perform the new test. The validation ensures that the new test will perform as expected with that blood bank's instrumentation, written procedures, personnel, and computer systems. The culmination of this validation process is a set of new procedures on which all personnel who will perform the new test must be trained. Training must be documented and personnel determined to be competent in the new process and procedures before they are implemented in the live environment.

Process Controls

It is essential to monitor a process to ensure that it is performing as required, to correct process problems before they affect output, and to improve processes to meet changing needs and technology. Routine process controls include:

- QC of test methods and reagents
- Reviews of work and QC records
- Capture of occurrences when the process did not perform as expected

These routine process controls monitor whether a process is functioning as needed.

Proficiency testing is another example of a process control. In proficiency testing, one laboratory's methods and procedures are compared with those of other laboratories for the ability to get the same result on a set of unknown specimens. Regulations require that all laboratories participate in proficiency testing for diagnostic laboratory testing. Blood bank proficiency test challenges include serologic testing for blood types, detection and identification of unexpected antibodies, compatibility of crossmatched blood, and tests for diseases transmitted through blood transfusion.

Other process controls include manual and automated steps to prevent the occurrence of errors. One common process control in serologic testing is the use of green-colored antiglobulin serum to ensure that the antiglobulin serum was indeed added at the antiglobulin phase of testing. Another common process control is the addition of IgG-coated reagent red blood cells after the antiglobulin phase reading to assure that the antiglobulin serum was indeed working. Computer process controls include automatic comparison of current blood type interpretation with the previous computer records on the same donor or patient to prevent ABO errors and warning signals when ABO-incompatible units are issued for transfusion.

Process Variations

The performance of a process can vary from day to day, but not every variation is cause for concern. Some minor variation is normal and results from causes that are not easily controlled or changed but that are predictable. Such common causes result from many factors, each of which may affect a process to a small extent but collectively have a minimal effect on the outcome. Certain factors such as changes in the marketplace, sharper competition, and technological improvements may require that a normally functioning process be fine-tuned because the common causes are limiting competitive advancement. Only process redesign removes common causes.

At other times, variations that exceed certain statistically determined operating limits are the results of special causes. The reason for special causes must be quickly determined and corrected because the process is out of control. Special causes can usually be found and eliminated and include variations resulting from malfunctioning equipment, untrained personnel, and defective reagents or supplies.

Control charts and trend analysis tools offer ways to measure and monitor a process and to determine whether process performance is in or out of control. For several decades, laboratories have been using control charts to monitor test assay performance by periodically testing standards or controls with known values and entering the results on a chart. Statistical calculations determine the upper and lower limits for the controls' values. Each time the controls are tested, the results determine whether the process is in control. If the values plotted on the control chart do not exceed the upper and lower limits, then the process is said to be in control. When the values exceed the control limits, the process is considered out of control. An investigation is performed to determine the special cause, and corrective action is taken and documented. Any patient tests associated with the out-of-range controls may need to be repeated after the process is brought back into control.

Control charts can be used for any repeatable process that can be measured over time. **Figure 24–5** is a sample of a control chart demonstrating upper and lower control limits and common and special causes of variation.

Documents and Records

Documents are approved information contained in a written or electronic format. *Documents* define the QS for external inspectors and internal staff. Examples of documents include written policies, process flowcharts, standard operating procedures (SOPs), forms, computer software, manufacturers' package inserts, operator manuals, and copies of regulations and standards. *Records* capture the results or outcomes of procedures and testing on written forms or electronic media such as manual worksheets, instrument printouts, tags, or labels. Both documents and records must be controlled to provide evidence that regulations and standards are being met.

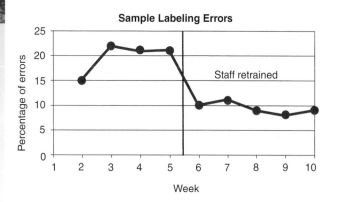

■ FIGURE 24–5 An example of a control chart used to monitor a process.

Document Control

A structured document control system links a facility's policies, processes, and procedures. A typical document control system is structured as a pyramid, as shown in **Figure 24–6**. The following example best illustrates how a blood bank should link its policies, processes, and procedures.

The blood bank should have a written policy document stating that the blood bank maintains a process and relevant procedures for correcting erroneous entries or results on a paper record or in the computer. A second document (such as a process flowchart) should describe the sequence of activities in identifying the need for a correction; obtaining any necessary approvals for the change; making the correction in the computer, on paper, or both; and notifying all appropriate parties of the correction. SOP documents instruct staff members how to record the need for a correction, how to obtain any necessary approvals for making the change, how to properly record a change to an entry on a paper record, how to properly record a change to an entry in a computer record, and how to notify appropriate parties of the change and document the notification. The process and procedures should be written in a way that ensures that all requirements to meet regulations and accreditation requirements are met. The documentation (written or electronic) of the actions taken provide a tracking record to provide evidence that the requirements were met.

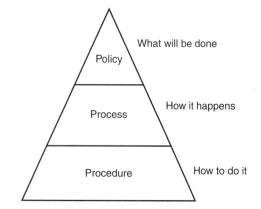

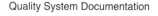

■ FIGURE 24–6 A simple structure for organizing QS documents.

There needs to be a mechanism that controls identification, approval, revision, and archiving of a facility's policies, process descriptions, procedures, and related forms. This mechanism includes instructions for writing SOPs in approved formats, assigning document identification numbers with version designation, approving new and revised documents, preparing a master document list, and maintaining document history files. This mechanism is called "change control" and usually requires the completion and routing of a form that contains information about the reason for a new document or a change to an existing one. Other important change information includes when the change was requested; who wants the change; what other documents, if any, are affected by this change; and approval, training, and in-use dates. A master copy of the new approved version is added to the master file, which contains copies of all previous versions of that same document. The hard copies in this master file capture the original signatures and provide a paper backup when electronic files cannot be accessed. The master list is updated with the new version number. When a revised version of a document is ready to be released, the distribution process needs to be controlled to ensure that copies of the obsolete document (e.g., procedures in a working manual) are replaced with the new version and then destroyed. Employees should not keep and refer to copies of procedures and forms stashed in lockers, drawers, and personal files. This helps to ensure that only the latest approved version of documents is available for use.

Records Management

Forms are specially designed documents—either paper or electronic—on which are recorded the results or outcomes of performing a given procedure. Forms are also controlled documents. The document numbering system should link the form to its respective procedure. Instructions for completion of forms, when needed, can be conveniently placed on the back side of the form. When a form is filled out, it becomes a record. Regulations and accreditation requirements mandate the review of records by supervisory personnel and specify the type of records and length of time they are to be stored for possible future reference. State, local, and facility requirements for record retention periods may also apply.

Occurrence Management

FDA regulations require that blood banks report any error or accident in the manufacture of blood components that may affect the safety, purity, potency, identity, or effectiveness of the component or that compromises the safety of the blood donor or recipient. Each blood bank must have a process for detecting, reporting, evaluating, and correcting deviations and nonconformances with its own procedures, products, or services. "Occurrence management" is one name for such a process.

Occurrence Reporting

Information about events involving the blood bank that deviate from accepted policy, process, or procedure should be captured and acted upon. Hospitals usually have in place a risk management program, but mostly this captures information about events involving patients and visitors that could result in financial loss to the facility. An internal blood bank occurrence management system captures and analyzes information about events that occurred across the entire path of workflow for blood collection and transfusion service activities.

It is convenient to use the generic terms *occurrence* or *event* to describe an unexpected happening until it is further classified as an error, accident, deviation, nonconformance, or other facility-determined definition. **Table 24–4** provides some definitions of terms used to further classify blood bank occurrences.

All employees are encouraged to participate in occurrence reporting. It is essential that occurrence reporting not be perceived by the staff as a tool for finger-pointing or disciplinary action. Instead, all staffers need to understand that occurrences represent blood banks processes that do not work as they should and, thus, occurrences provide opportunities for improvement. Occurrences may be identified either by staff in the course of routine activities or by supervisors during review of records. Information about all occurrences, including those identified before blood components are distributed or issued, is to be captured. In the reporting process, employees describe the "who," "where," and "when" and then briefly describe what happened and what they did at the time to remediate the problem. A standard report form can be used to capture information on all occurrences **(Fig. 24–7)**.

Investigation and Corrective Action

Supervisors and quality function personnel record the occurrences in a spreadsheet or database so that the resolution process can be tracked. The occurrences are reviewed, investigated, and further classified as errors, accidents, or another definition.

The immediate action, which is the initial quick-fix solution, is known as *remedial action*. Such remedial actions do not address the real cause of the problem, which can be determined only through investigation. Investigation of complaints or errors provides an opportunity to identify factors that contributed to the problem. Process improvement tools (discussed later in this chapter) are used to identify the contributing factors and to determine the best way to remove them through implementing corrective action.

Most corrective action involves making changes in the process. All employees performing that process must then be informed of the change and retrained when necessary. Sometimes the corrective action involves only retraining specific individuals who may not have been adequately trained initially or who have been taking unapproved personal deviations from established procedure.

The occurrence-reporting process must be clearly defined so that information is tracked and acted upon and feedback is provided. The person responsible for the QA function in the blood bank (called the QA officer or quality manager) reviews all occurrence reports, assigns an accession number, and forwards the occurrence form to the sections or departments that will be involved in the investigation. The completed report is returned to the quality officer, who reviews it for completeness and appropriateness of remedial and corrective action. If an identified error or accident must be reported to the FDA, the appropriate process is initiated.

In a good occurrence management program, occurrences are also mapped to the specific processes in the blood bank's path of workflow. This information is trended to determine which processes have the most problems. The trending information provides significant support for defending when a process needs to be changed. Facility staff must make a conscious decision not just to respond with remedial actions but to use occurrence information to take corrective action to remove the actual root cause of the problem and to make improvements that truly contribute to the safety and efficacy of transfusion medicine.

Internal Assessment

The blood bank needs to have an internal assessment process in place to continuously monitor the effectiveness of its QS. See **Figure 24–2** for a review of the QSEs supporting the blood bank's path of workflow. Both the quality essentials and the facility's specific operations need to be assessed. Compliance inspection and other checklists[6,7,9] can be used; however, they assess the adequacy of only the listed items. The quality indicators monitored by hospital-based blood banks and transfusion services as part of the laboratory's QA program are also helpful but do not usually cover all important aspects of each operation.

Each blood bank should review all its processes and ask the question, "What can we monitor on a scheduled basis to ensure that this process is working as needed?" Quantitative indicators can then be derived for which the numerator is the number of times the process did or did not work and the denominator is the total number of times the process was performed. Common transfusion service examples include the percentage of specimens received in the compatibility testing laboratory that was not acceptable for testing and the number of times the transfusion service met its established turnaround time for emergency release of uncrossmatched blood

TABLE 24–4	Common Classifications of Various Types of Occurrences
Occurrence Type	**Definition**
Accident	Occurrence generally not attributable to a person's mistake, such as a power outage or an aged instrument's malfunction
Adverse reaction	Complications that occurred to the donor during or after the donation process or to the recipient of transfused blood components
Complaint	Expression of dissatisfaction from internal customers (physicians, employees) or external customers (donors, patients)
Discrepancy	Difference or inconsistency in the outcomes of a process, procedure, or test results
Error	Occurrence attributable to a human or system problem, such as a problem from failure to follow established procedure or a part of a process that did not work as expected
Postdonation information	The receipt of information (call or letter) from a donor with additional details regarding his or her donation, such as subsequent illness or neglecting to mention an illness or medication

QUALITY ASSURANCE INCIDENT REPORT

ORIGINATOR　ACCESSION #_____ TODAY'S DATE _____

UNIT #(s) _____

DEPARTMENTS(s) _____

NAME OF ORIGINATOR _____

BRIEF DESCRIPTION OF INCIDENT (Attach additional paper, if needed) _____

_____

_____

_____

DATE SENT TO QA _____

INVESTIGATING DEPARTMENT _____

DATE RECEIVED _____ NAME OF INVESTIGATOR(s) _____

ADDITIONAL DESCRIPTION OF INCIDENT _____

_____

_____

INDICATE CORRECTIVE ACTION TO BE TAKEN (Attach additional paper if needed) _____

_____

_____

_____

_____

QUALITY ASSURANCE

SIGNATURE OF QA OFFICER _____ DATE _____

_____ REPORTABLE _____ NON-REPORTABLE

DATE SENT TO REGULATORY (If Reportable) _____

REGULATORY AFFAIRS

DATE RECEIVED _____ DATE INCIDENT REPORTED _____

RETURN FORM TO RESPONSIBLE QA OFFICER

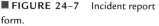 ■ **FIGURE 24–7**　Incident report form.

to the emergency department. See **Table 24–1** for additional examples of quality indicators.

Perhaps the best assessment tool is the internal audit. Unlike compliance inspections, audits review a specific facility process and determine, by examination of documents and records, whether the facility is meeting the applicable requirements. In a transfusion service, for example, an auditor could randomly select a unit number for a red blood cell component and track through each activity involved in how the component was received, tested, issued, and transfused. The training and competence assessment records of each employee involved in handling the component are reviewed, as are the QC records for the storage refrigerator and the reagents, centrifuges, and other instruments used in compatibility testing for that unit. The performance on the proficiency test most recent to the unit's testing is reviewed. Copies of procedures and forms used at the workstations for all testing and QC are examined to determine whether they are the most current version, according to the master list. Samples of records are reviewed for inclusion of all required information, interpretations, and required supervisory reviews.

For blood collection operations, a donor name or number could be randomly selected and the same process repeated for the donation record, computer files, all related SOPs, training and competence records, component production records, serologic and infectious disease testing records, and related QC, labeling, storage, and shipping records.

Audits should be conducted by personnel who have been trained to perform audits and to identify system problems. Auditors should not have responsibility for performing the procedures they are required to audit. In a hospital-based blood bank or transfusion service, there may be insufficient personnel to have a separate quality function, and the supervisor and/or senior personnel may have to perform some auditing activities. A free-standing blood center should have sufficient personnel to designate a quality officer and to separate the quality function from routine operations.

The auditor presents his or her findings to the appropriate management and operations personnel at the closing meeting on a form similar to that in **Figure 24–8**. The auditor may request corrective action for each finding. A process should be in place for the evaluation and review of the audit by management personnel to ensure that corrective actions will be implemented. The FDA requires that facilities prepare an annual summary of their audit findings and the corrective actions taken.[11]

QUALITY ASSURANCE INTERNAL AUDIT

Area/Function Assessed
Subject Area   Date:
Key Positive Findings:
Key Oppurtunity Areas:
Recommendations for Improvements:
Auditors: Date:
Response: Planned Actions and Completion Dates
Area Mgmt.:   Date:
Approved by: Date:

■ **FIGURE 24–8**   Internal audit form.

Process Improvement

Identifying Opportunities for Improvement

Opportunities for improvement for both blood collection facilities and transfusion services can be identified from at least six main sources:

- The occurrence trending process pointing to operational areas that are not functioning as well as intended
- Customer feedback: complaints, solicited feedback, or suggestions from external customers whom the organization serves and internal (employee) customers
- Information derived from monitoring quality indicators of operations, particularly when it is compared with that of peer groups in other institutions (a procedure known as benchmarking)
- Internal audit feedback, whereby objective evidence collected by the auditor should support the facility's understanding of why corrective action is needed and should be taken
- Feedback from periodic external compliance inspections (however, if the blood bank is already seriously involved in the previous four activities, there should be little new information learned of which the facility is not already aware)
- Reports from other departments in the hospital's organization-wide quality committee function, such as nursing or emergency department problems in dealing with the blood bank

Using Teams

The hospital blood bank or laboratory's quality committee, or the blood center's quality council, should set priorities for the problems that need the most immediate attention. Many organizations have successfully used teams to solve problems or to design process improvements. Names such as "process improvement teams," "quality action teams," "continuous improvement teams," and "corrective action teams" have all been used to refer to groups of people representing different parts of a given process who have been brought together to identify and to implement ways to remove the problem and to improve the process. Teams need good team skills to perform their assignments successfully. Members of teams should receive team-building and problem-resolution training to ensure the most effective outcome for the time and resources expended.[12] Common team "dos and don'ts" are shown in **Table 24–5**.

TABLE 24–5   Process Improvement Teams Should Focus on Opportunities to Improve Work Processes

Teams Should Improve Processes That Affect:	Teams Should Not Work on These Issues:
Quality of product	Problems governed by or directly related to union contracts
Quality and reliability of service to internal and external customers	Grievances and grievance procedures
Efficiency and accuracy of job performance	Seniority
Waste reduction, scrap, rework, and operating costs	Job assignments
Equipment performance, up-time, and reliability	Pay rates or benefits
Interdepartmental and intradepartmental communications	Job classifications
Improved process controls	
Safety, hygiene, and work environment	
SOPs and training	
Learning new skills, upgrading knowledge of the business, developing personal capabilities, team process	

Problem Resolution

Many approaches to the problem-solving process have been published. All the published problem-solving approaches contain essentially the same activities of problem identification, prioritization, selection, analysis, data collection, identifying possible solutions, implementation, monitoring, and evaluation. **Figure 24–9** depicts one common approach to managing the problem-solving process that includes these main activities:[13]

- Developing a customer-oriented action plan
- Putting the plan into action

Plan-Do-Check-Act (PDCA)
Plan

A mission-consistent, customer-oriented action plan
• Identify opportunities for improvement from data sources
• Prioritize improvement activities
• Develop an action plan for the selected activity, either
  - initiating a new process, or
  - improving an existing process
• Identify
  - customer needs
  - participants
  - timeframes
  - outcome measurements
  - success criteria

Do

Put the plan into action
• Implement the action plan
  - do a pilot project first
  - broaden only after success
• Collect performance data

Check
Has the planned and implemented change created intended improvement? • Analyze collected data • Compare performance data to established success targets and original performance data to determine if improvement was achieved • Identify any unexpected peripheral benefits • Identify unanticipated problems in other areas
Act

Decide what to do next
• Determine if customer needs were met
• Take action based on the results:
  • Success:
    - revise the processes for further improvements (optional), and
    - assess again to determine if improvement is maintained, and
    - if a pilot project, standardize to the bigger group
  • Lack of success—re-do the action plan and repeat

■ **FIGURE 24–9**   A common quality improvement process.

- Measuring and monitoring to determine effectiveness of the action
- Determining what to do based on the measurements

A formalized problem resolution process is just one piece of process improvement. **Figure 24–10** illustrates the whole cycle that encourages continuous improvement.

Facilities and Safety

In hospitals, the JCAHO mandates an environmental control program that addresses all significant environmental issues for facility management and maintenance such as temperature control, electrical safety, fire protection, and so forth.[5] The JCAHO also requires that hospital laboratories have training programs for all laboratory personnel on emergency preparedness, chemical hygiene, and infection control.[6] Therefore, hospital-based blood banks and transfusion services are already participating in facilities management and safety training. In addition, any blood bank that performs irradiation of blood components must also have a radiation safety program and document appropriate training.

A free-standing blood center must develop its own facility management program. All regulations and accreditation requirements for emergency preparedness, chemical hygiene, infection control, and radiation safety training and documentation also apply.

A Quality System (QS) for the Medical Laboratory

A laboratory-wide QS can be derived by simply replacing the blood bank path of workflow shown in **Figure 24–2** with the path of workflow of the medical laboratory **(Fig. 24–11)**. All the Quality Systems (QSEs) supporting the path of work flow remain the same because these quality elements are universal. In fact, at the point of Compatibility Testing in the blood bank path of workflow, the laboratory's (and transfusion service's) path of workflow is entered for all transfusion service testing.

A review of the International Organization for Standardization quality standards demonstrates that blood bank/laboratory QSEs are included in the international standards.[2] Therefore, all the discussion in the section on QSEs in this chapter applies equally to hospital laboratories. It is not only possible but also highly desirable to expand the blood bank's QS building efforts so that the entire laboratory benefits from improved organization, coordination, and effectiveness of its many processes.[14]

Summary

Today, working in a QS environment is required to achieve the standards of excellence necessary to survive the changes facing the nation's health care industry and to provide the level of patient safety that our patients both expect and deserve. Purchasers of health-care services want evidence that health-care providers such as hospitals and blood centers are involved in organization-wide quality improvement programs that increase the safety of donors and patients. Only those organizations demonstrating measurable quality improvements are approved for agreements for products and services. The cultural change needed to create a QS takes time, and organizations that have not started must begin immediately to keep pace. Consumers of hospital and laboratory services accept no less than total quality. Organizations that provide less will not survive.

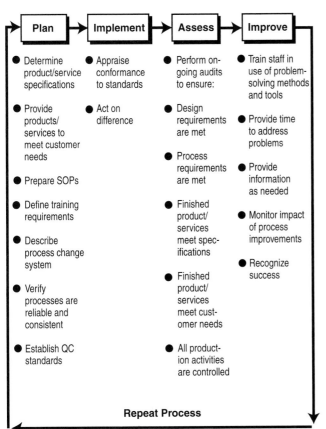

■ **FIGURE 24–10** The cycle of organization-wide QM.

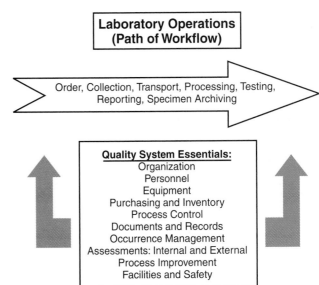

■ **FIGURE 24–11** A QS for the medical laboratory.

SUMMARY CHART:

Important Points to Remember (MT/MLT)

➤ Blood bank compliance with federal regulations and accreditation requirements is mandated by the FDA, JCAHO, AABB, and CAP.

➤ Compliance inspections measure the state of the facility's program with respect to the applicable requirements at a single point in time and are usually conducted every 1 to 2 years.

➤ Quality control procedures in blood banking may include daily testing of the reactivity of blood typing reagents, positive and negative controls in infectious disease testing, calibration of serologic centrifuges, and temperature monitoring of refrigerators, freezers, and thawing devices.

➤ QA is a set of planned actions to provide confidence that systems and elements that influence the quality of the product or service are working as expected individually and collectively.

➤ A QS provides a framework for uniformly applying quality principles and practices across all blood bank operations, starting with donor selection and proceeding through transfusion outcomes.

➤ Process control is a set of activities that ensures a given process will keep operating in a state that is continuously able to meet process goals without compromising the process itself.

➤ cGMP requires that facilities design their processes and procedures to ensure that blood components are manufactured consistently to meet the quality standards appropriate for their intended use.

➤ Process validation challenges all activities in a new process before implementation to provide a high degree of assurance that the process will work as intended.

➤ Routine QC procedures, review of records, and capture of occurrences when the process did not perform as expected are routine process control measures that monitor whether a process is functioning as needed.

➤ Occurrence management is a name for a process that detects, reports, evaluates, and corrects errors, accidents, deviations, and nonconformances in blood bank operations.

➤ An internal audit reviews a specific facility process and determines by examination of documents and records whether the facility is meeting applicable requirements and its own policies, processes, and procedures.

➤ A process improvement team is a group of people who represent different activities in a given process and who have been brought together to identify and implement ways to solve problems.

REVIEW QUESTIONS

1. A QS is:
   a. Synonymous with compliance
   b. Active and continuous
   c. Part of quality control
   d. An evaluation of efficiency

2. QSEs are applied to:
   a. Just the blood bank's management staff
   b. Blood bank quality control activities
   c. Only blood component manufacturing
   d. The blood bank's path of work flow

3. cGMP refers to:
   a. Regulations pertaining to laboratory safety
   b. Validation of testing
   c. Occurrence reporting
   d. Manufacturing blood components

4. Common causes of variation are:
   a. Constant and controllable
   b. Random and uncontrollable
   c. Constant and uncontrollable
   d. Random and controllable

5. Which *one* statement below is correct?
   a. A process describes how to perform a task
   b. A procedure simply states what the facility will do
   c. A procedure informs the reader how to perform a task
   d. A policy can be flowcharted

6. A blank form is a:
   a. Record
   b. Procedure
   c. Flowchart
   d. Document

7. An example of a remedial action is:
   a. Applying the problem-solving process
   b. Starting a process improvement team
   c. Resolving the immediate problem
   d. Performing an internal audit

8. The PDCA cycle is used for:
   a. Problem resolution
   b. Process control
   c. Validation
   d. Auditing

9. The difference between the blood bank and laboratory QSs is that:
   a. The laboratory has a different path of work flow
   b. The blood bank does not include computer systems
   c. The QSEs are different
   d. The blood bank excludes testing

10. The QSEs for the blood bank QS can be used for the laboratory because:
   a. The paths of work flow are identical

b. Both the laboratory and blood bank experience accreditation inspections

c. The QSEs are universal

d. They are required by international standards

REFERENCES

1. Food and Drug Administration, Center for Biologics Evaluation and Research: Guideline on General Principles of Process Validation. Food and Drug Administration, Rockville, MD, 1987.
2. International Organization for Standardization: ISO 9000: Quality management systems—Fundamentals and vocabulary. International Organization for Standardization, Geneva, 2000.
3. Food and Drug Administration, Department of Health and Human Services: Code of Federal Regulations, Title 21, Parts 200–299. U.S. Government Printing Office, Washington, DC, revised annually.
4. Food and Drug Administration, Department of Health and Human Services: Code of Federal Regulations, Title 21, Parts 600–799. U.S. Government Printing Office, Washington, DC, revised annually.
5. Joint Commission on Accreditation of Healthcare Organizations: Hospital Accreditation Standards. Oakbrook Terrace, IL, 2004.
6. Joint Commission on Accreditation of Healthcare Organizations: Laboratory and Point-of-care Testing Accreditation Standards. Oakbrook Terrace, IL, 2004.
7. College of American Pathologists: Inspection Checklists for Laboratory Accreditation. Northfield, IL, 2004.
8. American Association of Blood Banks: Standards for Blood Banks and Transfusion Services, ed 22. Bethesda, MD, 2003.
9. Ziebell, L, and Kavemeier, K: Quality Control: A Component of Process Control in Blood Banking and Transfusion Medicine. American Association of Blood Banks, Bethesda, MD, 1999.
10. Food and Drug Administration, Center for Biologics Evaluation and Research: Guideline on Quality Assurance in Blood Establishments (Docket No. 91N-0450). Food and Drug Administration, Rockville, MD, 1995.
11. Nevalainen, DE, Berte, LM, and Callery, MF: Quality Systems in the Blood Bank Environment, ed 2. American Association of Blood Banks, Bethesda, MD, 1998.
12. Scholtes, PR, et al: The Team Handbook, ed 3. Goal-QPC, Salem, MA, 2003.
13. McCloskey LA, and Collet DN: TQM: A Primer Guide to Total Quality Management. GOAL/QPC, Methuen, MA, 1993.
14. Berte, LM, and Nevalainen, DE: Quality Systems for the Laboratory. Chicago, IL, 2000.

BIBLIOGRAPHY

Berte, LM (ed): Transfusion Service Manual of SOPs, Training Guides and Competence Assessment Tools. American Association of Blood Banks, Bethesda, MD, 1996.

Clinical Laboratory Technical Procedure Manuals, ed 4. Approved guideline GP2A-4. NCCLS, Wayne, PA, 2002.

Galloway, D: Mapping Work Processes. ASCQ Press, Milwaukee, 1994.

Tague, NR: The Quality Toolbox. ASQC Press, Milwaukee, 1995.

Training Verification for Laboratory Personnel, ed 2. Approved guideline GP21-A2. NCCLS, Wayne, PA, 2003.

twenty-five

Transfusion Safety and Federal Regulatory Requirements

**Judy Ellen Ciaraldi, BS, MT(ASCP)SBB, CQA(ASQ), and
Alan E. Williams, Ph.D**

Introduction

History of Biologics Regulation
Public Health Service (PHS) Act
Federal Food, Drug, and Cosmetic
(FD&C) Act
Food and Drug Administration (FDA)

Regulatory Process
Manufacturers, Manufacturing, and
Biological Products
Statutes, Laws
Regulations
Recommendations
CBER

Registration and Licensure
Registration
Licensure

Unregistered and Unlicensed
Manufacturers

**Overview of the FDA's Inspection
Process**
Inspection Authorities
Inspection Procedures

Enforcement Actions
Advisory Actions: Warning
Letter
Administrative Actions: Suspension,
Revocation
Judicial Actions: Seizure, Injunction,
Prosecution

cGMP Regulations
Quality Control Unit
Quality Reviews

**Additional Requirements of
Biologics Manufacturing**
Variances
Contract Manufacturing
Short Supply Agreements
Biological Product Deviation
Reporting
Product Recalls
Fatality Reporting

**Summary Chart: Important Points
to Remember (MT/MLT)**

Review Questions

References

═══ **OBJECTIVES** ═══

On completion of the chapter, the learner should be able to:

1. Describe why laws governing regulation of biologics were
enacted.
2. Define a biologics manufacturer.
3. Describe the regulatory process.
4. List the requirements for and responsibilities of the United
States Food and Drug Administration (FDA) registration.
5. List the requirements for and responsibilities of FDA licensure.

6. Describe the FDA's inspectional authority of biologics manufacturers.
7. Distinguish between licensed-registered, unlicensed-regis-
tered, and unlicensed-unregistered blood establishments.
8. Describe the role of the FDA current Good Manufacturing
Practices (cGMP) in blood establishment operations.
9. List the possible enforcement actions.
10. List the FDA's five layers of safety

Introduction

The Public Health Service (PHS) is the principal health
agency of the federal government. The mission of PHS is to
protect, improve, and advance the health of the American
people. The Centers for Disease Control and Prevention
(CDC) and the FDA are agencies of the PHS.

In addition to food and veterinary products, the FDA
enforces regulations to ensure the safety and efficacy of bio-

logics, drugs, and devices, which include blood and blood
components, blood collection supplies and machines, and
blood bank reagents and infectious disease test kits.[1] The regulations for blood products promulgated under the PHS Act
and the federal Food, Drug, and Cosmetic (FD&C) Act are
found in Parts 210, 211, and 600 to 680 of Title 21, Code of
Federal Regulations (CFR). These regulations mandate adherence to cGMP. In addition, the regulations address the statutory requirements regarding product licensing and facility

registration as well as product-specific standards for human blood and blood components.

This chapter describes the history of the biologics regulations, FDA's regulatory process and requirements, and FDA's inspection and enforcement activities and quality assurance (cGMP) regulations. We have included the appropriate regulation citation next to the topic. We have also included commonly used abbreviations for this chapter in **Box 25–1**.

History of Biologics Regulation

Public Health Service (PHS) Act

Early in the 1900s, biological drugs came into widespread use in the United States after having met with great success in Europe and Russia. Countries such as France, Germany, Italy, and Russia had instituted regulatory controls for biologics as early as 1895. The regulation of biological products in the United States began when Congress passed the Biologics Control Act of 1902 (also known as the Virus-Toxin Law[2]).

In 1901, there was a serious epidemic of diphtheria, which resulted in a great demand for the diphtheria antitoxin. At the time, there were no requirements for safety testing. The horse from which the antitoxin was obtained had contracted tetanus. The Biologics Control Act was passed following the deaths of 13 children who had received injections of diphtheria antitoxin contaminated with tetanus.[3]

The 1902 Act required biological products to be manufactured in a manner that ensured the safety, purity, and potency of the product. The Act included provisions for licensing products, suspending or revoking the license for violations, labeling requirements, and authorize entry into facilities to conduct inspections.

The Act was expanded to Public Health Service Act (PHS Act) in 1944. The new Act requires a license to be in effect before a biological product enters into interstate commerce.[4] A biologics product license can be issued only after the manufacturer demonstrates that both the product and the manufacturing facility meet standards to ensure the continued safety, purity, and potency of the products.

The 1902 Act did not include all biological products; specifically, it did not address the regulation of blood and blood components. The PHS Act of 1944 expanded the defini-

tion of a biological product to include human blood and blood components.

Federal Food, Drug, and Cosmetic (FD&C) Act

The FD&C Act was passed in 1938 to further define the government's regulatory authority. This Act requires that manufacturers prove a drug is safe before marketing it. In addition, it authorizes facility inspections of drug manufacturers and requires drug manufacturers to register. The FD&C Act prohibits the interstate commerce of misbranded and adulterated products.[5] Misbranding is any false or misleading labeling, such as false therapeutic claims on the label. Adulteration is defined as manufacturing without adherence to cGMP in a manner that may render the product injurious to health. In 1976, the FD&C Act was amended to strengthen the FDA's authority to regulate medical devices. The FDA now requires manufacturers of certain new medical devices to demonstrate that they are safe and effective before they can be marketed.

Food and Drug Administration (FDA)

Originally, the National Institutes of Health (NIH) were charged with enforcing the PHS and FD&C Acts and regulating biological products. The FDA began in 1927 as the Food, Drug, and Insecticide Administration, a law enforcement agency within the U.S. Department of Agriculture. The name was changed to FDA in 1930. In 1972, the oversight of biologics regulation was transferred to the FDA. The FDA was moved to the U.S. Department of Health and Human Services in 1979.[6]

The FDA oversees the safety of the U.S. blood supply by ensuring that blood and blood component manufacturers conduct their operations and manufacture their products consistent with applicable laws, regulations, and cGMP. Reorganization within the FDA in 1988 created the Center for Biologic Evaluation and Research (CBER) to oversee and enforce biologics regulations. The Office of Blood Research and Review (OBRR) and the Office of Compliance and Biologics Quality (OCBQ) in the CBER are responsible for the regulation and enforcement of biological products, including human blood and blood components. The Office of Regulatory Affairs (ORA) is responsible for performing FDA inspections and other surveillance activities.

The FDA has identified five overlapping layers of safety that work together to prevent an unsuitable blood product from being released to a patient. Blood and blood component manufacturers must ensure that they have processes in place to perform and monitor each of these procedures:

- Donor eligibility
- Donor deferral and registries
- Infectious disease testing
- Quarantine of unsuitable products
- Investigation of adverse events

Regulatory Process

Manufacturers, Manufacturing, and Biological Products

Biological product manufacturers are defined as any legal person or entity engaged in the manufacture of biological products subject to licensure under the PHS Act (21 CFR

BOX 25–1
Commonly Used Abbreviations in this Chapter

- BLA: Biologics License Application
- CBER: Center for Biologics Evaluation and Research
- CFR: Code of Federal Regulations
- cGMP: Current Good Manufacturing Practice
- FDA: Food and Drug Administration
- FD&C Act: Food, Drug, and Cosmetic Act
- FR: Federal Register
- OBRR: Office of Biologics Research and Review
- OCBQ: Office of Compliance and Biologics Quality
- ORA: Office of Regulatory Affairs
- PHS: Public Health Service

600.3[t]). Manufacturing activities include the collection, preparation, processing, compatibility testing, labeling, testing, control procedures, repackaging, and other procedures of any biological product that meets the definition of a drug (21 FR 607.3). In 1997 the definition of "manufacturer" was changed. Previously the manufacturer had to perform all the manufacturing process on the product. The new definition states that the manufacturer may or may not own the facilities in which the product is manufactured. This change allows for a contractor to perform the manufacturing steps, with the original product manufacturer taking full responsibility for compliance of the product.

Biological products are medical products derived from living sources. They are defined in Section 351 of the PHS Act as "any virus, therapeutic serum, toxin, antitoxin, vaccine, blood, blood component or derivative, allergenic product, or analogous product applicable to the prevention, treatment, or cure of diseases or injuries of man" (21 CFR 600.3[b]). Biologics, including blood and blood components, are unique in that they are viewed as biological products under the PHS Act and as drugs under the FD&C Act. Biologics are used to prevent, treat, or cure diseases or injuries. This means that blood and blood components must meet the cGMP in the drug regulations (21 CFR 210 and 211) and the biological product regulations (21 CFR 600—680) **(Table 25–1)**.

There are a variety of tools used by FDA to communicate and enforce the requirements and product standards. These include statutes, regulations, and recommendations.

Statutes, Laws

Statutes are the laws and acts passed by Congress granting FDA the authority to fulfill its mission. The PHS Act and the FD&C Act require biologics, drug, and device manufacturers to prove that their product is safe before it is marketed. They also require that all biologics, drug, and device manufacturers follow cGMP and label their product correctly. The Acts grant the FDA the authority to oversee and enforce the requirements in the Acts, including inspecting the manufacturing facilities and imposing penalties for violations when appropriate. Over the years, there have been several amendments to the Acts to further define the regulatory authority and address technological advancements.

Regulations

Regulations are a standard or requirement of conduct set by the federal government under the statutory authority granted by Congress (21 CFR 10.90). These rules are an interpretation of the statutes and laws; like laws, they are legally binding on both the manufacturing industry and the government agencies charged with enforcing the laws. The regulations define and list specific minimum standards that manufacturers must meet. They do not provide specific procedures on how to meet the standard. This was done because the government realized that there are many acceptable ways to achieve the required objective. Regulations are codified in the CFR.

FDA regulations are found in Title 21 of the CFR. The blood and blood component regulations are found in Subchapter F of Title 21 of the CFR **(Table 25–2)**. Proposed and final regulations are published in the *Federal Register* (FR), the official news bulletin of the federal government.

Recommendations

Recommendations are practices that are acceptable to the FDA (21 CFR 10.90). They are not legally binding on the manufacturing industry or the government agencies. In spite of this, recommendations often become manufacturing industry cGMP and have been used in court to demonstrate a necessary practice or standard.

Recommendations are published in guidance documents (called memoranda up to 1996). Specifically, guidance documents are published to (21 CFR 10.115):

- Establish principles, practices, procedures, or standards
- Assist the manufacturing industry and government agencies by clarifying the regulations
- Explain how the manufacturing industry may comply with the regulations
- Provide application review and enforcement approaches

Guidance documents are developed and published under Good Guidance Practices (GGP) regulations (21 CFR 10.115). GGP regulations allow for two types of guidance documents: level 1 and level 2. Level 1 documents are first published as draft guidance for public comment only. Anyone can submit comments to public docket for the draft document. At the end of the comment period, the submitted comments are evaluat-

TABLE 25–1 Comparison of Biological Products and Drugs		
	Biological Products	**Drugs**
Definition	Medical products derived from living sources that are used to prevent, treat, or cure diseases or injuries in man	Finished dosage form (pill, solution, cream, etc.) that contains an active pharmacological ingredient and is used to prevent, treat, or cure diseases or injuries in man
Examples of products	• Blood and blood components • Tissues, cellular therapies • Vaccines, antitoxins • Plasma derivatives (e.g., albumin, clotting factors)	• Over-the-counter medications • Prescription medications • Chemotherapies
Regulatory authority	Public Health Service Act	Federal Food, Drug, and Cosmetic (FD&C) Act
cGMP regulations	21 CFR 210, 211, 606	21 CFR 210, 211
Regulatory center in FDA	Center for Biologics Evaluation and Research (CBER)	Center for Drugs Evaluation and Research (CDER)

TABLE 25–2   Regulations Pertaining to Blood and Blood Components

Title 21 CFR, Subchapter F, Parts	
600	General
601	Licensing
606	Current Good Manufacturing Practices
607	Registration
610	General Biological Product Standards
630	General Requirements for Blood
640	Additional Standards for Blood and Blood Products

ed, and the draft document is revised as necessary. The final guidance document is published for implementation by biological product manufacturers. Level 2 guidance documents are initially published as final documents for implementation. These documents describe current practices or policies that should be implemented immediately in the interest of public health. The public may comment on any document after final publication, and the FDA will determine if a revised guidance should be published. Guidance documents applicable to blood and blood components can be found on the CBER Web site at http://www.fda.gov/cber/guidelines.htm

CBER

The CBER uses laws, regulations, and recommendations to regulate the following manufacturers and products:

- Blood establishments that collect, manufacture, and test blood products for transfusion and for further manufacture into plasma derivatives
- Blood and blood components for transfusion: Whole Blood, Red Blood Cells, platelets, Fresh Frozen Plasma, Cryoprecipitated antihemophiliac factor (AHF)
- Blood components for further manufacturing: Source Plasma, Source Leukocytes, recovered plasma
- Devices used for blood product collection (including anticoagulants and preservative solutions), nondiagnostic blood bank reagents, infectious disease test kits for screening blood donors, and blood establishment computer systems and the device manufacturing facilities
- Biological drugs and vaccines used to treat and prevent diseases and the manufacturing facilities

Questions about the regulation of blood and blood components should be sent to: Division of Blood Applications, OBRR, CBER (HFM-370), 1401 Rockville Pike, Suite 400N, Rockville, MD 20852-1448.

Registration and Licensure
Registration

The FD&C Act requires food, drug, and cosmetic manufacturers to register their manufacturing facilities with the FDA. This part of the Act has been expanded and now includes all biological product and device manufacturers. Regulations for facility registration are found in the CFR (21 CFR 607.7). The following blood and blood component facilities are required to register with the FDA:

- Collection centers
- Community blood banks
- Component preparation facilities
- Hospital blood banks
- Plasmapheresis centers
- Product testing laboratories
- Storage and distribution centers
- Brokers who take possession and manipulate and/or relabel the product

Manufacturing facilities must register within 5 days after beginning their manufacturing operations. They may register by one of two methods: by completing a hard copy of the registration form (Form FDA-2930) and submitting it to FDA or by completing an electronic registration form found on the CBER Web site. The manufacturer must list on the registration form all products and manufacturing processes performed at the facility and complete a form for each manufacturing facility. Registered manufacturers are required to update their registration each year. In addition, registered manufacturers are responsible for complying with FDA regulations, cGMP, and applicable product standards and are inspected by ORA investigators.

The regulations exempt some blood and blood component manufacturers from registration. These manufacturers, listed below, do not perform the manufacturing steps that require registration:

- Transfusion services that do not collect blood products and only perform crossmatching, pooling of platelets and Cryopreciptitated AHF, and bedside filtration and transfusion
- Carriers that transport blood products
- Brokers who do not take possession, manipulate, or relabel the product.

Table 25–3 summarizes the registration of manufacturing facilities. Additional information about registration can be found on the CBER Web site at http://www.fda.gov/cber/blood/bldreg.htm

TABLE 25–3   Summary Table of the Registration of Manufacturing Facilities

The following facilities are required to register:	The following facilities are exempt from registration:
• Collection centers • Community blood banks • Component preparation facilities • Hospital blood banks • Plasmapheresis centers • Product testing laboratories • Storage and distribution centers • Brokers (take possession and manipulate and/or relabel product)	• Transfusion services (do not collect blood; only perform crossmatching, pooling of platelets and Cryoprecipitated AHF, bedside filtration and transfusion) • Brokers (do not take possession, manipulate, or relabel product) • Carriers (only transport product)

Licensure

The PHS Act requires a biologics license to be in effect if a manufacturer wants to engage in the interstate commerce of a biological product. A biologics license will be issued only after the manufacturer proves that the product is safe, pure, potent, and effective and that the facility where the product is manufactured meets cGMP standards. As of 2003, 85% to 90% of blood and blood components manufactured for blood transfusions and 100% of products collected for further manufacture in the United States are prepared in licensed blood and plasma centers.

All biological product manufacturers must be registered. If they want to engage in interstate commerce of the product, they must also apply for a U.S. biologics license. The Biologics License Application (BLA) process involves two steps: a desk review of submitted documents (e.g., standard operating procedures, forms, labels, product quality control, etc.) and an inspection of the manufacturing facility. The applicant for the license submits the necessary application forms and information about their operations to the CBER (21 CFR 601.2).[7] Consumer safety officers (CSOs) in the CBER review the application and supporting documents. CBER CSOs will inform the applicant if additional information is needed to complete the desk review of the documents. As part of the application review, CBER CSOs and ORA investigators will conduct a pre-license inspection of the facility. The investigators will observe the manufacturing process to determine if the product is prepared according to the regulations, cGMP, product standards, and commitments made in the application. The manufacturer must correct any deficiencies observed by the investigators. When the applicant has addressed all deficiencies noted during the desk review and the inspection, a U.S. license will be issued. The license number must appear on the label of the licensed product, and the product may enter into interstate commerce. Licensed manufacturers are responsible for complying with FDA regulations, cGMP, and applicable product standards and are inspected by ORA investigators.

Licensed applicants are required to inform the FDA about each change in manufacturing from what was submitted in the original application (21 CFR 601.12). Originally, when an applicant submitted a change to the FDA, the applicant had to wait for the CBER to approve the submission before being able to distribute the product made using the change into interstate commerce. In 1997, a new law, the Food and Drug Administration Modernization Act (FDAMA), was passed to streamline some of FDA activities and reduce the reporting burden by the manufacturing industry.[8] Regulations in the CFR were revised to include the requirements in the FDAMA. One revised regulation addresses how licensed applicants report their manufacturing changes to the FDA. The manufacturing changes are now divided into the following three categories as determined by the potential of the change to adversely affect the safety, purity, and potency of the product. Applicants determine the appropriate reporting category for the change. The CBER has published guidance to assist applicants with making this determination.[9]

- Major changes are reported as a Prior Approval Supplement. These submissions must be approved before the applicant can distribute the product made using the change into interstate commerce.
- Moderate changes are reported as a Changes Being Effected in 30 Days Supplement. These submissions must be sent to

the FDA for review and approval. The applicant may distribute the product made using the change 30 days after the FDA has received the submission, unless the FDA has informed the applicant not to distribute because of deficiencies in its submission. The 30-day wait is waived for some moderate changes. With these types of submissions, the product is distributed before the FDA has approved the change. Therefore, implementation of the change and distribution of the product made using the change are performed at the manufacturer's own risk. The FDA will review the submission and, if deficiencies are identified, will notify the manufacturer to submit the necessary information. In some cases, the FDA may require that the manufacturer stop distribution until the deficiencies have been corrected.

- Minor changes are reported to the FDA in an annual report. Minor changes do not need to be approved by the FDA before the product made using the minor change can be distributed into interstate commerce. The FDA will review the annual report to determine if the changes have been reported in the proper category. The FDA will notify the manufacturer if the annual report contains changes that should be submitted as a supplement for FDA approval. In some cases, the FDA may require that the manufacturer stop distribution until the supplement is reviewed and approved.

Unregistered and Unlicensed Manufacturers

The regulations exempt some manufacturers from registering with the FDA because they do not perform the manufacturing steps requiring registration. The manufacturers also do not need to be licensed because they do not distribute products into interstate commerce. The majority of these manufacturers operate as transfusion services that only perform crossmatching, pooling of platelets and Cryoprecipitated AHF, and bedside filtration and transfusion. Even though they are not registered or licensed, these manufacturers must still comply with FDA regulations, cGMP, and applicable product standards. There are rare instances when the FDA will inspect these facilities, but these are usually limited to "for cause" inspections, such as investigating a transfusion fatality.

In 1983 the FDA entered into an agreement with the Health Care Financing Administration, now called the Centers for Medicare and Medicaid Services (CMS).[10] The Memorandum of Understanding (MOU) between the FDA and CMS reduced the number of federal agencies inspecting the same facility. Transfusion services are now inspected under the authority of the CMS. Because the CMS does not have a cadre of inspectors to perform inspections, the CMS has delegated the inspections to a number of deemed status organizations, such as the College of American Pathologists, the American Association of Blood Banks, and state health departments.

Table 25–4 summarizes the regulatory oversight of blood and blood component manufacturing facilities.

Overview of the FDA's Inspection Process

Inspection Authorities

The laws granting the FDA the authority to enter manufacturing facilities for the purposes of conducting inspections

TABLE 25–4   Summary Table of the Regulatory Oversight of Blood and Blood Component Manufacturing Facilities

	Manufacturers that engage in interstate and intrastate commerce	Manufacturers that engage in intrastate commerce only	Manufacturers that do not engage in interstate or intrastate commerce
Requirements for registration	Must be registered	Must be registered	Exempt from registration
Requirements for licensure	Must hold active biologics license application	Do not need to be licensed	Do not need to be licensed
Required cGMP regulations	21 CFR 210, 211, 606	21 CFR 210, 211, 606	21 CFR 210, 211, 606
Inspections	Conducted by FDA: CBER (pre-license) and ORA investigators	Conducted by FDA: ORA investigators	Conducted by CMS deemed status organizations
Regulatory oversight	FDA	FDA	CMS, FDA (for cause and variance requests)

are found in both the PHS and FD&C Acts. Originally, the investigators came from various government organizations before this task was finally assigned to the FDA.

Previously, FDA investigators were responsible for conducting inspections on a variety of manufacturing facilities, including device, food, drug, and blood and blood component manufacturers. The process for inspecting biological product manufacturers underwent a change in 1997 after an audit showed that inspections were often conducted by untrained investigators who did not consistently detect serious deficiencies.[11] The investigators now receive intensive training in the technical and regulatory aspects of the products and manufacturing facilities they inspect. The biologics investigators are also specialized into two teams: the Core team is responsible for inspecting plasma derivative and reagent manufacturers, and the Blood Cadre inspects blood, plasma, and tissue centers. This reorganization has resulted in inspections with improved consistency and more appropriate citations.

Inspection Procedures

CBER and ORA investigators conduct pre-license inspections in manufacturing facilities that are applying for a biologics license application. Once a license has been issued, ORA investigators will inspect the manufacturing facility on a biennial basis. ORA investigators also inspect unlicensed, registered manufacturing facilities. All FDA inspections are conducted according to the same procedures.

The FDA inspection policies and procedures are described in compliance programs and compliance policy guides. The compliance programs provide guidance to investigators on how to conduct the inspection and specify the process for determining appropriate regulatory actions.[12] The compliance policy guides inform investigators and compliance officers about FDA policies and interpretations on specific regulatory issues.[13] These documents can be found on the ORA Web site at http://www.fda.gov/compliance_ref.

Each FDA inspection will cover some or all of the following manufacturing operations at the manufacturing facility to ensure that cGMP standards are being followed.

- Donor eligibility, deferral, and reactions
- Product collection
- Component preparation and labeling
- Storage and distribution
- Donor/product testing
- Disposition of unsuitable products
- Computer systems
- Equipment

- Personnel and training
- Records and documentation
- Quality control procedures
- Physical facilities
- Quality assurance procedures
- Transfusion reaction investigations

Investigators discuss their observations with the manufacturer as the inspection progresses. At the end of the inspection, investigators evaluate their observations and document the significant deficiencies on the Form FDA-483, Inspectional Observations. Investigators present the Form FDA-483 to the manufacturer and listen to the proposed corrective actions. Investigators may also discuss less serious observations with the manufacturer to point out areas that could potentially cause significant problems. Both significant and less serious observations, as well as any discussions with the manufacturer, are included in the investigators' Establishment Inspection Report. Most of the inspections result in voluntary compliance by the manufacturer to take corrective action, but inspections with numerous significant deficiencies have resulted in administrative and legal actions, such as license suspension, injunction, and prosecutions. Each year the FDA conducts an average of 1,700 inspections of blood and blood component manufacturers.[14]

Enforcement Actions

When a biological product manufacturer violates any of the laws the FDA enforces, the manufacturer is usually given an opportunity for voluntary correction before the FDA pursues enforcement actions. Enforcement actions are tools used by the FDA to bring biological product manufacturers that violate FDA laws into compliance. There are three types of enforcement actions: advisory, administrative, and judicial actions.

Advisory Actions: Warning Letter

The FDA will issue a warning letter to a biological product manufacturer if the FDA determines that deficiencies observed during an inspection are deviations from the regulations that could result in harm to the donor or distribution of an unsafe blood product or that represents a continuing pattern of noncompliance. A warning letter is a written communication from the FDA to the manufacturer notifying them that its product, practice, or other activity is in violation of the law.[15] The warning letter serves as a prior notice should the FDA decide to take further actions. The warning letter offers the manufacturer an opportunity to correct the deficiencies listed in the letter. The FDA will conduct a follow-up inspection of the manufacturing facility to determine if corrective actions have been implemented. Each year, the FDA issues an average of 20 warning letters to blood and blood component manufacturers.[14]

Administrative Actions[15]: Suspension, Revocation

Administrative actions apply only to licensed manufacturers. The FDA may suspend a manufacturer's license if there is a potential danger to the health of the donor or recipient as a result of the manufacturing operations at the facility (21 CFR 601.6). The FDA can administer this action immediately, and the manufacturer must take appropriate corrective actions. The manufacturer may not engage in interstate commerce of the product while taking corrective actions. Each year the FDA suspends the license of one or two blood and blood component manufacturers.[14]

A manufacturer's license will be revoked for several reasons: the FDA's inability to gain access to the facility to conduct an inspection; or if the FDA discovers significant cGMP deficiencies; or when the FDA determines that the product is not safe or effective for its intended use (21 CFR 601.5). The FDA may revoke a license when it observes that the deficiencies have been ongoing and have not been corrected after numerous inspections and warning letters. Revocation will prohibit the manufacturer from distributing the product into interstate commerce. Revocation is a lengthy process because the manufacturer has an opportunity for a hearing to show reasons why the license should not be revoked. Even so, the FDA revokes the license of one or two blood and blood component manufacturers each year.[14]

Judicial Actions[15]: Seizure, Injunction, Prosecution

Seizure is a civil action to condemn violative products and remove them from distribution channels. The FDA takes possession of the product under a court order. The court usually gives the owner of the seized product 30 days to decide on a course of action. The FDA will dispose of the product if the owner does not communicate proposed actions. The owner may contest the charges and litigate in court to have the seized products returned. The owner is required to provide a monetary deposit (e.g., a bond) to ensure that the orders of the court will be carried out and must pay for FDA supervision of any compliance procedure.

The FDA may consider an injunction when there is a current health hazard or the manufacturer has a history of uncorrected deviations despite past warnings, and the evidence suggests that serious violations will continue. The traditional injunction used by the FDA is the prohibitory injunction. Once ordered by the court, this civil action prohibits the manufacturer from operating until adequate corrections are made and verified by FDA investigators. The other type of injunction is a mandatory injunction. The court allows the manufacturer to operate while addressing certain specified conditions. An injunction may be used when the manufacturer does not hold a U.S. license. If there is no license to suspend or revoke, this is the only remedy left to

obtain the necessary corrective action. As of September 2003, two blood and blood component manufacturers were under consent decree of injunction.

A prosecution is a criminal action directed against a manufacturer or responsible individual(s) or both. The FDA may consider prosecution when fraud, health hazards, or continuing significant violations are encountered. The FD&C Act allows individuals for whom prosecution is being considered to be given an opportunity to present their views. Prosecution will proceed without a hearing if the violations are fraudulent or the responsible individuals are likely to flee.

Table 25–5 summarizes the different enforcement actions.

cGMP Regulations

The FDA defines a cGMP as a sound and feasible method that is current in the manufacturing industry that will either ensure or contribute to the manufacturing of a quality product.[16] A cGMP need not be widely prevalent in order to be a good manufacturing practice, but the cGMP regulations require all manufacturing facilities to implement and follow cGMP. Each step of the manufacturing process must be controlled to maximize the probability that the final product will be acceptable and meet quality and design specifications.

The FDA published the first drug cGMP regulations in 1963 after noticing that unsuitable products were being released.[17] The FDA believed that this was due to an increase in number and complexity of the tests being performed and untrained or undertrained personnel deviating from established standards. During inspections, the FDA observed that there were often no controls in place to monitor the whole manufacturing practice. The cGMP regulations were published to provide directions for this control and include the elements of quality assurance, quality control, and process validation. The cGMP regulations for blood and blood components were published in 1975.[18] Blood and blood component manufacturers must follow both the drug and blood cGMP regulations.

Quality Control Unit

The cGMP regulations require each manufacturer to designate an individual or group of individuals, known as a unit, to be responsible for ensuring that manufacturing controls are in place so that products will function as intended. The regulations identify this unit as a "quality control unit" (21 CFR 211.22). Today, many manufacturers identify this unit as a quality assurance unit.

The quality control unit's responsibilities must be described in writing and, at a minimum, include the following tasks:

- Approve and reject supplies, product, etc.
- Review records for accuracy and completeness
- Investigate errors and deviations from standards
- Review and approve standard operating procedures

The cGMP regulations do not require that the quality control unit perform all quality control functions, but the unit must ensure that all functions are performed properly. The cGMP regulations do not prescribe how each manufacturer should develop its quality control unit or program. This is to allow flexibility for each manufacturer to develop a program that will work best in its own manufacturing environment. The

TABLE 25–5   Summary Table of Enforcement Actions

Advisory actions	Warning letter	• Could cause harm to donor or distribution of unsafe product • Continuing pattern of noncompliance • Notice of possible further action • Manufacturer has opportunity to correct deviations
Administrative actions	Suspension	• Applied on licensed manufacturers only • Continuing pattern of noncompliance • Potential danger to health of donor or recipient • Manufacturer cannot engage in interstate commerce until deviations are corrected • FDA can take action quickly
	Revocation	• Applied to licensed manufacturers only • FDA cannot gain access to facility to inspect • Product is not safe or effective • Continuing pattern of noncompliance • Manufacturer cannot engage in interstate commerce • Lengthy process
Judicial actions	Seizure	• Civil action; court order needed • Condemn violative products and remove from distribution • FDA takes possession and could dispose product • Manufacturer can contest changes
	Injunction	• Civil action • Health hazard due to product or collection procedures • History of uncorrected deviations; violations will continue • Manufacturer can operate while correcting deviations • Applied on both licensed and unlicensed manufacturers
	Prosecution	• Criminal action • Fraud, health hazards, continuing significant violations • Applied to both licensed and unlicensed manufacturers

FDA has published a guidance document to assist blood and blood component manufacturers in developing quality programs.[19] The FDA does expect the quality control functions to be separate from the manufacturing operations because both have their own objectives that may sometimes conflict.

Quality Reviews

The FDA's quality assurance guidance document identifies the systems in a blood and blood component manufacturing operation and the critical control points that should be reviewed. The cGMP regulations require that the manufacturing records be reviewed at least annually (21 CFR 211.180). The quality control unit or other assigned individuals may perform this review. The FDA does not consider this required review an audit; records of these reviews may be requested during an FDA inspection.

The purpose of the review is to determine compliance with written procedures and cGMP. Specifically, the review should identify trends that could lead to the release of an unsuitable product. The quality control unit must investigate any errors or trends that could affect the manufacture of a quality product. The FDA expects that the outcome of such investigations will be the development and implementation of corrective and/or preventive actions. Implementing corrective and preventive actions could result in changes to product specifications or manufacturing or control procedures. The quality control unit must monitor these changes to ensure that they adequately address the error and will result in the manufacture of a quality product. The review, investigation, and corrective actions must be documented. The quality control unit must have the authority to stop production if it determines that the quality of the product is being adversely affected. The

quality control unit should share the results of the review with the management of the manufacturing operations in order to affect the necessary changes to correct and prevent ongoing problems.

Additional Requirements of Biologics Manufacturing

All biologics manufacturers must comply with all the biologics regulations in the CFR. This section lists some of the additional elements of biologics regulation.

Variances

The regulations allow for blood and blood component manufacturers to perform procedures that vary from what is required in the CFR (21 CFR 640.120). Specifically, manufacturers may request to vary from a regulation in Subchapter F of the CFR (Parts 600—680). Manufacturers that want to implement a procedure that varies from the regulations in these parts must submit a written request to the CBER. This requirement applies to all manufacturers, including licensed and unlicensed manufacturers and transfusion services. Manufacturers cannot implement an alternate procedure until they have received approval from the CBER. Examples of a variance include:

● Allowing collection of blood from hereditary hemochromatosis patients who meet all the other donor eligibility criteria and using this blood for allogeneic transfusion without specific labeling
● Allowing collection of plasmapheresis donors less than once every 8 weeks without monitoring donors' plasma protein levels or performing a physical examination

Contract Manufacturing

The change in the definition of a manufacturer has allowed the original manufacturer to employ the services of a contract manufacturer to perform some or all of the manufacturing steps.[20] The contractor is not under the direct control of the original manufacturer, but the original manufacturer is responsible for the compliance of the product being manufactured by the contractor. Contract manufacturers must be registered because they are performing a manufacturing step on a regulated product. In addition, the contractor must perform the manufacturing procedures according to regulations, cGMP, and product standards. Contractors must notify the original manufacturer of any changes in their operations because these changes could affect the product. The original manufacturer's quality control unit must ensure that the manufacturing steps performed by the contract manufacturer result in a quality product that meets product specifications. Examples of contract manufacturing include: (1) an outside testing laboratory performing infectious disease testing on donors or products; (2) another blood center irradiating blood products for transfusion.

Short Supply Agreements

A short supply agreement is an example of a cooperative manufacturing agreement. Short supply was introduced in 1948, and the provisions governing short supply are found in the CFR (21 CFR 601.22). The short supply regulations allow for an exemption from licensure in limited areas and under controlled conditions. Short supply agreements are usually arranged when a blood or blood component manufacturer wants to market recovered plasma. While the recovered plasma is not in short supply, the final products made from recovered plasma, such as factor VIII concentrates, can be in short supply. The short supply provision allows unlicensed source material, e.g., recovered plasma, to be shipped interstate and used to manufacture a licensed product. The short supply agreement must be in writing and is between the supplier of the recovered plasma, the blood and blood component manufacturer, and the licensed final product manufacturer. The written agreement specifies the necessary manufacturing procedures and labeling.

Brokers frequently act as intermediaries between suppliers and licensed final product manufacturers. Selling plasma to a broker does not relieve the supplier of the responsibility of obtaining a short supply agreement. Plasma brokers may act as authorized agents and should be identified in the agreement. Brokers that take physical possession of plasma must register with the FDA.

Biological Product Deviation Reporting

The regulations require all manufacturers, including licensed and unlicensed manufacturers and transfusion services, to report to the FDA any event that resulted in the distribution of a unsuitable product. Specifically, a manufacturer must report if it discovers a deviation in a manufacturing operation that adversely affects the safety, purity, or potency of the product and that product was distributed outside the manufacturer's control (21 CFR 606.171). The biological product deviation report (BPDR) must be submitted to the CBER within 45 calendar days of the date the event was discovered. Manufacturers may submit a hard copy report or report the

BPDR electronically at http://www.fda.cber/biodev/biodev.htm For additional information on BPDRs, contact the Division of Inspections and Surveillance, OCBQ, CBER (HFM-650), 1401 Rockville Pike, Suite 400S, Rockville, MD 20852-1448.

In 2002 the CBER received 33,370 BPDRs from blood and blood component manufacturers.[21] This represents 98.6% of the BPDRs reported to the CBER. The majority of the reports (69.2%) involved post donation information **(Table 25–6)**. Post donation information is information received from donors following the collection of the product. In many instances, this information is known by the donor at the time of donation and would have caused the donor to be deferred had the donor given the information to the blood center.

On occasion, the products from these donors are still at the blood center, but often they have already been distributed. The manufacturer should take appropriate action after reviewing the impact of the donor's information on product safety. The manufacturer may need to identify each affected product collected from a donor who is now determined to be unsuitable and recall these products.

Product Recalls

Product recalls are the manufacturer's removal or correction of a marketed product that the FDA considers to be in violation of the laws (21 CFR 7.3 and 7.40). Recalls are:

- Initiated by the manufacturer
- Requested by the FDA if the product represents a risk of illness or injury or there is misrepresentation to the consumer
- Ordered by the FDA if the product will cause imminent danger to the public health.

The manufacturer is responsible for developing a recall strategy and conducting the recall. The manufacturer must contact customers with information identifying the affected products and prescribe appropriate actions to take (21 CFR 7.49). The FDA will monitor the recall, assessing the manufacturer's efforts to notify the appropriate parties. A recall is classified as completed or closed when all reasonable efforts have been made to remove or to correct the product. The FDA may seize the product if it determines that the recall is ineffective.

Recalls of blood and blood components are different from most drug products because the unit of blood or blood component may already have been transfused. There can be no

TABLE 25–6   Biological Product Deviations Reported to the CBER in 2002

Manufacturing System	% of Total (33,370)
Post donation information	69.2
Quality control and distribution	11.6
Labeling	7.1
Donor screening	6.1
Routine testing (ABO, Rh, Antibody screen)	3.1
Component preparation	1.3
Blood collection	0.6
Miscellaneous	0.5
Donor deferral	0.4
Infectious disease testing	0.2

physical recall or return of the unit. When blood or a blood component has already been transfused, a recall is really a notification that the product did not meet product standards for safety, purity, and potency.

Recalls are accompanied by a health hazard evaluation of the recalled product by FDA scientists, usually physicians and nurses who work for the FDA, to determine if the product caused or could cause harm to a recipient (21 CFR 7.41). The recall will be classified based on the potential for the recalled product to cause serious health problems. In 2002, the CBER classified 2,052 recalls.[22] Blood and blood components represent the majority of the recalls (93.4%). Most of the recalls involved products that were either not likely to cause an adverse reaction or could cause only temporary health problems. About 5.4% of the recalls were for products that would predictably cause serious health problems or death.

Fatality Reporting

Blood and blood component manufacturers should initially notify the CBER of any transfusion-related fatalities or donation-related deaths as soon as possible after the incident is detected. The regulations require that the blood and blood component manufacturer notify the CBER within 7 days after the incident is detected (21 CFR 606.170).[23] The 7-day written report should describe all information related to the fatality. Collection facilities are required to report donation fatalities, and the facility that performed the compatibility tests must report the transfusion death. Fatalities are reported to the CBER to:

- Ensure that the incidents are thoroughly investigated
- Determine if appropriate corrective actions have been taken to prevent a recurrence
- Determine if there are trends that may warrant action by the FDA

FDA investigators will visit the reporting facility to follow up on the fatality reports. In 2002, the CBER received 85 transfusion-related fatality reports and 10 donation-related fatality reports.[22] Hemolytic transfusion reactions continue to be the most common cause of transfusion fatalities, and occult heart disease appears to be the most frequent cause of donation deaths. Additional information on reporting fatalities can be found on the CBER Web site at http://www.fda.gov/cber/transfusion.htm

Additional information about the FDA and regulatory issues related to blood and blood components can be found at http://www.fda.gov/cber

SUMMARY CHART:
Important points to remember (MT/MLT)

➤ The FDA enforces regulations to ensure the safety and efficacy of biologics, drugs, and devices, which include blood and blood components, blood collection supplies and machines, and blood bank reagents and infectious disease kits.

➤ Misbranding is defined as any false or misleading labeling, such as false therapeutic claims on the label.

➤ Adulteration is defined as manufacturing without adherence to cGMP in a manner that may render the product injurious to health.

➤ The ORA is responsible for performing FDA inspections and other surveillance activities.

➤ The FDA's five overlapping layers of safety include donor eligibility, donor deferral and registries, infectious disease testing, quarantine of unsuitable products, and investigation of adverse events.

➤ Biological products are defined as any virus, therapeutic serum, toxin, antitoxin, vaccine, blood, blood component or derivative, allergenic product, or analogous product applicable to the prevention, treatment, or cure of diseases or injuries of man.

➤ Statutes are the laws and acts passed by Congress granting the FDA the authority to fulfill its mission.

➤ The facilities required to register with the FDA under the FD&C Act include collection centers, community blood banks, component preparation facilities, hospital blood banks, plasmapheresis centers, product testing laboratories, storage and distribution centers, and brokers who take possession and manipulate and/or relabel the product.

➤ Seizure is a civil action to condemn violative products and remove them from distribution channels.

➤ The FDA defines a cGMP as a sound and feasible method that is current in the manufacturing industry that will either ensure or contribute to the manufacturing of a quality product.

➤ A variance allows a manufacturer of a blood product to perform an alternate procedure that deviates from requirements contained in certain sections of the CFR. An example of a variance is allowing collection of blood from a patient with hereditary hemochromatosis who meets all other donor eligibility criteria and using this blood for allogeneic transfusion without specific labeling.

➤ A product recall is the removal or correction of a marketed product that the FDA considers to be in violation of the laws.

➤ In the event of a fatality involving blood or a blood component, the manufacturer who performed the compatibility test must notify the CBER as soon as possible and provide a written report within 7 days of the incident.

REVIEW QUESTIONS

1. Which of the following is responsible for the safety of the nation's blood supply?
   a. Health Care Financing Administration
   b. Food and Drug Administration
   c. College of American Pathologists
   d. Occupational Safety and Health Administration

2. Where are the regulations for blood and blood products published?
   a. The AABB Technical Manual
   b. CAP Inspection Checklist

c. The Code of Federal Regulations

d. State Inspectional Guidance Documents

3. What was the tragedy that prompted passage of the Public Health Service Act?

 a. Three patients contracted hepatitis C following transfusion

 b. A child died following transfusion of hemolyzed red blood cells

 c. A group O patient received group A blood

 d. Thirteen children died after receiving diphtheria antitoxin contaminated with tetanus

4. What is required to ship blood and blood products across state lines (interstate)?

 a. AABB accreditation

 b. State license

 c. HCFA certification

 d. U.S. biologics license

5. Which enforcement action serves as an initial notification that the FDA has observed the manufacturer making violative products?

 a. Revocation

 b. Recall

 c. Warning letter

 d. Suspension

6. Which of the following is true about cGMP?

 a. cGMP need not be prevalent in the manufacturing industry

 b. A U.S. biologics license will be issued to a manufacturer who does not have a quality control plan

 c. The quality control unit must perform the entire quality function

 d. Blood and blood components do not have to comply with the drug cGMP regulations

7. A donor calls the blood bank and informs them that within a year prior to his donation he had had intimate contact with a person diagnosed with HIV. Which of the following actions is NOT required by FDA?

 a. Identify and recall all products from the donor

 b. Report the biological product deviation to the CBER if the product was distributed

 c. Enter the donor in a deferral registry

 d. Notify the AABB

8. A patient dies following transfusion of ABO-incompatible blood. To whom should this event be reported?

 a. The Center for Biologics Evaluation and Research

 b. The Health Care Financing Administration

 c. The AABB Central Office

 d. The Occupational Safety and Health Administration

9. Which federal group inspects a transfusion service that does not collect blood?

 a. Food and Drug Administration

 b. Centers for Medicare and Medicaid Services

 c. Occupational Safety and Health Administration

 d. State health department

10. Which of the following is NOT one of FDA layers of safety?

 a. Donor eligibility

 b. Biological license application

 c. Investigation of adverse events

 d. Infectious disease testing

REFERENCES

1. Code of Federal Regulations, Title 21, FDA. US Government Printing Office, Washington, DC, April 1, 2003.

2. Commemorating 100 Years of Biologics Regulation. Science and the Regulation of Biological Products from a Rich History to a Challenging Future, Center for Biologics Evaluation and Research, FDA, March 2002. (www.fda.gov/cber/inside/centennial.htm)

3. The Coroner's Verdict in the St. Louis Tetanus Cases. 1901 New York Medical Journal 74; Special Article: Fatal results from diphtheria antitoxin. Minor comments: Tetanus from antidiphtheria serum. JAMA, 1901; 37:1255, 1260

4. Public Health Service Act. Regulation of Biological Products. Title 42 United States Code, Chapter 6A, Part F, Section 262 (42USC262). (www.fda.gov/opacom/laws/phsvcact/phsvcact.htm)

5. Federal Food, Drug and Cosmetic Act. Drugs and Devices. Chapter V, Subchapter A. (www.fda.gov/opacom/laws/fdcact/fdctoc.htm)

6. History of the FDA. (www.fda.gov/oc/history/default.htm)

7. FDA Guidance for Industry: For the Submission of Chemistry, Manufacturing and Controls and Establishment Description Information for Human Blood and Blood Components Intended for Transfusion or for Further Manufacture and For the Completion of the Form FDA 356h "Application to Market a New Drug, Biologic or an Antibiotic Drug for Human Use," May 1999. (www.fda.gov/cber/guidelines.htm)

8. The FDA Modernization Act of 1997, November 21, 1997. (www.fda.gov/opacom/backgrounders/modact.htm)

9. FDA Guidance for Industry: Changes to an Approved Application: Biological Products: Human Blood and Blood Components Intended for Transfusion or for Further Manufacture, August 2001. (www.fda.gov/cber/guidelines.htm)

10. Memorandum of Understanding between the Health Care Financing Administration and the Food and Drug Administration. FDA Compliance Policy Guide – 7155e.03, Chapter 55E, September 1, 1983.

11. Blood Supply: FDA Oversight and Remaining Issue of Safety. U.S. General Accounting Office Report to the Ranking Minority Member; Committee on Commerce, House of Representatives, GAO/PEMD-97-1, February 1997.

12. FDA Compliance Program Guidance Manual. FDA Office of Regulatory Affairs, August 23, 2003. (www.fda.gov/ora/cpgm/default.htm)

13. FDA Compliance Policy Guides. FDA Office of Regulatory Affairs, July 8, 2003 (www.fda.gov/ora/compliance_ref/cpg/)

14. CBER's Regulatory Direction. Presentation by Steven M. Masiello, Director, Office of Compliance and Biologics Quality, CBER, FDA. FDA and the Changing Paradigm of Blood Regulations; January 15, 2003; New Orleans, LA.

15. FDA Regulatory Procedures Manual. FDA Office of Regulatory Affairs, August 1997. (www.fda.gov/ora/compliance_ref/rpm/default.htm)

16. Federal Register. 61 FR 20104, May 3, 1996.

17. Federal Register. June 20, 1963; 6385-6387.

18. Federal Register. 40 FR 53532, November 18, 1975.

19. FDA Guideline for Quality Assurance in Blood Establishments, July 11, 1995. (www.fda.gov/cber/guidelines.htm)

20. FDA Draft Guidance for Industry: Cooperative Manufacturing Agreements for Licensed Biologics, August 1999. (www.fda.gov/cber/guidelines.htm)

21. CBER Biological Product Deviation Reports, FY02 Summary, April 23, 2003. (www.fda.gov/cber/biodev/bpdrfy02.htm)

22. CBER Annual Report FY 2002 (October 1, 2001 through September 30, 2002). (www.fda.gov/cber/inside/annrpt.htm)

23. FDA Draft Guidance for Industry: Notifying FDA of Fatalities Related to Blood Collection or Transfusion, June 2002. (www.fda.gov/cber/gdlns/bldfatal.htm)

twenty-six

Informational Systems in the Blood Bank

Ann Tiehen, MT(ASCP)SBB, and Melissa Volny, MT(ASCP)SBB

OBJECTIVES

On completion of this chapter, the learner should be able to:

1. Describe the purpose of an information system in the blood bank.
2. Correlate the hardware components of a blood bank information system with their functions.
3. Illustrate a blood bank information system hardware configuation.
4. Describe the functions of the software components of a blood bank information system.
5. List the responsibilities for operating and maintaining a blood bank information system.
6. Identify regulatory and accrediting agency requirements pertaining to blood bank information systems.
7. Apply the functions of blood bank software applications to blood bank processes.

8. Describe the purpose of a truth table.
9. Construct a truth table for a routine blood bank test.
10. Name the standard operating procedures (SOPs) needed to manage a blood bank information system.
11. Describe and justify the kinds of testing that should be included in the validation of a blood bank information system.
12. Interpret the results of a software validation test.
13. Identify the times at which validation testing must be performed.
14. Define control function and differentate between process control and decision support.
15. Evaluate a validation test plan and identify its component parts.

Introduction

Information processing plays a vital role in blood banking practice. Proper management of information related to blood donors, blood components, and patients receiving transfusions is crucial to ensuring the safety and traceability of blood products. Blood bank personnel are relying more and more on computerized information systems to assist in the handling of this important information. Regulatory and standard-setting agencies have put increasing pressure on blood banks to be able to store information in a safe manner and to be able to retrieve it in a timely fashion. It must be pos-

sible to track a blood component from the time of its donation, through all of the processing steps, to the patient who receives it. It is also essential to be able to perform that trace in reverse order, from the recipient back to the donor. Before computerized information systems were available, all blood bank data were stored on paper, or "hard copy," records requiring labor-intensive and sometimes error-prone procedures to retrieve it. As blood bank information systems have become more sophisticated, they have made recovery of the information much more efficient and have offered the industry a great variety of process controls to reduce errors. Several acronyms unique to the specialty of information

TABLE 26–1	COMMON ACRONYMS
CPU:	Central processing unit
HIS:	Hospital information system
LIS:	Laboratory information system
PC:	Personal computer
RAM:	Random access memory
ROM:	Read-only memory
SOP:	Standard operating procedure

systems will be used throughout this chapter and are listed in **Table 26–1**.

Computerized blood bank information systems are available in many different configurations, but they comprise three general categories. They may take the form of a highly complex system like that found in a community blood center; they may be a small part of a complete clinical laboratory information system (LIS); or they may exist as a stand-alone system usually found in a hospital blood bank or transfusion service. The functionality of these systems varies from category to category and from vendor to vendor within each category. Some systems may act merely as record keepers, whereas others have the ability to use the information in such a way as to prevent errors in donor acceptance, blood component release, or patient transfusion. For example, a basic system used in a hospital transfusion service may simply allow the entry of an ABO group and Rh type in a patient's record with subsequent generation of a charge for the test. A more complex system in a hospital blood bank can record the donation of an autologous unit in the donor room and then make the transfusion service technologist aware of its presence when the patient is admitted for a type-and-screen test at the time of surgery.

System Components

A computer system includes three major components: hardware, software, and people. Hardware components are the physical pieces of equipment. Software is a set of instructions written in special computer language that tells the computer how to operate and manipulate the data. The people interface with the hardware to enter the data that are manipulated by the software. Just as there are many different kinds of people who enter data, so there are many different kinds of hardware and software.

Hardware

Most of the hardware components of a computer system are readily identifiable because they can be seen and touched, although some are hidden inside a case or a central system unit. Each piece of hardware performs a specific function in the handling of information. The three main functions performed by hardware components are processing, input/output, and storage.

Hardware components include a central system unit, sometimes referred to as the "box," and a number of different peripheral devices that send or receive information through the system unit. Peripheral devices include display terminals, keyboards, bar code readers, scanners and wands, pointing devices such as mice, printers, and modems. The hardware components and the way in which they are connected to each

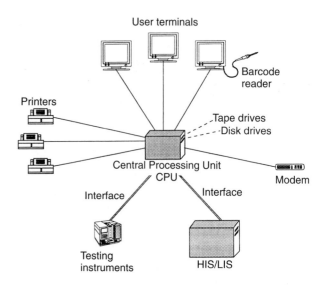

■ **FIGURE 26–1** Example of a blood bank information hardware configuration.

other is the system configuration. **Figure 26–1** illustrates one such configuration.

Processing Hardware

The central hardware component of a computer system is the central processing unit (CPU), which is an electric circuit or silicon "chip" that processes information. The CPU, also called a *processor,* is the core of the machine. It controls the interpretation and execution of instructions provided by the software. Other pieces of processing hardware that exist in the system unit are the ROM and RAM chips. ROM stands for *read-only memory* and contains the "start-up" instructions for the computer. *Random access memory* (RAM) is an array of chips where data are temporarily entered while they are being processed. When a computer is turned on, these chips interact with each other and the operating system software to prepare the computer to accept data and instructions from its users.

Input and Output Devices

Although users can occasionally be seen shouting at their computer systems, most blood bank information systems cannot recognize voice instructions. Commands and data must be entered in a format that the computer can understand. This requires tools that are connected to the system's CPU such as keyboards, pointing devices, bar code readers, and testing instruments. Keyboards are used to type instructions that tell the computer what to do or to enter data such as donor demographic information or patient test results. Many systems also accept bar-coded information from sources such as blood component labels or test tubes. Blood component labels contain many pieces of bar-coded information, including the unit number, blood type, product type, facility identification number, and expiration date. Entry of this information by a bar code reader is much more accurate than when done by manual entry methods. **Figure 26–2** shows a blood component label with this bar-coded information. Scanning the bar codes with an optical or laser device allows efficient entry of the blood component data.

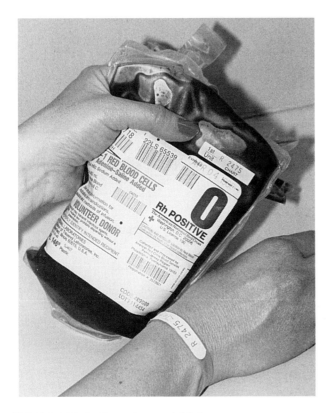

■ FIGURE 26–2   Bar codes on unit label.

The most common output device is the monitor, which displays information as it is typed on the keyboard. Together, the monitor and the keyboard make up the user terminal. The monitor may also display historical information at the request of the user.

Another commonly used output device is the printer, which provides hard-copy output on paper. Printers can produce labels, donor registration records, compatibility tags, management reports, patient chart reports, and donor correspondence. The kind of printer chosen for any of these applications depends on the quality of print desired. For example, a bar code label printer requires a high-resolution printing capability for accurate interpretation by the bar code reader. Management reports, which are usually used internally, can be of lower quality print.

A modem is an example of a combined input and output device. Modems allow computer systems to communicate with each other via telephone lines. Blood banks can use this mechanism to connect remote facilities to the main computer system so that all sites have access to the system's databases. This configuration is found in blood centers with several collection or testing locations or in a system of hospital affiliates. The technical support staff of software vendors uses modems to investigate and to solve system problems and to transfer files to the customer.

Information Storage Hardware

All computer systems have hardware that allows long-term storage of data. This is sometimes referred to as "memory" but should not be confused with RAM, which is only temporary and active when the system is turned on. Long-term memory is data saved on a medium from which they can later be retrieved, such as a hard disk. Most systems contain a hard disk controlled by a hard drive. The disk is made of metal coated with a magnetic film and contains software applications (programs) and user-entered data. The hard disk is often contained in the main system unit, but it may also be a peripheral device. The information on the disk is accessed by entering commands, usually with a keyboard connected to a display terminal. Other information storage hardware may be used for archiving old information that has been removed from the hard disk.

Software

Software tells the computer what to do with all of the information it has received. Minimally, every computer system has two kinds of software—operating system software and application software. Some systems may also use interface software, which allows the system to communicate with other computer systems.

Application Software

An application is software that has been designed to perform specific tasks. Personal computers (PCs) can be equipped with application programs such as word processing, spreadsheets, and databases. In a blood bank information system, the application software allows users to perform tasks that are specific to blood bank operations. In a donor setting, some of these tasks might include entry of donor demographic information and test results, confirmation of blood component labeling, and generation of donor recruitment lists. In a transfusion service, the computer may help with tasks such as searching for a blood component of a particular ABO group, entering blood component modification information, and issuing blood for transfusion. These tasks are very distinctly connected to blood banking and would be difficult, if not impossible, to perform in an application not specifically designed for blood bank use. One of the most important functions performed by blood bank applications is maintaining a database of donors, blood components, and transfusion recipients. A database is an organized set of information divided into files and then further subdivided into records. Files exist in one of two ways: they may be static or dynamic. The dynamic files contain records related to a specific donor, patient, or blood component. These records are frequently changed as updated information is added to them. For example, the status of a blood component can go from "quarantined" to "transfused," with many intermediate statuses during its shelf life. The static files contain information that is updated infrequently, such as the list of blood products used in the facility. These files, which look different in each blood bank, define the terminology that the blood bank uses. When a new blood bank information system is installed, the static files must be defined before the system can be put into use. One of the most important functions of the static files is to provide a "dictionary" of coded terms that the information system can use to sort and organize the tremendous amount of data entered into it. For example, two static files, one containing codes for physicians and the other codes for blood products, can allow the system to sort information regarding the crossmatch-to-transfusion (C:T) ratio of each physician who ordered blood within a particular period of time.

Figure 26–3 shows how the parts of a database relate to

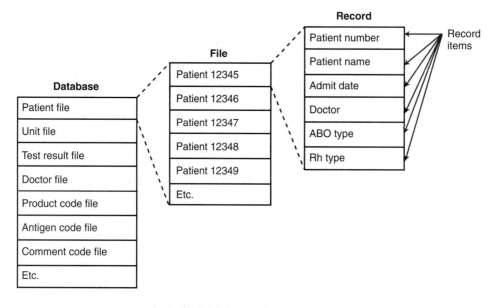

■ **FIGURE 26–3**   Database components.

each other. The database itself can be considered a file cabinet containing folders or files that, in turn, contain specific records. This illustration is of a dynamic file containing patient records. A static file illustrated in this way, for example, for blood product codes would list a separate file for each blood product code used in the facility. The associated records would include such information as the official name of the blood component, its maximum allowable shelf life, and whether it contains red blood cells (RBCs), thus requiring crossmatching.

Operating System Software

The tasks performed by the operating system are fairly invisible to users because this software works in the background. It is a set of instructions that controls the computer's hardware, manipulates the application software, and coordinates the flow of data to and from disks and memory. When new data are entered into one of the application programs, it is the operating system that places those data on the disk for storage; when a request for those data is made through the application program, the operating system retrieves them and sends them to the application software for display on a monitor or printed report.

Interface Software

Frequently, different information systems must be allowed to share data with each other to take full advantage of their functionality. Because different systems communicate in different computer languages, they need an interpreter that will allow data to flow between the two systems in a controlled manner. The interpreter is another set of software called an interface. Interface software may be used to allow data to flow between a hospital information system (HIS) and the blood bank system, or the LIS and the blood bank. For example, an interface between the HIS and the blood bank information system can allow flow of patient demographic information from the HIS to the blood bank system and allow test results and blood

component information to flow from the blood bank system to the HIS, where they can be displayed on terminals in patient care areas.

People

The human components of a blood bank information system are the users and at least one person designated the system manager. Users have access to the technical applications needed to perform daily blood bank operations. System managers require access to a wider range of applications, including system maintenance functions.

Users

Entry of commands and data into the system is performed by the users. The success with which a blood bank computer system can be used depends not only on its ease of use but also on the training provided to its users. Most systems are equipped with both a "live" or production database and a "test" database. The static files in both databases are identical, but their dynamic files contain different information. The production database contains real information, whereas the test database consists of fictitious records. The test database offers the user an opportunity to practice the applications of the system (and to make mistakes) without corrupting the database containing actual donor and patient information. Users should be trained in every application they will be expected to use.

System Managers

The configuration and location of the information system will determine the identity and quantity of people performing this task. In a large community blood center, there may be an entire staff dedicated to the management of the system. In a hospital blood bank or transfusion service that uses the blood bank module of a complete clinical LIS, the laboratory system manager is likely to have responsibility for the entire system, but there should also be a designated blood bank system manager. In blood banks equipped with a stand-alone blood bank computer, designated system managers may also have other supervisory, technical, or quality assurance duties as part of their job description.

Whatever the duties of the system manager, the manager also oversees the maintenance of the system's hardware and software. Some specific duties include adding or deleting items from the static database files, assigning access codes to new users, and implementing software upgrades from the vendor. In addition, the system manager will be required to investigate problems encountered by the users and to report them to the system vendor.

Blood Bank Software Applications

The kinds of data that must be managed by a particular blood bank information system depend on the types of services provided by the blood bank. Most community blood centers focus on donations and distribution of the donated blood components to customer hospitals. In the hospital transfusion service, the primary concern is the transfusion of patients. However, a community blood center or a hospital blood bank with both a transfusion service laboratory and a donation center must address issues of both donor and patient management. Application programs exist for every task, from scheduling donors to assigning a transfused status to a blood component. Many of the typical blood bank information system applications currently available are discussed in this section.

Donation Facility

Donor Management

The system should allow the capture of donor demographic information necessary for definitive donor identification, telephone contact for recruitment, and notification in the event that abnormal laboratory testing results are obtained. In addition, the system should have a means for preventing a donation from a deferred individual or from one attempting to donate before the required waiting period between donations.

Donor Registration

When a potential donor registers at a donation facility, several pieces of demographic data must be provided, such as social security number, name, date of birth, phone number, and mailing address. When this information is entered into the donor database, the system can search for a previous donation record from the same donor. If none is found, a new donor record is created. If there is a record of a previous donation, the system can review the donor's eligibility status. This would include calculating the length of time elapsed since the last donation and examination of the record for a deferral because of medical history or disease testing results. If the donor is ineligible because of an inadequate amount of time since the last donation or a previous deferral, the system can alert the registrar and prevent an unsuitable donation from occurring. If the registration is taking place at a location that does not have immediate access to the electronic database, as happens on a mobile blood drive, the registrars can be equipped with a printed list of eligible and ineligible donors.

Alternatively, the database can be downloaded to a portable PC and transported to the mobile site.

Donation Data

Information regarding the donation event can also be entered into the system. This data entry is usually performed after the donation but can include such important information as the unique identification number applied to the collection container, the type of donation made (e.g., whole blood or apheresis), the collection time, and the occurrence of a donor reaction. If the donation is intended for a specific recipient, as in the case of an autologous or designated donation, data regarding the intended recipient can be entered.

Donor Recruitment

The capture of donor demographic information at registration allows the collecting facility to recruit the donor from a system-generated list of eligible donors. Mailing labels can be generated for recruitment efforts. Once laboratory testing is associated with the donor's record, lists of donors meeting special needs can be printed. Such lists may include donors with a specific ABO group, other RBC antigen type, or cytomegalovirus (CMV) seronegativity.

Blood Component Management

Component Production

After a whole blood unit has been collected, it is usually delivered to a component-processing laboratory where it is separated into different components, including RBCs, fresh frozen plasma, and platelets, and labeled appropriately. Data on the new components created are entered into the system with the unique donation identification number assigned at the time of donation, new blood product codes, time of preparation, and expiration dates.

Laboratory Testing

Samples of the donor's blood that were collected at the time of donation and labeled with the same unique donation identification number are tested for ABO, Rh, atypical antibodies, and markers of transfusion-transmitted diseases such as hepatitis and human immunodeficiency virus. The results of all of these tests are entered into the system so that they are associated with the unique donation identification number as well as with the donor. In larger community blood centers, the results of testing performed on automated instruments can be sent directly from the instrument to the system via an instrument interface.

Label Application and Verification

After completion of component production and laboratory testing, the blood products are labeled with the ABO/Rh type. This is a crucial step and must be controlled stringently so that no unsuitable blood products are released into the blood supply. After the label has been applied, the unique donation identification number and ABO/Rh type bar codes on the blood component label can be scanned into the system with a bar code reader. This allows the system to perform a final check on donor suitability and blood type. If the component "passes" this verification, the blood component can be placed in the available inventory.

Inventory Management and Product Shipping

The collection facility staff members who are responsible for product distribution to customer hospitals must have access to the entire inventory of available blood products. As transfusion services place requests for quantities and ABO/Rh types of blood components, the distribution staff can monitor and control distribution to optimize blood use within the community. For example, blood products nearing their expiration date can be sent to active transfusion services where there is a high probability of transfusion before expiration. As products are shipped to transfusing facilities, their status is updated in the system, along with the identification of the facility to which they were shipped.

Transfusing Facility

Blood Component Management

Product Receipt and Entry

When the products are received at the transfusing facility, they are entered into the blood bank information system, where the entire inventory of blood components is maintained. If ABO/Rh confirmation is required, as in the case of components containing RBCs, a status of quarantine will be assigned by the system until confirmation testing is completed. Components not requiring ABO/Rh confirmation testing may be assigned a status of "available" on entry into the system.

Inventory Management

A computerized inventory makes it easy for blood bank staff members to monitor inventory levels so that levels do not drop below predefined minimums. Most systems sort the inventory by product code, ABO/Rh, and expiration date, and output it to a display monitor or printed report. When a selection list of blood components is indexed in this way, the products that are closer to the end of their shelf lives can be chosen for patients with a high likelihood of transfusion.

Blood Component Modification

Many components require modification to meet the special transfusion needs of a particular patient. Modifications include irradiation, leukocyte reduction, aliquoting (dividing), washing, and pooling. As these physical modifications are performed in the blood bank, the steps associated with them are captured by the information system, either by changing the product name or by adding a special attribute to the component data. Some of these steps may also require a shortening of the shelf life of the component, and the system can enter the new expiration date and time, if applicable. Attributes may also be added to components that have undergone special testing, such as tests for antibodies to CMV or specific RBC antigens.

Component Status Tracking

After blood components are received in the transfusion service, they are assigned various statuses, ending with a final dis-

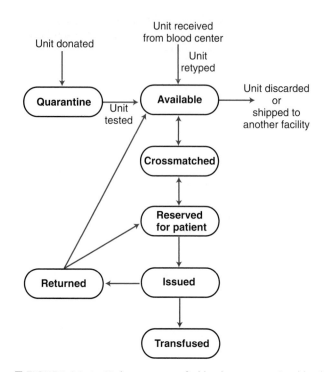

■ **FIGURE 26–4** Various statuses of a blood component in a blood bank information system.

position of "transfused" or "discarded." Each blood component record in the information system should contain a complete status history. **Figure 26–4** illustrates the various statuses that a blood component may be ascribed throughout its shelf life.

Patient Management

Patient Identification

A blood bank information system used by a facility issuing blood for transfusion should have the capability of capturing patient demographic information such as name and unique facility identification number. Other essential data include previous ABO/Rh type, transfusion history, previously identified clinically significant antibodies, and transfusion instructions such as the need for irradiated or leukocyte-reduced cellular components.

Order Entry

On receipt of a specimen for patient testing, the system can retrieve previous test results and alert the technologist to special transfusion requirements of the patient. For example, the record for a patient with a history of a clinically significant antibody can alert the technologist to the need for specific antigen-negative RBC components. Physicians' orders for blood components can also be entered.

Patient Testing

Some systems allow direct entry of test results into the system, thus replacing paper worksheets. If appropriate "truth tables" have been set up in the system, the entered test results can be compared with those of the truth tables for accuracy. Truth tables define the combination of results considered

TABLE 26–2   ABO TRUTH TABLE

Anti-A	Anti-B	A₁ Cells	B Cells	Interpretation
0	0	+	+	O
+	0	0	+	A
0	+	+	0	B
+	+	0	0	AB

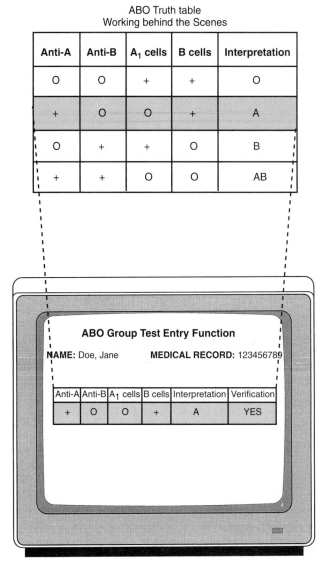

ABO Truth table
Working behind the Scenes

Anti-A	Anti-B	A₁ cells	B cells	Interpretation
O	O	+	+	O
+	O	O	+	A
O	+	+	O	B
+	+	O	O	AB

ABO Group Test Entry Function

NAME: Doe, Jane   MEDICAL RECORD: 123456789

Anti-A	Anti-B	A₁ cells	B cells	Interpretation	Verification
+	O	O	+	A	YES

■ FIGURE 26–5   Display monitor: entry of a valid ABO group.

valid for a particular test. This can prevent the release of invalid results such as nonmatching forward and reverse types. **Table 26–2** shows how such a truth table might look. Each row represents one combination of individual test results and an interpretation, which the system will allow in its ABO test entry function. In the case of the ABO test, there are only four valid result combinations, and the system warns the user if any other combination is entered. When the results are entered correctly and match one of the valid combinations in the truth table, the results are accepted and verified. Other tests, such as $Rh_0(D)$ and antibody screen, may also have to meet their own truth table requirements. **Figure 26–5** illustrates what a user would see on the display monitor when a valid ABO group is entered. Invisible to most users is the truth table, which in this figure is highlighted where the valid combination of results has been found to indicate the match with the valid ABO results entered and displayed on the monitor. Truth tables make their presence known when an invalid combination of results is entered. **Figure 26–6** illustrates what a user might see when invalid ABO results are entered. In this example, an incorrect result has been entered for the reaction of the patient's plasma or serum with group B reagent RBCs. When the technologist attempts to verify the results, the computer responds with a warning message, indicating that it was not able to find a match in the truth table for this particular combination of results.

The most critical test performed in the blood bank is the patient ABO/Rh type, and it is required that previous test results be compared with current results. When this comparison, performed by the system, reveals a discrepancy, a warning alerts the technologist to the possibility of a mislabeled specimen or incorrect test results.

Blood Component Reservation

The system can aid in the selection of blood components that will satisfy special transfusion needs and that are compatible with the patient's ABO/Rh. Selections may be made by manual entry, bar code entry, or from an indexed selection list. If autologous or designated blood components are available for a patient, the system can alert the user. As blood components are selected and either crossmatched or reserved for a patient, the system links those products to the patient record and prints compatibility tags.

A fairly recent application available on some systems is the computer crossmatch. It allows electronic verification of recipient and donor compatibility and dispenses with the serologic crossmatch test. A patient is eligible for the computer crossmatch when his or her records indicate that two criteria have been met: (1) there is no current or past history of clinically significant antibodies, and (2) there are at least two concordant ABO grouping test results. In addition, the system must contain the donation identification number, component name, component ABO group and Rh type, the interpretation of the component ABO confirmatory test, and recipient information including ABO group and Rh type. The system must process this information to alert the user when there are discrepancies between donor unit labeling and blood group confirmatory test interpretation and when ABO incompatibilities exist between the recipient and donor unit. Finally, the system must require verification of correct entry of data before release of blood components. These stringent requirements for a computer crossmatch must be in place to prevent the issue of ABO-incompatible components.

Result Reporting

Information regarding patient test results and any products linked to the patient should be accessible to the patient's caregivers. This may be in the form of printed reports and/or monitor displays. The status of linked products should be updatable. That is, as the products go from crossmatched or reserved, to issued, to transfused or returned, the status should be reported.

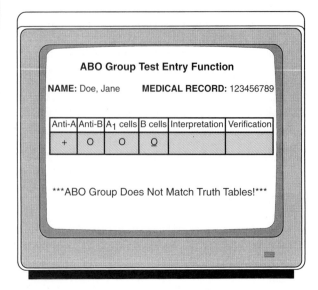

■ **FIGURE 26–6**   Display monitor: entry of an invalid ABO group.

Blood Component Issue

When blood components are requested for transfusion, the system can assist in issuing them appropriately. For example, if both an autologous RBC and an allogeneic RBC have been reserved for the same patient, it is essential that the autologous unit be issued first. Many systems alert the issuer if he or she attempts to issue the allogeneic unit first. In addition, the system can warn if a special transfusion need is not being met by the product being issued. Verification of unit inspection before issue can also be recorded in the system. When a product is issued, the system updates its status in the inventory.

General System Applications

In addition to the requirements specific to a collection or transfusion facility, there are general applications that are found in all blood bank information systems. These functions assist with system security, quality assurance, and management reports.

Security

It is critical for only authorized users to have access to the information contained in a blood bank computer system. Access is obtained through the use of assigned user codes and passwords, and it is the responsibility of the users to keep their passwords confidential. A second level of security restricts some users to some of the system's functions. This is important for two reasons: donor/patient confidentiality and protection of data from accidental or unauthorized destruction or modification. Sensitive information, such as test results for markers of transfusion-transmitted disease, should be available only to the medical director and selected supervisory personnel. The system manager has access to most or all of the functions, including those that allow modification of the static database files. Technical staff members can access those functions that are specific to their jobs, such as test result entry, labeling, or component production. Clerical staff members may be restricted to inquiry functions that allow them to answer questions from patients or physicians but not to enter or to modify patient data. In addition to providing system security, user codes capture the identity of each person performing each step in the information system.

Quality Assurance

Control Functions

One of the most useful features that a blood bank information system can offer is assistance to users in ensuring safe transfusion. When blood bank personnel depend on this assistance in making decisions at critical points in the selection of donors and release of blood products for transfusion, the system is said to be exerting "control functions." Control functions can be placed in two general categories: (1) process control and (2) decision support. Process control functions are decisions made by the system without human intervention. Decision support control functions occur when the system displays information to the user, who then decides on the next course of action. **Table 26–3** shows some examples of control functions.

Corrected or Amended Results

Sometimes it is necessary to correct or amend incorrect or incomplete information that was entered into the system. This need arises when errors are made in testing or when testing is performed on a mislabeled specimen so that results are associated with the wrong patient. When corrections must be made, both the original erroneous results and the corrected results must be clearly specified as such on monitor displays and printed reports. **Figure 26–7** illustrates one method for

TABLE 26–3   EXAMPLES OF CONTROL FUNCTIONS

Application	Process Control	Decision Support
Donor management	Prevention of registration of permanently deferred donor	Warning of current ABO/Rh not matching previous results
Blood component management: Collection facility	Prevention of unit release if testing unacceptable	Calculation of component expiration date
Blood component management: Transfusing facility	Prevention of entry of donation indentification number that already exists in the system	Warning of entry of an expiration date that exceeds the possible shelf life of a blood component
Patient management	Prevention of issue of outdated unit	Warning of product not meeting special transfusion needs

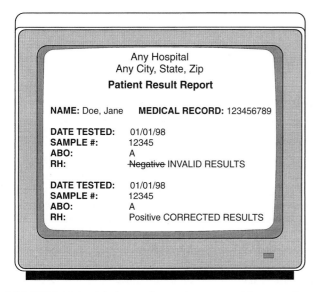

Any Hospital
Any City, State, Zip
Patient Result Report

NAME: Doe, Jane   **MEDICAL RECORD:** 123456789

DATE TESTED: 01/01/98
SAMPLE #:   12345
ABO: A
RH: ~~Negative~~ INVALID RESULTS

DATE TESTED: 01/01/98
SAMPLE #:   12345
ABO: A
RH: Positive CORRECTED RESULTS

■ **FIGURE 26–7**   Display monitor: patient report with corrected result.

correcting erroneous results. This method of error correction alerts caregivers who may have made clinical decisions based on the incorrect results. The information system should make it impossible to simply delete the erroneous result and substitute a corrected result.

Blood Product Utilization Review

Transfusion services are required by several accrediting agencies to monitor the utilization of blood products within the facility. This includes both blood ordering and transfusing practices of physicians. An information system can be of tremendous help in sorting and reporting utilization data. C:T ratios can be reported for individual physicians and for services such as surgery and obstetrics.

Management Assistance

Enormous amounts of different kinds of data can be entered into the blood bank information system. When appropriate reporting capabilities are designed into the system, they can provide valuable information to assist in management decisions. Reports of the number of donors drawn and deferred or blood products transfused and expired can help evaluate productivity and future resource needs. In addition, patient or hospital billing can be done more accurately and consistently than with manual systems.

Regulatory and Accreditation Requirements

Over the last 15 years, blood bank computer systems have been the subject of increasing regulatory oversight. In the late 1980s, the United States Food and Drug Administration (FDA) recognized that unsuitable blood components were being released into the blood supply because of inadequately controlled and validated computer systems. In 1988 and 1989, the FDA issued memoranda to registered blood establishments to provide guidance on the use of computer systems. In 1993 the FDA issued a draft guideline for the validation of

blood establishment computer systems, which outlined a validation program in compliance with current good manufacturing practices. After that, in 1994 and 1995, memoranda were sent to blood establishment computer software manufacturers, advising them that the FDA intended to regulate blood bank software as a medical device under the Safe Medical Devices Act of 1990. These regulatory initiatives have had significant impact on the availability and implementation of blood bank information systems. Both software vendors and users must follow prescribed guidelines in the introduction of new software. Vendors must perform thorough validation testing before making software available for purchase, and users must document validation procedures on site before using such a system.

Voluntary accreditation agencies, such as the Joint Commission on Accreditation of Healthcare Organizations, the American Association of Blood Banks (AABB), and the College of American Pathologists, also have standards or inspection checklist items that emphasize the responsibilities of operating an information system. A blood bank must have documented evidence of validation of its system as well as written procedures for all aspects of system management so as to comply with regulatory and accreditation requirements.

System Management

Many responsibilities are associated with the operation and maintenance of a computerized blood bank information system. The bulk of these responsibilities occur when a system is first installed as new SOPs are written, the system is validated, and personnel are trained. After a system is established, routine maintenance procedures are performed to ensure the ongoing operation of the system.

SOPs

Written procedures for every blood bank operation are required by all regulatory and accreditation agencies, and computer operations are no exception. The computer-related tasks associated with each of the blood bank's technical operations can be incorporated into each technical procedure or can be addressed in a separate section of the procedures manual. In addition, there are a number of computer-specific SOPs that must also be available. The subjects of these are included in the following discussions.

Archiving Data

As the system's databases grow in size, the hard disk becomes crowded with this stored information. As a result, the response time of the computer reaches an undesirably slow pace, and the hard disk is no longer able to store new data. When this happens, additional hard disks may be added to the system, or old data may be removed from the hard disk and placed in archival storage. Removing old data frees up space on the hard disk so that new data can be placed on it. Old data may be archived to long-term storage media as such as tape, disk, microfiche, or even paper. A procedure for periodic assessment of hard disk space should be instituted so that data can be archived in an orderly fashion before the hard disk becomes full. Procedures for archiving must also be written and should adhere to applicable regulatory and standard-setting agency requirements for data retention. For example,

AABB standards require that each donor's ABO group and Rh type be retained for a minimum of 5 years, and patient records of adverse reactions to transfusion must be retained indefinitely. Written procedures for retrieval of archived data must ensure that records can be retrieved within a reasonable period to maintain patient care.

Backup of Software Programs and Data

Blood banks have come to depend heavily on their information systems, but systems are not infallible. Unexpected, and sometimes inexplicable, failures of software or hardware can occur. Worse, a natural disaster such as a fire or flood can destroy parts or all of an information system. Software and databases should be routinely copied to some storage medium, such as tape or another set of disks. The copies can then be used to restore any corrupted or lost information. The frequency with which this backup routine is performed depends on an individual blood bank's data volume and the recommendations of the software vendor. The copies should be stored in a safe location separate from the information system so that they will not be affected by disastrous events such as fire or flooding. There should also be a procedure to identify and restore any information that was not included in the backup copies. This can be done by manually reentering data that was input between the time of the most recent backup and the disaster.

Computer Downtime

Every computer system, at some period, experiences downtime. Sometimes the downtime is planned, as when the system must undergo maintenance procedures, system backup, or software enhancement. Other downtimes are unplanned and usually unpleasant, because the system is experiencing some difficulty, such as a power outage. In either case, there must be a written procedure that will allow blood bank operations to continue. The procedure must address the need for historical patient and donor data as well as systems for recording new data obtained during the downtime. Transfusion service staff must be able to compare current patient test results with previous records before blood components are issued. Donor center staff must have access to permanently deferred donor files. This essential information may be in the form of paper records or may be available to personnel on a PC where the information has been previously downloaded from the blood bank information system. New data generated during downtime—such as test results, blood donations, and distribution or issuance of blood products—can be recorded on hard-copy worksheets or forms and then "backloaded" into the computer when it becomes functional.

Hardware Maintenance

Information system hardware, like all pieces of equipment, requires periodic cleaning, lubrication, and replacement of parts to ensure continued operation. Maintenance procedures usually require that the system be "taken down" or turned off for a period. For that reason, regular maintenance procedures should be scheduled and posted so that blood bank staff members can prepare for downtime. When possible, maintenance should be scheduled to minimize interruption of service, such as during usual periods of low activity.

As the system's databases grow in size, the response time of the computer may reach an undesirably slow pace. Procedures should be established for removing the data from the disk. The software will contain programs for purging and archiving older data. Vendors may also offer support services that can examine the system disk(s) to identify potential problems.

Maintenance of Security

A procedure for adding users to a system must be established, including the basis on which security levels will be assigned. For example, the list of functions or applications to which a user will have access can be created for each job description. It is also important to have a method for deleting the access codes of users who leave the facility. An additional level of security can be obtained by requiring users to change their passwords periodically; many security applications can be programmed to require this at specified intervals.

Tracking and Correction of Errors

Error management, required by regulatory and accrediting agencies, has become an integral part of blood bank operations. It includes detection, documentation, investigation, implementation of corrective actions, and reporting to appropriate agencies. Errors in the operation of a blood bank information system may be caused by inadequate training, incomplete or cumbersome written procedures, or system problems. In any case, tracking and categorization of errors is essential if corrective actions are to be taken. Identified information system problems should be reported to the software vendor so that other users can be notified and remedies can be included in a future software revision.

Personnel Training

The most elegant and user-friendly information system can be a disaster if staff members are inadequately trained in its use. Training programs should address every function and procedure that each user will be expected to perform. Flowcharts and checklists are useful training tools. Training modules can be designed that present users with the situations that they will encounter in their work. The competence of each staff person must be documented before allowing routine use of the computer. Competence assessment methods can include direct observation, review of system-generated records, and written examinations. Once initial competence has been demonstrated, an ongoing program of periodic assessment must be established to document the continued competence of blood bank staff to use the information system appropriately. As previously discussed, it is most beneficial to allow users access to a test database for training purposes. If one is not available, test data can be used in the production database.

Validation of Software

Software validation is the establishment of documented evidence that provides a high degree of assurance that the system will consistently function as expected. It is the responsibility of the software vendor to validate, to the extent possible, the functionality of a software product before it is marketed to blood banks. However, software vendors cannot simulate the conditions in which each system will be used. Differences in environment, hardware, databases, SOPs, and people require that each blood bank perform on-site validation testing to prove that the system will perform appropriately under those unique conditions.

Validation testing must be performed before a new system can be implemented and whenever new software, databases, or hardware is added to the system. When validation is to be performed on an existing system, the testing should be done in the test database, where it will not affect the production data.

Test Plan

Proper validation of the system requires careful planning. Each system function that the blood bank will use must be included in the test plan. A test plan should be created for each function or operation that the computer will perform. Test plans should include the following items:

- Control functions
- Data entry methods (keyboard, bar code reader, instrument interface, LIS, or HIS interface)
- Specific test cases
- Documentation methods
- Acceptance criteria (expected outputs)
- Result review
- Corrective action (if necessary)
- Acceptance

Most of these items will be different in each of the system's applications, so a separate test plan for each application may be necessary. Control functions should be defined by the vendor, but data entry methods will be selected by the user; some applications may have multiple data entry methods. Specific tests cases are discussed below. Screen printouts, written logs, or printed reports can be used to document the testing. After the testing is completed, the results should be compared with acceptance criteria to determine acceptability. If unacceptable results are obtained, they should be investigated, and corrective action should be implemented. When corrective action is necessary, testing should be repeated until it is found acceptable.

Test Cases

The validation test cases include the specific steps to be followed by those performing the testing. Test cases should assess the system under normal operating conditions but must also offer challenges to the system. The goal is to make sure that the system repeatedly performs intended functions and does not perform unintended functions. The types of testing that should be performed are termed normal, boundary, invalid, special, and stress cases.

1. Normal testing uses typical blood bank inputs to produce normal, or routine, outputs.
2. Boundary testing involves forcing the system to evaluate data that are slightly below or slightly above valid ranges. This kind of testing might be used for disease test results.
3. Invalid test cases assess the system's ability to recognize and to reject incorrect inputs. Examples of invalid inputs include entry of Q for an ABO interpretation or entry of a blood product code that has not been defined in the static database file.
4. Special cases are those that make the system react to unusual inputs. A special case could be designed to see how the system responds when more than one person attempts to add or edit special transfusion instructions in the same patient's record.
5. Stress testing involves pushing the system to its physical limits. This might be accomplished by allowing large volumes of data to be entered into the system via all available input devices.

Not every type of test case may be appropriate for each function to be tested. For example, boundary test cases will probably not be applicable in a donor registration function. Another kind of validation testing is parallel testing. This involves running two systems in parallel and comparing the outputs of both. For a blood bank switching from a manual to a computerized system, every procedure would be performed manually and in the computer.

Validation of a blood bank information system is a very lengthy and labor-intensive process, but it provides great benefits if undertaken in a thorough manner. Extensive testing will identify potential problems in the way that the blood bank intends to use the system. Sometimes workarounds have to be created, but when it is done as part of validation testing, staff members can be properly trained before going "live" on the new system or software. The creation and performance of comprehensive and detailed validation test cases require allocation of significant resources to the project, but the end result, a well-validated blood bank information system, is worth the resource costs.

SUMMARY CHART:
Important points to remember (MT/SBB)

➤ Blood bank information systems assist in the management of data and can allow tracing of a blood component through all processing steps from donation through transfusion (final disposition).

➤ A computer system is composed of three main components: hardware, software, and people.

➤ Hardware components perform functions related to input and output, processing, and storage of data.

➤ Software tells the computer what to do with the information it has received.

➤ Application software allows users to perform tasks that are specific to blood bank operations.

➤ Donor, patient, and blood component information is maintained in databases, which are divided into files and further subdivided into individual records.

➤ Static database files define the terminology that the blood bank will use and provides a dictionary of coded terms that the system can use to sort data.

➤ Operating system software controls the hardware, manipulates the application software, and coordinates the flow of information between the disks and memory.

➤ The system manager oversees the maintenance of the system's hardware and software, including adding or deleting items from the static database files, assigning access codes to new users, implementing software upgrades from the vendor, and investigating and reporting problems encountered by the users.

➤ A blood bank information system can have numerous specific applications related to the management of donors, patients, and blood components.

➤ User codes and passwords prevent unauthorized use of the system and provide a means for capturing the identity of each person who performs a task on the information system.

➤ Control functions assist in making decisions at critical points in the selection of donors and release of blood components for transfusion.

➤ When results must be corrected or amended, they must be clearly designated as such on printed reports and monitor displays used by patient caregivers.

➤ A blood bank must have documented evidence of validation of its system as well as written procedures for all aspects of system management in order to comply with regulatory and accreditation requirements.

➤ Blood bank SOPs must address computer tasks related to blood bank technical duties as well as computer-specific procedures such as computer downtime, backup of software programs and data, system maintenance, security, error management, and personnel training.

➤ On-site software validation must provide documented evidence that provides a high degree of assurance that the system will function consistently as expected under the unique combination of hardware, databases, environment, SOPs, and people at the site.

REVIEW QUESTIONS

1. Components of an information system consist of all of the following except:
   a. Hardware
   b. Software
   c. Validation
   d. People

2. Compliance with regulatory and accreditation agency requirements for blood bank information systems requires blood banks to maintain SOPs for all of the following except:
   a. Vendor validation testing
   b. Computer downtime
   c. System maintenance
   d. Personnel training

3. A validation test case that assesses the system's ability to recognize an erroneous input is called:
   a. Normal
   b. Boundary
   c. Stress
   d. Invalid

4. An example of interface software functionality is:
   a. The entry of blood components into the blood bank database
   b. The transmission of patient information from the HIS into the blood bank system
   c. The printing of a workload report
   d. Preventing access to the system by an unauthorized user

5. Backup copies of the information system:
   a. Can be used to restore the information system data and software if the production system is damaged
   b. Are used to maintain hardware components
   c. Are performed once a month
   d. Are created any time changes are made to the system

6. User passwords should be:
   a. Shared with others
   b. Kept confidential
   c. Posted at each terminal
   d. Never changed

7. The prevention of the issue of an incompatible blood component is an example of:
   a. Inventory management
   b. Utilization review
   c. System security
   d. Control function

8. Information is stored in a collection of many different files called the:
   a. Database
   b. Configuration
   c. Hardware
   d. Disk drive

9. Application software communicates with this type of software to retrieve data from the system disks:
   a. Interface
   b. Operating system
   c. Security
   d. Program

10. Validation testing for software should consider all of the following items except:
    a. Data entry methods
    b. Control functions
    c. Performance of testing in production database
    d. Invalid data

11. Complete the truth table below for a negative antibody screen using two screening cells (SCI, SCII) at the immediate spin (IS), 37°C (37), and antihuman globulin (AHG) phases.

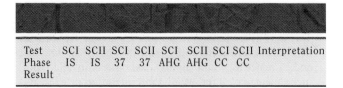

Test	SCI	SCII	SCI	SCII	SCI	SCII	SCI	SCII	Interpretation
Phase	IS	IS	37	37	AHG	AHG	CC	CC	
Result									

12. During validation testing a computer user entered the following results for an antibody screen test.

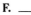

SCI	IS	37	AHG	CC	Interpretation
Result	0	0	0	+	**Negative**

After the user verified the entries, the monitor displayed the following message: "Invalid Test Results." What caused the error message to display?

A. An invalid entry was made in the check cells (CC) column.

B. The truth table was set up incorrectly.

C. The interpretation does not correlate with the test entries.

D. The interface to the laboratory computer system is down.

13. The following test plan has been created to validate the blood bank computer function used to update the status of blood units that have been transfused. The test plan contains each of the sections, lettered A through H, required for a thorough test plan. Evaluate each section and, using the list below, assign a name to each section.

Section Names

- Acceptance
- Acceptance criteria
- Control functions
- Corrective action
- Data entry methods
- Documentation methods
- Result review
- Test cases

TEST PLAN
FUNCTION: ASSIGNING TRANSFUSED STATUS

DESCRIPTION

This function is used to change the status of issued units to a transfused status. All records pertaining to the unit and patient will be updated.

A. _____

1. Prevention of assignment of transfused status to a quarantine blood unit.
2. Prevention of assignment of transfused status to a blood unit that has already been transfused.
3. Prevention of assignment of transfused status to a blood component that has not been issued.

B. _____

1. The computer will beep and display **Unit Has Not Been Issued** when a blood unit number that has not been issued is entered.
2. The computer will beep and display **Unit Is in Quarantined Status** when a blood component that is in quarantine status is entered.
3. The computer will beep and display **Unit Has Been Transfused** when a blood component that has already been transfused is entered.
4. The Transfusion History screen display will indicate the patient has been transfused and will display the date of the last transfusion.
5. Printed reports will indicate relevant units were assigned transfused status

C. _____

1. Attempt to assign transfused status to the following units:
   a. Quarantined blood component
   b. Selected (but not issued) blood component
   c. Transfused blood component
2. Selection of units from Issued inventory list
3. Manual entry of issued blood components

D. _____

1. Operator will input blood component information and select blood components.
2. Operator will input selected patient information.
3. Blood Bank computer will update the patient and unit record.

E. _____

The following screen displays and printed reports will be verified for accuracy.

Screen Displays	*Printed Reports*
Patient Information	Patient History Report
Unit Information	Transfusion Listing
Unit History	
Transfusion History	

F. _____

The acceptability of the results of each test case will be determined by the blood bank manager and documented on the Validation Documentation form.

G. _____

If the software does not perform as expected, the problem must be recorded on a Computer Problem Report and reported to a supervisor. A remedial action plan will be devised with the assistance of Blood Bank computer system vendor.

H. _____

Blood Bank Director Signature: _____ Date:_____
Comments:_____

_____

BIBLIOGRAPHY

Aller, R:. FDAs efforts frazzling many in blood bank field. CAP Today 12:50, 1998.

Aller, R: Blood bank information systems. CAP Today 13:38, 1999.

American Association of Blood Banks: Blood Bank/Transfusion Service Computer Systems User Validation Guidelines. Association Bulletin 93–2, August 27, 1993.

Brenner, ET: Computerizing the transfusion service department: One laboratory's experience. Med Lab Obs 30:44, 1998.

Butch, SH: Computer software quality assurance. Lab Med 22:18, 1991.

Butch, SH, et al: Electronic verification of donor-recipient compatibility: The computer crossmatch. Transfusion 34:105, 1994.

Butch, SH, and Judd, WJ: Letter to the editor. Transfusion 34:187, 1994.

Butch, SH: Innovation slows to trickle but ISBT 128 gains steam. CAP Today, 14:48, 2000.

Butch, SH: The blood bank software of your dreams. CAP Today 15:30, 2001

Butch, SH: Need for software savvy in push for patient safety. CAP Today 16:56, 2002.

Food and Drug Administration: Recommendation for implementation of computerization in blood establishments: Memo to all registered blood establishments, April 6, 1988.

Food and Drug Administration: Requirements for computerization of blood establishments: Memo to all registered blood establishments, September 8, 1989.

Food and Drug Administration: Draft guideline for the validation of blood establishment computer systems, September 28, 1993.

Food and Drug Administration: Guideline for quality assurance in blood establishments, July 11, 1995.

Hoffstadter, LK: Blood Bank Information Systems. Lab Med 25:110, 1994.

Kasten, BL. Bar coding: the ideal system. Med Lab Obs 25: 40, 1993.

Leavitt, J, and Smith, LE: Administrative workshop on quality assurance and the blood bank computer system. American Association of Blood Banks annual meeting, San Diego, November 1994.

American Association of Blood Banks: Responsibilities in Implementing and using a blood bank computer system. Washington, DC, 1989.

twenty-seven

Medicolegal and Ethical Aspects of Providing Blood Collection and Transfusion Services

Kathleen Sazama, MD, JD, MS, MT(ASCP)

═══════ OBJECTIVES ═══════

On completion of this chapter, the learner should be able to:

1. Understand the legal and ethical parameters for providing blood collection and transfusion services.
2. Know the legal bases for liability for providing transfusion medicine services.
3. Define the necessity for establishing and following standard operating procedures similar to those of other comparable facilities throughout the United States.

4. Identify and list the evolving legal and ethical concerns likely to accompany the increasing complexity of providing blood during the early 21st century.
5. List the two reasons why patients sue for transfusion injury.
6. List the steps that blood bank professionals can take to avoid or minimize litigation.

Introduction

In this chapter, after a brief discussion of the sources of law, theories of liability are discussed along with practical hints for reducing likelihood of being found liable, when possible. Emerging concerns for the 21st century are also identified. This chapter is not intended as a substitute for legal advice,

which is necessary in particular situations; rather, it is intended to provide the reader with some general principles and definitions so that ethically and legally sound practices continue within transfusion medicine.

Legal issues for the transfusion medicine professional in the early 2000s center around bacterial contamination of platelets, ABO errors, and patient privacy. There are also concerns about possible transfusion-transmitted viruses, including West Nile Virus (WNV), transfusion-transmitted acquired immunodeficiency syndrome (TTAIDS), and the hepatitis viruses, especially hepatitis C (HCV). Concern has also focused on issues regarding transfusion indications, informed consent, and other medically relevant topics.

However, even before TTAIDS became the basis for numerous lawsuits (probably more than 800 since 1985) against blood centers, hospitals, and physicians, there was litigation because of death and serious injury caused by transfusion-transmitted hepatitis B virus (HBV)* (*Perlmutter v. Beth David Hospital*, 308 NY 100, 123 N.E.2d 792 [1954]) and a few because of donor injury.[1] The HBV cases stimulated nearly every state legislature to enact protection for blood banks through "blood shield statutes."[2] (California was the first state to enact such protection for blood banks in 1955. Only New Jersey lacks such a law, but it provides similar protection solely through judicial decisions.) Because of these blood shield statutes, most of which extended protection without amendment or modification for TTAIDS and HBV, many TTAIDS lawsuits have been either dismissed or unsuccessful for the person suing (the plaintiff). Recently, however, this premise has come under new challenge in the courts. As most TTAIDS cases have been unsuccessful in compensating plaintiffs (usually patients or their families), new theories of liability are increasingly being raised. When questions of appropriateness of transfusion, availability of blood components, and informed consent arise, the ethical bases of transfusion medicine practice are focused more sharply.

Although blood shield statutes generally protect against application of strict liability, tort liability remains the basis for most lawsuits.

CASE STUDIES

Case One

A 26-year-old woman is critically injured in a two-car collision. She is rushed via helicopter to the nearest trauma center, where 10 units of uncrossmatched O-negative red blood cells (RBCs), 12 units of crossmatch-compatible A-negative RBCs, 4 A-negative apheresis platelet packs, and 8 units of group A fresh frozen plasma are administered within the first 24 hours of her care. Soon after her admission, she is taken to the operating room, where splenectomy is performed, liver and left kidney lacerations are repaired, numerous fractures of both lower extremities are reset, and a chest tube is placed for a collapsed left lung. She requires only 4 more units of A-negative RBCs during the next several days in the intensive care unit and recovers sufficiently to be discharged home 15 days after the accident to recuperate. Two years later, during her first prenatal visit for a second pregnancy, she tests positive for HIV. Her obstetrician tells her that the blood center reported that one of the units she received came from a donor who was test-positive for HIV a month ago.

---

*The court decided that transactions involving blood were not sales but were incidental to the provision of medical services. The effect of this decision was to preclude application of commercial law, particularly that of warranties, to blood transfusions.

Questions:

1. Was the blood center negligent?
2. Was the physician who transfused the patient negligent?
3. Would using an "ordinary" versus a "professional" standard of care yield a different answer?

Sources of Law

Laws are created by society through legislation called statutes (passed by either the U.S. Congress or by individual state legislatures) or by court decisions (in federal courts, including the U.S. Supreme Court, or in state courts through their own highest state court).

Statutes and Regulations

Frequently, federal law (enacted by Congress or by decision in federal courts, including the Supreme Court) supersedes state law, but both federal and state laws can be and often are applied in particular instances. The details of how laws are to be put into action are provided in regulations. Regulations, both federal and state, can be applied only if they have been established according to a formal process called the Administrative Procedure Act (APA).[3] Federal regulations that apply specifically to blood banking are found in the Title 21, Code of Federal Regulations, Parts 600–699, and to some extent in Parts 200–299 and 800–899, published annually on April 1.[4] Blood banks are also federally regulated by provisions of the Clinical Laboratories Improvement Act of 1988 and the Medicare provisions of the Social Security Act. In addition, the 1996 federal law protecting health information (Health Insurance Portability and Accountability Act [HIPAA]) should also be extended to protect donor health information.

State legislatures also enact laws and publish explanatory regulations about blood banking, clinical laboratories, and transfusion practices, principally covering licensure of facilities and personnel.

Case Law

Law is also established by court decisions, sometimes related to interpretations and applications of statutes and regulations. Patients generally believe that medical treatment administered to them (after obtaining their informed consent) will, on balance, be beneficial. When transfusion causes harm (e.g., through infectious agents, ABO mistransfusion, etc.), patients have understandably reacted by seeking redress in the courts. The legal bases for such suits are generally civil (not criminal) actions for tort. Tort is defined as any wrongdoing for which action for damages may be brought.

United States civil law depends on each adult person in our society behaving reasonably (i.e., not negligently and not aggressively) toward every other person, respecting other people's rights. Civil lawsuits arise because someone disrespects another's rights by:

1. Striking or threatening to strike another person (battery and assault)
2. Being careless or reckless (negligence)
3. Failing to complete an agreement (breach of contract)
4. Intruding on another's property or privacy
5. Misbehaving in other similar ways

Civil suits can also arise because of violation of specific statutes or regulations that require certain types of actions.

Basis of Liability: Torts

Intentional Tort of Battery

Any unconsented touching (including deliberate blows and intentional striking) is legally defined as battery. For transfusion medicine, this concept is used when a donor or a patient claims that he or she never agreed to have the needle placed in his or her arm. If significant harm occurs as a result of the needle, this legal theory may be upheld. Generally, however, the fact that the donor or patient allowed the needle to be placed is sufficient evidence that he/she agreed to the procedure. Informed consent is generally not an issue in battery but is fundamental in the tort of negligence.

Doctrine of Informed Consent

Particularly in the special circumstances of the practice of medicine, the issue of whether a patient (or, in the case of blood collection, a donor) agreed to undergo the procedure actually performed, with full knowledge of the possible benefits, alternatives, and harm that may accompany it, has come to be known as the doctrine of informed consent. This doctrine protects the patient (or donor) by requiring that information be provided in a manner understandable to the patient under circumstances that permit the patient to ask questions and to receive answers to any questions or concerns he or she may have (*Canterbury v. Spence,* 464 F.2d 772 [DC Cir 1972]).

For TTAIDS transfusion recipients, this issue first came into sharp focus in the case of *Kozup v. Georgetown University,* 663 F. Supp. 1048 (DC 1987), 851 F.2d 437 (DC Cir 1988), 906 F.2d 783 (DC Cir 1990). In this case, an infant brought by his parents to Georgetown University Hospital for medical care contracted TTAIDS and died. His parents argued that they were insufficiently informed about the harm of the transfusions and did not specifically agree to transfusions as part of the care given their child. The District of Columbia court ruled that their actions in bringing the child to the hospital and not objecting to transfusions at the time of infusion amounted to tacit consent. The issue of whether specific consent is required for transfusion and who should obtain such consent (generally physicians have been held responsible [*Ritter v. Delaney,* 790 S.W.2d 29 (Tex. App. San Antonio, 1990) and *Howell v. Spokane,* 785 P.2d 815 (Wash 1990)]) remains controversial (*Hoemke v. New York Blood Center,* 90–7182 [2d Cir. 1990] and *Gibson v. Methodist Hospital,* 01-89-00645-CV [Tex. Ct. App. 1991]). However, in 1996, the Joint Commission on Accreditation of Healthcare Organizations (JCAHO) specifically required hospitals to obtain informed consent for transfusion in some situations.[5]

Another arena in which the informed consent is the key to resolving disputes is donor rights. With the onset of AIDS, the language of donor histories has been subjected to continuous revising and updating to include information about the disease, how it is acquired, and under what circumstances a person should donate blood. Federal and voluntary requirements for the way in which the history is obtained have emphasized more face-to-face oral questioning, not just self-administra-

tion of these questionnaires. One part of the donation process has always been for donors to sign a statement of consent to donate.

Until the late 1980s, donors were protected from subpoena in cases of transfusion-transmitted diseases. However, an increasing number of plaintiffs in state courts are insisting that the donor be subject to questioning regarding his or her donation. This questioning may completely or partially protect a donor's identity or may require that donor to appear in open court. Because no one donates blood expecting to have to defend that altruistic act at some future date, the impact of these decisions on the future availability of blood for transfusion is uncertain.

Case Two

A 43-year-old man received a one-unit transfusion of RBCs during an emergency coronary artery bypass operation. He experienced sudden unexplained hemolysis, uncontrollable coagulopathy, and renal shutdown, from which he could not be resuscitated despite massive efforts by the cardiac surgeon and anesthesiologist. During the course of the resuscitation, when a new blood sample was sent for additional crossmatch, it was discovered that the patient's blood group was O-positive; the original unit of RBCs was A-positive. His spouse sued his cardiologist for lack of informed consent and negligence and the hospital and transfusion service physician for negligence.

Questions:

1. Which issue is likely to be successful for this plaintiff?
2. Would the result be different if ordinary rather than a professional standard of care were applied?

Negligence

Elements

Liability for negligence is found when all of the following factors are satisfied:

1. A duty was owed to the injured party.
2. The duty was not met by the injuring party.
3. Because the duty was not met, the injured party was harmed.
4. Failure to meet the duty owed was directly responsible for or could have been predicted to cause the harm suffered by the injured party.
5. Some measurable (compensable) harm (called "damages") occurred. **(Box 27–1)**

To be successful in a negligence action, the plaintiff has the responsibility to prove all these factors against the person being sued (the defendant).

BOX 27–1
Elements of Negligence

- Duty owed
- Breach of duty
- Harm/injury
- Causation
- Damages

Standard of Care

Ordinary Standard of Care

When the negligence involves ordinary things that anyone may encounter in daily life (e.g., injuries caused by traffic accidents, fist fights, etc.), a jury (or judge) can consider the facts and decide whether the behavior of the defendant was reasonable; that is, did the defendant meet the standard of care required in the situation? For ordinary negligence, this standard of care depends only on what the average person (e.g., a juror) believes is acceptable in our society. That is, the jury decides whether a reasonable person, in the same circumstances as the defendant, would have acted the same way as (or differently from) the way the defendant did. If the defendant acted reasonably in the circumstances, the plaintiff will be unsuccessful in the lawsuit and vice-versa.

In situations in which larger organizations are involved, the question of who is liable for the actions of employees has been resolved under the doctrine of *respondeat superior*. Under this doctrine, the actions of employees are attributable to the employer or person who directs their actions. The person responsible for transfusion services has been defined by federal regulation and general practice to be a physician, a definition that has been reinforced by judicial decision in many states for blood centers as well as for hospitals. The advantage of having a physician as the responsible employer is that the principles and regulations related to medical malpractice usually apply, including the requirement for establishing a professional standard of care.

Professional Standard of Care

When the negligence lawsuit involves professionals such as physicians and scientists, including laboratory professionals, nurses, or other allied health practitioners, the definition of what is reasonable, the "standard of care," depends on expert testimony from other professionals in the same field (e.g., physicians, nurses, or scientists) about what should have been done by other reasonable practitioners (usually of the same specialty). The law makes an extra requirement; that is, that in discharging his or her duty to the plaintiff, the defendant apply the special knowledge and ability he or she possesses by virtue of the profession. This increased "professional standard of care" is not just what a reasonable person such as the judge or members or the jury would have done but what other professionals (so-called expert witnesses) testify should have been done. The judge or jury is not permitted to decide what they would have done but must depend upon testimony by expert witnesses of the same profession as the defendant who define what that reasonable professional standard of care is. For the complex scientific, technical, and medical issues involved in TTAIDS litigation, this distinction has been a key element in protecting blood bankers.

Voluntary and Mandatory Standards

The testimony of experts should generally be supportable by authorities such as statutes, regulations, or other bodies of published knowledge, including published scientific articles and texts. The existence of voluntary standards—particularly those provided by the American Association of Blood Banks (AABB)[6] but also those from the College of American Pathologists (CAP), the American Association of Tissue Banks, the American Society for Histocompatibility and Immunogenetics, the Joint Commission on Accreditation of Healthcare Organizations (JCAHO), and other organizations—are helpful in establishing the professional standard of practice for transfusion medicine. In fact, some state and federal regulations cross-reference the AABB standards specifically. Blood bankers and transfusion services that can show that they acted in conformance with these standards are more likely to be found nonnegligent than those who do not follow such guidelines. (However, this safeguard has now been challenged in several states, notably Colorado and Texas.)

Is Blood Banking a Medical Profession?

The question of whether blood banking is a medical profession is being relitigated in courts today, with conflicting results.[7] One possible chilling result is that collecting, processing, and distributing blood may be considered differently from the crossmatching, issuance, and transfusion of blood to individual patients. Redefining blood banking as *not* medical practice removes the extra protection provided by the requirement for expert medical testimony to establish the standard of care, leaving defendants to be judged by the ordinary negligence standard. There is little dispute that loss of medical professional stature would significantly alter the practice of blood banking. None of the protections of medical malpractice reform would be available, and blood centers may even find themselves subject to strict liability.

Strict Liability

Manufacturers and distributors of goods used in everyday life have been defined by law to have certain responsibilities in their activities to protect consumers. Among other requirements, there are certain warranties that the product purchased—for example, a television set—will actually work and will continue to do so for some fixed period, with small risk of harm from such things as electric shock or blowing up. These warranties, actual or implied, exist for virtually anything a consumer buys and uses. If a product fails to perform as expected or creates harm when none was expected, the consumer has the right to have a replacement or, if the manufacturer denies responsibility, to sue for negligent manufacturing or distribution.

In addition, for some items (such as dynamite), the danger from proper use is so great that manufacturers are legally liable for *all* harm that occurs, so-called "strict" liability. This means that anyone who is harmed when properly using dynamite does not have to prove that the manufacturer or distributor was negligent; he or she has only to show that he or she was injured while properly using it. Imagine how rare and expensive blood transfusions would become if these theories were allowed to be applied to this medical practice. Instead, nearly every state has enacted specific protection, the blood shield statutes described previously, to exclude harm from blood transfusions from suit under these legal theories. It is important that blood bankers avoid implying or stating that blood transfusion is completely safe, because such statements may be construed as creating a warranty, invoking these theories of liability.

Case Three

A 32-year-old male repeat whole blood donor is found to test positive for HIV by nucleic acid testing, having been test-negative for HIV 1/2 antibodies and for HIV p24 antigen on several prior donations. Before all testing is completed, he returns to the blood collection center to donate HLA-matched platelets. At registration, the staff person notices that his prior record indicates his deferral status. She informs the donor that he is not eligible to donate the platelets. The donor is shocked and embarrassed by the news and storms out of the center. Two weeks later, the donor sues the blood center for intentional infliction of emotional distress.

Questions:

1. Is the donor likely to be successful?
2. Are there other bases on which suit can be brought?
3. Are there established standards for preventing such an occurrence?

Intentional Infliction of Emotional Distress

As this phrase suggests, a plaintiff must show that what the defendant did to cause actual and severe emotional distress was intentional, usually some extreme or outrageous conduct that was calculated to deliberately cause harm to the plaintiff. This can take the form of a claim for wrongful death of the plaintiff's relative, particularly in some TTAIDS cases.

Invasion of Privacy Under Civil Case Law

Healthcare providers, including blood bankers, are required to respect personal privacy and to maintain patient and donor confidentiality. Plaintiffs may claim remuneration for loss of privacy under four theories:

1. Intrusion upon plaintiff's seclusion or solitude or into his or her private affairs
2. Public disclosure of embarrassing facts
3. Placing plaintiff in a "false light" in public
4. Appropriation of plaintiff's name or likeness for defendant's benefit

These categories protect a patient or donor from illegal or inadvertent disclosure of his or her personal information, of particular concern with HIV because of the risk of loss of employment, housing, insurance, and other benefits of society. When information is exciting or noteworthy, the media may become aware of and publish private information.

Basis of Liability: Federal or State Law

HIPAA: The Federal Statute and Regulations

In 1996 the U.S. Congress responded to the information age by enacting a law specifically directed to the protection of personal medical information: the Health Information Portability and Accessability Act (HIPAA). The regulations implementing the provisions of this act have been coming out in segments since 1996, with the full provision for protected health information (PHI) becoming effective on April 7, 2003. With this new federal requirement, information about donors and patients must be kept in such a manner that inadvertent "use or disclosure" does not occur. Exceptions for healthcare providers, insurers, and government scrutiny have been specified, but safeguards should be in place even for these exceptions. Because the HIPAA is so new, no cases have as yet arisen.

However, blood banks and transfusion services will be involved in suits under the preexisting civil cases if they are responsible (through negligence or by intention) for release of confidential data identified to an individual donor or patient. Great care should be exercised by blood banking professionals to ensure that private information (whether about donors, patients, or relatives) be kept confidential and not released without written authorization. Procedures to safeguard such release should include proper use of copying and facsimile machines as well as direct electronic transfer via information systems.

Case Four

A 59-year-old man was notified in 1999 that he had received a unit of RBCs in 1989 that was negative by first-generation HCV antibody testing, but the donor was found to be positive when subsequently tested by second-generation methods. He was tested by the blood center in late 1999 and found to be HCV-positive. He filed a lawsuit against the treating physician, the hospital, and the blood center in 2002.

Questions:

1. What legal theory can this man use?
2. What is the likely outcome of this lawsuit?

Restrictions on Plaintiff Suits and Recovery

Statutes of Limitations

Some protection for defendants arises because of a statutorily defined limit of time during which a lawsuit can be filed. States often have different limits, depending on the legal requirements for initiating suits. Statutes of limitations for medical malpractice are generally shorter (approximately 2 years from the date that the injury should have been discovered in adults) than limitations for other kinds of negligence (2 to 6 years is common).

Doctrine of Charitable Immunity

Historically, courts provided immunity for nonprofit organizations such as hospitals from excess liability because they performed charitable acts. Many state legislatures have enacted and continue to support statutes to provide protection for boards of directors and/or volunteers using this common law rationale. A 1996 decision in New Jersey redefined this protection in that state (*Snyder v. AABB,* 144 N.J. 269 [1996]). Fortunately for blood bankers, other states have been loathe to accept the Synder decision. Also, many healthcare institutions rely less on this doctrine and more on insurance for protection.

Tort Reform

State legislatures, recognizing the need to protect some specialties such as obstetrics, have been active in seeking limits on damages against physicians, protecting them from abusive litigation. For transfusion practices, it is vital that these protections be afforded.

Risk Management

Avoiding liability for TTAIDS and other possible harm from practicing transfusion medicine, whether in hospitals or blood centers, depends on having well-established policies and procedures that are consistent with quality principles and that comply with recognized authorities, regulations, and statutes and that have some measurement of how persons engaged in all activities actually follow those procedures. Complying with accreditation requirements (e.g., AABB, Joint Commission on Accreditation of Healthcare Organizations, College of American Pathologists, and states) for quality systems will assist in limiting risk. To avoid being negligent, one must behave reasonably. Reasonable behavior for transfusion medicine practice includes continually obtaining and applying new knowledge from all possible sources that will safeguard the donor during collection, the component during handling and delivery, and the patient before and during transfusion.

Case Five

A 67-year-old woman crippled by degenerative arthritis requests that her own blood and blood from members of her family be used during her hip replacement surgery. The blood center describes its donation procedures, which do not permit directed donations. Although she is disappointed, she agrees to donate for herself. When her first unit is tested, it is reactive for hepatitis B surface antigen and for antibody to hepatitis B core antigen. The patient-donor is advised that she may no longer donate for herself and that the unit she has already donated will not be available for her surgery. Surgery proceeds. She receives 4 units of volunteer blood and develops TTAIDS 3 years later. She sues the blood-collecting organization.

Questions:

1. On what legal grounds can this suit be brought?
2. What is the current standard of care regarding patient-directed donations?
3. Can/should healthcare organizations deny autologous donor-patients access to their own test-reactive blood?

Specific Donor Issues

Screening

What the AIDS epidemic has taught us is that every person who volunteers to donate does not have an unqualified right to do so. In fact, for several years before March 1985 (the date when a test for HIV antibodies in blood was first available), the best safeguard against TTAIDS was improved donor education and more pertinent questioning regarding behaviors that might put that donor at risk for acquiring HIV. Although numerous lawsuits have been filed against blood collection agencies for improper donor screening, few have been successful when collecting facilities could show that they had implemented written procedures and had properly trained employees who followed those procedures and that proper

documentation of each screen occurred. Problems occurred when breaches in procedure, typically failures to follow or to properly document actual practice, were discovered. However, with several state courts demanding release of donor identity or access to donors for questioning, further attention to the process of donor screening is appropriate. Balancing the real threat of lack of availability of blood with the serious nature of litigation will continue to challenge blood banking professionals.

Donations Requested by Patients

Several monetary settlements in the range of hundreds of thousands to millions of dollars have resulted from either failing to offer directed donor services or from improperly characterizing them. With the advent of the HIPAA, patient-requested donations from friends and family require close attention to ensure that inadvertent or overt disclosure of protected health information does not occur.

Untimely Notification

When recipients received notification in years, rather than weeks or months, after blood centers knew (or should have known) that the recipient had received an HIV-reactive unit, many of them or their families were angry enough to file suit on the basis that they should have been informed sooner. Procedures for lookback and recipient notification were not well established for several years following application of specific testing in most blood collection organizations. It was not until 1996 that the federal government, through the Center for Health Care Financing Administration (now called Center for Medicaid and Medicare Services) and the FDA, issued specific regulations for HIV lookback notification by hospitals. Parallel requirements for HCV are proposed but not yet finalized.

Component Collection

Occasionally, lawsuits have occurred from injury to donors during the collection process. Generally, the injuries are more severe than a simple bruise at the needle site and involve such things as nerve damage, slip-and-fall incidents, and severe reactions. Also, although donor deaths continue to be reported at a rate of approximately two per year, these infrequently result in litigation.

Processing, Labeling, and Distribution

No Standard Protocol for Implementing Testing

Several successful TTAIDS lawsuits awarded millions of dollars against blood-collecting organizations (*Belle Bonfils Memorial Blood Bank v. Denver District Court*, 723 P.2d 1003 [Colo. 1988]) because they had no standard protocol for implementing new testing to ensure that all available components (including those distributed or in active inventory) were test-negative before transfusion, once the test kits and equipment was received by the collection facility. The lack of a written plan to implement such testing, including training of personnel, validating instrumentation and reagents, and establishing the necessary information service support, was seen as negligent by the jury (even *with* expert testimony to the contrary).

Failure to Perform Surrogate Testing

Despite concerted efforts, rarely has a plaintiff prevailed when alleging that blood collection facilities should have performed more or different surrogate tests between 1983 and 1985, when a specific test was first available (*Baker v. JK and Susie Wadley Research Institutes and Blood Bank, aka The Blood Center at Wadley*, 86-2728-C [Tex. Jud. Dist. Ct. 1988] and *Clark v. United Blood Services*, CV 88–6981 [Nev. 2d Jud. Dist. Ct. 1990]).

Failure to Properly Perform Testing

Testing personnel should be constantly alert to proper performance and documentation of all required testing of blood components. There are multiple opportunities for errors to occur during the processes of collecting and transfusing blood components. In addition to mistakes in doing the required   testing, failure to document is as damning as failure to perform at all. Considerable effort has been expended by the FDA to inform and to enforce requirements for proper testing for virally transmissible diseases in blood components. Private accrediting organizations, likewise, emphasize proper performance and documentation of these activities.

Informed Consent

In TTAIDS cases arising in the early 1980s, it was frequently alleged that patients were insufficiently warned of the hazards of transfusion because transfusion experts failed to warn hospitals and ordering physicians about them. Few cases were successful because the state of scientific knowledge, established by expert testimony relying on published data, was limited. Also, the early HBV cases had established a record that supported the defense position that transfusions were already known by hospitals and other physicians to be unavoidably unsafe, particularly for transfusion-transmitted viral diseases. Some states (e.g., California) enacted specific legislation about informed consent for transfusion.

Medical Malpractice

Several multimillion-dollar lawsuits, decided for the plaintiff, resulted from successful allegations that either the patient did not give adequate informed consent, did not need a transfusion at all, could have waited until test-negative blood was available before receiving a transfusion, or required transfusion solely because of something the physician did. In all these cases, the basis for fault was negligence by the treating physician.

Ethics and Transfusion Medicine

Case Six

On July 5, a Monday afternoon, two trauma victims, both group O-negative, arrive in the same hospital emergency room. Both patients have massive injuries requiring large-volume RBC transfusions. Because of the time of year, the hospital transfusion service is low on O-negative RBCs. As the requests for RBCs rise, units crossmatched for tomorrow's elective surgery are taken to be used for the trauma patients. The transfusion medicine physician (TMP) contacts the department of surgery to cancel elective surgery cases for Tuesday, July 6. The transfusion service manager (TSM) puts in an emergency call to the regional blood center. The blood center informs the TSM that it, too, is short of O-negative RBCs but that it will canvas the neighboring hospitals and put in an emergency request to the blood exchange network.

As several hours pass, during which the trauma surgeons and OR team work diligently to correct the injuries and restore vital organs, it is clear that there will be sufficient RBCs available to adequately support only one patient. The TMP contacts the chair of the hospital ethics committee for assistance in determining how to proceed.

Additional information available to the TMP and the ethics committee includes: One patient is a 55-year-old bank president who is the sole financial support for his spouse, two college-age children, and widowed mother; the other is a 28-year-old gas service attendant who is unmarried. Both patients are critically injured, but, with adequate transfusion support, both are deemed likely to recover by their treating physician.

Questions:

1. Which ethical principle is being emphasized?
2. How will a decision favoring one patient over the other be viewed ethically? Legally?

Ethical Principles

Biomedical ethical principles that must be balanced when considering appropriateness of and informed consent for transfusion include autonomy, beneficence, and justice (see definitions in **Box 27–2**). In transfusion medicine, autonomy is increasingly important as patients become more aware of the harm, as well as the benefit, of transfusions and insist on the right to choose the type of therapy and the source of the blood they receive. Although autonomy is not unrestricted, it must form part of the healthcare relationship. When transfusions are offered, patients expect that the treatment will benefit them. When the benefit is marginal or even questionable and, in particular, if something harmful occurs, the decision of the healthcare professional may be challenged both legally and ethically. The ethical principle of beneficence will be balanced against auton-omy in every instance. Fortunately, the ethical principle of justice is rarely invoked because there are only rare instances in which transfusions are inequitably distributed, generally because of shortage of collections. In times of blood shortages, rationing begins with canceling of elective surgical procedures for which transfusion may be indicated and rarely reaches a point at which emergency needs are compromised. An example of balancing ethical principles that has caused legal action is when patients have suffered serious or fatal consequences and were denied access to a choice of donating for themselves or selecting their own blood donors from among family members, church or social groups, or coworkers.

Emerging Issues

In addition to the concerns listed previously, there are new ones surrounding patient safety related to adequacy of patient identification, the changing practices of transfusion medicine, such as responsibilities for out-of-hospital (specifically

BOX 27–2
Ethical Principles

Autonomy

The right of each person to make decisions based on that person's values and beliefs, having adequate information and an understanding of the choices available to him or her and lacking any compulsion by external forces.

Beneficence

In the healthcare setting, professionals seek the well-being of each patient.

Justice

Patients should be treated fairly, with equal, need-based access to beneficial treatment.

---

at home) transfusions, issues surrounding provision of autologous services (crossover of unused units, transfusion of reactive components, freezing of unused reactive units, informed consent, etc.), use of newer therapies such as oxygen therapeutics and recombinant erythropoietin, standards for provision of perioperative blood collection and reinfusion, and control over use of gene therapy to treat certain transfusion-dependent illnesses. In the TTAIDS area, suits have been filed for reporting false AIDS test results and for fear of AIDS because of exposure through transfusion or via a healthcare worker, plus ongoing concerns over handling of lookback. New concerns about bacterial contamination, fueled by the still-unexplained upsurge in *Yersinia* growth in RBCs, and newer issues surrounding hepatitis C and other transfusion-transmissible agents, e.g., WNV and, potentially, SARS, will surface.

Summary

The lessons learned from transfusion-related litigation underscore the fact that every blood collection facility and transfusion service needs complete, comprehensive, and current written procedures and policies that conform with quality principles. When such procedures and policies conform to federal and state statutes and regulations as well as meet private voluntary standards, such as those of the CAP, AABB, and JCAHO, the organization can have a higher assurance that it will meet the standard of care required to avoid being found negligent and thus liable for the damages the patient or donor suffered. Patients are demanding, on ethical grounds, the right to have greater control over the use of human blood for treatment, including appropriate informed consent. Pending and future issues will redefine the legal and ethical aspects of transfusion medicine.

SUMMARY CHART:
Important points to remember (MT/MLT)

➤ Tort liability is the basis for most lawsuits.

➤ Federal regulations that apply specifically to blood banking are found in Title 21, Code of Federal Regulations.

➤ Claims of the intentional tort of battery is used in transfusion medicine when a donor or a patient claims that he or she never agreed to have the needle placed into his or her arm.

➤ The doctrine of informed consent protects the patient (or donor) by requiring that information be provided in a manner understandable to the patient under circumstances that permit the patient to ask questions and to receive answers to any questions or concerns.

➤ The elements of negligence include:
  ● A duty was owed to the injured party.
  ● The duty was not met by the injuring party.
  ● Because the duty was not met, the injured party was harmed.
  ● Failure to meet the duty owed was directly responsible for or could have been predicted to cause the harm suffered by the injured party.
  ● Some measurable (compensable) harm occurred (damages).

➤ Under the doctrine of *respondeat superior,* the actions of employees are attributable to the employer or person who directs their actions; that is, in transfusion medicine, a physician.

➤ The concept of strict liability implies that a warranty exists for virtually any product a consumer buys, and if the product fails to perform or creates harm when none was expected, the consumer has a right to a replacement or, if denied a replacement, to sue for negligent manufacturing or distribution.

➤ Blood centers may be liable for invasion of privacy lawsuits if confidentiality is breached via public disclosure of embarrassing facts (e.g., HIV-positive results) or for violation of federal law (the HIPAA).

➤ Traditionally, hospitals and other nonprofit organizations are protected under the doctrine of charitable immunity from excess liability because they perform charitable acts.

➤ Biomedical ethical principles that must be balanced when considering appropriateness of and informed consent for transfusion include autonomy, beneficence, and justice.

REVIEW QUESTIONS

1. Transfusion-transmitted diseases can result in lawsuits claiming:
   a. Battery
   b. Invasion of privacy
   c. Negligence
   d. A and B
   e. A, B, and C

2. Laws applicable to blood banking and transfusion medicine can arise:
   a. In state and federal courts
   b. In the U.S. Congress, state legislatures, and state and federal courts
   c. In state legislatures and courts
   d. In state legislatures and the U.S. Congress

3. The reasons patients have sued for transfusion injury include:
   a. Failure to perform surrogate testing
   b. Failure to properly test blood components
   c. Failure to properly screen donors
   d. Unnecessary transfusion
   e. All of the above

4. Blood banking professionals can avoid litigation by:
   a. Following published regulations and guidelines
   b. Knowing the legal bases for liability
   c. Disclosing all information about patients and donors
   d. Practicing good medicine
   e. None of the above

5. All issues about transfusion-transmitted diseases:
   a. Have already been litigated
   b. Frequently result in plaintiff verdicts
   c. Rarely provide for any protection for defendants
   d. Are known and avoidable
   e. Are evolving and will continue to result in litigation in the foreseeable future

REFERENCES

1. Randall, CH, Jr: Medicolegal Problems in Blood Transfusion. Joint Blood Council, Washington, DC, 1962. Reprinted by Committee on Blood, American Medical Association, Chicago, 1963.
2. Rabkin, B, and Rabkin, MS: Individual and institutional liability for transfusion-acquired disease: An update. JAMA 256:2242, 1986.
3. Administrative Procedure Act, 60 Statutes 237–244, 5 USC Sections 551–559, 1988.
4. Code of Federal Regulations: Food and Drugs, Title 21, Parts 200–299 and 600–699, Title 42, Part 482. U.S. Government Printing Office, Washington, DC, 1997.
5. Sazama, K: Practical issues in informed consent for transfusion. Am J Clin Pathol 107:572, 1997.
6. Klein, HG (ed): Standards for Blood Banks and Transfusion Services, ed 17. American Association of Blood Banks, Bethesda, MD, 1996.
7. Kelly, C, and Barber, JP: Legal issues in transfusion medicine: Is blood banking a medical profession? Clin Lab Med 12:819, 1992.

BIBLIOGRAPHY

Cooper, JS, and Rodrigue, JE: Legal issues in transfusion medicine. Lab Med 23:794, 1992.
Crigger, B-J (ed): Cases in Bioethics, ed 2. St. Martin's Press, New York, 1993.
Klein, HG (ed): Standards for Blood Banks and Transfusion Services, ed 18. American Association of Blood Banks, Bethesda, MD, 1997.
Prosser, WL, Wade, JW, and Schwartz, VE: Torts: Cases and Materials, ed 7. Foundation Press, Mineola, NY, 1980.
Rabkin, B, and Rabkin, MS: Individual and institutional liability for transfusion-acquired disease: An update. JAMA 256:2242, 1986.
Stowell, C (ed): Informed Consent for Transfusion. American Association of Blood Banks, Bethesda, MD, 1997.

Polyagglutination

Phyllis S. Walker, MS, MT(ASCP)SBB

Introduction

Polyagglutination refers to the agglutination of altered red blood cells (RBCs) by a large proportion of ABO-compatible adult human sera. Alterations in the RBC membrane may be acquired after microbial (bacterial or viral) activity, associated with certain forms of aberrant erythropoiesis, or inherited. In the microbially induced forms of polyagglutination, microbial enzymes alter the structure of the normal RBC membrane by removing carbohydrate residues and thus exposing cryptic (hidden) antigens, or *cryptantigens*. Naturally occurring IgM antibodies (polyagglutinins) found in normal adult human sera react with these cryptantigens, causing the altered cells to be polyagglutinable. Polyagglutinins are considered "naturally occurring," but their production is probably stimulated by intestinal flora, particularly gram-negative organisms, which have antigenic similarities to the RBC cryptantigens. Cryptantigen exposure can be detected before polyagglutination by testing the RBCs in vitro with specific lectins.[1] Polyagglutination, which requires significant cryptantigen exposure, is a rare condition; however, detectable cryptantigen exposure is not. Microbially induced polyagglutination may occur in vitro or in vivo. When polyagglutination occurs in vivo, the condition is usually transient. The microbial organisms may be present in the bloodstream, or the enzymes may enter the bloodstream from an extravascular site of infection. For polyagglutination to occur, the enzymes must be present in excess of the amount required to neutralize normal plasma enzyme inhibitors.[1] Microbially induced forms of polyagglutination include T, Th, Tk, Tx, acquired B, acquired microbial polyagglutination caused by passive adsorption, and probably VA. A nonmicrobial form of acquired polyagglutination, Tn, is caused by the somatic mutation of a faulty hematopoietic stem cell clone. This form of polyagglutination is usually a persistent condition. Finally, some forms of polyagglutination are inherited, including Cad, hemoglobin M-Hyde Park, hereditary erythroblastic multinuclearity with a positive acidified serum (HEMPAS), and NOR. The inherited forms of polyagglutination are permanent conditions.

Historically, polyagglutination was first described as an in vitro phenomenon caused by bacterial contamination of RBC suspensions. The first report, by Hübener, appeared in 1926.[2] Later, polyagglutination was described by Thomsen and Friedenreich,[3] and it became known as the Hübener-Thomsen-Friedenreich phenomenon. The cryptantigen exposed by the action of the bacterial enzyme became known as the T receptor (in honor of Thomsen). Over the past 70 years, other forms of polyagglutination have been described.

Recognition and classification of polyagglutinable cells may be complicated by variations in the strength of the antigens and antibodies. Also, it is not uncommon to find several forms of polyagglutination existing simultaneously in vivo. This appendix discusses the most common types, including the serologic recognition of polyagglutination and the classification of polyagglutinable RBCs by using lectins.

Categories of Polyagglutinable Cells

Microbially Associated

T Polyagglutination

T transformation is a transient, acquired form of polyagglutination, usually found in patients with septicemia, gastrointestinal lesions, or wound infections. Occasionally, T transformation has been observed in apparently healthy blood donors[4]; however, it is usually considered a pathologic finding—possibly an early symptom of a latent disease condition. It has been more frequently observed in infants and children than in adults. T activation of RBCs is caused by the action of neuraminidase, which is produced by bacteria, such as pneumococci, *Clostridium perfringens,* and *Vibrio cholerae,* and viruses such as the influenza virus.[5] Neuraminidase cleaves terminal *N*-acetylneuraminic acid (NeuNAc) residues from RBC membrane glycoproteins and glycolipids, exposing the subterminal T receptor.[6] One structure on the RBC membrane that can be altered to express the T receptor is the alkali-labile tetrasaccharide of Thomas and Winzler.[7] These tetrasaccharides are found on the MN-sialoglycoprotein (SGP), the Ss-SGP, other minor RBC SGPs, and on gangliosides.[8] **Figure A–1** illustrates the biochemical structures of the tetrasaccharide of Thomas and Winzler and the neuraminidase-modified structure that expresses the T receptor. T activation may occur in vitro or in vivo. In vitro, T activation may be produced by bacterial contamination of blood samples or by the deliberate addition of neuraminidase to RBC suspensions. When T receptors on RBCs are exposed, the cells are agglutinated by almost all normal adult sera, which contain naturally occurring anti-T. Patients who have T polyagglutination generally lack anti-T in their sera and therefore are expected to have negative autologous controls. The extent of T activation or cryptantigen exposure depends on the amount of neuraminidase that gains access to the bloodstream, the amount of inhibitor present in the patient's plasma, and the number of NeuNAc residues that are removed by the enzymes.[9] In addition to RBCs, T receptors may be found as cryptantigens on leukocytes,[10] platelets,[10] tissue

Alkali-labile tertrasaccharide of Thomas and Winzler:

Gal-β (1–3) - GalNAc----α----Serine or Threonine

α (2–3)   α (2–6)

NeuNAc   NeuNAc

T receptor:

Gal-β (1–3) - GalNAc----α----Serine or Threonine

Gal=Galactose
GalNAc=N-acetylgalactosamine
NeuNAc=N-acetylneuraminic acid

■ **FIGURE A–1.**   Structure of the alkali-labile tetrasaccharide of Thomas and Winzler and the neuraminidase-modified structure that expresses the T receptor in the terminal position.

cells,[11] and in body fluids.[12] T activation is a transient condition in vivo. When the microbial organism is eliminated, the polyagglutinable property of the RBCs usually disappears.

Th Polyagglutination

Th polyagglutination is probably another microbially induced form of polyagglutination. This form of polyagglutination was first observed in septic patients by Bird and coworkers in 1978.[13] Several microbial organisms were isolated from these patients, including Clostridia, Bacteroides, *Escherichia coli,* and Proteus. Because the polyagglutinins anti-T and anti-Tk were found in normal amounts in the sera of these patients, it was apparent that Th polyagglutination is different from T polyagglutination and Tk polyagglutination. In an in-vitro experiment, Sondag-Thull and associates[14] produced Th-transformed RBCs using the neuraminidase produced by *Corynebacterium aquaticum.* They showed that the neuraminidase associated with Th transformation is weaker than the neuraminidase that produces T transformation, and they concluded that Th-transformed RBCs express a weakened expression or an early stage of the T transformation.

Tk Polyagglutination

Like other forms of microbially associated polyagglutination, Tk transformation is a transient, acquired form of polyagglutination usually found in patients with septicemia, gastrointestinal lesions, or wound infections. Initially, enzymes produced by a certain strain of *Bacteroides fragilis* were associated with Tk polyagglutination.[15] Later, cultures of *Serratia marcescens, Aspergillus niger,* and *Candida albicans* were also shown to produce endo-β-galactosidases and exo-β-galactosidases that are capable of producing Tk transformation. The enzymes cleave a galactose residue from the paragloboside structure, exposing *N*-acetylglucosamine

(GluNAc), the Tk receptor.[16,17] Paragloboside is a precursor in the biosynthetic pathways of the ABH, Lewis, Ii, and P1 antigens. Thus, Tk-polyagglutinable RBCs may have altered expressions of these antigens, resulting in decreased antigen expression.[18] **Figure A–2** illustrates the biochemical structures of paragloboside and the Tk receptor. Tk transformation can be produced in vitro or in vivo.[16] When Tk receptors on RBCs are exposed, the cells are agglutinated by almost all normal adult sera, which contain naturally occurring anti-Tk. When the microbial organism is eliminated, the polyagglutinable property of the RBCs usually disappears.

Tx Polyagglutination

Tx transformation was first described in children with pneumococcal infections.[19] The mechanism of Tx transformation has not been explained. A second report of Tx transformation described a child with acute hemolytic anemia.[20] Tx transformation of the child's RBCs was observed, but no direct association with the anemia could be proved. Examination of family members showed Tx polyagglutination of the RBCs of two siblings. The polyagglutination was transient, lasting 4 to 5 months. The Tx transformation could have been caused by an unidentified bacterial or viral infection; however, blood, nasopharyngeal, urine, and rectal culture results were all negative.

Acquired-B Polyagglutination

Like T activation, acquired B is considered a transient, acquired form of polyagglutination, usually found in patients with septicemia, gastrointestinal lesions, or wound infections. Also like T activation, acquired B has been found in apparently healthy blood donors,[21] but the condition is considered a pathologic finding. The acquired-B antigen is caused by enzymes produced by certain strains of *E. coli,*[22] *Clostridium tertium,*[22] and probably by certain strains of *Proteus vulgaris.*[23] The microbial enzyme causes deacetylation of α-*N*-acetyl-D-galactosamine (group A determinant) with the

Paragloboside:

Gal-β (1–4) - GluNAc-β (1–3) - Gal-β (1–3) - Glu - Ceramide

Tk receptor:

GluNAc-β (1–3) - Gal-β (1–3) - Glu - Ceramide

Gal=Galactose
GluNAc=N-acetylglucosamine
Glu=Glucose

■ **FIGURE A–2.**   Structure of paragloboside and the enzymatically modified structure that expresses the Tk receptor in the terminal position.

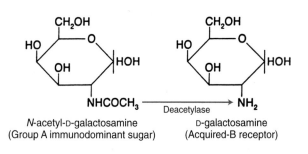

■ **FIGURE A–3.** Structure of the group A determinant (*N*-acetyl-D-galactosamine) and the enzymatically modified structure (D-galactosamine) that expresses the acquired-B receptor.

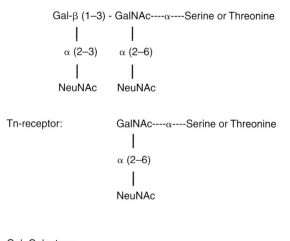

Alkali-labile tertrasaccharide of Thomas and Winzler:

Gal=Galactose
GalNAc=*N*-acetylgalactosamine
NeuNAc=*N*-acetylneuraminic acid

■ **FIGURE A–4.** Structure of the alkali-labile tetrasaccharide of Thomas and Winzler and the incomplete structure that expresses the Tn receptor in the terminal position.

production of α-D-galactosamine. α-D-Galactosamine is similar to α-D-galactose (group B determinant) and can cross-react with human anti-B typing sera and some monoclonal anti-B typing reagents.[24,25] **Figure A–3** illustrates the biochemical structures of α-*N*-acetylgalactosamine and α-D-galactosamine, the acquired B determinant. Acquired B may be produced in vitro or in vivo. In vitro, acquired B can be produced by coating group A or O RBCs with lipopolysaccharides from *E. coli* O$_{86}$ or *P. vulgaris* O$_{19}$. In vivo, acquired B is a transient condition, occurring only on RBCs that have the A antigen. When the microbial organism is eliminated, the cross-reactivity with anti-B typing reagent usually disappears.

Passive Adsorption of Bacterial Products

Very rarely, polyagglutination may be caused by the passive adsorption of bacterial products onto RBCs. Such coated cells can be polyagglutinable because human sera sometimes contain antibodies to the bacteria. Chorpenning and Dodd reported a severe transfusion reaction that was probably caused by this mechanism.[26]

VA Polyagglutination

VA polyagglutination is rare, and it has not been well characterized. It was first described in a 20-year-old man from Vienna, Virginia (VA), who had had hemolytic anemia most of his life.[27] The H antigens of VA polyagglutinable RBCs are significantly depressed. The action of a microbial α-fucosidase could account for the depressed H antigens; however, the presence of a microbial enzyme has not been proved.[9] VA polyagglutinability appears to be a persistent condition.

Nonmicrobially-Associated

Tn Polyagglutination

Tn polyagglutinability is believed to be caused by a mutation in the hematopoietic tissue. The mutation gives rise to a clone of cells that lack β-3-D-galactosyltransferase,[28] the transferase that is needed to complete the biosynthesis of the normal structure of the alkali-labile tetrasaccharide of Thomas and Winzler.[7] This tetrasaccharide structure is found on the MN-SGP and the Ss-SGP.[29] Inasmuch as this form of polyagglutination is caused by a mutation, it is considered permanent and irreversible. The mutant clone coexists with normal hematopoietic tissue and, therefore, this form of polyagglutination is characterized by a mixed-field appearance.[30] Only the cells produced by the mutant clone are agglutinated by the naturally occurring anti-Tn, which is found in normal adult sera. Tn polyagglutination occurs only in vivo, and it may occur in apparently healthy people. When the transferase is absent, the crypt Tn antigen (α-GalNAc) is exposed. In addition to RBCs, the Tn receptor may be found as a cryptantigen on leukocytes,[31] platelets,[31] and tissue cells.[11] **Figure A–4** illustrates the biochemical structures of the tetrasaccharide of Thomas and Winzler and the incomplete structure that expresses the Tn receptor.[32]

Inherited Forms of Polyagglutination

Cad

Cad polyagglutination was first described in 1968 by Cazal and coworkers.[33] Cad is an inherited autosomal dominant condition that gives rise to a permanent polyagglutinable state. The amount of Cad antigen varies on RBCs and, based on the amount of Cad antigen present, RBCs can be divided into four Cad phenotypes.[34] In 1971, Sanger and associates[35] reported that Cad-positive RBCs are agglutinated by anti-Sd^a. It is known that the structure that includes the Cad determinant is a potent inhibitor of anti-Sd^a; however, it is not clear whether this means that Cad and Sd^a are identical or that a concentrated isolate of a structure similar to Sd^a, with GalNAc as the terminal residue, has the ability to cross-react with anti-Sd^a.[36] Inasmuch as anti-Sd^a is present as an autoantibody in most normal adult sera, Cad cells can be classified as polyagglutinable. Cad polyagglutination is quite uncommon. This form of polyagglutination appears to have little clinical significance; however, Cad-positive cells show considerable resistance to invasion by merozoites of *Plasmodium falciparum*.[37] Cad polyagglutinable RBCs have normal sialic acid

Alkali-labile tertrasaccharide of Thomas and Winzler:

Gal-β (1–3) - GalNAc----α----Serine or Threonine

| |
α (2–3)   α (2–6)
| |
NeuNAc   NeuNAc

Cad receptor:

GalNAc-β (1–4) - Gal-β (1–3) - GalNAc----α----Serine or Threonine

| |
α (2–3)   α (2–6)
| |
NeuNAc   NeuNAc

Gal=Galactose
GalNAc=*N*-acetylgalactosamine
NeuNAc=*N*-acetylneuraminic acid

■ **FIGURE A–5.** Structure of the alkali-labile tetrasaccharide of Thomas and Winzler and the modified structure that expresses the Cad receptor.

levels. The Cad determinant on the RBC membrane and the Sd^a antigen isolated from Sd(a+) urine share a nonreducing trisaccharide.[38–40] The Cad receptor, a pentasaccharide, is produced when an additional sugar is added to the alkali-labile tetrasaccharide of Thomas and Winzler.[38] **Figure A–5** illustrates the biochemical structures of the tetrasaccharide of Thomas and Winzler and the modified structure that expresses the Cad receptor.

Hemoglobin M-Hyde Park

Polyagglutination associated with hemoglobin M-Hyde Park was initially reported in a South African family of mixed race.[41] The RBCs of 12 members of the family were weakly agglutinated, often mixed-field pattern, by many ABO-compatible human sera. All 12 family members who had hemoglobin M-Hyde Park had polyagglutinable RBCs; however, polyagglutination was absent in 23 other family members who had normal hemoglobin. Because all of the family members were apparently healthy, it is unlikely that the polyagglutinability was caused by in-vivo bacterial or viral activity. King and others[42] reported that the polyagglutinability associated with M-Hyde Park RBCs is caused by two unrelated abnormalities. They found heterogeneity in the molecular size of SGPs and a mild reduction in the sialylation of O-linked oligosaccharide chains on the M-Hyde Park membrane components. Also, these RBCs showed incomplete biosynthesis with exposure of terminal GluNAc on polylactosamine-type, *N*-linked carbohydrate chains of band 3.

HEMPAS

HEMPAS is also known as congenital dyserythropoietic anemia type II (CDA II). HEMPAS is an autosomal-recessive condition that is characterized by abnormal RBC membranes, multinucleated erythroblasts in the bone marrow, and RBCs that have a second membrane internal and parallel to the external membrane.[43,44] HEMPAS RBCs have increased amounts of i-antigen and decreased amounts of H antigen and sialic acid, and they show increased susceptibility to lysis by anti-i and anti-I in the presence of complement. Many normal human sera contain a naturally occurring IgM complement-binding alloantibody that reacts with HEMPAS cells. For this reason, HEMPAS cells are considered polyagglutinable.[9] A specific HEMPAS determinant has not been described.

NOR

NOR, an inherited dominant form of polyagglutination, was discovered when the RBCs of a 19-year-old blood donor from Norfolk, Virginia, were unexpectedly incompatible with the majority of adult sera tested. NOR cells were compatible with cord sera. Tests with lectins and other reagents ruled out other known forms of polyagglutination, and this donor's serum contained the expected naturally occurring antibodies to other forms of polyagglutination. No lectin has been found that agglutinates NOR cells. Possibly NOR polyagglutination is related to the P blood group system, inasmuch as it has been observed that anti-NOR is inhibited by hydatid cyst fluid and avian P1 substance. Anti-NOR is a naturally occurring IgM antibody that is found in approximately 75 percent of normal adult sera.[45] The NOR determinant has not been described.

Laboratory Testing: Detection, Confirmation, and Classification

Detection

In the past, cryptantigen expression and polyagglutination were sometimes detected by ABO discrepancies in which polyagglutinins in the typing sera reacted with polyagglutinable cells. Similarly, false-positive direct antiglobulin tests (DATs) were sometimes observed when polyagglutinins in the antiglobulin reagent reacted with polyagglutinable cells. When minor crossmatches were commonly performed, incompatible minor crossmatches could lead to the detection of polyagglutination, resulting from polyagglutinable recipient's cells reacting with polyagglutinins in the donor's serum.

Today, monoclonal antisera have replaced human ABO reagents, and these antisera fail to recognize polyagglutination because they lack the naturally occurring polyagglutinins that are found in adult human serum. Similarly, monoclonal antiglobulin reagents lack the polyagglutinins, and the minor crossmatch is rarely performed. Cyptantigen exposure would not be detected during routine compatibility testing unless the donor's cells demonstrated cryptantigens. If donor samples became bacterially contaminated in vitro, the samples could become polyagglutinable, and sometimes apparently healthy donors have Tn or one of the inherited forms of polyagglutination. In these cases, if the number of receptors on the donor cells and the amount of antibody in the patient's serum are adequate, polyagglutination can be detected; especially, if the immediate-spin, room temperature crossmatch is used.

The Tn receptor in Tn polyagglutination, which is produced by a mutant clone of hemopoietic cells, is *N*-acetylgalactosamine. This is the same sugar that defines the A antigens on group A cells. In the past, human anti-A reagent was used, and Tn polyagglutination was sometimes detected, when the anti-A antiserum cross-reacted with the Tn receptors. These reactions appeared like an "acquired A"—a mixed-field population of A cells in a group O individual or a weak subgroup of AB in a group B individual. Although some monoclonal antibodies have been produced that react with A cells and Tn polyagglutinable cells, commercial manufacturers of monoclonal anti-A reagents have formulated their typing sera to avoid this cross-reactivity [personal communication].

Acquired B is a relatively rare form of polyagglutination that is produced when bacterial deacetylase enzymatically converts the A antigen, N-acetylgalactosamine, into galactosamine, which cross-reacts with anti-B reagents. When monoclonal reagents replaced the human antisera, there was a sharp increase in the detection of acquired B by one particular clone, ES4.[46] ES4 detected many examples of acquired B that were previously nonreactive when tested with human anti-B reagents. Because the transfusion of group AB blood to a group A recipient who had acquired-B polyagglutination could result in a serious transfusion reaction, the three manufacturers who currently produce ES4-containing anti-B reagents quickly reformulated their antisera to avoid detecting acquired B. The detection of acquired B by ES4 is avoided by lowering the pH of the reagent; however, it is possible to reverse the pH inadvertently if unwashed RBCs are typed with ES4 reagents.

Because many monoclonal reagents are used in the transfusion laboratory today and the minor cross-match is rarely performed, it is unlikely that polyagglutination would be detected during testing. It is more likely that unexplained hemolysis following a blood transfusion would be the first clue that the patient has polyagglutination.

Confirmation

When polyagglutination is suspected, the RBCs should be tested with several cord blood sera and with several normal group AB adult sera. If the RBCs are agglutinated by most of the adult sera and are not agglutinated by the cord sera, polyagglutination has been established. The cord sera used for polyagglutination studies must be pretested to determine that

they lack maternal alloantibodies, which might produce misleading results. The adult sera must be pretested to determine that they are free of unexpected antibodies.

Polyagglutinins are naturally occurring antibodies in adult serum; however, the amount of antibody varies from one individual to another. For this reason, several adult sera should be used. Polyagglutinins usually react best at lower temperatures by direct agglutination. Because polyagglutinins are unstable, it is important to use fresh adult sera. The auto-control in individuals who have polyagglutinable RBCs is usually nonreactive. Polyagglutinins in most normal adult sera are low-titered. As polyagglutinable RBC transformation begins, the polyagglutinin antibodies are adsorbed onto the transformed cells until the antibodies have been completely removed from circulation. At that time, the auto-control is expected to be negative.

N-acetylneuraminic acid (sialic acid) is a normal component of the RBC membrane. Certain forms of polyagglutination (T and Tn) show decreased amounts of sialic acid. It is possible to quantitate sialic acid levels, but such testing is not practical in routine serology laboratories. Instead, sialic acid levels are usually determined qualitatively with Polybrene and *Glycine soja* lectin. Polybrene, a positively charged polymer, acts by neutralizing the negative charge on normal RBCs and causing them to aggregate nonspecifically. Because the negative charge is almost entirely caused by sialic acid groups, cells that lack sialic acid (T and Tn) are not aggregated by Polybrene. Conversely, *G. soja* lectin does not react with normal cells, but it strongly agglutinates sialic acid–deficient RBCs (T and Tn) as well as Cad cells.

Classification

Enzymes

Enzymes may be useful in the classification of polyagglutinable RBCs. Generally, agglutination of Tk-, Cad-, and NOR-polyagglutinable cells is enhanced following enzyme treatment. HEMPAS, VA-, and T-polyagglutinable cells show no change in their agglutination by normal adult sera following enzyme treatment. Tn- and Th-polyagglutinable cells show decreased agglutinability following enzyme treatment. Table A–1 summarizes the findings with normal cells versus polyagglutinable cells.

TABLE A–1   Normal versus Polyagglutinable Cells

| | Screening Methods | | | | |
	FRESH ADULT SERA	CORD SERA	POLYBRENE	AGGLUTINATION AFTER PAPAIN TREATMENT	DURATION
Normal group O	0	0	+	Usually enhanced	—
T	+	0	0	No effect	Transient
Tn	+	0	0/ + mf	Decreased	Persistent
Tk	+	0	+	Enhanced	Transient
Cad	Sometimes +	0	+	Enhanced	Permanent
Acquired-B	+	0			Transient
VA	+w	0	+	No effect	Persistent
Th	+	0	+	Decreased	Transient
NOR	+	0	+	Enhanced	Permanent

0 = no reactivity; + = reactivity/aggregation; +w = weak reactivity/aggregation; +mf = mixed-field reactivity; Transient = cells revert to normal state after primary condition is resolved; Persistent = essentially permanent, but rare cases have been reported in which the cells returned to normal; Permanent = cells remain permanently altered and polyagglutinable.

TABLE A–2   Differentiation of Polyagglutinable Cells Using Lectins

	GLYCINE SOJA	ARACHIS HYPOGAEA	DOLICHOS BIFLORUS	SALVIA SCLAREA	SALVIA HORMINUM	GRIFFONIA SIMPLICIFOLIA (GS II)*	VICIA GRAMINEA (N_{VG} RECEPTOR)
Normal group O	0	0	0	0	0	0	—
T	+	+	0	0	0	0	Enhanced
Tn	+	0	+	+	+	0	Depressed
Tk	0	+	0	0	0	+	No effect
Cad	0/+w	0	+	0	+	0	
Acquired-B	0	0	+/−	0	0	0	
VA	0	0	0	0	0	0	
Th	0	+	0	0	0	0	
NOR	0	0	0	0	0	0	

*Previously known as *Bandeiraea simplicifolia* (BS II).

Lectins

Lectins are routinely included in the classification of polyagglutinable RBCs. Lectins are proteins present in plants (usually seeds), invertebrate animals, and lower vertebrates. Lectins bind specifically to carbohydrate determinants; agglutinating erythrocytes by binding their cell surface oligosaccharide. Highly concentrated lectins may react nonspecifically with all RBCs; however, with careful standardization a battery of lectin reagents will permit the accurate classification of most forms of polyagglutination. Table A–2 summarizes the differentiation of polyagglutinable cells using lectins.

Typing Polyagglutinable RBCs

Typing polyagglutinable RBCs is usually uncomplicated when monoclonal reagents are used. These antisera contain antibodies that are specific for the desired antigen, and they lack contaminating polyagglutinins that are found in normal human-derived antisera. Typing polyagglutinable RBCs may be difficult if the cells are strongly polyagglutinable and only human, polyclonal antisera are available. Several approaches to typing cells under these conditions are available and are described in the following discussions.[47]

Adsorption

Some polyagglutinable cells can be prepared in vitro (T, Th, Tk, Tx, and acquired B), and these cells may be used to adsorb the polyagglutinins from human typing reagents.

Enzymes

Some polyagglutination receptors are destroyed by enzymes (Tn and Th). In these forms of polyagglutination, the polyagglutinable cells may be enzyme-treated before typing. This approach would be limited to typing the cells for antigens that are not destroyed by enzymes, and controls must be used carefully to avoid false interpretations caused by unexpected, enzyme-reactive antibodies in the human typing sera.

Cord Sera

ABO-compatible cord sera that contain the desired antibody specificity may be used as typing reagents. Polyagglutinins are expected to be absent from cord sera.

Aged Sera

Polyagglutinins are unstable, and time-expired or aged human sera often lack the polyagglutinins. Such sera may be used as typing reagents if the desired antibodies are still demonstrable.

Dilution

It may be possible to dilute human antisera beyond the endpoint of the polyagglutinins and still retain the desired specificity.

Sulfhydryl Compounds

If the desired antibody in the human antiserum is IgG, it may be possible to treat the typing serum with 2-mercaptoethanol or dithiothreitol to destroy IgM antibodies, such as the polyagglutinins, without affecting the desired IgG antibody.

Adsorption and Elution

Adsorption and elution techniques may be used to determine the correct blood type of polyagglutinable RBCs. After incubating the polyagglutinable RBCs with typing serum, an elution is performed. If the specificity of the typing serum is demonstrable in the eluate, the cells may be considered positive for the antigen.

Clinical Significance

Polyagglutination is a condition with both serologic and clinical significance. When cells are altered to expose cryptantigens, they are susceptible to agglutination by most adult sera. The reaction between the cryptantigens and the naturally occurring polyagglutinins produces antibody-coated cells that may have clinical significance. In addition to sepsis, polyagglutination has been associated with leukemia, breast cancer, and other malignancies.

Sepsis

Polyagglutination has been reported in patients with sepsis, upper respiratory infections, wound infections, intestinal infections, and malignancies. Some of the bacterial and viral organisms that have been associated with polyagglutination are *A. niger, B. fragilis, C. albicans, C. perfringens, C. tertium,*

C. aquaticum, E. coli, pneumococci, *P. vulgaris, S. marcescens, V. cholerae,* and viruses such as the influenza virus. Bird[9] pointed out that microbes do not have to be in the bloodstream to cause polyagglutination and that an extravascular site of infection can produce enzymes that enter the bloodstream in amounts greater than can be neutralized by normal serum inhibitors.

In infants with suspected necrotizing enterocolitis (NEC), cryptantigen exposure provides diagnostic information and may serve as an early guide to the causative organism and to antibiotic therapy. A simple test for cryptantigen exposure using a two-lectin panel (*A. hypogaea* and *G. soja*) should be performed using cells from any infant that is suspected of NEC. Positive test results for cryptantigen exposure should be quantified because the amount of exposure correlates with the severity of the NEC and the likelihood of intestinal perforation.[48]

Case Report

A 7-month-old girl was admitted to the hospital with acute intestinal obstruction. The child's hematocrit level was 22 percent (reference range 33 to 43 percent), and a 90-mL transfusion of packed RBCs was ordered. Immediately after the transfusion, hemoglobinemia and hemoglobinuria were noted; however, immediate surgery was performed to remove a segment of necrotic small intestine. During surgery, 250 mL of whole blood was administered. Following the transfusion, the patient's temperature rose from 37° to 39°C, and evidence of hemolysis persisted. A transfusion reaction work-up was ordered. The results of the laboratory tests indicated that the child's pretransfusion and post-transfusion antibody screen and crossmatches were nonreactive. The DAT was negative pretransfusion, but post-transfusion the patient's RBCs were weakly coated with complement. An antibody identification panel using the pretransfusion serum was nonreactive, and an eluate from the patient's post-transfusion RBCs was also nonreactive. Because the source of the hemolysis was unexplained, a lectin panel was performed to test for possible polyagglutination. The patient's RBCs were strongly agglutinated by *A. hypogaea* and *G. soja* lectins. T transformation was confirmed.

Hemolytic Anemia and Hemolytic Uremic Syndrome

When cryptantigen exposure occurs in vivo, the patient's own IgM, complement-binding polyagglutinins can initiate intravascular hemolysis by binding to the transformed cells. In addition, the transfusion of plasma products containing normal levels of polyagglutinins may intensify the hemolysis. In rare cases, disseminated intravascular coagulation (DIC) and hemolytic uremic syndrome have been reported.[49,50] Hemolytic anemia has been more commonly reported in T polyagglutination[51-54]; however, Th polyagglutination[55] has also been implicated in severe intravascular hemolysis and DIC. The presence of cryptantigens on RBCs, white blood cells, platelets, and tissue cells accounts for the anemia, thrombocytopenia, and renal dysfunction. Naturally occurring polyagglutinins are absent in newborns, and because these antibodies are IgM, they do not cross the placenta.[56] Consequently, hemolysis is not seen in newborns with NEC or

other cryptantigen-exposing conditions unless they are transfused with plasma products.

Leukemia, Breast Cancer, and Other Malignancies

Tn polyagglutination has been found in apparently healthy people; however, it has also been reported in patients with acute myelocytic leukemia.[57-59] One apparently healthy person who was found to have Tn polyagglutination later developed acute leukemia. In two of the leukemia patients, chemotherapy resulted in a clinical remission of the leukemia and the disappearance of the Tn-polyagglutinable RBCs.[58] Thus, it could be concluded that Tn may be a preleukemic state. Although several healthy individuals are known who have had Tn polyagglutination for a number of years, Ness and coworkers[58,59] recommend that these individuals be monitored hematologically. Monoclonal antibody FBT3 is a mouse IgM monoclonal antibody that reacts specifically with Tn-transformed RBCs by hemagglutination and by direct immunofluorescence. Roxby and colleagues[60] recommended using immunohistochemical staining with FBT3, which is far more sensitive than hemagglutination, to detect Tn antigen expression in bone marrow aspirates and peripheral blood. By using FBT3 to monitor bone marrow aspirates and peripheral blood from patients who have leukemia, it may be possible to detect small numbers of leukemic cells and to predict relapse.

The cryptantigens T and Tn have been found on malignant tissue cells from breast, colon, and urinary bladder and in metastatic lesions.[11] The presence of these cryptantigens on malignant tissue has been attributed to the incomplete synthesis of MN glycoproteins.[61] The amount of the expressed antigen usually parallels the cancer malignancy and invasiveness.[60,62] The finding of T and Tn cryptantigens and/or a decrease in their respective serum antibodies may serve as an immunologic marker, with diagnostic and therapeutic implications.

Cryptantigens in the Absence of Apparent Infection

Two cases of transient Tn polyagglutination were described in apparently healthy neonates.[63] Delayed maturation of the sialyltransferase system was postulated as the cause of the cryptantigen exposure. Similarly, both Tn and Th cryptantigens were detected in a patient with myelodysplasia.[64] These cryptantigens were detectable over a 5-year period, and the patient showed no apparent bacterial or viral infection. In a study of maternal and cord bloods, Wahl and others[65] reported that a significant number of normal mothers and their newborn infants had Th-activated RBCs without polyagglutination. This study suggested that Th activation could be a normal change in pregnancy and that the Th antigen could be a marker for fetal hematopoiesis that is enhanced by some conditions during pregnancy and in utero development. Similarly, Rodwell and Tudehope[48] reported that T, Th, and Tn are all expressed on fetal RBCs during the first trimester and that Th and Tn are thought to be developmental markers. Herman and colleagues[66] reported that Th activation may be a RBC developmental marker present in congenital hypoplastic anemias. This study suggested that Th is a more specific marker for congenital hypoplastic anemia than i antigen expression or other fetal RBC characteristics.

Case Report

A 19-year-old woman donated blood for the first time at a company-sponsored blood drive. She was apparently healthy, her medical history was unremarkable, and all the results of tests performed on her blood by the laboratory were normal. These tests included ABO typing, Rh typing, screening for unexpected antibodies, a serologic test for syphilis, and viral marker tests for HBsAg, anti-HBc, anti-HCV, anti-HIV-1/2, HIV p24 antigen, and anti-HTLV-I/II. However, the hospital transfusion service discovered that her unit of blood was incompatible with three patients who had no unexpected antibodies using an immediate-spin, room temperature compatibility test. A DAT, which is not included in the routine testing, was performed on the unit, and the results were negative. Finally, testing for polyagglutination was performed using the two-lectin panel (*A. hypogaea* and *G. soja*). The RBCs of the unit were agglutinated by *G. soja* but not by *A. hypogaea*. Tn polyagglutination was confirmed with an additional lectin, namely, *S. sclarea*.

Blood Transfusion

In conclusion, polyagglutination is a rare condition; however, cryptantigen exposure is not. Cryptantigen exposure can be detected before polyagglutination develops by testing the patient's RBCs in vitro with specific lectins. A screening test using a two-lectin panel of *A. hypogaea* and *G. soja* is simple to perform and detects most of the causes of polyagglutination: T, Th, Tk, Tn, and Tx.[53] Patients with a potential risk of developing cryptantigen exposure and polyagglutination (i.e., patients with various infections, malignancies,[67] and unexplained anemias, and infants with necrotizing enterocolitis[48,68]) should be screened for cryptantigen exposure with the two-lectin panel. When cryptantigen exposure is detected, Rodwell and Tudehope[48] recommend quantitating the amount of exposure to serve as a guide for transfusion options. If there is marked (3 to 4+) activation, washed RBCs should be supplied to avoid potentially fatal intravascular hemolysis. If the activation is only moderate (1 to 2+), it may be possible to select plasma-containing products for transfusion using the minor crossmatch technique.[48,67–70] The minor crossmatch using the patient's RBCs and potential donors' plasma would detect plasmas containing the specific polyagglutinin and identify compatible units that could be selected for transfusion.

SUMMARY CHART:

➤ Polyagglutination refers to the agglutination of altered RBCs by a large proportion of ABO-compatible adult human sera caused by microbial (bacterial or viral) activity, certain forms of aberrant erythropoiesis, or inherited alterations in the RBC membrane.

➤ Microbially associated forms of polyagglutination include T, Th, Tk, Tx, acquired-B, and VA. Nonmicrobial forms of polyagglutination include Tn, Cad, hemoglobin M-Hyde Park, HEMPAS, and NOR.

➤ In acquired-B polyagglutination, enzymes produced by *E. coli*, *C. tertium*, and *P. vulgaris* cause deacetylation of the group A determinant on RBCs (α-*N*-acetyl-D-galactosamine) to produce a structure similar to the group B determinant (D-galactose), which cross-reacts with human anti-B typing reagents.

➤ In T polyagglutination, the enzyme neuraminidase produced by bacteria such as pneumococci cleaves terminal *N*-acetylneuraminic acid residues from the RBC membrane, exposing the (hidden) T antigen.

➤ Tk polyagglutination may lead to decreased expression of the ABH, Ii, Lewis, and P1 antigens because of microbial enzymatic action on galactose present on the paragloboside structure.

➤ HEMPAS RBCs have increased amounts of i antigen and decreased amounts of H antigen and sialic acid and are susceptible to lysis by anti-i and anti-I in the presence of complement.

➤ Polyagglutination is investigated by using cord blood sera, fresh group AB adult sera, an auto-control, enzymes, and lectin studies. Polyagglutinins are naturally occurring and react best at lower temperature via direct agglutination.

➤ The clinical significance of polyagglutination is most related to sepsis, leukemia, and breast cancer.

➤ Blood transfusion options for persons exhibiting polyagglutinable RBCs include washed RBCs and minor crossmatch techniques to detect plasma-compatible units that do not contain the polyagglutinin.

REFERENCES

1. Bird, GWG: Clinical aspects of red blood cell polyagglutinability of microbial origin. In Salmon, CH (ed): Blood Groups and Other Red Cell Surface Markers in Health and Disease. Masson, New York, 1982.
2. Hübener, G: Untersuchungen über Isoagglutination mit besonderer Berücksichtigung scheinbarer Abweichungen vom Gruppenschema. Zeitschrift für Immunitäts Forschung 45:223, 1926.
3. Friedenreich, V: Production of a Specific Receptor Quality in Red Cell Corpuscles by Bacterial Activity: The Thomsen Hemagglutination Phenomenon. Levin and Munskgaard, Copenhagen, 1930.
4. Stratton, F: Polyagglutinability of red cells. Vox Sang 4:58, 1954.
5. Levene, C, et al: Red cell polyagglutination. Transfus Med Rev 2:176, 1988.
6. Uhlenbruck, G, et al: On the specificity of lectins with broad agglutination spectrum. II. Studies on the nature of the T antigen and the specific receptors for the lectin *Arachis hypogaea* (ground nut). Zeitschrift für Immunitäts Forschung 138:423, 1969.
7. Thomas, DB, and Winzler, RJ: Structural studies on human erythrocyte glycoproteins: Alkali-labile tetrasaccharides. J Biol Chem 244:5943, 1969.
8. Anstee, DJ: Blood group MNSs: Active sialoglycoproteins of the human erythrocyte membrane. In Sandler, SG, et al (eds): Immunobiology of the Erythrocyte: Progress in Clinical Biological Research. Liss, New York, 1980.
9. Bird, GWG: Lectins and red cell polyagglutinability: History, comments, and recent developments. In Beck, ML, and Judd, WJ (eds): Polyagglutination. American Association of Blood Banks, Washington, DC, 1980.
10. Hicklin, BL, and Beck, ML: Latent polyagglutinable receptors on leukocytes and platelets (abstract). Transfusion 14:508, 1974.
11. Anglin, Jr, JH, et al: Blood group-like activity released by human mammary carcinoma cells in culture. Nature 269:254, 1977.
12. Kline, WE, and Issitt, CH: T substance in body fluids (abstract). Transfusion 16:527, 1976.
13. Bird, GWG, et al: Th, a "new" form of erythrocyte polyagglutination. Lancet 1:1215, 1978.
14. Sondag-Thull, D, et al: Characterization of a neuraminidase from *Corynebacterium aquaticum* responsible for Th polyagglutination. Vox Sang 57:193, 1989.
15. Inglis, G, et al: Effect of *Bacteroides fragilis* on the human erythrocyte membrane: Pathogenesis of Tk polyagglutination. J Clin Pathol 28:964, 1975.
16. Dôinel, C, et al: Tk polyagglutination produced in vitro by an endo-beta-galactosidase. Vox Sang 38:94, 1980.

17. Judd, WJ: The role of exo-β-galactosidases in Tk-activation (abstract). Transfusion 20:622, 1980.

18. Andreu, G, et al: Induction of Tk polyagglutination by *Bacteroides fragilis* culture supernatants: Associated modifications of ABH and Ii antigens. Revue Française de Transfusion et Immuno-hématologie 22:551, 1979.

19. Bird, GWG, et al: Tx, a "new" red cell cryptantigen exposed by pneumococcal enzymes. Proceedings of the 16th Kongress Deutsche Gesamte Hämatologie 25:215, 1982.

20. Wolach, B, et al: Tx polyagglutination in three members of one family. Acta Haematol 78:45, 1987.

21. Kline, WE, et al: Acquired-B antigen and polyagglutination in a healthy blood donor. Transfusion 19:648, 1979.

22. Gerbal, A, et al: Immunologic aspects of the acquired-B antigen. Vox Sang 28:398, 1975.

23. Garratty, G, et al: Acquired-B antigen associated with *Proteus vulgaris* infection. Vox Sang 21:45, 1971.

24. Salmon, C, and Gerbal, A: The acquired-B antigen. In Handbook of Clinical Laboratory Science. CRC Press, Cleveland, 1977, vol 1, sect D, p 193.

25. Judd, WJ: Review: Polyagglutination. Immunohematology 8:58, 1992.

26. Chorpenning, FW, and Dodd, MC: Polyagglutinable erythrocytes associated with bacteriogenic transfusion reactions. Vox Sang 10:460, 1965.

27. Graninger, W, et al: "VA": A new type of erythrocyte polyagglutination characterized by depressed H receptors and associated with hemolytic anemia. I. Serological and hematological observations. Vox Sang 32:195, 1977.

28. Dahr, W, et al: Cryptic A-like receptor sites in human erythrocyte glycoproteins: Proposed nature of Tn-antigen. Vox Sang 27:29, 1974.

29. Lee, LT, et al: Immunochemical studies on Tn erythrocyte glycoprotein. Blood 58:1228, 1981.

30. Myllylä, G, et al: Persistent mixed-field polyagglutinability: Electrokinetic and serological aspects. Vox Sang 20:7, 1971.

31. Beck, ML, et al: Observations on leukocytes and platelets in six cases of Tn-polyagglutination. Med Lab Sciences 34: 325, 1977.

32. Dahr, W, et al: Molecular basis of Tn-polyagglutinability. Vox Sang 29:36, 1975.

33. Cazal, P, et al: Polyagglutinabilitié héréditaire dominante: antigène privé (Cad) correspondant à un anticorps public et à une lectine de *Dolichos biflorus*. Revue Française de Transfusion et Immuno-hématologie 11:209, 1968.

34. Cazal, P, et al: Les antigènes Cad en 1976. Revue Française de Transfusion et Immuno-hématologie 20:165, 1977.

35. Sanger, R, et al: Plant agglutinin for another human blood group. Lancet i:1130, 1971.

36. Herkt, F, et al: Structure determination of oligosaccharides isolated from Cad erythrocyte membranes by permethylation analysis and 500-MHz ^{1}H-NMR spectroscopy. Eur J Biochem 146:125, 1985.

37. Issitt, PD: The antigens Sd^a and Cad. In Moulds, JM, and Woods, LL (eds): Blood Groups: P, I, Sd^a and Pr. American Association of Blood Banks, Arlington, VA, 1991.

38. Blanchard, D, et al: Comparative study of glycophorin A–derived O glycans from human Cad, Sd(a+), and Sd(a−) erythrocytes. Biochem J 232:813, 1985.

39. Donald, ASR, et al: The human blood group Sd^a determinant: A terminal non-reducing carbohydrate structure in N-linked and mucin type glycoproteins. Biochem Soc Trans 12:596, 1984.

40. Williams, J, et al: Structural analysis of the carbohydrate moieties of human Tamm-Horsfall glycoprotein. Carbohydr Res 134:141, 1984.

41. Bird, AR, et al: Haemoglobin M-Hyde Park associated with polyagglutinable red blood cells in a South African family. Br J Haematol 68:459, 1988.

42. King, MJ, et al: Enhanced reaction with *Vicia graminea* lectin and exposed terminal N-acetyl-D-glucosaminyl residues on a sample of human red cells with Hb M-Hyde Park. Transfusion 28:549, 1988.

43. Crookston, JH, et al: Red cell abnormalities in HEMPAS (hereditary erythroblastic multinuclearity with a positive acidified serum test). Br J Haematol 23:83, 1972.

44. Gockerman, JP, et al: The abnormal surface characteristics of the red blood cell membrane in congenital dyserythropoietic anemia type II (HEMPAS). Br J Haematol 30:383, 1975.

45. Harris, PA, et al: An inherited RBC characteristic, NOR, resulting in erythrocyte polyagglutination. Vox Sang 42:134, 1982.

46. Beck, ML, et al: High incidence of acquired-B detectable by monoclonal anti-B reagents (abstract). Transfusion 32:17S, 1992.

47. Issitt, PD: Applied Blood Group Serology, ed 3. Montgomery Scientific Miami, 1985, pp 456–476.

48. Rodwell, R, and Tudehope, DI: Screening for cryptantigen exposure and polyagglutination in neonates with suspected necrotizing enterocolitis (editorial comment). J Paediatr Child Health 29:16-18, 1993.

49. Fischer, K, et al: Neuraminidase-induzierte Alteration der Erythrozyten und Gefässendothelium—eine Ursache des hämolytische urämischen Syndroms. Proceedings of the 16th Kongress Deutsche Gesamte Hämatologie, Bad Neuheim, 1972.

50. Rumpf, KW, et al: Hemolytic-uremic syndrome in an adult with T-cryptantigen liberation. Deutsche Medizinische Wochenschrift 115:1270, 1990.

51. van Loghem, Jr, JJ, et al: Polyagglutinability of red cells as a cause of a severe haemolytic transfusion reaction. Vox Sang 5:125, 1955.

52. Moores, P, et al: Severe hemolytic anemia in an adult associated with anti-T. Transfusion 15:329, 1975.

53. Levene, C, et al: Intravascular hemolysis and renal failure in a patient with T polyagglutination. Transfusion 26:243, 1986.

54. Judd, WJ, et al: Fatal intravascular hemolysis associated with T-polyagglutination. Transfusion 22:345, 1982.

55. Levene, NA, et al: Th polyagglutination with fatal outcome in a patient with massive intravascular hemolysis and perforated tumor of colon. Am J Hematol 35:127, 1990.

56. Novak, RW: The pathobiology of red cell cryptantigen exposure. Pediatr Pathol 10:867, 1990.

57. Bird, GWG, et al: Erythrocyte membrane modification in malignant disease of myeloid and lymphoreticular tissues. I. Tn-polyagglutination in acute myelocytic leukemia. Br J Haematol 33:289, 1976.

58. Ness, PM, et al: Tn polyagglutination preceding acute leukemia. Blood 54:30, 1979.

59. Ness, PM: The association of Tn and leukemia. Haematologia (Budap) 16:93, 1983.

60. Roxby, DJ, et al: Expression of the Tn antigen in myelodysplasia, lymphoma and leukemia. Transfusion 32:834–838, 1992.

61. Buskila, D, et al: Exposure of cryptantigens on erythrocytes in patients with breast cancer. Cancer 61:2455, 1988.

62. Springer, GF: T and Tn, general carcinoma autoantigens. Science 224:1198, 1984.

63. Rose, RR, et al: Transient neonatal Tn-activation: Another example (abstract). Transfusion 23:422, 1983.

64. Janvier, D, et al: Concomitant exposure of Tn and Th cryptantigens on the red cells of a patient with myelodysplasia. Vox Sang 61:142, 1991.

65. Wahl, CM, et al: Th activation of maternal and cord blood. Transfusion 29:635, 1989.

66. Herman, JH, et al: Th activation in congenital hypoplastic anemia. Transfusion 27:253, 1987.

67. Sigler, E, et al: Polyagglutination: A rare mechanism for intravascular hemolysis (letter). Am J Med 92:113, 1992.

68. Marshall, LR, et al: A fatal case of necrotizing enterocolitis in a neonate with polyagglutination of red blood cells. J Paediatr Child Health 29:63–65, 1993.

69. Buskila, D, et al: Polyagglutination in hospitalized patients: A prospective study. Vox Sang 52:99, 1987.

70. Adams, M, et al: Exposure of cryptantigens on red blood cell membranes in patients with acquired immune deficiency syndrome or AIDS-related complex. J Acquir Immune Defic Syndr Hum Retrovirol 2:224, 1989.

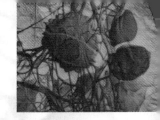

Answer Key for Review Questions

Chapter 1

1. C, 2. A, 3. B, 4. D, 5. D, 6. C, 7. D, 8. D, 9. A, 10. A, 11. B, 12. C, 13. D, 14. C, 15. C

Chapter 2

1. B, 2. B, 3. C, 4. D, 5. D, 6. D, 7. B, 8. A, 9. C, 10. A, 11. B, 12. A, 13. A, 14. A, 15. C

Chapter 3

1. C, 2. C, 3. C, 4. B, 5. B, 6. A, 7. D, 8. C, 9. B, 10. D, 11. C, 12. D, 13. A, 14. D, 15. A, 16. B, 17. D, 18. D, 19. C, 20. A, 21. D, 22. A, 23. B, 24. D, 25. A, 26. A, 27. A, 28. B, 29. D, 30. B

Chapter 4

1. A, 2. C, 3. C, 4. B, 5. D, 6. A, 7. D, 8. D, 9. C, 10. B

Chapter 5

1. D, 2. C, 3. A, 4. A, 5. B, 6. B, 7. D, 8. A, 9. B, 10. A, 11. C, 12. C

Chapter 6

1. D, 2. A, 3. D, 4. B, 5. C, 6. B, 7. A, 8. A, 9. C, 10. B

Chapter 7

1. A, 2. C, 3. B, 4. A, 5. C, 6. C, 7. D, 8. C, 9. E, 10. C, 11. D, 12. C

13.
R_1r	DCe/cde	Rh:1,2,-3,4,5
R_2R_0	DcE/cDe	Rh:1,-2,3,4,5
R_zR_1	DCE/DCe	Rh:1,2,3,-4,5
r^yr	CE/cde	Rh:-1,2,3,4,5

(*see* Table 7–3)   DCE/cde 1,2,3,4,5

14. E

Chapter 8

1. D, 2. A, 3. B, 4. B, 5. A, 6. A, 7. D, 8. C, 9. A, 10. D, 11. A, 12. D, 13. B

Chapter 9

1. A, 2. C, 3. D, 4. C, 5. B, 6. C, 7. B, 8. C, 9. C, 10. D, 11. A, 12. C

Chapter 10

1. D, 2. B, 3. A, 4. A, 5. D, 6. C, 7. C, 8. B, 9. C, 10. A = 1, E = 2, F = 3, C = 4, B = 5, D = 6, G = 7, I = 8, B = 9, F = 10

Chapter 11

1. C, 2. D, 3. E, 4. A, 5. A, 6. E, 7. A, 8. B, 9. C, 10. E, 11. A, 12. E, 13. B, 14. B, 15. A, 16. D, 17. C, 18. A, 19. C, 20. C

Chapter 12

1. D, 2. A, 3. C, 4. B, 5. C, 6. C, 7. D,
8. A, 9. B, 10. C

Chapter 13

1. C, 2. A, B, C, D, 3. D, 4. A, C, 5. B,
6. D, 7. B, 8. A, B, C, D, 9. D, 10. C,
11. B, 12. C, D, 13. B, D, 14. A, C,
15. A, B, C

Chapter 14

1. D, 2. C, 3. C, 4. C, 5. A, 6. B, 7. B, 8. A

Chapter 15

1. A, 2. D, 3. B, 4. C, 5. C

Chapter 16

1. D, 2. C, 3. C, 4. C, 5. A, 6. A, 7. A,
8. I A, II N, III B, IV D, V E, VI C,
VII B, VIII D, IX G, X H, XI F, XII J,
XIII I, XIV K

Chapter 17

1. B, 2. A, 3. B, 4. A, 5. C, 6. D, 7. B,
8. C, 9. C, 10. E

Chapter 18

1. D, 2. C, 3. B, 4. E, 5. A, 6. E, 7. B,
8. E, 9. C, 10. A, 11. C, 12. D, 13. B,
14. C, 15. D, 16. B, 17. A, 18. E, 19. D,
20. A, 21. D, 22. E, 23. A, 24. B, 25. C,
26. E, 27. E, 28. A, 29. D, 30. B

Chapter 19

1. A, 2. B, 3. D, 4. A, 5. C, 6. B, 7. C,
8. B, 9. D, 10. C, 11. C, 12. D, 13. A,
14. D, 15. A, 16. C, 17. A, 18. D, 19. C,
20. A, D, 21. B, 22. C, 23. A, 24. D, 25. B

Chapter 20

1. C, 2. A, 3. B, 4. D, 5. C, 6. A, 7. D,
8. D, 9. B, 10. B, 11. A, 12. B, 13. C

Chapter 21

1. D, 2. B, 3. A, 4. C, 5. A, 6. D, 7. B,
8. B, 9. C, 10. A, 11. D, 12. B, 13. D,
14. A, 15. C, 16. B, 17. C, 18. D

Chapter 22

1. C, 2. D, 3. C, 4. A, 5. D, 6. C, 7. E, 8. B

Chapter 23

1. B, 2. A, 3. B, 4. A

Chapter 24

1. B, 2. D, 3. D, 4. B, 5. C, 6. D, 7. C,
8. A, 9. A, 10. C

Chapter 25

1. B, 2. C, 3. D, 4. D, 5. C, 6. A, 7. D,
8. A, 9. B, 10. B

Chapter 26

1. C, 2. A, 3. D, 4. B, 5. A,
6. B, 7. D, 8. A, 9. B, 10. C,

11. Test	SCI SCII	SCII SCI	SCI SCII	SCII	SCI Interpretation
Phase	IS	IS	37	37	
	AHG	AHG	CC	CC	
Result	O	O	O	O	
	O	O	+	+	Negative

12. B
13. A. Control functions
    B. Acceptance criteria
    C. Test cases
    D. Data entry methods
    E. Documentation methods
    F. Result review
    G. Corrective action
    H. Acceptance

Chapter 27

1. E, 2. B, 3. E, 4. A, 5. E

Abruptio placentae: Premature detachment of normally situated placenta.

Absorbed anti-A$_1$: If serum from a group B individual that contains anti-A plus anti-A$_1$ is incubated with A$_2$ cells, the anti-A will adsorb onto the cells. Removal of the cells yields a serum containing only anti-A$_1$; thus, absorbed anti-A$_1$.

Absorption: Removal of an unwanted antibody.

Acid-citrate-dextrose (ACD): An anticoagulant and preservative solution that was once used routinely for blood donor collection but now used only occasionally.

Acid phosphatase (ACP): A red blood cell enzyme used as an identification marker in paternity testing and criminal investigation.

Adenosine deaminase (ADA): A red blood cell enzyme used as an identification marker in paternity testing and criminal investigation.

Adenosine triphosphate (ATP): A compound composed of adenosine (nucleotide containing adenine and ribose) and three phosphoric acid groups, which, when split by enzyme action, produces energy that can be used to support other reactions.

Adenylate kinase (AK): A red blood cell enzyme used as an identification marker in paternity testing and criminal investigation.

Adjuvant: One of a variety of substances that, when combined with an antigen, enhance the antibody response to that antigen.

Adsorption: Providing an antibody with its corresponding antigen under optimal conditions so that the antibody will attach to the antigen, thereby removing the antibody from the serum; often used interchangeably with absorption.

Agammaglobulinemia: A rare disorder in which gamma globulin is virtually absent.

Agglutination: The clumping together of red blood cells or any particulate matter resulting from interaction of antibody and its corresponding antigen.

Agglutinin: An antibody that agglutinates cells.

Agglutinogen: A substance that stimulates the production of an agglutinin, thereby acting as an antigen.

Agranulocytosis: An acute disease in which the white blood cell count drops to extremely low levels, and neutropenia becomes pronounced.

Albumin: Protein found in the highest concentration in human plasma; used as a diluent for blood typing antisera and a potentiator solution in serologic testing to enhance antigen-antibody reactions.

Aldomet: See Methyldopa.

Alkaline phosphatase (ALP): A red blood cell enzyme used as an identification marker in paternity testing and criminal investigation.

Allele: One of two or more different genes that may occupy a specific locus on a chromosome.

Allo-: Prefix indicating differences within a species (e.g., an alloantibody is produced in one individual against the red blood cell antigens of another individual).

Allogeneic: Transplant donor who is related or unrelated to the recipient.

Allograft: A tissue transplant between individuals of the same species.

Allosteric change: A change in conformation that exposes a new reactive site on a molecule.

Alpha-adrenergic receptor: A site in autonomic nerve pathways wherein excitatory responses occur when adrenergic agents such as norepinephrine and epinephrine are released.

Alum precipitation: A method for obtaining an enhanced response when producing an antibody; see also Adjuvant.

Amniocentesis: Transabdominal puncture of the amniotic sac, using a needle and syringe, in order to remove amniotic fluid. The material may then be studied to detect genetic disorders or fetomaternal blood incompatibility.

Amniotic fluid: Liquid or albuminous fluid contained in the amnion.

Amorph: A gene that does not appear to produce a detectable antigen; a silent gene, such as *Jk, Lu, O*.

Anamnestic response: An accentuated antibody response following a secondary exposure to an antigen. Antibody levels from the initial exposure are not detectable in the patient's serum until the secondary exposures, when a rapid rise in antibody titer is observed.

Anaphylaxis: An allergic hypersensitivity reaction of the body to a foreign protein or drug.

Anastomosis: A connection between two blood vessels, either direct or through connecting channels.

Anemia: A condition in which there is reduced oxygen delivery to the tissues; may result from increased destruction of red blood cells, excessive blood loss, or decreased production of red blood cells. Aplastic anemia: Anemia caused by aplasia of bone marrow or bone marrow's destruction by chemical agents or physical factors. Autoimmune hemolytic anemia: Acquired disorder characterized by premature erythrocyte destruction owing to abnormalities in the individual's own immune system. Hemolytic anemia: Anemia caused by hemolysis of red blood cells, resulting in reduction of normal red blood cell lifespan. Iron-deficiency anemia: Anemia resulting from a greater demand on stored iron than can be met. Megaloblastic anemia: Anemia in which megaloblasts are found in the blood. Sickle cell anemia: Hereditary, chronic hemolytic anemia characterized by large numbers of sickle-shaped red blood cells occurring almost exclusively in black people.

Angina pectoris: Severe pain and constriction about the heart caused by an insufficient supply of blood to the heart.

Anion: An ion carrying a negative charge.

Antecubital: In front of the elbow, at the bend of the elbow; usual site for blood collection.

Antenatal: Occurring before birth.

Anti-A$_1$ lectin: A reagent anti-A$_1$ serum produced from the seeds of the plant *Dolichos biflorus;* reacts with A$_1$ cells but not with A subgroup cells, such as A$_2$, A$_3$, and so on; reacts weakly with A$_{int}$ cells.

Anti-B lectin: A reagent anti-B serum produced from the seeds of the plant *Bandeiraea simplicifolia.*

Antibody: A protein substance secreted by plasma cells that is developed in response to, and interacting specifically with, an antigen. In blood banking, it is found in serum, from either a commercial manufacturer or a patient. Cross-reacting antibody: Antibody that reacts with antigens functionally similar to its specific antigen. Fluorescent antibody: Antibody reaction made visible by incorporating a fluorescent dye into the antigen-antibody reaction and examining the specimen with a fluorescent microscope. Maternal antibody: Antibody produced in the mother and transferred to the fetus in utero. Naturally occurring antibody: Antibody present in a patient without known prior exposure to the corresponding red blood cell antigen.

Antibody screen: Testing the patient's serum with group O reagent red blood cells in an effort to detect atypical antibodies.

Anticoagulant: An agent that prevents or delays blood coagulation.

Anticodon: A sequence of three bases that is found on transfer RNA, which also carries an amino acid residue; recognizes its complementary codon on messenger RNA at the ribosome and deposits the amino acid on the ribosome, generating the amino acid sequence of the protein.

Anti-dl: An antibody implicated in warm autoimmune hemolytic anemia, which reacts with all Rh cells including Rh$_{null}$ and Rh-deleted cells.

Antigen: A substance recognized by the body as being foreign, which can cause an immune response. In blood banking, antigens are usually, but not exclusively, found on the red blood cell membrane.

Antihemophilic factor: *See* Hemophilia A.

Antihemophilic globulin: *See* Hemophilia A.

Antihistamine: Drug that opposes the action of histamine.

Anti-H lectin: A reagent anti-H produced from the seeds of the plant *Ulex europaeus.*

Antihuman globulin or antiglobulin: *See* Antihuman serum.

Antihuman globulin or antiglobulin serum: *See* Antihuman serum.

Antihuman globulin test antiglobulin or (AGT): Test to ascertain the presence or absence of red blood cell coating by immunoglobulin G (IgG) or complement or both; uses a xenoantibody (rabbit antihuman serum) to act as a bridge between sensitized cells, thus yielding agglutination as a positive result. Also referred to as antiglobulin test. Direct antihuman globulin test (DAT): Used to detect in-vivo cell sensitization. Indirect antihuman globulin test (IAT): Used to detect antigen-antibody reactions that occur in vitro.

Antihuman serum: An antibody prepared in rabbits or other suitable animals that is directed against human immunoglobulin or complement or both; used to perform the antihuman globulin or Coombs' test. The serum may be either polyspecific (anti-IgG plus anti-complement) or monospecific (anti-IgG or anti-complement).

Anti-M lectin: A reagent anti-M serum produced from the plant *Iberis amara.*

Anti-nl: An antibody implicated in warm autoimmune hemolytic anemia, which reacts with all normal Rh cells except Rh$_{null}$ cells and deleted Rh cells.

Anti-N lectin: A reagent anti-N serum produced from the plant *Vicia graminea.*

Anti-pdl: An antibody implicated in warm autoimmune hemolytic anemia, which reacts with all normal Rh cells and deleted Rh cells but not with Rh$_{null}$ cells.

Antipyretic: An agent that reduces fever.

Antiserum: A reagent source of antibody, as in a commercial antiserum.

Antithetical: Referring to antigens that are the product of allelic genes (e.g., Kell [K] and Cellano [k]).

Apheresis: A method of blood collection in which whole blood is withdrawn, a desired component separated and retained, and the remainder of the blood returned to the donor. *See also* Plateletpheresis and Plasmapheresis.

Aplasia: Failure of an organ or tissue to develop normally.

Arachis hypogaea: A peanut lectin used to differentiate T polyagglutination from Tn polyagglutination.

Asphyxia: Condition caused by insufficient intake of oxygen.

Asthma: Paroxysmal dyspnea accompanied by wheezing caused by a spasm of the bronchial tubes or by swelling of their mucous membrane.

Atypical antibodies: Any antibody other than anti-A, anti-B, or anti-A,B.

Australia antigen: Old terminology referring to the hepatitis B–associated antigen.

Auto-: Prefix indicating *self* (e.g., an autoantibody is reactive against one's own red blood cell antigens); usually associated with a disease state.

Autoabsorption: A procedure to remove a patient's antibody, using the patient's own cells.

Autologous: Donor and recipient are the same person.

Autologous control: Testing the patient's serum with his or her own cells in an effort to detect autoantibody activity.

Autosome: Any chromosome other than the sex (X and Y) chromosomes.

Bactericidal: Destructive to or destroying bacteria.

Bandeiraea simplicifolia: *See* Anti-B lectin.

Bar code reader: An optical input device that reads and interprets data from a bar code for entry into a computer system.

Bilirubin: The orange-yellow pigment in bile carried to the liver by the blood; produced from hemoglobin of red blood cells by reticuloendothelial cells in bone marrow, spleen, and elsewhere. Direct bilirubin: The conjugated water-soluble form of bilirubin. Indirect bilirubin: The unconjugated water-insoluble form of bilirubin.

Bilirubinemia: Pathologic condition in which excessive destruction of red blood cells occurs, increasing the amount of bilirubin found in the blood.

Binding constant: The "goodness of fit" in an antigen-antibody complex.

Biphasic: Reactivity occurring in two phases.

Blood bank information system: Computer system that has

been developed specifically to assist blood bank professionals in the management of the patient, donor, and blood component information.

Blood gases: Determination of pH, Pco_2, Po_2, and HCO_3; performed on a blood gas analyzer.

Blood group–specific substances (BGSSs): Soluble antigens present in fluids that can be used to neutralize their corresponding antibodies; systems that demonstrate BGSSs include ABO, Lewis, and P blood group systems.

Bombay: Phenotype occurring in individuals who possess normal *A* or *B* genes but are unable to express them because they lack the gene necessary for production of H antigen, the required precursor for A and B. These persons often have a potent anti-H in their serum, which reacts with all cells except other Bombays. Also known as O_h.

Bovine: Pertaining to cattle.

Bradykinin: A plasma kinin.

Bromelin: A proteolytic enzyme obtained from the pineapple.

Buffy coat: Light stratum of a blood clot seen when the blood is centrifuged or allowed to stand in a test tube. The red blood cells settle to the bottom, and between the plasma and the red blood cells is a light-colored layer that contains mostly white blood cells.

Burst-forming unit committed to erythropoiesis (BFU-E): A primitive progenitor cell committed to erythropoiesis and believed to be a precursor to the CFU-E.

C3a: A biologically active fragment of the complement C3 molecule that demonstrates anaphylactic capabilities upon liberation.

C3b: A biologically active fragment of the complement C3 molecule that is an opsonin and promotes immune adherence.

C3d: A biologically inactive fragment of the C3b complement component formed by inactivation by the C3b inactivator substance present in serum.

C4: A complement component present in serum that participates in the classic pathway of complement activation.

C5a: A biologically active fragment of the C5 molecule, which demonstrates anaphylactic capabilities as well as chemotactic properties upon liberation. This fragment is also a potent aggregator of platelets.

Cadaveric: Source of organs and tissues from a person who has been declared dead.

Cardiac output: The amount of blood discharged from the left or right ventricle per minute.

Catecholamines: Biologically active amines, epinephrine and norepinephrine, derived from the amino acid tyrosine. They have a marked effect on nervous and cardiovascular systems, metabolic rate, temperature, and smooth muscle.

Cathode ray tube (CRT): A display device in an information system.

Cation: An ion carrying a positive charge.

CD34: Cell membrane marker of stem cells.

Central processing unit (CPU): The part of a computer that contains the semiconductor chips that process the instructions of the computer programs.

Central venous pressure: The pressure within the superior vena cava reflecting the pressure by which the blood is returned to the right atrium.

Chemically modified anti-D: IgG anti-D reagent antisera in which the immunoglobulin has been chemically modified to react in the saline phase of testing by breaking disulfide bonds at the hinge region of the molecule, converting the Y-shaped antibody structure to a T-shaped form through the use of sulfhydryl-reducing reagents.

Chemotaxis: Movement toward a stimulus, particularly that movement displayed by phagocytic cells toward bacteria and sites of cell injury.

Chimera: An individual who possesses a mixed cell population.

Chloroquine diphosphate: Substance that dissociates IgG antibody from red blood cells with little or no damage to the red blood cell membrane.

Chromogen: Any chemical that may be changed into coloring matter.

Chromosome: The structures within a nucleus that contain a linear thread of DNA, which transmits genetic information. Genes are arranged along the strand of DNA and constitute portions of the DNA.

Cis position: The location of two or more genes on the same chromosome of a homologous pair.

Citrate: Compound of citric acid and a base; used in anticoagulant solutions.

Citrate-phosphate-dextrose (CPD): The anticoagulant preservative solution that replaced ACD in routine donor collection. It has been replaced by CPDA-1 in routine use.

Citrate-phosphate-dextrose-adenine (CPDA-1): The anticoagulant preservative solution in current use. It has extended the shelf life of blood from 21 days (ACD and CPD) to 35 days.

Clone: A group of genetically identical cells.

Codominant: A pair of genes in which neither is dominant over the other; that is, they are both expressed.

Codon: A sequence of three bases in a strand of DNA that provides the genetic code for a specific amino acid. The complementary triplets are found on messenger RNA, which is synthesized from the DNA and then proceeds to the ribosomes for protein synthesis.

Colloid: A gluelike substance, such as protein or starch, whose particles, when dispersed in a solvent to the greatest possible degree, remain uniformly distributed and fail to form a true solution.

Colony-forming unit committed to erythropoiesis (CFU-E): A progenitor cell that is committed to forming cells of the red blood cell series.

Colony-forming unit—culture (CFU-C): Generation of stem cells using tissue culture methods. Current synonym is CFU-GM, which is a colony-forming unit committed to the production of myeloid cells (granulocytes and monocytes).

Colostrum: Thin yellowish breast fluid secreted 2 to 3 days after birth but before the onset of true lactation; it contains a great quantity of proteins and calories as well as antibodies and lymphocytes.

Complement: A series of proteins in the circulation that, when sequentially activated, causes disruption of bacterial and other cell membranes. Activation occurs via one of two pathways; once activated, the components are involved in a great number of immune defense mechanisms including anaphylaxis, chemotaxis, and phagocytosis. Red blood cell antibodies that activate complement may be capable of causing hemolysis.

Complement fixation (CF): An immunologic test.

Component therapy: Transfusion of specific components (e.g., red blood cells, platelets, plasma) rather than whole blood to treat a patient. Components are separable by physical means such as centrifugation.

Compound antibody: An antibody whose corresponding antigen is an interaction product of two or more antigens.

Compound antigen: Two or more antigens that interact and are recognized as a single antigen by an antibody.

Configuration: The physical layout and design of the central processing unit and the peripheral devices of an information system.

Conglutinin: A substance present in bovine serum that will agglutinate sensitized cells in the presence of complement.

Constant region: The portion of the immunoglobulin chain that shows a relatively constant amino acid sequence within each class of immunoglobulin. Both light and heavy chains have these constant portions, which originate at the carboxyl region of the molecule.

Convulsion: Involuntary muscle contraction and relaxation.

Coombs' serum: *See* Antihuman serum.

Coombs' test: *See* Antihuman globulin test (AGT).

Cord cells: Fetal cells obtained from the umbilical cord at birth; may be contaminated with Wharton's jelly.

Coumarin (Coumadin): A commonly employed anticoagulant that acts as a vitamin K antagonist to prolong prothrombin time.

Counterelectrophoresis (CEP): An immunologic procedure.

Crossmatch: The testing of the patient's serum with the donor red blood cells, including an antiglobulin phase or simply an immediate spin phase to confirm ABO compatibility. Computer crossmatch: Comparison of recent serologic results and interpretations on computer file for both the donor and the recipient being matched, establishing compatibility based on the comparison.

Cryoprecipitate: A concentrated source of coagulation factor VIII prepared from a single unit of donor blood; it also contains fibrinogen, factor XIII, and von Willebrand's factor.

Cryopreservation: Preservation by freezing at very low temperatures.

Cryoprotectant: A substance that protects blood cells from damaged caused by freezing and thawing. Glycerol and dimethyl sulfoxide are examples.

Cryptantigens: Hidden receptors that may be exposed when normal erythrocyte membranes are altered by bacterial or viral enzymes.

Crystalloid: A substance capable of crystallization; opposite of colloid.

Cyanosis: Slightly bluish or grayish skin discoloration resulting from accumulations of reduced hemoglobin or deoxyhemoglobin in the blood caused by oxygen deficiency or carbon dioxide buildup.

Cytomegalovirus (CMV): One of a group of species-specific herpesviruses.

Cytopheresis: A procedure performed using a machine by which one can selectively remove a particular cell type normally found in peripheral blood of a patient or donor.

Cytotoxicity: Ability to destroy cells.

Cytotoxicity testing: Procedure commonly used in HLA typing and crossmatching.

Dane particle: Hepatitis B virion.

Database: An organized group of files in which information is stored in an information system.

Deglycerolization: Removal of glycerol from a unit of red blood cells after thawing has been performed; required to return the cells to a normal osmolality.

Deletion: The loss of a portion of chromosome.

Deoxyribonucleic acid (DNA): The chemical basis of heredity and the carrier of genetic information for all organisms except RNA viruses.

Dexamethasone: A topical steroid with anti-inflammatory, antipruritic, and vasoconstrictive actions.

Dextran: A plasma expander that may be used as a substitute for plasma; can be used to treat shock by increasing blood volume. Rouleaux may be observed in the recipient's serum or plasma.

Diagnosis-related group (DRG): Classification system that organizes short-term, general hospital inpatients into statistically stable groups based on age and illness.

Diaphoresis: Profuse sweating.

Diastolic pressure: The point of least pressure in the arterial vascular system; the lower or bottom value of a blood pressure reading.

Dielectric constant: A measure of the electrical conductivity of a suspending medium.

Differential count: Counting 100 leukocytes to ascertain the relative percentages of each.

2,3-Diphosphoglycerate (2,3-DPG): An organic phosphate in red blood cells that alters the affinity of hemoglobin for oxygen. Blood cells stored in a blood bank lose 2,3-DPG, but once infused, the substance is resynthesized or reactivated.

Diploid: Having two sets of 23 chromosomes, for a total of 46.

Disk drive: A hardware device in an information system that contains a disk on which data are stored; provides for quick access to storing or retrieval of data.

Disseminated intravascular coagulation (DIC): Clinical condition of altered blood coagulation secondary to a variety of diseases.

Dithiothreitol (DTT): A sulfhydryl compound used to disrupt the disulfide bonds of immunoglobulin M, yielding monomeric units rather than the typical pentameric molecule.

Diuresis: Secretion and passage of large amounts of urine.

Diuretic: An agent that increases the secretion of urine, either by increasing glomerular filtration or by decreasing reabsorption from the tubules.

Dizygotic twins: Twins who are the product of two fertilized ova (also called fraternal twins).

DMSO: Dimethyl sulfoxide, a cryoprotectant used for hematopoietic progenitor cells.

DNA polymerase: An enzyme that catalyzes the template—dependent on synthesis of DNA. Also known as the HBeAg of the hepatitis B virion.

Dolichos biflorus: *See* Anti-A$_1$ lectin.

Domain: Portions along the immunoglobulin chain that show specific biologic function.

Dominant: A trait or characteristic that will be expressed in the offspring even though it is only carried on one of the homologous chromosomes.

Donath-Landsteiner test: A test usually performed in the blood bank to detect the presence of the Donath-Landsteiner antibody, which is a biphasic immunoglobulin G antibody with anti-P specificity found in patients suffering from paroxysmal cold hemoglobinuria.

Donor: An individual who donates a pint of blood.

Dopamine: A catecholamine synthesized by the adrenal gland, used especially in the treatment of shock.

Dosage: A phenomenon whereby an antibody reacts more strongly with a red blood cell carrying a double dose (homozygous inheritance of the appropriate gene) than with a red blood cell carrying a single dose (heterozygous inheritance) of an antigen.

Dyscrasia: An old term now used as a synonym for disease.

Ecchymosis: A form of macula appearing in large irregularly formed hemorrhagic areas of the skin; first blue-black, then changing to greenish brown or yellow.

Edema: A local or generalized condition in which the body tissues contain an excessive amount of tissue fluid.

Electrolyte: A substance that in solution conducts an electric current; common electrolytes are acids, bases, and salts.

Electrophoresis: The movement of charged particles through a medium (paper, agar gel) in the presence of an electrical field; useful in the separation and analysis of proteins.

Eluate: *See* Elution.

Elution: A process whereby cells that are coated with antibody are treated in such a manner as to disrupt the bonds between the antigen and antibody. The freed antibody is collected in an inert diluent such as saline or 6% albumin. This antibody serum then can be tested to identify its specificity using routine methods. The mechanism to free the antibody may be physical (heating, shaking) or chemical (ether, acid), and the harvested antibody-containing fluid is called an eluate.

Embolism: Obstruction of a blood vessel by foreign substances or a blood clot.

Embolus: A mass of undissolved matter present in a blood or lymphatic vessel, brought there by the blood or lymph circulation.

Endemic: A disease that occurs continuously in a particular population but has a *low* mortality; used in contrast to epidemic.

Endogenous: Produced or arising from within a cell or organism.

Endothelium: A form of squamous epithelium consisting of flat cells that line the blood and lymphatic vessels, the heart, and various other body cavities; derived from mesoderm.

Endotoxemia: The presence of endotoxin in the blood; endotoxin is present in the cells of certain bacteria (e.g., gram-negative organisms).

Engraftment: The successful establishment, proliferation, and differentiation of transplanted hematopoietic stem cells.

Enzyme: A substance capable of catalyzing a reaction; proteins that induce chemical changes in other substances without being changed themselves.

Enzyme-linked immunosorbent assay (ELISA): An immunologic test.

Enzyme treatment: A procedure in which red blood cells are incubated with an enzyme solution that cleaves some of the membrane's glycoproteins, then washed free of the enzyme, and used in serologic testing. Enzyme treatment cleaves some antigens and exposes others.

Epistaxis: Hemorrhage from the nose; nosebleed.

Epitope: The portion of the antigen molecule that is directly involved in the interaction with the antibody; the antigenic determinant.

Equivalence zone: The zone in which antigen and antibody concentrations are optimal and lattice formation is most stable.

Erythroblast: A precursor form of nucleated red blood cell that is not normally seen in the circulating blood.

Erythroblastosis fetalis: *See* Hemolytic disease of the newborn (HDN).

Erythrocyte: The blood cell that transports oxygen and carbon dioxide; a mature red blood cell.

Ethylenediaminetetraacetic acid (EDTA): An anticoagulant useful in hematologic testing and preferable when direct antihuman globulin testing is indicated.

Euglobulin lysis: Coagulation procedure testing for fibrinolysins.

Exogenous: Originating outside an organ or part.

Extracorporeal: Outside of the body.

Extravascular: Outside of the blood vessel.

Factor assay: Coagulation procedure to assay the concentration of specific plasma coagulation factors.

Factor VIII concentrate: A commercially prepared source of coagulation factor VIII.

Febrile reaction: A transfusion reaction caused by leukoagglutinins that is characterized by fever; usually observed in multiply transfused or multiparous patients.

Fibrin: A whitish filamentous protein or clot formed by the action of thrombin on fibrinogen, converting it to fibrin.

Fibrinogen: A protein produced in the liver that circulates in plasma. In the presence of thrombin, an enzyme produced by the activation of the clotting mechanism, fibrinogen is cleaved into fibrin, which is an insoluble protein that is responsible for clot formation.

Fibrinolysin: The substance that has the ability to dissolve fibrin; also called plasmin.

Fibrinolysis: Dissolution of fibrin by fibrinolysin, caused by the action of a proteolytic enzyme system that is continually active in the body but that is increased greatly by various stress stimuli.

Fibroblast: Cells found throughout the body that synthesize connective tissue.

Ficin: A proteolytic enzyme derived from the fig.

Ficoll: A macromolecular additive that enhances the agglutination of red blood cells.

Ficoll-Hypaque: A density-gradient medium used to separate and harvest specific white blood cells, most commonly lymphocytes.

Formaldehyde: A disinfectant solution.

Forward grouping: Testing unknown red blood cells with known reagent antisera to determine which ABO antigens are present.

Fresh frozen plasma (FFP): A frozen plasma product (from a single donor) that contains all clotting factors, especially the labile factors V and VIII; useful for clotting factor deficiencies other than hemophilia A, von Willebrand's disease, and hypofibrinogenemia.

Freund's adjuvant: Mixture of killed microorganisms, usually mycobacteria, in an oil-and-water emulsion. The material is administered to induce antibody formation and yields a much greater antibody response.

Furosemide (Lasix): An oral diuretic.

G-CSF: Granulocyte-colony stimulating factor, filgrastim.

GM-CSF: Granulocyte macrophage–colony stimulating factor, sargramostim.

G6PD (glucose-6-phosphate dehydrogenase): A red cell enzyme involved in the glucolytic pathway.

Gamete: A mature male or female reproductive cell.

Gamma globulin: A protein found in plasma and known to be involved in immunity.

Gamma marker: Allotypic marker on the gamma heavy chain of the IgG immunoglobulin.

Gel test: A blood group serology test method that uses a microtube containing gel (with or without antisera or antiglobulin sera) that acts as a reaction vessel for agglutination.

Gene: A unit of inheritance within a chromosome.

Genotype: An individual's actual genetic makeup.

Gestation: In mammals, the length of time from conception to birth.

Globin: A protein constituent of hemoglobin. There are four globin chains in the hemoglobin molecule.

Glomerulonephritis: A form of nephritis in which the lesions involve primarily the glomeruli.

Glutamic pyruvate transaminase: A liver enzyme used to monitor liver function; also called serum glutamic pyruvate transaminase (SGPT) or alanine transferase (ALT).

Gluten enteropathy: A condition associated with malabsorption of food from the intestinal tract.

Glycerol: A cryoprotective agent.

Glycerolization: Adding glycerol to a unit of red blood cells for the purpose of freezing.

Glycine soja: Soybean extract or lectin used to differentiate different forms of polyagglutination.

Glycophorin A: A major glycoprotein of the red blood cell membrane. MN antigen activity is found on it.

Glycophorin B: An important red blood cell glycoprotein: SsU antigen activity is found here.

Glycosyl transferase: A protein enzyme that promotes the attachment of a specific sugar molecule to a predetermined acceptor molecule. Many blood group genes code for transferases, which reproduce their respective antigens by attaching sugars to designated precursor substances.

Goodpasture's syndrome: A disease entity that represents a rapidly progressive glomerulonephritis associated with pulmonary lesions. Usually the patients possess an antibody to the basement membrane of the renal glomeruli.

Graft-versus-host (GVH) disease: A disorder in which the grafted tissue attacks the host tissue.

Granulocytopenia: Abnormal reduction of granulocytes in the blood.

Hageman's factor: Synonym for coagulation factor XII.

Half-life: The time that is required for the concentration of a substance to be reduced by one half.

Haploid: Possessing half the normal number of chromosomes found in somatic or body cells; seen in germ cells (sperm and ova).

Haplotype: A term used in HLA testing to denote the five genes (*HLA-A, -B, -C, -D, -DR*) on the same chromosome.

Haptene: The portion of an antigen containing the grouping on which the specificity depends.

Haptoglobin: A mucoprotein to which hemoglobin released into plasma is bound; it is increased in certain inflammatory conditions and decreased in hemolytic disorders.

Hardware: Components of an information computer system that are the tangible, physical pieces of equipment, such as the central processing unit, cathode ray tube, and keyboard.

HBcAg: Hepatitis core antigen, referring to the nucleocapsid of the virion.

HBeAg: Hepatitis DNA polymerase of the nucleus of the virion.

HBsAg: Hepatitis B surface antigen.

Hemangioma: A benign tumor of dilated blood vessels.

Hemarthrosis: Bloody effusion into the cavity of a joint.

Hematinic: Pertaining to blood; an agent that increases the amount of hemoglobin in the blood.

Hematocrit: The proportion of red blood cells in whole blood, expressed as a percentage.

Hematoma: A swelling or mass of blood confined to an organ, tissue, or space and caused by a break in a blood vessel.

Hematopoietic progenitor cell: Stem cells that are committed to produce blood cells.

Hematuria: Blood in the urine.

Heme: The iron-containing protoporphyrin portion of the hemoglobin wherein the iron is in the ferrous (Fe^{2+}) state.

Hemodialysis: Removal of chemical substances from the blood by passing it through tubes made of semipermeable membranes that are continually bathed by solutions that selectively remove unwanted material; used to cleanse the blood of patients in whom one or both kidneys are defective or absent and to remove excess accumulation of drugs or toxic chemicals in the blood.

Hemodilution: An increase in the volume of blood plasma, resulting in reduced relative concentration of red blood cells.

Hemoglobin: The iron-conjugated protein in the red blood cells whose function is to carry oxygen from the lungs to the tissues. This protein contains heme plus globin.

Hemoglobinemia: Presence of hemoglobin in the blood plasma.

Hemoglobin-oxygen dissociation curve: The relationship between the percent saturation of the hemoglobin molecule with oxygen and the environmental oxygen tension.

Hemoglobinuria: The presence of hemoglobin in the urine freed from lysed red blood cells, which occurs when hemoglobin from disintegrating red blood cells or from rapid hemolysis of red blood cells exceeds the ability of the blood proteins to combine with the hemoglobin.

Hemolysin: An antibody that activates complement, leading to cell lysis.

Hemolysis: Disruption of the red blood cell membrane and the subsequent release of hemoglobin into the suspending medium or plasma.

Hemolytic disease of the newborn (HDN): A disease, characterized by anemia, jaundice, enlargement of the liver and spleen, and generalized edema (hydrops fetalis), that is caused by maternal IgG antibodies crossing the placenta and attacking fetal red blood cells when there is a fetomaternal blood group incompatibility (usually ABO or Rh antibodies). Synonym is erythroblastosis fetalis.

Hemolytic transfusion reaction (HTR): A reaction from red

blood cell destruction caused by patient's antibody(ies) directed to donor red blood cell antigen(s).

Hemophilia A: A hereditary disorder characterized by greatly prolonged coagulation time (↑PTT). The blood fails to clot, and bleeding occurs; caused by inheritance of a factor VIII deficiency, it occurs almost exclusively in males.

Hemophilia B: "Christmas disease," which is a hemophilia-like disease caused by a lack of factor IX.

Hemopoiesis: Formation of blood cells. Synonym is hematopoiesis.

Hemorrhage: Abnormal internal or external bleeding; may be venous, arterial, or capillary; from blood vessels into the tissues or out of the body.

Hemorrhagic diathesis: Uncontrolled spontaneous bleeding.

Hemosiderin: An iron-containing pigment derived from hemoglobin from disintegration of red blood cells; a method of storing iron until it is needed for making hemoglobin.

Hemostasis: Arrest of bleeding; maintaining blood flow within vessels by repairing rapidly any vascular break without compromising the fluidity of the blood.

Hemotherapy: Blood transfusion as a therapeutic measure.

Heparin: An anticoagulant used for collecting whole blood that is to be filtered for the removal of leukocytes.

Hepatitis: Inflammation of the liver.

Hepatitis-associated antigen (HAA): Older terminology currently replaced by HBsAg.

Hepatitis B immunoglobulin (HBIg): An immune serum given to individuals exposed to the hepatitis B virus.

Heterozygote: An individual with different alleles on a gene for a given characteristic.

Heterozygous: Possessing different alleles at a given gene locus.

High-frequency antigen: Also known as high-incidence antigen; antigen whose frequency in the population is 98% to 99%.

Histocompatibility: The ability of cells to survive without immunologic interference; especially important in blood transfusion and transplantation.

HLA: Human leukocyte antigen.

Homeostasis: State of equilibrium of the internal environment of the body that is maintained by dynamic processes of feedback and regulation.

Homozygote: An individual developing from gametes with similar alleles and thus possessing like pairs of genes for a given hereditary characteristic.

Homozygous: Possessing a pair of identical alleles.

Hormone: A substance originating in an organ or gland that is conveyed through the blood to another part of the body, chemically stimulating it to increase functional activity and increase secretion.

Hyaluronidase: An enzyme found in the testes; present in semen.

Hybridoma: A hybrid (cross) between a plasmacytoma cell and a spleen (or Ab-producing) cell that produces a monoclonal antibody, resulting in a cell line that can grow indefinitely in culture and can produce high quantities of Ab. This antibody is monoclonal because only one Ab-producing cell combined with the plasmacytoma cell is present.

Hydatid cyst fluid: Source of P_1 substance.

Hydrocortisone: A corticosteroid with anti-inflammatory properties.

Hydrops fetalis: *See* Hemolytic disease of the newborn (HDN).

Hydroxyethyl starch (HES): A red blood cell sedimenting agent used to facilitate leukocyte withdrawal during leukapheresis.

Hypertension: Increase in blood pressure.

Hyperventilation: Rapid breathing that results in carbon dioxide depletion and that accompanies hypotension, vasoconstriction, and fainting.

Hypogammaglobulinemia: Decreased levels of gamma globulins seen in some disease states.

Hypotension: Decrease in blood pressure.

Hypothermia: Having a body temperature below normal.

Hypovolemia: Diminished blood volume.

Hypoxia: Deficiency of oxygen.

Iberis amara: See Anti-M lectin.

Icterus: A condition characterized by yellowish skin, whites of the eyes, mucous membranes, and body fluids caused by increased circulating bilirubin resulting from excessive hemolysis or from liver damage due to hepatitis. Synonym is jaundice.

Idiopathic: Pertaining to conditions without clear pathogenesis, or disease without recognizable cause, as of spontaneous origin.

Idiopathic thrombocytopenic purpura (ITP): Bleeding owing to a decreased number of platelets; the etiology is unknown, with most evidence pointing to platelet autoantibodies.

Idiothrombocythemia: An increase in blood platelets of unknown etiology.

Idiotype: The portion of the immunoglobulin variable region that is the antigen-combining site, which interacts with the antigenic epitope.

Immune response: The reactions of the body to substances that are foreign or are interpreted as being foreign. Cell-mediated or cellular immunity pertains to tissue destruction mediated by T cells, such as graft rejection and hypersensitivity reactions. Humoral immunity pertains to cell destruction response during the early period of the reaction.

Immune serum globulin: Gamma globulin protein fraction of serum-containing antibodies.

Immunoblast: A mitotically active T or B cell.

Immunodeficiency: A decrease from the normal concentration of immunoglobulins in serum.

Immunodominant sugar: In reference to glycoprotein or glycolipid antigens, the sugar molecule that gives the antigen its specificity (e.g., galactose, which confers B antigen specificity).

Immunogen: Any substance capable of stimulating an immune response.

Immunogenicity: The ability of an antigen to stimulate an antibody response.

Immunoglobulin (Ig): One of a family of closely related though not identical proteins that are capable of acting as antibodies: IgA, IgD, IgE, IgG, and IgM. IgA is the principal immunoglobulin in exocrine secretions such as saliva and tears. IgD may play a role in antigen recognition and the initiation of antibody synthesis. IgE, produced by the cells lining the intestinal and respiratory tracts, is important in forming reagin. IgG is the main immunoglobulin in human serum. IgM is formed in almost every immune response during the early period of the reaction.

Immunologic memory: The development of T and B memory

cells that have been sensitized by exposure to an antigen and that respond rapidly under subsequent encounters with the antigen.

Immunologic unresponsiveness: Development of a tolerance to certain antigens that would otherwise evoke an immune response.

Immunoprecipitin: An antigen-antibody reaction that results in precipitation.

Incubation: In-vitro combination of antigen and antibody under certain conditions of time and temperature to allow antigen-antibody complexes to occur.

Initiation: The deposition of N-formylmethionine on the ribosome, which begins the synthesis of all proteins.

In Lu: A rare dominant gene that inhibits the production of all Lutheran antigens as well as i, P_1, and Au^a (Auberger). The quantity of antigen on the red blood cell is markedly reduced in the presence of In Lu; it may be virtually undetectable.

Interface: Software that allows a computer system to send data to or receive data from another computer system.

Intraoperative salvage: A procedure to reclaim a patient's blood loss from an operation by reinfusion.

Intravascular: Within the blood vessel.

In utero: Within the uterus.

Inversion: The breaking of a chromosome during division, with subsequent reattachment occurring in an inverted or upside-down position.

In vitro: Outside the living body, as in a laboratory setting.

In vivo: Inside the living body.

Ion exchange resin: Synthetic organic substances of high molecular weight. They replace certain positive or negative ions, which they encounter in solutions.

Ionic strength: Refers to the number of charged particles present in a solution.

Ir genes: Immune response genes found within the region of the major histocompatibility complex. Ir genes in humans are likely to exist; preliminary evidence shows genes at the D-related locus may be analogous to the Ir genes of mice.

Irradiation: Gamma or electron treatment of a cellular blood product for protection against graft-versus-host disease.

Ischemia: Local and temporary deficiency of blood supply caused by obstruction of the circulation to a cell, tissue, or organ.

Isogglutinins: The ABO antibodies anti-A, anti-B, and anti-A,B.

Isoimmune: An antibody produced against a foreign antigen in the same species.

Isotype: The subclasses of an immunoglobulin molecule.

Jaundice: *See* Icterus.

Karyotype: A photomicrograph of a single cell in the metaphase stage of mitosis that is arranged to show the chromosomes in descending order of size.

Kernicterus: A form of icterus neonatorum occurring in infants, developing at 2 to 8 days of life; prognosis poor if untreated. This condition is due to an increase in unconjugated bilirubin.

Kinin: A group of polypeptides that have considerable biologic activity (e.g., vasoactivity).

Kleihauer-Betke technique: Quantitative procedure used to determine the amount of fetal cells present in the maternal circulation.

Km: Light chain marker on the kappa light chains of IgG (formerly known as InV).

Labile: Capable of deteriorating rapidly upon storage.

Lectin: Proteins present in plants (usually seeds), which bind specifically to carbohydrate determinants and agglutinate erythrocytes through their cell surface of oligosaccharide determinants.

Leukemia: Malignant proliferation of leukocytes, which spill into the blood, yielding an elevated leukocyte count.

Leukoagglutinins: Antibodies to white blood cells.

Ligature: Process of binding or tying; a band or bandage; a thread or wire for tying a blood vessel or other structure in order to constrict it.

Linkage: The association between distinct genes that occupy closely situated loci on the same chromosome, resulting in an association in the inheritance of these genes.

Linkage disequilibrium: Genes associated in a haplotype more often than would be expected on the basis of chance alone.

Locus: The site of a gene on a chromosome.

Low-frequency antigen: Also known as low-incidence antigen; antigen whose frequency in a random population is very low—less than 10%.

Low ionic-polycation test: A compatibility test that incorporates both glycine (low ionic) and protamine (polycation) in an effort to obtain maximal sensitivity and to minimize the need for antibody screening.

Low ionic strength solution (LISS): A type of potentiating medium in use for serologic testing. Reducing the ionic strength of the red blood cell–suspending medium increases the affinity of the antigen for its corresponding antibody such that sensitivity can be increased and incubation time decreased. LISS contains glycine or glucose in addition to saline.

Lymphocyte: A type of white blood cell involved in the immune response. Lymphocytes normally total 20% to 45% of total white blood cells. T lymphocytes mature during passage through the thymus or after interaction with thymic hormones; these cells function both in cellular and humoral immunity. Subsets include helper T-cells (T_h), which enhance B-cell antibody production, and suppressor T-cells (T_s), which inhibit B-cell antibody production. B-lymphocyte cells are not processed by the thymus. Through morphologic and functional differentiation, they mature into plasma cells that secrete immunoglobulin.

Lymphoma: A solid tumor of lymphocyte cells.

Lysosomes: Part of an intracellular digestive system that exists as separate particles in the cell. Even though their importance in health and disease is certain, all the precise ways lysosomes effect changes are not understood.

Macroglobulinemia: Abnormal presence of high-molecular-weight immunoglobulins (IgM) in the blood.

Macrophages: End-stage development for the blood monocyte; these cells can ingest (phagocytose) a variety of substances for subsequent digestion or storage and are located in a number of sites in the body (e.g., spleen, liver, lung), existing as free mobile cells or as fixed cells. Functions include elimination of senescent blood cells and participation in the immune response.

Major ABO incompatibility: ABO antibody in the recipient that is incompatible with the donor.

Major histocompatibility complex (MHC): Present in all mammalian and ovarian species; analogous to HLA complex. HLA antigens are within the MHC at a locus on chromosome 6.

Malaria: An acute and sometimes chronic infectious disease caused by the presence of a parasite within red blood cells. The parasite is *Plasmodium* (*P. vivax, P. falciparum, P. malariae, P. ovale*), which is introduced through bites of infected female *Anopheles* mosquitoes or through blood transfusion.

Meiosis: Type of cell division of germ cells in which two successive divisions of the nucleus produce cells that contain half the number of chromosomes present in somatic cells.

Menorrhagia: Excessive menstrual bleeding, in number of days or amount of blood, or both.

2-Mercaptoethanol (2-ME): A sulfhydryl compound used to disrupt the disulfide bonds of immunoglobulin M, yielding monomeric units rather than the typical pentameric units.

Metastasis: Movement of bacteria or body cells, especially cancer cells, from one part of the body to another; change in location of a disease or of its manifestations or transfer from one organ or part of another not directly connected. Spread is by the lymph or blood circulation.

Methemoglobin: An abnormal form of hemoglobin wherein the ferrous (Fe^{2+}) iron has been oxidized to ferric (Fe^{3+}) iron.

Methyldopa (Aldomet): Common drug used to treat hypertension; frequently the cause of a positive direct Coombs' test result.

Microaggregates: Aggregates of platelets and leukocytes that accumulate in stored blood.

Microglobulin (β_2): A protein synthesized by all nucleated cell types; an integral part of the class I MHC antigens.

Microspherocytes: Red blood cells, small and spherical, in certain kinds of anemia (i.e., hereditary spherocytosis).

Minor ABO incompatibility: ABO antibody in the donor that is incompatible with the recipient.

Mitosis: Type of cell division in which each daughter cell contains the same number of chromosomes as the parent cell. All cells except sex cells undergo mitosis.

Mixed field: A type of agglutination pattern in which numerous small clumps of cells exist amid a sea of free cells.

MLC: Mixed lymphocyte culture.

MLR: Mixed lymphocyte reaction.

Modem: Hardware device that provides the ability to attach to a computer system via telephone communication lines.

Monoclonal: Antibody derived from a single ancestral antibody-producing parent cell.

Monocytes: *See* Macrophage.

Monozygotic twins: Two offspring that develop from a single fertilized ovum.

Mosaic: An antigen composed of several subunits, such as the $Rh_0(D)$ antigen. A mixture of characteristics that may result from a genetic crossover or mutation.

Multiparous: Having borne more than one child.

Multiple myeloma: A neoplastic proliferation of plasma cells, which is characterized by very high immunoglobulin levels of monoclonal origin.

Mutation: A change in a gene potentially capable of being transmitted to offspring. Point mutation: A change in a base in DNA that can lead to a change in the amino acid incorporated into the polypeptide; identifiable by analysis of the amino acid sequences of the original protein and its mutant offspring. Frameshift mutation: A change in which a message is read incorrectly either because a base is missing or an extra base is added, which results in an entirely new polypeptide because the triplet sequence has been shifted one base.

Myelofibrosis: Replacement of bone marrow by fibrous tissue.

Myeloproliferative: An autonomous, purposeless increase in the production of the myeloid cell elements of the bone marrow, which includes granulocytic, erythrocytic, and megakaryocytic cell lines as well as the stromal connective tissue.

N-acetylneuraminic acid (NANA): *See* Sialic acid.

Neonate: A newborn infant up to 4 months of age.

Network: Configuration of personal computers linked together with cables; allows all of the personal computers to access common data and software located on a file server.

Neuraminidase: An enzyme that cleaves sialic acid from the red blood cell membrane.

Neutralization: Inactivating an antibody by reacting it with an antigen against which it is directed.

Neutrophil: A leukocyte that ingests bacteria and small particles and plays a role in combating infection.

Nondisjunction: Failure of a pair of chromosomes to separate during meiosis.

Nonresponder: An individual whose immune system does not respond well in antibody formation to antigenic stimulation.

Normal serum albumin: *See* Albumin.

O_h: *See* Bombay.

Oligonucleotide: A short synthetic segment of DNA, approximately 20 nucleotides in length, used as a probe.

Oliguria: Diminished amount of urine formation.

Opsonin: A substance in serum that promotes immune adherence and facilitates phagocytosis by the reticuloendothelial system.

Orthostatic: Concerning an erect position.

Osmolality: The osmotic concentration of a solution determined by the ionic concentration of dissolved substances per unit of solvent.

Ouchterlony diffusion: An immunologic procedure in which antibody and antigen are placed in wells of a gel medium plate and allowed to diffuse in order to visualize the reaction by a precipitin line.

Oxyhemoglobin: The combined form of hemoglobin and oxygen.

P_{50}: The partial pressure of oxygen or oxygen tension at which the hemoglobin molecule is 50 percent saturated with oxygen.

Pallor: Paleness; lack of color.

Panagglutinin: An antibody capable of agglutinating all red blood cells tested, including the patient's own cells.

Pancytopenia: A reduction in all cellular elements of the blood, including red blood cells, white blood cells, and platelets.

Panel: A large number of group O reagent red blood cells that are of known antigenic characterization and are used for antibody identification.

Papain: A proteolytic enzyme derived from papaya.

Paragloboside: The immediate precursor for the H and P antigens of the red blood cell.

Paroxysm: A sudden, periodic attack or recurrence of symptoms of a disease.

Paroxysmal cold hemoglobinuria (PCH): A type of cold autoimmune hemolytic anemia usually found in children suffering from viral infections in which a biphasic immunoglobulin G antibody can be demonstrated with anti-P specificity. *See also* Donath-Landsteiner test.

Paroxysmal nocturnal hemoglobinuria (PNH): An intrinsic defect in the red blood cell membrane, rendering it more susceptible to hemolysins in an acid environment; characterized by hemoglobin in the urine following periods of sleep.

Passenger lymphocytes: Donor lymphocytes in the transplanted organ or HPC product. (HPC: hereditary progenitor cell)

Perfusion: Supplying an organ or tissue with nutrients and oxygen by passing blood or another suitable fluid through it.

Perioral paresthesia: Tingling around the mouth occasionally experienced by apheresis donors, resulting from the rapid return of citrated plasma, which contains citrate-bound calcium and free citrate.

Peroxidase: An enzyme that hastens the transfer of oxygen from peroxide to a tissue that requires oxygen; this process is essential to intracellular respiration.

Phagocytosis: Ingestion of microorganisms, other cells, and foreign particles by a phagocyte.

Phenotype: The outward expression of genes (e.g., a blood type). On blood cells, serologically demonstrable antigens constitute the phenotype, except those sugar sites that are determined by transferases.

Phenylthiocarbamide (PTC): A chemical used in studying medical genetics to detect the presence of a marker gene. About 70% of the population inherits the ability to taste PTC, which tastes bitter; the remaining 30% finds PTC tasteless. The inheritance of this trait is due to a single dominant gene of a pair.

Phlebotomy: The procedure used to draw blood from a person.

Phosphoglyceromutase: A red blood cell enzyme.

Phototherapy: Exposure to sunlight or artificial light for therapeutic purposes.

Plasma: The liquid portion of whole blood, containing water, electrolytes, glucose, fats, proteins, and gases. Plasma contains all the clotting factors necessary for coagulation but in an inactive form. Once coagulation occurs, the fluid is converted to serum.

Plasma cell: A B lymphocyte–derived cell that secretes immunoglobulins or antibodies.

Plasmapheresis: A procedure using a machine to remove only plasma from a donor or patient.

Plasma protein fraction (PPF): Also known as Plasmanate; sterile pooled plasma stored as a fluid or freeze-dried and used for volume replacement.

Plasminogen: A protein in many tissues and body fluids important in preventing fibrin clot formation.

Plasmodium: See Malaria.

Plasmodium knowlesi: A parasite that causes malaria in monkeys.

Platelet: A round or oval disc, 2 to 4 μm in diameter, that is derived from the cytoplasm of the megakaryocyte, a large cell in the bone marrow. Platelets play an important role in blood coagulation, hemostasis, and blood thrombus formation. When a small vessel is injured, platelets adhere to each other and to the edges of the injury, forming a "plug" that covers the area and initially stops the blood loss.

Platelet concentrate: Platelets prepared from a single unit of whole blood or plasma and suspended in a specific volume of the original plasma; also known as random-donor platelets.

Plateletpheresis: A procedure using a machine to remove only platelets from a donor or patient.

Platelet refractoriness: Failure to yield an increase in recipient's platelet count on transfusion of suitably preserved platelets. HLA alloimmunization is a common cause.

Polyacrylamide gel: A type of matrix used in electrophoresis upon which substances are separated.

Polyagglutination: A state in which an individual's red blood cells are agglutinated by all sera, regardless of blood type.

Polyagglutinins: Naturally occurring immunoglobulin antibodies that are found in most normal human adult sera.

Polybrene: A positively charged polymer that causes normal red blood cells to aggregate spontaneously by neutralizing the negative surface charge contributed by sialic acid.

Polyclonal: Antibodies derived from more than one antibody-producing parent cell.

Polycythemia vera: A chronic life-shortening myeloproliferative disorder involving all bone marrow elements, characterized by an increase in red blood cell mass and hemoglobin concentration.

Polymer: Combination of two or more molecules of the same substance.

Polymerase chain reaction (PCR): An in-vitro method of amplification of a specific DNA or RNA segment.

Polymorphism: A genetic system that possesses numerous allelic forms, such as a blood group system.

Polyspecific Coombs' sera: A reagent that contains antihuman globulin sera against immunoglobulin G and C3d.

Polyvinylpyrrolidone (PVP): A neutral polymeric substance used to increase blood volume in patients with extensive blood loss; also used to enhance antigen-antibody reactions in vitro.

Portal hypertension: Increased venous pressure in the portal vein as a result of obstruction of the flow of blood through the liver.

Postpartum: Occurring after childbirth.

Potentiator: A substance that, when added to a serum and cell mixture, will enhance antigen-antibody interactions.

Precipitation: The formation of a visible complex (precipitate) in a medium containing soluble antigen (precipitinogen) and the corresponding antibody (precipitin).

Precipitin: An antibody formed in the blood serum of an animal by the presence of a soluble antigen, usually a protein. When added to a solution of the antigen, it brings about precipitation. The injected protein is the antigen; the antibody produced is the precipitin.

Precursor substance: A substance that is converted to another substance by the addition of a specific constituent (e.g., a sugar residue).

Pretransfusion compatibility testing: Series of testing procedures and processes with the ultimate objective of ensuring the best possible results of a blood transfusion, including recipient and donor identification, ABO testing, clerical checks, etc.

Primer: A short segment of single-stranded DNA, usually 17

to 25 nucleotides long, used to initiate DNA replication in PCR.

Private antigen: An antigenic characteristic of the red blood cell membrane that is unique to an individual or a related family of individuals and, therefore, is not commonly found on all cells (usually less than 1% of the population).

Probe: A fragment of DNA that is labeled and hybridized to diagnostic material to locate a complementary strand of DNA.

Prodrome: A symptom indicative of an approaching disease.

Propositus: The initial individual whose condition led to investigation of a hereditary disorder or to a serologic evaluation of family members. Feminine form is proposita. Synonyms are proband and index case.

Prospective validation: Validation testing of software; done before implementation of the computer system.

Prosthesis: An artificial substitute for a missing part, such as an artificial extremity.

Protamine: A polycation with applications similar to those of polybrene.

Protamine sulfate: A substance used to neutralize the effects of heparin.

Prothrombin complex: A concentrate of coagulation factors II, VII, IX, and X in lyophilized form.

Prozone: Incomplete lattice formation caused by an excess of antibody molecules relative to the number of antigen sites, resulting in false-negative reactions.

PRP: Platelet-rich plasma.

Public antigen: An antigen characteristic of the red blood cell membrane found commonly among individuals, usually more than 98% of the population.

Pulmonary artery wedge pressure: Pressure measured in the pulmonary artery at its capillary end.

Pulse pressure: The difference between the systolic and the diastolic pressures.

Quality assurance (QA): A set of planned actions to provide confidence that systems and elements that influence the quality of the product or service are working as expected, individually and collectively.

Radioimmunoassay (RIA): A very sensitive method for determination of substances present in low concentrations in serum or plasma by using specific antibodies and radioactively labeled or tagged substances.

Rapid passive hemagglutination assay (RPHA): A third-generation procedure used in hepatitis testing.

Rapid passive latex assay (RPLA): A second-generation procedure used in hepatitis testing.

Raynaud's disease: A peripheral vascular disorder characterized by abnormal vasoconstriction of the extremities upon exposure to cold or emotional stress. A history of symptoms for at least 2 years is necessary for diagnosis.

Recessive: A type of gene that, in the presence of its dominant allele, does not express itself; expression occurs when it is inherited in the homozygous state.

Recipient: A patient who is receiving a transfusion of blood or a blood product.

Refractory: Obstinate; stubborn; resistant to ordinary treatment; resistant to stimulation (said of a muscle or nerve).

Respiratory distress syndrome (RDS): A condition, formerly known as hyaline membrane disease, accounting for more than 25,000 infant deaths per year in the United States.

Clinical signs, including delayed onset of respiration and low Apgar score, are usually present at birth.

Reticulocyte: Also known as neocyte, the last stage of development before becoming a mature erythrocyte. The reticulocyte has lost its nucleus but retains some residual RNA in its cytoplasm, which is stainable by special techniques. It may be slightly larger than the mature red blood cell.

Reticuloendothelial system (RES): The fixed phagocytic cells of the body, such as the macrophage, having the ability to ingest particulate matter.

Retrospective validation: Validation testing of software, which is done after the computer system has been implemented.

Reverse grouping: Testing a patient's serum with commercial or reagent A and B red blood cells to determine which ABO antibodies are present.

Rh immunoglobulin (RhIg): A concentrated, purified anti-$Rh_0(D)$ prepared from human serum (of immunized donors) that is given to $Rh_0(D)$-negative mothers after they have given birth to an $Rh_0(D)$-positive baby or after abortion or miscarriage. It acts to prevent the mother from becoming immunized to any $Rh_0(D)$-positive fetal cells that may have entered her circulation and thereby prevents formation of anti-$Rh_0(D)$ by the mother.

Rh_{null}: A rare Rh phenotype in which no Rh antigens are expressed on the red blood cell; may result from the action of an inhibitor gene that is inherited independently from the *Rh* genes or caused by the rare genotype $\overline{rr}$, which is the *Rh* amorphic gene.

Ribonucleic acid (RNA): A nucleic acid that controls protein synthesis in all living cells. There are three different types, and all are derived from the information encoded in the DNA of the cell. Messenger RNA (mRNA) carries the code for specific amino acid sequences from the DNA to the cytoplasm for protein synthesis. Transfer RNA (tRNA) carries the amino acid groups to the ribosome for protein synthesis. Ribosomal RNA (rRNA), which exists within the ribosomes, is thought to assist in protein synthesis.

Ribosome: A cellular organelle that contains ribosomal RNA and protein and functions to synthesize protein. Ribosomes may be single units or clusters called polyribosomes or polysomes.

Rickettsia: Any of the microorganisms belonging to the genus *Rickettsia.*

Ringer's lactated injection: An aqueous solution suitable for intravenous use.

Rouleaux: Coinlike stacking of red blood cells in the presence of plasma expanders or abnormal plasma proteins.

Saline anti-D: A low-protein (6% to 8% albumin) immunoglobulin M anti-D reagent.

Salvia horminum: Plant lectin used in the differentiation of various forms of polyagglutination.

Salvia sclarea: Plant lectin with anti-Tn activity, used in the differentiation of various forms of polyagglutination.

Screening cells: Group O reagent red blood cells that are used in antibody detection or screening tests.

SD: Serologically defined antigens.

Secretor: An individual who is capable of secreting soluble, glycoprotein ABH-soluble substances into saliva and other body fluids.

Sensitization: A condition of being made sensitive to a specific substance (e.g., an antigen) after the initial exposure to that substance. This results in the development of immunologic memory that evokes an accentuated immune response with subsequent exposure to the substance.

Sepsis: Pathologic state, usually febrile, resulting from the presence of microorganisms or their toxins in the bloodstream.

Septicemia: Presence of pathogenic bacteria in the blood.

Serologic test for syphilis (STS): First developed in 1906 by Wassermann, present tests are of three main types based on complement fixation, flocculation, and detection of specific antitreponemal antibodies.

Serotonin: A chemical present in platelets that is a potent vasoconstrictor.

Serum: The fluid that remains after whole blood has clotted.

Sex chromosome: Chromosomes associated with determination of sex.

Sex linkage: A genetic characteristic located on the X or Y chromosome.

Shelf life: The amount of time blood or blood products may be stored upon collection.

Shock: A clinical syndrome in which the peripheral blood flow is inadequate to return sufficient blood to the heart for normal function, particularly transport of oxygen to all organs and tissues. Shock may be caused by a variety of conditions, including hemorrhage, infection, drug reaction, trauma, poisoning, myocardial infarction, or dehydration. Symptoms include paleness of skin (pallor), a bluish gray discoloration (cyanosis), a weak and rapid pulse, rapid and shallow breathing, or blood pressure that is decreased and perhaps unmeasurable.

Sialic acid: A group of sugars found on the red blood cell membrane attached to a protein backbone; the major source of the membrane's net negative charge.

Sickle trait: Blood that is heterozygous for the gene coding for the abnormal hemoglobin of sickle cell anemia.

Siderosis: Increase of iron in the blood that can lead to organ damage.

Single-donor platelets: Platelets collected from a single donor by apheresis.

Sodium dodecyl sulfate (SDS): An anionic detergent that renders a net negative charge to substances it solubilizes.

Software: Written instructions for a computer, which result in information being stored, manipulated, and retrieved.

Solid phase test: A blood group serology test method that uses red blood cell adherence on an endpoint instead of agglutination.

Specificity: The affinity of an antibody and the antigen against which it is directed.

Splenomegaly: Enlargement of the spleen.

Steatorrhea: Increased secretion of the sebaceous glands.

Stem cell: An unspecialized cell, capable of self-renewal, that gives rise to a group of differential cells, such as the hematopoietic cells.

Steroid hormones: Hormones of the adrenal cortex and the sex hormones.

Stertorous: Pertaining to laborious breathing.

Storage lesion: A loss of viability and function associated with certain biochemical changes that are initiated when blood is stored in vitro.

Stroma: The red blood cell membrane that is left after hemolysis has occurred.

Subgroup: Antigens within the ABO group that react less strongly with their corresponding antisera than do A and B antigens.

Survival studies: A measure of the in-vivo survival of transfused blood cells; usually performed with radioactive isotopes. Normal red blood cells survive approximately 100 to 120 days in circulation.

Syngeneic: Possessing identical genotypes, as monozygotic twins.

Synteny: Genes that are closely situated on a chromosome but cannot be shown to be linked.

System manager: A specially trained person who is responsible for the maintenance of an information system.

Systemic lupus erythematosus (SLE): A disseminated autoimmune disease characterized by anemia, thrombocytopenia, increased immunoglobulin G levels, and the presence of four immunoglobulin G antibodies: antinuclear antibody, antinucleoprotein antibody, anti-DNA antibody, and antihistone antibody; believed to be caused by suppressor T-cell dysfunction.

Systolic pressure: Maximum blood pressure that occurs at ventricular contraction; upper value of a blood pressure reading.

Tachycardia: Abnormally rapid heart action, usually defined as a heart rate greater than 100 beats per minute.

Tachypnea: Abnormally rapid respirations.

Template bleeding time: The elapsed time a uniform incision made by a template and blade stops bleeding, which is a test of platelet function, assuming a normal platelet count.

Tetany: A nervous affliction characterized by intermittent spasms of the muscles of the extremities.

Thalassemia major: The homozygous form of deficient beta-chain synthesis, which is very severe and presents itself during childhood. Prognosis varies; however, the younger the child at disease onset, the less favorable the outcome.

Thermal amplitude: The range of temperature over which an antibody demonstrates serologic and/or in-vitro activity.

Thrombin: An enzyme that converts fibrinogen to fibrin so that a soluble clot can be formed.

Thrombocytopenia: A reduction in platelet count below the normal level, which is associated with spontaneous hemorrhage.

Thrombotic thrombocytopenic purpura (TTP): A coagulation disorder characterized by (1) increased bleeding owing to a decreased number of platelets, (2) hemolytic anemia, (3) renal failure, and (4) changing neurologic signs. The characteristic morphologic lesion is thrombotic occlusion of small arteries or capillaries in various organs.

Thymidine: An essential ingredient used in DNA synthesis and incorporated by T lymphocytes undergoing blast transformation in response to foreign HLA-D antigens in the mixed lymphocyte culture test.

Titer: A measure of the strength of an antibody by testing its reactivity at increasing dilutions against the appropriate antigen. The reciprocal of the highest dilution that shows agglutination is the titer.

Titer score: A method used to evaluate more precisely than simple dilution by comparing the titers of an antibody. Agglutination at each higher dilution is graded on a continuous scale; the total is the titer score.

Trait: A characteristic that is inherited.

Trans: The location of two or more genes on opposite chromosomes of a homologous pair.

Transcription: The process of RNA production from DNA, which requires the enzyme RNA polymerase.

Transferase: An enzyme that catalyzes the transfer of atoms or groups of atoms from one chemical compound to another.

Transfuse: To perform a transfusion.

Transfusion: The injection of blood, a blood component, saline, or other fluids into the bloodstream. Autologous transfusion: blood taken from a patient to be used for the same patient. Direct transfusion: Transfer of blood directly from one person to another. Exchange transfusion: Transfusion and withdrawal of small amounts of blood, repeated until blood volume is almost entirely exchanged; used in infants born with hemolytic disease. Indirect transfusion: Transfusion of blood from a donor to a suitable storage container and then to a patient. Intrauterine transfusion: Transfusion of blood into a fetus in utero.

Transfusion reaction: An adverse response to a transfusion.

Translation: The production of protein from the interactions of the RNAs.

Translocation: Transfer of a portion of one chromosome to its allele.

Transposition: The location of two genes on opposite chromosomes of a homologous pair.

Trypsin: A proteolytic enzyme formed in the intestine.

Type and screen: Testing a patient's blood for ABO, Rh, and unexpected antibodies (antibody screen). If no abnormalities exist in the ABO and Rh and no unexpected antibodies are detected in the antibody screen, then the recipient blood sample is retained in the event that subsequent serologic crossmatching is necessary.

Ulex europaeus: See Anti-H lectin.

Ultracentrifugation: Rapid and prolonged centrifugation, used to separate by density gradient, substances of various specific gravities.

Urticaria: A vascular reaction of the skin similar to hives.

Vaccine: A suspension of infectious organisms or components of them that is given as a form of passive immunization to establish resistance to the infectious disease caused by that organism.

Validation: A systematic process of testing the hardware, software, and user components of an information system to ensure that they are functioning correctly for their intended purpose.

Valvular: Relating to or having a valve.

Variable region: That portion of the immunoglobulin light and heavy chains where amino acid sequences vary tremendously, thereby permitting the different immunoglobulin molecules to recognize different antigenic determinants. In other words, the variable region determines the antigen against which the antibody will react, thus providing each antibody molecule with its unique specificity. The variable region is located at the amino terminal region of the molecule.

Vasculitis: Inflammation of a blood or lymph vessel.

Vasoconstriction: Constriction of blood vessels.

Vasodilation: Dilation of blood vessels, especially small arteries and arterioles.

Vasovagal syncope: Syncope resulting from hypotension caused by emotional stress, pain, acute blood loss, fear, or rapid rising from a recumbent position.

Venesection: *See* Phlebotomy.

Venipuncture: Puncture of a vein for any purpose.

Veno-occlusive disease: Disease involving the veins of the liver associated with GVHD.

Venule: A tiny vein continuous with a capillary.

Viability: Ability of a cell to live or to survive for a reasonably normal lifespan.

Vicia graminea: See Anti-N lectin.

Virion: A complete virus particle; a unit of genetic material surrounded by a protective coat that serves as a vehicle for its transmission from one cell to another.

von Willebrand's factor: Coagulation factor VIII.

von Willebrand's disease: A congenital bleeding disorder.

WAIHA: Warm autoimmune hemolytic anemia. A hemolytic anemia caused by the patient's autoantibody that reacts at 37°C.

Wharton's jelly: A gelatinous intercellular substance consisting of primitive connective tissue of the umbilical cord.

X chromosome: The chromosome that determines female sex characteristics. The normal female has two X chromosomes, and the normal male has an X and a Y chromosome.

Xeno-: Prefix indicating differing species. For example, a xenoantibody is an antibody produced in one species against an antigen present in another species. Synonym is hetero-.

Xenogeneic: Transplantation between species.

Yaws: An infectious nonvenereal disease caused by a spirochete, *Treponema pertenue,* and found mainly in humid equatorial regions.

Zeta potential: The difference in charge density between the inner and outer layers of the ionic cloud that surrounds red blood cells in an electrolyte solution.

index

Boxed material is identified by page numbers ending with b.
Page numbers followed by f indicate figures; page numbers followed by t indicate tables; and page numbers followed by d refer to definitions of glossary entries.

ANTIGEN–ANTIBODY CHARACTERISTIC CHART*

ANTIGENS

Antigen System	Antigen Name	ISBT Number	Antigen Freq. % W	Antigen Freq. % B	RBC Antigen Expression at Birth	Antigen Distrib. Plasma/RBC	Demonstrates Dosage	Antigen Modification Enzyme/Other
Kidd	Jk^a	JK1	77	91	strong	RBC only	yes	Enz. ↑
	Jk^b	JK2	73	43	strong	RBC only	yes	Enz. ↑
		JK3	100	100	strong	RBC	no	Enz. ↑
Lewis	Le^a	LE1	22	23	nil	Plasma/RBC	no	Enz. ↑
	Le^b	LE2	72	55	nil	Plasma/RBC	no	Enz. ↑
†P	P_1	P1	79	94	moderate	RBC, platelets, WBC	individual variation	Enz. ↑ AET → ZZAP ↑
	P		100	100	moderate	RBC, platelets, WBC	no	Enz. ↑ AET → ZZAP ↑
	‡p^k		100	100	?	RBC, platelets, fibroblast	no	no
MNS	M	MNS1	78	70	strong	RBC only	yes	Enz. ↓ AET → ZZAP ↓
	N	MNS2	72	74	strong	RBC only	yes	Enz. ↓ AET → ZZAP →
	S	MNS3	55	37	strong	RBC only	yes	Enz. ↓ AET → ZZAP ↓
	s	MNS4	89	97	strong	RBC only	yes	Enz. ↓ AET → ZZAP ↓
	U	MNS5	100	100	strong	RBC only	no	Enz. → AET → ZZAP →
Lutheran	Lu^a	LU1	7.6	5.3	poor	RBC only	yes	Enz. → AET → ZZAP ↓
	Lu^b	LU2 LU3	99.8 >99.8	99.9	poor	RBC only	yes	Enz. → AET → ZZAP ↓

*This chart is to be used for general information only. Please refer to the appropriate chapter for more detailed information.

AET = 2-aminoethylisothiouronium bromide; ↑ = enhanced reactivity; → = no effect; ↓ = depressed reactivity; occ = occasionally; HDN = hemolytic disease of the newborn; HTR = hemolytic transfusion reaction; NRBC = non-red blood cell; RBC = red blood cell; WBC = white blood cell; ZZAP = dithiothreitol plus papain. PCH = paroxysmal cold hemoglobinuria; ↑ = enhanced reactivity;

† In the P system, phenotype P_1 contains both P_1 and P antigens; phenotype P_2 contains only P antigens; phenotype p lacks both P_1 and P antigens.

‡ The P^k antigen is typically converted to P; therefore there is no P^k antigen detectable on adult cells. There are rare individuals (P_1^k, P_2^k) where pk antigen is not converted to P.